For Reference

Not to be taken from this room

HANDBOOK OF RESEARCH
IN PERSONALITY PSYCHO

Handbook of
Research Methods
in Personality Psychology

edited by

Richard W. Robins
R. Chris Fraley
Robert F. Krueger

ℊp

THE GUILFORD PRESS
New York   London

© 2007 The Guilford Press
A Division of Guilford Publications, Inc.
72 Spring Street, New York, NY 10012
www.guilford.com

Printed in the United States of America

This book is printed on acid-free paper.

Last digit is print number: 9   8   7   6   5   4   3   2   1

Library of Congress Cataloging-in-Publication Data

Handbook of research methods in personality psychology / edited by Richard W. Robins,
R. Chris Fraley, Robert F. Krueger.
     p. cm.
   Includes bibliographical references and index.
   ISBN-10: 1-59385-111-1   ISBN-13: 978-1-59385-111-8 (hardcover)
   1. Personality—Research—Methodology.   I. Robins, Richard W.   II. Fraley, R.
Chris.   III. Krueger, Robert F.
   BF698.4.H28 2007
   155.2072—dc22

                                                                    2006035429

About the Editors

Richard W. Robins, PhD, is Professor of Psychology at the University of California, Davis. His research focuses on personality, emotion, and the self. Dr. Robins is coeditor of two forthcoming books, *Handbook of Personality* and *The Self-Conscious Emotions*, and served as Associate Editor of the *Journal of Personality and Social Psychology*. He was awarded the American Psychological Association's Distinguished Scientific Award for Early Career Contribution to Psychology and the Society for Personality and Social Psychology's Theoretical Innovation Prize.

R. Chris Fraley, PhD, is Associate Professor of Psychology at the University of Illinois at Urbana–Champaign. His research focuses on adult attachment dynamics, personality processes and development, and research methods. Dr. Fraley serves as Associate Editor of *Personality and Social Psychology Bulletin*. He received the American Psychological Association's Distinguished Scientific Award for Early Career Contribution to Psychology.

Robert F. Krueger, PhD, is McKnight Presidential Fellow and Associate Professor in the Department of Psychology at the University of Minnesota. His major interests lie at the intersection of research on personality, psychopathology, disorders of personality, behavior genetics, and quantitative methods. Dr. Krueger was the recipient of the Early Career Award from the International Society for the Study of Individual Differences, the American Psychological Association's Distinguished Scientific Award for Early Career Contribution to Psychology, and the American Psychological Foundation Theodore Millon Award for midcareer contributions to personality psychology.

Contributors

Leona S. Aiken, PhD, Department of Psychology, Arizona State University, Tempe, Arizona

Andrew T. Ainsworth, PhD, Department of Psychology, University of California, Los Angeles, California

Michael C. Ashton, PhD, Department of Psychology, Brock University, St. Catharines, Ontario, Canada

Rachel Bachner-Melman, MA, Scheinfeld Center of Human Genetics for the Social Sciences and Department of Psychology, Hebrew University, Jerusalem, Israel

Lisa Feldman Barrett, PhD, Department of Psychology, Boston College, Boston, Massachusetts

Jennifer S. Beer, PhD, Department of Psychology, University of California, Davis, California

Verónica Benet-Martínez, PhD, Department of Psychology, University of California, Riverside, California

Tim Bogg, PhD, Department of Psychology, University of Illinois at Urbana–Champaign, Champaign, Illinois

William F. Chaplin, PhD, Department of Psychology, St. John's University, Jamaica, New York

Rand D. Conger, PhD, Department of Human and Community Development, University of California, Davis, California

Tamlin S. Conner, PhD, Department of Psychiatry and Neuropsychiatric Institute, University of Connecticut Health Center, Farmington, Connecticut

Kenneth H. Craik, PhD, Department of Psychology, University of California, Berkeley, California

Phebe Cramer, PhD, Department of Psychology, Williams College, Williamstown, Massachusetts

Lisa M. Diamond, PhD, Department of Psychology, University of Utah, Salt Lake City, Utah

Audrey S. Dickey, BA, Department of Pharmacology, University of Iowa, Iowa City, Iowa

M. Brent Donnellan, PhD, Department of Psychology, Michigan State University, East Lansing, Michigan

Richard P. Ebstein, PhD, Scheinfeld Center of Human Genetics for the Social Sciences and Department of Psychology, Hebrew University, Jerusalem, Israel

Alan C. Elms, PhD, Department of Psychology, University of California, Davis, California

William Fleeson, PhD, Department of Psychology, Wake Forest University, Winston-Salem, North Carolina

R. Chris Fraley, PhD, Department of Psychology, University of Illinois at Urbana–Champaign, Champaign, Illinois

David C. Funder, PhD, Department of Psychology, University of California, Riverside, California

R. Michael Furr, PhD, Department of Psychology, Wake Forest University, Winston-Salem, North Carolina

Samuel D. Gosling, PhD, Department of Psychology, University of Texas at Austin, Austin, Texas

James W. Grice, PhD, Department of Psychology, Oklahoma State University, Stillwater, Oklahoma

Inga Gritsenko, MS, Scheinfeld Center of Human Genetics for the Social Sciences and Department of Psychology, Hebrew University and Sarah Herzog Memorial Hospital, Jerusalem, Israel

Rick H. Hoyle, PhD, Department of Psychology and Neuroscience, Duke University, Durham, North Carolina

Salomon Israel, MS, Department of Psychology, Hebrew University, Jerusalem, Israel

Oliver P. John, PhD, Department of Psychology, University of California, Berkeley, California

Robert F. Krueger, PhD, Department of Psychology and Institute of Child Development, University of Minnesota, Minneapolis, Minnesota

Nathan R. Kuncel, PhD, Department of Psychology, University of Illinois at Urbana–Champaign, Champaign, Illinois

Kibeom Lee, PhD, Department of Psychology, University of Calgary, Calgary, Alberta, Canada

Michael V. Lombardo, BA, Department of Psychology, University of California, Davis, California

Michael J. Marks, PhD, Department of Psychology, University of Illinois at Urbana–Champaign, Champaign, Illinois

Dan P. McAdams, PhD, Department of Psychology, Northwestern University, Evanston, Illinois

Robert R. McCrae, PhD, National Institute on Aging, National Institutes of Health, Baltimore, Maryland

Julien Morizot, PhD, Department of Psychology, University of Montreal, Montreal, Quebec, Canada

Daniel K. Mroczek, PhD, Department of Child Development and Family Studies, Purdue University, West Lafayette, Indiana

Lubov Nemanov, MD, Sarah Herzog Memorial Hospital, Jerusalem, Israel

John B. Nezlek, PhD, Department of Psychology, College of William & Mary, Williamsburg, Virginia

Kimberly D. Otter-Henderson, MA, Department of Psychology, University of Utah, Salt Lake City, Utah

Daniel J. Ozer, PhD, Department of Psychology, University of California, Riverside, California

Jennifer L. Pals, PhD, Foley Center for the Study of Lives, School of Education and Social Policy, Northwestern University, Evanston, Illinois

Joyce S. Pang, PhD, Department of Psychology, Nanyang Technological University, Singapore

Delroy L. Paulhus, PhD, Department of Psychology, University of British Columbia, Vancouver, British Columbia, Canada

Steven P. Reise, PhD, Department of Psychology, University of California, Los Angeles, California

William Revelle, PhD, Department of Psychology, Northwestern University, Evanston, Illinois

Brent W. Roberts, PhD, Department of Psychology, University of Illinois at Urbana–Champaign, Champaign, Illinois

Richard W. Robins, PhD, Department of Psychology, University of California, Davis, California

Michael D. Robinson, PhD, Department of Psychology, North Dakota State University, Fargo, North Dakota

Steven J. Schapiro, PhD, Department of Veterinary Sciences, M. D. Anderson Cancer Center, University of Texas, Houston, Texas

Oliver C. Schultheiss, PhD, Department of Psychology, University of Michigan, Ann Arbor, Michigan

Jeffrey W. Sherman, PhD, Department of Psychology, University of California, Davis, California

Yuichi Shoda, PhD, Department of Psychology, University of Washington, Seattle, Washington

Leonard J. Simms, PhD, Department of Psychology, University at Buffalo, Buffalo, New York

Dean Keith Simonton, PhD, Department of Psychology, University of California, Davis, California

Anna V. Song, PhD, Center for Tobacco Control Research and Education, University of California, San Francisco, California

Christopher J. Soto, AB, Department of Psychology, University of California, Berkeley, California

Jennifer L. Tackett, PhD, Department of Psychology, University of Toronto, Toronto, Ontario, Canada

Aaron B. Taylor, MA, Department of Psychology, Arizona State University, Tempe, Arizona

Howard Tennen, PhD, Department of Community Medicine, University of Connecticut Health Center, Farmington, Connecticut

Jessica L. Tracy, PhD, Department of Psychology, University of British Columbia, Vancouver, British Columbia, Canada

Michele M. Tugade, PhD, Department of Psychology, Vassar College, Poughkeepsie, New York

Simine Vazire, PhD, Department of Psychology, Washington University in St. Louis, St. Louis, Missouri

Wolfgang Viechtbauer, PhD, Department of Methodology and Statistics, University of Maastricht, Maastricht, The Netherlands

David Watson, PhD, Department of Psychology, University of Iowa, Iowa City, Iowa

Alexander Weiss, PhD, National Institute on Aging, National Institutes of Health, Baltimore, Maryland

Stephen G. West, PhD, Department of Psychology, Arizona State University, Tempe, Arizona

Barbara A. Woike, PhD, Department of Psychology, Barnard College, Columbia University, New York, New York

Wei Wu, MA, Department of Psychology, Arizona State University, Tempe, Arizona

Preface

One of the hallmarks of the field of personality psychology is the breadth and sophistication of its methods. Thumbing through a typical issue of a personality journal, one encounters a rich array of research designs, assessment procedures, and statistical techniques. Indeed, there is no standard personality study—instead, one finds longitudinal studies of personality development, experimental studies of motivational processes, twin and molecular genetic studies, and narrative studies of individual life stories. Just as personality psychologists appreciate the complexity of human nature and individual variability, so too do we appreciate the diverse ways in which that complexity can be assessed, quantified, and examined. It is this diversity that first attracted us to the field.

However, as aspiring personality psychologists, we quickly realized that there was no single source to which we could turn for guidance in how to design and implement a personality study. Instead, we learned about personality methods through a hodgepodge of articles, conference presentations, workshops, and seminars, as well as through direct mentoring from our seemingly all-knowing advisors. An earlier generation of researchers learned the ins and outs of personality methods from Wiggins's (1973) classic work, *Personality and Prediction: Principles of Personality Assessment*, but this book is long outdated and was never intended to be comprehensive.

The idea for the *Handbook of Research Methods in Personality Psychology* came from the recognition that one of the most noteworthy strengths of the field—the diversity of its research methods—was not represented in a single volume that could serve as a guide for researchers interested in conducting personality research. Our goal was simple: To create a "one-stop" source that describes, in a straightforward and practical manner, all of the resources in the methodological toolkit of the personality psychologist. This volume includes overviews of classic topics, such as how to construct a personality scale, as well as more recent innovations, such as neuroimaging and molecular genetic techniques. Each chapter provides a general introduction to a particular method and then explains, in a step-by-step manner, how the method can be used to address common research questions in the study of personality.

The book is divided into three sections, which collectively serve to guide the reader through all phases of conducting a personality study. The first section covers the various research designs used in the field, and helps readers determine the optimal type of study for addressing their particular research questions. The second section focuses on methods for assessing or measuring personality; chapters cover all of the most common methods used by personality researchers, as well as more recent but as yet less widely used methods. The third section covers the variety of procedures personality researchers use to analyze and interpret personality data; the chapters in this section help readers determine what to do with their data after they have conducted a personality study. This section also includes several chapters that address some methodological debates and challenges that are relevant to researchers in personality psychology and related fields.

Each chapter (1) provides an overview of a particular research design, assessment method, or statistical/data-analytic procedure; (2) summarizes the uses and applications of the method; (3) describes in detail (but with as little esoteric language as possible) the step-by-step procedure one would follow to implement the method in a study; (4) provides concrete examples of how the method has been used in personality research; and (5) discusses the practical and theoretical complexities that arise in using the method. The overarching goal of each chapter is to provide enough background so that readers will understand the method well enough to apply it thoughtfully and correctly in a specific research context.

The contributors are an elite group of researchers who are known as much for their substantive contributions to the field as for their innovative and sophisticated approaches to research. They understand the kinds of challenges that real-world researchers face in their ongoing research endeavors, and consequently the chapters do not get bogged down in technical details, but instead focus on the practical and theoretical complexities that arise in actually using each method.

Collectively, the chapters in this volume reflect the diversity that characterizes personality psychology, while at the same time revealing a field that is united by a common set of methodological themes, issues, and approaches, including an emphasis on multimethod assessment and the search for convergence across methods; the integration of laboratory and real-world studies; the study of diverse populations in naturalistic contexts; an emphasis on individual differences as well as general processes; and an attempt to understand personality at the level of intrapsychic processes and as it unfolds over time and across life contexts.

We thank Seymour Weingarten, editor-in-chief of The Guilford Press, for his encouragement and guidance throughout the project, and for his long-standing support of personality psychology. We also thank Carolyn Graham, Laura Specht Patchkofsky, and the other members of the Guilford staff who efficiently and effectively created a final product of which we and the contributors feel quite proud.

We hope that this volume will become an indispensable reference for students, researchers, and teachers interested in personality research. The task of assembling a large and diverse set of chapters for a volume of this nature can sometimes seem like a bit of a chore, but not so in this case. Since the inception of the project, we quickly realized that the contributors were just as enthusiastic as we were about the importance of creating a volume that captures the methodological breadth and sophistication of the field. We have been happy to serve as agents of a research community eager to share its accumulated knowledge and expertise. We learned a great deal from reading the chapters contained in this volume, and we trust that others will as well.

Reference

Wiggins, J. S. (1973). *Personality and prediction: Principles of personality assessment.* Reading, MA: Addison-Wesley.

Contents

II. METHODS FOR ASSESSING PERSONALITY AT DIFFERENT LEVELS OF ANALYSIS

III. ANALYZING AND INTERPRETING PERSONALITY DATA

HANDBOOK OF RESEARCH METHODS IN PERSONALITY PSYCHOLOGY

PART I

Designing a Personality Study

## CHAPTER 1

The Role of Theory in Personality Research

Dan P. McAdams
Jennifer L. Pals

Theory is at the heart of science. A common misconception has it that scientists mainly gather objective facts about the world. The truth of the matter, though, is that scientists traffic in theory, and shamelessly so. They formulate theories to describe and explain their interactions with the world, be those interactions the observations of cancer cells or interviews of people with schizophrenia. Over and over, scientists critically evaluate theories, eventually refining their conceptions to better reflect what they see, and sometimes throwing out their theories altogether when the data suggest that they are downright wrong. In the broadest terms, scientific theories deeply influence how scientists approach their observations (data), and their observations (data) ultimately come to influence the nature of the theories that scientists construct. It is an intricate dialectic: Observations lead to theories, which lead to new observations, which change theories, which result in yet newer observa-

tions, and on and on. Ideally, the process is open and progressive. The most secure theory can, in principle, be shot down in a hurry when new and repeated observations show it to be flawed. Over the long haul, the ongoing dialectic between observation and theory should lead to greater understanding, or what is often called "scientific progress."

The general process described above, however, plays itself out differently in different scientific fields. Physicists, for example, display different practices and adhere to different scientific conventions than biologists. What passes for theory in cultural anthropology may strike an organic chemist as odd. The purpose of this chapter is to consider some of the common and peculiar ways in which scientific theory relates to research in the particular subdiscipline of *personality psychology*. Like all scientists, personality psychologists have traditionally sought to develop the best possible theories for making sense of their observations.

And like all scientists, personality psychologists have developed a wide array of methods for observation and analysis to test hypotheses drawn from those theories. Nonetheless, the particular ways in which they have done these things and the problems they have historically faced are especially characteristic of the field they have pursued (Caprara & Cervone, 2000; Wiggins, 2003). Put differently, when it comes to the role of theory in research, personality psychology has its unique virtues and challenges.

In what follows, we first identify the characteristic features of personality psychology and consider the kinds of theories the field has historically offered. We next argue that a main function of these personality theories is to propose scientific *constructs* that help to describe and explain psychological individuality. Accordingly, the validation of constructs is a central task for personality research. The many different constructs that personality psychologists have examined may be grouped into three broad levels or domains—(1) dispositional traits, (2) characteristic adaptations, and (3) integrative life stories. In three successive sections of the chapter, we focus on one particular construct from each of these three levels. We examine the original theory behind the construct, the development of research methods to operationalize the construct, and important theoretical and empirical issues that have arisen as the construct has evolved over time. We end the chapter by considering the ways in which different theoretical constructs and the research programs they inspire each approach the study of psychological individuality in a different way, asking different questions and finding answers in different kinds of causal arguments. Although some might look with dismay upon the theoretical and empirical diversity in personality psychology today, we see it as a sign of a vibrant and dynamic science.

Personality Psychology and Personality Theory

What is personality psychology? In the field's first authoritative textbook, Allport (1937) considered 49 different definitions of the term *personality* before he settled on one he liked. Since then, many other definitions have been offered. Rather than propose our own, we prefer to consider what it is that personality psy-

chologists *do*. What makes the work of personality psychologists different from what other psychologists do? A survey of conceptual trends in the history of personality psychology suggests that the field has traditionally distinguished itself from other branches of psychology with respect to three different emphases: individual differences, motivation, and holism (McAdams, 1997).

First and probably most important, personality psychologists have always prioritized *individual differences* between people. Whether considering Freud's oral and anal types, Eysenck's traits of extraversion and neuroticism, or the self-report scales that make up the California Psychological Inventory (CPI; Gough, 1987), variability in human responding has traditionally captured the imagination of personality psychologists. To paraphrase a canonical passage in the history of personality psychology, every person is (1) like all other persons, (2) like some other persons, and (3) like no other person (Kluckhohn & Murray, 1953, p. 53). If the first panel in this famous triptych applies to common features of human nature, numbers 2 and 3 speak to what makes people different from each other—in particular those dimensions that make for recurrent and consistent differences between people. Beginning with Bernreuter's (1931) multitrait inventory, personality psychologists have designed hundreds of paper-and-pencil measures to assess individual differences on such dimensions as dominance, self-sufficiency, sociability, and neuroticism. The conceptual emphasis on inherent variations among persons and the development of instruments to assess these consistent variations have traditionally rendered the *correlational method* an especially suitable research strategy for studies focused on individual differences. In the correlational method, presumably stable and consistent individual differences in basic dimensions of personality can be related to corresponding variations in important behavioral outcomes.

A second traditional emphasis is *motivation*. More than most other fields in the social sciences, personality psychology concerns itself with the internal engines of human behavior and experience. This orientation is evident even in textbooks written before Allport (1937): "It is surely in the springs of human action, if anywhere, where the key to the problem of personality is to be found" (Garnett, 1928, p. 14). From Freud's drives to Murray's needs to Rogers's self-actualizing tendencies, most influential personality theories have tried to identify the internal factors that energize and give direction to human behavior. Motivational approaches focus on the dynamics of action, the forces that move people to do what they do—be those forces biological drives, evolved brain modules, cognitive schemas, or emotional scripts. Personality psychologists interested in human motivation have often shown a research preference for the *experimental method*. Motivational states may be readily aroused or activated under controlled laboratory conditions, and their effects on important dependent measures may be observed (see, e.g., Atkinson & Birch, 1978). Of course, experiments have been used in all branches of empirical psychology, and personality psychologists of many different stripes have employed the experimental method. But controlled laboratory experiments have traditionally been a favorite methodological choice for personality researchers who examine the internal forces responsible for energizing and directing human behavior.

Third, personality psychologists have long claimed that, unlike most other kinds of psychologists, they focus their attention on *the whole person*. The conceptual implications of this claim are at least twofold. First, personality psychologists have long sought to encompass a broad range of factors operating at many different levels in an effort to do justice to the complexity of the single individual's life. Second, many personality theories have shown a fondness for integrative concepts, terms like Allport's *proprium* and Erikson's *ego identity*, designed to explain how whole persons themselves find or construct wholeness, how their very lives suggest some degree of unity, purpose, and integration. Stern (1924) argued that a person is a *multiform dynamic unity*. Murray (1938) believed that many lives exhibit a *unity thema*. More recently, Deci and Ryan (1991) have described organismic needs for autonomy, competence, and relatedness—each of which serves an integrative function while expressing an authentic wholeness of self. These conceptual commitments to holism and integration have opened the methodological door to case studies of individual lives (Runyan, 1982). Correlational and experimental studies typify *nomothetic* research in personality psychology—that is, research examining propositions that apply to persons at large, or to some identifiable group of persons. In contrast, case studies typify *idiographic* research—the study of one particular person. It is only through the intensive examination of the single case, some have argued, that the holistic and integrative nature of personality can be fully seen and appreciated (Nasby & Read, 1997; Schultz, 2005).

As summarized in Table 1.1, personality psychologists develop theories and conduct research on individual differences, human motivation, and the whole person. Personality psychologists study those broad and socially consequential features of a person's psychological makeup that account for his or her individuality. In that human beings are goal-directed organisms, furthermore, it is impossible to articulate such an accounting without paying careful attention to motivation. In a nutshell, personality psychologists focus their attention

TABLE 1.1. Three Traditional Emphases in Personality Theory and Research

Emphasis	Questions	Traditional concepts	Method preferred
Individual differences	How are persons different from each other? What is the *structure* of human individuality?	Temperament, traits, types	Correlational studies
Motivation	Why do persons do what they do? What do persons want? What energizes and directs the person's behavior? What are the *dynamics* of human action?	Instincts, needs, values, goals, conflicts, complexes, defenses, self-actualizing tendencies	Laboratory experiments
Holism	How do we understand the whole person? What does a person's life mean? What integrates a life?	Ego, self, proprium, style of life, unity thema, identity, life structure	Case studies

on the *agential (goal-directed) individuality of whole persons*. They seek ultimately to make sense of individual persons as integrated and intentional agents living in a complex social world (Caprara & Cervone, 2000). Accordingly, personality theories address intriguing questions about the most socially consequential features of psychological individuality, questions like these: What makes individual persons different from each other? Why does this particular person do what he does (as opposed to doing something else), or live the way she lives (as opposed to living some other way)? Psychologically speaking, what is *this* individual person—and *any* individual person—fundamentally about?

In the first half of the 20th century, personality psychologists formulated a large number of grand theories designed to describe and explain the agential individuality of whole persons (Hall & Lindzey, 1957). Freud, Jung, Adler, Allport, Murray, Angyal, Goldstein, Murphy, Horney, Fromm, Erikson, Sullivan, Rogers, Maslow, Kelly, and a few others drew widely from case studies, clinical experience, philosophy and literature, common sense, and their own personal stories to develop all-purpose personality theories. More influenced by the conventions of laboratory science, Miller and Dollard, Rotter, Cattell, and Eysenck developed grand theories whose inspirations came largely from existing research findings and/or the general tenets of midcentury behaviorism.

Following World War II, personality researchers began to encounter important limitations in the grand theories developed only a few years before. For one, many of the statements articulated by Freud, Jung, and a number of other theorists proved too general or too ambiguous for empirical tests. How do you measure Freud's Oedipus complex? How do you evaluate the Jungian claim that all persons share a collective unconscious? In other instances, researchers found ways to test specific hypotheses derived from these theories, and the hypotheses received little support (Mendelsohn, 1993; Robins, Gosling, & Craik, 1999). Nonetheless, the grand theories helped to generate and sustain distinctive research programs, identified with particular personality researchers, their students, and their laboratories. For example, Murray's (1938) personological theory gave birth to McClelland's (1961) and Winter's (1973) more focused research programs for studying achievement and power

motivation, which ultimately came to influence research on personal strivings, goals, and projects (see, e.g., Emmons, 1986; Little, 1999).

The theories developed by personality psychologists in the past 30 years are more focused on circumscribed domains of human individuality and much more closely tied to systematic empirical observation than were most of the classic grand theories. Among the many examples of influential midlevel theories in personality psychology today are attachment theory (Bowlby, 1969; Fraley, 2002), socioanalytic theory (Hogan, 1982), self-determination theory (Deci & Ryan, 1991), various theories of self-regulation (e.g., Carver & Scheier, 1981), cognitive-affective systems theory (Mischel & Shoda, 1995), Loevinger's (1976) theory of ego development, Block's (1981) theory of ego control and resiliency, Tomkins's (1979) script theory, the life story model of identity (McAdams, 1985, 2001), and (despite its name) the Big Five trait taxonomy (Goldberg, 1993; McCrae & Costa, 1997). Although many of these theories offer relatively broad perspectives on human individuality, they tend not make the sweeping and untestable claims that were so common in the grand personality theories from the first half of the 20th century. Some contemporary observers lament the field's inability to merge these many new theories into one megatheory of everything. Yet many scholars have argued that science is often best served by a proliferation of many different theories, some competing with others, operating at different levels of analysis and seeking to explain somewhat different aspects of reality (Lakatos, 1970; Leary, 2005).

Formulating Constructs

A central function of personality theories is to propose measurable features of individual variation. These features are often called *constructs* (Wiggins, 1973), and the effort expended in developing appropriate measures for these features and exploring the meanings of these measures in research is essentially the process of *construct validation* (Cronbach & Meehl, 1955; Loevinger, 1957; Ozer, 1999). Constructs are convenient fictions that help us to describe and explain what cannot be directly assessed. Nobody has ever seen, heard, smelled, touched, or tasted the constructs of extraversion or the need for achievement. Instead, influential communities of like-minded behavioral scientists have essentially agreed to talk about psychological individuality in terms of constructs such as extraversion and the need for achievement. Even though constructs are socially consensual fictions, some constructs turn out to be extraordinarily useful in describing and explaining reality. And some do not. Rorer (1990) articulates a widely shared understanding of personality constructs:

> I believe that one can reasonably argue for an ontological realism while holding a pragmatic constructivist epistemology. Given this view, constructs are admittedly constructed, but reality, which we cannot know directly, places limits on the extent to which different constructions will work. Those that work, we keep. With respect to psychological constructs in particular, there are probably many that will work to varying degrees. (p. 713)

Research suggests that many personality constructs *do* work to varying degrees, and some better than others. Those that appear to work best are usually the ones that have generated the greatest amount of research activity. As more and more empirical studies are conducted on a given construct, the corpus of scientific findings builds up and the scientific community's understanding of the construct is further articulated. The construct becomes embedded in what Cronbach and Meehl (1955) called a *nomological network* of research findings. The overall usefulness and validity of the construct itself, therefore, is a function of the richness and extensiveness of the nomological network. The nomological network tells the scientific community "what we now know" about the construct, with the caveat that knowledge in science (and especially in personality psychology) is always provisional. In principle, each new study on the construct makes a small contribution to what we know, offers a further extension of or connection within the nomological network. In this way, the nomological network (what we know) is always developing.

There currently exists no broad theory or conceptual system that elegantly integrates *all* of the useful and valid personality constructs formulated by personality theorists and researchers. But most of the constructs can be provisionally arranged according to three broad conceptual domains or levels (Hooker & McAdams, 2003; McAdams, 1995, 2006a; McAdams & Pals, 2006; Sheldon, 2004). As shown in Table 1.2, level 1 encompasses *dispositional traits*, such as those organized within the popular Big Five framework. Dispositional traits account for broad individ-

TABLE 1.2. Three Levels of Personality Constructs

Level	Definition	Examples
Dispositional traits	Broad dimensions of psychological individuality that describe assumedly internal, stable, and global individual differences in behavior, thought, and feeling. Traits account for consistency in individual functioning across different situations and over time.	The Big Five Cattell's (1943) 15 personality traits Gough's (1987) folk concepts (the CPI) Ego resiliency and ego control
Characteristic adaptations	More particular features of psychological individuality that describe personal adaptations to motivational, social-cognitive, and developmental challenges and tasks. Characteristic adaptations are usually contextualized in time, place, situation, or social role.	Motives, goals, and projects Values and beliefs Cognitive schemas and styles Ego and psychosocial stages Relational modes and styles Identity statuses Coping strategies, defense mechanisms
Life stories	Internalized and evolving narratives of the self that people construct to integrate the past, present, and future and provide life with some sense of unity, purpose, and meaning. Life stories address the problems of identity and integration in personality—problems especially characteristic of modern adulthood.	Self-defining memories Nuclear scripts Recurrent life narrative themes: agency and communion The redemptive self

ual differences in behavioral trends across situations and over time. Typically assessed via self-report questionnaires, traits sketch an outline of psychological individuality. Level 2 brings together a wide assortment of *characteristic adaptations*, such as motives, goals, interests, values, strategies, and developmental tasks. Contextualized in time, place, or social role, characteristic adaptations address what people want in life and how they go about getting what they want, and avoiding what they do not want, during particular developmental periods, in particular situations and contexts, and with respect to particular social roles. Characteristic adaptations fill in many of the details of psychological individuality. Level 3 encompasses the individual's integrative *life story*. The life story consists of the person's internalized and evolving self-narrative(s), serving to reconstruct the past and imagine the future in such a way as to provide life with meaning, unity, and purpose. Life stories speak directly to what a whole life, situated in time and society, means and how the person believes that meaning has changed over time.

Personality constructs at each of the three levels in Table 1.2 have attracted active and vigorous research programs in personality psychology over the past few decades. In what follows, we examine how one particular construct at each of these three levels has been formulated, measured, and validated, with an emphasis on the research methods employed.

Dispositional Traits: The Case of Extraversion

The most extensively validated construct in all of personality psychology is probably *extraversion*. The classic example of a broad dispositional trait, extraversion refers to how outgoing, sociable, spontaneous, and energetic a person generally is, with individuals low on extraversion (that is, high on introversion) seen as generally withdrawn, retiring, quiet, and deliberate. Folk conceptions of extraversion can be traced back at least as far as Galen's (200 C.E.) ancient typology of the four temperaments (sanguine and choleric individuals were relatively extraverted; phlegmatic and melancholic persons were relatively introverted). In modern times, such pioneers in psychological science as Wundt, Pavlov, Heymans, Spearman, Guilford, and Cattell all studied the extraversion–introversion dimension in one way or another, and Jung popularized the distinction between extraverted and introverted types in his clinical writings. The one personality psychologist, however, who is most responsible for turning extraversion into a valid scientific construct is Hans J. Eysenck (1947, 1967, 1973).

Eysenck began with a clear and simple theory of extraversion drawn from folk wisdom and the results of a small body of previous research. He conceived of the trait as a general, bipolar, and linear continuum on which each person may be positioned, with the end points saved for those relatively pure or extreme types—the most extraverted or most introverted people of all. How might this individual difference be measured? Eysenck followed what may be called a *commonsense theory of trait manifestation*. According to this well-accepted view, people know themselves well enough to produce accurate self-reports regarding the ways in which they are similar to and different from other people. There is nothing deep, dark, or disguised about extraversion, Eysenck reasoned. Its manifestations should be readily observed in social behavior. Therefore, individual differences in extraversion should emerge clearly when people are asked to *observe themselves*.

Hogan (1976, 1987) distinguishes between personality from the standpoint of the observer (*Personalichkeit*) and personality from the standpoint of the actor (*Personalitiät*). Dispositional traits, like extraversion, are framed mainly in terms of the former, as dimensions of a person's social reputation in the eyes of others (observers). In self-report questionnaires, like those Eysenck developed to assess extraversion, individuals implicitly adopt the standpoint of observer vis-à-vis their own individuality. Their target of observation is the self. They evaluate each item with reference to the target, implicitly comparing themselves to others they know (or imagine) in order to come up with an accurate response. The test asks, "Do you enjoy yourself at lively parties?" Making a quick self-observation, I say, "Well, sometimes but not usually, not as much as many people I know." I answer "no." The test demands, "Rate yourself on a 1–7 scale with respect to how *energetic* you are." I think: "More than most people I know (and observe), certainly more than most people my age, though not as energetic as my wife." I answer "6."

Critics of trait theory love to poke fun at the items on trait inventories. For those dichotomous response formats wherein one is asked to answer either "yes" or "no" to each item, critics argue that an accurate answer would most surely be something like "sometimes" or "it depends" or even "what a dumb question this is!" However, most people have little trouble responding. In taking the commonsense role of self-observer, they realize that each item is asking about a simplified generality, a broad trend (Funder, 1995). They realize it is okay to ignore the specifics ("it depends on who is at the party") and the exceptions ("I really did enjoy myself *one time* at a lively party"). They know that they could rate other people they know on these same kinds of items, so why not rate the self? After all, the logic goes, the most accurate observer of the self is probably the self, given all the opportunities the self has had to observe what it usually does, how it usually thinks, what it usually feels.

Working from the premise that people are able to report accurately on their own traits, Eysenck followed well-accepted psychometric conventions in designing and validating trait questionnaires. The first step is to generate items that cover the substantive content of the trait domain (Jackson, 1971; Loevinger, 1957). Each item on the trait scale covers a small piece of what theory suggests is the content domain for the trait. When they are taken together, however, the items converge on the construct from a multitude of angles. The many items are then administered to large samples of respondents. Responses are factor analyzed and subjected to other statistical procedures in order to refine the scale and determine its structural features. In the process, some items are dropped and new ones added. In Eysenck's case, the results of these procedures showed that scales measuring extraversion yielded two related factors: sociability and impulsivity. Eysenck came to view these as the two faces of extaversion. Factor analyses of larger item pools led Eysenck to conclude further that extraversion and *neuroticism* are two broad and independent dimensions of personality, a conclusion that was originally suggested by Spearman (1927). In recent years, the Big Five trait taxonomy has appropriated versions of these as the first two dimensions in its five-factor scheme.

Once items have been generated and the structural features of the scale identified, researchers then look for evidence of the scale's predictive power. Drawing from theory, researchers deduce hypotheses and then test them

in experiments and correlational studies. The results of these studies come to comprise the nomological network for the construct. Construct validation largely depends on the extent to which studies are able to document empirical association between the construct and *external criteria* (Loevinger, 1957; Wiggins, 1973). Ozer (1999) spells out the logic of this step:

> Construct validity arguments must have a hard criterion core. Although there will rarely, if ever, be a single unequivocal external criterion for test validation purposes, there will nearly always exist a set of external variables, be they behavioral outcomes, group memberships, age changes, or assessment results using quite different sources of data (e.g., relation of a self-report scale to observer ratings), that collectively constitute a set of appropriate criteria. (p. 681)

Beginning with Eysenck, researchers have published hundreds of studies documenting associations between extraversion and a wide range of cognitive, emotional, and social variables. For example, extraverts talk more and sooner in a variety of social interactions than do introverts; they engage in more eye contact; they enjoy larger friendship networks and more social support; they seek out social activities for leisure time pursuits; they do more gambling; they engage in more sexual activity; and they are more likely to reside in households with other people rather than to be living alone. In the occupational realm, extraverts are more drawn to and tend to excel in jobs that involve dealing directly with other people, such as sales, marketing, personnel work, and teaching. By contrast, individuals scoring lower in extraversion (toward the introversion pole) tend to prefer jobs and professions in which they are more likely to work alone or in which social interaction is less sustained and intense, sharing interests with artists, mathematicians, engineers, researchers, and the like.

A significant body of research has found that extraversion is positively associated with reports of feeling good about life. In other words, extraverts report greater levels of positive emotion in everyday life than do introverts. This is most strongly shown when extraversion scale scores are correlated with reports of mood and affect *aggregated* across situations and over time (see, e.g., Emmons & Diener, 1986). Extraversion is consistently and positively associated with measures of subjective well-being. Typically, subjective well-being includes assessments of both positive and negative affect. Extraversion tends to predict positive emotions, but tends to be unrelated to negative emotions. (In contrast, the trait of neuroticism tends to predict individual differences in negative emotional states, but not positive emotions.) The empirical associations between extraversion and positive emotionality have proven to be so strong and consistent that some researchers now argue that extraversion is not so much about social interaction but is fundamentally instead a tendency to experience positive affect, or a tendency to approach situations that offer opportunities for experiencing positive affect (Watson & Clark, 1997). Although other researchers take issue with this line of reasoning, it is clear that the meaning of extraversion as a personality construct has changed since the time when Eysenck began his work. Over the past 50 years, the notion of impulsivity has migrated to the periphery of the broad extraversion construct (indeed, some conceptions see impulsivity to be part of [low] conscientiousness) whereas positive affectivity and energy level have tended to move more to the center. This kind of development is a common pattern in personality psychology, suggesting that as new findings come in, the theory behind a construct may change. Over time, a construct comes to be defined and understood primarily in terms of the evolving nomological network within which it is embedded.

Beginning with Eysenck, research on extraversion was strongly influenced by the behaviorist theories of learning and conditioning so popular among empirical psychologists in the 1930s, 1940s, and 1950s. Eysenck believed that Pavlov's description of the *weak nervous system* in dogs characterized the nature of the central nervous system for individuals low in extraversion (introverts). Dogs with weak nervous systems experienced a higher state of resting arousal, rendering them more readily conditionable in Pavlov's classical conditioning experiments. Midcentury behaviorists, such as Hull (1943), argued that higher arousal, or drive, enhanced the acquisition of stimulus–response (S–R) associations. Such dogs, furthermore, could tolerate only modest increases in stimulus arousal before S–R connections began to break down and they began to withdraw from the stimulation (what Pavlov called the threshold of transmarginal inhibition). Dogs with *strong nervous systems*, by contrast, re-

quired more stimulus trials or more potent stimuli to make classical conditioning happen. In their cases, lower drive levels retarded the acquisition of S–R connections. In addition, they could tolerate greater levels of stimulation increase before they reached the point of transmarginal inhibition. Correspondingly, Eysenck figured that extraverts experienced less resting-state arousal and therefore required stronger stimulation for conditioning. Laboratory experiments involving the classical conditioning of eyeblink responses in introverts and extraverts provided some initial support for Eysenck's view.

Eysenck eventually expanded his conception of extraversion to suggest a cortical explanation for differences in arousal levels between introverts and extraverts. He suggested that the brain's ascending reticular activating system (ARAS)—a network of nerve fibers ascending from the spinal cord to the thalamus and assumed to govern attention and general arousal levels—is responsible for the differences. For introverts, the ARAS is dispositionally set at a relatively high level. More aroused to begin with, introverts are more sensitive to any kind of stimulation. They can tolerate only relatively small increases in arousal (think: relatively little social stimulation) before they reach an optimal level of arousal. Once they reach that level, they are likely to engage in withdrawal behaviors to reduce arousal. In contrast, the extravert is endowed with an ARAS that is dispositionally set at a relatively low level. Less aroused to begin with, the extravert needs considerably more stimulation than does the introvert in order to reach a level of optimal arousal. The extravert is stimulus hungry—on the lookout for opportunities for social stimulation.

Eysenck's theory of cortical arousal produced many interesting hypotheses, which led to hundreds of experiments. Among the most famous were studies done with what Eysenck called *the lemon drop test*. Based on the general hypothesis that introverts should react more strongly to small increments in stimulation as compared with extraverts, Eysenck predicted that drops of lemon juice on the tongue should elicit greater salivation (a stronger response) for introverts than extraverts. Amazingly, Eysenck (1973) obtained a correlation of −.71 between amount of salivation produced and self-report extraversion scores in one study (*N* = 100). The finding has been replicated in subsequent studies, though with less statistical magnitude. Other studies with different conditions and stimuli provide some support for the overall idea that introverts are more physiologically reactive to stimulation at low-to-moderate levels of arousal. Support has also been garnered for the general prediction that extraverts seek out higher levels of stimulation as compared with introverts. However, studies have not provided support for the basic idea that introverts and extraverts differ in resting-state arousal to begin with. Furthermore, many researchers today are skeptical about the viability of the concept of general cortical arousal, pointing out that while one region of the brain may appear underaroused, other regions may be highly aroused at the same time (Geen, 1997).

As researchers have developed more sophisticated methodologies for studying brain activity, recent efforts to articulate a brain-based explanation for extraversion have shifted from Eysenck's arousal theory to the conception of a *behavioral approach system* (BAS). As a functional system of the brain, the BAS is hypothesized to govern positive approach behaviors in response to incentives. Important components of the BAS may be dopamine pathways and electrical activity in the left anterior portion of the brain. A small but growing body of research evidence links dopaminergic activity (Depue, Luciana, Arbisi, Collins, & Leon, 1994) and frontal-left brain activity (Davidson, 1992; Sutton & Davidson, 1997) to positive affect and approach behavior in some animals and humans. It has been proposed that individuals with a relatively strong BAS, being more sensitive and responsive to positive incentives for reward, may be more likely to be highly extraverted (and/or highly impulsive). Scientists have yet to flesh out an articulated picture of the BAS or to offer compelling evidence linking the BAS to extraversion directly. Nonetheless, this line of investigation may offer promising leads for future research on the biological origins of extraversion.

In sum, Eysenck formulated a clear descriptive theory of extraversion and developed measures of the construct based on a commonsense conception of trait assessment. Strongly influenced by one brand of midcentury behaviorism, Eysenck eventually expanded his theory of extraversion to encompass psychophysiological features. This second theoretical move led to hundreds of studies conducted by many different scientists and helped to establish a strong research tradition in personality psychology dedicated to exploring the cortical underpinnings of basic personality traits. As findings accrued over many years, the meaning of extraversion changed substantially and in ways that Eysenck may not have predicted. The history of the construct, therefore, shows how a strong initial theory can shape research methodology and design, but also how the findings of research often feed back to reshape the theory, which in turn stimulates new research.

Characteristic Adaptations: Loevinger's Stages of Ego Development

There exists a large and varied collection of personality constructs whose theoretical underpinnings resist their being viewed as broad, stable, linear, decontextualized, and noncontingent dimensions of human individuality accounting for cross-situational consistencies in behavior, feeling, and thought. Following Costa and McCrae (1994), we use the term *characteristic adaptations* for these important motivational, social-cognitive, and developmental concepts.

The key factor that keeps us from categorizing a number of concepts in personality psychology as dispositional traits is *context*. Context may refer to situation, domain, or role. For example, personality psychologists often propose constructs that are meant to apply only to particular settings in a person's life, rather than to broad consistencies across many settings (Cervone & Shoda, 1999; Mischel & Shoda, 1995). A person may be dominant only in the presence of family members or when interacting with children, or anxious only in the presence of people who remind him of his father or in the presence of snakes (Thorne, 1989). Characteristic adaptations may spell out a pattern of consistent individuality that manifests itself only within a particular social role—the authoritarian father, the bleeding-heart liberal (MacDermid, Franz, & De Reus, 1998). Many other characteristic adaptations are contextualized in *time*. Motivational concepts like goals (Roberts & Robins, 2000), strivings (Emmons, 1986), and personal projects (Little, 1999) are contextualized in time, for they all spell out how a person is *currently* orienting his or her life *for the future*. A developmental task or stage—for example, Marcia's (1980) *iden-

tity status—qualifies in the same way. A young adult may be in the *moratorium* status during a particular period in his or her life. During that time period, identity moratorium is a key aspect of his or her personality makeup. A decade later, however, the developmental issues of identity may no longer be relevant for construing the same person's psychological individuality.

One of the most influential developmental constructs in personality psychology is Jane Loevinger's (1976, 1979, 1983, 1987) *ego development*. Drawing from theoretical traditions in cognitive-developmental psychology (see, e.g., Kohlberg, 1969) and interpersonal psychodynamic psychology (Sullivan, 1953), Loevinger conceived of ego development as the sequence of changes that plays itself out in the way people make sense of themselves and the world over the human life course. The ego is one's overall interpretive frame and existential stance vis-à-vis the world at any given point in developmental time (Westenberg, Blasi, & Cohn, 1998). The interpretive frame encompasses many content domains. Loevinger (1976, p. 26) wrote that "what changes during the course of ego development is a complexly interwoven fabric of impulse control, character, interpersonal relations, and cognitive complexity, among other things."

Loevinger's full conception of ego development came many years after she began research on the construct. Equipped with only vague expectations regarding how people's sense of themselves and the world might change over time, Loevinger looked for a research method that might tap directly into sense making. She rejected the kind of self-report questionnaires used by Eysenck and other trait researchers in favor of a *sentence completion test* (SCT). On the SCT, a person actively constructs meanings in response to sentence stems. The researcher's challenge is to interpret the constructions in a psychologically useful way. Eysenck and Loevinger, therefore, followed very different research paths. Whereas Eysenck began with a clear conception of a stable personality feature, Loevinger began with general observations of developmental change. Whereas Eysenck wrote self-report test items to cover the content domain of the feature, Loevinger created opportunities for individuals to express different frames for making meaning (through the SCT) so that she could ultimately derive a conception of the construct in the developmental differ-

ences she observed. "My conception of ego development did not precede its measurement by the SCT; rather, the stages of ego development that developed from our many studies with the SCT embody and shaped my conception of ego development" (Loevinger, 1998, p. 353). Put differently, whereas Eysenck began with theory and moved to method, Loevinger began mainly with method (and some general observations about change) and eventually moved to theory. Only after administering the SCT to many subjects in a number of different studies did she eventually come to see what the method was indeed measuring.

Although Loevinger's concept of the ego is broad, like a dispositional trait, it is specifically contextualized in time. Over time, Loevinger argues, people move through a series of qualitatively distinct stages of meaning making. Young children see the world from a very egocentric point of view. Their framework is driven by impulses, the exigencies of the here and now, and such superficial concerns as physical appearance. As they grow up, however, they become better able to adopt the perspectives of others and, eventually, of society as a whole. In these middle stages of ego development, therefore, people's ways of making meaning are highly sociocentric and conventional; their views conform to and are defined by social convention and consensus. Later (higher) stages (which many people do not reach) show a kind of return to the self, but now from a more principled and autonomous perspective. Meaning making becomes especially complex and involves efforts to balance conflicting perspectives in light of deeply held convictions about self and world (see Hy & Loevinger, 1996).

Results from the SCT show that children tend to score lower than adolescents on ego development, and adolescents lower than adults. But among adults, one may still find the full range of stage scores represented. Therefore, the construct and the measure ultimately yield a developmental typology in adulthood. Stage scores are estimates of where on the ego developmental road an adult may be located at a particular time in the adult's life, with each stage suggesting a distinct type of interpretive frame or approach for making sense of self and world.

Loevinger's theory of ego development and the corresponding SCT method of measurement have stimulated a substantial body of personality research over the past three decades. Testing straightforward predictions about links between ego stages and discrete behaviors, however, can be tricky. Unlike extraversion, ego development is not a linear continuum with a clearly defined low end. Among well-educated adults, for example, "low" ego development may be the conformist stage, or even one stage above that. Among junior high students, however, the conformist stage may represent a relatively high level of ego development. Relatedly, many predictions about ego development are curvilinear. In examining the entire range of stages, for example, obedience to authority would be expected to be low at both the very low and very high stages of ego development and to peak in the middle. Among midlife women, John, Pals, and Westenberg (1998) found that those scoring at the lowest stages of ego development tended to present a *conflicted* personality prototype, those at the middle levels were rated as especially *traditional*, and those scoring in the highest region of the scheme manifested what the researchers called an *individuated* pattern of personality.

The construct of ego development has proven especially congenial for researchers more interested in patterns of thought and interpretation than in discrete behaviors per se. For example, studies have documented positive associations between ego development and stages of moral reasoning (Lee & Snarey, 1988), but research on how ego development predicts prosocial, moral, or altruistic behaviors is sparse. McAdams, Booth, and Selvik (1981) found that among religious college students, those who reported they had never gone through a period of strong religious doubt and those who described such a period but who suggested they had gotten "back on track" tended to score in the conformist range of ego development. By contrast, those scoring at higher levels of ego development tended to say that they were currently experiencing a period of religious questioning or that they had once done so and now saw questioning as integral to a lifelong journey of faith. Helson and Roberts (1994) showed that women high in ego level were open to thinking about difficult life experiences in new ways; apparently, high ego levels lead people to construct new schemas in the face of challenging life experiences. Studies like these suggest that among young and middle-aged adults, higher stages of ego development predict a more complex understanding of life, a

greater tolerance for change and ambiguity, and an appreciation for life's challenges as opportunities for growth (King & Raspin, 2004; Pals & John, 1998).

Given that ego development taps into how people *think* about and make sense of things, one would expect the construct to overlap with the general idea of intelligence. Studies have shown low but (often) significantly positive correlations (between +.15 and +.30) between IQ and ego scores on the SCT. The potential overlap between ego stage and intelligence raises the important issue of *discriminant validity* in personality research (Campbell & Fiske, 1959). A measure should measure what it says it measures, and not anything else. If IQ and ego scores are highly correlated, then one wonders if in fact the SCT is but an alternative measure of intelligence. The problem is a thorny one for ego development research, because the SCT is a verbal measure and more than a modicum of verbal intelligence seems to be required to produce sentences that are complex enough to score for higher stages of ego development. The current view has it that ego development measures may indeed tap partly into a general factor of intelligence, but the overlap seems modest and the problem is probably endemic to any personality measure that relies so heavily on verbal construction.

Life Stories: The Redemptive Self

Narrative theories of personality first made their appearance in the late 1980s. Although a few of the classic theories (e.g., Adler, 1927; Murray, 1938) intimated that human lives seem to take a storylike shape, it was not until Tomkins (1979; Carlson, 1981) articulated his *script theory* and McAdams (1985) proposed a *life-story model of identity* that personality psychologists began to take seriously the idea that the stories people tell about their lives are not simply reflections of personality trends but are instead *features of personality itself*. Rejecting approaches to personality that emphasize drives, motives, and even traits, Tomkins argued that from birth onward human beings unconsciously arrange their lives into affectively charged scenes and organizing scripts, which themselves become the structural features of psychological individuality. McAdams (1985) asserted that the development of what Erikson (1963) called ego identity is largely a matter of constructing and internalizing an integrative self-narrative to provide life with some sense of unity, purpose, and meaning. According to McAdams, people living in modern societies begin to arrange their lives into self-defining life stories—complete with settings, scenes, characters, plots, and themes—in the emerging adulthood years (see also Hermans, 1996; Singer & Salovey, 1993).

Life narrative constructs provide a stark conceptual counterpoint to dispositional traits (McAdams & Pals, 2006). The contrast mirrors the distinction in cognitive psychology between *episodic* and *semantic* memory. Life stories are framed in episodic terms. They package information about the self within an episodic frame, specifying when and where something happened (setting), who was involved (characters), how the action unfolded over time (plot), and what the significance of the episode might be (meaning). Life stories largely consist of the self-defining episodes of a person's life—both those from the past and those imagined for the future—and their arrangement into a broader narrative structure that provides what the narrator him- or herself believes to be a convincing explanation for how he or she came to be and where his or life may be going in the future. Life stories are expected to change markedly over the life course. In contrast, dispositional traits like extraversion and conscientiousness are framed as semantic categories of the self, and their framing emphasizes stability over time. An extravert sees him- or herself as generally outgoing, lively, and spontaneous. In the same semantic sense in which I "know" my phone number or the number of elements in the periodic table (not needing to recall the episodes from my past in which I learned this information), I may also "know" that I am lively and outgoing and respond accordingly on a self-report trait questionnaire. Some cognitive scientists have argued that episodic and semantic information about the self are processed in very different ways and with respect to different systems in the brain (see Klein, Loftus, & Kihlstrom, 1996). It should not be surprising, then, if dispositional constructs (level 1 in personality) and narrative constructs (level 3) do not map neatly onto each other.

Life narrative constructs are typically assessed through interviews or open-ended questionnaires wherein respondents are given an opportunity to describe key scenes, characters, and plots in the stories of their lives. The chal-

lenge for researchers is to develop reliable coding systems for analyzing the structural and content features of the narrative responses. One method used in a number of studies is McAdams's (1985) life story interview. The life story interview is a 2-hour procedure wherein an individual provides a narrative account of his or her life—past, present, and imagined future—by responding to a series of open-ended questions. The procedure begins by asking the respondent to divide his or her life into chapters and provide a brief plot outline for each. Next, the interview asks for detailed accounts of eight key scenes in the story, including a high point, low point, and turning point scene. The interview protocol goes on to cover main characters in the story, conflicts and challenges in the plot, imagined future chapters, and the basic values and beliefs on which the story's plot is developed.

Let us briefly consider one particular research program on life stories, a line of study that led to McAdams's (2006b) conception of *the redemptive self*. The program began with this question: What kinds of life stories do especially caring and productive adults in their midlife years construct? The researchers used self-report measures of generativity—an adult's concern for and commitment to promoting the well-being of future generations—to identify especially generative and less generative midlife adults, who then participated in individual life story interviews.

The researchers then examined carefully the interview transcripts produced by a small number of highly generative adults and a matched subsample of less generative adults. They compared and contrasted the two groups of stories in an attempt to discern the main thematic differences between them. The researchers were guided, in part, by the theoretical literature on generativity available at the time and by their own hunches regarding what kinds of life stories these two groups might produce. Mainly, though, they were guided by the rich narrative data. The researchers followed guidelines for what qualitative sociologists call *grounded theory methodology*, which basically involves constructing thematic categories to characterize groups and then refining those categories through successive readings of new data and repeated efforts to compare and contrast (Glaser & Strauss, 1967). After many meetings and discussions, the researchers settled on a small set of themes that seemed to differentiate between the two groups. They designed coding systems to operationalize these themes, and they trained new coders to achieve high levels of intercoder reliability.

The project then moved to a hypothesis-testing phase. Blind to identifying information for the respondents, the new coders analyzed a new sample of 70 life story interviews, 40 told by adults high in generativity and 30 told by adults scoring low in generativity. Some coding adjustments needed to be made along the way as some of the original categories proved difficult to apply to the new data. Once all of the coding was completed, the researchers employed standard statistical procedures to evaluate the extent to which the two groups showed statistically significant differences on the thematic categories hypothesized to differentiate between the two groups. Some of the categories did show the predicted differences, and some did not. The most interesting and robust category was what the researchers called a *redemption sequence* (McAdams, Diamond, de St. Aubin, & Mansfield, 1997). In a redemption sequence, a bad or affectively negative (sad, humiliating, fearful, shameful, guilt-provoking) scene gives way to a positive outcome or interpretation. The negative scene is saved, salvaged, or redeemed by a positive turn of events or by the narrator's conclusion that some redemptive meaning eventually emerged. Highly generative adults told life stories containing significantly more redemption sequences as compared with the life stories told by less generative adults.

Subsequent studies have shown that the redemptive pattern in life narratives can be reliably observed and scored in written accounts of self-defining memories, including those provided by college students (McAdams, Reynolds, Lewis, Patten, & Bowman, 2001). Redemptive imagery in life narratives is positively associated with self-report measures of subjective mental health for both college students and midlife adults. A related line of research has examined how individuals who have faced difficult life experiences construct stories to suggest they learned lessons, gained insights, or experienced positive psychological growth as a result (Bauer & McAdams, 2004; King, Scollon, Ramsey, & Williams, 2000; Pals, 2006; Thorne & McLean, 2003). These studies underscore the importance of (1) acknowledging and fully expressing strong negative emotions with respect to a negative life scene and

(2) constructing a narrative ending or meaning for the scene that affirms personal growth or greater integration of the self (Pals, 2006). The most redemptive narrative accounts in life plumb the depths of human experience before they eventually affirm growth and hope for the future.

McAdams and Bowman (2001) conducted a second intensive study of life stories told by highly generative adults. In this study the researchers sampled about 260 community adults, ranging in age from 35 to 65 years, approximately half of whom were African American and half White. Coding of 74 life story interviews chosen from the larger sample, half from adults scoring high in generativity and half from adults scoring low, replicated and extended the findings from McAdams and colleagues (1997). Again, redemption sequences differentiated between the two groups. In addition, a set of related narrative features again emerged as significant differences between the stories told by highly generative and less generative adults. These features included (1) early memories of enjoying a special *advantage* in life, (2) early memories of witnessing the *suffering or oppression of others*, (3) *moral steadfastness* and clarity stemming from ideological commitments made in adolescence, and (4) *prosocial life goals* for the future.

Along with the redemption theme, this suite of four narrative features converges on a general life story prototype, called the redemptive self, that is especially characteristic of the narrative identities constructed by highly generative adults, both Black and White, male and female. According to McAdams (2006b), the redemptive self is an especially well-designed narrative identity for supporting a generative approach to life in midlife. The redemptive self functions to affirm hope and commitment in the face of the many difficulties and challenges generativity poses for midlife adults. For example, believing one enjoyed an early advantage in childhood while others suffered may motivate a person to give back to others for the good fortune he or she has enjoyed. Expecting that bad things will ultimately be redeemed may help highly generative adults make the daunting investments of time, energy, and money that are often required to make a long-term, positive contribution to family or community. Holding to firm beliefs and values consolidated in adolescence may help keep away those nagging doubts and uncertainties that might compromise one's best generative efforts in the midlife years.

Most recently, McAdams (2006b) has reinterpreted the redemptive self in cultural terms, arguing that this particular life narrative prototype has a distinctively American flavor. In American cultural history and in contemporary popular culture, the most powerful stories of redemption employ the discourses of Christian atonement (from sin to salvation), political emancipation (from slavery to freedom), upward social mobility (from rags to riches), lifelong recovery (from illness/addiction to health), and individual self-development (from immaturity to the full actualization of the inner self). Drawing from a rich storehouse of cultural scripts, the redemptive self is a characteristically American kind of life story, well designed to support a generative life for midlife American adults. Caring and productive midlife adults living in very different cultural contexts are likely to construct different kinds of narratives to make sense of their lives and support their generative strivings. McAdams suggests that culture is most closely implicated in personality at the level of life narrative. More so than may be the case with dispositional traits and characteristic adaptations, life narrative studies push the personality psychologist to consider the many complex ways in which psychological individuality is intimately tied with society, history, and culture.

Conclusion: When Theories (and Their Constructs) Compete

We have argued that an important function of personality theory is to propose constructs to account for socially consequential aspects of psychological individuality. Most constructs proposed by personality theories may be located in one of three different conceptual levels or domains: dispositional traits, characteristic adaptations, and integrative life stories. We have examined the ways in which theory informs research and research informs theory with respect to representative constructs from each of these three levels. Research programs examining extraversion, ego development, and the redemptive self, respectively, illustrate many of the challenges and opportunities that personality psychologists have traditionally encountered and continue to encounter today.

At the present time, personality psychology is a field wherein many different theories, with their corresponding constructs and preferred methods, continue to develop, interact, and sometimes compete. Whereas some research programs focus exclusively on a single construct, many others attempt to relate different constructs to each other, to examine patterns of constructs in individual lives, and/or to chart the development of patterns over time. Even though no single grand theory exists to synthesize these many different strands of inquiry, the field of personality psychology continues to grow and flourish. We believe the field is best seen today as a broad and diverse set of somewhat overlapping programs of inquiry, each attracting a corresponding community of scientists who combine theory and research in a characteristic way (Wiggins, 2003). Different programs and their intellectual communities have different strengths to offer. No program or community can do it all, so the judicious scientist or student is well-advised to sample broadly, to acquaint him- or herself with a wide range of theories and research traditions.

One of the reasons that different programs of theory and research have different strengths to offer is that each asks somewhat different questions and sets forth somewhat different forms of scientific argument. One of the main functions of any program of research and theory in personality psychology is *to suggest what kinds of causal arguments will be convincing to a particular scientific/scholarly community*. Different theoretical traditions favor particular kinds of causal explanations that just seem "right" to those scientists who consider themselves part of, or at least strongly influenced by, the tradition. For example, proponents of social learning theories and related situationist approaches (e.g., Mischel & Shoda, 1995) have never been impressed with the evidence for cross-situational consistency in behavior linked to broad personality traits. Their disdain for trait theories has relatively little to do with empirical findings but instead reflects their commitment to arguments that privilege proximal determinants of particular behaviors displayed in particular social situations—arguments about process and context—rather than arguments about what general forms behavioral continuities take from one situation to the next. (But see Fleeson's, 2004, effort to reconcile trait and situationist approaches.) From the standpoint of situationist approaches, conceptions of personality that privilege broad trait continuities are asking the wrong questions and posing the wrong causal arguments. Of course, proponents of trait theories, who aim to describe and explain the basic tendencies that broadly differentiate people from each other, are quick to return the favor (McCrae & Costa, 1997). They find little of interest in questions asked by social learning theories and related approaches, and they find their causal arguments unconvincing and even irrelevant.

Going back to Aristotle, Rychlak (1981) asserts that the different causal arguments to be found in personality psychology may be classified into four groups: (1) *material*-cause arguments, which explain a phenomenon in terms of what substances make it up; (2) *efficient*-cause arguments, which explain a phenomenon in terms of the events that lead up to it; (3) *formal*-cause arguments, which specify the design or form of a phenomenon; and (4) *final*-cause arguments, which focus on the function or ultimate reason for a phenomenon. Most theories and their corresponding programs of construct validation research address all four of Aristotle's explanations in one way or another. Nonetheless, each approach seems to privilege one or two of the four, attracting scientists who find those corresponding kinds of arguments to be especially convincing.

The different preferences are quite apparent in the three programs of research reviewed in this paper. One of the reasons the construct of extraversion has enjoyed so much research attention in the past 50 years is that, beginning with Eysenck, scientists have proposed and tested intriguing arguments about material cause. Whether considering Eysenck's early hypotheses regarding arousal and the ARAS or more recent formulations that foreground a behavioral approach system in the brain, a strong research tradition in personality psychology has focused on the psychobiological underpinnings of extraversion. For scientists attracted to this tradition, the most interesting theoretical questions are about brain circuitry, neurotransmitters, and the patterns of cortical activity that essentially make up the basic material stuff of extraversion. Of course, the brain is surely involved in ego development, redemptive life narratives, and any other well-validated personality construct one may name. But the research programs that have developed with respect to these constructs have had little to say about material-cause issues.

As a developmental construct, Loevinger's ego stages chart a kind of efficient-cause sequence for the life course. People's overall perspectives for making sense of themselves and the world develop according to a predictable sequence. In addition, the particular stage one finds oneself in at any given point in the life course provides the basic form or structure, Loevinger argues, for psychological individuality at that stage. Loevinger's research program, therefore, seems to privilege efficient-cause and formal-cause arguments. Scientists attracted to her program find especially appealing questions like these: What is the sequence of stages through which people develop over time? How do people get to a particular developmental level? At any given stage in life, what form does a person's understanding of self and world assume?

Life narrative approaches seem to privilege formal-cause and final-cause explanations. Beginning in the emerging adulthood years, McAdams argues, people put their lives together into narrative forms. An especially compelling form, and one that seems to support a highly caring and productive life at midlife in contemporary American society, is the redemptive self. In a final-cause sense, life stories are constructed for the sake of personal integration. People find unity, purpose, and meaning in life through the psychosocial construction of life narrative. Furthermore, certain life stories function to support certain kinds of lives. Scientists attracted to life narrative research may find questions like these to be especially interesting: What do people think their lives mean? What kinds of narrative forms do people articulate in making sense of their lives? Do some life stories work better than others?

Personality psychologists pursue a great many questions in their efforts to account for the psychological individuality of persons. The different accounts they ultimately offer privilege certain kinds of arguments over others. One might imagine an ultimate, fully satisfying accounting of the individual person as providing compelling arguments regarding material-cause, efficient-cause, formal-cause, and final-cause explanations. To understand a person's individuality is ultimately to identify the essential substances of which that individuality is made, to chart the developmental sequences that account for how that individuality has come to be, to formulate a compelling picture of the design of that individuality, and to explain fully the ends or functions for which that particular form of individuality exists. What is the person made up of? How did the person come to be? What is the person's design or form? What purpose does that design fulfill? If we knew the full and unequivocal answers to these questions, we would no longer need personality psychology, its theories, its constructs, and its research. But we will likely never know all we need to know. Or if we ever do, that day is surely far in the future. In the meantime, we have personality theory and research.

Recommended Readings

McAdams, D. P., & Pals, J. L. (2006). A new Big Five: Fundamental principles for an integrative science of personality. *American Psychologist, 61,* 204–217.

Ozer, D. J. (1999). Four principles of personality assessment. In L. A. Pervin & O. P. John (Eds.), *Handbook of personality: Theory and research* (2nd ed., pp. 671–686). New York: Guilford Press.

References

Adler, A. (1927). *The practice and theory of individual psychology.* New York: Harcourt Brace World.

Allport, G. W. (1937). *Personality: A psychological interpretation.* New York: Henry Holt.

Atkinson, J. W., & Birch, D. (1978). *An introduction to motivation* (2nd ed.). New York: Van Nostrand.

Bauer, J. J., & McAdams, D. P. (2004). Personal growth in adults' stories of life transitions. *Journal of Personality, 72,* 573–602.

Bernreuter, R. G. (1931). *The personality inventory.* Stanford, CA: Stanford University Press.

Block, J. (1981). Some enduring and consequential structures of personality. In A. I. Rabin, J. Aronoff, A. M. Barclay, & R. A. Zucker (Eds.), *Further explorations in personality* (pp. 27–43). New York: Wiley.

Bowlby, J. (1969). *Attachment.* New York: Basic Books.

Campbell, D. T., & Fiske, D. W. (1959). Convergent and discriminant validation by the multitrait–multimethod matrix. *Psychological Bulletin, 56,* 81–105.

Caprara, G. V., & Cervone, D. (2000). *Personality: Determinants, dynamics, and potentials.* New York: Cambridge University Press.

Carlson, R. (1981). Studies in script theory: I. Adult analogs to a childhood nuclear scene. *Journal of Personality and Social Psychology, 40,* 501–510.

Carver, C. S., & Scheier, M. F. (1981). A control systems approach to behavioral self-regulation. In L. Wheeler & P. Shaver (Eds.), *Review of personality and social psychology* (Vol. 2, pp. 107–140). Beverly Hills, CA: Sage.

Cattel, R. B. (1943). The description of personality: Basic traits resolved into clusters. *Journal of Abnormal and Social Psychology, 38,* 476–506.

Cervone, D., & Shoda, Y. (1999). Beyond traits in the study of personality coherence. *Current Directions in Psychological Science, 8,* 27–32.

Costa, P. T., Jr., & McCrae, R. R. (1994). Set like plaster? Evidence for the stability of adult personality. In T. F. Heatherton & J. L. Weinberger (Eds.), *Can personality change?* (pp. 21–40). Washington, DC: American Psychological Association Press.

Cronbach, L. J., & Meehl, P. E. (1955). Construct validity in psychological tests. *Psychological Bulletin, 52,* 281–302.

Davidson, R. J. (1992). Emotion and affective style: Hemispheric substrates. *Psychological Science, 3,* 39–43.

Deci, E., & Ryan, R. M. (1991). A motivational approach to self: Integration in personality. In R. Dienstbier & R. M. Ryan (Eds.), *Nebraska Symposium on Motivation: 1990* (pp. 237–288). Lincoln: University of Nebraska Press.

Depue, R. A., Luciana, M., Arbisi, P., Collins, P., & Leon, A. (1994). Dopamine and the structure of personality: Relationships of agonist-induced dopamine activity to positive emotionality. *Journal of Personality and Social Psychology, 67,* 485–498.

Emmons, R. A. (1986). Personal strivings: An approach to personality and subjective well-being. *Journal of Personality and Social Psychology, 51,* 1058–1068.

Emmons, R. A., & Diener, E. (1986). Influence of impulsivity and sociability on subjective well-being. *Journal of Personality and Social Psychology, 50,* 1211–1215.

Erikson, E. H. (1963). *Childhood and society* (2nd ed.). New York: Norton.

Eysenck, H. J. (1947). *Dimensions of personality.* London: Routledge & Kegan Paul.

Eysenck, H. J. (1967). *The biological basis of personality.* Springfield, IL: Charles C. Thomas.

Eysenck, H. J. (1973). *Eysenck on extraversion.* New York: Wiley.

Fleeson, W. (2004). Moving personality beyond the person–situation debate. *Current Directions in Psychological Science, 13,* 83–87.

Fraley, R. C. (2002). Attachment and stability from infancy to adulthood: Meta-analysis and dynamic modeling of developmental mechanisms. *Personality and Social Psychology Review, 6,* 123–151.

Funder, D. C. (1995). On the accuracy of personality judgment: A realistic approach. *Psychological Review, 102,* 652–670.

Garnett, A. C. (1928). *Instinct and personality.* New York: Dodd, Mead.

Geen, R. C. (1997). Psychophysiological approaches to personality. In R. Hogan, J. A. Johnson, & S. Briggs (Eds.), *Handbook of personality psychology* (pp. 387–414). San Diego, CA: Academic Press.

Glaser, B. G., & Strauss, A. L. (1967). *The discovery of grounded theory.* Chicago: Aldine.

Goldberg, L. R. (1993). The structure of phenotypic personality traits. *American Psychologist, 48,* 26–34.

Gough, H. G. (1987). *California Psychological Inventory.* Palo Alto, CA: Consulting Psychologists Press.

Hall, C. S., & Lindzey, G. (1957). *Theories of personality.* New York: Wiley.

Helson, R., & Roberts, B. W. (1994). Ego development and personality change in adulthood. *Journal of Personality and Social Psychology, 66,* 911–920.

Hermans, H. J. M. (1996). Voicing the self: From information processing to dialogical interchange. *Psychological Bulletin, 119,* 31–50.

Hogan, R. (1976). *Personality theory: The personological tradition.* Englewood Cliffs, NJ: Prentice-Hall.

Hogan, R. (1982). A socioanalytic theory of personality. In M. Page (Ed.), *Nebraska Symposium on Motivation: 1981* (pp. 55–89). Lincoln: University of Nebraska Press.

Hogan, R. (1987). Personality psychology: Back to basics. In J. Aronoff, A. I. Rabin, & R. A. Zucker (Eds.), *The emergence of personality* (pp. 79–104). New York: Springer.

Hooker, K. S., & McAdams, D. P. (2003). Personality reconsidered: A new agenda for aging research. *Journal of Gerontology: Psychological Sciences, 58B,* 296–304.

Hull, C. L. (1943). *Principles of behavior.* New York: Appleton Century Crofts.

Hy, L. X., & Loevinger, J. (1996). *Measuring ego development* (2nd ed.). Mahwah, NJ: Erlbaum.

Jackson, D. N. (1971). The dynamics of structured personality tests. *Psychological Review, 78,* 229–248.

John, O. P., Pals, J. L., & Westenberg, P. M. (1998). Personality prototypes and ego development: Conceptual similarities and relations in adult women. *Journal of Personality and Social Psychology, 74,* 1093–1108.

King, L. A., & Raspin, C. (2004). Lost and found possible selves, subjective well-being, and ego development in divorced women. *Journal of Personality, 72,* 603–632.

King, L. A., Scollon, C. K., Ramsey, C., & Williams, T. (2000). Stories of life transition: Subjective well-being and ego development in parents of children with Down syndrome. *Journal of Research in Personality, 34,* 509–536.

Klein, S. B., Loftus, J., & Kihlstrom, J. F. (1996). Self-knowledge of an amnesic patient: Toward a neuropsychology of personality and social psychology. *Journal of Experimental Psychology: General, 125,* 250–260.

Kluckhohn, C., & Murray, H. A. (1953). Personality formation: The determinants. In C. Kluckhohn, H. A. Murray, & D. Schneider (Eds.), *Personality in nature, society, and culture* (pp. 53–67). New York: Knopf.

Kohlberg, L. (1969). Stage and sequence: The cognitive-developmental approach to socialization. In D. A. Goslin (Ed.), *Handbook of socialization theory and research* (pp. 347–480). Skokie, IL: Rand McNally.

Lakatos, I. (1970). Falsification and the methodology of scientific research programmes. In I. Lakatos & A. Musgrave (Eds.), *Criticism and the growth of knowledge* (pp. 91–196). Cambridge, UK: Cambridge University Press.

Leary, M. R. (2005). The scientific study of personality. In V. J. Derlega, B. A. Winstead, & W. H. Jones (Eds.), *Personality: Contemporary theory and research* (pp. 2–26). Belmont, CA: Thomson Wadsworth.

Lee, L., & Snarey, J. (1988). The relationship between ego and moral development: A theoretical review and empirical analysis. In D. K. Lapsley & F. C. Power (Eds.), *Self, ego, and identity: Integrative approaches* (pp. 151–178). New York: Springer-Verlag.

Little, B. R. (1999). Personality and motivation: Personal action and the conative evolution. In L. A. Pervin & O. P. John (Eds.), *Handbook of personality: Theory and research* (2nd ed., pp. 501–524). New York: Guilford Press.

Loevinger, J. (1957). Objective tests as instruments of psychological theory. *Psychological Reports, 3,* 635–694.

Loevinger, J. (1976). *Ego development.* San Francisco: Jossey-Bass.

Loevinger, J. (1979). Construct validity of the sentence-completion test of ego development. *Applied Psychological Measurement, 3,* 281–311.

Loevinger, J. (1983). On ego development and the structure of personality. *Developmental Review, 3,* 339–350.

Loevinger, J. (1987). *Paradigms of personality.* New York: Freeman.

Loevinger, J. (1998). Completing a life sentence. In P. M. Westenberg, A. Blasi, & L. D. Cohn (Eds.), *Personality development: Theoretical, empirical, and clinical investigations of Loevinger's conception of ego development* (pp. 347–354). Mahwah, NJ: Erlbaum.

MacDermid, S. M., Franz, C. E., & De Reus, L. A. (1998). Generativity: At the crossroads of social roles and personality. In D. P. McAdams & E. de St. Aubin (Eds.), *Generativity and adult development* (pp. 181–226). Washington, DC: American Psychological Association Press.

Marcia, J. E. (1980). Identity in adolescence. In J. Adelson (Ed.), *Handbook of adolescent psychology* (pp. 159–187). New York: Wiley.

McAdams, D. P. (1985). *Power, intimacy, and the life story: Personological inquiries into identity.* Homewood, IL: Dorsey Press.

McAdams, D. P. (1995). What do we know when we know a person? *Journal of Personality, 63,* 365–396.

McAdams, D. P. (1997). A conceptual history of personality psychology. In R. Hogan, J. Johnson, & S. Briggs (Eds.), *Handbook of personality psychology* (pp. 3–39). San Diego, CA: Academic Press.

McAdams, D. P. (2001). The psychology of life stories. *Review of General Psychology, 5,* 100–122.

McAdams, D. P. (2006a). *The person: A new introduction to personality psychology* (4th ed.). New York: Wiley.

McAdams, D. P. (2006b). *The redemptive self: Stories Americans live by.* New York: Oxford University Press.

McAdams, D. P., Booth, L., & Selvik, R. (1981). Religious identity among students at a private college: Social motives, ego stage, and development. *Merrill-Palmer Quarterly, 27,* 219–239.

McAdams, D. P., & Bowman, P. J. (2001). Narrating life's turning points: Redemption and contamination. In D. P. McAdams, R. Josselson, & A. Lieblich (Eds.), *Turns in the road: Narrative studies of lives in transition* (pp. 3–34). Washington, DC: American Psychological Association Press.

McAdams, D. P., Diamond, A., de St. Aubin, E., & Mansfield, E. (1997). Stories of commitment: The psychosocial construction of generative lives. *Journal of Personality and Social Psychology, 72,* 678–694.

McAdams, D. P., & Pals, J. L. (2006). A new Big Five: Fundamental principles for an integrative science of personality. *American Psychologist, 61,* 204–217.

McAdams, D. P., Reynolds, J., Lewis, M., Patten, A., & Bowman, P. J. (2001). When bad things turn good and good things turn bad: Sequences of redemption and contamination in life narrative, and their relation to psychosocial adaptation in midlife adults and in college students. *Personality and Social Psychology Bulletin, 27,* 208–230.

McClelland, D. C. (1961). *The achieving society.* New York: Van Nostrand.

McCrae, R. R., & Costa, P. T., Jr. (1997). Personality trait structure as a human universal. *American Psychologist, 52,* 509–516.

Mendelsohn, G. (1993). It's time to put theories of personality in their place, or, Allport and Stagner got it right, why can't we? In K. H. Craik, R. Hogan, & R. N. Wolfe (Eds.), *Fifty years of personality psychology* (pp. 103–115). New York: Plenum Press.

Mischel, W., & Shoda, Y. (1995). A cognitive-affective systems theory of personality: Reconceptualizing situations, dispositions, dynamics, and invariance in personality structure. *Psychological Review, 102,* 246–268.

Murray, H. A. (1938). *Explorations in personality.* New York: Oxford University Press.

Nasby, W., & Read, N. (1997). The life voyage of a solo circumnavigator. *Journal of Personality, 65*(3).

Ozer, D. J. (1999). Four principles of personality assessment. In L. A. Pervin & O. P. John (Eds.), *Handbook of personality: Theory and research* (2nd ed., pp. 671–686). New York: Guilford Press.

Pals, J. L. (2006). Constructing the "springboard effect": Causal connections, self-making, and growth within the life story. In D. P. McAdams, R. Josselson, & A. Lieblich (Eds.), *Identity and story.* Washington, DC: American Psychological Association Press.

Pals, J. L., & John, O. P. (1998). How are dimensions of adult personality related to ego development? An application of the typological approach. In P. M. Westenberg, A. Blasi, & L. D. Cohn (Eds.), *Personality development: Theoretical, empirical, and clinical investigations of Loevinger's conception of ego development* (pp. 113–131). Mahwah, NJ: Erlbaum.

Roberts, B. W., & Robins, R. W. (2000). Broad dispositions, broad aspirations: The intersection of personality traits and major life goals. *Personality and Social Psychology Bulletin, 26,* 1284–1296.

Robins, R. W., Gosling, S. D., & Craik, K. H. (1999). An empirical analysis of trends in psychology. *American Psychologist, 54,* 117–128.

Rorer, L. G. (1990). Personality assessment: A conceptual survey. In L. A. Pervin (Ed.), *Handbook of personality: Theory and research* (pp. 693–720). New York: Guilford Press.

Runyan, W. M. (1982). *Life histories and psychobiography: Explorations in theory and method.* New York: Oxford University Press.

Rychlak, J. F. (1981). *Introduction to personality and psychotherapy: A theory-construction approach.* Boston: Houghton Mifflin.

Schultz, W. T. (Ed.). (2005). *Handbook of psychobiography.* New York: Oxford University Press.

Sheldon, K. (2004). *Optimal human being: An integrated, multilevel perspective.* Mahwah, NJ: Erlbaum.

Singer, J. A., & Salovey, P. (1993). *The remembered self: Emotion and memory in personality.* New York: Free Press.

Spearman, C. (1927). *The abilities of man.* London: Macmillan.

Stern, W. (1924). *Die menschliche Personalichkeit.* Leipzig: J. A. Barth.

Sullivan, H. S. (1953). *The interpersonal theory of psychiatry.* New York: Norton.

Sutton, S. K., & Davidson, R. J. (1997). Prefrontal brain asymmetry: A biological substrate of the behavioral approach and behavioral inhibition systems. *Psychological Science, 8,* 204–210.

Thorne, A. (1989). Conditional patterns, transference, and the coherence of personality across time. In D. M. Buss & N. Cantor (Eds.), *Personality psychology: Recent trends and emerging directions* (pp. 149–159). New York: Springer-Verlag.

Thorne, A., & McLean, K. C. (2003). Telling traumatic events in adolescence: A study of master narrative positioning. In R. Fivush & C. Haden (Eds.), *Autobiographical memory and the construction of a narrative self* (pp. 169–185). Mahwah, NJ: Erlbaum.

Tomkins, S. S. (1979). Script theory. In H. E. Howe & R. A. Dienstbier (Eds.), *Nebraska Symposium on Motivation: 1978* (pp. 201–236). Lincoln: University of Nebraska Press.

Watson, D., & Clark, L. A. (1997). Extraversion and its positive emotional core. In R. Hogan, J. Johnson, & S. Briggs (Eds.), *Handbook of personality psychology* (pp. 767–793). San Diego, CA: Academic Press.

Westenberg, P. M., Blasi, A., & Cohn, L. D. (Eds.). (1998). *Personality development: Theoretical, empirical, and clinical investigations of Loevinger's conception of ego development.* Mahwah, NJ: Erlbaum.

Wiggins, J. S. (1973). *Personality and prediction: Principles of personality assessment.* Reading, MA: Addison-Wesley.

Wiggins, J. S. (2003). *Paradigms of personality assessment.* New York: Guilford Press.

Winter, D. G. (1973). *The power motive.* New York: Free Press.

## CHAPTER 2

Designing and Implementing Longitudinal Studies

M. Brent Donnellan
Rand D. Conger

Drawing good conclusions from bad data is a lot like reassembling Humpty Dumpty after his big fall—largely impossible. Thus, researchers strive to design and implement studies that have the potential to yield high-quality data. In those areas of psychology where laboratory experimentation is not the method of first resort for logistical or ethical reasons, longitudinal studies are often recommended. Indeed, we believe that it is imperative to observe what happens as time passes and lives unfold. However, there are many challenges that face the researcher who decides to use this method. In short, it is difficult to maintain the rigor, relevance, and vitality of a study that may take years to produce even partial answers to once burning questions.

Accordingly, the goal of this chapter is to provide personality researchers with some of the insights that we have gained for ensuring data quality through the conduct of a nearly 20-year study of individual development. We discuss procedures that have worked well and confess to errors that have been made so that other researchers might learn from both. We hope that the final product will be a useful guide for designing and implementing longitudinal studies in a fashion that increases the probability that future studies will yield high-quality data.

At the outset, it is worth noting that there is an interesting asymmetry in the methodological literature surrounding longitudinal studies. On one hand there are numerous resources that describe how to appropriately analyze data from longitudinal research (e.g., Collins & Sayer, 2001; Ferrer & McArdle, 2003; Mroczek, Chapter 31, this volume; Nagin, 2005; Raudenbush, 2001; Singer & Willett, 2003), yet on the other hand there are fewer resources offering guidance on designing and running longitudinal studies (Taris, 2000; but see Cauce, Ryan, & Grove, 1998; Friedman & Haywood, 1994; Hartmann, 2005;

Stouthamer-Loeber, van Kammen, & Loeber, 1992). This deficit in information may contribute to a situation in which the intense planning and management required for collecting the raw material for these sophisticated analyses is overlooked. Thus, our overarching purpose is to add to the limited literature that provides practical advice for conducting longitudinal research.

This chapter is organized into three major sections. First, we outline and discuss four critical design decisions that should be addressed when planning to study lives over time. Second, we offer practical advice for running these kinds of studies. Finally, we describe some techniques for reducing attrition, one of the most pernicious threats to the health of a longitudinal investigation. An integral part of each of these sections is a recounting of experiences from our own longitudinal research to illustrate the points we wish to make. We draw on the Family Transitions Project, a prospective study of more than 500 participants and their families (see Conger & Conger, 2002), as a case study that helps to illustrate both the successes that accrue when appropriate procedures are followed and the problems that occur when they are not. Prior to addressing these issues, we briefly consider why researchers should ever bother conducting longitudinal research in the first place.

Why Bother Studying Personality the Long Way?

This question seems reasonable, given the cost and time commitment associated with a longitudinal study, particularly one that lasts several years. Despite these difficulties, our view is that longitudinal designs are better able to capture the dynamic aspects of human lives as compared with alternative approaches such as cross-sectional studies or laboratory experiments. For instance, long-term research in the natural environment has the capacity to evaluate the influence of major events, such as the birth of child or the loss of a job, on trajectories of individual development. Consider that Costello, Compton, Keeler, and Angold (2003) found remarkable, positive changes in the personal dispositions of children when their families experienced significant increases in economic well-being as a result of the introduction of a new industry in an economically depressed

region of the country. This kind of discovery would not have been possible without longitudinal inquiry. Indeed, cross-sectional studies cannot begin to disentangle consequences from causes, and potentially life-altering events are rarely created in the laboratory of the social psychologist.

To be sure, Block (1993) contends that longitudinal studies are necessary to answer the "big" questions that come to mind when most people (i.e., nonacademics) think about psychology. These are the questions that spark human curiosity, such as whether childhood characteristics influence adult personality, whether personality is fixed by age 30, or whether happiness is something that changes in response to life events. For instance, consider just three controversial issues in personality psychology that are also of public interest.

1. Are adult life experiences related to changes in personality traits (e.g., McCrae & Costa, 2003; Neyer & Asendorpf, 2001; Roberts, Caspi, & Moffitt, 2003)?
2. How stable are individual differences in attachment security across the lifespan (e.g., Fraley & Brumbaugh, 2004)?
3. Does low self-esteem have real-world consequences (e.g., Baumeister, Campbell, Krueger, & Vohs, 2003; Trzesniewski et al., 2006)?

It is difficult to see how these theoretically and practically important issues could be adequately addressed without longitudinal research. Therefore, we believe that longitudinal designs are essential for answering fundamental questions in personality psychology. However, before attempting to use this type of costly and time-consuming research strategy, a researcher needs to carefully consider several issues involved in the design, implementation, and maintenance of such an effort.

Initial Design Decisions: Answering Four Basic Questions

Before outlining the most pressing questions that face investigators who are conceptualizing and designing a longitudinal study (see also Taris, 2000), we think it is useful to provide our broad perspective on conducting longitudinal research. First, we propose that longitudinal designs need to be driven by conceptual and theoretical concerns and not simply by the desire to apply a "hot" methodological technique to repeated measures data (e.g., Hartmann, 2005). There are too many decisions that cannot be made without theoretical guidance. Second, longitudinal studies should be designed with more than a single mode of data analysis in mind. Accordingly, we urge researchers to think about collecting the most flexible kinds of data they can. Often this will involve a much closer scrutiny of measures than is involved in cross-sectional research. For instance, in dealing with correlations, the actual metrics of scales are often given little attention. As long as there is variability in measures of X and Y, then the analyses can often proceed. However, the metric used to measure variables matters a great deal for many of the types of analyses central to longitudinal studies, such as mean-level comparisons over time. Indeed, the most flexible longitudinal measures need to do more than just capture individual differences at one point in time; they need to be suitable for capturing individual differences in change over time and perhaps intraindividual differences in change over time. This need places much more stringent requirements on the types of measures selected for longitudinal studies.

Finally, the overarching theme of this chapter is that longitudinal studies require careful planning, deliberation, and management. Quite frankly, there are individual differences in the ability to carry out longitudinal studies, inasmuch as this kind of research typically requires a great deal of foresight, patience, diligence, leadership, and the ability to work well with others under stressful conditions. Indeed, most major longitudinal studies require the work of fairly large teams of researchers who are supported by federal grants. Working together to pursue the research agenda and to maintain public investments in an ongoing study become central aspects of the scientific enterprise. In short, personality traits matter in conducting this kind of research, and not everyone has the personality profile that fits well with these requirements. Investigators contemplating this kind of research should first ask themselves if they are suited for the task. A little self-insight will go a long way in channeling personal resources to the most productive research pursuits. With this background in mind, we turn to the four questions that need to be addressed in designing a prospective, longitudinal study of personality (see Table 2.1).

TABLE 2.1. Summary of Recommendations Regarding Initial Design Decisions

Question 1: Decide what to measure and how to measure it

1. Assess important constructs.
2. Anticipate statistical analyses.
3. Use well-validated and reliable instruments.
4. Pilot test all measures.
5. Use the exact same measure at every wave.

Question 2: Decide on the number and timing of assessments.

1. Strive for three or more waves of data collection.
2. Let conceptual issues dictate the timing of assessments.

Question 3: Decide on sources of data.

1. Strive for multiple informant studies.

Question 4: Decide on a sample and sample size

1. Engage in the thought experiment of defining the population of interest and select an appropriate sampling strategy.
2. Determine an adequate sample size that takes into account the reality of attrition.

Question 1: Decide What to Measure and How to Measure It

Specific answers to the "what" question will naturally depend on the particulars of a given project. At the most fundamental level, answers to this question depend on the theoretical and conceptual concerns of the longitudinal investigation. However, when a long-term study is launched, investigators must be both focused and yet relatively open in their conceptualization of needed areas of assessment. The reason for this approach rests on the fact that the theoretical reasoning of the moment may not prove to be the most fruitful; therefore, the researcher needs to consider potentially worthwhile alternatives to his or her preferred theoretical framework. This strategy reduces dogmatism and creates the possibility of maximal scientific payoff for the time and resources invested. Simply put, given the inevitable lag between the time the research begins and the time when results are ready for publication, the best advice is to focus on a range of constructs of relatively wide interest to the field. It would be very unfortunate to invest the effort required to design and implement a longitudinal study that, in the long run, produces results that make only limited scientific contributions. A good eye for distinguishing between the research fad of the moment and the fundamental topics of enduring interest is a valuable asset at this stage.

Once the constructs have been selected, then researchers must decide on specific measures that can be used to represent those constructs. At this step it is important to select psychometrically strong instruments that are well validated. As noted above, there is a time commitment involved in longitudinal studies, which introduces an element of risk. It is quite tragic if, shortly after data collection commences, there appears convincing evidence in the literature that a particular measure used in a longitudinal study is severely flawed. The best strategy for minimizing such risks is to conduct extensive literature reviews of the measures to be used and, to the degree possible, conduct pilot tests on all of these measures. There is no substitute for firsthand knowledge of the psychometric properties of all instruments used in the study. It is also worthwhile to solicit advice from other experts in the field about recent advances in the measurement of specific constructs. Often, other investigators have already conducted extensive evaluations of measures of potential interest and have a great deal of unpublished information that would be valuable for project planning. Finding such consultants can greatly improve measurement decisions and save substantial amounts of time and money in the planning process. This discussion also underscores the need for more published papers providing critical evaluations of existing assessments. Our suspicion is that evidence of psychometric flaws in particular instruments goes into the so-called file drawer far too often.

Decisions about "how" to measure particular constructs also require the researcher to anticipate data analyses, because many of the recent advances in longitudinal statistical techniques offer sophisticated ways to study individual differences in absolute change. As such, these techniques make assumptions about the variables used in the analyses. For example, standard growth models assume that variables are measured with interval level scales where "a given value of the outcome on any occasion [represents] the 'same' amount of the outcome on every occasion" (Singer & Willett, 2003, p. 13). This requirement has important implications for how constructs are measured.

For example, a commonly used instruction in personality research is to have respondents rate how they compare with other people of their age and gender on a specific characteristic. This instruction renders the data largely inappropriate for studying absolute changes in personality. For example, consider that Sally absolutely increased in self-control from ages 18 to 30 but retained the same relative position with respect to her age-mates at both time points. Under these circumstances, Sally should report the same self-control score at both assessments even though her absolute level of self-control increased. Put differently, the value of 3.75 on this scale represents a different absolute amount of self-control at ages 18 and 30. This fact renders this hypothetical measure of self-control inappropriate for growth curve modeling.

Thus, it should be clear that longitudinal studies require close attention to how items and instructions are worded and what response options are used. This work must be completed in the pilot and planning stages of the research because measures of a specific construct should remain the same from one wave to the next. As Willett, Singer, and Martin (1998) note, "The time for instrument modification is during pilot work, not data collection" (p. 411). Put simply, the same exact instrument should be used at each wave (Willett et al., 1998).[1] Nonetheless, administering the same instrument at each wave does not guarantee that the instrument will measure the same latent construct in exactly the same way at each wave. This is the issue of measurement invariance (e.g., Hartmann, 2005) or measurement equivalence (e.g., Baltes, Reese, & Nesselroade, 1977), and it deserves some comment because it is so important in longitudinal research.

Measurement equivalence is required to draw valid inferences about continuity or change across time from longitudinal data (e.g., Horn & McArdle, 1992). For example, measurement invariance or equivalence is a prerequisite for growth modeling (Chan, 1998; Vandenberg & Lance, 2000) because this technique assumes that the same construct is being measured in the same way at each wave—otherwise, differences between measures at one wave and another "may be tantamount to comparing apples and spark plugs" (Vandenberg & Lance, 2000, p. 9). Unfortunately, measurement equivalence is infrequently tested despite several accessible tutorials on this topic (e.g., Ployhart & Oswald, 2004; Raykov & Marcoulides, 2000; Vandenberg & Lance, 2000; Widaman & Reise, 1997). Thus, we recommend that researchers examine existing evidence for measurement equivalence for measures they are considering for a longitudinal study.

To this point the scenario for deciding how to measure constructs seems relatively straightforward: For each construct, pick the best available measure or measures and make sure there is evidence that these assessments demonstrate measurement equivalence over time. Unfortunately, things are rarely this simple in the real world. First, some experts may believe that measure *A* is a state-of-the-art instrument whereas other experts believe that measure *B* is the best possible assessment instrument. Partisans for measure *A* anticipate rejecting any study that uses measure *B*, and vice versa. In some cases a researcher may choose to use both measures; however, this practice may result in irritated participants who have to complete several similar questionnaires. Here the investigator must rely on professional judgment to determine which measurement strategy is likely to yield the greatest gain for the particular project. Tradeoffs and compromises are a reality of longitudinal studies. Researchers must accept the fact that they will occasionally make the wrong choice and have to live with that decision. Even Tiger Woods makes the occasional bogey.

Second, sometimes the content of measures needs to be modified over time, particularly in a study focused on change over relatively long spans of time that cross developmental periods. For example, an investigator may be interested in evaluating the degree to which aversive or challenging life events exacerbate tendencies toward aggressive behavior during late childhood, adolescence, and the early adult years. The problem lies in the fact that valid indicators of both negative life events and aggressive actions may reasonably vary across these developmental periods. One might, for instance, ask about violence toward a romantic partner as an indicator of aggressiveness during early adulthood, but this item would be inappropriate during late childhood. Similarly, physical abuse by a parent or interparental conflict would be an especially important stressor during childhood and adolescence, but would be less appropriate during the adult years. The researcher is faced with a dilemma and will

certainly need to rely on strong theoretical conceptualizations about heterotypic continuity (e.g., Caspi, 1998) and may well need to seek the advice of experts in measurement and substantive areas to deal with these complex situations. Nevertheless, we believe that investigators should measure constructs of central theoretical interest as well as they possibly can, even if they cannot be certain at the time of study onset that they have fully solved all of the problems related to measurement equivalence.

With regard to the issue of conceptualization and selection of measures, some experiences from the Family Transitions Project (FTP) are informative. The FTP was initially concerned with how a severe downturn in the agricultural economy of the 1980s affected rural families in Iowa and, in particular, seventh-grade children living in those families (Conger & Conger, 2002). For that reason, the domains of measurement were relatively broad and included, among others, economic experiences, related stressful life events, and the quality of family relationships. The psychosocial problems and competencies of the focal adolescents in the study were also assessed. The theoretical models that guided the research were developed with the idea that they would be tested using cross-lagged panel models. When pretesting occurred in 1987 and 1988, growth modeling was used only rarely in the literature, and we were not as sensitive then as we are today about the issue of maintaining the same metric at each point in time. In some cases, we did not take sufficient time to adequately scour all of the relevant literatures or to contact measurement experts who might have helped identify emerging measures of constructs that would provide the best possible information over the next two decades of the study. A few times, the crystal ball simply malfunctioned.

In truth, we did not expect that the initial findings would be so valuable that they would lead to an investigation that would span all of adolescent and the early adult years. However, it seems advisable for any investigator contemplating a longitudinal study to consider the possibility that it might last longer than an initial 2–5 years, the usual time period for a federal grant award. On the basis of these lessons, it behooves the researcher to take the exceptional kinds of care in measurement planning that we advocate here. Indeed, we would have done so ourselves if we had realized the long-term possibilities for the study. As it turned out, we were able to maintain the metric across time for many of our measures, and as a result we have been able to take advantage of growth modeling in several instances (e.g., Cui, Conger, & Lorenz, 2005; Kim, Conger, Lorenz, & Elder, 2001).

Experiences with the FTP have also added to our understanding of how to deal with the problem of measurement design in relation to developmental change. As noted earlier, the appropriate indicators for a construct may vary over the years, especially across crucial life course transitions such as from childhood to adolescence and adolescence to adulthood. As needed, many of the measures used in the FTP have been altered to reflect these life changes. In this process, however, we learned that many core items could be maintained in most measures so that we could achieve an equivalent metric for at least some scores over time. For example, aggression toward other family members that involves hitting, pushing, or grabbing may differ in force with age, but may be functionally equivalent whether the person is a child or an adult. At each stage of the research the investigator should seek to maintain a sample of core items in relation to each construct, even if some items need to be added or deleted for the final measure to be appropriate for a given time of life. Another important area for consideration is the use of IRT (see Morizot, Ainsworth, & Reise, Chapter 24, this volume) to determine which items measured at one time may be replaced by more developmentally appropriate items at a later point in time and still maintain measurement equivalence. We are only beginning to use this technique in the FTP; thus, we do not have any specific examples regarding its usefulness from this study.

All told, the selection of measures for a longitudinal project requires the researcher to anticipate how assessment procedures will stand the test of time to reveal processes of change and continuity across the years of the study. Moreover, as previously noted, the investigator also needs to be concerned about the measurement of constructs that may not be central to the initial focus of the study, but that may prove important as the research proceeds. For example, the initial concern in the FTP was the relatively immediate response of family members to economic difficulties, and there was little emphasis on more enduring traits or dispositions. However, the research team suspected that relatively stable personality characteristics

play an important role in the long-term development of the cohort of youth in the study. As it turned out, this early expectation proved to be quite accurate, and the personality measures collected during the adolescent phase of the research are proving to be important predictors of long-term developmental outcomes (e.g., Donnellan, Larsen-Rife, & Conger, 2005).

Indeed, it is important to keep in mind that casting a wide net often provides data that can be used to rule out rival hypotheses for particular findings. This strategy is crucial for advancing scientific knowledge and counteracting confirmation biases. In short, it is important to think carefully about alternative explanations for potential findings and incorporate measures of these constructs at the outset. This strategy may lead to so-called critical tests and will help optimize the scientific payoff from a longitudinal study.

This suggestion underscores the importance of having a group of investigators with complementary sets of expertise for any long-term study. A single investigator will be hard pressed to adequately survey the myriad possibilities for conceptualization, assessment, and later data analysis that will be important for the initiation and conduct of a first-rate longitudinal study. Collaborations across disciplines and subdisciplines are almost a necessity and will provide fertile ground for novel scientific advances. This point brings us back to the importance of being able to work well with a group of scientists and research staff. A successful investigator will need to have the ability to engage with others in the give and take of considering alternative possibilities for the design and implementation of the research. Although difficult at times, this process is also one of the most exciting and productive aspects of this type of inquiry.

Question 2: Decide on the Number and Timing of Assessments

It is axiomatic in longitudinal research that two-wave studies provide an impoverished picture of change (e.g., Rogosa, 1995). Consider Rogosa's comment that "two waves of data are better than one, but maybe not much better (Rogosa, Brandt, & Zimowski, 1982, p. 744). To be fair, two-wave studies are useful and informative, especially in new research areas. However, two-wave studies do not provide enough information to assess patterns of individual growth using anything other than a straight line and therefore provide a limited picture of change (individuals can only increase, decrease, or remain constant on a given measure). In addition, if rates of change fluctuate over time, then estimates provided by two-wave studies may be quite biased.

The situation improves with three waves of data because then it is possible to test the adequacy and appropriateness of a linear conception of change. Moreover, the precision of parameter estimates in individual growth models and the reliability of the estimate of the rate of change for the sample increases with additional waves (Willett et al., 1998). These increases are particularly pronounced when there are a few waves of data, such that adding a 4th wave to a 3-wave study produces greater gains than adding the 19th wave to an 18-wave study (see Willett et al., 1998, Fig. 4). Thus, we simply echo the admonishment to "collect extra waves of data at all costs" (Willett et al., 1998, p. 409).

The timing of assessments deserves more attention than it is normally given in designing longitudinal research. Often the decision of when to assess participants is based on practical considerations, such as once a semester or once a year, rather than deriving from theoretical or conceptual concerns. This is likely to be a big mistake, especially for researchers who are designing longitudinal studies to test the plausibility of causal hypotheses or to test mediational models (e.g., Cole & Maxwell, 2003). The reason is that causes produce effects that play out over time and the sizes of these causal effects may vary over time (Gollob & Reichardt, 1987). Thus, a lack of attention to the timing of assessments in the design phase of the study can have severe consequences.

To illustrate these concerns, we borrow the example of the effects of aspirin on pain reduction from Gollob and Reichardt (1987). Assume that there is no effect in the immediate few minutes after the drug is taken but that pain-reducing effects are noticeable 30 minutes after ingesting an aspirin. Further assume that the effects peak about 3 hours later and then diminish to zero after 6 hours. Given this state of affairs, it is clear that the time intervals selected by researchers will influence the conclusions drawn from a particular study. The researcher who spaces assessments at 10-hour intervals will find little evidence that aspirin has any pain-relieving properties, whereas the researcher who spaces assessments at 1-hour intervals will find evidence for the substantial pain-relieving properties of aspirin that diminish over time. Thus, when designing a longitudinal study, it greatly helps to have some understanding of how aspirin should work. In the absence of that kind of conceptual guidance, more frequent assessments with shorter time lags would lead to fewer Type II errors with respect to whether or not aspirin has any effect at all on pain relief.

The broad point is that the lag between assessments is an important design consideration that should be tied to the theoretical and conceptual issues under study. Our view is that more frequent assessments are needed during periods of rapid change, such as the transition from elementary school to junior high or during the initial phases of a romantic relationship. More frequent assessments are also important in those cases in which the investigator has little insight into the underlying causal processes of interest. Naturally, careful attention to this issue will increase the power of a given study to find particular effects and help researchers to answer more nuanced questions concerning how effects vary with time. We consider this issue to be a major challenge in designing a well-crafted longitudinal study.

As a practical matter, however, we note that the number of assessments may be constrained by the availability of funding for a project, especially after a study has already been ongoing for a period of time. For example, the FTP has been supported by a series of renewal grants which, when resources have been limited, have required adjustments in the number of planned assessments and in the scope of the assessments at any given point in time. When such circumstances arise, investigators need to be flexible and have alternative scenarios for how they might achieve the goals of the study. Should they cut the scope of assessments within given time periods, or should they reduce the number of assessments across the years of the project? These questions need to be considered and planned for as part of the ongoing study. In the FTP, we have sometimes maintained the full assessment battery in alternate years and collected more limited information via telephone interviews in the off years. This strategy has allowed us to get annual information on core constructs every year even while cutting activities to meet budgetary limitations. This kind of adjustment must be anticipated during the course of any longitudinal study.

Question 3: Decide on Sources of Data

According to Caspi (1998), longitudinal studies should rely "on multiple measures gathered from multiple sources using multiple methods" (p. 369). Accordingly, we recommend that researchers supplement self-reports with informant reports or behavioral observations whenever possible. Indeed, self-report studies are so common that Funder (2004) lamented that "some investigators seem to have forgotten that other kinds of data even exist" (p. 27). To be sure, the problem is that any one source of data is limited and subject to particular weaknesses; self-reports are by no means a uniquely bad approach to obtaining data. Thus, when planning research, we believe that researchers should strive for "gold standard" designs that use multiple sources of data. This strategy will ultimately increase the scientific rigor of personality psychology.

It is especially important to note that an entire study based on self-reports will always be susceptible to the criticism that shared method variance, rather than a "true" causal relation, is responsible for the observed associations between constructs. Critics of personality research often offer this as a reasonable alternative explanation for positive findings in the literature. For example, Gottman (1998) noted that the link between personality and marital functioning may be an artifact of method variance. Fortunately, there is a compelling solution to this problem, as noted by Podsakoff, MacKenzie, Lee, and Podsakoff (2003) in their comprehensive review of common method biases and remedies: "If the predictor and criterion variables can be measured from different sources, then we recommend that this be done." (p. 897). We believe that personality researchers can and should follow this strategy whenever possible. With regard to Gottman's critique, Donnellan, Larsen-Rife, and Conger (2005) used FTP data to show that parent reports of adolescent personality were robust predictors of the quality of their early adult children's romantic relationships as reported by the romantic partners and trained observers. Findings of this type provide very strong evidence that personality traits have an association with outcome variables that cannot be attributed to a singular reliance on self-reported data.

A particularly rigorous but, we hope, attainable goal is to obtain three separate sources of data for each construct, especially when researchers plan to use latent variable models. Three sources of data should strike an appropriate balance between construct coverage and resource constraints for use in structural equation models (Little, Lindenberger, & Nesselroade, 1999). In longitudinal studies of personality, informant reports may be a particularly important alternative source of data. Moreover, there are also suggestions that informant reports of personality may have increased predictive validity as compared with self-reports of personality for certain criteria such as job performance ratings (e.g., Mount, Barrick, & Strauss, 1994). Thus, we strongly endorse the practice of obtaining informant reports and note that informant reports may have even greater power to detect personality effects than self-reports for some criterion variables.

Moreover, collecting observational data is another possibility that should be considered. For example, we have been interested in how personality traits are associated with interactions in family and other close relationships (e.g., Donnellan et al., 2005; Ge & Conger, 1999). Thus, we have used videotaped family interactions in the FTP to assess how individuals behave in those intimate settings. Indeed, a fundamental interest in personality research is the degree to which emotional, behavioral, and cognitive dispositions either result from or lead to social relationships of varying types and styles (Caspi, 1998). A particularly good way to gain insight into social relationships is to actually observe them. In addition, there is growing evidence that observed interactions in families and other types of dyads provide particularly sensitive markers of change over time (Conger, Lorenz, & Wickrama, 2004; Kim et al., 2001). As such, they are well suited to longitudinal studies, and the observational data completely overcome potential method biases that result from a singular reliance on self-reports by study participants.

Question 4: Decide on a Sample and Sample Size

Sampling is arguably the Achilles' heel of psychology (Caspi, 1998) because convenience samples dominate so much of the literature. The problem is that the biases introduced by convenience samples often go unrecognized and are nearly impossible to estimate (Hartmann, 2005). This renders claims about the generalizabilty of findings very tenuous and makes an honest consideration of external validity difficult. We concur with Hartmann (2005), who suggests that researchers should engage in the thought experiment of imagining the target population to which they wish to generalize. After identifying the population or populations of interest, the ideal step would be to draw a random sample from this group or groups. However, this step is not feasible for many studies and there are alternatives that can be considered (Hartmann, 2005; see Cook & Campbell, 1979, pp. 75–80).

The first is the model of deliberate sampling for heterogeneity (or purposive sampling of heterogeneous instances; Shadish, Cook, & Campbell, 2002). The objective here is to select for a wide variety of individual differences to maximize variation in the constructs of interest. This approach will be the strategy that is selected in most personality research. An alternative approach is the impressionistic modal instance model (or the purposive sampling of typical instances; Shadish et al., 2002). In this approach, the researcher identifies the kinds of people to which he or she most wants to generalize and then constructs a sample that contains cases or instances that are "impressionistically" similar to these kinds of people. For instance, a team of researchers may want to generalize about the developmental course of self-esteem in relatively economically advantaged and relatively economically disadvantaged older populations, so they then select a sample that contains both wealthy older individuals and impoverished older individuals.

The most important point of this discussion is that issues of sampling should be approached in a thoughtful and deliberate fashion. Hartmann (2005) noted, "Whichever of these alternative models of sampling is selected, you as investigator . . . will have *reflected* [italics in original] about population definitions, desired generalization, and sampling" (p. 331). Indeed, a thorough consideration of sampling issues and an honest assessment of the generalizability of findings from particular samples are far too often ignored in actual practice. Just engaging in this exercise will place the researcher in relatively rare company.[2]

The last initial issue to decide is the size of the sample. Watson (2004) noted that samples used to estimate short-term retest correlations for personality measures were often unacceptably small. For example, less than 10% of the studies he reviewed contained samples of 200 or more participants. The situation was somewhat better for longer-term stability studies reviewed by Roberts and DelVecchio (2000), but samples were still relatively small, especially after considering participant attrition. The problems with small samples are well known—statistical power is unacceptably low, and there is very little precision in parameter estimates (i.e., confidence bands are quite large). These limitations tend to impede scientific progress and frequently lead to needless debates over whether effects are truly present.

It is also important to recognize that some attrition will occur over the course of a study, such that the sample size at the last assessment will be smaller than the sample size at the first assessment. Consider that Roberts and DelVecchio (2000) reported that the average attrition rate in studies of personality consistency was 42% in their meta-analytic review. Although we believe that an attrition rate of 42% is unacceptably high for high-quality studies, this figure underscores the reality of attrition in longitudinal studies. Accordingly, researchers need to carefully select a sample size that takes into account the unpleasant fact that a certain number participants will drop out of even the best-designed studies.

Once the investigators have designed the study by answering these four critical questions regarding what to measure, how to measure it, how frequently to collect information, and the size and nature of the study sample, they are ready to launch the investigation. Of course, as a first step, they must secure the funds necessary to conduct the research. But assuming that both the design and the resources are in place, it is time to consider some practical guidelines for ensuring the successful implementation of a longitudinal project that is ready to go into the field.

Practical Issues in Managing the Study

In managing the study, we have two perspectives that guide our specific recommendations.

The first is that it is helpful to think about a study as a factory for collecting, processing, and analyzing data. In a real sense, a well-run longitudinal study is very much like a well-run team or company. For instance, Stouthamer-Loeber and colleagues (1992) argued that "a large study has to be run like a production business whose function is to deliver high-quality data on time and within a predetermined budget" (p. 64). This viewpoint applies equally well to any longitudinal study, big or small, short-term or long-term. A well-run longitudinal study should have an overarching philosophy that places the project before individual egos and, likewise, should have clearly defined roles for project staff. In the following sections we use the term *project staff* inclusively to refer to all sorts of assistance, ranging from a cadre of undergraduates to a full-time paid professional staff.

The second general perspective on running a study concerns the importance of keeping detailed records as the study is progressing. Block (1993) offered clear guidance in this regard: "A longitudinal study should make public and communicable just what was done" (p. 17). Likewise, Stouthamer-Loeber and colleagues (1992) stated, "We cannot overemphasize the necessity of monitoring and *making visible* [italics in original] all aspects of a study's progress. Only when errors and actual or potential problems are made visible can action be taken" (p. 77). This philosophy of transparency should extend to all aspects of data collection, analyses, and write-ups. Perhaps the best way to approach this issue is by imagining that the data will be immediately archived and outside researchers will demand high-quality documentation regarding everything about the study to adequately use the resource. Put differently, the "memory" of the project should exist in tangible documents rather than in the minds of project staff members. This dedication to documentation will redress the natural limitations of human memory and greatly reduce any damage caused by staff turnover. Moreover, thorough documentation as the study is progressing will greatly enhance the accuracy of write-ups from the project.

An Aside on Data Collection Basics

A good piece of general advice is that researchers must allocate adequate time and resources to collecting data and reducing attrition (e.g.,

Stouthamer-Loeber et al., 1992). Charting realistic timelines is an important step in the planning and implementation of the project, which ensures that the ultimate "product" of the longitudinal study will be of sufficiently high quality. Data can be collected from participants in a number of ways, ranging from pencil-and-paper surveys to computer-mediated techniques such as computer-assisted in-person interviewing or Internet-based surveys. All methods have both strengths and limitations, which need to be carefully evaluated.

A notable advantage of computer-assisted techniques is that these methods avoid the error-prone task of data entry by project staff. Internet-based surveys are also particularly convenient for participants who have ready access to a computer. The disadvantages of these techniques are that computers are expensive, machines can fail, and websites can crash. The advantages of pencil-and-paper surveys are that they require no special equipment and there is always a hard copy to serve as a backup of last resort. The disadvantages are that surveys can be lost and that data entry is a large task that will also have to be managed. No matter what method is selected, it is important to have well-established procedures for thoroughly checking the data for accuracy and backing up computer files to guard against catastrophic loss. This is all the more important in longitudinal studies, in which the prolonged time span increases the probability that some computer-related problems with data entry and management will arise.

In some cases an investigator will be well served by using a professional unit within or outside a university to actually collect data. These units have as their full-time work the collection and management of high-quality survey data. For example, the survey unit within the Institute for Social and Behavioral Research at Iowa State University provides state-of-the-art services in terms of recruitment, interviewing, and data entry for the FTP. Because of the high caliber of its work, which is similar to the expertise of survey organizations across the country, the FTP has experienced a very high rate of sample retention (about 90% after 16 years) and the quality of the resulting data has proven to be quite good. In many cases, investigators will profit from working with such a group in the conduct of a long-term study, especially when it involves a community sample.

The Importance of Codebooks and Variable Labeling Conventions

An important way to facilitate transparency and adequate documentation is through the creation of a good codebook that provides information about the data that have been collected and the names of specific variables maintained in a computer file. The codebook should also include copies of the original assessments as well as the source of all instruments used in the study, with extensive notation concerning any deviations in the measures from their original sources. This last function greatly facilitates manuscript writing. A good codebook should serve as the "bible" for all analyses and can help further the goals of transparency and good recording keeping.

The codebook should provide the labels for all variables as well as response categories. In designing the codebook, we believe that it is useful to establish variable naming conventions at the outset of the study, perhaps even before any data are collected. A good system for naming variables will assist with smoother data analyses and prevent errors. Specifically, it may help facilitate accuracy if variable labels reflect the wave of data collection and source of the data and when the same items measured at different waves have common elements in their labels.

For example, consider a study in which Negative Affect is measured with a 10-item scale at three time points by self-report. A reasonable scheme for wave 1 could be something like this: W1NA1S, W1NA2S, to W1NA10S for the 10 Negative Affect items. In this case "W1" refers to wave 1, "NA1" to "NA10" refers to the item on the Negative Affect scale, and "S" refers to self-report. Following these conventions, the same 10 items administered at wave 2 would be labeled W2NA1S, W2NA2S, to W2NA10S, and likewise the same 10 items at wave 3 would be labeled W3NA1S, W3NA2S, to W3NA10S. Moreover, if an informant report was solicited, then "I" could be substituted for "S" at each wave.

This scheme is useful because it can facilitate the writing of computer syntax, such as commands to compute the reliabilities of the Negative Affect measures and routines to compute scales at each wave. Using such a scheme also makes debugging syntax easier because the variable labels have intrinsic meaning. It is our experience that haphazard labels for variables or labels that carry very little intrinsic meaning increase the probability that data analysts will make errors. Indeed, recognition of this issue came late in the FTP, and many extra hours of data analyst time and effort were generated by not having this type of codebook scheme. We are certain as well that the error rate in the computation of specific scales for different years of the study likely increased as a result of failing to take this approach.

The Importance of Open Communication and Defined Project Roles

Stouthamer-Loeber and colleagues (1992) noted that "large longitudinal studies are clearly team efforts whose success depends largely on how well staff members work together" (p. 77). Thus, things must be done to facilitate teamwork and open communication. Having regular meetings is a good way to develop the cohesion necessary for sustained data collection and managing the project. It is helpful if someone is given the responsibility of taking detailed notes and then archiving them in a centralized location. This record can then be accessed by new project staff to provide them with a complete picture of the natural history of the study. Thus, there is an important role for a historian in any longitudinal project to facilitate both communication and documentation.

Likewise, another important role is that of the project librarian. It is typically more efficient to place centralized resources in a library that is housed on a computer network. For example, if more than one person will be conducting data analyses, then it helps to construct a centralized repository for syntax to conduct item analyses and scale construction. This saves individual analysts from having to reinvent the wheel and generally reduces mistakes because the "open source" encourages the detection of errors. Moreover, fully annotating each routine with detailed comments, including dates when the file was constructed and modified, will help in managing the library of routines. It is important, however, that each data analyst who is using a scale for the first time goes back and verifies the original syntax for scale construction. This procedure ensures that errors will be identified over time. Once errors are detected and corrected, the central library should be updated and all staff should be alerted. The point is to recognize that a few errors will be made in the initial stages of data analysis and to adopt a team philosophy that it is necessary to identify and fix errors quickly and efficiently. Everyone, including the primary investigator, must be aware that errors will always occur in a large, complex study. The important point is that adequate procedures must be in place to find and remedy such errors in all phases of the research.

The alternative to this "open source" approach is to have one person act as a gatekeeper for all analyses. The individual is given responsibility for constructing all variables and providing each analyst with a very circumscribed dataset. This approach has the advantage of creating greater control over who is working on what project and provides uniformity in how variables are scored across the project. The downside is that this data manager must be entrusted with a large amount of responsibility, which may prove overwhelming. Moreover, this system may lead to mistakes in constructing datasets that go undetected for a longer period of time. There may also be a greater tendency for mistakes to go unreported.

In academic settings one source of friction and conflict among staff members with research career aspirations stems from disagreements over authorship and intellectual property. Thus, depending on the size of the project, it may be very helpful to establish formal procedures for deciding authorship on all papers. A clear and reasonable method for assigning authorship is likely to prove very useful to the extent that it reduces friction among project staff members. One approach is to use a concept paper model.[3] In this model, anyone working on analyses from the project must submit a formal document, to senior project staff, that includes a short write-up of the idea, what variables will be used, a list of authors, a justification of the authorship order, timelines, and potential publication outlets. This document thus formalizes expectations and authorship order at the outset and is therefore particularly useful when managing collaborations between faculty members and graduate students (see also Fine & Kurdek, 1993). It also provides for a formal record of who is working on what project and thus fulfills the dual objectives of adequate recording keeping and increased team cohesion.

We should note that with the FTP, and probably most other longitudinal studies, the biggest problem is finding enough people to pursue all of the interesting topics that can be addressed with the resulting dataset. An agreement of the type described can also be used as a document that assigns responsibility for completing certain publishable papers. Such papers are extremely important both to the scientific community and to funding agencies that expect to see significant scientific contributions from the research they are funding. Without demonstrating a strong record of publication, it is unlikely that a longitudinal study will receive continuing support and last long enough to fulfill its full potential.

Ways to Reduce Attrition

One of the greatest threats to the health and scientific vitality of a longitudinal study is participant attrition. Nonrandom attrition compromises the external validity of longitudinal research because it limits the generalizability of research findings (e.g., Ribisl et al., 1996; Shadish et al., 2002). Likewise, nonrandom attrition within experimental conditions undermines the internal validity of a longitudinal study (e.g., Shadish et al., 2002). Thus, maintaining the sample over time should be a major focus of the business of running a longitudinal study. To be sure, impressive retention rates are possible, even with "high-risk" samples (e.g., Capaldi & Patterson, 1987). A comprehensive list of strategies for preventing attrition is provided in Ribisl and colleagues (1996; see also Kessler, Little, & Groves, 1995), and a large portion of this section borrows from their excellent review. We focus on three issues: making the experience of participating pleasant, creating an atmosphere in which participants develop a connection to the project, and collecting adequate tracking information.

First, it is important to make the experience of participating in the study relatively pleasant. One of the easiest ways to do this is to provide compensation (e.g., Ribisl et al., 1996; Stouthamer-Loeber et al., 1992). This often takes the form of money, but it can take other forms such as gift certificates (e.g., Amazon.com) or toys for children. It is important that participants are compensated in a timely fashion if not immediately upon completion of the first assessment. It can also help to offer bonuses for completing all waves of a study or to increase the level of compensation at subsequent follow-ups.

Attention to the length of the assessment protocol is also important when considering the pleasantness of a particular study. Researchers naturally want to be as comprehensive as possible in creating assessments, but this can lead to the use of survey packages and procedures that are far too long and tedious to complete in a reasonable time period. Researchers must balance their desire for exhaustive information with the needs of participants who have limited attention spans and real lives to lead. It is helpful to consider the experience of completing the assessment protocol from the perspective of study participants (Donnellan, Oswald, Baird, & Lucas, 2006). Little things, like making questionnaires visually appealing or using large fonts, can help reduce the burden on respondents. Few people enjoy looking at pages of questions written in a 10-point font. It is also possible that short forms of personality or other types of measures can be employed to reduce respondent burden (e.g., Donnellan et al., 2006). Moreover, there are instances when in-person interviews rather than questionnaires will make the assessment procedures more palatable to participants.

Ultimately, conducting a focus group with individuals who completed a potential assessment package can pay large dividends in preventing attrition. Be as receptive as possible to any feedback from members of this group about their experiences. Do not ignore their feedback! If the group conveys the message that the assessment is too long, then items must be cut. Reducing the length of the assessment may seem painful, but it is far less painful than running a longitudinal study that implodes because of skyrocketing attrition rates.

A second factor is the need to create a project identity (Ribisl et al., 1996). The goal is to create a connection to the project on the part of participants so that they are more motivated to continue their participation at each wave. It helps to give the project a snappy title with a catchy acronym and to create a formal project logo for use on all correspondence (Ribisl et al., 1996). However, be sure to select a name that does not stigmatize participants or somehow indicate research hypotheses. Another important way to form a connection to the project is

to send birthday cards and regular newsletters to all study participants (Stouthamer-Loeber et al., 1992). This simple technique is especially helpful.

The third and perhaps most important strategy to reduce attrition is the collection of extensive contact information from participants (Ribisl et al., 1996). The idea is to initially obtain all the information needed to adequately track participants. Tracking information should include names, addresses, telephone numbers, e-mail addresses, and permanent addresses (for students), as well as contact information for families or friends. This latter kind of information can be very helpful in tracking participants who have moved since the last wave of data collection. It is also very efficient to include address change procedures inside project newsletters and birthday cards if these features are incorporated into the project (Stouthamer-Loeber et al., 1992). In rare instances special tracking services can be used to local participants who cannot be found any other way.

Two other considerations are worth noting. First, it is useful to try to ascertain why individuals drop out of the project. Thus, collecting even brief information from dropouts is helpful. For example, if participants explain that the assessment procedures were too long, this should provide insights for future designs. Second, it is useful to note that participants may rejoin the project at a subsequent wave. Stouthamer-Loeber and colleagues (1992) reported that a large number of participants who refused at one wave would participate again in subsequent waves. Thus, the message is not to give up on participants. Individuals may refuse to participate in one wave because it coincides with a particularly busy time in their lives. Asked again at a less busy time, they may be willing to be involved.

In the FTP, we have used all of these procedures to maintain the participation of members of the original study cohort and their families. Retention rates vary, depending on the length of an assessment at a particular wave of data collection; however, we have consistently re-interviewed between 85 and 95% of the participants across the almost 20 years of the study. We have every confidence that these procedures work and strongly recommend them to researchers interested in conducting longitudinal studies.

Concluding Comment

We believe that well designed and managed longitudinal studies have the potential to make contributions to the study of human lives that are just not possible with cross-sectional studies or laboratory experiments. Indeed, questions about antecedents, consequences, and stability of personality characteristics almost require longitudinal study. Accordingly, this design should have a central place in the technology of personality psychology. To borrow from Jack Block (1993), we hope that researchers will continue to be committed to studying personality "the long way." Longitudinal research is not rocket science, but it does require creativity, planning, and patience, and we hope that our advice proves useful for those considering this kind of study.

Acknowledgments

Support for the Family Transitions Project and writing of this chapter has come from multiple sources, including the National Institute of Mental Health (Grant No. MH51361), the National Institute on Drug Abuse (Grant Nos. DA017902 and HD047573), the National Institute of Child Health and Human Development (Grant No. HD047573), and the National Institute on Alcohol Abuse and Alcoholism (Grant No. DA017902). Richard E. Lucas, Kimberly K. Assad, and Greg Fosco provided helpful comments on a draft of this chapter.

Notes

1. It is possible that item response theory methods (see, e.g., Morizot et al., Chapter 24, this volume; Reise, Ainsworth, & Haviland, 2005) could be used to identify a latent metric from different measures of the same trait at different waves for use in growth models. However, these methods are not particularly easy to implement (as of this moment), and therefore the best advice is to use the exact same measure at each wave.
2. Of course, much more elaborate approaches to sampling are possible such as those that involve various clustering or stratification algorithms. In these situations a sampling expert should be consulted in the design of the research.
3. This discussion borrows from procedures used by Terrie Moffitt and Avshalom Caspi (principal investigators of several longitudinal projects) to manage their collaborations.

Recommended Readings

Block, J. (1993). Studying personality the long way. In D. C. Funder, R. D. Parke, C. Tomlinson Keasy, & K. F. Widaman (Eds.), *Studying lives through time: Personality and development* (pp. 9–41). Washington, DC: American Psychological Association.—This chapter provides a personal look at the design and implementation of a particularly influential longitudinal study. It also details nine desiderata for longitudinal studies from a pioneer personality psychologist.

Conger, R. D., & Conger, K. J. (2002). Resilience in Midwestern families: Selected findings from the first decade of a prospective longitudinal study. *Journal of Marriage and the Family, 64,* 361–373.—This article provides additional background and substantive results from the Family Transitions Project.

Singer, J. D., & Willett, J. B. (2003). *Applied longitudinal data analysis: Modeling change and event occurrence.* New York: Oxford University Press.—This book is an accessible introduction to growth modeling and survival analysis. An understanding of these techniques is invaluable in designing longitudinal studies that plan to take advantage of these powerful techniques.

Stouthamer-Loeber, M., van Kammen, W., & Loeber, R. (1992). The nuts and bolts of implementing large-scale longitudinal studies. *Violence and Victims, 7,* 63–78.—This article offers guidance for running large-scale longitudinal studies that stresses practical considerations such as budgeting and managing personnel. This article contains great tips that are applicable to all longitudinal studies.

Ribisl, K. M., Walton, M. A., Mowbray, C. T., Luke, D. A., Davidson, W. S., & Bootsmiller, B. J. (1996). Minimizing participant attrition in panel studies through the use of effective retention and tracking strategies: Review and recommendations. *Evaluation and Program Planning, 19,* 1–25.—This article offers an extensive list of strategies for reducing attrition and describes statistical techniques for accounting for attrition.

Willett, J. B., Singer, J. D., & Martin, N. C. (1998). The design and analysis of longitudinal studies of development and psychopathology in context: Statistical models and methodological recommendations. *Development and Psychopathology, 10,* 395–426.—This article offers a very readable account of growth modeling and survival analysis. It also offers important recommendations for designing longitudinal studies and selecting measures for these studies. In many ways this is essential reading for anyone conducting or even evaluating longitudinal research using these techniques.

References

Baltes, P. B., Reese, H. W., & Nesselroade, J. R. (1977).

Life-span developmental psychology: Introduction to research methods. Monterey, CA: Brooks/Cole.

Baumeister, R. F., Campbell, J. D., Krueger, J. I., & Vohs, K. E. (2003). Does high self-esteem cause better performance, interpersonal success, happiness, or healthier lifestyles? *Psychological Science in the Public Interest, 4,* 1–44.

Block, J. (1993). Studying personality the long way. In D. C. Funder, R. D. Parke, C. Tomlinson Keasy, & K. F. Widaman (Eds.), *Studying lives through time: Personality and development* (pp. 9–41). Washington, DC: American Psychological Association.

Capaldi, D., & Patterson, G. R. (1987). An approach to the problem of recruitment and retention rates for longitudinal research. *Behavioral Assessment, 9,* 169–178.

Caspi, A. (1998). Personality development across the life course. In W. Damon (Ed.), *Handbook of child psychology: Vol. 3. Social, emotional, and personality development* (5th ed., pp. 311–388). New York: Wiley.

Cauce, A. M., Ryan, K. D., & Grove, K. (1998). Children and adolescents of color, where are you? Participation, selection, recruitment, and retention in developmental research. In V. C. McLoyd & L. Steinberg (Eds.), *Studying minority adolescents: Conceptual, methodological, and theoretical issues* (pp. 147–166). Mahwah, NJ: Erlbaum.

Chan, D. (1998). The conceptualization and analysis of change over time: An intergrative approach incorporating longitudinal mean and covariance structures analysis (LMACS) and multiple indicator latent growth modeling (MLGM). *Organizational Research Methods, 1,* 421–483.

Cole, D. A., & Maxwell, S. E. (2003). Testing mediational models with longitudinal data: Questions and tips in the use of structural equation modeling. *Journal of Abnormal Psychology, 112,* 538–577.

Collins, L. M., & Sayer, A. G. (Eds.). (2001). *New methods for the analysis of change.* Washington, DC: American Psychological Association.

Conger, R. D., & Conger, K. J. (2002). Resilience in Midwestern families: Selected findings from the first decade of a prospective longitudinal study. *Journal of Marriage and the Family, 64,* 361–373.

Conger, R. D., Lorenz, F. O., & Wickrama, K. A. S. (2004). Studying change in familyrelationships: The findings and their implications. In R. D. Conger, F. O. Lorenz, & K. A. S. Wickrama (Eds.), *Continuity and change in family relations: Theory, methods, and empirical findings* (pp. 383–403). Mahwah, NJ: Erlbaum.

Cook, T. D., & Campbell, D. T. (1979). *Quasi-experimentation: Design and analysis issues for file settings.* Chicago: Rand McNally.

Costello, E. J., Compton, S. N., Keeler, G., & Angold, A. (2003). Relationships between poverty and psychopathology: A natural experiment. *Journal of the American Medical Association, 290,* 2023–2029.

Cui, M., Conger, R. D., & Lorenz, F. O. (2005). Predicting change in adolescent adjustment from change in marital problems. *Developmental Psychology, 41,* 812–823.

Donnellan, M. B., Larsen-Rife, D., & Conger, R. D. (2005). Personality, family history, and competence in early adult romantic relationships. *Journal of Personality and Social Psychology, 88,* 562–576.

Donnellan, M. B., Oswald, F. L., Baird, B. M., & Lucas, R. E. (2006). The Mini-IPIP Scales: Tiny-yet-effective measures of the Big Five factors of personality. *Psychological Assessment, 18,* 192–203.

Ferrer, E., & McArdle, J. J. (2003). Alternative structural equation models for multivariate longitudinal data analysis. *Structural Equation Modeling, 10,* 493–524.

Fine, M. A., & Kurdek, L. A. (1993). Reflections on determining authorship credit and authorship order on faculty–student collaborations. *American Psychologist, 48,* 1141–1147.

Fraley, R. C., & Brumbaugh, C. C. (2004). A dynamical systems approach to conceptualizing and studying stability and change in attachment security. In W. S. Rholes & J. A. Simpson (Eds.), *Adult attachment: Theory, research, and clinical implications* (pp. 86–132). New York: Guilford Press.

Friedman, S. L., & Haywood, H. C. (Eds.). (1994). *Developmental follow-up: Concepts, domains, and methods.* New York: Academic Press.

Funder, D. C. (2004). *The personality puzzle* (3rd ed.). New York: Norton.

Ge, X., & Conger, R. D. (1999). Adjustment problems and emerging personality characteristics from early to late adolescence. *American Journal of Community Psychology, 27,* 429–459.

Gollob, H. F., & Reichardt, C. S. (1987). Taking account of time lags in causal models. *Child Development, 58,* 80–92.

Gottman, J. M. (1998). Psychology and the study of the marital processes. *Annual Review of Psychology, 49,* 169–197.

Hartmann, D. P. (2005). Assessing growth in longitudinal investigations: Selected measurement and design issues. In D. M. Teti (Ed.), *Handbook of research methods in developmental science* (pp. 319–339). Malden, MA: Blackwell.

Horn, J. L., & McArdle, J. J. (1992). A practical and theoretical guide to measurement invariance in aging research. *Experimental Aging Research, 18,* 117–144.

Kessler, R. C., Little, R. J. A., & Groves, R. M. (1995). Advances in strategies for minimizing and adjusting for survey nonresponse. *Epidemiologic Reviews, 17,* 192–204.

Kim, K. J., Conger, R. D., Lorenz, F. O., & Elder, G. H., Jr. (2001). Parent–adolescent reciprocity in negative affect and its relation to early adult social development. *Developmental Psychology, 37,* 775–790.

Little, T. D., Lindenberger, U., & Nesselroade, J. R.

(1999). On selecting indicators for multivariate measurement and modeling latent variables: When "good" indicators are bad and "bad" indicators are good. *Psychological Methods, 4,* 192–211.

McCrae, R. R., & Costa, P. T. (2003). *Personality in adulthood: A five-factor theory perspective* (2nd ed.). New York: Guilford Press.

Mount, M. R., Barrick, M. R., & Strauss, J. P. (1994). Validity of observer ratings of the Big Five personality factors. *Journal of Applied Psychology, 79,* 272–280.

Nagin, D. S. (2005). *Group-based modeling of development.* Cambridge, MA: Harvard University Press.

Neyer, F. J., & Asendorpf, J. B. (2001). Personality–relationship transaction in young adulthood. *Journal of Personality and Social Psychology, 81,* 1190–1204.

Ployhart, R. E., & Oswald, F. L. (2004). Applications of mean and covariance structure analysis: Integrating correlational and experimental approaches. *Organizational Research Methods, 7,* 27–65.

Podsakoff, P. M., MacKenzie, S. B., Lee, J., & Podsakoff, N. P. (2003). Common method biases in behavioral research: A critical review and recommended remedies. *Journal of Applied Psychology, 88,* 879–903.

Raudenbush, S. W. (2001). Comparing personal trajectories and drawing causal inferences from longitudinal data. *Annual Review of Psychology, 52,* 501–525.

Raykov, T., & Marcoulides, G. A. (2000). *A first course in structural equation modeling.* Mahwah, NJ: Erlbaum.

Reise, S. P., Ainsworth, A. T., & Havilan, M. G. (2005). Item response theory: Fundamentals, applications, and promise in psychological research. *Current Directions in Psychological Science, 14,* 95–101.

Ribisl, K. M., Walton, M. A., Mowbray, C. T., Luke, D. A., Davidson, W. S., & Bootsmiller, B. J. (1996). Minimizing participant attrition in panel studies through the use of effective retention and tracking strategies: Review and recommendations. *Evaluation and Program Planning, 19,* 1–25.

Roberts, B. W., Caspi, A., & Moffitt, T. E. (2003). Work experiences and personality development in young adulthood. *Journal of Personality and Social Psychology, 84,* 582–593.

Roberts, B. W., & DelVecchio, W. F. (2000). The rank-order consistency of personality traits from childhood to old age: A quantitative review of longitudinal studies. *Psychological Bulletin, 126,* 3–25.

Rogosa, D. (1995). Myths and methods: "Myths about longitudinal research" plus supplemental questions. In J. M. Gottman (Ed.), *The analysis of change* (pp. 3–67). Mahawah, NJ: Erlbaum.

Rogosa, D., Brandt, D., & Zimowski, M. (1982). A growth curve approach to the measurement of change. *Psychological Bulletin, 92,* 726–748.

Shadish, W. R., Cook, T. D., & Campbell, D. T. (2002). *Experimental and quasi-experimental designs for generalized causal inference.* New York: Houghton Mifflin.

Singer, J. D., & Willett, J. B. (2003). *Applied longitudinal data analysis: Modeling change and event occurrence.* New York: Oxford University Press.

Stouthamer-Loeber, M., van Kammen, W., & Loeber, R. (1992). The nuts and bolts of implementing large-scale longitudinal studies. *Violence and Victims, 7,* 63–78.

Taris, T. W. (2000). *A primer in longitudinal analysis.* Thousand Oaks, CA: Sage.

Trzesniewski, K. H., Donnellan, M. B., Moffitt, T. E., Robins, R. W., Poulton, R., & Caspi, A. (2006). Low self-esteem during adolescence predicts poor health, criminal behavior, and limited economic prospects during adulthood. *Developmental Psychology, 42,* 381–390.

Vandenberg, R. J., & Lance, C. E. (2000). A review and synthesis of the measurement invariance literature: Suggestions, practices, and recommendations for organizational research. *Organizational Research Methods, 3,* 4–69.

Watson, D. (2004). Stability versus change, dependability versus error: Issues in the assessment of personality over time. *Journal of Research in Personality, 38,* 319–350.

Widaman, K. F., & Reise, S. P. (1997). Exploring the measurement invariance of psychological instruments: Applications in the substance use domain. In K. J. Bryant, M. Windle, & S. G. West (Eds.), *The science of prevention: Methodological advances from alcohol and substance abuse research* (pp. 281–324). Washington, DC: American Psychological Association.

Willett, J. B., Singer, J. D., & Martin, N. C. (1998). The design and analysis of longitudinal studies of development and psychopathology in context: Statistical models and methodological recommendations. *Development and Psychopathology, 10,* 395–426.

CHAPTER 3

Experimental Approaches to the Study of Personality

William Revelle

Personality is an abstraction used to explain consistency and coherency in an individual's pattern of affects, cognitions, desires, and behaviors. What a person feels, thinks, wants, and does changes from moment to moment and from situation to situation but shows a patterning across situations and over time that may be used to recognize, describe, and even to understand that person. The task of the personality researcher is to identify the consistencies and differences within and between individuals (what one feels, thinks, wants, and does) and eventually to try to explain them in terms of a set of testable hypotheses (why one feels, thinks, wants, and does).

Personality research is the last refuge of the generalist in psychology: It requires a familiarity with the mathematics of personality measurement, an understanding of genetic mechanisms and physiological systems as they interact with environmental influences to lead to development over the lifespan, an apprecia-

tion of how to measure and manipulate affect and cognitive states, and an ability to integrate all of this into a coherent description of normal and abnormal behavior across situations and across time.

Although the study of personality is normally associated with correlational techniques relating responses or observations in one situation or at one time with responses in other situations and other times, it is also possible to examine causal relations through the use of experimental methods. This chapter outlines some of the challenges facing personality researchers and suggests that an experimental approach can be combined with more traditional observational techniques to tease out the causal structure of personality.

Central to this analysis is the distinction between personality traits and personality states. Experimental studies do not change trait values, but rather combine (and perhaps interact) with traits to affect the current state. States can be thought of as the current values of a person's affects, behaviors, cognitions, and desires, whereas traits have been conceptualized as average values of these states or, alternatively, the rates of change in these states (Ortony, Norman, & Revelle, 2005). In more cognitive terms, traits are measures of chronic accessibility or activation, and states are levels of current activation. (Although many personality theorists do not include intellectual ability in their theories, those of us who do consider ability traits as reflecting maximal performance and noncognitive traits of personality as reflecting typical or average behavior.) It is perhaps useful here to think analogically and to equate states with today's weather and traits as long-term characteristics of weather, that is, climate. On any particular day, the weather in a particular location can be hot or cold, rainy or dry. But to describe the climate for that location is more complicated, for it includes among other aspects a description of the seasonal variation in temperature and the long-term likelihood of draught, blizzards, or hurricanes. Extending this analogy, climatologists explain differences in climate between locations in terms of variations in solar flux associated with latitude and proximity to large bodies of water, and changes in climate in terms of long-term trends in, for example, greenhouse gases in the atmosphere. The role of the personality researcher is analogous to those of the meteorologist and climatologist, trying to predict someone's immediate states as well as understanding and explaining long-term trends in feelings, thoughts, and actions.

Integrating Two Alternative Research Approaches

Psychological research has traditionally been described in terms of two contrasting approaches: the correlational versus the experimental (see, e.g., the influential papers by Cronbach, 1957, 1975, and Eysenck, 1966, 1997). Francis Galton and his associate Karl Pearson introduced the correlation coefficient as an index of how individual differences on one variable (e.g., the height of one's parents or one's occupation) could be related to individual differences in another variable (e.g., one's own height or one's reaction time). Correlational approaches have been used in personality research since Galton to predict a multitude of

outcomes (e.g., adjustment, career choice, health, leadership effectiveness, marital satisfaction, romantic preferences, school achievement, and job performance) and when combined with known family structures (e.g., parents and their offspring, monozygotic or dizygotic twins with each other, adopted and biological siblings) and structural equation models, have allowed for an examination of the genetic basis of personality. Applying structural techniques such as factor analysis to covariance or correlation matrices of self and other descriptions has led to taxonomic solutions such as the Giant Three or Big Five trait dimensions. The emphasis in correlational research is on *variability, correlation*, and *individual differences*. Central tendencies are not important; variances and covariances are. The primary use of correlational research is in describing how people differ and how these differences relate to other differences. Unfortunately for theoretical inference, that two variables are correlated does not allow one to infer causality. (For example, that foot size and verbal skill are highly correlated among preteens does not imply that large feet lead to better verbal skills, because a third variable, age, is causally related to both. Similarly, that yellowed fingers, yellowed teeth, and bad breath are associated with subsequent lung cancer should not lead to a run on breath fresheners or gloves, but rather to stopping smoking.)

A seemingly very different approach to research meant to tease out causality is the use of experimental manipulation. The psychological experiment, introduced by Wundt (1904) and then used by his students and intellectual descendants, allows one to examine how an experimental manipulation (an independent variable, IV) affects some psychological observation (the dependent variable, DV) that, in turn, is thought to represent a psychological construct of interest. The emphasis is on *central tendencies*, not variation, and indeed, variability not associated with an experimental manipulation is seen as a source of noise or error that needs to be controlled. Differences of means resulting from different experimental conditions are thought to reflect the direct causal effects of the IV on the DV. Threats to the validity of an experiment may be due to confounding the experimental manipulation with multiple variables or poor definition of the dependent variables or an incorrect association between observation and construct.

One reason that correlational and experimental approaches are seen as so different is that they have traditionally employed different methods of statistical analysis. The standard individual differences/correlational study reports either a regression weight or a correlation coefficient. Regression weights are measures of how much variable Y changes as a function of a unit change in variable X. Correlations are regressions based on standard scores or, alternatively, the geometric mean of two regression slopes (X on Y and Y on X). A correlation is an index of how many *standardized* units Y changes for a *standardized* unit of X. (By converting the raw Y scores into standardized scores, $z_y = (Y - \overline{Y})/SD_Y$, one removes mean level as well as the units of measurement of Y.) Experimental results, however, are reported as the differences of the means of two or more groups, with respect to the amount of error within each group. Student's t-test and Fisher's F-test are the classic ways of reporting experimental results. Both t and F are also unit free, in that they are functions of the effect size (differences in means expressed in units of the within-cell standard deviation) and the number of participants.

But it is easy to show that the t-test is a simple function of a correlation coefficient where one of the variables is dichotomous. Similarly, the F statistic of an analysis of variance is directly related to the correlation between the group means and a set of contrast coefficients.

The use of meta-analysis to combine results from different studies has forced researchers to think about the size and consistency of their effects rather than the statistical significance of the effects. Indeed, realizing that $r = \sqrt{F/(F + df)}$ or $\sqrt{t^2/(t^2 + df)}$ (where df = degrees of freedom) did much to stop the complaint that personality coefficients of .3 were very small and accounted for less than 10% of the variance to be explained (Ozer, 2006). For suddenly, the highly significant F statistics reported for experimental manipulations in other subfields of psychology were shown to be accounting for even a smaller fraction of the variance of the dependent variable.

The realization that statistics that seemed different are actually just transformations of each other forced experimentalists and correlationalists to focus on the inferences they can make from their data, rather the way in which the data are analyzed. The problem is, what kind of inferences can one draw from a particular design, not whether correlations or experiments are the better way of studying the problem. That is, recognizing that correlations, regressions, and t and F statistics are all special cases of the general linear model has allowed researchers to focus on the validity of the inferences drawn from the data, rather than on the seeming differences of experimental versus correlational statistics.

Latent Constructs, Observed Variables, and the Problems of Inference

Fundamental to the problem of inference is the distinction between the constructs that we think about and the variables that we measure and observe. This distinction between *latent* (unobserved) constructs and *measured* (observed) variables has been with us at least since Plato's allegory of the cave in Book VII in *The Republic*. Consider prisoners shackled in a cave and able to see only shadows (observed scores) on the cave wall of others (latent scores) walking past a fire. The prisoners attempt to make inferences about reality based upon what they can observe from the length and shape of the shadows. Individual differences in shadow length will correctly order individual differences in height, although real height cannot be determined. To make this more complicated, as people approach the fire, their shadow lengths (the observed scores) will increase, even though their size (the latent score) has not changed. So it is for personality research. We are constrained to make inferences about latent variables based on what we measure of observed variables.

The problem may be shown diagrammatically (Figures 3.1 and 3.2), with boxes representing observed variables, circles latent constructs, and triangles experimental manipulations. Figure 3.1 is a simplified version of Figure 3.2 and shows how the relationship between an observed person variable and outcome variables (path A), when combined with an experimental manipulation (path B) and a potential observed interaction between the manipulation and the person variable (path C), reflects the interrelationships of latent variables as they are affected by an experimental manipulation (paths a, b, c, respectively) and

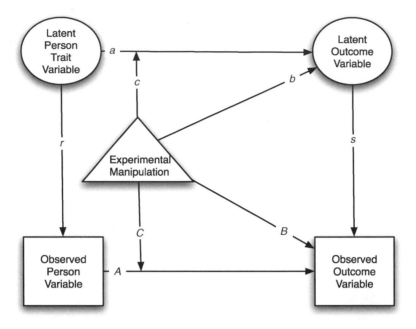

FIGURE 3.1. The problem of inference—Case 1: no state variables: Observed Person and Experimental and Outcome Variables represent the effect of Latent Person Variables and Experimental Variables on Latent Outcome Variables. The strength of latent relationships (a, b, c) are estimated by the strength of observed relationships (A, B, C) and reduced by the validities (r, s) of the measures. (Paths c and C represent the interaction of the experimental manipulation with either the Latent (c) or Observed (C) Variables. Paths r and s reflect the square roots of the reliabilities of the observed variables but also any nonlinearities in the Latent to Observed Variables.

attenuated by the reliability of measurement (*r* and *s*). Thus, A = ras and B = bs and C = rcs. Our goal is to solve these equations for the unknowns (*a*, *b*, *c*, *r*, and *s*) in terms of the knowns (A, B, C). Figure 3.2 extends this analysis by adding in intervening Latent and Observed State Variables. From the observed pattern of correlations or *t*-tests (paths A–H), we attempt to make inferences about the relationships between the latent variables (*a*, *d*, *e*), the effect of manipulations on those latent variables (*b*, *f*), interactions between experimental and latent variables (*c*, *g*, *h*) as well as the quality of measurement relating the latent and observed variables (*r*, *s*, *t*).

There are at least three challenges that we face when making inferences about relationships between latent variables: the *shape* of the functional relationship between observed and latent variables, the *strength* of the functional relationship between observed and latent variables, and the *proper identification of the latent variables* associated with observed variables and manipulation. Experimental design,

when combined with conventional psychometric techniques, helps facilitate these inferences.

Consider the following two hypothetical studies that show the importance of the *shape* of the observed to latent variable relationship. Both are field studies of the effect of education on student outcomes. In study 1, students from a very selective university, a less selective university, and a junior college are given a pretest exam on their writing ability and then given a posttest exam at the end of the first year. The same number of students are studied in each group, and all students completed both the pretest and posttest. Although there were differences on the pretest between the three student samples, the posttest differences were even larger (Figure 3.3a). Examining Figure 3.3a, many who see these results conclude that students at the highly selective university learn more than students at the less selective university, who change more than the students at the junior college. Some (particularly faculty members) like to conclude that the high tuition and faculty salaries at the prestigious and selective university lead to this greater gain. Others believe that the teaching methods at the more selective university are responsible for the gains, and if used at the other institutions, would also lead to better outcomes. Yet others (particularly students) point out that the students in the prestigious university were probably smarter and thus more able to learn than the students in the junior college.

Hypothetical study 2 was similar to study 1, in that it was done at the same three institutions during the first year, but this time the improvement on mathematics achievement was examined (Figure 3.3b). Here we see that stu-

dents at the most selective school, although starting with very high scores, did not improve nearly as much as the students at the less selective university, who improved even less than the students at the junior college. Most faculty members and students who see these results immediately point out that the changes for the selective university students were limited by a "ceiling effect" and that one should not conclude that the selective university faculty used less effective techniques nor that the students there were less able to learn.

The results and interpretations from these two hypothetical studies are interesting, for, in

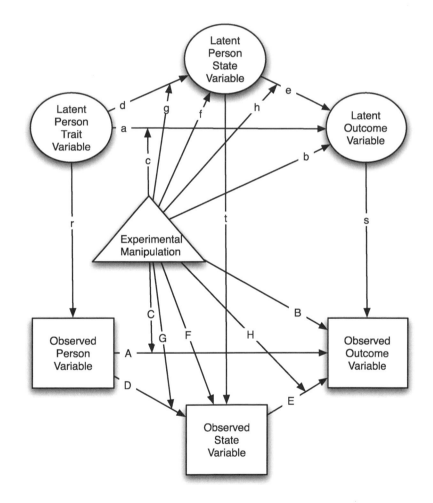

FIGURE 3.2. The problem of inference—Case 2: intervening state variables: Observed Person, State, and Outcome Variables reflect the effect of Latent Person Variables and Experimental Variables on the Latent State and Outcome Variables. The strength of latent relationships (a–h) are estimated by the strength of observed relationships (A–H) and reduced by the validities (r, s, t) of the measures. (Paths c, g, h and C, G, H represent the interaction of the experimental manipulation with either the Latent (c, g, h) or Observed (C, G, H) variables. Paths r, s, and t reflect the square roots of the reliabilities of the Observed Variables but also any nonlinearities in the Latent to Observed Variables.

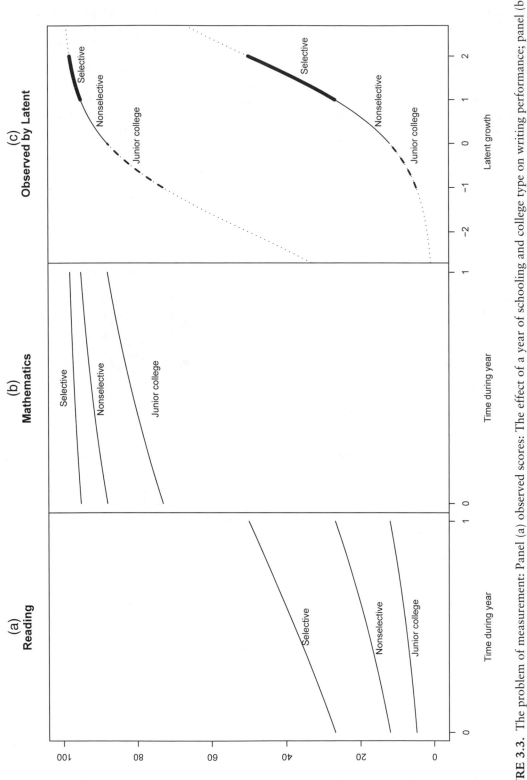

FIGURE 3.3. The problem of measurement: Panel (a) observed scores: The effect of a year of schooling and college type on writing performance; panel (b) observed scores: The effect of a year of schooling and college type on mathematics performance; panel (c) latent scores: The effect of a year of schooling, college type, and performance measure. The two curves represent a difficult test (bottom line) and an easy test (top line) corresponding to the writing and mathematics tests of panels (a) and (b). The groups are assumed to start at different locations (−1, 0, and 1) on the latent scale, and all groups improve equally (1 point from 0 to 1 on the latent score). The seeming interactions in panels (a) and (b) are due to the difficulty of the measures.

fact, one is the inverse of the other. After reversing the groups, scores in study 2 are merely the scores in study 2 subtracted from 100. The results from both studies 1 and 2 can be seen as representing equal changes on an underlying latent score, but using tests that differ in their difficulty. Study 1 used a difficult test in which improvements of the students at the less selective institution were masked; study 2 used an easy test in which improvements of students at the more selective institution were masked. This is shown more clearly in Figure 3.3c, where observed scores are plotted as a function of latent scores. It is assumed that although the three groups differ in their original latent scores (−1, 0, 1 for the junior college, nonselective college, and selective college, respectively), that all groups gain one unit on the latent scale for a year of college. If the observed score is a monotonic, but nonlinear function of the latent score (e.g., is a logistic function),

$$\text{Observed} = 100/(1 + \exp[\text{difficulty} - \text{latent score}])$$

with difficulties of −2 and 2, then the observed scores have different amounts of change from the beginning to the end of the year, even though the latent scores for all groups go up the same amount. That people tend to explain differences in outcome in study 1 by ability, but by scaling effects (in this case, a ceiling effect) in study 2, exemplifies the need to examine one's inferences carefully and to avoid a confirmation bias of accepting effects that confirm one's beliefs and searching for methodological artifacts when facing results that are disconfirming.

The discussion revisits this problem of how the *shape* of latent to observed relationship can cause scaling artifacts which can distort our inferences of differential effects of personality and situational manipulations when it considers the appropriate interpretation of interactions of personality and situations.

A second problem in inferring differences in latent scores based on changes in observed score is the *strength* of the relationship between latent and observed scores. This is the problem of reliability of measurement. Although addressed more completely in other chapters, the basic notion of reliability is that any particular observed score reflects some unknown fraction of the latent score as well as a (typically much larger) fraction of random error. By aggregating observations across similar items or situations, the proportion of the observed score due to the latent score will increase asymptotically toward 1 as a function of the number of items being used and the similarity of the items. Assuming that items are made up of a single latent score and random error, the proportion of latent score variance in a test with k items and an average inter-item correlation of r is alpha = $k*r/(1 + (k − 1)*r)$ (Cronbach, 1951). Furthermore, whereas r is the average correlation between any two items and is equal to the ratio of latent score variance in an item to total item variance, alpha is equal to the percentage of total test variance that is due to latent score variance. More generally, the reliability of a measure of individual differences is a function of what we are trying to generalize across (e.g., items, people, raters, situations, etc.) and the structure of our measures (Zinbarg, Revelle, Yovel, & Li, 2005).

Strong Inference: Confirmatory versus Disconfirmatory Designs

Although it is very tempting (and unfortunately extremely common) to test a hypothesis by looking for evidence that is consistent with the hypothesis (e.g., "testing" the hypothesis "all swans are white" by looking for white swans), in fact disconfirming evidence is the only test of a hypothesis (even after seeing 1,000 white swans, seeing 1 black swan disconfirms the hypothesis.) The use of strong inference (Platt, 1964), to ask what hypothesis a finding can *disconfirm*, should be the goal of all studies. For science is the process of refining theories by excluding alternative hypotheses.

> I will mention one severe but useful private test— a touchstone of strong inference—that removes the necessity for third-person criticism, because it is a test that anyone can learn to carry with him for use as needed. It is our old friend the Baconian "exclusion," but I call it "The Question." Obviously it should be applied as much to one's own thinking as to others.' It consists of asking in your own mind, on hearing any scientific explanation or theory put forward, "But sir, what experiment could disprove your hypothesis?"; or, on hearing a scientific experiment described, "But sir, what hypothesis does your experiment disprove? (Platt, 1964, p. 352)

Consider the following sequence of numbers that have been generated according to a certain rule: 2, 4, 8, X, Y, . . . What is that rule? How do you know that is the rule? One can test the hypothesized rule by generating an X and then a Y and seeing if they fit the rule. Many people, when seeing this sequence will believe that the rule is successive powers of 2 and propose $X = 16$ and then $Y = 32$. In both cases they would be told that these numbers fit the rule generating the sequence. These people will think that they have confirmed their hypothesis. A few people will infer that the rule is actually increasing even numbers and test the rule by proposing $X = 10$ and then $Y = 12$. When told these numbers fit the rule, they will conclude they have confirmed their hypothesis (and disconfirmed the powers of 2 hypothesis). A few will suspect the rule is merely an increasing series of numbers (which is in fact the rule used to generate the numbers) and try $X = 9$ and $Y = 10.92$, and conclude that they have discovered the rule (and disconfirmed the even number hypothesis). Even fewer will propose that the rule is any series of numbers and try to test the rule by proposing $X = 7$ or that $Y = \sqrt{43}$. These terms do not fit the rule and allow us to reject the hypothesis that any number will work. This simple example shows the need to consider many alternative hypotheses and to narrow the range of possible hypotheses by disconfirmation. For, as that great (but imaginary) scientist Sherlock Holmes reasoned, "When you have eliminated the impossible, whatever remains, however improbable, must be the truth" (Doyle, 1929, Chap. 6).

Although it is nice to think of theories as mutually incompatible, with evidence for one disconfirming a second, in fact most theoretical descriptions of personality make predictions for only a limited range of phenomena and are silent about others. In this case, it is helpful to make a table with phenomena as rows, theories as columns, and entries as +, 0, −, or blank. Although many cells of this table will be empty, and some rows will all make the same prediction, there will be some rows that show real differences between the theories. These are the phenomena to test (see, e.g., Anderson & Revelle, 1982, for tests of alternative theories of impulsivity and arousal; Leon & Revelle, 1985, for tests of alternative theories of anxiety and performance; and Zinbarg & Revelle, 1989, for tests of alternative theories of impulsivity and conditioning).

Experimental Manipulations as Tests of Theories of Causality

In the mid-1500s, a revolutionary technique was added to the armamentarium of scientific reasoning. Rather than using arguments based on assumptions and logical reasoning, the process of empirical observation and, more important, experimental manipulation was introduced (see Shadish, Cook, & Campbell, 2002, for a wonderful discussion of the development of experimentation and causal reasoning. See also the webpage of the Carnegie Mellon Curriculum on Causal and Statistical Reasoning at *www.cmu.edu/CSR/index.html*). By observing the results of experimental manipulations, it became possible to tease apart alternative hypotheses and to address issues of causality. Although statistically there is little to differentiate experimental and correlational data, the importance of experimental techniques is that they provide the ability to make statements about causality and to exclude possible explanations by experimental control.

In addition to testing the range of generalization, experimental techniques allow for tests of causal hypotheses. That is, if we believe that X causes Y and that if and only if X occurs will Y occur, we can test this by doing both X and not X and seeing when Y occurs. To show that X leads to Y, it is not enough to merely observe that X and Y occur together, we also need to know what happens when we do not do X.

Note the following table of possible outcomes for X and Y and consider which observations are necessary to test the hypothesis that X causes Y:

Hypothesis: $X \rightarrow Y$ (read, X implies Y)

Two states of X	Two states of Y	
	Y	Not Y
X	a	b
Not X	c	d

Four possible observations:
  a. Do X, observe Y
  b. Do X, observe not Y
  c. Do not do X, observe Y
  d. Do not do X, observe not Y

Observing outcome a when we do X, and outcome d when we do not do X supports our hypothesis. Observing b when we do X or c when we do not do X provides disconfirming evidence.

But more typically, our causal theories are somewhat weaker and we claim that doing X increases the probability or strength of Y occurring. Then we need to compare the values of Y associated with doing X to those associated with not doing X. Comparing the probability of Y following X, written as $p(Y|X)$, to the probability of Y following not X ($p(Y|{\sim}X)$) allows us to test whether there is an association between X and Y. If $p(Y|X) > (p(Y|{\sim}X)$, then X and Y are related. But if X is not manipulated, but merely an observation, this relationship is not necessarily causal. Although it is easy to believe that two variables are causally related whenever we observe that a particular outcome was preceded by a particular condition, mere temporal sequencing does not imply causality. That cocks crow before the sun rises does not imply that roosters cause dawn.

Inference and the Problem of Conditional Probabilities

It is important to determine how often a condition occurs and how frequently that condition is followed by the outcome. But high postdictive prevalences do not necessarily imply high predictive power. Examples include such important issues as the relationship between depression and suicide, between smoking and lung cancer, and between sexual intercourse and pregnancy. Consider depression and suicide. Although almost all individuals who commit suicide were depressed before the act, the lifetime risk for suicide, given prior depression, is only 2% for depressed outpatients and goes up to 6% for patients hospitalized for suicidal tendencies. This compares to a base rate of suicide of 0.5% for the total population (Bostwick & Pankratz, 2000). That is, the conditional probability of depression, given suicide, is many times higher than that of suicide, given depression.

Perhaps the most striking example of the problems of inferring and testing causality is to consider is the relationship between sexual intercourse and pregnancy: If someone is pregnant, she has had intercourse (outcome a in the 2×2 table above); if someone has not had intercourse, she will not become pregnant (outcome d). However, not being pregnant does not imply not having had intercourse (column 2),

nor does having intercourse necessarily imply pregnancy (row 1). Although intercourse is causally related to pregnancy, it is not sufficient. (It is interesting to note that even with such a well-known causal relationship of sex with pregnancy, that with the reasonable assumption of frequency of intercourse twice a week for 20 years resulting in two children, the correlation coefficient for two dichotomous variables (phi) is .026, and goes up to only .059 for the case of 10 children over 20 years.)

Personality Variables and Experimental Designs

The fundamental requirement of an experiment is that there are at least two levels of a manipulated variable (the independent variable, IV). With the additional requirement that that assignment to those two (or more) levels is independent of any possible prior conditions, we have a true experiment. Observations on some outcome measure of interest (the dependent variable, DV) are then related to the states of the IV to detect whether variation in the IV caused changes in the DV.

Subject variables or person variables (PVs) reflect prior and stable characteristics of the individual and are not subject to manipulation. That is, one cannot manipulate the age, extraversion, intelligence, or sex of a participant. Although person variables are seen as nuisance variables to many cognitive and social psychologists, to personality researchers, person variables are of greatest import. Excellent personality research can be done using correlations rather than experimental manipulation, but with the use of experimental techniques, we are able to test the range of generality of our person variables and test causal hypotheses.

The generic experimental personality study (Figure 3.1) can be thought of as examining how one or more stable personality traits (the person variables, or PVs) combine (either additively or interactively) with one or more experimental manipulations (the experimental variables, or EVs) to affect some hypothetical (but unobserved) states, the effects of which are then observed on at least one measure (the observed variable, or OV). In some designs, measures of the intervening state are also taken and used either as manipulation checks or as part of the theoretical and statistical model (Figure 3.2).

Experiments allow one to test the range of generality of a particular personality variable. In the most basic design of a single PV and a single EV, if the EV has an effect but does not interact with the PV, then we are able to extend the generality of the PV across at least the conditions of the EV. If the EV does interact with the PV, then the range of generalization of the PV is reduced. In both cases, we know more about the range of the PV–OV relationship. In the more complex case of multiple PVs or multiple EVs, interactions between the PVs or higher-order interactions with several EVs constrain the limits of generalization even more.

It should be noted that experimental techniques do more than just limit the extent of inferences about personality. The use of personality in experimental designs allows one to achieve a greater range of the underlying state constructs (e.g., arousal, fear, positive or negative affect) than would be achievable by simple manipulations. That caffeine increases arousal is well known, but the range of arousal can be increased by choosing subjects known to have high or low arousal in certain situations (evening people in the morning and morning people in the evening will have very low arousal, morning people in the morning and evening people in the evening will have very high arousal). Similarly, when studying mood effects on memory, by choosing very depressed versus nondepressed participants, the range of negative affective state is greatly enhanced.

A correlational study examines the relationship between a (presumably stable) PV and some observed outcome variable of interest (OV). For instance, the hypothesis that trait extraversion (E) is related to positive mood is supported by a positive correlation of .4 between E as measured by scales from the International Personality Item Pool (IPIP; Goldberg, 1999; Goldberg et al., 2006) and positive mood as measured by items such as happy and cheerful. What is unclear from such an observed relationship is whether some people are chronically happy and cheerful and that this leads to the outgoing and energetic behavior of extraversion, whether the behavioral approach exhibited by the more chronically extraverted results in higher positive mood, or whether more extraverted individuals are more responsive to positive stimuli.

The introduction of an experimental manipulation of mood, where we find that showing a comedy increases positive affect more than showing a control movie, and that in both movie conditions, extraversion is still related to positive affect (PA), allows us to simultaneously increase the range of generalization of the E–PA relationship (Rogers & Revelle, 1998).

The range of potential person variables and potential manipulations is limited by one's imagination, but it is possible to list a number of the more common trait and state personality variables that have been examined in an experimental context (Table 3.1). The variables shown in this table reflect the influence of two major proponents of experimental approaches to personality research, J. W. Atkinson and H. J. Eysenck. Both of these pioneers in personality research emphasized the importance of integrating studies of individual differences with experimental procedures. A strength of their models was that, with proper experimental design, hypotheses could be specified with enough detail that they could be rejected (e.g., Anderson & Revelle, 1994; Leon & Revelle, 1985; Zinbarg & Revelle, 1989).

Arousal-based models of the introversion–extraversion (I-E) dimension (Eysenck, 1967) made two strong theoretical statements: Introverts are chronically more aroused than are extraverts, and arousal is curvilinearly related (with an inverted U-shaped function) to cognitive performance. Thus, typical tests of the model involve manipulations of arousal by giving stimulant or depressant drugs (e.g., amphetamine, caffeine, barbiturates), putting participants in arousing situations (e.g., under time pressure, noise, large groups), or varying the time of day. Confirmatory tests of this hypothesis showing interactive effects on complex cognitive performance of caffeine and introversion–extraversion (Revelle, Amaral, & Turriff, 1976) were followed up with studies that more precisely limited the effects by showing that these earlier results also interacted with time of day and were limited to a subcomponent of I-E, impulsivity (Revelle, Humphreys, Simon, & Gilliland, 1980).

More recent conceptualizations of introversion–extraversion have focused on the relationship of extraversion with positive affect and have examined the effects of positive mood-inducing stimuli (e.g., movies, pictures, autobiographical memories) on subsequent mood (Larson & Ketelaar, 1989), performance (Rog-

TABLE 3.1. Examples of Experimental Personality Research

Person variable	Experimental variable	Hypothetical state variable	Observed variable
Introversion/ extraversion	Caffeine Time of day Time limits Noise	Arousal	Cognitive performance: total correct, attention decrements over trials, reaction time, accuracy, speed–accuracy tradeoffs
	Movies	Positive affect	Cognitive performance: reaction time to valenced words
	Autobiographical memory		Mood ratings
	Affective pictures		MRI activation
Impulsivity	Cues for reward/ punishment	Behavioral activation	Learning
	Time of day Caffeine	Arousal	Cognitive performance: total correct, attention decrements over trials, reaction time, accuracy, speed–accuracy tradeoffs
Achievement motive	Success versus failure feedback	Achievement motivation	Task choice
	Task difficulty		Persistence
Emotional stability/ neuroticism	Movies	Negative affect	Cognitive performance
	Affective pictures		MRI activation
Anxiety	Success versus failure feedback	State anxiety	Learning
	Task difficulty		
	Memory load		Cognitive performance: speed–accuracy tradeoff
	Cues for reward/ punishment	Behavioral inhibition	Learning
	Autobiographical memory	State anxiety Negative affect	Emotional "Stroop" task Dot probe task
	Fearful pictures	State anxiety	Illusory correlation
Chronic promotion focus/prevention focus	Cues for reward/ punishment	Activation of promotion Focus/prevention Focus	Cognitive performance: reaction time to valenced words
Conscientiousness/ obsessive– compulsive	Global versus local stimuli	Breadth of attention	Reaction time

ers & Revelle, 1998) and psychophysiological (Canli, Sivers, Whitfield, Gotlib, & Gabrieli, 2002) measures.

Early tests of theories of achievement motivation theory (Atkinson, 1966) focused on the effect of perceived task difficulty and success and failure feedback on task choice (Hamilton, 1974), persistence following failure, and changes in effort over time (Kuhl & Blankenship, 1979). More recent work has emphasized interactions between achievement goals and task feedback (Elliot & Thrash, 2002).

Studies of Neuroticism and Anxiety have focused on ways of manipulating negative affect and inducing state anxiety. Manipulations similar to those used for inducing positive affect have been used for inducing negative affect and fear (e.g., sad or frightening movies, pictures of feared objects such as snakes or spiders; Öhman & Mineka, 2002).

Although framed in more social-psychological than personality terms, studies of "motivational focus" emphasize chronic goals to promote gains (promotion focus) or to prevent losses (prevention focus) and how these chronic conditions interact with manipulations to affect activated states of eagerness and vigilance (seemingly alternative terms for approach and inhibitory motivations), which in turn affect cognitive and affective processing (Higgins, Idson, Freitas, Spiegel, & Molden, 2003).

Cognitive approaches to personality assume that individuals differ in their response to objectively similar situations because of differences in the way they process those situations. Models of obsessiveness and conscientiousness suggest that highly conscientious individuals have a narrow range of attentional focus and thus should be better at detecting details in a display mixing global and local information. The global–local paradigm uses large letters (e.g., H and T) made up of little letters (also H and T but one-eighth as large). Using a within-subjects paradigm, obsessive–compulsivity interacted with reaction times to locally inconsistent versus locally neutral stimuli (Yovel, Revelle, & Mineka, 2005). Although this study reports the data in terms of correlations of obsessive–compulsivity with the difference between locally inconsistent versus locally neutral stimuli, this is equivalent to testing the interaction of these two sets of variables.

Avoiding Confounds through Experimental Control, Randomization, Counterbalancing, and Theoretical Analysis

Many seemingly different designs (one EV with two levels, one EV with multiple levels, two EVs, etc.) all have a similar requirement: the need to assign subjects to experimental conditions with no relationship to another existing condition. That is, the only expected variation between participants in the different conditions should be due to those conditions and not some other, *confounded* variable.

Perhaps the clearest way of thinking of the problem is to consider a hypothetical data matrix in which the rows are the participants, and the columns include the person variables, experimental variables, and observed variables of interest, as well as other, extraneous person and context variables (CVs). The inferential problem for the researcher is to know that the observed relationship between the PV, EV, and OV is not due to any other source of variance—that is, that the effect is not due to the extraneous PVs or CVs. These extraneous variables, if correlated with either the PVs or the EVs are said to be confounded with the variables of interest and invalidate any causal inferences we try to make. The (unreachable) goal of good design is to eliminate all possible confounding variables.

There is, of course, an infinite number of such possible confounding variables. Confounding person variables include individual differences in intelligence, socioeconomic status (SES), broad personality trait dimensions such as the Big Five, narrow trait dimensions such as impulsivity or anxiety or achievement motivation, and prior experience with the task. Confounding context variables range from the obvious effects of time of day, time of week, and time of year, to effects of experimenter characteristics including gender, formality of clothing, friendliness, ethnicity, and age, as well as possible participant–experimenter interactions, of which among college students important interactions to consider are those between participant gender and ethnicity and experimenter gender and ethnicity.

Quasi-experimental designs typically associated with field studies are rife with these potential confounds. Indeed, issues of differential selection, attrition, age, and experience are the topics of entire texts on quasi-experiments

(Shadish et al., 2002). Our challenge as researchers is to eliminate the effect of these potential confounds. Unfortunately, we can not control for the effect of extraneous PVs by experimental design, but rather need to worry about them when trying to make inferences about the specific PVs of interest. We can, however, eliminate the effect of CVs by ensuring that their correlations with the EVs are 0.

It is possible to control explicitly for some confounding variables by making them part of the design. Thus, it is possible to avoid time of day and experimenter characteristics as sources of variation by having a sole experimenter conduct the test with all participants and all experimental conditions at the same time of day. While avoiding confounds with time of day and experimenter characteristics, and reducing the amount of variation within experimental conditions, this procedure also reduces the generalizability of the findings to that particular combination of time of day and experimenter. Generalization can be increased at the cost of increasing within-condition variability by having multiple experimenters test subjects at multiple times of day (but to avoid confounding time of day with experimenter, each experimenter needs to test an equal number of participants in each condition at all the different times of day). Explicit control for confounds by restricting the experimental conditions thus increases the power of the design at the cost of reducing the generalization of the findings.

A statistically less powerful but much more generalizable control for confounds is to use random assignment. The technique of random assignment of participants to conditions will, *on average*, yield no correlation between the experimental conditions and extraneous, confounding variables. It is important to note that although randomization has an expected value of no relationship, it does not guarantee no relationship in any particular study. (My colleagues and I once found that impulsivity and caffeine had an interactive effect on cognitive performance on a pretest, before the caffeine was administered. We had either confirmed precognition or had observed a failure of randomization to equate the groups.)

Random assignment of participants to conditions is easier to say than to do, for there are problems that arise with randomization. For a given number of participants, statistical analysis will have the greatest power when an equal number of participants are assigned to each condition. But simple randomization (e.g., flipping a coin or rolling a die) will normally not achieve this goal, for there is random variation in the outcome. (Assume you want 10 participants in each of two cells; there is only about an 18% chance that a coin flip will result in equal size samples, and about a 26% chance that there will be 7 or fewer in one group. Indeed, as the sample size increases, the probability of exactly equal numbers per condition decreases, even though the chance of large variations from equality also decreases.)

A seeming solution to this problem is to randomly assign participants to the two conditions until the desired number is achieved in one condition, and then assign the remaining participants to the other condition. Unfortunately, this will normally result in an overabundance of later arriving participants in one condition than in the other. If there is any reason (and there are many—for example, early arriving subjects are likely to be more anxious, conscientious, and introverted than late arriving subjects) to expect that participant arrival is correlated with extraneous variables, then the condition effect is confounded with arrival time (which, for studies in a single day, is confounded with time of day as well).

A solution that guarantees equal numbers of subjects per condition, but also has no expected correlation with other variables, is to block randomize—that is, to divide the n participants into n/k blocks, where k is the number of conditions. Then, within each block, randomly assign participants to conditions by choosing the condition for a participant by sampling without replacement from the set of all conditions.

With random assignment of participants to conditions, the expected correlation of experimental manipulation with other possible confounds is 0. However, if not all participants complete the assigned conditions, problems can arise. For instance, highly impulsive subjects tend to be not very wide awake in the morning and are much more likely to drop out of studies when assigned to morning versus evening conditions. Randomly assigning them to morning or evening avoids problems with differential volunteering, but the problem of differential attrition still needs to be considered.

Random assignment of participants to conditions tends to eliminate confounds of the EV with extraneous variables, but even the best of randomization and counterbalancing cannot control for confounds introduced by the EVs. Avoiding such confounds requires a theoretical understanding of the task rather than just a mechanical consideration of design. Consider the interactive effect of task difficulty and anxiety on performance in list learning. Although more than 20 studies have shown that anxious subjects learn easy lists more rapidly than do less anxious subjects, but learn difficult lists more slowly than do the less anxious subjects (e.g., Spence, Farber, & McFann, 1956) this effect was shown to be due to a confound of task difficulty and implicit feedback (Weiner & Schneider, 1971). The traditional list-learning task used a serial anticipation procedure in which each participant would be shown a cue word, recite his or her answer, and then be shown the correct answer. Although no feedback was explicitly given, implicitly, participants could judge how well they were doing whenever they made an incorrect response. Weiner and Schneider (1971) used the same procedure, but added explicit feedback—"Compared to other students, you are doing very well (or not very well)." Feedback interacted with anxiety such that highly anxious participants with either difficult or easy lists to learn did better when told they were doing better than average, but did less well when they were told they were doing worse than average. As is true with most interactions, the Weiner and Schneider study may also be interpreted as limiting the generality of the anxiety by task difficulty effect to situations where no feedback is given.

Basic Experimental Designs

There are two broad classes of experimental designs used in personality research. In both of these, of course, the primary variable of interest is the person variable. The first, the *between-subjects* design, randomly assigns participants to conditions, but each person is in just one condition. The second, the *within-subjects* design, assigns each person to all conditions. These two broad types of designs can be combined into mixed designs whereby participants are assigned to multiple but not all conditions. Although the examples discussed below use just one PV and one EV, the generalization to multiple PVs and multiple EVs is straightforward.

Between Subjects

The classic experiment is to administer an experimental variable to two groups of randomly assigned participants. Unfortunately, by ignoring individual differences, the classic experiment cannot test any hypothesis about personality. But with the addition of a person variable to the study, we have the basic between-subject PV × EV study. Until recently the person variable was some dichotomously scored trait, resulting in two levels of the PV and two levels of the EV, and the analysis was a classic analysis of variance. With a greater understanding of the general linear model, more recent studies have treated the PV as a continuous variable and analyzed the data in terms of a moderated regression analysis. Some studies, in order to increase power to detect effects of the PV, give a pretest and then select participants with extreme scores on the PV. This extreme groups design is typically then analyzed using conventional analysis of variance.

An example of a between-subjects study is the examination of the effect that extraversion and mood induction have on positive affect (Rogers & Revelle, 1998). Contemporary models of introversion–extraversion claim that extraverts are either more likely to be in a positive mood or are more sensitive to positive mood inductions. These hypotheses may be examined by a simple PV × EV experiment in which extraversion is indexed by a self-report questionnaire and a mood induction, such as showing a short film clip with humorous content (e.g., the birthday party scene from *Parenthood*) versus a control film clip with neutral content (e.g., a National Geographic film about African wildlife). Positive affect may be assessed with a short rating scale including items such as happy and pleased. Alternative measures and manipulations may include peer ratings of extraversion and instructions to think about a positive event (e.g., finding $20 while walking on a beach) or a neutral event (e.g., studying in the library).

Within Subjects

A way of controlling for large between-subjects variation in response, particularly when examining interactions with cognitive or psychophysiological variables, is to use a within-subject design in which all levels of the experimental variable are presented to each subject.

For instance, testing the hypothesis that there is cerebral lateralization of the response to positive stimuli and that this should depend on levels of extraversion, Canli and colleagues (2002) examined the BOLD response (blood oxygen level dependent changes) in a functional magnetic resonance imagining (fMRI) paradigm. Correlations of the BOLD response to positive versus negative stimuli as a function of extraversion showed left lateralization of the response to positive stimuli as a function of extraversion. The within-subject design examined the response to affectively valenced stimuli as compared with neutral stimuli to control for the very large variation between subjects in the amount of brain activation measured.

Similar within-subject designs are necessary when using reaction time as the dependent variable. There are large between-subjects differences in reaction time that reflect both extraneous state variables (e.g., time of day, sleep deprivation) and extraneous trait variables (age, intelligence). The effects of these extraneous variables can be minimized by using each subject as his or her own control. Thus, when examining the relation of anxiety or neuroticism to the cognitive impairment induced by fearful or negative stimuli using the "dot probe" paradigm, or using the "emotional Stroop" paradigm, each participant serves as his or her own control by giving responses to valenced and nonvalenced stimuli (Gilboa & Revelle, 1994).

A potential confound in all such within-subject studies is the effect of trial order, because for some, the effect of some manipulations can persist well beyond the experiment. This requires testing participants on multiple occasions rather than in rapid sequence. Examples of such possible carryover manipulations are the effects of alcohol, caffeine, or nicotine. To use any of these potent arousal manipulations in a within-subject design requires doing the study over multiple days rather than in one session.

If many observations are collected for the same subject across different conditions, block randomization can still be used to avoid confounding condition with order. If there are only a few (e.g., two) observations per participant, then randomly assigning participants to one of two counterbalanced orders avoids possible order effects (e.g., if there are two experimental conditions, half the participants are given the conditions in the order ABBA, and the other half are given BAAB.) With three, four, or more

levels of a within-subject variable, the use of Latin squares removes simple order and first order sequential effects: Participants can then be randomly blocked into each of the orders. For example, for a study with four conditions, participants are randomly assign to each of the four orders:

	Trial			
Order	1	2	3	4
1	A	B	C	D
2	B	D	A	C
3	C	A	D	B
4	D	C	B	A

Both the ABBA and Latin squares techniques force the correlation of order and experimental condition to be 0. Note that in the Latin square, not only does every condition appear in every trial position, but first order sequential effects (e.g., the frequency with which A precedes versus follows B) is also controlled. (See Fisher & Yates, 1963, for tables of Latin squares.)

Examples of Experiments and Data Analysis

This section gives a brief overview of how to analyze the data from several prototypical personality experiments. To allow the reader to compare alternative analytic strategies, the data are simulated using the R computer language (R Development Core Team, 2005), with the R code included as Appendix 3.1. Further details on R and much more extensive analyses may be found in an online appendix at the Personality Project (*personality-project.org/r/ simulating-personality.html*). The online appendix includes the R code for each analysis discussed below, as well as additional analyses. By showing the R code for generating simulated data, as well as the code for analysis, it encourages readers to try out some of the techniques for themselves rather than just passively reading yet another chapter.

In all the simulations, data are generated on the basis of a model indicating that positive affect is an interactive and nonlinear function of extraversion and rewarding cues in the environment, that negative affect is an additive but nonlinear function of neuroticism and punishing cues in the environment, that arousal is an additive function of stimulant drugs and introversion, and that cognitive performance is a curvilinear function of arousal. This model is the "truth" that the analyses hope to uncover. Unlike the situation in real studies, in all simulations we have access to the latent (but unobserved) "true" variables as well as the observed person and outcome variables. (The simulations are based on somewhat simplified summaries of a number of studies conducted over the past years at the Personality, Motivation and Cognition lab at Northwestern University, but are idealizations and simplifications of the actual results of those studies.) Readers are encouraged to try the simulations and analyses for themselves, varying the sample sizes and the strength of the relationships. By presetting the seed for the random number generator to a memorable constant value (Adams, 1979), the results obtained in these simulations and reported below should match those carried out by copying the code in Appendix 3.1 and running the simulations.

The first study considers a single person variable, neuroticism, and a single manipulation, a negative versus a neutral movie. The observed variable is negative affect. In the simulation, the true model is that latent negative affect is a simple additive function of neuroticism and the movie condition, but that the observed score is a nonlinear but monotonic effect of the latent score. That is, negative affect = $1/(1 + \exp(-\text{movie} - \text{neuroticism}))$. This particular equation is the logistic function commonly used in item response theory (IRT) analyses of responses to personality and ability items.

The second study considers a single person variable, extraversion, and a single manipulation, a positive versus a neutral movie. The observed variable is positive affect. In the simulation, positive affect is a monotonically increasing function of the interaction of extraversion and the mood induction. That is: Positive affect = $1/(1 + \exp[-\text{extraversion} * \text{movie}])$.

The third study is just a combination of the first two and analyzes the data from studies 1 and 2 as part of one larger regression model.

The fourth study examines the effects of two levels of caffeine-induced arousal on the performance of introverts and extraverts in a within-subject design. The underlying model is that performance is an inverted-U-shape function of arousal and that arousal is a decreasing function of extraversion. (Ignoring the time-of-day effects that are most interesting, see Revelle et al., 1980.)

Study 1

Study 1 examined the effect of neuroticism and a negative mood induction on negative affect. One hundred participants, differing in neuroticism, were block randomly assigned to one of two movie conditions. Neuroticism was assessed by the Eysenck Personality Questionnaire (Eysenck & Eysenck, 1975), and the movie conditions were 9-minute selections from a PBS *Frontline* episode (May 1985) depicting the allies' liberation of Nazi concentration camps and a National Geographic film depicting animals in their natural habitat, grazing. (See Rafaeli & Revelle, 2006, or Rogers & Revelle, 1998, for actual results using these manipulations.)

The analysis used the general linear model procedure from R with the model

$$\text{Negative affect} = \beta_1 \text{neuroticism} + \beta_2 \text{movie} + \beta_3(\text{neuroticism} * \text{movie})$$

Movie was made a categorical "factor" and neuroticism was "centered" around the mean. Centering is required when doing regression models with interaction terms for proper interpretation of the main effects. The three regression coefficients ($\beta_1, \beta_2, \beta_3$) were estimated using the Linear Model command, and the magnitude of a t-statistic (the ratio of the estimate to the standard error of the estimate) gives the investigator confidence in the estimates. The summary statistics for the model show that both the neuroticism slope (.72) with a standard error of .09 and the movie slope (1.09) with a standard error of .11 are reliable effects (t's > 8.0, $p < .001$), but that the interaction effect, with a negligible slope (.02) and a much larger standard error (.13), does not differ from 0. The model fit is shown graphically and is compared to the true model in Figure 3.4.

Study 2

Study 2 examined the effect of extraversion and a positive mood induction on positive affect. One hundred participants, differing in introversion–extraversion, were block randomly assigned to one of two movie conditions. Extraversion was assessed by a short

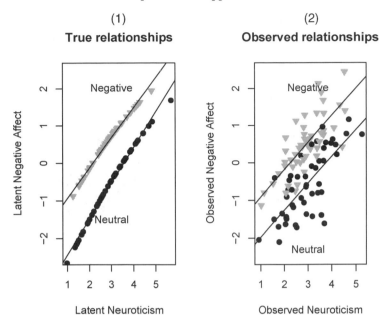

FIGURE 3.4. Analysis of simulated study 1. Negative Affect is an additive function of Neuroticism and a Negative Affect manipulation. Panel (1), latent scores; panel (2), observed scores.

measure of the Big Five, using items from the IPIP (Goldberg et al., 2006), and the movie conditions were 9 minutes taken from the 1989 film *Parenthood* and a National Geographic film depicting animals in their natural habitat, grazing. (See Rafaeli & Revelle, 2006, or Rogers & Revelle, 1998, for actual results using these manipulations.)

The analysis used the general linear model procedure from R with the model

$$\text{Positive affect} = \beta_1\text{extraversion} + \beta_2\text{movie} + \beta_3\text{extraversion * movie})$$

Movie was made a categorical "factor" and extraversion was "centered" around the mean. The three regression coefficients ($\beta_1, \beta_2, \beta_3$) were estimated using the Linear Model command, and the magnitude of a *t*-statistic gives the investigator confidence in the estimates. The summary statistics for the model show that there is no effect for extraversion ($\beta_1 = -.06$ with a standard error of .07), but there is a strong effect for the movie (1.6, $SE = .11$) and for the interaction (.37 with $SE = .10$). As seen in Figure 3.5, the observed interaction suggests that the slopes in the two conditions go in opposite directions, but this is due to sampling error.

Study 3

Study 3 examined the effects of extraversion and neuroticism and positive and negative mood inductions on positive and negative affect. These are just the data from studies 1 and 2 combined into one analysis, noting that the affect measures are repeated within participants. Because of the within-subject design, the analysis is slightly more complicated and can be done either as a repeated measures analysis of variance (ANOVA) or as mixed effects analysis (Pinheiro & Bates, 2000).

The data are organized as a function of subject, movie conditions, extraversion, and neuroticism. Although some statistical packages (e.g., SPSS and SYSTAT) treat repeated measures as separate columns in the data matrix, in R it is necessary to "stack" the repeated measures so that regressions with the categorical condition variable may be found. (See the online appendix for details.) The model is

$$\begin{aligned}
\text{Response} = &\ \beta_1\text{AffectMeasure} + \beta_2\text{Extraversion}\\
&+ \beta_3\text{Neuroticism} + \beta_4\text{PositiveMovie}\\
&+ \beta_5\text{Negative Movie} + \ldots\\
&+ \beta_{15}\text{AffectMeasure*Extraversion}\\
&\ \text{*Neuroticism*PositiveMovie}\\
&\ \text{*NegativeMovie} + \text{error(subject)}
\end{aligned}$$

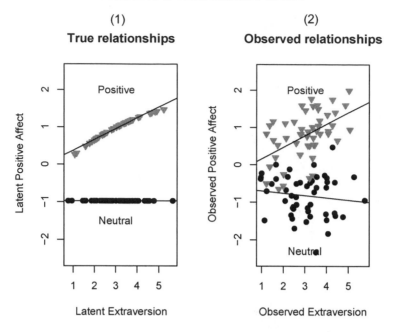

FIGURE 3.5. Analysis of simulated study 2. Positive Affect is an interactive function of Extraversion and a Positive Affect manipulation. Panel (1), latent scores; panel (2), observed scores.

As would be expected, the results show effects of the positive and negative movie conditions, neuroticism, and interactions of the positive mood condition with extraversion, as well as interactions of type of affect with positive and negative movies and a triple interaction of affect type with positive movies and extraversion. To show these effects graphically is somewhat more complicated, and the graph becomes a four-panel graph (Figure 3.6).

Study 4

Study 4 examined the effect of extraversion and drug-induced arousal on cognitive performance. This is a conceptual simulation of Revelle and colleagues (1976), which showed that practice Graduate Record performance was an interactive effect of caffeine-induced arousal and introversion–extraversion. This study simulates a within-subject manipulation of arousal induced by either placebo or 4 mg/kg body weight of caffeine.

The analysis used the general linear model procedure from R with the model

$$\text{Performance} = \beta_1\text{Extraversion} + \beta_2\text{Condition} + \beta_3\text{Extraversion} * \text{Condition})$$

The error term in this model is more complicated in that the conditions are within subjects. Once again, we need to make condition a categorical variable, center extraversion around its mean, and stack the two repeated measures conditions. Thus, there is a between-subjects analysis of the effects of extraversion and a within-subject comparison of the drug conditions and the interaction of the drug conditions with extraversion.

The within-subject interaction of extraversion × drug condition ($F = 10.79, p < .01$) indicated that performance decreases with extraversion with a placebo but increases with caffeine. Figure 3.7 demonstrates two graphic techniques for showing this interaction, the first just plotting the linear trends for both conditions, the second plotting the "lowess" fit (a locally optimized running fit). The curvilinear nature of the results is much clearer with the lowest fit. The online appendix includes additional graphics to help explain these and other results.

All four simulations are sensitive to the number of subjects simulated, as well as the quality of measurement (the reliability of the measures). The reader is encouraged to vary these and other parameters to explore the sensitivity

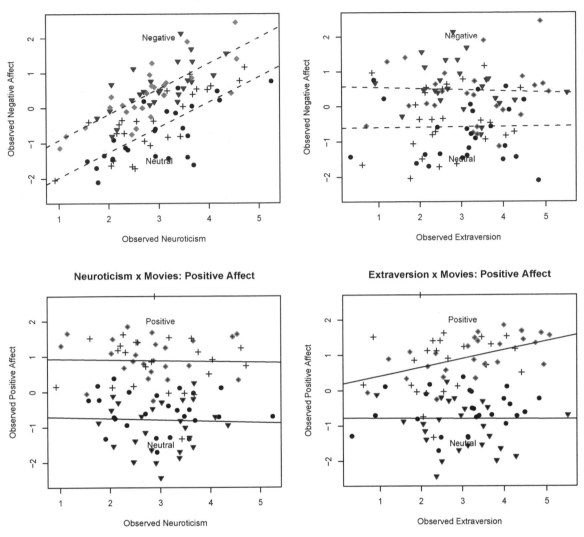

FIGURE 3.6. Analysis of simulated study 3. Affect is an interactive function of affect type (Positive versus Negative), mood manipulation (Positive, Neutral, or Negative movies), and personality (Introversion–Extraversion and Neuroticism–Stability).

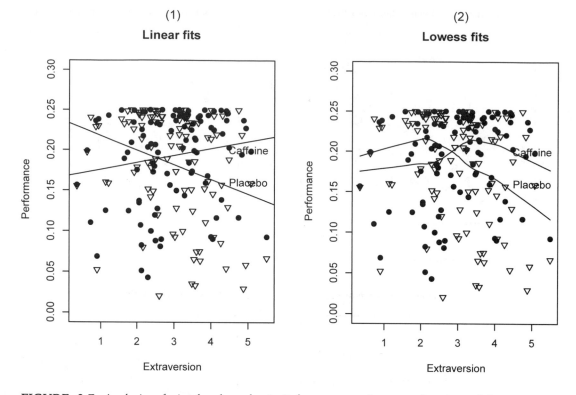

FIGURE 3.7. Analysis of simulated study 4. Peformance varies as a function of Introversion–Extraversion and drug condition. Panel (1) shows the two best-fitting linear fits, panel (2) shows "lowess" fits. The lowess fits better reflect the true curvilinear nature of the data.

of the analytical techniques for detecting real effects (those built into the model) and not detecting artificial effects (those not in the model but detected because of random error). By doing multiple simulations, one quickly becomes aware of the distinction between Type I errors (falsely detecting effects) and Type II errors (failing to detect true effects).

Conclusion

All research involves the detection of associations between observed variables as a way of inferring relationships between latent variables. With the introduction of experimental techniques, it is possible to go beyond mere structural models of the data and to test causal hypotheses as well. The process of experimental inference involves a concern with the quality of how well observed data represent latent constructs and how particular manipulations either affect these latent constructs directly or moderate the relationship between latent constructs.

This familiar research endeavor becomes much more challenging, and exciting, with the introduction of individual differences in personality. Stable individual differences combine with experimental manipulations to affect temporary states of affect, cognition, and desire. These temporary states, in turn, affect ongoing behavior. The emphasis in experimental design in personality research is to control for extraneous, confounding variables by minimizing the expected value of their correlation with the person variables and experimental variables of interest. The detection of personality by experimental variable interactions specifies the limits of generalization of our theories.

The study of personality can benefit from the combination of the finest multivariate methodologies with good experimental design. With this combination, it is possible to move forward in developing and testing causal explanations of how individual differences in personality combine with the environmental and developmental context to produce the complex patterning of behavior that we see around us.

Recommended Readings

Platt, J. R. (1964). Strong inference. *Science, 146,* 347–353.

Revelle, W., & Anderson, K. J. (1992). Models for the testing of theory. In A. Gale & M. W. Eysenck (Eds.), *Handbook of individual differences: Biological perspectives* (pp. 81–113). Chichester, UK: Wiley.

Shadish, W. R., Cook, T. D., & Cambell, D. T. (2002). *Experimental and quasi-experimental designs for generalized causal inference.* Boston: Houghton Mifflin.

References

Adams, D. (1979). *Hitchhiker's guide to the galaxy.* New York: Harmony Books.

Anderson, K. J., & Revelle, W. (1982). Impulsivity, caffeine, and proofreading: A test of the Easterbrook hypothesis. *Journal of Experimental Psychology: Human Perception and Performance, 8,* 614–624.

Anderson, K. J., & Revelle, W. (1994) Impulsivity and time of day: Is impulsivity related to the decay of arousal? *Journal of Personality and Social Psychology 67,* 334–344.

Atkinson, J. W. (1966). Motivational determinants of risk-taking behavior. In J. W. Atkinson & J. T. Feather (Eds.), *A theory of achievement motivation* (pp. 11–31). New York: Wiley.

Bostwick, J. M., & Pankratz, V. S. (2000). Affective disorders and suicide risk: A reexamination. *American Journal of Psychiatry, 157,* 1925–1932.

Canli, T., Sivers, H., Whitfield, S. L., Gotlib, I. H., & Gabrieli, J. D. E. (2002). Amygdala response to happy faces as a function of extraversion. *Science, 296,* 2191.

Cronbach, L. J. (1951). Coefficient alpha and the internal structure of tests. *Psychometrika, 16,* 297–334.

Cronbach, L. J. (1957). The two disciplines of scientific psychology. *American Psychologist, 12,* 671–684.

Cronbach, L. J. (1975). Beyond the two disciplines of scientific psychology. *American Psychologist, 30,* 116–127.

Doyle, A. C. (1929). *Sherlock Holmes: The complete long stories by Arthur Conan Doyle.* London: J. Murray.

Elliot, A. J., & Thrash, T. M. (2002). Approach–avoidance motivation in personality: Approach–avoidance temperaments and goals. *Journal of Personality and Social Psychology, 82,* 804–818.

Eysenck, H. J. (1966). Personality and experimental psychology. *Bulletin of the British Psychological Society, 19,* 1–28.

Eysenck, H. J. (1967). *The biological basis of personality.* Springfield, MO: Charles C. Thomas.

Eysenck, H. J. (1997). Personality and experimental psychology: The unification of psychology and the possibility of a paradigm. *Journal of Personality and Social Psychology, 73,* 1224–1237.

Eysenck, H. J., & Eysenck, S. B. G. (1975). *Manual of the Eysenck Personality Questionnaire (Adult and Junior).* London: Hodder & Stoughton.

Fisher, R. A., & Yates, F. (1963). Statistical tables for biological, agricultural and medical research (6th ed.). New York: Macmillan.

Gilboa, E., & Revelle, W. (1994). Personality and the structure of emotional responses. In S. Van Goozen, N. E. Van de Poll, & J. A. Sargent (Eds.), *Emotions: Essays on current issues in the field of emotion theory* (pp. 135–159). Hillsdale, NJ: Erlbaum.

Goldberg, L. R. (1999). A broad-bandwidth, public-domain, personality inventory measuring the lower-level facets of several five-factor models. In I. Mervielde, I. Deary, F. De Fruyt, & F. Ostendorf (Eds.), *Personality psychology in Europe* (Vol. 7, pp. 7–28). Tilburg, The Netherlands: Tilburg University Press.

Goldberg, L. R., Johnson, J. A., Eber, H. W., Hogan, R., Ashton, M. C., Cloninger, C. R., et al. (2006). The International Personality Item Pool and the future of public-domain personality measures. *Journal of Research in Personality, 40,* 84–96.

Hamilton, J. O. (1974) Motivation and risk-taking behavior: A test of Atkinson's theory. *Journal of Personality and Social Psychology, 29,* 856–864.

Higgins, E. T., Idson, L. C., Freitas, A. L., Spiegel, S., & Molden, D. C. (2003). Transfer of value from fit. *Journal of Personality and Social Psychology, 84,* 1140–1153.

Kuhl, J., & Blankenship, V. (1979). The dynamic theory of achievement motivation: From episodic to dynamic thinking. *Psychological Review, 86,* 141–151.

Larsen, R. L., & Ketelaar, T. (1989). Extraversion, neuroticism and susceptibility to positive and negative mood induction procedures. *Personality and Individual Differences, 10,* 1221–1228.

Leon, M. R., & Revelle, W. (1985) The effects of anxiety on analogical reasoning: A test of three theoretical models. *Journal of Personality and Social Psychology, 49,* 1302–1315.

Öhman, A., & Mineka, S. (2002). The malicious serpent: Snakes as a prototypical stimulus for an evolved model of fear. *Current Directions in Psychological Science, 12,* 5–9.

Ortony, A., Norman, D. A., & Revelle, W. (2005). Effective functioning: A three level model of affect, motivation, cognition, and behavior. In J. M. Fellous & M. A. Arbib (Eds.), *Who needs emotions?: The brain meets the machine* (pp. 173–202). New York: Oxford University Press.

Ozer, D. (2006) Personality and the prediction of consequential outcomes. *Annual Review of Psychology, 57,* 401–422.

Pinheiro, J. C., & Bates, D. M. (2000). *Mixed-effects models in S and S-plus.* New York: Springer.

Platt, J. R. (1964). Strong inference *Science, 146,* 347–353.

Rafaeli, E., & Revelle, W. (2006). A premature consensus: Are happiness and sadness truly opposite affects? *Motivation and Emotion, 30,* 1–12.

R Development Core Team. (2005). *R: A language and environment for statistical computing.* Vienna, Austria: R Foundation for Statistical Computing, *www.R-project.org.*

Revelle, W., Amaral, P., & Turriff, S. (1976). Introversion/extroversion, time stress, and caffeine: Effect on verbal performance. *Science, 192,* 149–150.

Revelle, W., & Anderson, K. J. (1992). Models for the testing of theory. In A. Gale & M. W. Eysenck (Eds.), *Handbook of individual differences: Biological perspectives* (pp. 81–113). Chichester, UK: Wiley.

Revelle, W., Humphreys, M. S., Simon, L., & Gilliland, K. (1980). The interactive effect of personality, time of day, and caffeine: A test of the arousal model. *Journal of Experimental Psychology: General, 109,* 1–31.

Rogers, G., & Revelle, W. (1998). Personality, mood, and the evaluation of affective and neutral word pairs. *Journal of Personality and Social Psychology, 74,* 1592–1605.

Shadish, W. R., Cook, T. D., & Campbell, D. T. (2002). *Experimental and quasi-experimental designs for generalized causal inference.* Boston: Houghton Mifflin.

Spence, K. W., Farber, I. E., & McFann, H. H. (1956). The relation of anxiety (drive) level to performance in competitional and non-competitional paired-associates learning. *Journal of Experimental Psychology, 52,* 296–305.

Weiner, B. & Schneider, K. (1971). Drive versus cognitive theory: A reply to Boor and Harmon. *Journal of Personality and Social Psychology, 18,* 258–262.

Wundt, W. (1904). *Principles of physiological psychology* (E. B. Titchener, Trans.). London: Swan Sonnenschein.

Yovel, I., Revelle, W., & Mineka, S. (2005). Who sees trees before forest? The obsessive–compulsive style of visual attention. *Psychological Science, 16,* 123–129.

Zinbarg, R., & Revelle, W. (1989). Personality and conditioning: A test of four models. *Journal of Personality and Social Psychology, 57,* 301–314.

Zinbarg, R. E., Revelle, W., Yovel, I., & Li. W. (2005). Cronbach's alpha, Revelle's beta, McDonald's omega: Their relations with each and two alternative conceptualizations of reliability. *Psychometrika, 70,* 123–133.

APPENDIX 3.1. ABBREVIATED R CODE FOR SIMULATING
PERSONALITY × SITUATION EFFECTS

Also available in a much more complete form at http://personalilty project.org/r/simulating personality.html

```
set.seed(42) #random number seed is fixed to produce identical "random" sequences
          #remove to allow each run to be different

#first set some parameters of the model
#change these to try different models

num <- 100            #number of people to simulate
weightreward<- .5 #an index of how strong is the effect of reward on positive affect
weightpunish<- .4 #how strong is the effect of punishment on negative affect
weight_e<- .0             #how strong is the effect of extraversion on positive affect
weight_n<- .3             #how strong is the effect of neuroticism on negative affect?
weight_er <- 4            #how strong is the interaction of e x reward on positive
affect
weight_np <- 0            #how strong is the interactionof n * punish on negative
affect
reliability_e <- .7  #the reliability of the observed extraversion score
reliability_n <- 8 #the reliability of the observed neuroticism score
reliability_P <- 7 #the reliability of observed measures of Postive Affect
reliability_N <- .8 #the reliability of observed measures of Negative Affect
weight_arousal <- .7 #relationship between extraversion and arousal
reliability_arousal <- .8 #reliability of arousal
weight_caff <- .5 #within subject weight of effect of caffeine
mean_E <- 3          #mean of true extra<- ver<- sion
mean_N <- 3                #mean of true neuroticism

#generate the data using the random normal distribution

                          #first simulate true (latent) scores
true_e <- rnorm(num,mean_E) #true trait extraversion is normally distributed with
sigma=1
true_n <- rnorm(num,mean_N) #true trait neuroticism is normally distributed
true_arousal_plac <- rnorm(num) - weight_arousal * (true_e - mean_E) -weight_caff
true_arousal_caff <- rnorm(num) - weight_arousal * (true_e - mean_E) + weight_caff
          #observed E and N are a mixture of true and error scores
extraversion<- sqrt(reliability_e)*(true_e-mean_E) + sqrt(1-reliability_e)*rnorm(num) +
mean_E
neuroticism<- sqrt(reliability_n)*(true_n -mean_N)+ sqrt(1-reliability_n)*rnorm(num) +
mean_N
arousal_plac <- sqrt(reliability_arousal) * (true_arousal_plac) + sqrt(1-
reliability_arousal)*rnorm(num)
arousal_caff <- sqrt(reliability_arousal) * (true_arousal_caff) + sqrt(1-
reliability_arousal)*rnorm(num)
performance_plac <- (1/(1+exp(-true_arousal_plac)))*(1/(1+exp(true_arousal_plac)))
#inverted u function of arousal
performance_caff <- (1/(1+exp(-true_arousal_caff)))*(1/(1+exp(true_arousal_caff)))
#inverted u function of arousal

                                   #experimental conditions are block randomized
reward <- rep(c(0,1),num/2) #reward vector of 0 or 1
punish <- rep(c(0,0,1,1),num/4) #punishment vector
block <- sort(rep(seq(1:(num/4)),4)) #block the data to allow for block randomization
temp.condition <- data.frame(reward,punish,block,rand =rnorm(num)) #experimental
conditions ordered by block
condition <- temp.condition[order(temp.condition$block,temp.condition$rand),1:2]
#conditions are now block randomized
```

```
#true affect measures are a function of a trait, a situation, and their interaction
TruePosAffect <- 1/(1+exp(-(weight_e * true_e + weightreward * condition$reward
+weight_er * true_e * condition$reward)))
TrueNegAffect <- 1/(1+exp(-(weight_n * true_n + weightpunish * condition$punish
+weight_np * true_n * condition$punish)))
TruePosAffect <- scale(TruePosAffect) #standardize TruePosAffect to put on the same
metric as the error scores
TrueNegAffect <- scale(TrueNegAffect) #standardize TrueNegAffect to put on the same
metric as the error scores

#observed affect is a function of true affect and errors in measurement
PosAffect <- sqrt(reliability_P) * TruePosAffect+sqrt(1-reliability_P)*rnorm(num)
NegAffect <- sqrt(reliability_N) * TrueNegAffect+sqrt(1-reliability_N)*rnorm(num)
#organize all the data in a data frame to allow for analysis

#organize all the data in a data frame to allow for analysis
#because it is also possible to do repeated measures as ANOVA on sums and differences
#the between effects are found by the sums
#the within effects are found the differences

PosplusNeg = PosAffect+NegAffect
PosminusNeg <- PosAffect - NegAffect
affect.data <-
data.frame(extraversion,neuroticism,PosAffect,NegAffect,PosplusNeg,PosminusNeg,true
_e,true_n,TruePosAffect,TrueNegAffect,reward =
as.factor(condition$reward),punish=as.factor(condition$punish))
centered.affect.data <- data.frame(scale(affect.data[,1:10],scale=FALSE),reward =
as.factor(condition$reward),punish=as.factor(condition$punish))
drug.data <-
data.frame(extraversion,true_arousal_plac,true_arousal_caff,arousal_plac,arousal_caff,pe
rformance_plac,performance_caff)



#the first models do not use 0 centered data and are incorrect
#these are included merely to show what happens if the correct model is not used
#do the analyses using a linear model without centering the data—wrong
mod1w <- lm(PosAffect ~ extraversion+reward,data= affect.data) #don't exam
interactions
mod2w <- lm(NegAffect ~ neuroticism+punish,data = affect.data)
mod3w <- lm(PosAffect ~ extraversion*reward,data = affect.data) #look for interactions
mod4w <- lm(NegAffect ~ neuroticism*punish,data = affect.data)
mod5w <- lm(PosAffect ~ extraversion*neuroticism*reward*punish,data = affect.data)
                                        #show the results of these incorrect analyses
summary(mod1w,digits=2)
summary(mod2w,digits=2)
summary(mod3w,digits=2)
summary(mod4w,digits=2)
summary(mod5w,digits=2)


#do the analyses with centered data—this is the correct way—note the differences
#just look at main effects
mod1 <- lm(NegAffect ~ neuroticism+punish,data = centered.affect.data) #just main
effects
mod2 <- lm(PosAffect ~ extraversion+reward,data= centered.affect.data) #don't exam
interactions

#include interactions
# note that mod3 and mod4 are two different ways of specifying the interaction
mod3 <- lm(PosAffect ~ extraversion*reward,data = centered.affect.data) #look for
interactions
mod4 <- lm(NegAffect ~ neuroticism+ punish + neuroticism*punish,data =
centered.affect.data)
```

```
#go for the full models
mod5 <- lm(PosAffect ~ extra<- ver<- sion*neuroticism*reward*punish,data =
centered.affect.data)
mod6 <- lm(NegAffect ~ extra<- ver<- sion*neuroticism*reward*punish,data =
centered.affect.data)
mod6.5 <- lm(c(NegAffect,PosAffect) ~ extraversion*neuroticism*reward*punish,data =
centered.affect.data)
                    #show these analyses
summary(mod1,digits=2)
summary(mod2,digits=2)
summary(mod3,digits=2)
summary(mod4,digits=2)
summary(mod5,digits=2)
summary(mod6,digits=2)
```

## CHAPTER 4

Behavior Genetic Designs

Robert F. Krueger
Jennifer L. Tackett

If we want to understand an individual's characteristic ways of thinking, feeling, and behaving (his or her personality), the immediate family is an obvious place to look. We could, for example, assess the personalities of all the individuals in a sample of families and see if personality resemblance within the families is greater, on average, than resemblance between two unrelated persons. The limitation of this approach is that people within families probably have more similar personalities than two randomly matched people, for multiple reasons. For example, we may find that extraverted mothers tend to have more extraverted daughters, on average, but we would be hard-pressed to defend a specific account of how this came about. Did the mothers pass on genes associated with extraversion to their daughters? Did the daughters become extraverted by being exposed to the environments created by the extraverted mothers? Are both genetic and en-

vironmental influences contributing to the similarities seen between mothers and daughters? Are both influences combining in some way, and, if so, how are they combining?

A fundamental goal of merging ideas from behavior genetics with ideas in personality psychology is to sort out these possibilities. Other exciting work is also being conducted at this interface, for example, work aimed at characterizing genetic contributions to personality at a molecular level. Approaches to this molecular work are covered in another chapter of this handbook (Ebstein, Bachner-Melman, Israel, Nemanov, & Gritsenko, Chapter 23, this volume). In the current chapter, we focus primarily on studies of twins as a means of understanding the ways genes and environments transact in influencing human personality variation. Briefly, twins provide clarity in distinguishing genetic and environmental effects because expectations about the similarity of different kinds of twins vary systematically with the presence of different kinds of genetic and environmental effects in data.[1]

Before we delve into the body of this chapter, there is one additional point we wish to make at the outset. The approaches we discuss here, involving twins as research participants, emerged in the field of "behavior genetics," hence the title of our chapter. When psychologists in general think of the "behavior genetics of personality," they often seem to think of using twin studies to document the "heritability of personality," that is, to amass evidence that genes are relevant contributors to human personality variation. This was indeed an important contribution of twin research on personality; numerous studies document significant genetic influences on self-reports of personality (see, e.g., Plomin, DeFries, McClearn, & McGuffin, 2001).

This does not mean, however, that twin research on personality has outlived its usefulness. The challenge is no longer to document genetic influences on personality traits; any fair reading of the evidence indicates that this task has been accomplished. Rather, knowing that genes matter in understanding personality traits, we feel the challenge now lies in understanding how specific genetic and environmental forces transact in more diverse personality phenomena. As can be seen from the diversity of chapters in this handbook, self-reported personality traits, although bedrock constructs in personality psychology, do not exhaust the constructs of interest to personality psychologists. To pick one example, although genetic factors have not been a major focus of social-cognitive personality research, such approaches do not necessarily exclude genetic effects, and some even posit their potential relevance (see, e.g., Mischel, 2004).

We begin with a discussion of how twin studies help disambiguate genetic and environmental effects and how twin studies allow for the estimation of these effects. In the course of that discussion, we also outline some considerations (traditionally referred to as "assumptions") that are important in interpreting the meaning of putative genetic and environmental effects. With this conceptual understanding in place, we then lead the reader through some of the nuts and bolts of gathering twin data. We then turn to putting the first two sections together; with an understanding of genetic and environmental effects, and twin data relevant

to an investigator's interests, how can an investigator model those twin data? We focus here initially on the fundamental single-variable (univariate) model for twin data, and we then describe more elaborate model extensions. We also comment on basic aspects of power analysis for twin studies. We conclude by highlighting some emerging directions, which we see as particularly interesting, at the intersection of personality and behavior genetics.

Our goal in our presentation is to expose the reader to some of the ideas in this area at a level that we hope is sufficient to generate a basic understanding of and interest in twin methodology for studies of personality. It is not possible in a chapter of this length to instruct the reader in all aspects of twin research. Fortunately, we have the luxury of being able to refer the reader to a number of fine textbooks that provide a more in-depth treatment of the issues discussed in this chapter (Carey, 2003; Neale & Maes, 1999; Plomin et al., 2001).

Sources of Human Individual Differences: The Parameters of Biometrical Models

People are different from each other on a host of variables, such as height, intelligence, socioeconomic status, and so on. Personality is one of these variables—and the focus of this chapter—but the concepts described here are equally applicable to any other variable on which people differ.

The extent to which people differ from one another on an observable characteristic is termed the *variance*, which can be computed using the formulas given in any introductory statistics text. To be more precise, we will term this statistic the *phenotypic variance* because it describes the total, directly observable extent to which people differ. In populations of living things (e.g., humans), phenotypic variance is attributable to both genetic and environmental sources. Expressed algebraically, if P is the total phenotypic variance in a population, then

$$P = G + E \qquad (4.1)$$

An initial goal of a twin study is to estimate G and E. Later, we also describe ways of thinking about and modeling the possibility that G and E effects are not uniform for the entire population (a phenomenon that could be thought of colloquially as "gene–environment interaction"). For now, though, our goal is simply to convey an understanding of how twin studies allow estimation of *G* and *E* in this fundamental equation.

Types of Twins

There are two types of twins, and these distinct types are due to distinct biological processes that produce twins. Monozygotic (MZ), or identical twins, result from the splitting of a single fertilized egg (zygote) into two embryos. Monozygotic twins have the same DNA; as a result they are also of the same gender within pairs. Dizygotic (DZ) twins, in contrast, result from two separate eggs being fertilized by two separate sperms. As a result, dizygotic twins are as genetically similar as two siblings. Dizygotic twins can be of the same sex or of opposite sexes.

Zygosity Diagnosis

Twin pairs do not necessarily know their zygosity, and even if they suspect they are of a certain zygosity, they may be incorrect. In spite of this, zygosity diagnosis—correctly identifying MZ and DZ pairs in a sample—is a surprisingly straightforward process. For example, a number of very brief questionnaires exist for this purpose. Although the questions on these instruments seem very straightforward and simple (e.g., "Could you fool friends and family by pretending to be each other?"), they are extremely effective. In spite of the general challenge of identifying natural types on the basis of modestly valid indicators of category membership (cf. Waller & Meehl, 1998), the distributions of scores on zygosity questionnaires tend to be markedly and obviously bimodal, with the two modes corresponding to the two types of twins. Evidence that the two modes seen in the distributions of scores on these questionnaires correspond to MZ and DZ twins is provided by studies that have linked questionnaire scores to zygosity diagnoses via blood samples. For example, consider a report from Lykken, Bouchard, McGue, and Tellegen (1990). These researchers made zygosity diagnoses based on both blood samples and a five-item questionnaire for a sample of 74 twin pairs. They reported substantial agreement between the two methods, with only 3 pairs of

the 74 classified differently via questionnaire versus blood sample. Also helpful is the fact that the zygosity questions used by Lykken and colleagues are printed in their article, such that budding twin researchers can use their questionnaire simply by obtaining a copy of Lykken and colleagues.

Genetic Sources of Variance

Genetic variance refers to the amount of variance in the construct of interest that is attributable to genetic influences, that is, the extent to which genetic differences between people are associated with phenotypic, observable differences. In Equation 4.1, it is represented by *G*. In a sample of unrelated persons, without genotypic data, we have no way of distinguishing *G* and *E* (environmental variance). However, in a sample of twins, *G* and *E* effects are associated with distinct predictions about the similarity of MZ and DZ pairs of twins. For this brief introductory chapter, the nuts-and-bolts principles of quantitative (biometrical) genetics that lead to distinct predictions about the similarity of MZ and DZ pairs of twins cannot be reviewed, because this would require extensive introductory material on principles of quantitative genetics. For the interested reader, a good source for this material is Falconer (1990). For our purposes, the important concepts from quantitative genetics pertain to the fact that MZ and DZ twins differ systematically in their genetic similarity.

Complex traits such as personality are polygenic; they result from the actions of numerous genes. In regard to polygenic inheritance, genetic effects can be thought of as "adding up" across all the parts of the genome (loci) contributing to a phenotype. If individual differences in a phenotype such as a personality variable were entirely attributable to genetic influences, we would expect the observed similarity of MZ and DZ pairs to be entirely consistent with their genetic similarities. Specifically, under an additive and polygenic model of inheritance, MZ twins are genetically identical (they have the same forms of genes, or alleles, at all loci), whereas DZ twins are as genetically similar as siblings (Neale & Maes, 1999). Expressed as correlation coefficients, the "genetic correlation" for MZ pairs is 1.0 and the genetic correlation for DZ pairs is .5 (i.e., DZ pairs share half of the total additive genetic variance; this fact derives algebraically from the additive polygenic model; see, e.g., Plomin et al., 2001).

It is these distinct expectations for MZ and DZ pair similarity that allow for the estimation of G in Equation 4.1. If a personality phenotype were attributable entirely to additive genetic effects (typically abbreviated A), then twin pairs should be exactly as similar as predicted in a model containing only A. That is, the MZ twins should be exactly the same within pairs (as would be shown by a correlation of 1.0 between the phenotypes of the halves of the MZ pairs), and the DZ twins should be as similar as predicted by the additive polygenic model (as would be shown by a correlation of .5 between the phenotypes of the halves of the DZ pairs). Indeed, for some human phenotypes, this is what tends to be observed. For example, Plomin, DeFries, and McClearn (1990) reported MZ correlations of .93 and .91, respectively, for height and weight, with corresponding DZ correlations of .48 and .58. The correspondence of these correlations with the additive polygenic model suggests that height and weight are mostly genetic characteristics of persons and, moreover, that the relevant underlying genes are functioning in a polygenic, additive manner (many genes are involved and they each contribute interchangeable, "additive" bits to overall height and weight).

Technically speaking, G can be further decomposed into distinct types of genetic effects. For example, some alleles (forms of genes) are known to dominate over other alleles in their impact on phenotypes. Such "dominance" effects (typically abbreviated D) lead to a different expectation for DZ pair similarity ($r = .25$), a value again derived from the algebra underlying the field of quantitative genetics. It could even be the case that a phenotype is entirely attributable to the precise combination of alleles, as opposed to the number of relevant alleles. This situation, known as *epistasis*, again leads to a distinct prediction for the DZ pairs ($r = 0.0$, with the MZ pairs still expected to correlate 1.0 because they share the same combination of alleles across loci).

Environmental Sources of Variance

Expectations for various G effects are distinct from expectations for E effects, and it is this further fact that allows for the disambiguation of G and E in twin data. Expectations for E fol-

low from quantitative models of twin similarity under different environmental hypotheses in the same way that expectations for G follow from quantitative models of twin similarity under different genetic hypotheses. Two straightforward environmental hypotheses are typically articulated. *Shared environmental variance* refers to the amount of variance that is attributable to aspects of the environment that affect two siblings reared in the same family in the same way. Shared environment is also termed *common environment* and is typically abbreviated C. *Nonshared environmental variance* refers to the amount of variance that is attributable to aspects of the environment that are *unique* to each individual, or environments that affect each individual uniquely. This effect is typically abbreviated E. The expectations for C effects are $r(MZ) = 1.0$ and $r(DZ) = 1.0$. That is, if only common environmental effects are operating, then twins growing up together should be exactly the same, within pairs, and regardless of zygosity. In contrast, the expectations for E effects are $r(MZ) = r(DZ) = 0.0$. That is, if only nonshared environmental effects are operating, then twins within pairs should be no more similar than two randomly matched people.

Equal Environments Assumption

In theory, effects that are consistent with G effects could be observed for spurious reasons. For example, MZ pairs may be more similar than DZ pairs on personality characteristics because they are more similar in physical appearance. This consideration typically falls under the rubric of the *equal environments assumption* (EEA). Stated as an assumption, the EEA indicates that it can be safely assumed that MZ and DZ correlations consistent with G effects reflect actual G effects, as opposed to greater MZ than DZ within-pair similarity for nongenetic reasons.

It may be helpful to clarify use of the term *assumption* in this context. Specifically, we see the considerations that fall under the rubric of the EEA as something closer to a source of testable hypotheses, as opposed to an "a priori assumption" that may be "violated." Consider, for example, the hypothesis that greater MZ versus DZ similarity in personality is attributable to the greater physical similarity of MZ twins. This hypothesis may be evaluated by considering literature on how appearance predicts personality. Generally, physical attractiveness is weakly correlated with personality in nontwin participants, although physically attractive people are often perceived as having desirable characteristics they may not actually possess (Feingold, 1992). Thus, similarity in physical attractiveness is an unlikely explanation of actual personality similarity in MZ twins, given that physical attractiveness per se is not a major predictor of personality in general. The general point is that thinking through the issues under the rubric of the EEA may be more generative than imposing the concept of an "assumption" on such issues.

Along these lines, the EEA has been subject to various creative tests, and these tests tend to support the reasonability of interpreting twin correlations consistent with G effects as genetic in nature (Bouchard & Propping, 1993). By way of example, consider a test presented by Goldsmith, Lemery, Buss, and Campos (1999), investigators interested in temperament in infant twins. These investigators performed a thorough diagnosis of zygosity, but they also asked parents if they thought their twins were MZ or DZ. For a number of pairs, parents thought their twins were DZ but the zygosity diagnoses indicated they were MZ. Nevertheless, these "MZ thought to be DZ" pairs were no more or less similar in temperament, on average, than "MZ correctly thought to be MZ" pairs. In this study, actual zygosity was a better predictor of twin similarity, versus perceived zygosity.

Another issue to consider in regard to assumptions is the extent to which twins are representative of people in general. Essentially, for twin studies to generalize to the population at large, twins should be representative of people in general. In the case of personality traits, this issue was recently evaluated by Johnson, Krueger, Bouchard, and McGue (2002). In this study, across a number of personality trait measures, twins and singletons did not differ markedly. These findings support the idea of generalizing from twin research to research on other persons, at least where personality traits are concerned.

Gathering Twin Data

We hope that the previous section has convinced the reader about the unique value of twins in personality research. Essentially, in working with twins, G and E effects can be disambiguated. Indeed, once these effects are separated, they can then be recombined in ways that we feel are central to understanding personality (e.g., models can be evaluated that allow for G–E interaction). Before we turn to those topics, however, we first describe how an investigator interested in twins could go about gathering twin data.

Researchers who are interested in starting twin studies have numerous examples from which to draw. A variety of starting points for identifying twins have been employed, including birth records, birth announcements, school recruitment, newspaper and media announcements, and area twins organizations (e.g., Mothers of Twins clubs). Birth records are a popular and desirable means of ascertaining families of multiples, as they allow researchers to access a more representative sample. However, some states may not allow researchers to access birth records and even when this option is available, the researcher may still obtain a poor response rate (see, e.g., DiLalla, 2002). Researchers may choose to gather data from birth records or published birth announcements and later contact the families by mail or phone. However, it may also be possible for researchers to regularly gather birth record information in the hospital itself and approach the mothers during their stay for possible participation in the research (Strassberg et al., 2002). It is also common for researchers using the birth records/birth announcements approach to cross-reference their database with death records, such as to eliminate those twin pairs in which one or both of the twins does not survive past infancy.

Another recruitment strategy that varies by community in ease of implementation is school recruitment. In some areas, researchers may form direct relationships with the schools that enable them to access the database of enrolled students or distribute flyers at the schools. This approach also initially offers a more representative sample (although, again, response rates must be adequate to achieve good representation). It also allows researchers to more easily identify and even target certain demographic variables of scientific interest, such as ethnic representation, at the school-wide level.

Recruitment via other methods, such as media announcements, is perhaps less desirable because of the potential problems posed for personality researchers. To the extent that individual differences in personality influence rates of response to such announcements, one could be limiting the very information that forms the focus of personality research. Thus, some researchers have used various incentives to try to boost response rates, particularly among those who do not respond initially (Jang, Livesley, & Vernon, 2002; Krueger & Johnson, 2002). There are a number of popular recruitment strategies that, although they may struggle with this problem of limited variance, are nonetheless commonly used in current research. Such strategies include having researchers give presentations at Mothers of Twins clubs, researchers conducting interviews that appear on local television programs and in area newspapers, advertising on the researcher's lab website, recruiting families of multiples when they are encountered by the researchers in the community, and asking research participants for referrals to other families of multiples.

Although there are inherent challenges in all of the approaches described thus far, it is most important for researchers to be aware of potential biases that may exist in their samples resulting from their recruitment strategies. For example, school recruitment strategies may show different response rates based on the age of the target children (Hur, 2002). Thus, researchers may take a more aggressive or alternative approach to recruitment, depending on the age of interest. If researchers are interested in targeting adult participants, they may encounter more difficulties when utilizing birth records. For example, adult individuals are more likely to have moved at least once in their lives, which can complicate tracking them. Similarly, many female participants may have changed their names, and researchers may want to cross-reference marriage records to identify these individuals. In addition, many studies based on volunteer subjects show much greater response rates for females. Thus, recruitment strategies targeted at male participants may be desirable to increase representativeness. In general, it is always important to compare the characteristics of participants and nonparticipants to identify any potential limitations to generalizability.

As researchers are identifying the recruitment strategies they intend to use, they should also consider how their methods of assessment may influence recruitment. The most common methods of assessment are self-report paper-and-pencil measures, which can easily be filled out either in the lab or at home and returned by mail. This approach is typically cheaper and quicker, but may yield lower response rates (Hansen, Alessandri, Croft, Burton, & de Klerk, 2004). Some studies use interviews (Harris, Magnus, & Tambs, 2002; Mina Bergem, 2002), either in person or over the phone, or observational paradigms (DiLalla, 2002; Spinath, Angleitner, Borkenau, Riemann, & Wolf, 2002; Van Hulle, Lemery, & Goldsmith, 2002). Given the need to obtain large samples in twin studies, research that intends to employ more expensive assessment techniques may choose to recruit more aggressively in order to maximize response rates.

Fitting Models to Twin Data: Estimating the Parameters of Biometrical Models

With twin data in hand and the understanding that those data can be used to estimate the parameters of biometrical models (the components of G and E in Equation 4.1), the next step is to formally undertake this endeavor.

The Univariate ACE Model

Earlier, we described how G effects are typically subsumed under a polygenic-additive model, and how these effects in that model are abbreviated A to stand for additive genetic effects. We also described how E effects can be separated into common environmental (C) effects and nonshared environmental (E) effects. All three effects make distinct predictions about the similarity of MZ and DZ twins, and this distinctiveness in predictions allows the effects to be estimated simultaneously.[2]

An "effect" can be thought of as the extent to which the total phenotypic variance in a variable is consistent with the previously described hypotheses regarding the origins of individual differences. Real data tend not to fit the predictions of only a single effect (A, C, or E). More commonly, real data tend to reveal the simultaneous presence of both genetic and environmental effects. The extent of phenotypic variation in a variable consistent with a given prediction is the magnitude of that effect.

How does one move from observed twin data to estimating the magnitudes of ACE effects? This is the process of biometrical model fitting, and a good way to portray biometrical models is in terms of path diagrams. The *ACE* model for data obtained from MZ and DZ twins is portrayed in Figure 4.1. Path models are described in a number of commonly used text books (see, e.g., Loehlin, 2004), and these sources can be consulted for additional details about path models. For our current purposes, we describe some of the key features of Figure 4.1 as they pertain to biometric model fitting. First, consider the squares at the bottom of Figure 4.1. These squares represent observed variation in a phenotype, as observed in the first and second halves of the twin pairs in a sample. Twins can be divided into halves of pairs in any number of ways. For example, P_1 could correspond to the first-born twins and P_2 could correspond to the second-born twins.

Next consider the three arrows pointing at both P_1 and P_2. These arrows represent the magnitudes of the A, C, and E effects. Notice that they are connected with circles labeled A, C, and E, with separate A, C, and E circles for both halves of the twin pairs. In path diagrams, circles correspond with indirectly observed variables, as opposed to squares, which correspond with directly observed variables. That is, the A, C, and E variables are not observed directly (unlike the observed phenotypes of the twins); they are inferred from the observed phenotypes of the twins.

The curved lines at the top of the figure represent correlations.[3] These curved lines serve to define the A, C, and E effects in a manner consistent with our previous definitions. First consider the A effect. Notice that the curved line connecting the A_1 circle with the A_2 circle has a value of MZ 1.0/DZ .5. This notation is shorthand for the value of the correlation being 1.0 for MZ twins and .5 for DZ twins. Recall that this was the definition of an A effect. This part of the model is "known" in the sense that the expectations associated with the A effect are known. What is unknown is the value of *a* in the figure. This value is the extent to which the observed MZ and DZ twin data are consistent with an A effect. As with the A effect, the C and E effects are also defined by the correlations between the C and E circles in the figure. Notice that the C effect is defined by a correlation of 1.0 between the C_1 and C_2 circles (for both MZ and DZ pairs), and the E effect is defined by the absence of a correlation between the E_1 and E_2 circles (i.e., no line connects the E variables on the figure).

Figure 4.1 is a graphical representation of a statistical model for twin data. The process of estimating the unknown quantities in Figure 4.1 (*a*, *c*, and *e*) is known as model fitting and is conducted using computer software. A popular package for model fitting to twin data was developed by Mike Neale and his colleagues and is called "M_X" (Neale, Boker, Xie, & Maes, 1999). Biometrical models of the sort portrayed in Figure 4.1 are types of structural equation models (see Hoyle, Chapter 26, this volume), and hence could be fit by other commonly used structural equation modeling pack-

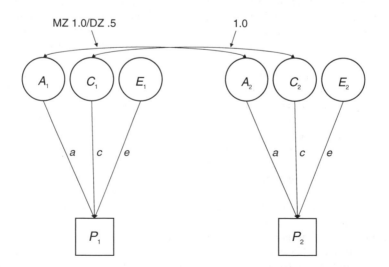

FIGURE 4.1. Univariate *ACE* model for data obtained from MZ and DZ twins.

ages. However, M_X has become popular for biometrical modeling because it is unusually flexible and therefore well suited to accommodating the technical aspects of biometrical modeling. M_X is also free and can be obtained from *www.vcu.edu/mx/*. A related URL (*www.vcu.edu/mx/examples.html*) allows access to many M_X scripts (computer instructions) for performing various types of statistical analyses.

The typical statistical approach employed in M_X (and other structural equation packages) is known as *maximum likelihood estimation*. The idea behind maximum likelihood estimation is to use information obtained from sample data to determine the most likely values of the unknown parameters of a statistical model in the population from which the sample was drawn. In the case of the *ACE* model, the unknown parameters are *a*, *c*, and *e*, as shown in Figure 4.1. For a straightforward model such as the *ACE* model, the sample data can be summarized in terms of six basic statistics. Within the MZ pairs of twins, there are two halves of the twin pairs, and the variance of the observed phenotype can be computed in both halves, yielding two statistics. The halves of the twin pairs can be formed either by making the first half the first-born twins, and the second half the second-born twins, or by randomly assigning twins within pairs to be twin 1 or twin 2. In addition, the covariance between the two halves of the MZ pairs can be computed.[4] Repeating this process for the DZ pairs yields three more statistics (the variance of the phenotype in the first half of the DZ pairs, the variance in the second half of the DZ pairs, and the covariance across the halves of the DZ pairs). These quantities can be computed using numerous standard statistical packages (e.g., SPSS or SAS) and the resulting values "plugged into" the M_X software to estimate the parameters of the *ACE* model.

An M_X script for fitting the *ACE* model to data obtained from MZ and DZ twins is given in Appendix 4.1. If the reader were to obtain twin data and compute the aforementioned six summary statistics, these values could be plugged into the script in the appendix, and executing the resulting script in M_X would provide *a*, *c*, and *e* estimates for the reader's data.

A complete account of what the script in Appendix 4.1 is designed to do would require that the reader have a background in matrix algebra. Although such a background is useful in

understanding the nuts and bolts of statistical modeling, it is not essential to being able to fit the *ACE* model to twin data. Nevertheless, the following discussion reviews some of the major features of the script in the appendix to give the reader some understanding of what the script is doing and how this relates to our previous description of *G* and *E* effects and the path model in Figure 4.1.

The script is divided into three "paragraphs" or blocks of computer code. The first paragraph defines basic quantities that will be used in setting up the model (note that although dominance effects, or *D*, are in the script, they are fixed at a value of 0.0). The second paragraph defines the model for the MZ twin pairs and reads the observed data in those pairs. In the "Data" line of the script, the number of MZ twin pairs is given, as are labels for the phenotype as observed in the MZ twin pairs. Under the command "CMatrix," the three aforementioned statistics for the MZ pairs are read: the MZ twin 1 variance, the MZ covariance, and the MZ twin 2 variance. The "Covariances" statement then defines the way in which the effects in the model predict the observed MZ sample statistics. This statement defines the expected covariance matrix for the MZ twins. A matrix is a way of arranging multiple numbers in a grid. In the case of this specific covariance statement, the expected variances of the phenotype in the MZ twins are given on the diagonal of the matrix (the upper left and lower right-hand cells of the matrix). These expected variances are derived from Figure 4.1. Notice that in Figure 4.1, all three effects (*A*, *C*, and *E*) contribute to the observed variation in the phenotype, as shown by all three effects having arrows connecting them to the observed phenotypes. This is the same idea expressed in Equation 4.1, with *G* being defined more specifically as *A*, and *E* broken into both *C* and *E* parts. Notice also that the predicted covariance in the MZ pairs is given on the off-diagonal cells of the matrix. This also relates directly to Figure 4.1. In the figure, the *A* effects are connected with a coefficient of 1.0 for the MZ pairs and the *C* effects are also connected with a coefficient of 1.0 for the MZ pairs, but the *E* effects are not connected across the halves of the pairs. Hence, *A* and *C* effects contribute to the covariance for the MZ pairs, but *E* effects do not. This relates back to the definition of the *E* effect. Recall that the *E* effect pertains to the uniqueness of each person, in spite of the fact that persons in twin pairs grew up together and share genetic material consistent with their zygosity. As a result, E effects contribute to variation among people, but not to similarities between people.

The third paragraph provides the observed data for the DZ twin pairs, as well as the expected covariance matrix for those pairs. Note the similarities and differences between the expected MZ and DZ matrices. Specifically, the expected variances in both groups are the same. This is because the same effects lead to variation in the population for all persons; that is, the variance in any given phenotype is a result of the A, C, and E effects. However, consistent with the model in Figure 4.1, the expected covariance between the DZ twins reflects the distinct genetic similarity of those pairs as compared with MZ pairs. In particular, the quantity .5 is multiplied by the A effect for the DZ twins (and .25 for the D effect, which would be relevant if the D effect were freely estimated). This is consistent with Figure 4.1 and our previously mentioned definition of the polygenic additive model.

The Multivariate *ACE* Model

The model in Figure 4.1 and the script in Appendix 4.1 can be expanded readily to encompass data from multiple phenotypes observed simultaneously in a sample of twins (see Neale & Maes, 1999). This multivariate extension of the univariate *ACE* model can be used to address some fundamental issues in personality psychology. For example, it is well known that personality constructs are capable of predicting external criteria. What, however, is the etiology of such predictive validity? For example, might the connections between personality constructs and outcomes be mediated genetically, so that both personality and its correlates may be thought of as alternate manifestations of linked, underlying genetic processes? Such questions can be addressed via multivariate extensions of the *ACE* model.

A particularly useful extension of the univariate *ACE* model to multiple phenotypes is known as the Cholesky model. An *AE* Cholesky model is portrayed in Figure 4.2 (we have dropped C from this model because the model is difficult to draw with C effects; if these effects were in the model, they would be drawn in the same way as the A effects, only the correlation across twins would be 1.0 for both MZ and DZ twins). The model is named after mathematician André-Louis Cholesky, who developed a method of solving equations such that the result would have an appealing mathematical property known as *positive definiteness*. Essentially, by performing multiplication of the matrix representing a set of effects in Figure 4.2 (e.g., the A effects) by what is known as the *transpose* of that same matrix (the matrix rearranged so that the rows are transposed with the columns), the result is a matrix representing the A variances and covariances of the variables that is also positive definite. Positive definite matrices are more directly amenable to various kinds of multivariate statistical procedures (e.g., factor analysis) than are matrices that lack this quality. For example, these properties of the Cholesky model have been put to use in studying the genetic and environmental bases of the structure of personality (see, e.g., Krueger, 2000; Livesley, Jang, & Vernon, 1998).

The model in Figure 4.2 can also be interpreted directly in terms of the paths shown on the figure, without the additional step provided by the aforementioned multiplication operation. Consider, for example, the model in Figure 4.2 with only two observed phenotypes (i.e., delete P_1 and its associated effects, leaving P_2 as the first variable and P_3 as the second variable). These phenotypes could be, for example, a personality trait (P_2) and a specific outcome such as work performance, or physical health, or any other phenotypic outcome variable (P_3). In this situation, the unique genetic effects on P_3 (represented in the model by the path a_{33}) represent the residual etiological contributions to P_3 not shared with P_2. One could test, for example, whether the unique A effect (path a_{33}) on P_3 is so small as to be negligible in its impact. This is essentially a test of the hypothesis that the genetic effects on P_2 are entirely in common with the genetic effects on P_3, such that both phenotypes can be conceived of as alternate manifestations of the same underlying genetic risk factors. The genetic effects on P_3 estimated to be in common with those effects on P_2 are represented in the model by the path a_{32}.

A brief note on model fit: Strictly speaking, almost all effects are non-zero, given a sufficient sample size (see Fraley & Marks, Chapter 9, this volume), but some effects are so trivial that they render models more complex than they need to be to account for data in a

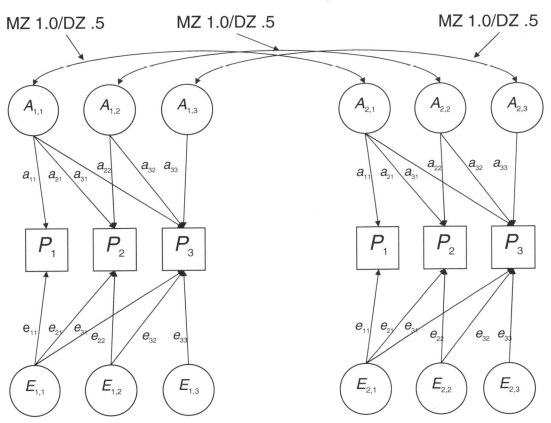

FIGURE 4.2. Multivariate *ACE* model for data obtained from MZ and DZ twins.

straightforward manner. Moreover, more complex models are less likely to be "true models" in the sense of being the correct model in the population from which a sample was drawn. This point has been appreciated in biometric modeling for some time, but Fraley and Marks (Chapter 9, this volume) suggest that the point is somewhat less appreciated in personality psychology more broadly. Along these lines, the fit of biometrical models has traditionally been evaluated using a criterion known as Akaike's information criterion (AIC; Akaike, 1987). When models are fit to covariance matrices, this criterion is easily computed from the output of standard statistical modeling packages as the chi-square value for the fitted model minus two times the degrees of freedom for that model (AIC = $\chi^2 - 2\ df$).

Larger, more negative values of AIC are associated with better-fitting models. This is because AIC balances the χ^2 value of a model with the degrees of freedom of a model in evaluating model fit. The χ^2 value of a model indexes its ability to reproduce the observed data, with larger χ^2 values being associated with poorer reproduction. The degrees of freedom for a model index its complexity, at least when complexity is understood simply as the number of unknown quantities that need to be estimated in fitting a model to sample data. Smaller degrees of freedom are associated with more complex models. Hence, models with smaller χ^2 values and larger df (less complexity) have larger, more negative AIC values.

One can formulate the evaluation of the need to model the unique etiological contributions to P_3 in this framework. One would ask: Does the AIC value for the model improve when various effects on P_3 are dropped from the model? Similarly, one can drop specific A and C effects from the model and see if the AIC value for the model improves (E effects are not dropped because they contain residual variation, and a model without residual variation makes little substantive sense). If the AIC improves when effects are dropped, it means that these effects are adding unnecessary complexity to the model. Other criteria that approach model fit in the same way as AIC have also been articulated; these derive from an area of statistical inquiry known as information theory. We see this area as exciting when applied to psychological phenomena because it leads to thinking about the ability of a model to capture data, as opposed to thinking about whether various individual effects are statistically significant. The latter is less appealing because it tends to lead to piecemeal empirical inquiry, as opposed to inquiry aimed at building scientific, quantitative models of psychological phenomena (see Fraley & Marks, Chapter 9, this volume). As an introduction to diverse information theoretic fit criteria in biometrical modeling, the reader may consult, for example, Markon and Krueger (2004), a simulation study of the performance of various information theoretic fit criteria in the context of multivariate biometric models.

The *ACE* Model Fit to Raw Data

Up to this point, we have focused on fitting the *ACE* model to covariance structures (see, e.g., the M_X script in Appendix 4.1). An exciting development in biometric modeling (and statistical modeling more generally) involves the ability to fit directly to the raw data. When summary statistics such as variances and covariances are computed, one is essentially collapsing over numerous details in the raw data obtained in a study. Such collapsing is reasonable if the summary statistics accurately represent all the information in a dataset. Nevertheless, to the extent that collapsing glosses over interesting details in a dataset, modeling the raw data becomes scientifically exciting and important. That is, the ability to model raw data opens up numerous fascinating possibilities for modeling more complex phenomena.

Consider again the fundamental univariate model shown in Figure 4.1. As we noted earlier, this model is traditionally fit to variances and covariances (see the MX script given in Appendix 4.1). As a result, the endeavor characterizes *ACE* effects in the entire population from which the sample was drawn. It assumes that the *ACE* effects are consistent for the entire population.

What would it mean if *ACE* effects are not consistent for the entire population? In particu-

lar, what if the *ACE* effects varied systematically as a function of some other variable? This "other variable" would then be considered a *moderator* of the *ACE* effects. A legitimate shortcoming of the *ACE* model fit to covariances is that it is not able to characterize such moderator effects because the covariances represent summary statistics for the entire sample as a whole (vs. characteristics of the data contingent on another variable). Colloquially, one could think of such moderator effects as a form of "gene × environment interaction" because the moderator is influencing the magnitude of genetic and environmental effects. This terminology is somewhat imprecise in the sense that the moderator is not actually an environment but, rather, a phenotype that may itself have both genetic and environmental aspects.

Models of this sort were recently described and evaluated by Purcell (2002). To give the reader a feel for these models, Figure 4.3 presents a variation on the *ACE* model fit to raw data that also takes into account the possibility of moderation of the *ACE* effects. For illustrative purposes, only part of the overall model is shown, that part being the model for only one twin and pertaining solely to the *ACE* effects. Note that the familiar *ACE* effects have been replaced by equations of the form effect + beta × moderator. In this model, overall *ACE* effects are still estimated, but in addition to these effects, moderating effects are also estimated. These later effects are represented by the beta terms in the figure. Per the equations in the figure, the betas characterize the "impact" of the moderator. These effects are constants, but they are weighted by (multiplied by) moderator values to determine overall *ACE* effects on the phenotype. Hence, with this model fit to data and values of *ACE* and the betas determined, model-predicted *ACE* components can be evaluated across various levels of the moderator variable.

Power Considerations in Twin Studies

At this point, we hope, the reader has some sense of why we see twin studies as scientifically exciting in personality psychology, especially given the possibilities opened up by raw data modeling. Nevertheless, we must pause for a moment to evaluate the issue of power. Power has traditionally been conceived of as the probability of concluding that an effect is nonzero, assuming it really is nonzero. Unfor-

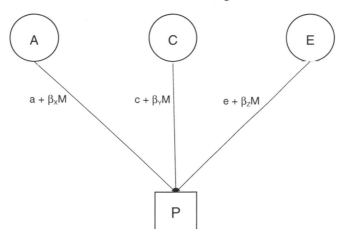

FIGURE 4.3. Univariate *ACE* model for data obtained from MZ and DZ twins taking into account potential moderation of *ACE* effects.

tunately, the confidence intervals around biometrical effects are often nontrivial, unless the sample sizes used in estimating these effects are relatively large by the traditional standards of psychological research. Hence, a large sample size is needed for the investigator to gain confidence about the size of an effect, or to confidently conclude that an effect is nonzero. To gain an intuitive feel for this phenomenon in the context of biometrical modeling, consider that biometrical effects rely on the comparison of correlation coefficients. Many readers have probably had the experience of formally comparing two correlations and discovering that relatively large samples (by psychological standards) are needed to conclude that the two correlations are different in the statistical sense.

Power considerations are a major reason why twin researchers often collaborate and rely on very large registries of twins in their work. We hope this does not discourage the reader from contemplating twin research, however. The scientific culture of behavior genetics, in our experience, is very open to collaboration and has frequently been enriched by contact between statistical modelers and researchers with various kinds of substantive interests. For example, the Institute for Behavioral Genetics at the University of Colorado (*ibgwww.colorado.edu/*) sponsors workshops on the methodology of twin and family studies. These workshops provide hands-on experience with the sorts of methods described in this chapter, and an opportunity for substantive researchers to

make contact with researchers developing biometric models.

Another point we wish to make concerning power has to do with reconceptualizing power in terms of the ability to distinguish models, as opposed to the ability to reliably detect univariate effects. To the extent that two models are very clearly distinguished in their empirical implications, the ability of information theoretic indices to pick up on these differences is enhanced. Nevertheless, power is still often conceptualized in terms of detecting specific univariate effects. For example, grant applications often characterize the "power to detect an *A* effect of small, medium, and large magnitude, given such and such values of *C* and *E*." This is probably a less useful way of thinking about study design, versus mapping theoretical models onto quantitative models and evaluating the ability to distinguish those quantitative models via information theoretic fit criteria, given various sample sizes and other design considerations. We see this as an important area for continued inquiry, which may lead to new and more scientifically generative ways of thinking about study design.

Finally, we wish to note that implementing traditional power analysis for biometric models is straightforward in MX. Essentially, one determines the observed covariance structures that would correspond with a model of interest and then fits to those data omitting the effect for which one wants to evaluate power, asking MX to report the power associated with this omission. We refer the reader to the M_X manual for the nuts and bolts of implementing this approach (Neale et al., 1999, p. 114)

Current and Future Directions: Beyond Traits and Beyond Heritability

Our goal in this chapter has been to expose the reader to some modern ideas in behavior genetics, in the hope that these ideas can continue to intersect with ideas in personality psychology. Along these lines, we return now to an issue that we introduced at the start of this chapter, namely, the tendency for behavior genetic research on personality to focus primarily on traits. Our own research has relied heavily on personality traits, and extensive data support the view that traits are critical in understanding diverse real-world outcomes (see, e.g., Krueger, Caspi, & Moffitt, 2000; Roberts & Pomerantz, 2004). Yet personality phenomena encompass much more than just traits. One need look no further than the diversity of chapters in this handbook to appreciate this point.

Nevertheless, self-reported personality traits have been the major foci of behavior genetic inquiry in personality psychology. This focus is consistent with the common intellectual origins of trait psychology and behavior genetics as fields of study under the broader rubric of the study of human individual differences. Yet extending behavior genetic inquiry beyond self-reports of personality traits opens up fascinating avenues of inquiry.

Consider, for example, a recent study that we feel helps to make this point concretely. Borkenau, Riemann, Spinath, and Angleitner (2006) collected extensive and detailed data on the performance of twin pairs in 15 distinct tasks, asking judges who had never met the twins to evaluate the twins' personalities based on videotapes of the twins' performance in these tasks. This design allowed Borkenau and colleagues to evaluate both genetic and environmental contributions to personality impressions aggregated across the tasks, as well as the extent to which there were residual genetic effects on task-specific impressions. Task-specific genetic influences were found, independent of aggregate cross-task genetic influences. That is, genetic effects were found not only on cross-situational "traits," but also on personality impressions as manifested in specific tasks (although it is also theoretically important to note that the cross-situational genetic effects were stronger).

In our view, the creative work of Borkenau and colleagues (2006) provides an appealing "ecumenical" perspective on the role of genetic factors in personality. Genetic factors do impact personality at the aggregate level, and this impact can be seen not only in self-reports, but also in personality impressions. Yet genetic effects on personality are not seen only at this level. The sorts of person × situation profiles more characteristic of social-cognitive theorizing in personality (Mischel, 2004) are also impacted by genetic factors. Our interpretation of this situation is that, ultimately, understanding the ways genes and environments influence behavior will require embracing diverse personality constructs beyond just traits.

We also argue that raw data modeling has similar potential to articulate richer personality processes, beyond genetic effects on cross-situational consistency. Along these lines, the reader may be wondering at this point why we have not yet formally defined certain better-known behavior genetic concepts such as heritability. The reason is that these concepts take on a more nuanced meaning, given the range of modeling options available. Heritability is the proportion of the total phenotypic variation in a trait attributable to genetic influences. In terms of Equation 4.1, heritability = $G/P = G/G + E$. Or, stated in terms of the ACE model, additive heritability = $A/A + C + E$.

Heritability is a fine index of overall extent of genetic contribution to P when G and E are consistent for a population. Indeed, as we noted at the outset, the understanding that G/P is far from 0% for self-reported personality traits was a critical intellectual contribution of behavior genetics. However, the meaning of heritability becomes more nuanced in the raw data context. Consider Figure 4.4, reprinted from Johnson and Krueger (2006). These authors examined how the A, C, and E components of variation in life satisfaction changed across levels of financial position in a sample of twins. They found that whereas A and C variances were constant across finances, E was not; rather, E variation was enhanced at low levels of financial position (see Figure 4.4). A reasonable psychological interpretation of this finding is that finances provide protection from random shocks to life satisfaction, as such random shocks would be sources of E variance.

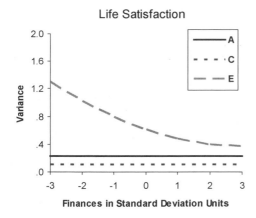

FIGURE 4.4. Genetic and environmental variance in life satisfaction as a function of finances. From Johnson and Krueger (2006). Copyright 2006 by the American Psychological Association. Reprinted by permission.

Now consider the meaning of the concept of heritability in the context of Figure 4.4. Although the amount of genetic variation (*A*) is constant, the heritability (*A*/*A* + *C* + *E*) increases with increasing financial position. Moreover, the total phenotypic variation (*A* + *C* + *E*) increases with decreasing financial position. Modeling the raw data and plotting the raw variance estimates (as opposed to the variance estimates as a proportion of total phenotypic variance) was critical in recognizing these phenomena, and they have interesting psychological interpretations. In particular, a reasonable interpretation elaborates on the interpretation of *E* variance offered above in noting that greater finances allow for greater clarity of expression of genetic effects on life satisfaction. One can think of heritability as "clarity" in the sense that if a greater proportion of *P* is *G*, then a greater proportion of an observed outcome is attributable to underlying genetic influences. The upshot is that finances might not lead in a direct, phenotypic sense to greater life satisfaction in developed nations (cf. Diener & Seligman, 2004), but the Johnson and Krueger (2006) study suggests that greater finances create a situation that buffers unforeseen shocks to life satisfaction, thereby allowing for underlying genetic influences on life satisfaction to be expressed with greater clarity.

Our general concluding point is that behavior genetic approaches continue to grow and develop. These approaches gain their intellectual vigor through their application to diverse psychological phenomena. Personality traits are heritable, but personality psychology is about more than just traits, and behavior genetic ideas and concepts are about more than just heritability. We hope the reader has gained some introduction to modern ideas in behavior genetics in the course of this chapter and may feel inspired to explore these ideas in the context of his or her own work in personality psychology.

Notes

1. Another design that can get at gene–environment transactions involves studying adoptees. Adoption research is also an important avenue to understanding gene–environment transactions because, like twin studies, adoption studies provide a handle on separating genetic and environmental effects. For example, children adopted into a family with biological offspring share a family environment with those biological offspring, but are no more likely to share genes with those biological offspring than are two randomly matched children, in the absence of selective placement. Typically, however, it is considerably more challenging to gather adoption data, and hence there is much less adoption research on personality than twin research on personality (Plomin, Corley, Caspi, Fulker, & DeFries, 1998). The good news for personality researchers contemplating twin research is that twins are plentiful, and many personality researchers can therefore seriously contemplate involving twins in their programs of research. Hence, we focus this chapter on twin research designs, as opposed to adoption designs. We note, however, that ideas that have emerged in the quantitative modeling of twin data can be readily extended to adoption data (see, e.g., Burt, McGue, Krueger, & Iacono, 2006).

2. At this point, the reader may wonder if additional effects discussed above (e.g., dominance or *D* effects) can also be estimated along with the *A*, *C*, and *E* effects. This is not mathematically possible with twin data alone. The problem here is known as *identification*. Essentially, an *ACED* model postulates more effects than can be identified in data coming from only MZ and DZ twin pairs reared together. However, one could replace one of the *ACE* effects, which would result in an identified model. For example, an *ADE* model is identified. Given that many phenotypes show little evidence of *C* effects, many investigators turn to fit an *ADE* model after fitting an *ACE* model and discovering that *C* effects are minimal.

3. Technically speaking, the curved lines in the figure represent covariances. For the current purposes, the indirectly observed variables in Figure 4.1 are "standardized" to a variance of 1.0 (this could be shown explicitly in the figure by inserting a curved arrow with "1.0" above each circle). The covariances in the figure can be interpreted as correlations because the latent variables in the figure have been standardized to unit variance (1.0).
4. Regarding the covariance, throughout this chapter thus far, we have quantified observed twin similarity using the correlation coefficient, which can be thought of as the standardized covariance (the correlation is the covariance standardized by the variances of the two variables being correlated; it is this property that allows the correlations among various variables to be compared directly). Thus, the reader may wonder why we are using the covariance instead of the correlation. This is essentially because biometrical models were developed for covariance structures, not correlation structures. For example, the variances of the phenotype in the halves of the twin pairs contain statistical information, but this information is lost when the variables are standardized.

Recommended Readings

Carey (2003) provides an excellent and very readable introduction to human genetics as applied to behavioral and social phenomena. From Carey (2003), the budding twin researcher could turn next to Neale and Maes (1999), who provide a hands-on introduction to biometrical modeling of twin data. With an understanding of the models described by Neale and Maes (1999) in place, we suggest that the reader next turn to Purcell (2002), who describes models that allow for moderation of *ACE* effects. As we described earlier, we see these moderation models as having great promise in unraveling the ways genes and environments work together to lead to psychological outcomes (see, e.g., Johnson & Krueger, 2006).

References

Akaike, H. (1987). Factor analysis and AIC. *Psychometrika, 52*, 317–332.

Borkenau, P., Riemann, R., Spinath, F. M., & Angleitner, A. (in press). Genetic and environmental influences on person × situation profiles. *Journal of Personality, 74*, 1451–1479.

Bouchard, T. J., Jr., & Propping, P. (Eds.). (1993). *Twins as a tool of behavioral genetics.* Chichester, UK: Wiley.

Burt, S. A., McGue, M., Krueger, R. F., & Iacono, W. G. (2006). *Environmental mediation of the association between parent–child relationships and adolescent delinquency: Findings from an adoption study.* Manuscript submitted for publication.

Carey, G. (2003). *Human genetics for the social sciences.* Thousand Oaks, CA: Sage.

Diener, E., & Seligman, M. E. P. (2004). Beyond money: Toward an economy of well-being. *Psychological Science in the Public Interest, 5*, 1–31.

DiLalla, L. F. (2002). Preschool social and cognitive behaviors: The Southern Illinois twins. *Twin Research, 5*, 468–471.

Falconer, D. S. (1990). *Introduction to quantitative genetics* (3rd ed.). New York: Longman.

Feingold, A. (1992). Good-looking people are not what we think. *Psychological Bulletin, 111*, 304–341.

Goldsmith, H. H., Lemery, K. S., Buss, K. A., & Campos, J. J. (1999). Genetic analyses of focal aspects of infant temperament. *Developmental Psychology, 35*, 972–985.

Hansen, J., Alessandri, P. T., Croft, M. L., Burton, P. R., & de Klerk, N. H. (2004). The Western Australian register of childhood multiples: Effects of questionnaire design and follow-up protocol on response rates and representativeness. *Twin Research, 7*, 149–161.

Harris, J. R., Magnus, P., & Tambs, K. (2002). The Norwegian Institute of Public Health Twin Panel: A description of the sample and program of research. *Twin Research, 5*, 415–423.

Hur, Y. (2002). Seoul Twin Family Study: Design, sampling, assessments, and future directions. *Twin Research, 5*, 389–393.

Jang, K. L., Livesley, W. J., & Vernon, P. A. (2002). The etiology of personality function: The University of British Columbia twin project. *Twin Research, 5*, 342–346.

Johnson, W., & Krueger, R. F. (2006). How money buys happiness: Genetic and environmental processes linking finances and life satisfaction. *Journal of Personality and Social Psychology, 90*, 680–691.

Johnson, W., Krueger, R. F., Bouchard, T. J., Jr., & McGue, M. (2002). The personalities of twins: Just ordinary folks. *Twin Research, 5*, 125–131.

Krueger, R. F. (2000). Phenotypic, genetic, and nonshared environmental parallels in the structure of personality: A view from the Multidimensional Personality Questionnaire. *Journal of Personality and Social Psychology, 79*, 1057–1067.

Krueger, R. F., Caspi, A., & Moffitt, T. E. (2000). Epidemiological personology: The unifying role of personality in population-based research on problem behaviors. *Journal of Personality, 68*, 967–998.

Krueger, R. F., & Johnson, W. (2002). The Minnesota Twin Registry: Current status and future directions. *Twin Research, 5*, 488–492.

Livesley, W. J., Jang, K. L., & Vernon, P. A. (1998). Phenotypic and genetic structure of traits delineating personality disorder. *Archives of General Psychiatry, 55*, 941–948.

Loehlin, J. (2004). *Latent variable models.* Mahwah, NJ: Erlbaum.

Lykken, D. T., Bouchard, T. J., Jr., McGue, M., & Tellegen, A. (1990). The Minnesota twin family registry: Some initial findings. *Acta Geneticae Medicae et Gemmellologiae, 39*, 35–70.

Markon, K., & Krueger, R. F. (2004). An empirical comparison of information-theoretic selection criteria for multivariate behavior genetic models. *Behavior Genetics, 34*, 593–610.

Mischel, W. (2004). Toward an integrative science of the person. *Annual Review of Psychology, 55*, 1–22.

Mina Bergem, A. L. (2002). Norwegian twin registers and Norwegian twin studies: An overview. *Twin Research, 5*, 407–414.

Neale, M. C., Boker, S. M., Xie, G., & Maes, H. (1999). *Mx: Statistical modeling* (5th ed.). Richmond: VA: Virginia Commonwealth University, Department of Psychiatry.

Neale, M. C., & Maes, H. (1999). *Methodology for genetic studies of twins and families*. Dordrecht, the Netherlands: Kluwer.

Plomin, R., Corley, R., Caspi, A., Fulker, D. W., & DeFries, J. (1998). Adoption results for self-reported personality: Evidence for nonadditive genetic effects? *Journal of Personality and Social Psychology, 75*, 211–218.

Plomin, R., DeFries, J. C., & McClearn, G. E. (1990). *Behavioral genetics* (2nd ed.). New York: Freeman.

Plomin, R., DeFries, J. C., McClearn, G. E., & McGuffin, P. (2001). *Behavioral genetics* (4th ed.). New York: Worth.

Purcell, S. (2002). Variance component models for gene–environment interaction in twin analysis. *Twin Research, 5*, 554–571.

Roberts, B. W., & Pomerantz, E. M. (2004). On traits, situations, and their integration: A developmental perspective. *Personality and Social Psychology Review, 8*, 402–416.

Spinath, F. M., Angleitner, A., Borkenau, P., Riemann, R., & Wolf, H. (2002). German Observational Study of Adult Twins (GOSAT): A multimodal investigation of personality, temperament and cognitive ability. *Twin Research, 5*, 372–375.

Strassberg, M., Peters, K., Marazita, M., Ganger, J., Watt-Morse, M., Murrelle, L., et al. (2002). Pittsburgh Registry of Infant Multiples (PRIM). *Twin Research, 5*, 499–501.

Van Hulle, C. A., Lemery, K. S., & Goldsmith, H. H. (2002). Wisconsin Twin Panel. *Twin Research, 5*, 502–505.

Waller, N. G., & Meehl, P. E. (1998). *Multivariate taxometric procedures*. Thousand Oaks, CA: Sage.

APPENDIX 4.1. AN M$_X$ SCRIPT FOR FITTING THE *ACE* MODEL TO DATA FROM MZ AND DZ TWINS

```
G1: Model parameters
Data Calc NGroups=3
Begin Matrices;
X Lower 1 1 Free
Y Lower 1 1 Free
Z Lower 1 1 Free
W Lower 1 1 Fixed
End Matrices;
Begin Algebra;
A= X*X';
C= Y*Y';
E= Z*Z';
D= W*W';
End Algebra:
End

G2: MZ twin pairs
Data NInput_vars=2 NObservations=500
Labels P1MZ P2MZ
CMatrix 1.0 0.5 1.0
Matrices= Group 1
Covariances A+C+D+E | A+C+D _
            A+C+D   | A+C+D+E /
Options RSidual
End

G3: DZ twin pairs
Data NInput_vars=2 NObservations=500
Labels P1DZ P2DZ
CMatrix 1.0 0.25 1.0
Matrices= Group 1
H Full 1 1
Q Full 1 1
Covariances A+C+D+E | H@A+C+Q@D _
            H@A+C+Q@D | A+C+D+E /
Matrix H .5
Matrix Q .25
Start .6 All
Options RSidual NDecimals=4
End
```

## CHAPTER 5

Idiographic Personality

The Theory and Practice of Experience Sampling

Tamlin S. Conner
Lisa Feldman Barrett
Michele M. Tugade
Howard Tennen

Since the early days of psychological research, scientists have promoted more personalized and contextualized approaches to understanding personality. These approaches, exemplified by theorists, including Allport, Mischel and many others, all share a commonality—they encourage the use of idiographic methods, which seek to identify patterns of behavior within an individual over time and within contexts, rather than to strictly identify patterns of behavior across individuals, as is the case with standard nomothetic approaches. In the science of personality, methods known as *experience sampling* are essentially modern-day tools for realizing a within-person, idiographic approach; these methods provide researchers with multiple snapshots of people's situated experiences over time in the context of daily life.

In this chapter, we review experience sampling methods (ESMs) as tools for use in the science of personality. We describe the basic method, give a brief history, and ground its rationale in several idiographic perspectives. We then give a short "how to" primer, admit some practical and theoretical complexities, and end by discussing exciting future directions for ESM and its contributions to personality theory. Throughout the chapter, we emphasize personality applications and pay special attention to computerized ESM using personal digital assistants (PDAs). In this way, we hope to supplement the excellent methodology reviews that currently exist (see Recommended Readings).

Experience Sampling Methods

ESM refers to a collection of procedures that are designed to allow respondents to report their thoughts, feelings, and behaviors over time in natural settings. Originally, "the Experience Sampling Method" (coined by Larson & Csikszentmihalyi, 1983) referred to a particular technique whereby participants reported on their experiences in response to a random signaling device like a pager. Today, ESM is often used more broadly to refer to any procedure that has three qualities—assessment of experiences in *natural settings*, in *real time* (or close to the occurrence of the experience being reported), and on *repeated time* occasions. Reports can be made in response to a random signaling device (e.g., Larson & Csikszentmihalyi, 1983), at predetermined times during the day (e.g., noon, 2:00 P.M., 4:00 P.M., nightly), or following a particular event (e.g., like a social interaction; Reis & Wheeler, 1991). Note that experience sampling methods are also referred to as *diary methods* (Bolger, Davis, & Rafaeli, 2003) or *daily process methods* (Tennen, Affleck, & Armeli, 2003). In health-related fields, the term *ecological momentary assessment* (EMA) is used (Stone & Shiffman, 1994) to refer to experience sampling, as well as to procedures that sample aspects of a person's physical state (e.g., ambulatory blood pressure or heart rate).

A History of Experience Sampling in Brief

The self-recording of everyday experiences began in the early years of social science. Precursors to modern-day experience sampling methods were sociological in nature and designed to gather detailed accounts of how people spent their time (for a detailed history, see Wheeler & Reis, 1991). Participants were given booklets of paper-and-pencil diaries and asked to keep a daily record of their activities each day. With the influence of behaviorism, early sampling methods in the science of psychology were used mostly for recording concrete behavioral events (cf. Wheeler & Reis, 1991). Later, as behaviorism waned, recording methods were applied to the study of internal subjective states, most notably mood.

The 1970s and early 1980s saw the development of modern-day experience sampling methods. Paper-and-pencil diaries were combined with audible beepers to allow for the spontaneous sampling of subjective experience (see, e.g., Csikszentmihalyi, Larson, & Prescott, 1977; Hurlburt, 1979). Researchers

also developed the Rochester Interaction Record (Nezlek, Wheeler, & Reis, 1983), which was the first formalized "event-contingent" sampling procedure that allowed people to record their experiences on paper-and-pencil records immediately following predefined events.

Personality researchers quickly added experience sampling methods to their methodological toolbox. During the 1980s and early 1990s, there was a threefold increase in the use of sampling procedures (Tennen, Suls, & Affleck, 1991), culminating in a 1991 special issue of the *Journal of Personality* dedicated to personality and daily experience (Tennen et al., 1991). Early applications included investigations of daily affective experience (e.g., Eckenrode, 1984; Zevon & Tellegen, 1982) and stress (e.g., Bolger & Schilling, 1991), as well as motivation, self-esteem, and interpersonal relations (see Tennen et al., 1991).

The 1990s saw two developments in the sophistication of the method. First, on the implementation side, technology and software became available to fully computerize sampling (e.g., the Experience Sampling Program, ESP; Barrett & Barrett, 2001). Computerized sampling was first accomplished with the use of handheld or "palmtop" computers (see, e.g., Penner, Shiffman, Paty, & Fritzsche, 1994) and, later, with the smaller personal digital assistants (PDAs; also called pocket PCs) (see, e.g., Oishi, 2002). Second, on the data analysis side, multilevel modeling procedures became more widely used, allowing for simultaneous modeling of idiographic (within-person) and nomothetic (between-persons) relationships in ESM data.

Rationale for Experience Sampling

There are several reasons why personality researchers adopted ESM. First, ESM is a powerful method that captures nuanced *within-person patterns* otherwise unattainable from standard cross-sectional or longitudinal designs in personality.[1] These nuanced patterns provide insight into the dynamic regularities of personality *in situ*, and they reveal, rather than assume, behavioral patterns that are true for a given individual. Second, ESM measures *experience in natural contexts*. By taking personality research out of the lab, researchers can study how people behave in their environments that really matter—as people work, play, and interact with those they love and loathe. Third, ESM provides better measurement of *situation-specific behavior*, revealing how personality is grounded in situations. Fourth, ESM measures *actual rather than recalled experience*. We address each of these points in turn.

Within-Person Patterns

By virtue of its intensive repeated measures design, ESM is a powerful idiographic method that can reveal within-person patterns in personality. In the modern usage of the term, *idiographic methods* aim to identify patterns of behavior *within the person* across time and in context; in contrast, *nomothetic methods* aim to identify general patterns of behavior *across people*.[2] The rationale for idiographic methods in personality research can be traced back to Gordon Allport, who, seven decades ago, rallied against the strict nomothetic approaches to personality of the time (Allport, 1937). He argued that conceptualizations of personality derived from across-individual analyses reflect the psychology of a nonexistent average individual that neglects the unique patterning of personality within the individual. As a modern method in personality research, ESM realizes an idiographic approach, not through the "low-powered" single case studies, as idiographic methods were sometimes conceived in the past, but through "high-powered" multiple, ongoing case studies that allow researchers to determine idiographic relations and then to make lawful generalizations. For example, using ESM data, researchers can generate an idiographic index for each person. This index may be a within-person average (reflecting a reliable aggregate of that person's experience over the sampling period; e.g., Epstein, 1983); it may be a within-person slope (reflecting change in a reported experience over time or the relation between two reported experiences for an individual; e.g., Bolger & Schilling, 1991); or it could be any other index that captures some meaningful pattern for that individual (within-person factor structure, e.g., Barrett, 1998; standard deviation, e.g., Eid & Diener, 1999; spectral density estimates, e.g., Larsen, 1987). Then, investigators can determine whether these indices vary across individuals. If indices vary, steps can be taken to model whether other factors such as demographic characteristics or personality traits account for

some of the variability. In this way, ESM weds the specificity of within-person idiographic analyses with the goal of nomothetic inference. This type of hybrid idiographic–nomothetic design has also been called *idiothetic* (Lamiell, 1981), as well as *ipsative–normative* (Lazarus, 2000), wherein *ipsative* refers to deviations around the individual mean and *normative* refers to deviations around the group mean.

Within-person analyses are as relevant to today's scientific investigation of the human personality as they were nearly 70 years ago. Within-person analyses aid theory building by avoiding the nomothetic fallacy (i.e., assuming that what is true for the "average" person is also true for each and every person). For example, many cross-sectional studies of affect have identified valence (pleasure–displeasure) as a basic property of affective experience (see, e.g., Russell, 1980), but only idiographic methods using ESM have demonstrated that valence is a property of each and every respondent's experience (for a review, see Barrett, 2006). Thus, idiographic methods are useful for testing when and for whom a theory is valid. Idiographic methods also yield patterns that cannot be assumed from cross-sectional designs. As a general rule, within-person associations and across-persons associations are conceptually and methodologically independent (Nezlek, 2001), so that one can never be inferred from the other. In fact, within- and across-persons associations can depart in both size and direction, as illustrated by Tennen and Affleck (1996). They describe a study in which participants reported on pleasant and unpleasant daily events over time. Two types of correlations were computed—a set of within-person correlations (the association between pleasant and unpleasant events over time for each person) and a between-persons correlation (the association between the aggregated number of pleasant and unpleasant events across persons). The within-person correlations were mostly negative, showing that on days when people experienced more pleasant events, they typically experienced fewer unpleasant events. But the between-persons correlation was positive (*r* = .50), showing that people who experienced more pleasant events on average also experienced more unpleasant events (i.e., they had eventful lives). Although informative for certain research questions, the between-persons correlation does not reveal the temporal patterning of events in individuals' lives.

Measurement of Experience in Natural Contexts

ESM takes personality research out of the lab and into real life, realizing Gordon Allport's vision that "psychology needs to concern itself with life as it is lived" (Allport, 1942, pp. 56; see also Bolger et al., 2003). Sampling experiences *in vivo* (in life) and *in situ* (in place) contrasts markedly with many standard ways of assessing personality that often neglect the varied and rich context of life. Having people fill out questionnaires about how they behave "in general" (called a *global self-report*) does not adequately capture behavior as it unfolds over time and across situations. Furthermore, laboratory-based experiments do not always approximate real life. Consider the value of natural reporting contexts in the study of intimate relationships. By using ESM, researchers have been able to measure how couples seek out and respond to each other emotionally in daily life, revealing systematic factors that promote feelings of intimacy (see, e.g., Laurenceau, Barrett, & Pietromonaco, 1998).

Better Measurement of Situation-Specific Behavior

By measuring people's experiences across situations, ESM allows for a more conditional conceptualization of personality. *Conditionality* refers to the way in which people interpret their surroundings to produce a psychological situation that is most potent for the expression of personality. From this perspective, personality reflects the tendency to behave in a particular way within certain situations rather than the tendency to behave the same way across all situations. As exemplified by Mischel and Shoda's situation-specific signatures, some individuals who are classified as "aggressive" may behave aggressively only when hassled by a peer, whereas others may show aggressive behaviors only when reproached by an adult (Shoda, Mischel, & Wright, 1994). Similarly, individuals high in neuroticism may not feel distressed all the time, but only when faced with situational press (such as a perceived threat) (Bolger & Schilling, 1991). With ESM, researchers can model these signatures by having respondents report on properties of the psychological situation (i.e., construals of current threat, stress, and so on) as well as physical surroundings (i.e., the location, the number of other people present, interacting with a peer or supervisor).

Measurement of Actual Experience Rather than Recalled Experience

ESM also captures experiences in real time, rather than relying on people's retrospective reports as proxy measures for momentary experiences. Retrospective questionnaires are pervasive in the science of psychology. Popular instruments such as the Beck Depression Inventory, the Positive and Negative Affect Schedule (PANAS), and numerous widely used quality-of-life surveys (e.g., Symptom Checklist-90—Revised, SF-36 Health Questionnaire) often ask people to reflect back on their affective and somatic experiences over the past 2 weeks, or even months. The validity of these measures rests on the assumption that people can accurately remember their experiences as they occurred during these intervals and summarize them by taking an average. Yet the assumption that people can both remember and summarize their prior experiences is not warranted. Consider what happens when we ask people to report on something like "How sad have you felt over the past 2 weeks?" To answer this question, respondents may first attempt to reflect back over the past 2 weeks, think about specific episodes of feeling sad, and then summarize them (a *recall-and-aggregate* strategy). In this process, however, summaries will be disproportionately influenced by the strongest experiences during the time frame (*peak effect*), by the most recent experience (*end effect*) (for a review, see Fredrickson, 2000), and by the respondent's current affective state.

Alternatively, people may not even attempt a recall-and-aggregate strategy when retrospecting on experiences over longer intervals, instead adopting a "semantic" strategy—reporting what they *believe* they felt (Robinson & Clore, 2002b). This shift to a semantic strategy was demonstrated in a study that measured the latency for individuals to judge their emotional experiences over increasingly longer (and more difficult) time frames (e.g., "To what extent do (did) you feel happy *at this moment*, the *last few hours, days, weeks, months, years, in general*?") (Robinson & Clore, 2002b). Response latencies increased in a linear fashion over the shorter intervals (moment, last few hours, days) as participants took time to recall and aggregate experiences; however, at the longer intervals (weeks, months, years, in general), response latencies sharply decreased, suggesting that participants stopped trying to recall and aggregate their past experiences and simply began accessing an already cached knowledge source. The knowledge appears to reflect people's stable, generalized beliefs about themselves and their experiences (reviewed in Robinson & Clore, 2002a).

Several examples illustrate the value of capturing experiences unfiltered from belief-based reconstruction. In studies of gender differences in emotional experience, for example, reports made using retrospective or global questionnaires often reveal strong gender differences consistent with the cultural stereotype that women are the more "emotional sex" (Barrett, Robin, Pietromonaco, & Eyssell, 1998). However, when immediate reports using ESM are used, these differences disappear (Barrett et al., 1998). Why would the depiction of the emotional lives of men and women differ depending on how we asked the questions? The reason is that in retrospect and in the abstract, people rely on knowledge other than what actually happened, including gender stereotypes and implicit theories, to help inform their self-reports of experience.

Belief-based reconstruction also has implications for studies of personality change. In some cases, the use of retrospective questionnaires may *overestimate* the amount of change that has actually occurred. For example, if people are asked to recollect how they were some time ago, they may remember themselves as being worse off so that their present-day self confirms a belief that they are improving (Ross & Wilson, 2003). In other cases, the use of retrospective inventories may *underestimate* change. Consider a study in which a depression inventory is administered before and after an intervention of some sort. If the inventory contains a retrospective component (e.g., "Reflect back on the past 2 weeks"), both reports will be infused with participants' beliefs about their depressed nature and, in turn, show high stability. But most interventions are not designed to change beliefs; they are designed to change the actual depressive symptoms in daily life. ESM provides the means to measure those symptoms directly.

Applying ESM to Personality Research

In this section, we review the primary ways in which ESM has been used in personality research. Because of space considerations, we highlight only selected examples of ESM studies that examine the *phenomenological content of daily life*, *daily processes*, the *structures of daily experience*, and *temporal changes in experience* as means of understanding personality.

Phenomenological Content Investigations

Phenomenological content investigations are those in which ESM is used to examine conscious representations of phenomenological experience in daily life (e.g., mood, daily events, pain, coping). In these investigations, participants report on their experience across time and situations; reports are then averaged and examined for their links to other variables of interest. Content investigations are often used to demonstrate the links between personality characteristics and situated experience. For example, studies using ESM have shown that stable personality factors such as neuroticism (e.g., Barrett & Pietromonaco, 1997), pessimism and optimism (Norem & Illingworth, 1993), and dispositional approach/avoidance-related motivations (Updegraff, Gable, & Taylor, 2004) all predict average levels of affective experience *in situ*.

Daily Process Investigations

In daily process investigations, ESM is used to investigate how two self-report variables covary within the person over time. The resulting "within-person slopes" capture the relations between situational, cognitive, or affective factors in daily life (e.g., the relation between stressful events and affective experience). Daily process research is extremely powerful and at the core of many ESM applications in personality. Such research has revealed strong within-person links between daily stressful events and negative affect (Bolger & Schilling, 1991), attributions of control and feelings of depression (Swendsen, 1998), and certain situations and the likelihood of behaviors detrimental to health (e.g., drinking; Mohr et al., 2001), among other notable applications. Daily process researchers also recognize that within-person slopes commonly vary in size or direction. In these situations, researchers typically ascertain whether there are other factors that might account for the variation (e.g., neuroticism predicts stronger stressor–affect slopes; Bolger & Schilling, 1991).

Structural Investigations

Structural investigations seek to discover the (often implicit) properties that characterize reports of momentary experience. In these applications, ESM is used to obtain reports of multiple experiences over time (e.g., current happiness, sadness, anger, etc), which are then factor analyzed for each person to determine the dimensions (or "structure") that account for regularities in experience (see, e.g., Barrett, 1998, 2005; Carstensen, Pasupathi, Mayr, & Nesselroade, 2000; Nesselroade, 2001). Such investigations have revealed common structures in momentary affective experience (e.g., valence and arousal dimensions; Feldman, 1995), as well as individual differences in the structure of experience (see, e.g., Barrett, 1998). For example, ESM research shows that some people are much more likely to characterize their affective experiences in broad, global terms (e.g., as good vs. bad), whereas others may make more complex distinctions—a difference termed *emotional granularity* (Barrett, 1998). It is important to note that such discoveries can be determined only through structural analysis of repeated measures reports and not by directly asking people what they believe the structure to be.

Temporal Investigations

In temporal investigations, ESM is used to measure changes in experience (e.g., mood, social behavior, coping) across time. Such investigations have revealed temporal patterns in mood (see, e.g., Larsen & Kasimatis, 1990), as well as individual differences in mood variability (Eid & Diener, 1999) and entrainment to normative cycles (Larsen & Kasimatis, 1990). Furthermore, important trait factors such as neuroticism and extraversion predict variance in these within-person patterns—for instance, higher neuroticism predicts greater variability (Eid & Diener, 1999) and greater extraversion predicts less entrainment to weekly mood cy-

cles (Larsen & Kasimatis, 1990). Temporal investigations have also shown that there are patternings across time in several personality markers, including Big Five characteristics (Fleeson, 2001) and trait mindfulness (Brown & Ryan, 2003). Moreover, research has shown that within-person variability in experiences is itself stable (Eid & Diener, 1999; Fleeson, 2001).

A Brief Primer on ESM

ESM is a valuable research tool, but it involves a design and implementation process that can be challenging to even the most seasoned researcher. In this section, we present several steps for successfully designing and launching an ESM study. These steps are part of a growing corpus of guidelines dedicated to sampling science (for other primers see Recommended Readings). Note that our discussion is mainly targeted to studies using "normal" adult samples (college students, community members) and we do not discuss the use of ESM for populations with specific needs (young children, elderly persons, individuals with psychopathology, and so on; see deVries, 1992, for uses of ESM in clinical populations).

Resources

The feasibility of conducting an ESM study depends on three primary resources. A *strong and conscientious research team* is integral to the success of any study, especially studies utilizing ESM. In addition, having the *resources to remunerate* participants is important because of the taxing nature of participation. It is useful to remunerate participants both as the study progresses (for meeting milestones during the observation period) and at the end of the study (usually with a cash payment). Offering enough incentive and remuneration throughout the sampling procedure (although not too much so as to be coercive) can proactively reduce attrition. There are a variety of potential remuneration sources, including research credits (if using college student participants), monetary payment, and other creative items such as weekly/monthly drawings (e.g., gift certificates to restaurants, university sweatshirts, tickets to functions) or larger "grand prizes" (e.g., PDAs). Also consider *resources for the sampling platform*. ESM platforms range in cost, from higher-cost computerized sampling (using palmtop computers or PDAs) to lower-cost paper-and-pencil options (see the section "Choosing the Platform" below). An awareness of resources early on allows you to choose the platform that accommodates your budget and, if possible, to find more financial support.

Designing the Sampling Protocol

The next step is to design the sampling protocol—how to sample experiences and how frequently to do it. These decisions must be based on how the phenomenon under study is thought to behave. If the phenomenon of interest is relatively rare, such as experiences surrounding unprotected sex, sampling at random moments during the day is inefficient and likely to miss the behavior of interest. Such behaviors can be recorded reliably after each event. If the behavior of interest is ongoing (e.g., mood), then sampling throughout the day will work better. Note that a critical function of ESM data is to represent a *population of occasions*, just as cross-sectional data functions to represent a population of individuals. Thus, researchers need to ensure that the data capture enough occasions with enough frequency to adequately represent the phenomenon under study.

One of the first decisions to make is whether to use an *event-based* versus *time-based* sampling protocol (Bolger et al., 2003). With event-based sampling, people make their reports following a predefined event. This type of protocol, also called event-contingent sampling (Wheeler & Reis, 1991), is best used for investigating experiences and behaviors surrounding specific events, especially those that are rare and may not be occurring if sampling is done at fixed or intermittent times during the day (e.g., instances of drinking, lying, smoking, social events). Event-contingent procedures can be challenging to participants especially if the events are frequent (e.g., every social interaction) or too broadly defined. It is important to set clear and appropriately inclusive criteria.

With time-based sampling, people make their reports at designated or varied times. Time-based sampling is more typical and is used for investigating experiences that occur frequently in a person's daily life (e.g., daily events, stressors, coping, etc.) or are ongoing (mood, stress). If using time-based sampling, consider whether to use a *fixed schedule* or

variable schedule. With a fixed schedule, also called interval–contingent sampling (Wheeler & Reis, 1991), people make their reports at fixed times throughout the day (e.g., at morning, afternoon, and evening intervals or at night daily). They may be asked to report on their experiences at that current moment (an immediate or "online" report) or, more typically, to report on their experiences that occurred during the time frame since the previous report (over the prior interval). This latter format requires some retrieval or reconstruction over a period of time and is best used for studying concrete events and behaviors that are less susceptible to memory bias (e.g., using a checklist of daily events). Fixed schedules are also well suited to time series (temporal) investigations. The fixed nature of observations allows one to make generalizations about time (e.g., diurnal or weekly patterns in mood) by statistically comparing responses within and between individuals. Finally, fixed schedules are also typically the least burdensome to participants—reports are made at standardized times and so participants can configure their schedules around these reports. This regularity can be a drawback, however. If people make their own reports, or initiate them in response to a signal at a fixed time, their reports will not reflect spontaneous contents in the stream of consciousness; reports may also be susceptible to mental preparation and/or self-presentation. If these issues are of concern, then a variable schedule can be used, or the fixed schedule "relaxed," so that prompts are delivered less predictably around specified times.

With a variable schedule, also called signal-contingent sampling (Wheeler & Reis, 1991), people make their reports in response to a signal that is delivered at unpredictable times, typically between 4 and 10 times per day. At each signal, people are typically asked about experiences occurring at that particular moment (i.e., How are you feeling *right now*?). Variable schedules are well suited for studying target behaviors that are ongoing and therefore likely to be occurring at a given signal (e.g., mood, pain, stress levels). They are also appropriate for studying states that are susceptible to retrospective memory bias (e.g., emotions, subjective well-being, or any experience quick to decay), as well as states that people may attempt to regulate if they could anticipate having to make a report (as with a fixed schedule). The main disadvantage of signal-contingent sampling is the burden to participants, who are interrupted by the signals. But participants typically become accustomed to the procedure rather quickly (within 2 days).

Other important decisions to make are the sampling parameters—the number of sampling moments per day and the length of the sampling period. These decisions can be made at the outset or later, after choosing the platform (computerized, paper-and-pencil, Web, etc.), and should first reflect the naturalistic incidence of target phenomena. For event-based procedures, the sampling period should be long enough to accommodate sufficient numbers of observations per person to provide a reliable estimate for that person. For time-based procedures, observations should be frequent enough during each day to capture important fluctuations in experience, but not so frequent as to inconvenience participants without any incremental gain (Reis & Gable, 2000). There are no set rules, but general guidelines have emerged. For example, Delespaul (2006) advises against sampling more than six times per day over longer sampling periods (i.e., 3 weeks +) unless the reports are especially short (i.e., 2 minutes or less) and additional incentives are provided. Variable schedules typically employ between 4 and 10 signals each day, and the signals are usually distributed throughout the day randomly within equal intervals. For example, in a study sampling eight times a day between the hours of 9:00 A.M. to 9:00 P.M., the first signal would come randomly between 9:00 and 10:30 A.M., the second signal would come randomly between 10:30 A.M. and 12:00 P.M., and so on, because there are eight 1½-hour intervals. Furthermore, if the experience of interest were hypothesized to be cyclical, the observations need to be frequent enough to catch the trough and peak of the cycle *at minimum*, although more observations are better. Otherwise, cycles will be missed or misidentified (an error known as *aliasing* in the time series literature).

Another consideration is statistical power, both in terms of the number of moments sampled and the number of participants involved. Power analysis programs are available for precisely determining the number of observations and sample size needed to estimate various effects (Bosker, Snijders, & Guldemond, 2003). In the absence of using these estimation procedures, we can offer several guidelines (see also Kreft & de Leeuw, 1998). In general, the number of observations needed for sufficient statistical power depends on the complexity of analysis. If using ESM to construct an aggregate measure (e.g., a mean across time), observations should be sufficient to achieve reliability, akin to constructing a reliable scale with multiple items. In published ESM research, aggregates are typically created with about 30 observations, although some studies have as few as 7 observations per person for a 1-week-long diary study.

Observations should be increased for more complex analyses that estimate both within (idiographic) and between (nomothetic) variance components (i.e., cross-level interactions using multilevel modeling procedures; Nezlek, 2001). For example, in their discussion of multilevel power, Kreft and de Leeuw (1998, pp. 125) reviewed several simulation studies suggesting that when testing cross-level interactions with small to moderate effect sizes, the study should include at least *30 people with 30 observations* in order to have sufficiently high power (.80). Presumably, these numbers can be adjusted up if using a more stringent alpha (e.g., .01). Kreft and de Leeuw also described research suggesting that increasing the number of people, rather than the observations, has a greater effect on the power to detect cross-level interaction effects. By these guidelines, ESM studies appear to be doing well in terms of power. Although normative estimates are hard to come by, the average number of observations for a variable schedule (signal-contingent) procedure is estimated to be between 56 and 168 (for studies that run for 1–2 weeks; Reis & Gable, 2000), with N ranging from 30 to 100. Moreover, to achieve adequate power, observations may have to be increased if the anticipated response rate is low. Generally, response rates tend to be highest (95% and above) for fixed scheduling procedures, especially those completed once daily. Response rates are typically lower (e.g., 70–85% on average) for variable schedules, employing computerized devices that signal multiple times per day.

Choosing the Platform

Next, choose the sampling platform. *Computerized sampling* uses palmtop computers or personal digital assistants (PDAs) outfitted with specialized configurable software that enables participants to answer questions about their experiences (for a discussion of computerized ESM, see Barrett & Barrett, 2001; Conner Christensen, Barrett, Bliss-Moreau, Lebo, & Kaschub, 2003). Computerized sampling can be used with any of the sampling protocols—people can initiate the report themselves (for event and fixed sampling) or respond when cued by the device (for fixed and variable sampling)—but computerized procedures are especially beneficial for time-based protocols. Time-based protocols rest on the assumption that respondents will complete their reports at fixed times or immediately in response to a variable audible signal. Computerized methods control these timing elements, ensuring that reports are made on time and not from memory.[3] When self-initiated, a report is automatically "time-date" stamped. And, when cued, there is a short window to make the report and, again, a report is time-date stamped. Note that computerized methods do not ensure compliance with event-based procedures in which participants initiate their own reporting. Although every report is time-date stamped, researchers cannot know how much time has elapsed since the event, which can potentially introduce memory bias.

There are several other advantages of computerized experience sampling procedures. First, they allow for flexibility in how the questions are presented (randomly or in fixed order), which can reduce response sets and order effects. Second, they reduce human error associated with data management because data can be transferred directly from the PDA to a master computer without being entered by hand. Third, they provide the ability to record ancillary information, like latencies to respond to each question, which is not attainable with paper-and-pencil reports.

The disadvantages to computerized ESM start with the upfront financial investment. The cost of units can vary considerably (at the time of this writing the least expensive PDA was $100, and the most expensive that was linked to physiological recording was $12,000). There is also the potential cost for sampling software (which range from free to very costly; see the following section, "Choosing Software and Purchasing Equipment"). Computerized ESM also imposes limits on the question format (open-ended or "free" responses are not easily incorporated). Moreover, the platform may not be amenable for all subject populations. For example, the human factors of PDAs can be poor for some older individuals—the screens are small and the prompts are at high frequencies, which can make them difficult to hear.

There are several alternatives to computerized ESM. *Web platforms* are increasingly popular and well suited to a daily diary procedure. Every day participants can log onto a secured website and complete their reports, which are time-date stamped. A Web diary can also easily accommodate free text entries, which are not currently possible with handheld PDAs. However, not everyone has easy or frequent access to the Web and these platforms are not always cost-effective. A *paper-and-pencil platform* is the lowest-cost alternative. Questionnaire sheets, booklets, or any type of rating form can be designed and given to participants (for helpful guidelines, see Reis & Gable, 2000). Participants can then fill them out following specific events, at designated times, or when signaled by lower-cost pagers or programmable watches. The advantages of paper-and-pencil methods include reduced cost, less overhead in terms of equipment, and the allowance of open-ended questions. The disadvantages include the inability to randomize item content and a greater risk of noncompliant responding (see Stone, Shiffman, Schwartz, Broderick, & Hufford, 2002). Noncompliant responding occurs if people forget to fill out their reports at designated times; if they fill them out at the wrong times; or if they complete multiple reports later from memory (called *back-filling*). Fortunately, more recent research suggests that such concerns may be overstated and that establishing good working relationships is the best strategy for improving compliance (see Green, Rafaeli, Bolger, Shrout, & Reis, 2006). So, although rapport with participants is important for all ESM studies, it is critical for ESM studies using paper-and-pencil measures.

Choosing Software and Purchasing Equipment

In running a computerized ESM study, the next step is to choose the software, purchase the hardware units, and configure the devices. A more detailed description of software and equipment considerations can be found in Conner Christensen and colleagues (2003). At the time of this writing, there are several free software programs available for running computerized ESM studies using PDAs. They include the Experience Sampling Program (ESP; *www.experience-sampling.org*), the Intel Experience Sampling Program (iESP; *seattleweb.intel-research.net/projects/esm/iESP.html*), and the Purdue Momentary Assessment Tool (PMAT; *www.cfs.purdue.edu/mfri/pages/PMAT/Index.html*). Each can accommodate event- or time-based sampling protocols, although they have slightly different features. See their online manuals for a complete and updated list of requirements and features.

After selecting the software, purchase the hardware devices (e.g., PDAs), taking into account several factors, the most important of which is the operating system. The devices must run on the same operating system for which the software was designed (e.g., Windows CE, Windows Mobile 2003, Palm OS) and in the specific version. Also consider the size of the screen, the brightness and resolution, the sound of the audible signal, the length of warrantees, and customer support. Prior to purchasing an entire fleet, purchase a test PDA to make sure the software works on that model. Install the software, configure it according to your design, and pilot. If all is well, then purchase the rest of your fleet.

Configuration of the fleet usually involves a day or two of work. Each software program has its own instruction manual and process for configuring the PDAs. Configuration typically involves specifying the sampling protocol, the frequency of signals (if using an audible signal), the length of the sampling period, and the questions and response options. Prior to running the study, researchers should test all of the PDAs to make sure they work; pilot test a smaller number of units through the full procedure (i.e., aided by research assistants); and solicit feedback about the clarity of questions, formatting, and response features.

If using Web-based sampling, there are several options. Most researchers hire their own programmer to design the website. There is also commercial software that can be tailored for a repeated measures nightly diary. Although we cannot recommend any specific vendors, we can note that some companies sell the diary survey software outright (for around $1,500) without a per-survey usage fee, which can be very helpful for repeated assessments (for one example, see *www.snapsurveys.com*). In the fu-

ture, we hope to see more freeware options available.

Implementing the ESM Study

Once participants are recruited, it is important to keep them motivated throughout the sampling period. There are several strategies for maintaining motivation, including having a complex remuneration structure with incentives such as money, research credits, and lotteries. Also crucial are positive attitudes on the part of the research team members, which translates into positive contact with participants. Through our own and others' experiences (see Green et al., 2006), we have observed that the data quality is highest when participants feel they are valued and have a sense of responsibility to their research assistant. Of course, participants should also clearly understand the study procedures. They should know how and when they will be asked to report and how to use the computerized device, if applicable. With such devices, it is best to have participants answer their first prompt in the lab, giving them an opportunity to ask questions and get comfortable with the device. In addition, during the study, feedback about response rates can increase the amount of usable data by making participants aware of any need to boost their response rates. Sometimes researchers tie payment to response rates (e.g., paying people for every report they make), which is a good strategy for daily diaries but may not work for more intensive signal-contingent sampling. Finally, if using computerized sampling, steps can be taken to minimize damage and wear of equipment. PDAs can be carried around in protective cases, and using top-of-the-line batteries can extend the life of the units because such batteries are less likely to corrode.

Preparing and Cleaning Data for Analysis

ESM yields volumes of data that must be entered, organized, and readied prior to any statistical analysis. Consider an ESM study with 100 participants. If each participant answers 40 items at 50 observation points, this study will potentially yield 200,000 data points! With paper-and-pencil sampling procedures, all data must be entered by hand—a lengthy and error-prone process, but certainly achievable. Computerized ESM bypasses this step because data are retrieved directly from the portable devices. This process eliminates manual data entry; however, careful steps must be taken not to inadvertently override or erase files. Once the data are entered, they are typically compiled and cleaned prior to analysis, with two steps unique to computerized ESM. First, the records are checked for duplicates (a common error is to compile the same data twice, leading to duplicate rows), and, second, trials with extremely fast reaction times are excluded and documented in the writeup (they typically indicate participant error such as an inadvertent screen tap).

Analyzing Data

After being compiled and cleaned, the data are ready to be analyzed according to the nature of the research question. If the goal is to understand something about each person (either an *average* for content investigations, or a *slope* for process investigations) and to examine how these indices might be moderated by other factors, then multilevel modeling may be especially useful (for primers, see Luke, 2004, as well as Kenny, Bolger, & Kashy, 2002; Kreft & de Leeuw, 1998; Nezlek, 2001). In multilevel modeling of ESM data, the "lower-level" data include all the self-reports obtained during sampling and the "upper-level" data include characteristics of the persons, typically measured separately from ESM (e.g., personality or cognitive variables), although not necessarily (e.g., an aggregate derived from ESM). The elegance of multilevel modeling is that it allows researchers to model certain patterns within each individual (using a lower-level equation), to test whether those patterns are the same or different (a variance test of the lower-level coefficients), and, if the patterns are different, to use upper-level predictors to account for that variance (so called cross-level interactions).

Multilevel modeling procedures echo the conceptual spirit of an idiographic framework. First, computing a lower-level regression equation for each person preserves the idiographic or intra-individual patterns. This equation might be simple (an *intercept only model* to estimate, for example, the average positive affect reported across 30 days for each person) or more complex (a *slope model* that regresses "affect" onto "per-

ceptions of stress" to determine their relation for each person). Even when it appears that simple aggregation is occurring (e.g., as with an *intercept-only model*), multilevel modeling takes into account individual variability in the reliability of these intercepts, because some people have more stable estimates (i.e., those with a higher response rate). Furthermore, a variance test of the lower-level coefficients is, essentially, a test of the nomothetic assumption (i.e., whether "the average" is a good fit for most of the people in the sample). If the coefficients are homogeneous, then the average fits well. If the coefficients are heterogeneous, then the average fits less well, suggesting that other between-subjects factors might account for heterogeneity across participants.

For structural investigations involving the analysis of multiple co-occurrences between states, *P-factor analyses* can be used (Nesselroade, 2001). In these analyses, a correlation matrix is computed for each person using his or her ESM reports. This matrix reflects the extent to which changes in reports of one state (e.g., nervous) accompany changes in reports of another state (e.g., angry) for that person over time. Each P-correlation matrix can then be factor analyzed to statistically extract the dimensions that account for the variability in that person's experience.

Finally, there are also numerous procedures for investigating temporal patterns. Researchers have measured within-person variability by taking the standard deviation of a person's ESM reports over time (which, technically, reveals the *extremity of experience*; see, e.g., Eid & Diener, 1999), by examining skew and kurtosis (to reveal the *density of distributions*; Fleeson, 2001), and by employing spectral analysis (to reveal *rate of change*; Larsen, 1987). *Time-series analyses* are also powerful tools for determining cyclic patterns as well as other lagged effects (see West & Hepworth, 1991). Depending on the researcher's statistical sophistication, time series can be incorporated into multilevel modeling procedures.

Practical and Theoretical Complexities

Beyond the standard issues of implementation and analysis, there are several practical and theoretical complexities to consider.

Practical Complexities

Resource-Intense Method

Money can be a considerable obstacle for conducting ESM studies, especially given the current state of highly competitive grant funding for social and personality research. For computerized ESM studies, much of the expense requires capital upfront before the study is underway. Funds are required to purchase PDAs, pagers, or other devices. Other costs include software (if applicable) and participant remuneration. Together, these can add considerable expenses to one's budget. The most extreme cost-effective strategy is to avoid computerized sampling and instead use a simple paper-and-pencil diary—but this platform can be used only when appropriate to the research question. Fortunately, there are a number of ways to minimize costs and make the most of resources for a computerized study. Researchers can collect data in waves to minimize the number of PDA units needed, collaborate with others to share expenses (e.g., embed numerous research questions into the same protocol), and remunerate with research credits rather than money, whenever possible. They can also consider purchasing replacement PDAs upfront to save resources in the long run. As the PDAs become damaged, fresh units taken out of reserve will extend the lifetime of the fleet. We recommend purchasing about 20% replacement PDAs (e.g., 10 extra to maintain a fleet of 50).

Constraints in the Window of Observation

Because of time and resource limitations, ESM studies are typically constrained to data collection over a period of a few weeks at most. This window of observation may be a concern for researchers interested in determining regularities in behavior across a time span. To deal with this concern, researchers have a couple of options: First, depending on the particular research question, the sampling period can be extended to several weeks or even months. This option should be taken with caution, however, as it can raise the risk of participants providing set responses (i.e., responses become more routinized). Second, once the study has concluded, researchers can probe how typical these past weeks were as compared with their normal experience (e.g., by using a Likert-type scale, usual = 0 to unusual = 7), and responses used as covariates in analyses. Constraints in the window of observation may also be an issue for researchers who use college students as their subject sample. It is important to be mindful of the time of year when data are collected, as the ends of semesters are typically associated with higher stress levels compared to the beginnings of semesters.

Psychometric Issues

The same psychometric issues are important in ESM as with other questionnaire-type measures. Investigators should be careful about the ways in which questions are asked (e.g., framed in a positive versus negative way) and take caution in selecting scale anchors (e.g., unipolar rather than bipolar mood scales should be used).

Reactivity

ESM is unique in that it requires people to actively attend to and verbalize their experiences repeatedly over time (often as much as 10 times per day over several weeks). This raises the question about whether the repeated self-reporting of experience changes the very experience being measured (reactivity). Whereas studies in the EMA literature appear to demonstrate that participant reactivity is modest, clinical research on self-monitoring suggests that there could be reactivity in several circumstances (Korotitsch & Nelson-Gray, 1999).[4] First, reactivity may be more likely when people monitor only one type of target behavior or experience, especially a behavior that is negative or socially undesirable. This condition could be a concern for certain event-based studies, but it may be less a concern for time-based studies in which people report on multiple experiences of different valences at each time point. Second, reactivity appears likelier when participants are motivated to change the target behavior. In a revealing study (cf. Korotitsch & Nelson-Gray, 1999), individuals recruited by advertisements looking for "people who want to quit smoking" showed greater change in their smoking behaviors over time during sampling, as compared with others who were recruited for the same study looking for "people who are cigarette smokers." Thus, if reactivity is a concern, ESM researchers should be mindful not to inadvertently recruit people who are motivated to change the primary experience being sampled (e.g., emotion researchers should not advertise their studies to those who "want to feel happier"). Third, reactivity may occur if people are asked to report on experiences that they find difficult to verbalize. Research has shown that processing is disrupted when people are asked to describe experience that is more sensually or less linguistically based (i.e., enjoying the beauty in a sunset or a favorite song; see Schooler, Ariely, & Loewenstein, 2003). Finally, there is the risk that ESM, especially signal-contingent sampling, takes people "out of the moment." Such prompting may make people temporarily self-aware, which could dampen or change their subjective states (Silva, 2002). Certainly this is a risk with ESM, but it may be ameliorated as people become accustomed to the sampling procedure (typically 1–2 days). Of course, some individuals may take some time to become accustomed to sampling and therefore have the greatest risk of reactivity (i.e., people with lower working memory capacity who are less flexible at allocating attention).

Theoretical Complexities

ESM Is Different, Not Better

ESM has developed a reputation as the "gold standard" of self-report procedures, suggesting that ESM is inherently better than other types of self-reports and should be used whenever possible. But ESM is not a better self-report procedure; it is just different. ESM measures immediate subjective states that fluctuate in response to changing events and conditions, and constitute a form of episodic experience, in contrast to global self-reports, which measure people's generalized conceptualizations of themselves, a form of self-related semantic knowledge (Robinson & Clore, 2002a). ESM should not be used in all circumstances—only when seeking to measure episodic experience.

In fact, there may be circumstances when it is entirely *in*appropriate to use immediate ESM reports in a study. Asking people about their experiences in the present moment does not reveal how people organize and retain their representations of experience over time. Sometimes it is how people *remember* their experiences, not necessarily what *actually* happened across various moments, that is the stronger predictor of future behavior. For example, retrospective pain more than real-time pain has been shown to predict people's deci-

sions about whether to undergo follow-up colonoscopies (Redelmeier, Katz, & Kahneman, 2003), and retrospective reports of enjoyment during a vacation, but not people's actual reported enjoyment during the vacation, have been shown to predict decisions about whether or not they would go on a similar trip in the future (Wirtz, Kruger, Napa Scollon, & Diener, 2003). These same effects may hold for other types of personality investigations, so it is important to consider what types of representations (immediate vs. retrospective vs. global) are best suited to the research question. Retrospective reports may be the "better measure" in studies in which people recollect their past to guide judgments and decisions.

ESM Does Not Always Eliminate the Influence of Memory

Many ESM studies use short-term retrospective reports (asking people about experiences *this morning*, these past *few hours, today*), which require retrieving past experiences from memory. Although short-term retrospective reports do not appear to be influenced by the belief-based reconstruction that occurs with longer-term retrospective reports, they can still be affected by the same retrieval biases that affect episodic memory, including "peak and end" effects as well as mood-congruent memory (for a discussion of short-term retrospective reports, see Robinson & Clore, 2002a, 2002b). Furthermore, these episodic biases will occur more when people are trying to recall fleeting states that are difficult to remember (like mood or pain), which is why immediate ESM reports are often used when sampling those states. Finally, even immediate reports can reflect stable beliefs if people are asked to report on some phenomenon to which they have no introspective access (e.g., self-perceptions of autonomic physiology, such as, "How fast is your heart beating?") (Robinson & Clore, 2002a).

ESM Is Bounded by the Conditions of Self-Report

ESM may bypass certain forms of memory bias, but it will not attenuate the issues associated with the self-report process, such as socially desirable responding or self-deception. Although the reporting conditions in ESM could possibly lessen socially desirable responding (people are outside the lab and away from cues reminding them that they are being evaluated on their responses), the reporting conditions are not likely to reduce self-deception or psychological defense, which are thought to color conscious experience. In fact, there is evidence that defensive processes affect ESM reports (Cutler, Larsen, & Bunce, 1996). As compared with those lower in defense, individuals higher in defense report less negativity and show more rigidity in their ESM reports. Findings like these remind us that ESM yields only that information a person is willing and able to represent in conscious awareness at the moment the report is made.

Future Directions

There are several exciting future directions both for the method itself and for applications to personality theory. In terms of method, computerized ESM should become even more accessible, as hardware costs remain low and software continues to be available without charge to the scientific community. We also anticipate a greater incorporation of indirect or performance-based measures into ESM. Already, researchers have the capacity to record response latency information and to administer a portable Implicit Association Test *in situ* (the P-IAT; Dabbs, Bassett, & Dyomina, 2003). In the future we may see other cognitive tasks incorporated into sampling, for example, measures of working memory or other indirect measures of cognitive processing. Thus *experience* sampling could incorporate *cognitive* sampling. Also exciting is the portable EAR (Electronically Activated Recorder) technique, which allows for the sampling of spontaneous audible expressions in daily life (Mehl, Pennebaker, Crow, Dabbs, & Price, 2001; *www.tipware.com*). This technique, developed by Mehl and Pennebaker, allows researchers to extract regularities and patterns in spontaneous conversations otherwise unattainable through standard experience sampling.

There are several other methodology trends. Although free software is still available, ESM appears to be becoming increasingly commercialized. There are a growing number of high-end consultation practices that specialize in all stages of design and implementation, as well as smaller vendors selling more affordable "software solutions" for implementing ESM-type studies on PDAs, the Web, and via phone systems (interactive voice response, or IVR). We expect websystems and IVR to become increasingly popular platforms. In terms of data gathering, look for continual data transmission over wireless networks. Increased use of the Web, phones, and continual data transmission may have unforeseen costs, however, such as reducing personal contact between participants and researchers. This disconnect could present new challenges for maintaining participant rapport, response rates, and integrity of data.

In terms of personality theory, ESM will likely play a role in mapping the complex relations between episodic experiences and personality characteristics. The field appears to be moving beyond documenting a simple relation between states and traits and toward better understanding of how states configure to produce a characterization of the human personality. Especially exciting is the reinvigoration of the idea that some individuals are much more "traited" on certain characteristics than are others. For example, recent research has capitalized on sampling procedures to show stronger state–trait relations for certain individuals (i.e., those who are more habitual in their processing tendencies; Robinson & Cervone, 2006).

ESM could also aid in the development of an experience-based typology with links to important outcomes such as physical health, marital success, and well-being. The field already has the Big Five factor model for the structure of semantic personality beliefs; however, understanding of the major "state dimensions" or "episodic signatures" is still underdeveloped. ESM can capture these regularities, but not without appropriate and well-thought-out analyses to tease apart the patterns. Such teasing may require idiographic *P*-factor analysis or other sophisticated procedures. Again, it would also be judicious to go beyond description to test whether these finer-grained behavioral signatures (more so than general traits) are stronger predictors of cardiovascular reactivity, interpersonal successes, and so on.

Paradoxically, ESM—which is an explicit self-report procedure—may also stimulate work on the implicit aspects of personality. Many of our well-learned habits and processing tendencies lie outside of our awareness, yet nonetheless influence our spontaneous, situated reactions (Robinson, 2004). The key here is that these implicit aspects of personality typically influence reactions that are *spontaneous and situated*, which ESM captures. In fact, researchers are now using indirect measures in the lab to predict ESM reports and the results are very promising. For example, one study has shown that implicit attitudes about the self (as measured by an Implicit Association Test) predict variance in people's real-time affective experience, above and beyond what is predicted by self-reported attitudes alone (Conner & Barrett, 2005). Another study links implicit evaluative processing to real-time affect, showing that individuals who are fast to distinguish between neutral and negative stimuli in the lab have a higher level of negative daily affect in daily life (Robinson, Vargas, Tamir, & Solberg, 2004, Study 3). If this trend continues, immediate experience, measured by ESM, may be an important intersection between implicit personality processes and spontaneous experience.

Conclusion

Experience sampling is a powerful tool for realizing a modern-day idiographic and contextualized approach to personality. It enables measurement of dynamic *within-person patterns*, behavior *as it occurs*, and experiences as people *live their lives*. Although ESM should not be undertaken lightly without proper consideration of rationale and resources, the method itself is becoming increasingly feasible with gains in technology and a growing body of methodological guidelines. We hope that this chapter serves as a useful resource for practitioners in the science of personality.

Notes

1. Longitudinal designs in personality often involve test–retest situations separated by long time intervals. Although these designs reveal within-person change on the end points, they do not capture dynamic within-person change between the end points.
2. Historically, the terms *nomothetic* and *idiographic* were never intended to refer to methods in psychology. They were proposed by German philosopher Wilhelm Windelband as an alternative way to classify academic disciplines. The goal of nomothetic disciplines, like physics, was to develop general laws and principles (*nomo* in Greek = "law"); whereas the goal of idiographic disciplines, like history, was to understand a single event (or person) situated in time or place without generalizing (*idio*, Greek = "one's own, private") (Windelband, 1894/1998). Windelband made this distinction, in part, to classify the emerging field of experimental psychology as a nomothetic science inasmuch as its goal was to develop general laws about people. Over time, the terms have changed in meaning and are now used to refer to methods.
3. Some sampling software programs allow respondents to delay their reports if signaled at an inconvenient time. This option should be used cautiously because it can introduce sampling bias, where the reports reflect moments of convenience.
4. *Self-monitoring* refers to a method used in clinical psychology that is similar to event-based sampling. People are asked to monitor the occurrence of a behavior (thought, feeling, or action) and document the behavior by either simply noting that it occurred (using a counter or a paper-and-pencil record) or noting it and providing other information surrounding the experience. This procedure is used in two ways—to obtain an accurate picture of behaviors *in situ* and as a means of therapeutic change. When used in therapy, reactivity vis-à-vis the reduction of the behavior is considered a good thing—it indicates a successful intervention.

Recommended Readings

Resources for Learning More about Experience Sampling

Bolger, N., Davis, A., & Rafaeli, E. (2003). Diary methods: Capturing life as it is lived. *Annual Review of Psychology, 54*, 579–616.

Conner Christensen, T., Barrett, L. F., Bliss-Moreau, E., Lebo, K., & Kaschub, C. (2003). A practical guide to experience-sampling procedures. *Journal of Happiness Studies, 4*(1), 53–78.

Hektner, J. M., Schmidt, J. A., & Csikszentmihalyi, M. (2006). *Experience sampling method: Measuring the quality of everyday life*. Thousand Oaks, CA: Sage.

Reis, H. T., & Gable, S. L. (2000). Event sampling and other methods for studying daily experience. In H. T. Reis & C. M. Judd (Eds.), *Handbook of research methods in social and personality psychology* (pp. 190–222). New York: Cambridge University Press.

Tennen, H., Affleck, G., & Armeli, S. (2005). Personality and daily experience revisited [Special issue]. *Journal of Personality, 73*, 1465–1483.

Examples of Empirical Studies Using Experience Sampling

Barrett, L. F. (2004). Feelings or words? Understanding the content in self-report ratings of emotional experience. *Journal of Personality and Social Psychology,* 87(2), 266–281.

Bolger, N., & Zuckerman, A. (1995). A framework for studying personality in the stress process. *Journal of Personality and Social Psychology,* 69(5), 890–902.

Conner, T., & Barrett, L. F. (2005). Implicit self-attitudes predict spontaneous affect in daily life. *Emotion,* 5(4), 476–488.

Fleeson, W. (2001). Toward a structure- and process-integrated view of personality: Traits as density distributions of states. *Journal of Personality and Social Psychology,* 80(6), 1011–1027.

Oishi, S. (2002). Experiencing and remembering of well-being: A cross-cultural analysis. *Personality and Social Psychology Bulletin,* 28, 1398–1406.

Wirtz, D., Kruger, J., Napa Scollon, C., & Diener, E. (2003). What to do on spring break?: The role of predicted, on-line, and remembered experience in future choice. *Psychological Science,* 14(5), 520–524.

References

Allport, G. W. (1937). *Personality: A psychological interpretation.* New York: Henry Holt.

Allport, G. W. (1942). The use of personal documents in psychological science. *Social Science Research Council Bulletin,* 49.

Barrett, L. F. (1998). Discrete emotions or dimensions? The role of valence focus and arousal focus. *Cognition and Emotion,* 2(4), 579–599.

Barrett, L. F. (2005). Feeling is perceiving: Core affect and conceptualization in the experience of emotion. In L. F. Barrett, P. M. Niedenthal, & P. Winkielman (Eds.), *Emotions: Conscious and unconscious* (pp. 255–284). New York: Guilford Press.

Barrett, L. F. (2006). Solving the emotion paradox: Categorization and the experience of emotion. *Personality and Social Psychology Review,* 10, 20–46.

Barrett, L. F., & Barrett, D. J. (2001). An introduction to computerized experience sampling in psychology. *Social Science Computer Review,* 19(2), 175–185.

Barrett, L. F., & Pietromonaco, P. R. (1997). Accuracy of the five factor model in predicting perceptions of daily social interactions. *Personality and Social Psychology Bulletin,* 23, 1173–1187.

Barrett, L. F., Robin, L., Pietromonaco, P. R., & Eyssell, K. M. (1998). Are women the "more emotional" sex? Evidence from emotional experiences in social context. *Cognition and Emotion,* 12(4), 555–578.

Bolger, N., Davis, A., & Rafaeli, E. (2003). Diary methods: Capturing life as it is lived. *Annual Review of Psychology,* 54, 579–616.

Bolger, N., & Schilling, E. A. (1991). Personality and the problems of everyday life: The role of neuroticism in exposure and reactivity to daily stressors. *Journal of Personality,* 59(3), 355–386.

Bosker, R. J., Snijders, T. A. B., & Guldemond, H. (2003). *PINT (Power IN Two-level designs): Estimating standard errors of regression coefficients in* hierarchical linear models for power calculations. *User's Manual.* Version 2.1. Groningen: Rijksuniversiteit Groningen.

Brown, K. W., & Ryan, R. M. (2003). The benefits of being present: Mindfulness and its role in psychological well-being. *Journal of Personality and Social Psychology,* 84(4), 822–848.

Carstensen, L. L., Pasupathi, M., Mayr, U., & Nesselroade, J. R. (2000). Emotional experience in everyday life across the life span, *Journal of Personality and Social Psychology,* 79, 644–655.

Conner, T., & Barrett, L. F. (2005). Implicit self-attitudes predict spontaneous affect in daily life. *Emotion,* 5(4), 476–488.

Conner Christensen, T., Barrett, L. F., Bliss-Moreau, E., Lebo, K., & Kaschub, C. (2003). A practical guide to experience-sampling procedures. *Journal of Happiness Studies,* 4(1), 53–78.

Csikszentmihalyi, M., Larson, R., & Prescott, S. (1977). The ecology of adolescent experience. *Journal of Youth and Adolescence,* 6, 281–294.

Cutler, S. E., Larsen, R. J., & Bunce, S. C. (1996). Repressive coping style and the experience and recall of emotion: A naturalistic study of daily affect. *Journal of Personality,* 64(2), 379–405.

Dabbs, J. M., Jr., Bassett, J. F., & Dyomina, N. V. (2003). The Palm IAT: A portable version of the Implicit Association Test. *Behavior Research Methods, Instruments, and Computers,* 35, 90–95.

Delespaul, P. A. E. G. (1992). Technical note: Devices and time-sampling procedures. In M. W. deVries (Ed.), *The experience of psychopathology: Investigating mental disorders in their natural settings* (pp. 363–373). New York: Cambridge University Press.

deVries, M. W. (1992). *The experience of psychopathology: Investigating mental disorders in their natural settings.* New York: Cambridge University Press.

Eckenrode, J. (1984). Impact of chronic and acute stressors on daily reports of mood. *Journal of Personality and Social Psychology,* 46(4), 907–918.

Eid, M., & Diener, E. (1999). Intraindividual variability in affect: Reliability, validity, and personality correlates. *Journal of Personality and Social Psychology,* 76(4), 662–676.

Epstein, S. (1983). Aggregation and beyond: Some basic issues on the prediction of behavior. *Journal of Personality,* 51, 360–392.

Feldman, L. A. (1995). Variations in the circumplex structure of emotion. *Personality and Social Psychology Bulletin,* 21, 806–817.

Fleeson, W. (2001). Toward a structure- and process-integrated view of personality: Traits as density distributions of states. *Journal of Personality and Social Psychology,* 80(6), 1011–1027.

Fredrickson, B. L. (2000). Extracting meaning from past affective experiences: The importance of peaks, ends, and specific emotions. *Cognition and Emotion,* 14(4), 577–606.

Green, A. S., Rafaeli, E., Bolger, N., Shrout, P. E., & Reis, H. T. (2006). Paper or plastic?: Data equivalence in paper and electronic diaries. *Psychological Methods, 11*, 87–105.

Hurlburt, R. T. (1979). Random sampling of cognitions and behavior. *Journal of Research in Personality, 13*(1), 103–111.

Kenny, D. A., Bolger, N., & Kashy, D. A. (2002). Traditional methods for estimating multilevel models. In D. S. Moskowitz & S. L. Hershberger (Eds.), *Modeling intraindividual variability with repeated measures data: Methods and applications* (pp. 1–24). Mahwah, NJ: Erlbaum.

Korotitsch, W. J., & Nelson-Gray, R. O. (1999). An overview of self-monitoring research in assessment and treatment. *Psychological Assessment, 11*(4), 415–425.

Kreft, I., & de Leeuw, J. (1998). *Introducing multilevel modeling.* Thousand Oaks, CA: Sage.

Lamiell, J. T. (1981). Toward an idiothetic psychology of personality. *American Psychologist, 36*(3), 276–289.

Larsen, R. J. (1987). The stability of mood variability: A spectral analytic approach to daily mood assessments. *Journal of Personality and Social Psychology, 52*, 1195–1204.

Larsen, R. J., & Kasimatis, M. (1990). Individual differences in entrainment of mood to the weekly calendar. *Journal of Personality and Social Psychology, 58*, 164–171.

Larson, R. W., & Csikszentmihalyi, M. (1983). The experience sampling method. *New Directions for Methodology of Social and Behavioral Science, 15*, 41–56.

Laurenceau, J. P., Barrett, L. F., & Pietromonaco, P. R. (1998). Intimacy as an interpersonal process: The importance of self-disclosure, partner disclosure, and perceived partner responsiveness in interpersonal exchanges. *Journal of Personality and Social Psychology, 74*(5), 1238–1251.

Lazarus, R. S. (2000). Toward better research on stress and coping. *American Psychologist, 55*(6), 665–673.

Luke, D. A. (2004). *Multi-level modeling.* Thousand Oaks, CA: Sage.

Mehl, M., Pennebaker, J. W., Crow, D. M., Dabbs, J., & Price, J. (2001). The Electronically Activated Recorder (EAR): A device for sampling naturalistic daily activities and conversations. *Behavior Research Methods, Instruments, and Computers, 33*, 517–523.

Mohr, C. D., Armeli, S., Tennen, H., Carney, M. A., Affleck, G., & Hromi, A. (2001). Daily interpersonal experiences, context, and alcohol consumption: Crying in your beer and toasting good times. *Journal of Personality and Social Psychology, 80*(3), 489–500.

Nesselroade, J. R. (2001). Intraindividual variability in development within and between individuals. *European Psychologist, 6*(3), 187–193.

Nezlek, J. B. (2001). Multilevel random coefficient analyses of event and interval contingent data in social and personality psychology research. *Personality and Social Psychology Bulletin, 27*, 771–785.

Nezlek, J. B., Wheeler, L., & Reis, H. T. (1983). Studies of social participation. *New Directions for Methodology of Social and Behavioral Science, 15*, 57–73.

Norem, J. K., & Illingworth, K. S. (1993). Strategy-dependent effects of reflecting on self and tasks: Some implications of optimism and defensive pessimism, *Journal of Personality and Social Psychology, 65*, 822–835.

Oishi, S. (2002). Experiencing and remembering of well-being: A cross-cultural analysis. *Personality and Social Psychology Bulletin, 28*, 1398–1406.

Penner, L. A., Shiffman, S., Paty, J. A., & Fritzsche, B. A. (1994). Individual differences in intraperson variability in mood. *Journal of Personality and Social Psychology, 66*, 712–721.

Redelmeier, D. A., Katz, J., & Kahneman, D. (2003). Memories of colonoscopy: A randomized trial. *Pain, 104*(1), 187–194.

Reis, H. T., & Gable, S. L. (2000). Event sampling and other methods for studying daily experience. In H. T. Reis & C. M. Judd (Eds.), *Handbook of research methods in social and personality psychology* (pp. 190—222). New York: Cambridge University Press.

Reis, H. T., & Wheeler, L. (1991). Studying social interaction with the Rochester Interaction Record. In M. P. Zanna (Ed.), *Advances in experimental social psychology* (Vol. 24, pp. 269–318). San Diego, CA: Academic Press.

Robinson, M. D. (2004). Personality as performance: Categorization tendencies and their correlates. *Current Directions in Psychological Science, 13*, 127–129.

Robinson, M. D., & Cervone, D. (2006). Riding a wave of self-esteem: Perseverative tendencies as dispositional forces. *Journal of Experimental Social Psychology, 42*, 103–111.

Robinson, M. D., & Clore, G. L. (2002a). Belief and feeling: Evidence for an accessibility model of emotional self-report. *Psychological Bulletin, 128*(6), 934–960.

Robinson, M. D., & Clore, G. L. (2002b). Episodic and semantic knowledge in emotional self-report: Evidence for two judgment processes. *Journal of Personality and Social Psychology, 83*(1), 198–215.

Robinson, M. D., Vargas, P. T., Tamir, M., & Solberg, E. C. (2004). Using and being used by categories: The case of negative evaluations and daily well-being. *Psychological Science, 15*(5), 521–526.

Ross, M., & Wilson, A. E. (2003). Autobiographical memory and conceptions of self: Getting better all the time. *Current Directions in Psychological Science, 12*(2), 66–69.

Russell, J. A. (1980). A circumplex model of affect. *Journal of Personality and Social Psychology, 39*, 1161–1178.

Schooler, J. W., Ariely D., & Loewenstein, G. (2003). The pursuit and assessment of happiness can be self-defeating. In I. Brocas & J. Carrillo (Eds.), *The psy-*

chology of economic decisions (pp. 41–70). Oxford, UK: Oxford University Press.

Shoda, Y., Mischel, W. & Wright, J. C. (1994). Intraindividual stability in the organization and patterning of behavior. Incorporating psychological situations into the idiographic analysis of personality. Journal of Personality and Social Psychology, 67(4), 674–687.

Silvia, P. J. (2002). Self-awareness and emotional intensity. Cognition and Emotion, 16(2), 195–216.

Stone, A. A., & Shiffman, S. (1994). Ecological momentary assessment (EMA) in behavioral medicine. Annals of Behavioral Medicine, 16, 199–202.

Stone, A. A., Shiffman, S., Schwartz, J. E., Broderick, J. E., & Hufford, M. R. (2002). Patient noncompliance with paper diaries. British Medical Journal, 324, 1193–1194.

Swendsen, J. D. (1998). The helplessness-hopelessness theory and daily mood experience: An idiographic and cross-situational perspective. Journal of Personality and Social Psychology, 74(5), 1398–1408.

Tennen, H., & Affleck, G. (1996). Daily processes in coping with chronic pain: Methods and analytic strategies. In M. Zeidner & N. S. Endler (Eds.), Handbook of coping: Theory, research, applications (pp. 151–177). Oxford, UK: Wiley.

Tennen, H., Affleck, G., & Armeli, S. (2003). Daily processes in health and illness. In J. Suls & K. A. Wallston (Eds.), Social psychological foundations of health and illness (pp. 495–529). Malden, MA: Blackwell.

Tennen, H., Suls, J., & Affleck, G. (1991). Personality and daily experience: The promise and the challenge [Special issue]. Journal of Personality, 59(3), 313–337.

Updegraff, J. A., Gable, S. L. & Taylor, S. E. (2004). What makes experiences satisfying? The interaction of approach–avoidance motivations and emotions in well-being. Journal of Personality and Social Psychology, 86(3), 496–504.

West, S. G., & Hepworth, J. T. (1991). Statistical issues in the study of temporal data: Daily experiences. Journal of Personality, 59, 609–662.

Wheeler, L., & Reis, H. T. (1991). Self-recording of everyday life events: Origins, types, and uses [Special issue: Personality and daily experience]. Journal of Personality, 59(3), 339–354.

Windelband, W. (1894/1998). Geschichte und naturwissenschaft [History and natural science; reprinted]. Theory and Psychology, 8(1), 5–22.

Wirtz, D., Kruger, J., Napa Scollon, C., & Diener, E. (2003). What to do on spring break?: The role of predicted, on-line, and remembered experience in future choice. Psychological Science, 14(5), 520–524.

Zevon, M. A., & Tellegen, A. (1982). The structure of mood change: An idiographic/nomothetic analysis. Journal of Personality and Social Psychology, 43(1), 111–122.

## CHAPTER 6

Psychobiography and Case Study Methods

Alan C. Elms

Rae Carlson (1971) famously asked, "Where is the person in personality research?" We may similarly ask, "Where is *a* person in personality research?" That is, looking beyond the broadly defined whole person of Carlson's question, where can we find research on any distinct and identifiable individual as examined by one or more personality psychologists? As our partially rhetorical question suggests, we seldom find such persons in the personality research literature. When we do find them, we are probably looking at an example of psychobiographical or case study research.

For one reason or another, most personality psychologists regard such a focus on a given individual as less than legitimate, whether that individual is enough of a public figure to be identified by name (as in psychobiography) or anonymous enough to be protected by standard confidentiality procedures (as in other kinds of case studies). Case studies may be accepted as part of the workaday world of clinical psychology, and perhaps as illustrative devices in textbooks and classroom lectures. But they are not seen as Real Science. Though psychologists are often attracted to the field initially because of an interest in a particular case (either someone known personally to the proto-researcher or an intriguing figure in culture, politics, or the sciences), they are quickly educated to think in terms of experimentation, prediction, control, and quantitative analysis of results. Given these common assumptions about what constitutes scientific psychology, psychologists have devoted relatively little attention to developing research methods applicable to individual case studies. With so little investment in improving such research methods, psychobiography and case history research continue to be seen as unscientific. Most psychologists are content to let this circular loop continue largely undisturbed.

However, a few personality psychologists have remained interested enough in studying individuals as individuals to focus on identifying appropriate research strategies, guidelines, and rules of thumb. Certain of these research approaches have been borrowed from clinical psychology, but most have been developed by researchers concerned with the psychology of specific public figures. *Psychobiography* is the term most often used for such research. Though some researchers prefer other terms, that one will continue to be used here. A few researchers (e. g., Robert W. White, 1975) have done nonclinical case studies of private individuals; their data collection may be more systematic, but otherwise their research methods differ little from psychobiographers'. The methods discussed in this chapter, though illustrated only by psychobiographical research, may be regarded as generally applicable to the study of individual lives.

Are these methods inherently unscientific? Even Sigmund Freud was uneasy about the scientific status of his case histories, sometimes comparing them to short stories. C. G. Jung's first contact with his internal archetypes happened, according to his autobiographical report (1963, pp. 185–187), when a feminine voice told him that what he was doing was not science but art. Freud and Jung may have been less precise in their collection and interpretation of data than the experimental psychologists of their day; and psychobiographers of our time, even if they have learned worthwhile lessons from the errors of Freud and Jung, may continue to press beyond standard scientific protocols in reaching their conclusions. But the data with which they deal, the specific facts of individual lives (whether observed or self-reported), are no more outside the boundaries of science than an ethologist's observations of a specific chimpanzee's behavior or a neuroscientist's collection of perceptual reports from a uniquely brain-impaired patient. The methodological strategies by which psychological data are collected, organized, and interpreted may differ substantially between the psychobiographer and the ethologist or neuroscientist. The scientific objectives may differ as well, as indicated by Gordon W. Allport's (1937) differentiation of idiographic research (concerned with unique patterns or outcomes) from nomothetic research (aimed at discovering general laws). But studying a specific individual with the methods best adapted to individual study does not automatically exclude such research from scientific psychology. Nor can it be

sharply differentiated from the broader sweep of science that also includes biology, geology, and astronomy as well as the more experiment-oriented fields of physics and chemistry. The proof is in the pudding, and a closer examination of psychobiographical research methods will show that the scientific kitchen can reliably produce individual puddings of considerable merit, as well as institutional dishes more suitable to cafeteria dining. (See Elms, 1994, Chaps. 1 and 15, and Schultz, 2005, Chaps. 1 and 2, for further discussions of psychobiography's scientific status. See also Barenbaum and Winter [2003] for a historical account of psychologists' long-term "ambivalence toward the study of individual lives.")

General Uses and Applications

Why would a psychologist turn to an individual case study approach, in view of the field's traditionally strong emphasis on nomothetic rather than idiographic research methods? The fact that various prominent figures in the history of psychology have explored the use of case studies at least briefly, as well as the persistence of case study research in a corner of the field even today, suggests that such an approach can serve certain useful functions. Several such functions can be discerned.

Understanding of Unique Personality Patterns

Citing a familiar dictum, Schultz recently observed that if Henry Murray and Clyde Kluckhohn were "correct in asserting that we are all in some respects like all other people, like some other people, and like no other people, then psychobiography and related case-study approaches work to fill in that last cell of information, namely, how people are unique" (2005, p. 4). Psychologists may on the whole prefer to study psychological processes and patterns that human beings share in common; indeed, many researchers appear uncomfortable with the very idea of psychological uniqueness. But among our common experiences as humans are our recognition of distinctive qualities in those around us and our feeling that we ourselves have personal histories and current characteristics that are not identical to those of our fellow humans. Though psychologists have often sought to discover commonalities shared even by the most radical creative artists, there comes a point when such reductive research must stop short before the artist's inescapably non-nomothetic uniqueness. At that point the resourceful psychobiographer comes into his or her own, seeking to locate those unmatchable experiences and talents that have shaped the artist's (or politician's, or scientific theorist's) originality. Within psychology itself, such efforts to study and understand the unique in human functioning may not be much valued. But when literary scholars, historians, political scientists, and biographers look to psychology to help them understand individual human beings, they seldom adopt our painfully established nomothetic laws and standard research approaches. Rather, they seek out the psychobiographical models and case history techniques most likely to reward them in their quest.

Clinical Diagnostics

As with such fields as evolutionary biology, paleontology, and archaeology, psychobiography is largely a postdictive enterprise. Typically, the psychobiographer begins with a limited range of information on the subject's public achievements in middle to later adulthood, then seeks information on the subject's private life, especially his or her earlier psychological development, in hope that such information will reveal how the particular pattern of public achievements came about. Clinical case studies likewise tend to be largely postdictive, linking the client's current symptoms to earlier life-history events. But if they are to be of any use to the clinician, case studies must be predictive as well.

The scientific status of clinical case studies has been challenged (e. g., by Spence, 1982) because they are largely dependent on the client's self-reported and therefore unreliable life-history data. Such critiques are largely inapplicable to psychobiography, which is likely to be based on such diverse sources as archival records, interviews with other individuals familiar with the subject, and the subject's self-reports at several life-historical intervals, rather than solely on memories retrieved by the subject during the early phases of a clinical interaction. It should also be noted that whereas the utility of the case study workup in terms of guiding subsequent therapy remains a point of contention among clinicians and their critics, psychobiography seldom if ever serves as a

guide to the therapeutic treatment of the subject (although some psychobiographers wish it were so). Thus, psychobiographers need only aim for a greater *understanding* of the subject's psyche, not for a *reworking* of that psyche.

Predicting Political Candidates' Performance in Office

One partially predictive psychobiographical enterprise involves the study of candidates for high political office. Political psychobiography has a long and checkered history, beginning in the 1920s. It moved from a postdictive to a predictive phase only with the publication of the first edition of James David Barber's *The Presidential Character* in 1972. Barber proposed a quadripartite typology for U.S. presidents and presidential candidates (active-positive, active-negative, passive-positive, and passive-negative), and suggested ways of interpreting psychobiographical data to assign each political figure to one of the four types. Barber presented fairly detailed psychobiographical sketches of the first four U.S. presidents and most 20th-century presidents, finding considerable postdictive prowess for his typology. He also proposed to use the typology in combination with psychobiographical data to predict the broad behavioral patterns of future presidents, beginning with Richard Nixon (who had not yet been reelected when Barber's book was published). His predictions about Nixon's second term in office were sufficiently validated by post-Watergate events to interest other political psychologists and, especially, political journalists. Journalists have continued to use Barber's predictive system, often rather crudely and with little serious psychobiographical support. At the same time, politicians (starting with Jimmy Carter) have learned to "game the system"—to exaggerate their possession of the characteristics that identify them as active-positives, the most desirable among Barber's four presidential categories. Nonetheless, further scholarly development of Barber's work remains a tantalizing possibility.

Source of Nomothetic Hypotheses and Theories

By their own accounts, several prominent psychological theorists first gained major insights into personality through psychobiographical research. Though Freud had begun to develop theories of homosexuality and sublimation before he began to study Leonardo da Vinci's life, his ideas about both those constructs shifted significantly as he assembled data on Leonardo (Elms, 1994, Chap. 3). Abraham Maslow first began to conceptualize self-actualization when he closely observed and compared the lives and personalities of Ruth Benedict and Max Wertheimer. Erik Erikson (1958) had written about identity crises before he set to work on Martin Luther, and about adult midlife generativity before he settled on Mohandas Gandhi as a prime example (1969). But as with Freud on Leonardo, Erikson grew to understand his own theoretical concepts much more fully as he examined those specific lives more closely. Other psychobiographers have reported similar experiences with psychobiography as a source of new ideas about personality (e.g., Elms, 1994, Chap. 1; Schultz, 1996).

Validation or Invalidation of Nomothetic Hypotheses and Theories

Mainstream personality psychologists have often been willing to grant that psychobiographical study may generate theoretical ideas worth further exploration. They have been more reluctant to grant psychobiography a role in the confirmation or disconfirmation of psychological constructs that were nomothetically derived. But psychobiography is to a large extent an empirical enterprise, and its accumulations of facts about individual lives can at times challenge a theorist's carefully structured theses or, conversely, can encourage mainly nomothetic researchers to feel they are on the right path. Rae Carlson's (1988) skillful psychobiographical demonstration of the utility of Silvan Tomkins' (1987) script theory, for instance, probably did more to encourage further development of script theory applications than any theoretical elaboration that Tomkins ever wrote.

Psychobiographical research that appears to disconfirm the researcher's favored theoretical concepts may not be carried much further, or may never reach publication. (Psychobiography is not unique in this regard; disconfirming studies of any kind suffer a high mortality rate before they find a publication outlet.) But sometimes an established theoretical construct may be substantially modified or even pushed into a distinctly different shape by

the pressure of psychobiographical evidence. Psychobiographical data and interpretations have also been used as ammunition in theoretical battles where the contenders assert the superiority of one conceptual system over another (e.g., the ongoing "Freud wars," in which data and speculation about Sigmund Freud's personal psychology are used to support or contradict his theories).

Step-by-Step Guide

Psychobiographical research does not follow any standard format. Depending on the subject, the researcher, the publication venue, and the length of the published work, the presentation of results may vary enormously, and the ways in which the research was conducted may vary even more. In *Gandhi's Truth*, Erik Erikson (1969) began with a visit to a provincial Indian city, where he learned about an obscure labor strike in which Gandhi had participated, before he embarked on a systematic collection of data about Gandhi's early history. Then Erikson interrupted his psychobiographical account in the middle to write a sternly worded "Letter" to the long-deceased Gandhi, taking up certain troubling ethical issues that Gandhi had not successfully confronted, before getting back to his relatively orderly psychobiographical account. In *No Ordinary Time*, Doris Kearns Goodwin (1994) offered a sophisticated psychobiography of Eleanor and Franklin Roosevelt, in the guise of a historical account of their personal and political responses to World War II, with hardly a mention of the theoretical constructs on which she depended for her psychobiographical analysis. In many briefer psychobiographical studies, the pattern of presentation is more reminiscent of an American Psychological Association journal's standard format (introductory literature survey, hypotheses, data, discussion, conclusion). Even in such cases, the actual research process will surely have been quite unlike a typical psychological experiment. In every psychobiographical study, however, certain matters need to be dealt with in roughly the order given in the following sections.

Choice of Subject

At the beginning of any psychobiographical study, the choice of whom to study may appear wide open—and certainly the range of possible subjects, across wide expanses of time and space, is much greater than that available to experimenters. The psychobiographer's choice is somewhat constrained by the general assumption that psychobiographies will focus on individuals who have attained some measure of accomplishment and/or fame in a given area of endeavor. (The researcher can instead decide to focus on an ordinary individual and call the result a case study.) Furthermore, the choice should be a subject worth substantial investments of time and energy, as well as possessing some appeal to potential readers. Beyond those commonsense requirements, the recommendation has sometimes been made (e.g., by Elms, 1994, p. 20) that the subject be a person about whom the psychobiographer initially feels substantial ambivalence. Either idealizing or demonizing a subject from the beginning makes for poor psychobiography. Even that recommendation may be waived in certain cases, however, as long as the psychobiographer remains alert to his or her personal biases. Psychobiographies of Adolf Hitler or Mother Teresa should not be entirely ruled out because of his bad or her good reputation.

Certain practical considerations regarding the choice of subject should be kept in mind. Assuming that the researcher plans to publish, matters of privacy and libel laws must be taken into account with regard to living subjects. Such considerations are less relevant for deceased subjects, especially for long-deceased subjects. For that reason among others, most psychobiographical subjects are chosen from the dead rather than the living. Even for deceased subjects, the feelings of surviving relatives and friends should be considered, as unpleasant revelations and distressing conclusions may become part of any psychobiography. Beyond matters of simple human kindness, the possibility of research assistance from those relatives and friends should be kept in mind. For subjects living and dead, the likely availability of biographical data is a very important consideration in subject choice. Living subjects may be unwilling to make their private papers or personal reminiscences available to the psychobiographer, and they may instruct friends and relatives to be similarly reticent. The papers of deceased subjects, and the reminiscences of those who knew them, may be of easier access; but for some subjects, crucial archival materials may be destroyed by the heirs,

sometimes at the subject's posthumous direction. The further back in time a subject has lived, the less likely that substantial life records have survived. For this reason many potential subjects cannot be given a full or even a sufficiently partial psychobiographical treatment: biblical figures, legendary heroes such as King Arthur or Robin Hood, and so on. Before settling on a subject, the psychobiographer needs to make a quick assessment of how much biographical data is likely to be available and how reliable it may be.

Formulation of Tentative Hypotheses

Like psychological researchers of nearly any stripe, the psychobiographer is likely to begin a project with only the vaguest of hypotheses about a potential subject. If the project is of any interest at all to the researcher or to a potential audience, the initial hypothesis is not likely to be "This person had an ordinary life, and his (her) achievements were mostly a matter of hard work and luck." Instead it will be, at a minimum, "This person achieved something remarkable, and that achievement was probably influenced by identifiable aspects of the person's life history," or perhaps a tentative insight that is already the subject of public speculation, such as "This person's distinguished political career appears to have been driven by competition with his father." Even better is the presence of a genuine mystery in the subject's life: a crucial act that seems hard to explain in terms of the subject's background or usual behavior, or perhaps a puzzling relationship with another individual. Keep in mind, too, that few if any lives have ever been fully explained. The fact that one or more other psychobiographers have already "done" a given subject's life doesn't necessarily mean that you need to turn elsewhere. New data turn up, new angles are always possible. Elvis Presley or Marilyn Monroe, Virginia Woolf or Sylvia Plath, Vincent van Gogh or Pablo Picasso, Adolf Hitler or Abraham Lincoln or George W. Bush—all remain ripe for further exploration.

Initial Data Collection from Varied Sources

Psychobiographical data collection usually begins with a reading of the chosen subject's available biographies, if any. Such biographies may range from obituaries and magazine articles to full-scale, single- or multiple-volume life histories. The subject's creative work, plus published memoirs, diaries, and correspondence by the subject and by others who knew the subject, may also be available. Psychologists who do psychobiography part-time often stop after exhausting these published sources, and indeed the published data may be sufficient for their purposes. (Carlson, 1988, for example, chose to study two prominent subjects by relying entirely on information from the best biography available for each.) But for many subjects, unpublished archival material may supplement the published biographical data in important and unanticipated ways. (See Anderson, 1981, and Elms, 1994, for discussion of the value of archival research.) Research in unpublished archives may necessitate travel to the archival site, but more and more archival material is coming online. Beyond formal archives, surviving relatives of a deceased subject often retain some archival material and may be willing to share it with a well-intentioned psychobiographer.

Revision of Tentative Hypotheses

By the time a researcher has explored the most readily accessible published and unpublished data on a subject, the original tentative hypotheses about the subject are likely to have been replaced by more focused or even quite different hypotheses. If you are such a researcher, you may have noted, within the huge mass of data that you have accumulated about your chosen subject, a previously unidentified but distinctively idiosyncratic pattern that is worth pursuing further. Or you may see a different way to organize the data in terms of certain familiar psychological constructs. It may be worth pausing to consider, at this point in your research, whether the usual Freudian suspects are at work: Oedipal feelings, oral or anal personality traits, unconscious defenses, and so on. But there are plenty of non-Freudian possibilities as well: Eriksonian issues of identity, intimacy, generativity; the patterns of motivation first named by Murray and explored by McClelland, Winter, and others, such as achievement, affiliation, and power; such empirically derived constructs as authoritarianism and Machiavellianism; personality patterns based on early attachment experiences; the basic emotional scripts described by Tomkins and Carlson; even those five factors so popular in recent personality assessment literature, swimming in the shallows of personality rather than its depths. This is by no means an exhaustive list of existing concepts that one might employ to organize a given body of life-historical data. The list is offered to suggest that the energetic and astute psychobiographer has many possible ways to organize the data and should try more than one of them at this investigational stage.

Increasingly Focused Data Collection

By this stage in your research, you will probably have new ideas about where to look for data on your subject and what kinds of data may be most salient in supporting or contradicting your modified hypotheses. But while you bring your data-collection focus more precisely to bear on those hypotheses, you need to remain alert to the possibility that newly discovered data may reveal yet other perspectives—perhaps perspectives that will prove more productive than your current focus. How do you decide which of those data points now coming into view you should pursue further?

One method that increasing numbers of researchers have found useful is to stay alert for the *primary indicators of psychological saliency* developed by Irving Alexander (1990; see also Elms, 1994, pp. 245–247, and Schultz, 2005, pp. 43–47). In reading what a subject has written or listening to what the subject has recorded, Alexander suggests that we pay particular attention to those things the subject mentions *first*, mentions *most often*, repeatedly *rejects*, repeatedly *misspeaks* about, repeatedly *starts* talking about but *doesn't finish*—and so on through nine distinct indicators. Some of these indicators look obvious, others perhaps less so (e. g., "isolation," in which a discordant element briefly intrudes into the subject's remarks and then is not heard about again). But they all serve to sensitize the researcher to look in productive directions. Furthermore, consistent groupings of the subject's especially salient remarks may identify what Schultz (2005, p. 48) describes as a " 'supersaliency,' a single scene encapsulating all the core parameters of a life story." Such a *prototypical scene* in a subject's verbal accounts may provide a focus not only for the subject's own life story, but also for the psychobiographer's further development of hypotheses (Schultz, 2003).

Dealing with Discrepancies across Data Sources

When you are working with biographical data from multiple sources (as you should be), it does not take long to run into contradictory information. The contradictions are often trivial, involving such things as slightly different dates of birth or death. But at times the contradictions may bear directly on central issues in the subject's life. In most instances the discrepancies cannot be resolved by any method of statistical analysis known to psychologists. (Though certain literary scholars have developed quantitative techniques for resolving questions of authorship—for example, Foster, 2000—their methods remain controversial and in any case rarely bear on psychobiographical matters.) In order to continue with some confidence, the psychobiographer must develop rationales for trusting certain sources of information more than others. Several rules of thumb concerning contradictory data are familiar to mainstream biographers and historians and can reasonably be adopted by psychobiographers as well. They include:

1. Reliance on primary sources where possible. Use of secondary sources allows additional degrees of factual error to intrude into a biographical account. Primary sources, such as the subject's own writing and oral testimony, may not always be totally accurate, but at a minimum they convey an impression of what the subject believes to be true about his or her life, or at least about what the subject wishes to convey to others about the life story. Secondary sources process that material through other viewpoints and thus remove the psychobiographer from the intimate contact with a life that is needed to make psychological sense of that life.

2. When the primary data come not from the subject but from others who have directly interacted with the subject, the psychobiographer needs to ask whether the observers were in the right place at the right time to make the reported observations. Spouses, for instance, can be remarkably inaccurate about a late husband's or wife's life before they met. Others who claim to have been firsthand observers of important events in a subject's life may, upon closer examination, prove to have exaggerated their closeness to the subject and the frequency or time span of their contacts—

as with, for instance, Laurens van der Post's often repeated claims of close friendship with C. G. Jung (Jones, 2002). Van der Post is a good example of why the psychobiographer needs to make a further check in assessing data: How *generally* reliable is the source whose specific reports about the subject are to be used? According to his main biographer, van der Post was verifiably a liar about important aspects of his life beyond his relationship with Jung. Therefore, his reports about Jung are probably less trustworthy than those that come from sources with better reputations for general reliability.

3. In instances of conflicting testimony between two sources who presumably observed the same events, the psychobiographer should ask Cicero's penetrating question, *"Cui bono?"* (To whose advantage?) Even without a conscious intention to bias their testimony, those who make self-serving reports about the subject should generally be regarded as less dependable observers than those who make no attempt to benefit. For instance, two individuals claimed to have first "discovered" the talents of Elvis Presley when he came in to make an amateur recording at the Sun Records studio in Memphis. Sam Phillips, the Sun Records owner and producer, made his claims of discovery repeatedly, publicly, and in a floridly self-promoting manner. Marion Keisker, Phillips's assistant at the studio, made her claim of recognizing Elvis's talent (and of then encouraging Phillips to record him professionally) only when biographers directly asked for her account, and never in any way that benefited her financially. Whom should we trust here? *Cui bono?*

Extending the Iterative Research Process

In mathematics, certain values can be arrived at only by successively closer approximations. A square root, for instance, must be derived through such an iterative process (unless you have an electronic calculator or a slide rule to do the work for you). Likewise in psychobiography, most research is iterative: Instead of accumulating every possible bit of data on a subject into one big pile and then pulling conclusions out of that pile, a conscientious psychobiographer will engage in a more or less continuous process of examining preliminary data, framing tentative hypotheses, looking for more data to confirm or disconfirm those initial hypotheses, narrowing or shifting the direction of the hypotheses, looking for yet more evidence (independent of those data from which the main hypotheses were derived) to confirm or disconfirm—and so on, until a point is reached where the data in hand convincingly support the most recently framed set of hypotheses and further iterations only add to that support. Even then, the psychobiographer's cessation of the search to write up and publish the results may well turn out to be only a temporary pause in the iterative process. More data may come into view that stimulate the psychobiographer to resume the search, or other psychobiographers may propose different ways to interpret the data already at hand, and a renewed search is then directed toward finding support or disconfirmation for the competing hypotheses.

Psychologists who are accustomed to doing their research one experimental study at a time, followed by intense data analysis with probability values aimed at confirming or disconfirming a previously stated set of hypotheses, may see such iterative research as too open to manipulation of data. But biographical data seldom arrive in one neat package. Fresh archival material becomes available; previously silent or unknown witnesses begin to speak. The resourceful psychobiographer remains alert for additional data on either side (or on one of several sides) of the constantly emerging and evolving hypotheses about the subject's motives and acts. Protection against data manipulation comes partly from the psychobiographer's open presentation of the evidence for and against specific hypotheses, and partly from the safeguards described in the two following sections. (It is also worth noting that experimental research involves its own long-running iterative processes, as researchers set up experiments that are most likely to support their hypotheses or general theoretical orientations, while other researchers work to devise experiments that are intended to challenge the results of the first set, and so on. See any detailed history of research on attitude change for examples of sustained experimental iteration.)

Identifying and Delimiting Valid Conclusions

Given that each iterative sequence in a psychobiographical study ends with no statistical probability values to point toward the truth, the researcher may appear relatively free to choose from a variety of possible conclusions. Critics of psychobiography seem to assume that this is typically the case, and indeed various incautious psychobiographers (starting with Freud) have given them reason to think so. But responsible psychobiographers are careful to consider alternative explanations for the behavior of their subjects, assessing the amount of data support for each explanation or hypothesis. Even when they are not as careful as they might be in assessing the data at hand, other psychobiographers are likely to do the critical assessments for them. In a well-known illustration of such assessments, Runyan (2005) considers various published explanations of van Gogh's assault on his own ear. As Runyan points out, certain explanations can be definitively ruled out by contradictory factual evidence, whereas other explanations may be judged as more or less probable, depending on how strongly they are sustained by a "tree of explanatory inquiries, with the trunk representing the initial question or puzzle, each limb representing an explanatory conjecture, and smaller branches off the limb representing tests of that particular hypothesis or conjecture" (p. 100).

Further Iterative Study of Subject by Other Researchers

The final and most definitive check on whether a psychobiographical study has been responsibly conducted, and whether alternative explanations for its results have been adequately explored, is the extension of the iterative process by other researchers. As successive studies of a particular subject are published, it is up to the reader—or to the psychobiographical referees, namely, the critics and synthesizers in the field—to decide which interpretations are best supported by the available biographical facts and explanatory inquiry trees. Some subjects never attract the attention of more than a single psychobiographer. But those subjects of most interest to a broader audience are likely, over the years, to receive close attention by multiple psychobiographers, and out of such close attention by contentious and ingenious scholars, solidly supported psychological truths about the subject may emerge. By now, such multiple and iterative psychobiographical studies have been made of subjects ranging from Lincoln to

Hitler to Nixon, from Dickinson and Twain to Nietzsche and Wittgenstein, from Freud and Jung to Skinner and Allport. The interested reader can locate the key psychobiographical studies of most of these and other figures through such reference sources as Schultz's annual annotated bibliography (in the journal *Biography* and on the website *psychobiography.com*). One particular iterative research line, that on Gordon W. Allport, is considered as an illustrative example below.

Case Example

Choice of Subject

Psychobiographical research projects seldom arise from a single stimulus. At the broadest level, I began to pursue the case of Gordon Allport and his encounter with Sigmund Freud through my teaching of an undergraduate course in personality theory. From the time I first taught the course in the summer of 1966, Allport was always one of the seven or eight theorists I considered in detail. I introduced each theorist with salient biographical information; as the course developed over time, these biographical introductions became increasingly psychobiographical. I also showed filmed interviews of the theorists when available, mainly from Richard Evans's Notable Contributors to the Psychology of Personality series. Evans's interview of Allport (transcribed in Evans, 1970) begins with Allport telling the story of his single meeting with Sigmund Freud. As a young man, Allport happened to be in Vienna for other reasons and decided to see Freud mainly out of curiosity. When he entered Freud's office, the famous analyst sat waiting for him to explain himself. Allport responded to Freud's silence by recounting his observation, on the tramcar coming over, of a little boy who appeared to have a severe dirt phobia. Freud asked, "And was that little boy you?" Allport, greatly flustered, changed the subject. Whenever he told the story afterward (as he did many times), he insisted that the little boy was *not* himself. He also insisted that Freud was much too concerned with finding unconscious and "dirty" motives, in that instance and others, when he should have been paying attention to conscious and worthy motives. After several years of teaching the personality theory course, I was very familiar with that story and with Allport's style of presenting it in the film.

Then I came across another version of Allport's story, in his brief autobiography (1967) for the History of Psychology in Autobiography series. It was not much different from the film version, so initially I paid it little attention. But soon I came across a brief paper on the Allport–Freud encounter, written by a psychoanalytic scholar, M. D. Faber (1970). Faber interpreted the interaction between Allport and Freud as largely a matter of Allport assuming that Freud "was the sort of human being who liked to hear 'dirty stories,' " and of Freud "tweaking good-humoredly the nose of his naughty visitant," at which point Allport defensively denied to himself (and later to others) that he "had been a naughty boy."

Faber's quick-and-dirty analysis of the situation was the sort of thing an analyst might offer a patient to initiate a deeper discussion of motives. But Faber made no effort to be psychobiographical. He did not look for any life-history basis for Allport's choice of what to tell Freud, or of Allport's defensive reaction to Freud's response. Faber's interpretation was clever, but what I already knew of Allport's long-term reaction to the Freud encounter suggested that much more was involved here than a temporary social awkwardness. As Allport described the meeting in his autobiography, it was "an event of pungent significance," "a traumatic developmental episode," which taught him that "depth psychology, for all its merits, may plunge too deep, and that psychologists would do well to give full recognition to manifest motives before probing the unconscious" (1967, p. 8). He said much the same thing in his filmed interview with Richard Evans. Considering nothing but Allport's vivid descriptions, 40 to 50 years later, of a 2-minute-or-so verbal exchange with Freud, I decided at the broadest possible level: Here are a man and a mystery worth studying psychobiographically.

Formulation of Tentative Hypothesis

It didn't take me long to formulate a rather more specific hypothesis, one that seemed sufficient for the short paper I began to think about. Allport said little about his personal life in his short autobiography, but what he did say struck me as dovetailing remarkably well with his choosing to tell Freud about a little boy with a dirt phobia, and with his quick defensiveness when Freud asked, "And was that little boy you?" In the autobiography's single paragraph about his childhood, Allport described an early home life of "plain Protestant piety and hard work"—a very religious mother, a sternly hardworking physician father, and the workaday obligations of little Gordon himself: "Since my father lacked adequate hospital facilities for his patients, our household for several years included both patients and nurses. Tending office, washing bottles, and dealing with patients were important aspects of my early training" (1967, pp. 4–5).

This limited information on Allport's childhood suggested to me that he might have had grounds for developing obsessive–compulsive tendencies, even perhaps for developing the broad pattern that Freud saw as most closely associated with obsessive–compulsive traits: an anal personality. But I didn't know enough about Allport to go that far. What I did have was at least an indication of childhood cleanliness concerns: clean thinking (encouraged by his mother) and clean behavior (encouraged by his physician father). The story Allport told Freud also involved cleanliness concerns, as exhibited both by the little boy on the tramcar and by Allport's choosing to tell that particular story to Freud. So by now my minimal research hypothesis had evolved this far: There was a connection between Allport's early cleanliness concerns, his choice of story to tell to Freud, and his strong reaction to Freud's question, "Was that little boy you?"

Initial Data Collection from Varied Sources

At this point I had Allport's brief autobiography and my transcript of his filmed interview. What else did I need? I didn't know of other sources for biographical data on Allport—and indeed no such sources were readily available at that time. Allport had died several years earlier, too recently for his personal papers to be archived. But I could collect more information about his ideas. From my previous reading of Allport and my teaching of his theories in class, I already knew a good deal about his general orientation toward personality theory. Now I began to look through his published writings for signs of his attitudes toward Freud and Freudian theory. I quickly found that such signs were rather uniform in orientation: He saw Freud as too insistent on digging below the surface of personality, as too interested in the dirty

and the sexual. More broadly, Allport (in my published summation) "rejected psychological data on such unsavory creatures as rats, children, and neurotics as being largely irrelevant to an understanding of the mature personality" (Elms, 1972, pp. 630–631). Instead he proposed that most adult motives achieve *functional autonomy*, independence from their lower origins, and that truly mature adults develop a unifying philosophy of life, preferably a deep religious faith.

Revision of Tentative Hypotheses

I suggested in my brief published paper that Allport's view of human psychology could be "appropriately described as 'The Clean Personality,' " and that its foundation was Allport's early training in cleanliness and related concerns (Elms, 1972, p. 630). I cautiously observed that "our knowledge of Allport's childhood is so slight that we must not push our speculations further" and that "Allport's theoretical formulations are clearly the immediate product of much intellectual effort of the highest quality" (p. 631). Nonetheless, I concluded that "when a personality theorist finds it easy to believe the worst of another theorist, perhaps on the basis of no more than a single brief response to an ambiguous stimulus, he should look not only at the other theorist's system but within himself for the reasons" (p. 631). Allport should not have kept denying that he was (at least by analogy) the little boy with the dirt phobia. He should instead have recognized that much of his theoretical system and his general rejection of Freudian theory was a defensive response to Freud's perceptive question.

Increasingly Focused Data Collection

For several years after my paper was published, I remained satisfied with that reformulation of my working hypothesis. I didn't plan to write any more on the Allport–Freud encounter, and I didn't go out of my way to seek further evidence. I had already started psychobiographical research on other personality theorists, including Freud, Skinner, and Murray, and I was thinking about eventually writing a psychobiographical book on these and other theorists, including Allport. Of course the chapter on Allport would make reference to his Freud encounter, but my net would be cast much more widely than that.

I felt somewhat nervous when the Allport paper appeared in print. I was afraid his colleagues and former students would denounce me for demeaning him, for reducing him to a psychoanalytic stereotype. Instead, several of them let me know, by mail or in person, that they felt I had captured an important part of his personality. They even offered further examples of his cleanliness concerns or his dirt phobia. Their positive reactions to my little paper encouraged me to persist in my broader psychobiographical exploration of personality theorists. As part of that broader exploration, I continued to read Allport's publications and looked for more information on his life history. But I still didn't feel motivated to examine the Allport–Freud encounter any further. I felt I had wrapped it up rather nicely.

Four years after my paper was published, another paper appeared that took a brief look at the Allport–Freud encounter. This paper, by George Atwood and Silvan Tomkins (1976), encouraged psychologists to do what I was already doing: "Every psychological theory arises from a background of personal factors and predisposing subjective influences. These influences can be studied by means of a psychobiographical method which systematically interprets the major ideas of personality theories in the light of the critical formative experiences in the respective theorists' lives" (p. 170). Atwood and Tomkins offered several brief examples of what they had in mind, from the lives and work of Jung, Freud, Allport, and Carl Rogers. They quoted Allport's description of the Freud encounter, then rather vaguely suggested that for Allport to have "fully acknowledged" the correctness of Freud's interpretation "would have meant risking being thrown back into the painful childhood feelings which played such an important role in [Allport's] development of his personality" (p. 177). I was disappointed that they cited neither my paper nor the indications of Allport's cleanliness concerns. Instead, their discussion of Allport's childhood focused on "an extended group of childhood experiences which made him feel painfully inferior to his older brothers"—inferiority feelings that later led him to devalue the "childhood qualities of egocentricity and selfish vanity" that he felt his brothers had displayed. It was in the process of rejecting his early identification with his brothers, according to Atwood and Tomkins, that Allport developed his theoretical emphasis on individual

uniqueness, higher motives, and the functional autonomy that separated those motives from the childish motives stressed by Freud (pp. 174–175).

If Atwood and Tomkins had cited my paper, and if I had then cited theirs in my further work on Allport, I could now offer this sequence of publications as an instructive example of the iterative research process in action. Instead, I present it as an example of how the iterative process sometimes goes astray. Atwood and Tomkins apparently failed to see my paper, which was published in a psychoanalytic journal not ordinarily indexed in *Psychological Abstracts*. I read their paper soon after publication and agreed with their general emphasis "on the subjectivity of personality theory" (as the paper was titled). But I soon forgot their discussion of Allport. Perhaps my forgetfulness was encouraged by the publication, 3 years later, of an important book by Atwood in collaboration with Robert Stolorow, borrowing its subtitle from the Atwood and Tomkins paper: *Subjectivity in Personality Theory* (Stolorow & Atwood, 1979; revised version by Atwood & Stolorow, 1993). That book offered further case history details on Freud and Jung and added chapters on Wilhelm Reich and Otto Rank, but completely dropped Allport (as well as Rogers) from discussion. Atwood and Tomkins's take on Allport dropped out of my memory as well.

Meanwhile, however, I kept running across new information about Allport, and sometimes about the Freud encounter, as I pursued several different lines of psychobiographical research. Sometimes the information appeared as I was looking for data on another theorist—for example, when I interviewed Henry Murray (Allport's long-time colleague and ambivalent friend) or while I was tracking down information on Abraham Maslow at the Archives of the History of American Psychology. At other times, I was looking for information on Allport but not on the Freud encounter, in the Harvard Archives' newly opened Allport Papers and in interviews with Allport's son and Allport's personal secretary. At still other times, information just popped up unexpectedly—for instance, when Dan Ogilvie, one of Allport's final graduate students, told me about a striking incident in which Allport's dirt phobia was on full display. At the Library of Congress, where I was looking for information on Freud, I came across the manuscript of an unpublished reminiscence by Allport, written specifically for the Freud Archives. He described his Freud meeting as usual but added previously undisclosed details on what happened *after* Freud asked the traumatic question "And was that little boy you?"

I still had no intention of writing further about the Freud encounter, until I was asked to participate in an American Psychological Association (APA) symposium marking the 50th anniversary of Allport's pioneering textbook, *Personality: A Psychological Interpretation* (1937). By then I had seen, in an unpublished interview transcript in the Harvard Archives, Allport's explanation of the personality textbook's genesis: "You can see the impact of my encounter with Freud as the origin of my idea that adult motivation is not necessarily a channeling, or conditioning, or overlay of cathected instincts or infantile motivations or fixations. . . . That is the focus of my concept of functional autonomy and in general of all the 1937 book, as well as much subsequent writing" (Allport, 1962).

Amazing! One perceptive but off-the-cuff remark by Freud, plus one defensive reaction by an embarrassed 22-year-old, equals a highly influential 600-page textbook 17 years later (with a lot of hard work in between). As I pointed out in my APA talk and elaborated in a later book chapter (Elms, 1993, 1994), Allport kept insisting throughout his life that he was *not* just a boy with a *dirt phobia*, but also that he was *not a little boy*, and that he was *not just anyone* Freud might compare him to. He was instead a *mature adult*, and indeed a *unique individual*. Along with the rejection of Freud's "dirty" psychology, those themes run throughout Allport's 1937 textbook.

In expanding my five-page 1972 paper into a 15-page book chapter, I was adding to my original emphasis on Allport's dirt phobia a discussion of his concerns about being perceived as an adult and as a unique individual. These latter concerns happened to be what Atwood and Tomkins had stressed in their 1976 paper, though they had not been very specific about the connections with the Freud encounter. I failed to cite their paper, but that wasn't in revenge for their not having cited my 1972 paper—it was sheer forgetfulness. And perhaps I should attribute the similarities between my 1993/1994 chapter and their 1976 paper to sheer cryptomnesia—the unrecognized influence of a hidden memory on one's current

thinking. But I had continued doing my own iterative research, which had turned up a variety of independent sources on Allport's difficult relationships with his brothers, his desires to be seen as unique and fully adult, and so on. So I would have discussed those points in my new paper even if I'd never read Atwood and Tomkins. (But I should have given them credit, and I'm pleased to have the opportunity to do so now.)

Dealing with Discrepancies across Data Sources

The data sources that I relied on in studying Allport were remarkably consistent. His retelling of the Freud encounter differed in only a few words across half a dozen printed, filmed, or recorded versions. The only substantially different version was the one I found in the Freud Archives, and it mainly differed by adding a description of what happened immediately after Freud asked the traumatic question "And was that little boy you?" The rest of the interaction, as Allport and Freud continued through what amounted to an initial analytic hour, struck me as involving further cleanliness issues (see Elms, 1994, p. 77). But I chose not to emphasize those issues in the later paper, because I felt that Allport's personality was considerably more complex and his achievements were far broader than were suggested by his simplistic criticisms of Freud's concerns with dirt.

Actually, the major "discrepancies across data sources" in Allport's case involved discrepancies between his self-concept and his visible behavior. Most obvious, of course, was his denial that he was the little boy with the dirt phobia, in spite of the perception of many people who knew him that he was indeed at some level that little boy. In a related matter, in spite of his pervasive cleanliness concerns, Allport was a heavy cigarette smoker throughout his adult life, and he died of smoking-related lung disease. (One very specific discrepancy across data sources was that when I asked Allport's longtime personal secretary about his smoking habits, she denied ever having known that he smoked! Other colleagues and friends were more forthcoming on this point.) Allport also refused to acknowledge that a variety of other Freudian concepts might be applicable to his personality. Henry Murray delighted in telling me funny stories about Allport's inability to recognize his own Freudian defensiveness. I accumulated enough information from other sources to indicate that Murray's stories, though probably exaggerated for humorous effect, were to a large extent accurate.

Extending the Iterative Research Process

I have gone about as far as I want to go in refining my hypotheses about Allport's Freud encounter. But other researchers have continued to contribute useful information and further hypotheses. In terms of useful information, the major recent contribution is a book-length biography of Allport written by Ian Nicholson (2003). Nicholson's book is not a psychobiography. He characterizes it instead as "part biography and part intellectual history," with particular attention to how Allport's personal life interacted with political and cultural variables to shape his ideas (p. 4). In keeping with Allport's own theoretical emphases, Nicholson seldom considers unconscious motives, instead stressing Allport's conscious inclinations, ruminations, intentions, and goals. But throughout the book there is plenty of information about Allport that strengthens the already established psychobiographical picture of a high-minded and work-oriented gentleman, unusually concerned with issues of cleanliness and dirt, and distressed that he was younger, weaker, and less masculine than his brothers.

Nicholson of course discusses Allport's Freud encounter and footnotes the "several scholars" who had argued that Freud's was-that-little-boy-you question "was not as wildly speculative as Allport would later claim" (p. 69). However, though he cites Allport's much later observation that the Freud encounter was "an event of pungent significance" that "started a deep train of thought," Nicholson fails to pursue in detail this direct link between Allport's denial of Freud's insight and his subsequent career as a personality theorist.

Nicholson obtained access to a key document that earlier researchers did not: Allport's "journal" or diary, including his immediate account of the meeting with Freud. According to Nicholson, the evidence of the diary shows that Allport was not

> particularly unsettled by Freud's probing analysis of the boy on the tram. Viewing the meeting as a rather routine affair, Allport did not even mention

the story of the boy, and he concluded his journal account of the discussion by casually mentioning that he and Freud "discussed also repressions and their mechanisms. To understand psychoanalysis one must, according to him, read German." (p. 70)

But most psychobiographers, instead of concluding that Allport was not "particularly unsettled" by this "rather routine" meeting, would instantly raise a simple question: Why did Allport *not* describe the story of the little boy and Freud's crucial response in his diary entry that day (or, apparently, on any other day of that year's journal)? He described it many times later, and he always stressed how *un*routine it was. Why the silence about it as he reflected on the day's events for his personal diary?

No one has yet taken up that question in print. But psychobiographical discussions of Allport's Freud encounter continue. William Todd Schultz (2003) used it, for instance, to illustrate one of his main criteria for a prototypical scene, that of *specificity*:

> The setting is foregrounded with confidence. In most cases dialogue also occurs. The actors are "quoted," and when the scene gets retold, their lines do not vary or else vary only slightly. . . . Freud's unsurprising punch line is given by Allport numerous times—in print, on film, and on audiotape—but the words hardly change. . . . These scenes have a certain frozen quality to them, like "pauses" in an ongoing movie. To the subject, they stand out—like agates in a bag of rocks.

Schultz reached no new conclusions about the Freud encounter. But Nicole Barenbaum, who had been working on other aspects of Allport's life and work, was intrigued by Schultz's description of the Allport–Freud meeting as a prototypical scene (N. Barenbaum, personal communication, July 17, 2005). Using biographical material from Nicholson's book as well as from her own study of the Allport Papers and other archives, she has developed the most nuanced analysis of the Freud encounter published so far (Barenbaum, 2005). She starts by identifying ways in which Allport's story meets all five of Schultz's criteria for the prototypical scene: not only *specificity* but *interpenetration* (Allport's telling of the tale on many occasions and in many media), *developmental gravity* (the event occurred at a crucial time in Allport's professional development, and with crucial effects on his occupational identity), *thrownness* (the subject finds him- or herself "in a situation that violates the status quo, in which something anomalous or surprising transpires," and has to cope somehow with "the anxiety it provokes"; Schultz, 2005, p. 51), and *family conflict*. That final criterion, as Barenbaum notes, is not immediately evident in Allport's repeated telling of the story, but Atwood and Tomkins (1976), Elms (1993, 1994), and Nicholson (2003) all provide evidence for such conflict, especially in terms of Allport's continuing distress about being a very junior brother in relation to his siblings.

This firm identification of the Freud encounter as a prototypical scene may be seen simply as another indication of its long-lasting personal importance to Allport. But Barenbaum goes further, proposing that the scene's basic script was played out repeatedly in Allport's life: "Having first approached older models and felt rejected and humiliated by them, Allport responded eventually by asserting his own independence and uniqueness" (Barenbaum, 2005, p. 227). He had done so numerous times before and after Freud, in encounters with one or all of his brothers; he did so as a graduate student in a painful encounter with the distinguished experimental psychologist E. B. Titchener (pp. 225–226); and, I might add, on the basis of my conversations with Henry Murray, Allport did so yet again on many occasions with his only-4-years-older but very patronizing friend Harry Murray.

In addition to identifying the repetitive nature of this personal script, Barenbaum suggests several other useful ways to look at Allport's reaction to Freud, and at his life and work more broadly. For one thing, Allport fits Frank Sulloway's theory of sibling role differentiation within the family, with Allport as the last-born tending to be "more rebellious and more open to new experiences," as well as "more sociable and more accommodating than first-born children" (Barenbaum, 2005, p. 228). Barenbaum also suggests that, especially in relation to his next-oldest brother, Floyd, who had already become a social psychologist of considerable distinction, Gordon Allport chose theoretical positions that showed "a contrast effect perhaps enhanced by a 'narcissism of minor differences,' the tendency for people who 'are otherwise alike' to exaggerate their differences" (itself a Freudian concept; p. 230). And, following Nicholson's evidence from Allport's journals and letters, she high-

lights Allport's divided personality: "Allport first embraced, and then struggled during much of his career to reconcile, a series of opposites—science and spirituality, American psychometric and German intuitive approaches to personality, the general and the unique" (Barenbaum, 2005, p. 233). These opposites were embodied partly in Allport's immediate responses to Freud (shock and denial in response to the crucial question, followed by Allport's attempts to get Freud to diagnose his problems and send him to a good analyst in America), and partly in his long-term reactions to the Freud encounter (rejection of Freud's deeper probings into personality, but a continuing fascination with individual case histories).

Identifying and Delimiting Valid Conclusions

Some three decades have passed since the publication of the first psychobiographical papers on Gordon Allport and his encounter with Freud. My initial and somewhat tentative conclusion (that his delayed but emphatic "No!" to Freud's question was a form of denial, and that his early family life had predisposed him to be a cleanliness-focused young man who naturally developed a theory of the Clean Personality) has not been substantially contradicted by evidence to the contrary. Indeed, the evidence bearing on Allport's cleanliness concerns has only increased over time. What else has increased is evidence that other issues also played an important part in his life and work. One major issue was his distress at being considered a "little boy" by his family, in contrast with his older brothers. Another issue was his insistence on being considered a unique individual, distinct from the little boy on the tramcar, distinct from his older brothers, distinct from anyone else. Again, these issues have been supported by increasing evidence, from the fairly limited biographical information available to Atwood and Tomkins (1976), to the archival and interview sources I consulted for my 1993/1994 chapter, to Ian Nicholson's ample archival and other sources for his 2003 biography, to Nicole Barenbaum's use of all the material available to those previous researchers plus her own archival investigations. Nicholson also makes a strong case that Allport's theoretical positions derived in part from his close study of the work of German psychological theorists, and in part from his responses to major cultural changes in America during his professional development. These intellectual and cultural influences should be taken into account by psychobiographers, but they do not contradict previous psychobiographical accounts of Allport's theoretical development. Indeed, those psychobiographical accounts help to answer a question that Nicholson never clearly addresses: Why did Allport, among all the psychologists of his generation, respond so enthusiastically to the German theorists' emphasis on uniqueness?

Allport's defenders may argue that his reactions to Freud's question did not bear significantly on his professional development and theory building, or that cleanliness concerns and inferiority feelings were not especially important personal issues for Allport. I think such defenders would have to ignore a good deal of Allport's own autobiographical comments, as well as the testimony of most of his professional colleagues and others who knew him well. These defenders would also need to trace Allport's theoretical development in ways that make the psychobiographical underpinning unnecessary or irrelevant. I would be interested in seeing such a case advanced and defended. But no one has offered to do it yet.

Further Iterative Study of Subject by Other Researchers

Nicole Barenbaum has indicated that she may someday do a longer paper about the Freud incident, in hopes of adding further depth to her already nuanced treatment (Barenbaum, personal communication, July 17, 2005). As she observes in her 2005 chapter (citing both my 1994 chapter and Nicholson's 2003 book), "Allport did not reject Freudian theory immediately after meeting Freud in 1920, as he implied in some accounts" (p. 235). She sketches several steps in the development of his profunctional-autonomy position between the Freud meeting and the writing of his 1937 textbook, and suggests that the details of this gradual development can be enlarged and expanded upon. The extensive Allport archives and other unpublished material (some still held by Allport's family) can surely be used by Barenbaum and others to examine more precisely the complementary roles of Allport's emotional and intellectual reactions to Freud over the course of his long career.

Future Directions

Moving from Individual Psychobiographies to Comparisons of "Similar" Cases

Most psychobiographical studies deal with a single life history. We need more of those, indeed lots more of them, given the avoidance of single cases that was characteristic of psychology in the 20th century. But methodological and conceptual advancements in 21st-century psychology will also include detailed psychobiographical comparisons of two or more individuals at a time, similar in some ways but differing in other crucial aspects. We already have a few examples of such studies, such as Alexander's comparison of Freud and Jung (1990), Atwood and Stolorow's examination of four personality theorists (1993), and my comparisons of two national leaders and four foreign policy advisers (Elms, 1994, Chaps. 13 and 14). Kate Isaacson (2005) has discussed the methodological issues involved in such multiple-case or parallel-iteration psychobiographies.

Building Larger Databases of Individual Cases for Cross-Case Comparisons within Biographical Categories

Henry Murray, who pioneered the multiple-case-study comparison of nonpathological subjects at the Harvard Psychological Clinic, once told me he looked forward to seeing the publication of more and more psychobiographies for nomothetic as well as idiographic reasons: "If you have 80 or 90 psychobiographies where the person had a business failure, and you did another study of a person who'd been a business failure, you'd have something to go on" (personal communication, May 24, 1986). As far as I know, our psychobiographical studies of business failure remain sparse. But we do have by now quite a few studies of creative writers, so maybe the more quantitatively oriented among our life history researchers can begin to draw statistically meaningful conclusions across them. It will remain important to look at each writer individually, to appreciate the unique qualities of his or her life and work. But there is no reason to protect our methodological purity by refusing to look also at data across a number of those individual and unique writers.

Developing Quantitative Analyses Appropriate for Study of Individual Cases

Likewise, there is no need to avoid statistics when we can apply such analysis to the individual. I have already mentioned Don Foster's (2000) studies of stylistic patterns in order to identify the authorship of a particular work as by one writer or another. Foster is not interested in psychobiographical issues, but such issues can sometimes be addressed quantitatively. Dean Simonton (2004), for instance, has done an ingeniously quantitative study of Shakespeare's plays and the political environment in which each was presumably written. His results not only indicate that the plays were indeed written by Shakespeare and not by Edward de Vere (as some scholars had argued), but that "artistic creativity is responsive to conspicuous political events." Simonton is statistically ingenious enough to develop ways to answer other carefully selected psychobiographical questions as well—though not, I suspect, the question of why Gordon Allport reacted with such long-lasting distress to Freud's ingeniously insightful question.

Acknowledgments

I would like to thank James William Anderson, Nicole B. Barenbaum, Richard W. Robins, and William McKinley Runyan for their helpful suggestions concerning an earlier draft of this chapter.

Recommended Readings

Alexander, I. (1990). *Personology: Method and content in personality assessment and psychobiography.* Durham, NC: Duke University Press.
Elms, A. C. (1994). *Uncovering lives: The uneasy alliance of biography and psychology.* New York: Oxford University Press.
Erikson, E. H. (1969). *Gandhi's truth.* New York: Norton.
McAdams, D. P., & Ochberg, R. (Eds.) (1988). *Psychobiography and life narratives.* Durham, NC: Duke University Press.
Runyan, W. M. (1982). *Life histories and psychobiography: Explorations in theory and method.* New York: Oxford University Press.
Schultz, W. T. (Ed.). (2005). *Handbook of psychobiography.* New York: Oxford University Press.

References

Alexander, I. (1990). *Personology: Method and content in personality assessment and psychobiography.* Durham, NC: Duke University Press.
Allport, G. W. (1937). *Personality: A psychological interpretation.* New York: Holt.
Allport, G. W. (1962). *My encounters with personality theory.* Unpublished manuscript, recorded and edited by W. G. T. Douglas, Boston University School of Theology, October 29. Gordon W. Allport Papers, Harvard University Archives, Cambridge, MA.
Allport, G. W. (1967). Autobiography. In E. G. Boring & G. Lindzey (Eds.), *A history of psychology in autobiography* (Vol. 5, pp. 3–25). Boston: Appleton Century Crofts.
Anderson, J. W. (1981). Psychobiographical methodology: The case of William James. *Review of Personality and Social Psychology, 2,* 245–272.
Atwood, G. E., & Stolorow, R. D. (1993). *Faces in a cloud: Intersubjectivity in personality theory,* revised edition. Northvale, NJ: Jason Aronson.
Atwood, G. E., & Tomkins, S. S. (1976). On the subjectivity of personality theory. *Journal of the History of the Behavioral Sciences, 12,* 166–177.
Barber, J. D. (1972). *The presidential character: Predicting performance in the White House.* Englewood Cliffs, NJ: Prentice-Hall.
Barenbaum, N. B. (2005). Four, two, or one? Gordon Allport and the unique personality. In W. T. Schultz (Ed.), *Handbook of psychobiography* (pp. 223–239). New York: Oxford University Press.
Barenbaum, N. B., & Winter, D. G. (2003). Personality. In I. B. Weiner (Series Ed.) & D. K. Freedheim (Vol. Ed.), *Handbook of psychology: Vol. 1. History of psychology* (pp. 177–203). New York: Wiley.
Carlson, R. (1971). Where is the person in personality research? *Psychological Bulletin, 75,* 203–219.
Carlson, R. (1988). Exemplary lives: The uses of psychobiography for theory development. *Journal of Personality, 56,* 105–138.
Elms, A. C. (1972). Allport, Freud, and the clean little boy. *Psychoanalytic Review, 59,* 627–632.
Elms, A. C. (1993.) Allport's *Personality* and Allport's personality. In K. M. Craik, R. T. Hogan, & R. N. Wolfe (Eds.), *Fifty years of personality psychology* (pp. 39–55). New York: Plenum Press.
Elms, A. C. (1994). *Uncovering lives: The uneasy alliance of biography and psychology.* New York: Oxford University Press.
Erikson, E. H. (1958). *Young man Luther.* New York: Norton.
Erikson, E. H. (1969). *Gandhi's truth.* New York: Norton.
Evans, R. I. (1970). *Gordon Allport: The man and his ideas.* New York: Dutton.
Faber, M. D. (1970). Allport's visit with Freud. *Psychoanalytic Review, 57,* 60–64.

Foster, D. (2000). *Author unknown: On the trail of Anonymous*. New York: Holt.

Goodwin, D. K. (1994). *No ordinary time: Franklin and Eleanor Roosevelt: The home front in World War Two*. New York: Simon & Schuster.

Isaacson, K. (2005). Divide and multiply: Comparative theory and methodology in multiple case psychobiography. In W. T. Schultz (Ed.), *Handbook of psychobiography* (pp. 104–111). New York: Oxford University Press.

Jones, J. D. F. (2002). *Teller of many tales: The lives of Laurens van der Post*. New York: Carroll & Graf.

Jung, C. G. (1963). *Memories, dreams, reflections* (Recorded and edited by A. Jaffé; trans. R. & C. Winston). New York: Pantheon.

Nicholson, I. A. M. (2003). *Inventing personality: Gordon Allport and the science of selfhood*. Washington, DC: American Psychological Association.

Runyan, W. M. (2005). How to critically evaluate alternative explanations of life events: The case of Van Gogh's ear. In W. T. Schultz (Ed.), *Handbook of psychobiography* (pp. 96–103). New York: Oxford University Press. (Original work published 1981)

Schultz, W. T. (1996). An "Orpheus complex" in two writers-of-loss. *Biography: An Interdisciplinary Quarterly, 19*, 371–393.

Schultz, W. T. (2003). The prototypical scene: A method for generating psychobiographical hypotheses. In R. Josselson, A. Lieblich, & D. P. Adams (Eds.), *Up close and personal: The teaching and learning of narrative research* (pp. 151–175). Washington, DC: American Psychological Association.

Schultz, W. T. (Ed.). (2005). *Handbook of psychobiography*. New York: Oxford University Press.

Simonton, D. K. (2004). Thematic content and political content in Shakespeare's dramatic output, with implications for authorship and chronology controversies. *Empirical Studies of the Arts, 22*, 201–213.

Spence, D. P. (1982). *Narrative truth and historical truth*. New York: Norton.

Stolorow, R. D., & Atwood, G. E. (1979). *Faces in a cloud: Subjectivity in personality theory*. Northvale, NJ: Aronson.

Tomkins, S. S. (1987). Script theory. In J. Aronoff, A. I. Rabin, & R. A. Zucker (Eds.), *The emergence of personality* (pp. 147–216). New York: Springer.

White, R. W. (1975). *Lives in progress* (3rd ed.). New York: Holt, Rinehart & Winston.

## CHAPTER 7

Mining Archival Data

Phebe Cramer

With the abundance of information currently available in our psychological journals, why would one want to spend time digging through reams of data collected in years past? In fact, mining archival data has certain similarities to the work of an archeologist, and likely shares some of the same motivations.

A most straightforward answer to the question, why do it? is that one has an interest in life as it was lived in earlier times. For students of human behavior, this may include a curiosity about family values, leisure time activities, religious beliefs, gender roles, or methods of discipline—related, perhaps, to a question such as whether children of an earlier era did in fact grow up without exposure to the violence and sex portrayed today in our national media. Or perhaps one is curious about what people thought, and thought about, at an earlier time, prior to the scientific discoveries and technological inventions that have forever changed

the world we live in. In this case, we study people from the past for their intrinsic interest.

A related, but different reason to study archival data is the intriguing question of whether people have changed, in some fundamental way, over the years. The archeologist has shown us how hominid morphology has evolved, and the anthropologist has described the evolution of social structures. Psychological archival data provide an opportunity to study the question of whether personality has evolved. Are the basic personality traits and dispositions the same today as they were in the past? Or is personality evolving into new, previously unknown dimensions? In this case, we study people of the past in comparison to those of the present day.

A third, and most important reason for "mining" archival data is that, in some cases, it allows us to study change within the same individual—that is, to study development. Although cross-sectional studies allow us to discover differences in children and adults at different ages, only longitudinal studies in which data have been collected from the same group of individuals over a period of years provide the opportunity to study personality change. In turn, we are able to investigate the factors that promote change. In this case, archival data allow us to study how personality develops.

Finally, a very important reason for using archival data is that it allows the individual investigator to benefit from the years of work of previous researchers. Carrying out a longitudinal study is a long and difficult process. It requires great skill to maintain the participant sample, which in turn requires staff, finances, laboratory and archival space, as well as the steadfast motivation of the investigator(s) to continue the study over a lengthy period of time. It is unlikely that an individual investigator would be able to collect such data.

In this chapter, I discuss how one might conduct research on personality development using archival longitudinal data. I describe the steps involved in this type of study, illustrating these with my own experience using data from the Intergenerational Study conducted at the Institute of Human Development (IHD), University of California, Berkeley. I consider the importance of clarifying certain assumptions at the beginning of such an enterprise, and deciding on the questions to be asked. Next, available sources for obtaining archival longitudinal data are discussed. I follow this with a more lengthy section that highlights the complexities of carrying out this type of work. These complexities include potential problems with the original data files, issues related to the existing measures, and important considerations regarding the participants in the study.

Step-by-Step Guide

Beginning a Longitudinal Study, Using Archival Data

Underlying Assumptions

In carrying out a longitudinal study with archival data, there are certain underlying assumptions that should be made explicit. A first assumption was well stated in the title of an article by Caspi (2000): "The child is father of the man." By studying the material from archi-

val files, one can determine if there are continuities between personality/behavior as assessed early in life and personality/behavior later in life. The opportunity to test this possibility underlies the interest in looking at archival data collected over a period of years.

Longitudinal research, in addition to addressing issues of continuity in personality characteristics, also provides a unique opportunity to address issues of personality stability and change. Whether personality remains stable, or whether it changes with age is a question that can be adequately answered only by looking at longitudinal data. As recent work has demonstrated (e.g., Caspi & Roberts, 1999), personality is best characterized as showing both continuity and change. The most adequate, unconfounded demonstration of this comes from longitudinal data. For example, using data from the Intergenerational files of the IHD, Haan, Millsap, and Hartka (1986) demonstrated that the rank order of individuals for six basic personality components was reasonably stable across the adult ages 30–40 and 40–55[1] (median r's = .52 and .55), but at the same time the mean levels of the traits changed significantly with age. Jones, Livson, and Peskin (2003), studying the same group of individuals, were able to demonstrate not only that change occurred in personality—this time assessed with the California Psychological Inventory (CPI) scales—but, more important, that it occurred in different ways for different individuals. Using hierarchical linear modeling analyses, they demonstrated that although the mean score for each personality dimension, based on the total group of participants, may not change from age 33 to age 75, some individuals show a steady increase and others show a steady decrease. In terms of underlying assumptions, both of these studies investigated the possibility that personality, as assessed at one age, would be related to personality assessed at a subsequent age.

Inevitably, the researcher's own basic assumptions will guide the work carried out with archival longitudinal data. These assumptions include, but are not limited to, the researcher's theoretical orientation, developmental knowledge, and personal experience. If, for example, one believes that early childhood personality will be continuous with personality and adjustment in adulthood, one will search the archival data for ways to demonstrate such connections. Based on this assumption, I had demonstrated in an earlier study (Cramer & Block, 1998) that the personality characteristics of 3- to 4-year-old children from the Block and Block longitudinal study, as assessed by the California Child Q-Set (CCQ; Block & Block, 1980) were predictive of defense mechanism use at age 23. On the basis of this knowledge, I looked in the Intergenerational files for further evidence that early child personality would predict adult defense use and would replicate my previous findings linking specific traits to particular defense mechanisms. In addition, as based on assumptions coming from theory, knowledge of previous research, and clinical experience, I expected that adult defense use would be related to adult adjustment and maladjustment. Thus, I used archival data to study the connections among child personality, later defense use, adult personality, and adult adjustment and maladjustment (Cramer & Tracy, 2005).

The main point here is that unless one's theoretical orientation, developmental knowledge, and/or personal experience includes the assumption that early childhood personality is connected, psychologically, with later personality and adjustment, a researcher would not look for such an association.

Deciding on the Questions to Be Asked

The richness of archival data—the multitude of variables, the variability of participants, the multiple ages of assessment—make it possible to ask seemingly endless questions about development. To avoid being overwhelmed by the myriad data, it is advisable to sort out the kinds of questions one wishes to raise and to be clear about their differences and the different types of data that will be relevant for each question. Here, I discuss three different types of questions that a researcher may wish to study.

First, one may be interested in concurrent personality relations. For example, we may ask the question of how, in early adulthood, Marcia's (1966) identity dimensions are related to the use of defense mechanisms. From the IHD archival files, measures of the four identity styles (Achieved, Moratorium, Foreclosed, and Diffused) may be constructed from the existing California Adult Q-sort (CAQ) (Block, 1971) early adult data. (See below for the construction of new measures.) The archival files also include typescripts of Thematic Apperception Test (TAT) stories from early adulthood, which

may be coded to assess the use of defense mechanisms.

As another example, which leads into the second type of question, we may ask how the Big Five trait of Extraversion relates to Conscientiousness, at early adulthood, at early middle age, and at late middle age. From the IHD archival data, after developing a measure of Big Five traits (see below), it is then possible to correlate the two traits at each age period. We may have some hypothesis that the relation between the two traits will change with age, because we know that the mean levels of the Big Five traits change with age. Or we may hypothesize that the concurrent relation between the two traits will be similar at different ages, because we know that there is stability in the trait across ages. For the Intergenerational data, the correlations between Extraversion and Conscientiousness at each age are found to be: age 30, $r = .17$, age 40, $r = .21$; age 55, $r = .37$. These results demonstrate the concurrent relation between the same variables at three different ages and show a change in the nature of these relations as participants grow older.

The previous analyses do not, however, address a second question—namely, do individual personality traits change with age? To answer this type of question, we rely on archival data in which the same personality variable is assessed in the same individual(s) at several different ages. The results of this type of study, using the IHD archival data and looking at the Big Five traits, are discussed below (see also Cramer, 2003).

The third type of question, and one uniquely amenable to study with longitudinal data from archival files, is whether one dimension of personality from an earlier age will predict a different dimension of personality at a later age. Often the question of prediction from one age to another is combined with the question of personality change. The research question then becomes, does personality variable X at an earlier age predict change over time in another dimension of personality (variable Y)?

Different types of archival data are required to answer the three different questions. To address questions of concurrent relations, data for two (or more) dimensions of personality must be available for the same age. To address questions of personality stability over time, data for the same dimension(s) of personality must be available for the same person(s) across two or more different ages. Data of this kind can be analyzed using repeated-measures analyses of variance or using multilevel or hierarchical linear modeling (HLM; Bryk & Raudenbush, 1987), which does not require having data from every participant at every age tested. To address questions concerning determinants of personality change, both of the above types of data must be available.

Obtaining Archival Data

Archival Sources

Very few investigators have the time or resources available to carry out a longitudinal study. Fortunately, archival data can be obtained in several ways. First, one may use a national repository, in which datasets from many different studies have been gathered together and cataloged. At the Henry A. Murray Research Center, Radcliffe Institute for Advanced Study, Harvard University, data from nearly 300 psychological studies have been archived, including the Intergenerational Study, Vaillant's longitudinal study of Harvard men (the Grant study), and numerous longitudinal studies of mental health. The entire collection may be viewed online at *murray.hmdc.harvard.edu*, and specific topics may be searched.

Another source of extensive data may be found at the American Psychological Society website (*www.psychologicalscience.org/observer*), which includes the National Longitudinal Study of Adolescent Health, the National Archive of Computerized Data on Aging, and a link to the Henry A. Murray Research Center of Radcliffe College.

Data files from early Head Start research are available at *www.childcareresearch.org*, which includes datasets from a multitude of studies. Topics may be searched either under "Datasets and Statistics," which may be downloaded, or under "Instruments and Measures." For example, a search under "Datasets" for the topic "IQ" takes one to a number of different studies of IQ, including the Carolina Abcedarian Project on the effectiveness of early childhood educational intervention for at-risk children. A similar search under the topic "Self" brings up nine different data sources, each with an abstract and directions for downloading.

Data from questionnaires administered as part of the National Longitudinal Surveys conducted with children, adolescents, and young and old adults from 1979 to 2000 are available

at *www.nslinfo.org*. Data from the Block and Block (1980) longitudinal study will soon be available to qualified researchers through the Henry Murray Research Center at *murray.hmdc.harvard.edu*.

For these types of data sources, there are often codebooks available that provide information about the sample, study design, and measures available, and sometimes even the original forms (questionnaires, tests, etc.) used to acquire the data. These codebooks are generally freely available; however, access to the data files typically requires further permission.

In addition to national repositories, there are local repositories in which individual research centers or investigators have maintained a database that includes information collected on the participants in their studies over the years. Examples of this type of archival data are found for the Intergenerational study and the Mills study, located at the University of California, Berkeley. Use of this type of archival data may be made available to sponsored researchers and requires the permission of the project director.

A third way in which archival data may be obtained is through direct contact with the original researcher or research center. Some important longitudinal studies have never been formally archived in a national or local repository but may nonetheless be available to investigators who were not part of the original research team. And even those that have been archived may not include all of the data collected, either because the data were never computerized or because only a subset of the original dataset was placed in the repository. Here are two examples from my own experience. First, in reading a paper by Caspi, Bem, and Elder (1989), it became apparent that the Intergenerational files included data on a range of behavioral problems for children ages 4–16, as they were growing up. These data were not part of the Murray Center computer files, but, through the help of the archivist at the IHD, they were retrievable from the Intergenerational IHD computer files.

Similarly, staff reports of the Intergenerational study, written in 1981 (see Eichorn, Clausen, Haan, Honzik, & Mussen, 1981), mentioned that TAT stories were obtained from the children on a regular basis as they were growing up. On the basis of this information, the TAT stories told by the participants during their childhood and early adolescent years, along with stories told at age 18, were retrieved from the archival data storage area at IHD.

In a second example, earlier research reports (Peskin, 1972) indicated that Q-set items had been used to construct an index of Psychological Health, which was calculated for study participants in adolescence and adulthood. These Psychological Health measures exist in the Murray Center files. However, subsequent study of the Q-sort data indicated that certain items of the original measure were found to be unreliable at some ages. In a recent publication (Jones & Meredith, 2000) the original measure of Psychological Health has been revised, using only the 73 reliable Q-set items. Again, the helpful cooperation of a colleague allowed me to construct this important measure by providing me with the Q-items and their rating weights.

Another type of problem that occurs is that measures used at different ages, although similarly named, may in fact not be identical. For example, the CPI data (Gough & Bradley, 2002) of the Intergenerational study collected at age 30/37 and 40/47 were based on different versions of the CPI than data from age 52/60. Consequently, the scale scores at the different ages are not strictly comparable. Again, colleagues brought this fact to my attention, as well as the existence of adjusted CPI data that make scale scores comparable across ages. These data are available in the IHD files, but not in the Murray files.

Further problems associated with archival data are discussed below in the section "Complexities."

Case Example

Description of the Intergenerational Study

Most of the examples I provide in this chapter come from the IHD Intergenerational study. At this point, I describe the main features of the study. Also, because I rely on the TAT to facilitate my research on defense mechanisms, I discuss how I obtained this information from the archival files and some of the associated problems.

The Intergenerational files consist of data from two separate longitudinal studies.[2] The first study, called the Guidance study, began by enlisting every third child born in Berkeley during the years 1928–1929. This initial sample was divided into a *Guidance* group and a *Control* group, with parents of the Guidance children receiving advice from the professional child development staff over the years of the study. The children in this Guidance/Control cohort were studied intensively from birth until late adolescence, with annual or semiannual behavioral and psychological assessments, including parent interviews, interviews with teachers, ratings by peers, and IQ tests. Projective tests, including the TAT, were also given at various ages.

In order to summarize the massive amount of data collected, experienced personality researchers (advanced graduate students and PhDs) subsequently read through the extensive dossier of each child for each age period (Early Childhood, ages 5–7; Late Childhood, ages 8–10; Early Adolescence, ages 11–14; Late Adolescence, ages 15–18) . Several raters then described the child for each period, using a 104-item Q-set (Eichorn et al., 1981). Their ratings were composited to create a reliable Q-sort for each child at each age period. Information from parent interviews and test results was not provided to the raters so that their assessments would be independent from this information. In addition, it is important to note that the same raters did not Q-sort a child at more than one age, so that ratings at one age were not influenced by ratings made at another age. Other ratings were made by the staff regarding the children's health and behavior problems, personality characteristics, family relations, and personality appraisals of family members. Extensive information regarding family variables, such as income, parent education and occupation, and number of siblings, was also collected and computerized. Much of this sociodemographic information is contained in the Murray Center files.

After adolescence, the participants were followed up at approximately ages 30, 40, and 52. In addition to engaging in extensive interviews, from which Q-sorts were subsequently made, the participants completed personality inventories, received physical examinations, were given IQ tests, and provided stories to TAT cards. A further wave of data is being collected as the participants move into the seventh decade of life.

The second sample that comprises the Intergenerational study was termed the "Oakland Growth" study. This study began at early adolescence as the children were about to enter junior high school in 1932. The school personnel were contributors to the study, and a special clubhouse for the participants was set up adjacent to the school. Most data collection took place in this clubhouse and in the classroom. In addition to the collecting of behavioral and test data, interviews with the parents were carried out. On the basis of the observational data, each participant was Q-sorted by several researchers, and the composite ratings for each Q-item, for early adolescence and again for late adolescence, were computed across raters. As was the case for the Guidance/Control study, different raters did the Q-sorts for early and late adolescence. As before, parent interview and test data were not provided to the raters. This group was also followed up at three points in adulthood—at approximately ages 37, 47, and 60, with comparable procedures as those used with the Guidance/Control group.

Because the Growth study began when the participants were early adolescents, there are no data available for their childhood years. Moreover, it appears that the TAT was not given until they were age 18, when a large group of cards was administered. In contrast, the Guidance/Control sample was given the TAT throughout childhood and early adolescence; however, only two cards were consistently administered when the participants were age 18.

In my own work, these differences between the Growth and Guidance/Control samples resulted in certain limitations. For example, the relations between childhood, adolescent, and adult personality variables, and between child and adult defense use can be carried out only with the Guidance/Control group. In contrast, the relation between adolescent and adult defense use, and the question of how adolescent defense use influences adult personality change, can be reliably assessed only with the Growth sample. There is a further problem encountered when trying to combine the TAT measures from the age 30/37 assessments. Of the six TAT cards used, only three were the same for both the Growth and the Guidance/Control groups; the other three cards differed by group.

Research with the Archival Data

In this section, I describe the course of my involvement with these data, from inception to the present.

My awareness of a substantial number of TAT stories told by the Intergenerational participants during the age 30/37 assessment (1958) occurred through my professional association with another personality psychologist who was aware of my research using the TAT and of my interest in longitudinal studies. He provided me with the typed protocols of a number of TAT stories, collected during the age 30/37 assessment of the Intergenerational study. When I contacted the sender about the arrival of these protocols, he indicated that these were from an earlier assessment of participants whom he had recently interviewed and that other longitudinal data for these participants, including personality, IQ, and family measures, could be obtained from the Murray Center. After determining that the protocols were appropriate for defense coding, I began the process of coding the stories and acquiring the computerized data.

This involved contacting the Murray Center to send me the standard request form. I provided a professional *vita*, indicating my qualifications to use the data, and the purposes for which the data would be used. In addition, I obtained the permission of the Director of the Institute of Human Development, where the data had been originally collected, and paid a fee to the Murray Center.

After my request and documents were approved, I received the computerized data files, codebooks that listed variable names and acronyms, and copies of the original tests, questionnaires, and interview rating forms that had been used to create these variables. Having this extensive information was critical to understanding the nature of the large number of variables included in the file. At this point, I spent considerable time reading the codebook, familiarizing myself with the method of variable designation, and in general getting a "lay of the land."

The next step was to merge my defense-coded TAT data with the data file that had been sent to me. Once this was done, I could begin looking at connections between the existing variables and the new defense scores. At this point, I discovered that there were longitudinal data for many more participants than those for whom I had TAT stories. I contacted the archivist at IHD and provided her with the case identification numbers of the participants with missing stories. She affirmed that in the paper archives of IHD there were stories available for a number of those participants, and she alerted me to the existence of stories from an earlier assessment (age 18). For a fee, I was provided with copies of the additional age 30/37 stories. After this new group of stories were coded, the additional defense scores were added to the computerized data file. Subsequently, during a stay in Berkeley, I obtained the age 18 stories.

With the data in place, I proceeded to investigate the three types of questions discussed earlier in the section "Deciding on the Questions to Be Asked." In a first study, I determined the concurrent relation between defense use at age 30/37 and Big Five personality traits (Cramer, 2003). For this purpose, it was necessary to create Big Five scores, as these did not exist in the data file (see below). After creating Big Five measures for each of the adult ages studied (30/37, 40/47, 52/60), I next addressed the question of whether the Big Five scores changed with age, analyzing the data for men and women separately. Finally, I investigated the question of whether defense use at early adulthood (age 30/37) would predict change in Big Five traits at subsequent ages (40/47, 52/60). The results of this study showed (1) significant correlations between defenses and Big Five traits at early adulthood; (2) significant change in Big Five traits with age; and (3) that defense mechanisms were significant predictors of Big Five change.

A second study demonstrated that defenses are related to adult identity and identity change (Cramer, 2004). An important finding was that the defenses that predicted identity change were different from those that predicted Big Five change. In addition, because identity is theoretically related to life experiences, the archival data were mined for relevant information about life experiences during adulthood. Specifically, identity theory posits that love and work (*lieben und arbeiten*) are essential elements in identity development. From the archival data, it was possible to extract a number of variables that would provide this information. Significant concurrent relations between these life experience variables and adult identity were found; life experiences were also shown to predict identity change.

A third study addressed the question of whether, and how, adult adjustment and maladjustment are related to early childhood personality (Cramer & Tracy, 2005). The hypothesized model is shown in Figure 7.1. Beginning with the adult archival data, measures of psychological health, depression, and anxiety were created from the existing early adult CAQ data (see below). Then, based on theory and evidence that adjustment and personality are often related, these adjustment/ maladjustment measures were correlated with early adult personality components, which had been previously created (Haan et al., 1986) and were part of the Murray Center computerized data file.

Next, the relations between the personality components and defense use were determined. Finally, the relations between defense use and early childhood personality components, also in the Murray data file, were ascertained. For each of these steps, significant and theoretically meaningful relations were found. Then, to determine the developmental pathways from early child personality to adult adjustment/ maladjustment, we conducted a path analysis and found significant pathways from childhood to adulthood, which helped explain how defense-mediated change in adult personality contributed to adult adjustment/maladjustment.

As mentioned above, previous reports of the childhood studies with the Intergenerational sample had mentioned the existence of TAT stories collected throughout childhood and adolescence. Furthermore, published research (Caspi et al., 1989) had indicated the existence of ratings for problem behaviors throughout this time. Because I was especially interested in tracing the development of defenses, personality, and adjustment across this age period, and relating these early markers of development to later adult functioning, I was eager to obtain this information from childhood and adolescence. For this purpose, I spent a semester at the IHD, where, with unending help from the archivist, it was possible to locate, from among the many archived paper files of the Intergenerational study, numerous binders containing typescripts of TAT stories told by these children at varying ages. After making copies of these stories, I began the lengthy process of coding the stories for defense use (see below). At the same time, the archivist was able to locate the computer files containing the Problem Behavioral Rating scales and the codebooks that defined these scales.

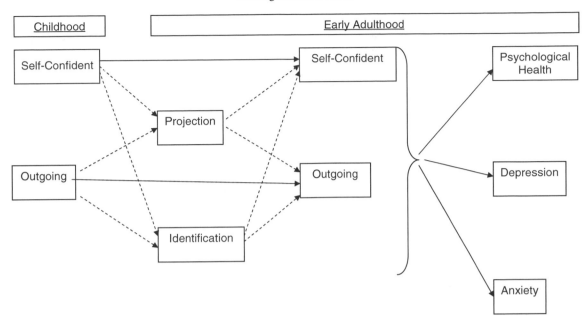

FIGURE 7.1. Conceptual model. Also modeled but not shown are the correlations between the personality constructs in childhood, between the defense mechanism disturbance terms, between the adult personality disturbance terms, and between the adjustment outcomes disturbance terms. Adjustment outcomes are regressed on all prior variables (childhood and adult personality and defense mechanisms).

Complexities

Problems Associated with the Original Data

When accessing information gathered in years past, there are inevitable complexities, and these problems likely increase as a function of the number of years elapsed since the data were collected. A recurring problem is that different types of data, or different forms of a test or questionnaire (e.g., the CPI), may have been used for different ages of data collection.

This issue immediately became evident once I began looking at the TAT stories, first collected around 1938 and continuing until 1946 (age 18), and again in early adulthood (1958). During the period that the TAT was being developed (1935–1943), the format of the test was modified. In several different versions, some pictures were changed and/or different identifying labels were used for the same pictures. As a result, some of the IHD stories collected in the 1930s–1940s had different pictures and different identifying labels than the stories told in 1958 (age 30/37). The IHD

typed protocols did not include the information needed to identify the specific TAT card that had elicited a particular story at each age. Fortunately, in the paper archives, there were copies of the old TAT pictures used at different ages, with their identifying labels, and information about the order of picture presentation. Examination of these pictures indicated that some had continued to be used in the final (and current) version of the TAT; others were dropped, and still others were created especially for the IHD assessment. I selected, for further study, those stories told in response to pictures that are part of the current version of the TAT, for which coding rules had been developed.

The Q-sort data also changed across assessments. A 104-item Q-set was used in the Childhood and Adolescent assessments. Beginning with age 30 and at each successive assessment, a 100-item Q-set was used. Ninety of the items in the child and adult versions of the Q-set have equivalent meanings (Eichorn et al., 1981). As mentioned above, subsequent analyses of the Q-sort data suggested that only 73 of the items were sufficiently reliable to be used for further study. This information is not provided in the codebooks for the computerized data file, but has been reported in published articles (Haan et al., 1986; Jones & Meredith, 2000).

Yet another type of problem with archival data points to the necessity of carefully reading the codebook. In the Intergenerational files, for the Behavioral Rating composite scores, the variable name (e.g., Selfishness) indicates the *low* end of the scale; that is, a score of 1 would indicate high Selfishness. However, for the same participants, the name of the Personality Component variables (e.g., Dependability) describes the *high* end of the scale.

Other types of problems may occur for the computerized data. Depending on the age of the archival data, it may have been created when punch cards and FORTRAN programming were used to create data files on mainframe computers. Most current researchers will wish to transform these mainframe raw data files to SPSS files. In the process of doing this, mistakes in the original FORTRAN programming and/or the original data entry may be found. These errors are easily corrected in the PC data file.

It is also a good idea to check the raw data file to determine if each participant has a unique case identification number. In the Intergenerational files, I discovered that a set of twins had been given the identical case number. In another instance, I found two different names associated with the same identification number. Fortunately, the presence of the archivist allowed this to be cleared up: The boy began using a different first name at age 18. In addition, when merging data files, it is important that all of the defining factors of the old data file, such as study group, case identification number, and sex (in the Intergenerational file sex is coded twice, as sex 1 and sex 2), are included in the new data files to be merged. If these factors do not match exactly (for example, if sex 2 is not specified), the new data will be entered as belonging to an additional participant with the same case identification number, with the result that the same participant is represented twice in the data file. Thus, after merging data, it is important to examine the raw data file to determine if a case identification number appears more than once and/or if the number of cases in the data file has changed from the premerged file.

Missing Data

In archival data, and especially in longitudinal studies, one encounters the problem of missing data. At any one age, some participants will not have scores available for all of the variables assessed at that age. Furthermore, not all of the participants who were assessed at one age will have participated in the assessment at a subsequent age. Thus, there are two types of missing data: within age and across age.

For the Intergenerational study, there were myriad variables assessed at each age during childhood, and again during the adult assessments. However, not all individuals who participated at any one age had information recorded for all the variables assessed at that age, for reasons unknown. For example, in childhood, there are children who have Behavioral Ratings for some, but not all of the 35 variables assessed at each age. In the case of the TAT data, although there was a standard set of cards to be administered at age 11 and again at age 12, there are some children who provided stories for only a subset of these cards, and this subset varies across children. My initial solution to this problem was to include in the data analytic sample only those children who had told at least four stories at a particular age, and then to take the mean across stories to represent their overall defense score. Other approaches to missing data within age may be used, such as substituting the group mean value for each missing data point, but this will reduce individual differences that may be of interest. More sophisticated procedures have also been developed that use regression and other statistical techniques to estimate missing data (see West, Aiken, Wu, & Taylor, Chapter 33, this volume).

Finding the Measures You Want

Measures Available in Computerized Data Files

Data from an extensive number of variables will be found in the computerized data files and will provide the possibility of an endless number of investigations. For example, the Intergenerational files from the Murray Center contain several thousand variables from more than 500 participants. Thus, having a general theoretical orientation and a set of flexible research questions is a necessity.

As a first step, acquiring and reading the codebooks describing the data files is crucial. These codebooks may also include the original rating or scoring sheets and the tests administered. To understand the meaning of the computerized data, it is helpful to immerse oneself in this information. I have found it helpful to print out a list of the variables in the file, which also provides information about the changing number of participants for whom data are available for each variable.

In addition, it is valuable to read earlier published papers and books based on these data. Information in these publications, even if not on the topic in which you are interested, may clarify aspects of the study and suggest new hypotheses. For example, in our study of childhood precursors of adult adjustment (Cramer & Tracy, 2005), a reading of an earlier report on psychological adjustment in this sample (Peskin, 1972) indicated that adolescent *change* in adjustment related to later psychological health. This finding contributed to my formulating a model in which defense use was hypothesized to mediate personality *change*, which in turn would predict adult adjustment.

In addition, information from the earlier publication may alert you to the existence of data that are not part of the national archival computer files, as in the case of the childhood behavioral ratings of the Intergenerational sample used by Caspi and colleagues (1989) (see above).

Once the dataset has been examined, there is the important question of which variables to select for study. For example, in the Intergenerational data for ratings of Behavior Problems, there are scores for 35 variables for each age from 4 to 16, although some variables were not rated at some ages. A decision must be made as to whether the score for each individual age will be used in subsequent analyses, or whether a composite score summed over several ages is a better, more stable representation of the child's functioning. In the IHD-based Intergenerational data files (but not in the Murray files) such composite scores have been created for ages 6, 9, 12, and 15. The same question arises with the defense mechanism scores, which are available for age 11 and for age 12. Should these scores be used separately, or combined across ages? This decision should depend on (1) whether one expects, theoretically, there to be a meaningful change over a period of 1 year

and (2) whether one finds, empirically, significant changes in the variable over the period of a year for the whole group, or for a subgroup of participants. Such variability may be an important predictor of other aspects of personality (Biesanz, West, & Kwok, 2003). Although the composite measure may be more stable, it also may obscure meaningful differences, such as change in the magnitude or direction of a correlation across the ages that have been combined. Using a composite measure will also reduce the number of participants if not all the participants were assessed at all the ages.

What to Do When the Measure You Want Is Not Part of the Dataset

As research interests change over time, personality dimensions that are currently of interest may not have been studied in the past; in this case no archival data for these dimensions will have been recorded. However, there are several ways to use the existing data to study the dimension of current interest.

First, if it is possible to identify subcomponents of the currently desired dimension, these may have been studied in the previous years. One example of this is found in the Caspi and colleagues (1989) study, in which their interest in assessing three aspects of personality not explicitly measured—moving toward, moving away, and moving against the world—was met by combining the existing variables of Dependency and Attention-Demanding (moving toward), Shyness and Excessive Reserve (moving away) and Severity plus Frequency of Temper Tantrums (moving against).

Another example of using existing variables to provide a measure of a dimension not previously assessed comes from the Intergenerational study of adult identity development (Cramer, 2004). Theoretically, the development of identity includes satisfaction in the areas of love and work and having found a "niche" in the social community (Erikson, 1968; Marcia, 1966). Inspection of the Intergenerational files indicated that information relevant to these dimensions had been collected from interviewer ratings and self-report questionnaires. Specifically, information on Work experience could be obtained from the *Hollingshead rating of occupational level*, and from the degree of *job satisfaction* as rated by the interviewer.

Love (marital and family relations) could be assessed from information regarding *satisfaction with marital relationship*, *length of marriage*, and *closeness of family relationships*. Social network was assessed from information regarding relationship with father, based on the interviewer's ratings of the *frequency of seeing father* plus ratings of the *quality* of the relationship; a similar method was used to create a measure of relationship with mother. Additional information regarding involvement with social and community groups added to this dimension. Further existing variables were used to assess other life experiences that were theoretically expected to be related to identity development.

For the purpose of this study, it was also necessary to have a measure of the four identity styles (Achieved, Moratorium, Foreclosed, Diffused). At the time that the data were collected, the concept of identity style was not part of the research literature; thus, a measure of identity was not part of the archival data. However, the existence of the CAQ data made it possible to create the needed measure. By correlating each participant's Q-scores with previously established prototype Q-sorts for each identity dimension (Mallory, 1989), it was possible to create identity scores for each Intergenerational participant. This method for establishing identity scores had previously been used successfully (e.g., Cramer, 1997; Helson, Stewart, & Ostrove, 1995). In other contexts, this use of experts to sort the CAQ items to represent different personality dimensions, such as ego control and ego resiliency, was pioneered by Block (1961) and has been used to create several new measures, including narcissism (Wink, 1992) and psychopathy (Reise & Oliver, 1994). Thus, if a measure of a desired personality dimension is not part of the data file, but CAQ data are present, a new measure can be created by having experts provide a prototype Q-sort for that dimension.

Another example of creating a desired measure comes from the study of Big Five traits in the adult assessments of the Intergenerational sample (Cramer, 2003). When these assessments were carried out, the Big Five traits had not been identified and so there were no measures of these dimensions. However, in previous research the CAQ had been factor analyzed, indicating how the 100 CAQ items comprise the five personality factors (McCrae, Costa, & Busch, 1986). To construct new CAQ-based measures of the Big Five, I created scales based on the CAQ items that had the strongest loadings on each factor. These scales could then be scored using the CAQ data available at each age (Cramer, 2003).

Another way in which existing Q-sort data may be used to produce desired measures is to create criterion-keyed scales. For example, in the study of childhood predictors of adult adjustment (Cramer & Tracy, 2005), adult measures of adjustment and maladjustment were needed. The recently revised CAQ-based Psychological Health Index (Jones & Meredith, 2000) could be used to create a measure of adjustment from the existing data files, but no variables assessing psychopathology were included in the files deposited at the Murray Center. In a previous publication with a different sample, Kremen (1996) had demonstrated that selected CAQ items correlated with criterion measures of anxiety and depression. This relation between the Q-items and the criterion pathology measures was used as the basis to create new, Q-sort item criterion-keyed measures of depression and anxiety to be used in our study.

Participant Issues

Cohort Considerations

When studying any archival data, it is important to be aware of the socioeconomic and sociocultural conditions that existed during the time that the original study was conducted. To understand the life circumstances of the participants who are preserved in archival data files, it is often informative to read earlier reports that describe the studies, such as Clausen's (1993), Elder's (1974), and Eichorn and colleagues' (1981) richly descriptive accounts of the Intergenerational studies.

The socioeconomic context may be particularly important for the Intergenerational study, because the Growth sample participants (born 1920–1921) were preadolescent and adolescent during the Great Depression, whereas the Guidance sample participants (born 1928–1929) were either in infancy or early childhood. In turn, we may expect that the Growth group had greater awareness and reaction to the tremendous economic distress of that period. Likewise, the advent of World War II, with the mobilization of troops and the ongoing wartime industry, occurred when members of the Growth group were early adults (ages 20–25), whereas the Guidance participants were in their adolescence (ages 12–17) during this time and thus not subject to direct participation in the war (Elder, 1981). Such differences in life experiences may have relevance for the development of certain personality dimensions. Interestingly, Elder (1981) concluded that because the members of the Growth group had experienced a "relatively secure phase of early development" (p. 3) and avoided joblessness by being conscripted into wartime armed services, they avoided the costs of the Great Depression. In contrast, he stressed that the Guidance participants experienced the difficult times during the "vulnerable years of early childhood . . . increasing their feelings of inadequacy during the war years" (p. 4). He suggested, however, that by middle age, the earlier differences in experiences of the two groups had little effect on development. In fact, in contrast to Elder's expectations, a comparison of the two groups at age 30/37 shows that the Growth cohort was significantly more anxious, although the two cohorts did not differ on six other personality components.[3]

Combining or Not Combining Subsamples

When archival data include participants from clearly distinguishable groups, as in the case of the Intergenerational data, the question naturally arises as to whether the groups should be combined or not. A clear advantage of combining is the increase in the number of cases available for study, whereas an advantage of keeping the samples separate is the possibility of replication. In some instances, the answer to the issue of combining participants will be determined by the research question. With the Intergenerational data, only the Guidance study includes data from childhood. Thus, any research question focusing on childhood variables will be restricted to this sample.

Furthermore, given the differences in the adolescent experience of the two samples, the two cohorts should be examined separately if one is studying variables that might be expected to be influenced by these experiences, such as financial distress, socioeconomic or educational level, but also, perhaps, personality factors such as optimism, self-confidence, or locus of control. If the findings for the two groups are comparable, then combining the two samples may be appropriate. But if noticeable differ-

ences emerge, then they are better kept separate, with the investigator looking for explanations of the differences.

In addition to there being cohort differences related to historical events, participants within a cohort are likely to have been differentially exposed to and/or affected by these conditions (cf. Olweus & Alsaker, 1991). Within the Berkeley group, participants were divided into a "Guidance" group, in which parents received advice from the professional staff, and a "Control" group. Although these participants are generally grouped together under the rubric *Guidance study*, a quick check of one personality component indicates that the Guidance group was significantly less Hostile than the Control group. This suggests (but does not prove) that the parental guidance received may have had beneficial effects for the children in that group.

Another point to consider is that what may appear to be cohort effects may be due to sampling or selection bias (Olweus & Alsaker, 1991). For the Intergenerational study, the Guidance/Control participants were originally selected to be part of a 6-year study of normal development including "the influence of intensive discussions with parents about child-rearing practices on children's problem behavior" (Eichorn et al., 1981, p. 33). Although family income was below the national average, the "parents were above average in education status and more likely to own their own homes" (Eichorn et al., 1981, p. 34). In contrast, the Oakland study was designed to investigate normal adolescence. Selection, which began at the end of elementary school, was based on the expectation that the children would attend a particular junior high school, where they could be observed; also the sample was lower in education level, relative to the Berkeley study. Thus, the basis for selection of these two cohorts was quite different, and this may have produced different patterns of findings that in retrospect appeared to be due to cohort effects.

Yet another issue arises when the purpose of the study is to compare cohorts. It may well be the case that different measures have been used for the different groups, even when similar personality constructs have been studied. For the Intergenerational sample, there is consistency across groups for certain measures, such as the CPI, CAQ, and CAQ-based measures. However, other variables, such as TAT stories and childhood and adolescent behavioral variables, differ across groups. When cohorts are composed of participants assessed at widely different time periods or research centers, the problem of different measures is more likely to occur. One example of this occurred in a study by Helson and colleagues (1995), which compared data from the California Mills College study of women (collected in 1982), the Radcliffe College study of women (collected 1991), and the Intergenerational Guidance study (collected 1969). Because Q-sort data were available for the participants in all three cohorts, it was possible to construct comparable identity style measures for all, based on Q-sort identity prototypes (see above). The authors also wished to control for possible cohort differences in intelligence, especially as these might affect identity, but the three cohorts did not share a common measure of this variable. Wechsler Adult Intelligence Scale (WAIS) scores were available for the Intergenerational cohort, Scholastic Aptitude Test (SAT) scores for the Mills cohort, and a measure of TAT-based verbal fluency was used to estimate intelligence in the Radcliffe cohort.

To determine if intelligence was differentially related to identity, the two measures were correlated within each cohort. The results showed no relation between the four identity styles and intelligence for the Guidance and Radcliffe cohorts, and only one (out of four) significant correlation for the Mills cohort. Thus, although comparable measures of intelligence were not available for all three cohorts, using different measures across cohorts and demonstrating that there was no systematic relation between intelligence and identity style in any cohort allowed the researchers to remove a possible concern about the effect of differences in intelligence.

What to Do about Participant Attrition?

It is inevitable in longitudinal studies that, over the years, participants will drop out of the sample. If one is interested in mean-level changes in a personality trait from one age to another, then different numbers of participants at each age may be used to determine the mean level of the trait at each age. However, assessing rank order stability requires data from the same participant across ages. Thus, if one wishes to study both forms of stability, only participants for whom data are available at all time periods should be included.[4] Alternatively, one might report mean-level scores both for the maximum number of participants at any one age, and for those participants (the "repeated" individuals) who were studied at all ages. Restricting analyses to the "repeated" participants can create a problem when the overall number of participants is small. For the Intergenerational data, this is not a problem for the three adult assessments. For example, considering the CAQ assessments, there are data available for 232 participants at age 30/37, 233 at 40/47, and 233 at 52/60. Of this group there are 177 participants with data at all three ages. However, there are far less data available for those who were assessed during early childhood and again at age 30. With the longer time gap and the greater number of changes in residence and other social factors between childhood and adulthood, of the 101 participants for whom childhood Q-sort data are available, only 74 have CAQ data available for age 30. Typical attrition rates for follow-up periods of 12 to 18 months are about 17–20%; attrition of 10–15%, found in some studies, is considered low. Over periods longer than 5 years, attrition may be expected to be 30% or greater.

Another point to consider is that participants drop out of longitudinal studies for various reasons, including moving away from the research area, loss of contact, loss of interest on the part of the participant, illness, and death. Moreover, attrition is greater when participants are of lower educational level and/or have been recruited by impersonal methods. The resulting change in the participant sample may, or may not, be an important factor to consider. In any case, it is important to determine if the participants differ in some significant way from nonparticipants, especially with relevance to the variables being investigated. Thus, participants and nonparticipants may be compared for their standing on relevant variables at the time of initial data collection (e.g., scores on personality variables at early childhood) to detect possible differences in the personality of those who continued in the study. However, even if there are no mean differences between participants and nonparticipants on any of the variables of interest, this does not guarantee that any observed results would have been the same if there had been no attrition.

Issues of Gender

In most archival datasets, there are data for both males and females. The question arises as to whether these data should be analyzed by gender or combined in a single analysis. If the data are analyzed by gender, then there is obviously a reduction in sample size, and consequently a reduction in power.

If there are theoretical reasons to expect gender differences, then clearly separate analyses are needed. If not, then testing for mean differences and gender interactions with the variables of interest will indicate whether separate analyses are needed. Failure to analyze separately by gender may obscure meaningful relations. For example, in the Guidance/Control sample, the correlation between use of the defense of Projection at ages 11–12 and the Behavior Rating of "Insufficient Appetite" is only .16, which is nonsignificant. However, separate gender analyses indicated that this correlation is $+.40$ for boys ($p < .05$) and $-.21$ for girls (nonsignificant). Such gender differences in the direction of the correlation are not uncommon.

Issue of Outliers

Having obtained archival data, it is important for the investigator to examine the data not only to determine missing or misidentified scores and duplicated cases (see above) but also to identify possible outlier participants, which is easily done by most statistical packages (e.g., using SPSS's Explore option). If there are such cases, it is necessary to decide whether these cases are meaningful or whether they represent measurement or data entry error. An extreme case that is due to error or other "fluke" factors may produce correlations that are not representative of the majority of the participants in the sample. If not due to error, such cases may represent meaningful deviations from the average, and so may be most informative for understanding the personality functioning of atypical or pathological cases. Eliminating a meaningful outlier restricts the range of observations, which decreases the likelihood of finding significant relations between the variables.

One way to decide whether to include the outliers is to look at statistical results with and without those participants. If the correlation is in the same direction, but perhaps not significant when they are omitted, that would be an indication to keep them in the sample. If, however, the results are in the opposite direction, the outliers might well be omitted.

Future Directions

Archival data offer myriad opportunities for continuing research. An interesting possibility is afforded by archival data to study different generations, with the possibility of disentangling maturational differences from sociohistorical differences. Because data are available for individuals of the same chronological age, but from different generations, it would be possible to study the personality, or character structure, of persons growing up during the Great Depression as compared with those identified as baby boomers, as Generation X, or Generation Y, or, most recently, as the "Millennial Generation." Archival data from the IHD Intergenerational study, the Block and Block study, and other more current investigations provide information about personality development in these different generations, which have been described in popular media as differing in personality characteristics. Despite variations in the design of these studies, creative researchers may find ways to devise measures of comparable personality constructs from the different databases and thus be able to study how personality has changed across different generations, or, alternatively, to reveal unsuspected consistency in personality structure regardless of sociohistorical change.

As an alternative to this variable-centered approach, an equally fascinating use of these multigenerational archival files might take a person-centered typological approach (e.g., Ozer & Gjerde, 1989) with the intent of determining whether there are personality types unique to each generation. This kind of cross-generational study could provide a response to the concern expressed by Block (1971)—"the possibility that longitudinal studies, by the time they are brought to some point of completion, may provide dependable results valid only about a time or circumstance that will never recur" (p. 276). If this does turn out to be the case, then these archival data are of considerable psychohistorical importance.

Acknowledgments

The cooperation of Dr. Pamela Bradley, archivist of the Intergenerational files, in obtaining both computerized and noncomputerized information from the archival files is greatly appreciated. Also, thanks to Dr. Paul Wink for providing the initial set of adult

TAT stories, and to Dr. Constance Jones for information regarding the revised version of the Psychological Health Index.

Some of the studies reported in this chapter come from the Intergenerational Longitudinal Study conducted by the Institute of Human Development at the University of California, Berkeley, and from the Intergenerational Studies datasets (made available in 1995, machine-readable data files). These data were collected by the Institute of Human Development and donated to the archives of the Henry A. Murray Research Center of Radcliffe College, 10 Garden Street, Cambridge, Massachusetts (Producer and Distributor).

Notes

1. These are the ages of the Berkeley cohort. Participants from Oakland, the second cohort of the Intergenerational study, were 7 years older.
2. A third study, the Berkeley Growth study, has far less data and did not include TAT stories.
3. These components had been identified on the basis of factor analyses of the CAQ items, and included Self-Confidence, Assertiveness, Cognitive commitment, Outgoingness, Dependability, and Warmth.
4. Use of the statistical technique of hierarchical linear modeling may overcome these problems.

Recommended Readings

Caspi, A. (2000). The child is father of the man: Personality continuities from childhood to adulthood. *Journal of Personality and Social Psychology, 78,* 158–172.

Clausen, J. (1993). *American lives: Looking back at the children of the Great Depression.* New York: Free Press.

Cramer, P., & Tracy, A. (2005). The pathway from child personality to adult adjustment: The road is not straight. *Journal of Research in Personality, 39,* 369–394.

Eichorn, D. H., Clausen, J. A., Haan, N., Honzik, M. P., & Mussen, P. H. (1981). *Present and past in middle life.* New York: Academic Press.

Elder, G. H. (1974). *Children of the Great Depression: Social change in life experience.* Chicago: University of Chicago Press.

Haan, N., Millsap, R., & Hartka, E. (1986). As time goes by: Change and stability in personality over fifty years. *Psychology and Aging, 1,* 220–232.

Jones, C. J., Livson, N., & Peskin, H. (2003). Longitudinal hierarchical linear modeling analyses of California Psychological Inventory data: From age 33 to age 75: An examination of stability and change in adult personality. *Journal of Personality Assessment, 80,* 294–308.

Magnusson, D., Bergman, L. R., Rudinger, G., & Torestad, B. (Eds.). (1991). *Problems and methods in longitudinal research: Stability and change.* Cambridge, UK: Cambridge University Press.

References

Biesanz, J. C., West, S. G., & Kwok, O-M. (2003). Personality over time: Methodological approaches to the study of short-term and long-term development and change. *Journal of Personality, 71,* 905–941.

Block, J. (1961). *The Q-sort method in personality assessment and psychiatric research.* Springfield, IL: Thomas.

Block, J. (1971). *Lives through time.* Berkeley, CA: Bancroft Books.

Block, J. & Block, J. H. (1969). *The California Child Q-Set.* Palo Alto, CA: Consulting Psychologists Press.

Block, J. H., & Block, J. (1980). The role of ego-control and ego-resiliency in the organization of behavior. In W. A. Collins (Ed.), *Development of cognition affect and social relations. Minnesota Symposia on Child Psychology* (pp. 39–101). Hillsdale, NJ: Erlbaum.

Bryk, A. S., & Raudenbush, S. W. (1987). Application of hierarchical linear modeling to assessing change. *Psychological Bulletin, 101,* 147–158.

Caspi, A. (2000). The child is father of the man: Personality continuities from childhood to adulthood. *Journal of Personality and Social Psychology 78,* 158—172.

Caspi, A., Bem, D. J., & Elder, G. (1989). Continuities and consequences of interactional styles across the life course. *Journal of Personality, 57,* 375–406.

Caspi, A., & Roberts, B. W. (1999). Personality continuity and change across the life course. In L. A. Pervin & O. P. John (Eds.), *Handbook of personality: Theory and research* (pp. 300–326). New York: Guilford Press.

Clausen, J. (1993). *American lives: Looking back at the children of the Great Depression.* New York: Free Press.

Cramer, P. (1997). Identity, personality and defense mechanisms: An observer-based study. *Journal of Research in Personality, 31,* 58–77.

Cramer, P. (2003). Personality change in later adulthood is predicted by defense mechanism use in early adulthood. *Journal of Research in Personality, 37,* 76—104.

Cramer, P. (2004). Identity change in adulthood: The contribution of defense mechanisms and life experiences. *Journal of Research in Personality, 38,* 280–316.

Cramer, P., & Block, J. (1998). Preschool antecedents of defense mechanism use in young adults. *Journal of Personality and Social Psychology, 74,* 159–169.

Cramer, P., & Tracy, A. (2005). The pathway from child personality to adult adjustment: The road is not straight. *Journal of Research in Personality, 39,* 369–394.

Eichorn, D. H., Clausen, J. A., Haan, N., Honzik, M. P., & Mussen, P. H. (1981). *Present and past in middle life*. New York: Academic Press.

Elder, G. (1974). *Children of the Great Depression: Social change in life experience*. Chicago: University of Chicago Press.

Elder, G. (1981). Social history and life experience. In D. H. Eichorn, J. A. Clausen, N. Haan, M. P. Honzik, & P. H. Mussen (Eds.), *Present and past in middle life* (pp. 3–31). New York: Academic Press.

Erikson, E. H. (1968). *Identity: Youth and crisis*. New York: Norton.

Gough, H. G., & Bradley, P. (2002). *The California Personality Inventory manual* (3rd ed.). Palo Alto, CA: CPP.

Haan, N., Millsap, R., & Hartka, E. (1986). As time goes by: Change and stability in personality over fifty years. *Psychology and Aging, 1*, 220–232.

Helson, R., Stewart, A. J., & Ostrove, J. (1995). Identity in three cohorts of midlife women. *Journal of Personality and Social Psychology, 69*, 544–557.

Jones, C. J., Livson, N., & Peskin, H. (2003). Longitudinal hierarchical linear modeling analyses of California Psychological Inventory data: From age 33 to age 75: An examination of stability and change in adult personality. *Journal of Personality Assessment, 80*, 294–308.

Jones, C. J., & Meredith, W. (2000). Developmental paths of psychological health from early adulthood to later adulthood. *Psychology of Aging, 15*, 351–360.

Kremen, A. M. (1996). Depressive tendencies and sus-ceptibility to anxiety: Differential personality correlates. *Journal of Personality, 64*, 209–242.

Mallory, M. E. (1989). Q-sort definition of ego identity status. *Journal of Youth and Adolescence, 18*, 399–411.

Marcia, J. E. (1966). Development and validation of ego-identity status. *Journal of Personality and Social Psychology, 3*, 551–558.

McCrae, R. R., Costa, P., & Busch, C. M. (1986). Evaluating comprehensiveness in personality systems: The California Q-set and the five-factor model. *Journal of Personality, 54*, 430–446.

Olweus, D., & Alsaker, F. D. (1991). Assessing change in a cohort-longitudinal study with hierarchical data. In D. Magnusson, L. R. Bergman, G. Rudinger, & B. Torestad (Eds.), *Problems and methods in longitudinal research: Stability and change* (pp. 107–132). New York: Cambridge University Press.

Ozer, D. J., & Gjerde, P. F. (1989). Patterns of personality consistency and change from childhood through adolescence. *Journal of Personality, 57*, 483–507.

Peskin, H. (1972). Multiple prediction of adult psychological health from preadolescent and adolescent behavior. *Journal of Consulting and Clinical Psychology, 38*, 155–160.

Reise, S. P., & Oliver, C. J. (1994). Development of a California Q-set indicator of primary psychopathy. *Journal of Personality Assessment, 62*, 130–144.

Wink, P. (1992). Three narcissism scales for the California Q-set. *Journal of Personality Assessment, 58*, 51–66.

## CHAPTER 8

Using the Internet for Personality Research

What Can Be Done, How to Do It, and Some Concerns

R. Chris Fraley

During the past few years, an increasing number of psychologists have begun to use the Internet as a tool for conducting personality research. It is easy to understand the appeal of using the Web for research purposes. Just about any study that can be conducted via traditional pencil-and-paper methods can be implemented online, but without the hassles of data entry by hand, the scheduling of participants, and paper costs. Moreover, researchers who use computers in their experiments for manipulating visual or narrative stimuli, randomizing trials, or creating customized assessments can easily implement their protocols online. Most important, although researchers can use the Web simply as an efficient way to collect data from undergraduates in their departmental subject pools, the Web allows us to open our laboratory doors to people from across the world.

In this chapter I discuss the potential of the Internet for the way psychologists collect data in personality research. One of the themes of this chapter is that the Internet provides a valuable medium through which researchers can implement traditional methods of data collection (e.g., questionnaires) as well as more complex methods (e.g., ideographic assessment) that would be difficult to realize without the interactive features of the Internet. Moreover, because the Internet is coming to play an enduring role in the way in which people work and communicate, one of the fundamental tasks for the next generation of personality scientists is to learn how to make the most of this rapidly expanding technology for the study of personality. I begin the chapter by reviewing some of ways in which the Internet can be used in personality research. Some of the methods and techniques I discuss will be familiar to those well versed in traditional paper-and-pencil techniques. Other methods are more inventive and have the potential to advance personality research in novel directions. Next, I provide a tutorial on how to create an online personality questionnaire. The tutorial describes how to obtain a Web server, as well as how to create an online questionnaire that provides feedback to participants and automatically records and stores the data. The tutorial is not designed to demonstrate all of the creative things that can be done using the Internet, but it will serve as a useful stepping stone for helping to get the interested reader started in collecting personality data online. Finally, I review and address some of the concerns that psychologists have about data collected over the Internet. I attend specifically to issues concerning sampling, the thoughtfulness of Internet respondents, and some of the ethical issues that arise when conducting Internet research (e.g., how should consent be obtained? how secure are Internet data?). I begin the chapter by explaining briefly how the Internet works and introducing some of the critical concepts that are relevant for understanding the role that the Internet can play in personality science.

How the Internet Works: Some Important Concepts and Definitions

Because so many researchers use the Internet on a regular basis, it is easy for them to take the process for granted. After all, the process seems relatively straightforward: You type in a Web address, click on various links, and, for the most part, sit back and enjoy the show. However, there are many complex things taking place beneath the surface that make this seemingly simple experience possible. First, when you type a *URL* (universal resource locator) or Web address (e.g., *www.psych.uiuc.edu/ ~rcfraley*) into your computer's browser, your computer sends a request to another computer "located" at that address. This computer is often called a *server*, and its job is to receive such requests and then "serve" the requested information back to you, the user. More often than not, the kind of information that is sent to your browser is a file that is coded in the form of *hypertext markup language*, or *HTML*. HTML has become one of the most commonly used means of sharing information over the Internet. Your Web browser translates the code in the HTML file that it receives from the server into the kinds of webpages with which we are familiar. Thus, as a Web user, you never see the HTML code per se, only the rendered version

of the code. (If you want to see the HTML code, you can right-click on the webpage in Windows and choose the "view source" option.)

In your typical day-to-day experience with the Web, you probably do little more than view your favorite webpages or link from one page to another in hope of discovering something new or interesting. Sometimes, however, your Web experience may be more complex than this. You may, for example, use the Web to order a book from an online retailer, such as Amazon.com. In this case, the server is doing something a bit more complex than simply serving you the same HTML files that it serves everyone. It may, for example, be storing your shipping address or tracking items you have purchased in the past in order to make recommendations for other products you might enjoy. The pages you see in these cases are typically created "on the fly," just for you.

In these situations, the server is performing a number of tasks that make your Web experience highly dynamic and interactive. This kind of interactivity is one reason that the Internet is such an exciting frontier for personality research. Consider, for example, an assessment paradigm in which the kinds of questions that are asked of a research subject are conditional upon the answers that the subject has given previously, much in the way that the "recommended book titles" that Amazon.com shows you are dependent on books you have purchased or viewed in the past. In Computerized Adaptive Testing (CAT; see Wainer, 1990) a person is administered items that are dynamically tailored to the person's evolving item response pattern—a procedure that would be extraordinarily difficult to implement via traditional paper-and-pencil methods. Researchers can use this kind of interactivity to create short, but powerful, assessment instruments, or to probe about certain constructs (e.g., marital satisfaction) only once other facts about an individual's life have been established (e.g., the person is married). This latter form of interactivity allows researchers to implement the kinds of "skip patterns" that are commonly used in questionnaire research without asking the subject to literally skip from one question to the next (a process that may lead to subject errors).

What enables this level of interactivity? This interactivity is made possible by programs called *CGI scripts* that run on the server. CGI, which stands for *common gateway interface*, is a method or protocol by which the server interacts with other software on the server (e.g., databases), as well as with other computers on the Web. There are a number of programming languages that can be used for writing CGI scripts (e.g., ASP, C++, Cold Fusion, Perl, PHP). Each of these languages has a steep learning curve, but there are only a few critical techniques that a researcher needs to understand in order to use each language. Once these basic techniques are mastered, it is quite easy to build complex, interactive webpages simply by combining those techniques in creative ways.

The Potential of the Internet for Research on Personality

There are many ways in which online research may benefit personality researchers. One of the most significant is that the use of the Internet allows researchers to study people using interactive-dynamic methods. This not only allows us to make the research more interesting for our research participants, it also allows us to create and use more innovative and flexible assessment protocols. In addition, using the Internet allows us to study people in a way that is relatively independent of location. People can participate in research at home, in the lab, in Internet cafés, at libraries, or anywhere else where an Internet connection is available. In fact, as wireless technology evolves, our ability to interface with our research subjects will continue to expand, allowing for increasingly innovative research opportunities.

In the following sections I briefly review some of the many techniques and research designs that can be implemented via the Internet. As the reader will notice, many of these techniques are not unique to the medium; they are what Skitka and Sargis (2005) call "transitional" applications of the Internet—online realizations of traditional research paradigms. In fact, many of the techniques I discuss can be realized via computers more generally, but implementing them online can be valuable because it provides a decentralized way to conduct research—a way that is less bounded by time and geography. Other techniques that I discuss are unique to the medium and simply cannot be done easily or in a cost-effective manner using traditional research tools. The fact that the Internet can be used for both traditional and novel purposes makes it a valuable methodological tool for personality researchers.

Collecting Questionnaire Data

The most obvious (and basic) use of the Internet for personality research is for the collection of questionnaire data. By placing questionnaires online, it is relatively easy to obtain a large amount of data that can be used for a variety of purposes, such as questionnaire development, item analyses, collecting norms, or doing correlational research. One of the key benefits of collecting questionnaire data online is that the responses can be automatically stored by the Web server. Thus, the use of the Internet eliminates the lackluster task of data entry. By automating this part of the process, research assistants have time free to contribute to the more meaningful and intellectually challenging phases of a research project. Moreover, because the data are stored automatically, they are immediately available to the research team. This allows researchers to monitor the progress of a study quite easily—a feature that can be valuable in the early stages of a research project.

Randomizing the Order of Stimuli

One of the limitations of the traditional paper-and-pencil format is that it does not allow the order of questionnaire items to be randomized across subjects. Randomization is a valuable tool because, theoretically, it eliminates any order effects that might be present in item responses. It is quite simple to create a CGI script that randomizes the order in which questions/stimuli are presented (or even to randomize the order in which different questionnaires are presented). An important feature is that the questions can be presented in a different order for each participant while still having the responses saved in the same order for all participants in the main dataset.

Random Assignment to Conditions

One of the advantages of random assignment to conditions is that it allows hypotheses about causal processes to be tested in a relatively rigorous manner. As one might imagine, it is possible to instruct the server to randomly assign people to different conditions of an experiment. For example, if one were interested in studying the way in which item responses are affected by different instructional sets, a CGI script can be written to randomly assign participants to different instructional conditions.

Substitution and Idiographic Assessment

In programming, the process of substitution refers to a programming language's ability to take information (e.g., information provided by a research subject) and substitute it into generic programming code, thereby producing output that is customized within certain constraints. The process of substitution can be valuable in personality research because it enables researchers to better study the idiosyncratic ways in which a person construes his or her social world. For example, Grice (2004) recently wrote a program for assessing personality structure, inspired by the repertory grids of George Kelly's personal construct theory (Kelly, 1955). In Grice's program, Ideogrid, people can nominate different selves or roles as well as different adjectives that may be used to describe themselves in these different contexts. The program then draws upon the user-supplied information to query the person about the way these roles and descriptors interface. In other words, the program uses the ideographic information provided by the subject in order to create an assessment protocol that is uniquely tailored to the subject. Although Ideogrid is currently available as a stand-alone application (i.e., one that can be installed and run on an individual computer) rather than as an Internet program, the ideas that inspired Ideogrid could be implemented online using CGI scripting.

Making the Debriefing Process Personally Meaningful to Research Subjects

In university settings, the use of student subject pools is often predicated on the research experience being an educational one for students. During a typical debriefing, however, we usually have nothing to tell our subjects about *their* personalities; the best we can do is explain the purpose of the research, summarize previous findings, and provide them with contact information in case they want to learn more when the study is complete. With Internet-based research, it is possible to provide the participant not only with an overview of the research field, but also with feedback about his or her personality and/or the aggregated results of the study to date. Indeed, the opportunity to learn more about themselves through the use of scientifically developed tests might be one of the primary reasons why people take the time to participate in research outside the laboratory.

If a researcher is assessing a construct for which a scoring method already exists, it is easy enough to instruct the CGI script to compute the subject's scale scores and then report those scores, along with a customized interpretation (using the substitution methods described previously), to the subject. Moreover, it is possible to instruct the server to perform simple analyses (e.g., compute means, SD's, correlations) on the data from the overall sample so that the results can be reported to the subject right away. The "automated data-analysis" feature can also be created so that it can be performed at a later date by the subject in case he or she wants to see how the study is progressing. In fact, this feature can be used by the researcher as a way to monitor the progress of the study as it is taking place.

Adaptive Testing

One of the disadvantages of traditional personality assessment is that more questionnaire items are used than are necessary to assess a person's trait score accurately. If a person high in Neuroticism has already endorsed items such as "I tend to worry a lot" and "I sometimes feel anxious for no apparent reason," administering an item such as "I do not worry a lot" does not provide much additional information for locating the person's score on the trait continuum. One of the objectives of computerized adaptive testing is to make the assessment process more efficient. By iteratively estimating a person's trait level and selecting items based on those estimates, it is possible to home in on a person's trait level much more efficiently than is possible in traditional paper surveys (Wainer, 1990; Waller & Reise, 1989). This enables the test to tailor itself to the person. Adaptive testing can be implemented online, thereby allowing researchers to assess traits using as few items as necessary. This has the benefit of allowing researchers to free up time for assessing additional constructs or to reduce the total number of questions a person has to answer.

The Measurement of Response Times

When a browser requests information from a Web server, the Web server is capable of recording the time at which the request was made. Thus, by instructing the server to track these times, it is possible to use simple subtraction to calculate the amount of time a person spends on any one page. For example, if a person submits a response to question 14 at 3:51:23 P.M. and submits his or her response to question 15 at 3:51:28 P.M., the participant's response time for question 15 would be calculated as 5 seconds.

This method, although relatively crude, can be useful for a variety of research purposes. Imagine a research situation in which one is interested in the recall of episodic memories. The subject is asked to recall a time from his or her past in which he or she felt happy and click a button when this memory is fully retrieved. The retrieval time can be estimated as the difference between the time when the page was originally delivered to the subject and the time when the response was submitted. If one were interested in studying the relationship between recall times and personality traits, for example, one could examine the association between these estimated retrieval times and a variety of individual differences constructs. The assessment of response times would, of course, be subject to more error than would be obtained in a laboratory session because of the variation in connection speeds, processor speeds, and server traffic, but, theoretically, those errors would be random and uncorrelated with experimental condition or personality traits.

This particular approach, although useful for a wide variety of circumstances, is not appropriate for studying psychological processes that occur very quickly because it can take anywhere from 1 to 3 seconds for a full transaction to take place between a user's browser and the Web server. If one wanted to assess response times with greater fidelity, it would be possible to do so by using *plug-ins*—programs that can be downloaded and run on the subjects' browsers. One of the most commonly used plug-ins is Macromedia's Flash. Once the plug-in is installed on the user's computer, the study can be run on the subject's computer itself; there does not need to be an active connection sustained between the subject and the server. When the session is complete, the data are transmitted back to the server for processing and storage.

Display Graphics, Animation, and Sound

Although it is possible to display graphics in traditional paper-and-pencil questionnaires, the kind of photocopying our budgets allow for rarely allow us to reproduce high-quality images. Online, however, it is possible to present images that both look good and download quickly, owing to advanced image compression techniques. More important, it is possible to present animated images or interactive features, such as sliding rating scales.

The use of plug-ins allows for an even more sophisticated use of graphics and sound. Niedenthal and her colleagues recently developed an interesting paradigm for studying the processing of emotional stimuli (Niedenthal, Brauer, Robin, & Innes-Ker, 2002). Using a computer, Niedenthal and colleagues asked participants to view a movie of a person experiencing a specific emotional state. In the movie, the person begins expressing an emotional state, such as sadness, but the image gradually evolves to a neutral expression. Participants are asked to press a button to stop the movie at the point at which they believe the actor is no longer experiencing the emotional state in question. There is quite a bit of interindividual variation in the point at which people stop the movie, suggesting that people may be differentially sensitive to emotional cues. In principle, this paradigm could be implemented online, allowing for a wide range of individual differences to be studied easily with respect to affective processing (see Fraley, Niedenthal, Marks, Brumbaugh, & Vicary, 2006).

Sound can also be used to advantage with a plug-in such as Flash. Baldwin and his colleagues have recently begun to adapt classic tone conditioning paradigms to condition specific tones to feelings of social acceptance and rejection (see Baldwin & Kay, 2003, for an example). Although there is some risk in conducting such a study online because it is difficult to control the ambient sounds in a person's environment, if the paradigm were to work online, it would open exciting new avenues for personality research.

Multiple Data-Gathering Inputs (Text, Rating Scales, Coordinates)

There are many ways in which data can be collected via traditional paper-and-pencil methods. One can collect open-ended responses, narratives, rankings, and ratings. Each of these formats is possible in an Internet survey as well. In fact, one of the valuable features of collecting open-ended responses from people is that these typed responses do not need to be transcribed. In addition, subjects can use "radio buttons," a special way of collecting ratings online, to provide ratings for response scales. It is also possible to provide a graphical representation of a response scale and have the coordinates of the mouse click used as the item response. This can be used to obtain more graded, continuous measurements, or to provide more creative input methods. (American corporate websites often have users indicate their state of residence by clicking on the appropriate state on a map of the United States. The server can easily process the coordinates of the mouse click to record the appropriate state.) With the use of a plug-in, one can even implement a card-sorting procedure online in order to gather Q-sort data.

Longitudinal Research

Because an increasing number of people have access to the Internet, via personal computer, wireless personal data assistants (PDAs), and phones, it is possible to study people more easily across time and in different life contexts. Park, Armeli, and Tennan (2004) conducted a daily Internet study in which participants logged onto a website and completed self-report measures of stress, coping, and affect once a day for 28 days. The use of usernames and passwords allowed the researchers to keep track of different people's data. This method provided an efficient way to study people across time. Moreover, because the Web server automatically records the time at which a response is submitted in Internet diary research, there is less ambiguity about the authenticity of responses than there is when traditional diary methods are used to study people over time (see Reis & Gable, 2000).

Internet Behavior

Although I have focused on using the Internet as a method, many writers have highlighted the use of the Internet as a genuine life context—one that can be revealing of social and personality processes in its own right. For example, Vazire and Gosling (2004) studied the way in which people's personalities might be manifested in their websites. They found that accurate personality judgments, particularly in the domains of Extraversion and Agreeableness, could be made about people based on nothing more than the information provided on those people's websites. Other writers have highlighted the potential value of studying online behavior as manifested in online discussion forums, social networks, and dating (for reviews, see McKenna & Bargh, 2000; McKenna, Green, & Gleason, 2002).

How to Collect Data over the Internet

How does one go about collecting data on the Web? In this section I explain some of the basics of collecting data over the Internet. I do not provide a comprehensive tutorial on how to implement all of the techniques discussed previously, but I explain how to perform some of the more basic steps in personality research, such as collecting self-report data, processing those data to provide feedback to the user, and storing the data on the server. As we move through the tutorial, I direct the reader to additional resources for learning more about Internet methods.

In this tutorial we create two kinds of files. The distinction between the two file types is critical. The first kind of file is an HTML file—a file that contains HTML code for a webpage designed to collect personality data. HTML files often end with the extension *.htm*. Thus, if you create a webpage using HTML called "mypage," the full file name will be *mypage.htm*. The second kind of file we discuss is a CGI script, written in the Perl programming language. We use the *.pl* extension for CGI scripts. Thus, if you create a CGI script called "processdata," its full file name will be *processdata.pl*. As I explain later, these distinct kinds of files, HTML and CGI files, must be stored in separate directories on your Web server.

In order to collect data over the Internet, the first thing one needs is access to a Web server. There are at least three ways to obtain such access. One could transform an old computer into a server by downloading and installing the appropriate software (e.g., Apache; see *www.apache.org*). This approach is rather advanced and is not recommended for people who are new to Internet research. A second approach is to use the server associated with your department, university, or organization. The advantage of this approach is that it does not require server maintenance on your part. You will, however, be constrained by the rules of the organization. Some universities, for example, will supply you with ready-made CGI scripts for performing some functions (e.g., processing forms via e-mail), but will not allow you to use scripts that you create. A third approach—the one I recommend—is to use a professional Web hosting service. There are many Web hosting companies that will allow you to use customized CGI scripts for a trivial fee. The hosting company I use, Netfirms (*www.netfirms.com*) offers Web space with CGI capacity for free, as long as you are willing to let it place small ads at the tops of your pages. For a small fee (about $5 per month) you can pay Netfirms to remove the ads. The advantage of using a professional hosting service is that the company will house and maintain the servers.

Setting Up a Netfirms Server

In this section I show you how to obtain a Web server through the Netfirms service. I show you how to obtain a free account so that we can work through the examples at no cost to you. If you find the techniques discussed to be useful, you should consider paying for the service so that you can have the Netfirms ads removed.

The first thing you will need to do is visit the Netfirms website at *www.netfirms.com*. Find a link labeled "Free Web Hosting" in the lower portion of the page and click it. After clicking the "signup now" button, you will be asked to choose a domain name. A *domain name* is like a street address—a label that allows your website to be kept distinct from others. Amazon's domain name, for example, is *amazon.com*. The domain name for the University of Illinois Department of Psychology is *psych.uiuc.edu*. If you would like to create a truly customized domain name, you will need to register it and pay a fee. If you would like your domain name to be a subdomain of *netfirms.com* (e.g., *amazon.netfirms.com* or *psychuiuc.netfirms.com*), you can choose a subdomain name for free by clicking the "I prefer a free Netfirms sub domain." Simply select a name and, if the name is not already in use, Netfirms will take you to the next stage in which you review and place your order. Once the registration process

is complete, Netfirms will e-mail you a username and password for accessing your new website.

Transferring Files to and from Your Website

Now that you have a Web server, you will need a way to transfer the files (both HTML files and CGI scripts) that you create to the server and vice versa. The file transfer process is one that many people find confusing. To make it seem as intuitive as possible, you will need to conceptualize the process as one that is analogous to transferring files from your office computer to your home computer and vice versa. If you work on a file called "*my_next_article.doc*" on your office computer, go home, and then open a previous draft of the file called "*my_next_article.doc*" on your home computer, you will discover that the file at home does not contain the changes that you made in the office. In order to keep the file up-to-date, you have to transfer the revised file from your office to your home computer via e-mail, disk, thumb drive, or some other means. Similarly, the next day when you return to the office, you need to ensure that you bring the most up-to-date version of the file with you from home.

The same logic applies to the file transfer process on the Internet. When you create a webpage for collecting personality data, you will be creating the appropriate file on *your* computer. However, in order for that file to function as a webpage, you will need to transfer it to the Web server. Because the Web server is not located in your home or office, you need to use a special interface in order to transfer the files correctly.

Fortunately, Netfirms provides an interface that allows you to upload files from your computer to the Web server (and vice versa). To access this interface, go the to main Netfirms website at *www.netfirms.com* and click on the "members" tab near the top. Doing so will take you to a log-in screen where you will enter your member name and your password. (This information was e-mailed to you by Netfirms when you created your account.) If you log in successfully, you'll be taken to a new page that provides you with basic page statistics (e.g., how much bandwidth you have used, how many visitors you have had to your site). Click on the option called "File Manager" on the left-hand side of the screen. This will open a Web-based file transfer interface application.

The File Manager application works in the same way that the My Computer application works in Windows. When the application is active, you will see a display of directories and files on your Netfirms server account. You can open a folder or directory by clicking on it. You can move up through a directory by clicking the "up" icon. To copy/transfer a file from your computer to the server, simply click the icon called "upload." Use the browse "button" option to find the file on your computer and then upload it to the server. To download a file from your server to your computer, find the file, check the box next to the file's name, and click the "download" icon to the far right of the line for that file.

The Structure of Your Netfirms Directories

When you log onto your Netfirms Web server, you should notice two directories or folders: one called "*www*" and one called "*cgi-bin*." The distinction between these directories is important. The www folder will be used to hold any webpages you create. Any file that you place in this directory can be viewed over the Web. Thus, if I were to transfer a file called "*researchproposal1.htm*" to my *www* directory, anyone could view it by going to the following URL: *fraleychapter.netfirms.com/ researchproposal1.htm*. The other directory, cgi-bin, will contain any CGI scripts you write for the purposes of creating interactive webpages. If I were to create a script called "*study1script.pl*," I would transfer it to my *cgi-bin* directory and it would have the following address: *fraleychapter.netfirms.com/ cgi-bin/study1script.pl*. Please note that although the "*cgi-bin*" appears as part of the Web address for CGI scripts, the "*www*" does not appear as part of the Web address for the documents placed in the www folder.

To review, there are three key ideas you need to keep in mind as you work with files on your server. First, your Web server has two folders, the *www* directory and the *cgi-bin* directory. Webpages that you create with the **.htm* extension should be transferred to the *www* directory of your Web server to be viewed or used by other people over the Internet. CGI scripts that you write should be transferred to the *cgi-bin* directory so that they can be run on the server. Second, when you create HTML and

CGI files on your computer, you will need to transfer them to the server before they can be used by others. Finally, the files you transfer to your server will automatically be given Web addresses. Any HTML file, such as mypage.htm, that you send to your www directory will have a URL of the following form: *myaccount.net-firms.com/mypage.htm*. Any CGI script, such as myscript.pl, that you send to the cgi-bin directory will have a URL of the following form: *myaccount.netfirms.com/cgi-bin/myscript.pl*.

Creating a Basic Personality Questionnaire Using HTML

Figure 8.1 shows a webpage for a simple four-item questionnaire designed to assess individual differences in attachment security. You can explore the questionnaire online at the following URL: *fraleychapter.netfirms.com/ study1.htm*. There are a few things to note about this questionnaire. First, there are several distinct ways of obtaining input from the user. One kind of input is text-based and is called a *text box*. Using a text box, users freely type information into the space provided. The second kind of input is a *pull-down menu*. For this input option, the user clicks on the menu to see the available response options and then chooses the most appropriate option. The third kind of input option is called a *radio button*, an input option commonly used in Likert-type rating scales. For this kind of input, the user simply clicks a button corresponding to his or her response. It is important to note that if the user changes his or her mind and chooses another option, the previous choice disappears; only one radio button within a set of buttons can be selected at once.

Figure 8.2 shows the HTML code used to generate this questionnaire. If you do not have any programming experience, some of this code may look intimidating, but I assure you that it is quite intuitive once you begin to study it. The actual HTML commands are given within the "<" and ">" signs and are called *tags*. For example, the first tag, <HTML>, instructs the user's browser to interpret the code to follow as if it is HTML code (which it is). Many HTML tags allow you to modify the appearance of text and images on a webpage. For example, the tag <B> allows you to set the text in bold. Some tags, such as the <B> tag, have what are called "closing tags," such as </B>. Closing tags are used when a command is rele-

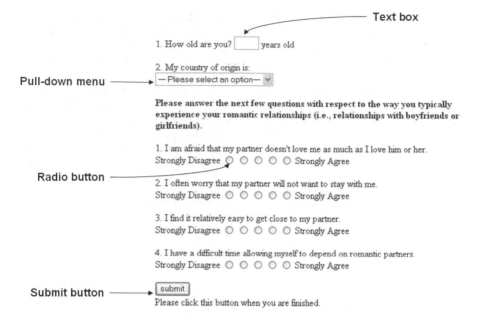

FIGURE 8.1. An illustration of various input devices on a webpage.

vant only to a certain portion of the page, as may be the case when only certain parts of the text should be printed in bold.

The tag for creating a radio button follows this generic form:

```
<INPUT TYPE = 'radio' NAME = 'v01' value='1'>
```

The TYPE attribute inside the Input tag instructs the browser as to which kind of response option to create (a radio button, in this case), the NAME attribute provides a name for the response option, and the VALUE attribute provides a numeric assignment for the option. Notice that for our first questionnaire item, we have several of these tags:

```
<INPUT TYPE = 'radio' NAME = 'v01' value='1'>
<INPUT TYPE = 'radio' NAME = 'v01' value='2'>
<INPUT TYPE = 'radio' NAME = 'v01' value='3'>
<INPUT TYPE = 'radio' NAME = 'v01' value='4'>
<INPUT TYPE = 'radio' NAME = 'v01' value='5'>
```

This set of commands crates five radio button options, each one corresponding to a different numeric value (which represents the subject's item response). Notice that each response option within a set, however, is assigned the same name (i.e., "v01"). This ensures that the variable v01 can assume only one value, despite the fact that five possible response options exist.

Notes on Use and Customization

To use this file, all you need to do is enter the HTML text into a blank document in a word processor and save it as "*study1.htm*." (I have made the code available at *fraleychapter.netfirms.com/* so that you can copy and paste it instead of typing it verbatim.) Unfortunately, Microsoft Word is not an ideal choice for this purpose because it often renders HTML code automatically (i.e., it displays the code as a webpage rather than an HTML file per se). Instead of using Microsoft Word, you may want to consider using Notepad—a free application that is installed with Windows. Notepad, however, has a nasty habit of adding "*.txt*" to all of your file extensions, so when you save the file, make sure it is saved with the appropriate extension.

The example HTML code shown in Figure 8.2 is designed to be a template to help you build webpages that will meet your needs. It is not designed to illustrate all of the things that can be accomplished with HTML; you will need to refer to additional sources for such purposes (see "Recommended Reading"). These resources discuss in more depth which HTML tags exist and how they can be used.

If you want to customize this file, you will need to consider the following:

```
<HTML>
<FORM ACTION = '/cgi-bin/study1results.pl' METHOD = post>

1. How old are you?
<INPUT TYPE = 'textbox' SIZE = '3' MAXSIZE = '3' NAME = 'age'> years old
<BR><BR>

2. My country of origin is: <BR>
<SELECT NAME = 'country' SIZE = '1'>
<OPTION VALUE = '0' SELECTED>-<197>Please select an option--</OPTION>
<OPTION VALUE = '1'>USA</OPTION>
<OPTION VALUE = '2'>CANADA</OPTION>
<OPTION VALUE = '3'>MEXICO</OPTION>
<OPTION VALUE = '4'>OTHER</OPTION>
</SELECT>
<BR><BR>

<B>Please answer the next few questions with respect to the way you typically experience
your romantic relationships (i.e., relationships with boyfriends or girlfriends).</B>
<BR><BR>

1. I am afraid that my partner doesn't love me as much as I love him or her. <BR>
Strongly Disagree
<INPUT TYPE = 'radio' NAME = 'v01' value='1'>
<INPUT TYPE = 'radio' NAME = 'v01' value='2'>
<INPUT TYPE = 'radio' NAME = 'v01' value='3'>
<INPUT TYPE = 'radio' NAME = 'v01' value='4'>
<INPUT TYPE = 'radio' NAME = 'v01' value='5'>
Strongly Agree
<BR><BR>

2. I often worry that my partner will not want to stay with me. <BR>
Strongly Disagree
<INPUT TYPE = 'radio' NAME = 'v02' value='1'>
<INPUT TYPE = 'radio' NAME = 'v02' value='2'>
<INPUT TYPE = 'radio' NAME = 'v02' value='3'>
<INPUT TYPE = 'radio' NAME = 'v02' value='4'>
<INPUT TYPE = 'radio' NAME = 'v02' value='5'>
Strongly Agree
<BR><BR>

3. I find it relatively easy to get close to my partner. <BR>
Strongly Disagree
<INPUT TYPE = 'radio' NAME = 'v03' value='1'>
<INPUT TYPE = 'radio' NAME = 'v03' value='2'>
<INPUT TYPE = 'radio' NAME = 'v03' value='3'>
<INPUT TYPE = 'radio' NAME = 'v03' value='4'>
<INPUT TYPE = 'radio' NAME = 'v03' value='5'>
Strongly Agree
<BR><BR>

4. I have a difficult time allowing myself to depend on romantic partners. <BR>
Strongly Disagree
<INPUT TYPE = 'radio' NAME = 'v04' value='1'>
<INPUT TYPE = 'radio' NAME = 'v04' value='2'>
<INPUT TYPE = 'radio' NAME = 'v04' value='3'>
<INPUT TYPE = 'radio' NAME = 'v04' value='4'>
<INPUT TYPE = 'radio' NAME = 'v04' value='5'>
Strongly Agree
<BR><BR>

<INPUT TYPE = 'submit' VALUE = 'submit'>
<BR>Please click this button when you are finished.

</FORM>
</HTML>
```

FIGURE 8.2. HTML code for the basic questionnaire illustrated in Figure 8.1.

1. You can easily copy-and-paste your items into this basic template. You will probably want to change the anchor labels, the questionnaire items, and the instructions. To add text to the webpage, you do not need to do anything more complicated than paste the text into the appropriate place in the file.

2. If you want to add a line break or a carriage return, you must insert special code. Simply pressing the "return" key won't work. The code for a line break is <BR>. You can use as many line breaks as you wish. In addition, if you want to insert more than one space (e.g., for the purposes of formatting your text), you will need to use a special piece of code, , which stands for "nonbreaking space." You can string several of these together to create a series of empty spaces.

3. When adding additional questionnaire items, be sure that the various radio buttons for a given item all have the same name.

4. When you save your file, remember that you need to use Netfirm's File Manager application to transfer it to the www directory of your Web server. If you do not transfer the file, the revised file will not be available to users on the Internet; the file will be on your personal computer only.

5. If the name of your HTML file is "study1.htm," you should be able to access it online by going to the following address: *yourdomain.netfirms.com/study1.htm*. If you submit your data at this point, however, you will get an error because we have yet to create a CGI script for processing those data. We will do this next. The line <FORM ACTION = '/cgi-bin/study1results.pl' METHOD = post> instructs the server as to which CGI script to run when the data are submitted, and that file name will need to be altered if you use a name different than "*study1results.pl*" in your own applications.

Creating a CGI Script to Process the Questionnaire Data

Now that we have an Internet questionnaire for collecting data, we need a way to process and save those data when they are submitted by the user. This processing can be accomplished with a CGI script. As mentioned before, it is possible to write CGI scripts in a number of languages; the script that I explain below is written in a language called Perl—a programming language that is quite flexible and relatively easy to use. Figure 8.3 shows the code for a CGI script called *study1results.pl* that will process our data. I have broken the script into distinct segments so that I can discuss the various tasks that the script will perform. The first few lines of code will be present in any CGI script that you write; they simply tell the server what kind of program the current file is and how to acquire the data submitted by the user. The next block of commands is designed to extract the data that were submitted by the participant and assign those data to variables that can be used within the CGI script itself. In English, the first of these Perl commands, $age= $query-param('age');, translates to "take the quantity submitted by the user labeled 'age' and call it '$age' within this CGI script." Notice that the name of the variables we used in the HTML file (e.g., age, country, v01) are used here too. Notice also that we have placed a dollar sign in front of the variable names that will be used in the CGI script itself. Thus, the age variable will be represented as $age. The use of the dollar sign allows Perl to distinguish easily between variables and nonvariables. It is also important to note that each line of commands ends with a semicolon.

The next set of commands will compute scale scores for the participant based on his or her item responses. The first two questionnaire items are measures of attachment-related anxiety. Because both items are keyed in the direction of anxiety, we can estimate the person's score simply by averaging his or her responses to these items. The command $anxiousAttachment = ($v01 + $v02)/2; instructs the Web server to create a new variable called $attachmentAnxiety and let it equal the sum of the values for items 1 and 2 (i.e., $v01 and $v02), divided by 2. The next line computes a score for attachment-related avoidance based on items 3 and 4 (i.e., $v03 and $v04). Because item 3 is keyed in the low anxiety or secure direction, we reverse-key it when we compute the average by subtracting 6 (one value higher than the highest value possible) from the actual response.

The next set of commands is designed to extract the date and time that the data were submitted, as well as the user's Internet protocol (IP) address. I will not explain these commands in depth because they are the kinds of commands you will use in any script you write. The only important—and quirky—things you need to know are that the variable "$year" repre-

```perl
#!C:/perl/bin/perl.exe
use CGI;
$query = new CGI;

# Import the submitted data into this script

$age= $query->param('age');
$country= $query->param('country');
$v01= $query->param('v01');
$v02= $query->param('v02');
$v03= $query->param('v03');
$v04= $query->param('v04');

# Compute the subject's scale scores for the two attachment dimensions

$anxiousAttachment = ($v01 + $v02)/2;
$avoidantAttachment = ((6-$v03) + $v04)/2;

# Obtain the date and time of the submission, as well as the user's IP address

($sec,$min,$hour,$mday,$mon,$year,$wday,$yday,$isdst) = localtime(time);
$ip= $query->remote_addr();

# Open a text file and save the user's data as a new row within the file

open(INFO, ">>$ENV{'DOCUMENT_ROOT_OLD'}/www/study1data.txt");
 print INFO "$mon/$mday/$year,";
 print INFO "$hour:$min:$sec,";
 print INFO "$ip,";
 print INFO "$age,$country,$v01,$v02,$v03,$v04,";
 print INFO "$anxiousAttachment,$avoidantAttachment";
 print INFO "\n";
close (INFO);

# Prepare to send HTML code to the browser

print $query->header;
print $query->start_html(-title=>'Thank You');

# Send the text within quotes as HTML code to the user's browser

print "<B>Results Page</B>
<BR><BR>
Thank you for completing this questionnaire. It is designed to measure your attachment
style—the way you relate to others in the context of intimate relationships. As you might
suspect, people differ greatly in the ways in which they approach close relationships. For
example, some people are comfortable opening up to others emotionally, whereas others are
reluctant to allow themselves to depend on others.

According to attachment theory and research, there are two fundamental ways in which
people differ from one another in the way they think about relationships. First, some
people are more anxious than others. People who are high in <B>attachment-related anxiety</
B> tend to worry about whether their partners really love them and often fear rejection.
People low on this dimension are much less worried about such matters. Second, some people
are more avoidant that others. People who are high in <B>attachment-related avoidance</B>
are less comfortable depending on others and opening up to others.

According to your questionnaire responses, your attachment-related anxiety score is
$anxiousAttachment, on a scale ranging from 1 (low anxiety) to 5 (high anxiety). Your
attachment-related avoidance score is $avoidantAttachment, on a scale ranging from 1 (low
avoidance) to 5 (high avoidance).

Please click <A HREF = 'http://www.psych.uiuc.edu/~rcfraley/attachment.htm'>here</A> to
learn more about adult attachment theory.";

# End of HTML code to be sent

print $query->end_html;
```

FIGURE 8.3. Perl/CGI code for a file that will process the questionnaire data.

141

sents the number of years since 1900. Thus, the value 102 stands in for 2002. Also, because Perl begins counting at 0 instead of 1, the value 2 for the month corresponds to March, not February.

The next block of commands is responsible for three things. First, it opens a text file called "*study1data.txt*" that is located on the server. (If the file does not exist, it will be created automatically.) Next, the data are printed to the file, with each piece of information separated by commas. The date (in month/day/year) form is entered first, followed by the time (hour:minute:second), followed by the user's IP address. Next, the response to each of the six questions is entered, along with the total scores for anxiety and avoidance that we created. Finally, we insert a line break ("\n") and close the data file. By inserting a line break at the end of the line, we ensure that the next time a subject submits data, the data will be placed on the line underneath that of the current subject.

The final section of code is quite simple. This section instructs the server to send some HTML code back to the user. In short, the CGI script will create a customized webpage for the subject to view. The text, which is placed within quotes of the `print ""` command, explains the study and—this is important—uses the process of substitution to tell the subject what his or her attachment scores were. Because the variable $anxiousAttachment contains the subject's attachment-related anxiety score, we can simply insert this variable into the text and the CGI script will automatically substitute the appropriate value. Thus, the user will see something like "your attachment-related anxiety score is 2.25, on a scale . . . " instead of literally seeing "your attachment-related anxiety score is $attachmentAnxiety, on a scale . . . ."

Notes on Use and Customization

To use this script, you will need to copy it into a blank file and save it as *study1results.pl*. (If your word processor does not allow you to use the .pl extension, save the file as a text file with the .txt extension and then manually change the extension by "renaming" the file using your My Computer application in Windows.) Once you have saved the file to your personal computer, you will need to transfer it to your Netfirms server. When you do so, be sure to transfer it to the *cgi*-directory and not the *www* directory.

There are many ways to customize this script. For example, you can modify the debriefing text in any way that is appropriate for your own research. If you change the names of the variables, simply make sure you have used those names consistently throughout the script (and the corresponding HTML file).

Here are a few additional points to keep in mind:

1. You will need to "read in" each piece of data submitted by your subject. Thus, if you have 20 questionnaire items with names such as v01 to v20, you will need 20 lines of the "`$v01= $query-param('v01');`" variety to read in those responses.

2. You can create as many (or as few) subscales as you wish. For example, if we wanted to create a scale for security (which, theoretically, is defined as the negatively weighted composite of the anxiety and avoidance items), we could use the following line of code: `$security = ((6- $v01) + (6 - $v02) + $v03 + (6 - $v04))/4;`.

3. Any data you wish to save to the data file should be included within the `print INFO "";` commands. Use a comma to separate each variable.

Downloading Your Data Files and Importing Those Files into SPSS

Once your questionnaire has been online for a while, you will want to download your data. The CGI script has been written to save the data in a "comma delimited" format—in a format in which each piece of data for a single subject is separated by a comma. Comma delimited files are easily imported into programs such as Excel and SPSS.

The CGI script we created earlier was written to save your data in a file called "*study1data.txt*," located in your *www* directory. Thus, to download your data, you can log in to your Netfirms account and open the File Manager. Locate the data file in your *www* directory and transfer it to your personal computer by clicking the icon labeled "download." To import the file into SPSS (version 12), follow these steps:

1. Open SPSS.
2. Open a new data file: File > Open > Data.
3. In the pull-down menu labeled "Files of Type," choose "Text (*.txt)."

4. Select the *study1data.txt* file.

5. Once you select a file, a new window called the "Text Import Wizard" should appear. Follow the instructions and go with all the defaults. The only exception is when the following question is asked: "Which delimiters appear between variables?" In this case, choose only "comma," inasmuch as we are using commas to separate different values of the variables within a row.

Using metaForm—a Webpage That Creates Webpages

There are several software packages that can be used to generate Web-based questionnaires for researchers who do not want to learn about coding HTML and CGI scripts firsthand. Unfortunately, these packages are proprietary, thereby making them costly for researchers and students. To facilitate research, I have been developing a free software program, metaForm2, that can be used for collecting basic questionnaire data, scoring responses, and providing feedback to users. metaForm2 is an Internet-based application that can be used to create questionnaires on-line and is available at *www.web-research-design.net/metaform2/ metaForm2.htm*. The program runs online (i.e., you do not have to download the program and run it on your computer) and is designed to create the CGI code that is needed to implement a questionnaire over the Internet. All the researcher needs to do is supply the questions, instructions, and debriefing information and then transfer the automatically generated CGI code to his or her own server. In addition to creating the CGI code, metaForm2 allows the user to edit existing questionnaires that were generated by metaForm2. I encourage you to explore metaForm2 if you are looking for a quick and simple way to create an online survey.

Making Your Research Study Known

If you want to recruit participants over the Internet, there are several cost-free ways to make your site known. First, you should create a home page for your lab that has an up-to-date list of the various online studies currently available at your Web lab. By having a stable page (i.e., one that will be around even as individual studies come and go), it is more likely that people will find your site and participate in

your research. Second, you should register the URL for the home page of your website with popular search engines. Yahoo!, for example, organizes its searches by subject areas. You will want to register the URL for your site under the area that is most relevant to your research (see *docs.yahoo.com/info/suggest/*). Third, you will want to make sure the title of your home page closely matches the kinds of keywords someone might use if he or she is interested in participating in online research. A good title might contain the phrase "free online research in psychology."

Many scientific organizations in psychology have webpages that list URLs to online research. For example, the American Psychological Society has a page maintained by John Krantz that keeps an up-to-date listing of online studies (*psych.hanover.edu/Research/ exponnent.html*). You might want to visit this site and submit the URL for your page. You should also visit the Web Experimental Psychology Lab (*www.psychologie.unizh.ch/sowi/ Ulf/Lab/WebExpPsyLab.html*), run by Ulf-Dietrich Reips, one of the pioneers in online psychological research.

Summary

This tutorial should provide you with enough information to get you started with collecting basic, self-report questionnaire data online. I have attempted to make the presentation as simple as possible and, as a consequence, I have not emphasized the many advanced techniques that can be used (e.g., skip patterns, randomization, hyperlinks). To learn more about these techniques, consult the sources listed in "Recommended Readings."

Concerns about Data Collected over the Internet

One of my goals in this chapter has been to highlight some of the ways in which collecting data over the Internet can be facilitate personality research. Despite some advantages of using the Internet, there are many psychologists who are suspicious of Internet data. In a recent article, Gosling, Vazire, Srivastava, and John (2004) outlined six preconceptions about Internet data and addressed each of them by comparing data collected over the Internet with data collected and reported in the 2002 volume of the premier journal in our field, the *Journal of Personality and Social Psychology* (*JPSP*). I summarize some of their key findings in the sections that follow.

Are Internet Participants Representative of the Population?

One of the common preconceptions about Internet research is that Internet samples represent only a narrow portion of the population—a group of people who are predominantly young, affluent, North American, and male. To determine whether this preconception is warranted, Gosling and his colleagues (2004) analyzed a sample of more than 361,000 people that had completed measures of the Big Five traits at their research site, *outofservice.com*. Approximately 43% of the *outofservice.com* sample was male, suggesting that research collected over the Internet is unlikely to be composed almost exclusively of men. It is worth noting that the 43% rate is relatively close to the desirable 50–50 split. As a point of comparison, Gosling and his colleagues also analyzed the nature of the samples reported in the 2002 volume of *JPSP*. Only 23% of participants in research published in *JPSP* were male. In other words, there is a strong female bias in traditional modern personality research, one that appears to be less severe in Internet research. With respect to race, the majority (77%) of respondents in the *outofservice.com* sample were White. This result, however, was comparable to that of *JPSP* samples (80%). The average age among participants 18 years old or older was 27.6 in the *outofservice.com* sample, whereas it was estimated to be 23 in *JPSP* samples.

Questions about socioeconomic status were administered to 116,800 of the participants in the *outofservice.com* sample. Of these people, 1,323 (1.1 %) reported being poor; 17,981 (15.4%) reported being working class; 6,405 (5.5%) reported being lower middle class; 53,669 (46%) reported being middle class; 34,105 (29.2%) reported being upper middle class; and 3,314 (2.8%) reported being upper class. These findings suggest that, on average, Internet participants are relatively well off, but it is noteworthy that there is still a wide range of socioeconomic groups represented. How does this compare to the samples typically used in *JPSP*? It is difficult to know for sure because,

of the studies Gosling and his colleagues surveyed, socioeconomic information was reported for only 5–10% of them. However, 85% of the samples were composed of university students, indicating that *JPSP* samples, on average, are more highly educated than the general population, of which only 27% are college graduates (Gosling et al., 2004, p. 98).

In summary, it is clear from these statistics that Internet samples are not representative of the population, even when that population is restricted to North Americans. However, perhaps the more important question is whether Internet samples are less representative than those composed of college students—a group that comprises approximately 85% of the research reported in our premier journal (Gosling et al., 2004). The analyses reported by Gosling and his colleagues (2004) is a resounding "no." In fact, Internet samples are generally more diverse than college samples, targeting more men and a more diverse range of ages and socioeconomic strata. Moreover, because of the large number of participants that can be recruited over the Internet, large absolute numbers of people from across the world can be studied, even when the relative proportion of people from other countries is low. For example, although the proportion of people from Albania was relatively small (less than one-tenth of a percent) in the *outofservice.com* sample, there were nonetheless 368 Albanians in the sample—a number that exceeds the sample size of a typical study published in *JPSP*.

Despite the fact that Internet samples are more diverse than college subject pools, one should not view Internet samples as representing anything more than a modest improvement over traditional sampling methods. As Skikta and Sargis (2005) recently noted, "Sampling from a biased portion of the population yields a biased sample, no matter how large the sample" (p. 13). Psychologists, in general, have paid insufficient attention to the nature of their sampling procedures and, as a result, it is not clear that the kinds of phenomena that have been studied are as pervasive as we tend to assume. Skikta and Sargis report, for example, that the fundamental attribution error—dispositional inferences made in circumstances in which situational factors are exclusively responsible for behavioral variation—is made by only White, wealthy, conservative men.

Careless Data

Another preconception about data collected over the Internet is that it is of poor quality. It is generally assumed that research participants will not take Web-based research seriously—that they will submit multiple responses or that they will be unmotivated to read the questions and instructions carefully.

These assumptions beg the question of why people would want to participate in research in the first place. In the case of the Internet, where participation is fully voluntary, the primary reason seems to be that people hope to learn something interesting about themselves—to gain some degree of self-insight, to allow their opinions to be known, or, perhaps, just to have a bit of fun. If this is true, then participants will be motivated to provide honest responses in order to receive useful feedback about themselves. It is hard to imagine any other reason to voluntarily participate in a research study, but, to the best of my knowledge, the question has not been systematically investigated.

If we assume that participants are, in fact, intrinsically interested in participating, this may resolve one issue but raise another. Namely, participants may submit responses multiple times in order to see how their feedback is affected. There are several ways to deal with this potential problem. One method is to record the user's IP address upon the submission of data. An *IP* (or *Internet protocol*) address is a number that is unique to each computer and is used to identify that computer on the network. In many organizations (e.g., universities), such IP addresses are "static" (i.e., permanent), but for many home users the IP addresses are "dynamic" and reassigned each time the person logs onto the Internet. In either case, if someone submits his or her responses twice and within the same general period of time (i.e., within an hour), it is possible to note this and remove those cases. (In the example questionnaire created in a previous section, the IP address of the user's computer was saved for this purpose.) This method, like any solution, will have some non-zero Type I error rate (i.e., cases will be deleted that were not from the same user, as might happen if someone invites his or her roommate to participate in the research), but, given the large number of participants that can be recruited, this conservative option should have no pragmatic disadvantages.

Another possible solution discussed by Gosling and colleagues (2004) is to provide links on the feedback page to a separate website where participants can "try again." These links lead to the same questionnaire (with the user's previous response preselected), but this time the data are not saved when the user presses the submit button. (If they are saved, they are saved to a different data file.) It is also possible to add a variable, unbeknownst to the user, that denotes the fact that the user has already submitted data and that the newly submitted data represent explorations on the part of the subject.

A third solution is to include a question that explicitly asks the subject whether he or she has participated in the research before. In the data our lab collects online, we include this question and have it set to "yes" by default so that the user has to actively choose the "no" option if he or she has not participated before. Thus, if the user were to go back and reanswer some of the questions, he or she would have to explicitly change this question to "no" again, which would be an unnecessary step for someone who is simply changing a few responses here and there.

Of course, it is always possible that someone might take the time to participate in your research for malevolent reasons—to provide you with bad data. I should note, however, that there is no reason to assume that this is more likely to happen in Internet research than in traditional laboratory research. In fact, if subjects are recruited through the human subjects pool, they may feel some resentment at having to participate in your research for course credit in their psychology classes. This may lead them to answer questions in a careless manner or even provide responses in a deliberately misleading way. It has yet to be empirically demonstrated that people are more malicious in an Internet context than in a traditional one.

It is possible to screen out careless responses by using techniques that are already widely used in traditional paper-and-pencil scales. As Gosling and colleagues (2004) discuss, one can easily study a subject's item response pattern to see if the person is simply endorsing all the items in the same manner or whether the person's responses are sensitive to items that are reverse keyed.

Ethical Concerns in Internet Research

Despite the opportunities provided by the use of the Internet in personality research, there are a number of ethical issues that need to be considered. For example, how should informed consent be obtained? How can we debrief participants effectively? How can we ensure the confidentiality of data collected online? Kraut and colleagues (2004) recently provided a thoughtful discussion on some of these matters. I summarize some of the key issues they raise below, but I direct the reader to their article for a more in-depth consideration of these issues (please see the "Recommended Readings" section).

Obtaining Informed Consent

According to federal guidelines (Title 45, Part 46 of the Code of Federal Regulations for the Protection of Human Subjects [45 CFR 46]; available online at *ohsr.od.nih.gov/guidelines/45cfr46.html*), the following kind of research on human subjects is "exempt":

> research involving the use of educational tests (cognitive, diagnostic, aptitude, achievement), survey procedures, interview procedures or observation of public behavior, unless: (i) information obtained is recorded in such a manner that human subjects can be identified, directly or through identifiers linked to the subjects; and (ii) any disclosure of the human subjects' responses outside the research could reasonably place the subjects at risk of criminal or civil liability or be damaging to the subjects' financial standing, employability, or reputation. (Title 45 Code of Federal Regulations § 46.101(b)(2))

By these standards, the vast majority of personality research that might be conducted over the Internet would be classified as exempt by Internal Review Boards (IRBs). (Please note, however, that the IRB, not the investigator, is charged with determining whether the proposed research is exempt.) The primary reason is that most research projects would not require the recording of information that allows subjects to be identified. Unless a researcher intends to follow people longitudinally, there is little need for obtaining identifying information. One potential exception to this rule concerns the use of IP addresses. As mentioned before, some IP addresses are static, which means

that an address is specific to a given machine. As such, it is possible to trace that IP address to a specific user, potentially compromising his or her anonymity. Many IP addresses, however, are dynamically assigned and thus cannot be used to identify a specific user, only a broader pool of machines (e.g., those of Ameritech/SBC customers in the Champaign-Urbana area). The best way to ensure confidentiality is by not recording the user's IP address. Tracking IP addresses is, of course, a useful way to determine whether a user has recently submitted the same data twice, but there are other ways to address this problem (see the section titled "Careless Data" above).

If the research is not deemed "exempt" by the IRB, it may be necessary to obtain informed consent. However, the traditional methods of obtaining written informed consent have the potential to violate the anonymity that would otherwise be assured to a research participant online. According to § 46.117(c) of the federal guidelines, consent can be waived if the research involves no more than minimal risk to subjects, where minimal risk is defined such that "the probability and magnitude of harm or discomfort anticipated in the research are not greater in and of themselves than those ordinarily encountered in daily life or during the performance of routine physical or psychological examinations or tests" (§ 46.102(i)). The probability of harm or discomfort is likely to be remarkably small in most forms of personality research. Moreover, the "risk" portion of the risk/benefit ratio is considerably reduced when that research is conducted online, because online research subjects are free to withdraw from the study at any time with no consequences whatsoever. Although this is technically true in research conducted in the laboratory, social norms are likely to discourage a research subject from withdrawing from a study even when that subject is uncomfortable with the procedures (e.g., Milgram, 1963).

An IRB may waive the requirement for written consent if "the only record linking the subject and the research would be the consent document and the principal risk would be potential harm resulting from a breach of confidentiality" (§ 46.117(c)(1)). In the case of online research, obtaining a standard written document of consent (e.g., a signature) would clearly compromise the confidentiality of the research. Kraut and his colleagues (2004) have stated, "We recommend that IRBs should waive the [written] document and allow a procedure in which subjects click a button on an online form to indicate they have read and understood the consent form" (p. 113). In light of this recommendation, it is probably wise to include, at the beginning of the study and with as little legalese as possible, a webpage that explains to the research participant what will be expected of him or her; how the data will be used; and that, by clicking a button, he or she is consenting to participate. An example consent form that I use in one of my studies is available at *fraleychapter.netfirms.com/*.

The Use of Deception in Online Research

Is deception advisable in an online study? I argue that using deception online is unwise for several reasons. First, some social science disciplines already have a bad reputation for misleading research participants. Although some research suggests that participants do not mind mild forms of deception in laboratory experiments (Epley & Huff, 1998), it is easier to explain the nature of the deceptive technique in face-to-face debriefing sessions than it is online. Moreover, in an educational institution, where a lot of behavioral research is conducted, it is probably easier for participants to appreciate the benefits of research and the necessity of deception in certain contexts. It is not clear whether a nonstudent visiting your website is going to appreciate the fact that mild deception is sometimes necessary in order to get more truthful answers to certain questions. Finally, without a face-to-face debriefing, it can be difficult to ascertain how the deception has affected the subjects.

Debriefing

The purpose of debriefing is to explain the nature of the research to participants. In most traditional psychological research, the debriefing takes place at the end of a study and usually involves a brief verbal summary of the aims of the study, the purpose of the methods, and the expected findings. The online version of debriefing should follow a similar structure. Moreover, the medium of the Internet allows you to make the debriefing process more educational for research subjects. For example, you can include links to additional online resources that are rele-

vant to your research. You can provide the participant with an automated analysis of the data to date, thereby allowing the participant to see how the study has been progressing. Finally, you can also allow for interactivity by providing an e-mail address in case the person has additional questions about the research. The debriefing context provides an opportunity for us to "give away" psychology (Miller, 1969). Given the large number of people we have access to in Internet research, this opportunity is not something that should be taken lightly. A thoughtful debriefing provides an important means for educating the public about psychological science.

Summary

The Internet offers many opportunities for students of personality. Not only can it be used as a new means for collecting data using tried-and-true methods in personality research (e.g., self-report questionnaires), it can be used in innovative ways—ways that allow us to bring computerized assessment to the homes, offices, and PDAs of our participants. Moreover, as wireless technology continues to advance, the potential for studying people in their natural contexts will develop as well. It is my hope that personality scientists will take advantage of these developments and play a role in finding innovative uses for Internet-based technologies in psychological science.

Recommended Readings

Useful Sources on Creating Webpages in HTML

Birnbaum, M. H. (2001). *Introduction to behavioral research on the Internet*. Mahwah, NJ: Prentice-Hall.

Castro, E. (2001). *HTML for the World Wide Web with XHTML and CSS: Visual Quickstart guide* (5th ed.). Berkeley, CA: Peachpit Press.

Fraley, R. C. (2004). *How to conduct behavioral research over the Internet: A beginner's guide to HTML and CGI/Perl*. New York: Guilford Press.

Further Reading on CGI Scripting

Castro, E. (2001). *Perl and CGI for the World Wide Web* (2nd ed.). Berkeley, CA: Peachpit Press.

Fraley, R. C. (2004). *How to conduct behavioral research over the Internet: A beginner's guide to HTML and CGI/Perl*. New York: Guilford Press.

Further Reading on Ethics and the Internet

Kraut, R., Olson, J., Banaji, M., Bruckman, A., Cohen, J., & Couper, M. (2004). Psychological research online: Report of Board of Scientific Affairs' advisory group on the conduct of research on the Internet. *American Psychologist, 59,* 105–117.

Nosek, B. A., Banaji, M. R., & Greenwald, A. G. (2002). E-research: Ethics, security, design, and control in psychological research on the Internet. *Journal of Social Issues, 58,* 161—176.

References

Baldwin, M. W., & Kay, A. C. (2003). Adult attachment and the inhibition of rejection. *Journal of Social and Clinical Psychology, 22,* 275–293.

Epley, N., & Huff, C. (1998). Suspicion, affective responses, and educational benefit as a result of deception in psychology research. *Personality and Social Psychology Bulletin, 24,* 759–768.

Fraley, R. C., Niedenthal, P. M., Marks, M. J., Brumbaugh, C. C., & Vicary, A. (2006). Adult attachment and the perception of emotional expressions: Probing the hyperactivating strategies underlying anxious attachment. *Journal of Personality, 74,* 1163–1190.

Gosling, S. D., Vazire, S., Srivastava, S., & John, O. P. (2004). Should we trust Web-based studies?: A comparative analysis of six preconceptions about Internet questionnaires. *American Psychologist, 59,* 93–104.

Grice, J. W. (2004). Bridging the idiographic–nomothetic divide in ratings of self and others on the Big Five. *Journal of Personality, 72,* 203–241.

Kelly, G. A. (1955). *The psychology of personal constructs.* New York: Norton.

Kraut, R., Olson, J., Banaji, M., Bruckman, A., Cohen, J., & Couper, M. (2004). Psychological research online: Report of Board of Scientific Affairs' advisory group on the conduct of research on the Internet. *American Psychologist, 59,* 105–117.

McKenna, K. Y. A., & Bargh, J. A. (2000). Plan 9 from cyberspace: The implications of the Internet for personality and social psychology. *Personality and Social Psychology Review, 4,* 57–75.

McKenna, K. Y. A., Green, A. S., & Gleason, M. E. J. (2002). Relationship formation on the Internet: What's the big attraction? *Journal of Social Issues, 58,* 659–671.

Milgram, S. (1963). Behavioral study of obedience. *Journal of Abnormal and Social Psychology, 67,* 371–378.

Miller, G. A. (1969). Psychology as a means of promoting human welfare. *American Psychologist, 24,* 1063–1075.

Niedenthal, P. M., Brauer, M., Robin, L., & Innes-Ker, A. H. (2002). Adult attachment and the perception of facial expression of emotion. *Journal of Personality and Social Psychology, 82,* 419–433.

Park, C. L., Armeli, S., & Tennen, H. (2004). Appraisal-coping goodness of fit: A daily internet study. *Personality and Social Psychology Bulletin, 30,* 558–569.

Reis, H. T., & Gable, S. L. (2000). Event sampling and other methods for studying daily experience. In H. T Reis & C. M. Judd (Eds.), *Handbook of research methods in social and personality psychology* (pp. 190–222). New York: Cambridge University Press.

Skitka, L. J., & Sargis, E. G. (2005). Social psychological research and the Internet: The promise and peril of a new methodological frontier. In Y. Amichai-Hamburger (Ed.), *The social net: Human behavior in cyberspace* (pp. 1–25). Oxford, UK: Oxford University Press.

Vazire, S., & Gosling, S. D. (2004). E-perceptions: Personality impressions based on personal websites. *Journal of Personality and Social Psychology, 87,* 123–132.

Wainer, H. (1990). *Computerized adaptive testing: A primer.* Hillsdale, NJ: Erlbaum.

Waller, N. G., & Reise, S. P. (1989). Computerized adaptive personality assessment: An illustration with the Absorption scale. *Journal of Personality and Social Psychology, 57,* 1051–1058.

## CHAPTER 9

The Null Hypothesis Significance-Testing Debate and Its Implications for Personality Research

R. Chris Fraley
Michael J. Marks

In 1915, Einstein published his now classic treatise on the theory of general relativity. According to his theory, gravity, as it had been traditionally conceived, was not a force per se, but an artifact of the warping of space and time resulting from the mass or energy of objects. Although Einstein's theory made many predictions, one that captured a lot of empirical attention was that light should bend to a specific degree when it passes by a massive object owing to the distortions in space created by that object. Experimental physicists reasoned that if an object's mass is truly capable of warping space, then the light passing by a sufficiently massive object should not follow a straight line, but rather a curved trajectory. For example, if one were to observe a distant star during conditions in which its light waves had to pass near the sun, the star would appear to be in a slightly different location than it would under other conditions.

Scientists had a challenging time testing this prediction, however, because the ambient light emitted by the sun made it difficult to observe the positioning of stars accurately. Fortunately, copies of Einstein's papers made it to Cambridge, where they were read by astrophysicist Arthur Stanley Eddington. Eddington realized that it would be possible to test Einstein's prediction by observing stars during a total eclipse. With the sun's light being momentarily blocked, the positioning of stars could be recorded more accurately than would be possible during normal viewing conditions. If Einstein's theory was correct, the angular deflection of the stars' light would be 1.75 seconds of an arc—twice that predicted by the then dominant theory of Sir Isaac Newton. Eddington was able to obtain funding to organize expeditions to Sobral, Brazil, and the island of Principe off the West African coast to take photographs of the sky during an eclipse. The expeditions, although not going as smoothly as Eddington had hoped, were productive nonetheless. The Sobral group obtained an angular deflection estimate of 1.98; the Principe group obtained an estimate of 1.61 (Kaku, 2004). In November 1919 the Royal Society announced that the observations gathered during the expeditions confirmed Einstein's predictions. The announcement immediately catapulted Einstein—both the scientist and the personality—onto the world's stage.

By many accounts, the 1919 test of Einstein's theory is one of the highlights of 20th-century science. It ushered in a new era of physical research and helped establish the theory of general relativity as one of the most significant theoretical advances since the publication of Newton's *Principia* in 1687. Consider, however, how these data would have been received if they had been presented in a 21st-century psychology conference. After the presentation, someone in the back of the room would raise a hand and ask, "Were those angular deflection estimates significantly different from zero?" Chances are that the audience would nod, signifying their approval of the question. Einstein's theory of relativity, lacking data with proper significance tests, would have sunk into obscurity.

We open with this anecdote because we want to underscore the fact that some of the major scientific discoveries of the past century were made without the use of significance tests. Indeed, some of these discoveries, such as that made in 1919, would likely have been impeded by significance testing.[1] The argument that significance testing is a Bad Thing should be a familiar one to readers. It resurfaces every 10 years or so in psychology, but fades away quickly as researchers convince themselves that, like other things, significance testing in moderation is okay. One of the goals of this chapter is to reopen the significance-testing debate, with an emphasis on the deleterious effects of the misuse of null hypothesis significance testing (NHST) on theoretical and empirical advances in personality science. Specifically, we argue that the field's reliance on significance testing has led to numerous misinterpretations of data, resulted in a biased research literature, and has hampered our ability to develop sophisticated models of personality processes.

We begin by reviewing the basics of significance tests (i.e., how they work, how they are used). Next we discuss some common misinterpretations of NHST as well as some of the criticisms that have been leveled at NHST even when understood properly. Finally, we make some recommendations on how personality

psychologists can avoid some of the pitfalls that tend to be accompanied by the use of significance tests. It is our hope that this chapter will help facilitate discussion of what we view as a crucial methodological issue for the field, while offering some constructive recommendations.

What Is a Significance Test?

Before discussing the significance-testing debate in greater detail, it will be useful to first review what a significance test is. Let us begin with a hypothetical, but realistic, research scenario. Suppose our theory suggests that there should be a positive association between two variables, such as attachment security and relationship quality. To test this hypothesis, we obtain a sample of 20 secure and 20 insecure people in dating and marital relationships and administer questionnaires designed to assess relationship quality.

Let us assume that we find that secure people score 2 points higher than insecure people on our measure of relationship quality. Does this finding corroborate our hypothesis? At face value, the answer is "yes": We predicted and found a positive difference. As statisticians will remind us, however, even if there is no real association between security and relationship quality, we are likely to observe *some* difference between groups due to *sampling error*— the inevitable statistical noise that results when researchers study a *subset* of cases from a larger population. Thus, to determine whether the empirical difference corroborates our hypothesis, we first need to determine the probability of observing a difference of 2 points or higher under the hypothesis that there is *no* association between these constructs in the population. According to this *null hypothesis*, the population difference is zero and any deviation from this value observed in our sample is due to sampling error.

Fortunately, statisticians have developed methods for quantifying the amount of sampling error that should be observed in different sampling conditions. In this case, the expected magnitude of sampling error for the difference between means, the *standard error of the difference* or SE_{DIFF}, is proportional to the sample size and the variance of the scores within the population. Mathematically, this relationship is given by the following equation:

$$SE_{DIFF} = \sqrt{\frac{\sigma_1^2}{N_1} + \frac{\sigma_2^2}{N_2}}$$

The standard error of the difference quantifies how much of a discrepancy there will be, on average, between an observed difference and the true difference due to sampling error. In order to determine the probability of observing a mean difference of 2 or higher, we need to evaluate the magnitude of this observed difference relative to the magnitude of the difference expected on the basis of sampling error (i.e., SE_{DIFF}).[2] This ratio, the t statistic, can be represented as follows:

$$t = \frac{(M_2 - M_1) - (\mu_2 - \mu_1)}{SE_{DIFF}}$$

where the numerator represents the discrepancy between the observed difference ($M_2 - M_1$) and the hypothesized difference ($\mu_2 - \mu_1$) between the two groups, and SE_{DIFF} represents the discrepancy that would be expected on the basis of sampling error. The distribution of this ratio describes a t-distribution—a distribution that closely approximates a normal distribution as the sample size increases. If we assume that the population variance for secure and insecure people is 10, then, in our example, $SE_{DIFF} = 1$ and $t = 2.00$. By consulting various statistical tables, or by using statistical software, a researcher can find the probability associated with the observed t-value under the null hypothesis. In this example, the probability of observing a t-value greater than or equal to 2 on 38 degrees of freedom is about .026.

Is .026 a large or small probability? Deciding whether the p-value associated with a test is small enough to make the result "unlikely" under the null hypothesis requires a subjective judgment. Thus, to make it less subjective, psychologists use a threshold for judging p-values. This threshold, called *alpha*, is set to .05 by convention. If the p-value associated with a test is less than alpha, the result is said to be "statistically significant" and the researcher concludes that the result is not simply due to chance fluctuations in the sample. If the p-value associated with the result is greater than alpha, the result is said not to be significant or "nonsignificant" and the researcher will either conclude that the null hypothesis offers a credible explanation for the results or that the data are not sufficient to reach a judgment.

In this example the p-value is less than .05; thus, we would reject the null hypothesis and conclude that attachment security and relation-ship quality are related to one another in ways anticipated by the theory. It is important to note that the general logic undying this example is common to the many kinds of significance tests that are used in psychology, whether they are analyses of variance (ANOVAs), tests of regression coefficients, or tests of correlations. The key question addressed by the use of a significance test is whether the result would have been likely if the null hypothesis were true. If the observed result is unlikely (i.e., the p-value is less than alpha), the null hypothesis is rejected.

Some Common Misinterpretations of Significance Tests and *P*-Values

Significance testing is widely used in personality psychology, despite the fact that methodologists have criticized those tests for several decades. One of the many claims that critics of NHST have made is that many researchers hold mistaken assumptions about what significance tests can and cannot tell us about our data. In this section we review some of the common misconceptions that researchers have concerning the meaning of p-values. Once we have clarified what p-values do and do not tell us about our data and hypotheses, we turn to the more controversial question of whether significance tests, even when properly understood, are a help or a hindrance in the scientific enterprise.

Statistically Significant = Substantively Significant

It is commonly assumed that the p-value is indicative of the meaningfulness or importance of a finding. According to this logic, the smaller the p-value (e.g., $p = .001$ vs. $p = .05$), the more important the finding. In practice, this logic is manifested not only in explicit statements celebrating the size of the p-value (e.g., "highly significant"), but also in the ornamentation of coefficients with multiple asterisks to denote just how significant they are.

Critics of NHST have argued that the meaningfulness or importance of a result can be evaluated only in the context of a specific theory or application. According to this perspective, although p-values can be useful for some purposes, they are not particularly informative for evaluating the theoretical significance of findings. To illustrate why, let us assume that researchers were to discover that power motivation was associated ($r = .30$) with increases in testosterone under certain conditions (e.g., see Schultheiss & Pang, Chapter 19, this volume). If the sample size was 50, the p-value associated with this correlation would be .03. If the sample size was 1,000, however, the p-value associated with the correlation would be <.001. One association is clearly more statistically significant than the other, but is one more important than the other? No. The actual magnitude of the correlations is the same in both cases; therefore, the two studies have identical implications for the theory in question. It is true that one finding is based on a larger sample size than the other and thus produces a smaller standard error. However, it would be better to conclude that one correlation estimates the true correlation with more precision than the other (i.e., one study is better designed than the other because it draws upon a larger sample size) than to conclude that one correlation is more substantively important than the other.

The key point here is that the way in which a finding is interpreted should depend not on the p-value but on the magnitude of the finding itself—the effect size or parameter value under consideration. Meehl (1990) argued that one reason researchers tend to look to p-values rather than effect sizes for theoretical understanding is that statistical training in psychology encourages students to equate "hypothesis testing" with NHST. When NHST is equated with hypothesis testing, it is only natural to assume that the size of the p-value has a direct relationship to the theoretical significance of the findings. But, in Meehl's view, this subtle equation has led psychologists to conflate two very distinct roles that mathematics and statistics play in science (see Figure 9.1). One function of mathematics is for the formalization of theories and the derivation of quantitative predictions that can be tested empirically. For example, if one works through the mathematics underlying Einstein's theory of general relativity, one can derive the angular deflection of light as it passes by an object of a given mass. The theoretical model can then be tested by comparing the theoretical values with the empirical ones. The other function of mathematics is for quantifying sampling error and estimating the degree to which empirical values deviate from population values. This latter function, which is more familiar to psychologists and statisticians, is useful for deriving the expected magnitude of sampling errors in different research sit-

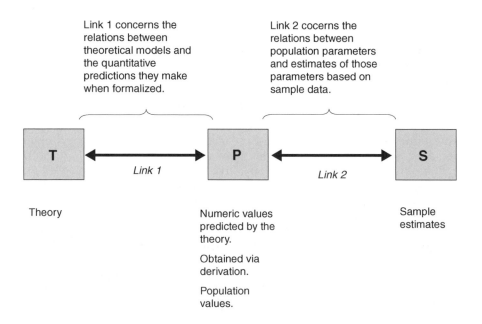

FIGURE 9.1. The relations between theory, population/predicted values, and statistical/empirical values. From Meehl (1990). Copyright 1990 by Lawrence Erlbaum Associates. Adapted by permission.

uations, but it is not directly relevant for testing psychological theories.

Given Meehl's (1990) distinction between hypothesis tests (i.e., the comparison of theoretical values to observed ones) and inferential statistics (i.e., the study of sampling distributions), why do psychologists assume that evaluating sampling error is the same thing as testing a substantive hypothesis? It is hard to say for sure, but both Meehl (1990) and Gigerenzer (1993) have speculated that is has something to do with the artificial sense of rigor that comes along with using the machinery of NHST.

To demonstrate just how ingrained this sense is in psychologists, Meehl (1990) challenged his readers to imagine how hypothesis testing would proceed if the sample values *were* the population values, thereby making sampling error and NHST irrelevant. In such a situation, theory testing would be relatively straightforward in most areas of psychology. If a theory predicts a positive correlation and, empirically, the correlation turns out to be positive, then the hypothesis would pass the test. Most psychologists would admit that this seems like a flimsy state of affairs. Indeed, from Meehl's perspective, it is not only flimsy, but it poses a huge problem for the philosophy of theory testing in psychology. Meehl (1978) argued that when a directional prediction is made, the hypothesis has a 50:50 chance of being confirmed, even if it is false. In his view, a test would be much more rigorous if it predicted a point value (i.e., a specific numerical value, such as a correlation of .50 or a ratio between parameters) or a narrow range of values. In such a case, the empirical test would be a much more risky one and the empirical results would carry more interpretive weight.

Meehl argues that researchers have created an artificial sense of rigor and objectivity by using NHST because the test statistic associated with NHST must fall in a narrow region to allow the researcher to reject the null hypothesis. The difficulty in obtaining a statistic in such a small probability region, coupled with the tendency of psychologists to make directional predictions, is one reason why researchers celebrate significant results and attach substantive interpretations to *p*-values rather than the effects of interest. (As discussed in a subsequent section, obtaining a significant result can be challenging not because of the rigor of the test, but because of the relative lack of attention psychologists pay to statistical power.)

Statistically Significant = The Null Hypothesis Provides an Unlikely Explanation for the Data

Another problematic assumption that researchers hold is that the *p*-value is indicative of the likelihood that the results were due to chance. Specifically, if *p* is less than .05, it is assumed that the null hypothesis is unlikely to offer a viable account for the findings. According to critics of NHST, this misunderstanding stems from the conflation of two distinct interpretations of probability: relative frequency and subjective probability. A *relative frequency* interpretation of probability equates probability with the long-run outcome of an event. For example, if we were to toss a fair coin and claim that the chances that the coin will land on heads is .50, the ".50" technically refers to what we would expect to observe over the long run if we were to repeat the procedure across an infinite number of trials. It is important to note that ".50" does not refer to any specific toss, nor does it reference the likelihood that the coin is a fair one. From a relative frequency perspective, the language of probability applies only to long-run outcomes, not to specific trials or hypotheses. A *subjective* interpretation of probability, in contrast, treats probabilities as quantitative assessments concerning the likelihood of an outcome or the likelihood that a certain claim is correct. Subjective probabilities are ubiquitous in everyday life. For example, when someone says, "I think there is an 80% chance that it will rain today," he or she is essentially claiming to be highly confident that it will rain. When a researcher concludes that the null hypothesis offers an unlikely account for the data, he or she is relying on subjective interpretations of probability.

The familiar *p*-value produced by NHST is a relative frequency probability, not a subjective probability. As described previously, it reflects the proportion of time that a test statistic (i.e., a *t*-value) would be observed if the same study were to be carried out ad infinitum *and* if the null hypothesis were true. It is also noteworthy that, because it specifies the probability (P) of an outcome (D) given a particular state of affairs (i.e., that the null hypothesis is true: H_0), the familiar *p*-value is a *conditional probability* and can be written as $P(D|H_0)$. An important point is that this probability does not indicate whether a specific outcome (D) is due to chance, nor does it indicate the likelihood that the null hypothesis is true (H_0). In other words, $P(D|H_0)$ does not quantify what researchers think it does, namely, the probability that null hypothesis is true given the data (i.e., $P(H_0|D)$).

Bayes's theorem provides a useful means to explicate the relationship between these two kinds of probability statements (see Salsburg, 2001). According to Bayes's theorem,

$$P(H_0|D) = \frac{P(H_0) \times P(D|H_0)}{P(H_0) \times P(D|H_0) + P(H_1) \times P(D|H_1)}$$

In other words, if a researcher wishes to evaluate the probability that his or her findings are due to chance, he or she would need to know the a priori probability that the null hypothesis is true, $P(H_0)$, in addition to other probabilities (i.e., the probability that the alternative hypothesis is true, $P(H_1)$, and the probability of the data under the alternative hypothesis, $P(D|H_1)$).[3] Because these first two probabilities are not relative frequency probabilities (i.e., probabilities based on long-run frequencies) but are subjective probabilities (see Oakes, 1986), they can be selected freely by the researcher or by a quantitative examination of the empirical literature (see Oakes, 1986, for an example).

To illustrate just how different the probability of observing the data, given the null hypothesis (i.e., the p-value or $P(D|H_0)$), can be from the probability that the null hypothesis is true, given the data (i.e., $P(H_0|D)$), consider Table 9.1. Example A in this table illustrates a situation in which, a priori, we have no reason to assume that the null hypothesis is any more likely to be true than the alternative. That is, $P(H_0) = P(H_1) = .50$. If we gather data and find that the p-value for our correlation is .05, we reject the null hypothesis and conclude, de facto, that the alternative hypothesis provides a better account of the data. However, we have failed to consider the probability of observing the data under the alternative hypothesis. Let us assume for a moment that this probability is also small (i.e., .01), indeed, smaller than that associated with the null hypothesis. If we substitute these quantities into Bayes's theorem, we find that the probability that the null hypothesis is true has increased from .50 to .83, in light of the data. In other words, our statistically significant finding, when considered in the context of Bayesian statistics, reinforces, not refutes, the null hypothesis.

Let us focus on one more scenario, one that is fairly common in personality research. In most studies, investigators are not testing hypotheses in a Popperian fashion (i.e., with the goal of disproving them); instead, they are trying to provide evidence to support their preferred hypotheses. In this scenario, it is probably unlikely that the values of $P(H_0)$ and $P(H_1)$ are equivalent, unless personality psychologists have but the most tenuous understanding of how the world works. For the purposes of discussion, let us assume that we have strong reasons to believe that the true correlation is not zero; thus, let us set $P(H_0)$ to .10 and $P(H_1)$ to .90 to reflect this assumption (see Example B in Table 9.1). We conduct the study, compute the correlation, and find a p-value of .15. The result is not statistically significant; thus, standard NHST procedures would lead us to "fail to reject" the null hypothesis. Does this mean that the null hypothesis is likely to be correct? If we assume that the data are equivocal with respect to the research hypothesis (i.e., $P(D|H_1)$), the probability of the null hypothesis being true, given the data, is actually .03. Thus,

TABLE 9.1. Conditions in Which the p-Value Does and Does Not Equal the Probability That the Data Are Due to Chance

| Example | Probability term | | | | |
	$P(H_0)$	$P(H_1)$	$P(D|H_0)$	$P(D|H_1)$	$P(H_0|D)$
A	.50	.50	.05	.01	.83
B	.10	.90	.15	.50	.03
C	.50	.50	.05	.95	.05
D	.90	.10	.05	.05	.90

Note. $P(H_0)$ = the a priori probability of the null hypothesis; $P(H_1)$ = the a priori probability of the research hypothesis; $P(D|H_0)$ = the probability of the data if the null hypothesis is true (i.e., the p-value); $P(D|H_1)$ = the probability of the data if the research hypothesis is true; $P(H_0|D)$ = the probability that the null hypothesis is true, given the data.

although the empirical result was not statistically significant, the revised likelihood estimate (which Bayesians call the *posterior probability*) that the null hypothesis is correct has dropped from .10 to .03. These data, in fact, undermine the null hypothesis, despite the fact that standard NHST procedures would lead us to not reject it.

Table 9.1 illustrates these and some alternative situations, including one in which the *p*-value *is* equal to the inverse probability (see Example C). The important thing to note is that, in most circumstances, these two quantities will not be identical. In other words, a small *p*-value does not necessarily mean that the null hypothesis is true, nor does a nonsignificant finding indicate that the null hypothesis should be retained. Within a Bayesian framework, evaluating the null hypothesis requires attention to more than just one probability. If researchers are truly interested in evaluating the likelihood that their results are due to chance (i.e., $P(H_0|D)$), it is necessary to make assumptions about other quantities and use the empirical *p*-value in combination with these quantities to estimate $P(H_0|D)$. Without doing so, one could argue that there are little grounds for assuming that a small *p*-value provides evidence against the null hypothesis.

Before closing this section, we should note that when researchers learn about subjective probabilities and Bayesian statistics, they sometimes respond that there is no place for subjective assessments in an objective science. Bayesians have two rejoinders to this point. First, some advocates of Bayesian statistics have argued that subjective probability is the *only* meaningful way to discuss probability. According to this perspective, when laypeople and scientists use probability statements, they are often concerned with the assessment of specific outcomes or hypotheses; they are not truly concerned with what will happen in a hypothetical universe of long-run experiments. No one really cares how often it would rain in Urbana, Illinois, on September 8, 2005, for example, if that date were to be repeated over and over again in a hypothetical world. When researchers conduct a study on the association between security and relationship quality or any other variables of interest, they are concerned with assessing the likelihood that the null hypothesis is true in light of the data. This likelihood cannot be directly quantified through long-run frequency definitions of probability, but, if the

various quantities are taken seriously and combined via Bayes's theorem, it is possible to attach a rationally justified probability statement to the null hypothesis. This brings us to the second rejoinder: Subjective assessments play an inevitable role in science, even for those who like to conceptualize science as an objective enterprise. Bayesian advocates argue that, so long as subjective appraisals are used in psychology, it is most defensible (i.e., more objective) to formalize those appraisals in a manner that is public and rational, rather than to allow them to seep into the scientific process through more idiosyncratic, and potentially insidious, channels. In other words, the use of subjective probabilities, when combined with Bayesian analyses, facilitates an objective and rational means for evaluating scientific hypotheses.

In summary, researchers often assume that a small *p*-value indicates that the null hypothesis is unlikely to be true (and vice versa: a nonsignificant result implies that the null hypothesis may provide a viable explanation for the data). In other words, researchers often assume that the *p*-value can be used to evaluate the likelihood that their data are due to chance. Bayesian considerations, however, show this assumption to be false. The *p*-value, which provides information about the probability of the data, given that the null hypothesis is true, does not indicate the probability that chance events can explain the data. Researchers who are interested in evaluating the probability that chance explains the data can do so by combining the *p*-value with other kinds of probabilities via Bayes's theorem.

Statistically Significant = A Reliable Finding

Replication is one of the cornerstones of science. The most straightforward way to demonstrate the reliability of an empirical result is to conduct a replication study to see whether or not the result can be found again. The more common approach, however, is to conduct a null hypothesis significance test. According to this tradition, if a researcher can show that the *p*-value associated with a test statistic is very low (less than 5%), the researcher can be reasonably confident that if he or she were to do the study again, the results would be significant.

The belief that the *p*-value of a significance test is indicative of a result's reliability is widespread (see Sohn, 1998, pp. 292–293, for examples). Indeed, authors often write about statistically significant findings as if the results are "reliable." However, as recent writers have explained, researchers hold many misconceptions about what p-values can tell us about the reliability of findings (Meehl, 1990; Oakes, 1986; Schmidt, 1996; Sohn, 1998). Oakes (1986), for example, surveyed 70 academic psychologists and found that 60% of them erroneously believed that a p-value of .01 implied that a replication study would have a 99% chance of yielding significant results (see Oakes, 1986, for a discussion of why this assumption is incorrect). Although recent advocates of significance tests have concurred that the probability of replicating a significant effect is not literally equal to 1 minus the p-value, they have defended researchers' intuition that p-values indicate *something* about the replicability of a finding (Harris, 1997; Krueger, 2001; Scarr, 1997).

Is this intuition correct? To address this question, we must first discuss which factors determine whether a finding is replicable. The likelihood of replicating an empirical result is directly related to the statistical power of the research design. *Statistical power* refers to the probability that the statistical test will lead to a significant result, given that the null hypothesis is false (Cohen, 1992). Statistical power is a function of three major factors: (1) the alpha level used for the statistical test (set to .05, by convention), (2) the true effect size or population parameter, and (3) the sample size. Thus, to determine whether a significant finding can be replicated, one needs to know the statistical power of the replication study. It is important to note that, because the statistical power is determined by the population effect size and that that effect is unknown (indeed, it is the key quantity to be inferred from an estimation perspective), one can never know the statistical power of a test in any unambiguous sense. Instead, one must make an assumption about the population effect size (based on theory, experience, or previous research) and, given the sample size and alpha level, compute the statistical power of the test.

For the sake of discussion, let us assume that we are interested in studying the correlation between security and relationship quality and that the population correlation is .30. Now, let us draw a sample of 100 people from the population, assess both variables, and compute the

correlation between them. Let us assume that the correlation we observe in our initial study is .20 and that the associated p-value is .04. Does this p-value tell us anything about the likelihood that if we were to conduct an exact replication study (i.e., another study in which we drew 100 people from the same population), we would get a significant result?

No. To understand why, it is necessary to keep in mind the way in which sampling distributions work and which factors influence statistical power. If we define the probability of replication as the statistical power of the test, the first thing to note is that in a series of replication studies, the key factors that influence the power of the test (i.e., alpha, N, and the population effect size) are constants, not variables. Thus, if the true correlation is .30 and the sample size used is 100, the power of the test is .80 in Study 1, .80 in Study 2, .80 in Study 3, and so on, *regardless of the* p-*value associated with any one test*. In other words, the p-value from any one replication study is irrelevant for the power of the test. More important, the p-value in any one study is statistically independent of the others because the only factor influencing variation in the observed correlations (on which the p-value is calculated) is random sampling error. Thus, the p-value observed in an initial study is unrelated to the likelihood that an exact replication study will yield a significant result.

There is one exception to this conclusion. Namely, if researchers are examining a large number of correlations (e.g., correlations between 10 distinct variables) in one sample, the correlations with the smaller p-values are more likely to be replicable than those with larger p-values (see Greenwald, Gonzalez, Harris, & Guthrie, 1996). This is the case because the larger correlations will have smaller p-values and larger correlations are more likely to reflect larger population correlations than smaller ones. Although one could argue that the p-values for the various correlations is associated with the replicability of those correlations (see Greenwald et al., 1996; Krueger, 2001), it would be inaccurate to assume that the p-value itself is responsible. It would be more appropriate to conclude that, holding sample size constant, it is easier to replicate findings when the population correlations are large as opposed to small. Larger effects are easier to detect for a given sample size.

The Potential Problems of Using Significance Tests in Personality Research

Although some of the major criticisms of NHSTs concern misinterpretations of *p*-values, several writers have argued that, even if properly interpreted, *p*-values and significance tests would be of limited use in psychological science. In the following sections we discuss some of these arguments, with attention focused on their implications for research in personality psychology.

The Asymmetric Nature of Significance Tests

Significance tests are used to evaluate the probability of observing data of a certain magnitude, assuming that the null hypothesis is true. When the test statistic falls within the critical region of a sampling distribution, the null hypothesis is rejected; if it does not, the null hypothesis is retained. When students first learn this logic, they are often confused by the fact that the null hypothesis is being tested rather than the research hypothesis. It would seem more intuitive to determine whether the data are unlikely under the research hypothesis and, if so, to reject the research hypothesis. Indeed, according to Meehl (1967), significance tests are used in this way in some areas of science, but this usage is rare in psychology.

When students query instructors on this apparent paradox, the common response is that, yes, it does seem odd to test the null hypothesis instead of the research hypothesis, but, as it turns out, testing the research hypothesis is impossible. (This is not an answer that most students find assuring.) When the research hypothesis leads to a directional prediction (i.e., the correlation will be greater than zero, one group will score higher on average than the other), there are an infinite number of population values that are compatible with it (e.g., $r = .01$, $r = .10$, $r = .43$, $r = .44$). It would not be practical to generate a sampling distribution for *each* possibility. Doing so would lead to the uninteresting (but valid) conclusion that the correlation observed is most likely in a case in which the population value is equal to the observed correlation.

The fact that only one hypothesis is tested in the traditional application of NHST makes sig-nificance tests inherently asymmetrical (see Rozeboom, 1960). In other words, depending on the statistical power of the test, the test will be biased either in favor of or against the null hypothesis. Consider the following example. Let us assume that the true correlation is equal to .30. If a researcher were to draw a sample of 40 cases from the population and obtain a correlation of .25 ($p = .12$), he or she would not reject the null hypothesis, thereby concluding that the null hypothesis offers a viable account of the data. If one were to generate a sampling distribution around the true correlation of .30, however, one would see that a value of .25 is, in fact, relatively likely under the true hypothesis. In other words, in this situation we cannot reject the null hypothesis, but, if we compared our data against the "true" sampling distribution instead of a null one, we would find that we cannot reject the research hypothesis either.

The important point here is that basic statistical theory demonstrates that the sample statistic (in some cases, following adjustment, as with the standard deviation) is the best estimate of the population parameter. Thus, in the absence of any other information, researchers would be better off to conclude that the population value is equal to the value observed in the sample regardless of the *p*-value associated with sample value. When significance tests are emphasized, focus shifts away from estimation and toward answering the question of whether the null hypothesis provides the most parsimonious account for the data. The use of a significance test implicitly gives the null hypothesis greater weight than is warranted in light of the fundamentals of sampling theory. If researchers want to give the null hypothesis greater credence than the alternatives a priori, it may be useful to use Bayesian statistics so that a priori weights can be explicitly taken into account in evaluating hypotheses.

Low Statistical Power

Statistical power refers to the probability that the significance test will produce a significant result when, in fact, the null hypothesis is false. (The Type II error is the complement of power; it is the probability of incorrectly accepting the null hypothesis when it is false.) As noted previously, the power of a test is a function of three key ingredients: the alpha level (i.e., the probability threshold for what counts as significant, such as .05), the sample size, and the true effect size. In an ideal world, researchers would make some assumptions when designing their studies about what the effect size might be (e.g., $r = .30$) and select a sample size that would ensure that, say, 80% of the time they will be able to reject the null hypothesis. In actuality, it is extremely rare for psychologists to consider statistical power when planning their research designs. Surveys of the literature by Cohen (1962) and others (e.g., Sedlmeier & Gigerenzer, 1989) have demonstrated that the statistical power to detect a medium-sized effect (e.g., a correlation of .24) in published research is about 50%. In other words, the power to detect a true effect in a typical study in psychology is not any better than a coin toss.

The significance of this point is easily overlooked, so let us spell it out explicitly. If most studies conducted in psychology have only a 50–50 chance of leading researchers to the correct conclusion (assuming the null hypothesis is, in fact, false), we could fund psychological science for the mere cost of a coin. In other words, by flipping a penny to decide whether a hypothesis is correct or not, on average, psychologists would be right just as often as they would be if they conducted empirical research to test their hypotheses. (The upside, of course, is that the federal government would save millions of dollars in research funding by contributing one penny to each investigator.)

Is statistical power a problem in personality psychology? To address this issue, we surveyed articles from the 2004 volumes of the *Journal of Personality and Social Psychology: Personality Processes and Individual Differences* (*JPSP:PPID*) and the *Journal of Personality* (*JP*) and recorded the sample sizes used in each study, as well as some other information that we summarize in a subsequent section. The results of our survey are reported in Table 9.2. Given that a typical study in personality psychology has an *N* of 120, it follows that a typical study in personality psychology has a power of 19% to detect a correlation of size .10 (what Cohen, 1992, calls a "small" effect), 59% to detect a correlation of .20 (a small to medium effect), 75% to detect a correlation of .24 (what Cohen calls a "medium" effect), and 98% to detect a correlation of .37 (what Cohen calls a "large" effect). This suggests that, for simple bivariate analyses, personality researchers are doing okay with detecting medium to large effects, but poorly for detecting small to medium ones.

TABLE 9.2. Typical Sample Sizes and Effect Sizes in Studies Conducted in Personality Psychology

	Mdn	*M*	*SD*	Range
N	120	179	159	15–508
r	.21	.24	.17	0–.96

Note. The absolute value of *r* was used in the calculations reported here. Data are based on articles published in the 2004 volumes of *JPSP:PPID* and *JP*.

It has long been recognized that attention to statistical power is one of the easiest ways to improve the quality of data analysis in psychology (e.g., Cohen, 1962). Nonetheless, many psychologists are reluctant to use power analysis in the research design phase for two reasons. First, some researchers are uncomfortable in speculating about what the effect size may be for the research question at hand. We have two recommendations that should make this process easier. One approach is to consider the general history of effects that have been found in the literature of interest. The data summarized in Table 9.2, for example, imply that the typical correlation uncovered in personality research is about .21. Thus, it would be prudent to use .21 as an initial guess as to what the correlation might be if the research hypothesis is true, and select a sample size that will enable the desired level of statistical power (e.g., 80%) to detect that size correlation. To facilitate this process, we have reported in Table 9.3 the sample sizes needed for a variety of correlations in order to have statistical power of 80%. As can be seen, if one wants to detect a correlation of .21 with high power, one needs a sample size of approximately 200 people.

Another way to handle the power issue is to ask oneself how large the correlation would need to be either to warrant theoretical explanation or to count as corroboration for the theory in question. Doing so may seem unduly subjective, but, we have found it to be a useful exercise for some psychologists. For example, if one determines that the correlation between conscientiousness and physical health outcomes is only worth theorizing about if it is .10 or higher, then one could select a sample size (in this case, an *N* of 618) that would enable a fair test of the research hypothesis. We call this the "choose your power to detect effects of interest" strategy, and we tend to rely on it in our own work when the existing literature does not

TABLE 9.3. Statistical Power for a Correlation Coefficient as a Function of Population Correlations and Sample Sizes

N	Population correlation							
	.10	.20	.30	.40	.50	.60	.70	.80
20	.06	.13	.24	.40	.60	.80	.94	.99
40	.09	.23	.46	.72	.91	.98	.99	.99
60	.11	.33	.64	.88	.98	.99	.99	.99
80	.14	.42	.77	.96	.99	.99	.99	.99
100	.16	.51	.86	.98	.99	.99	.99	.99
120	.19	.59	.92	.99	.99	.99	.99	.99
140	.22	.66	.95	.99	.99	.99	.99	.99
160	.24	.72	.97	.99	.99	.99	.99	.99
180	.27	.77	.98	.99	.99	.99	.99	.99
200	.29	.81	.99	.99	.99	.99	.99	.99
386	.50	.97	.99	.99	.99	.99	.99	.99

provide any guidance on what kinds of effects to expect.

The bottom line is that if power is not taken into consideration in the research design phase, one's labor is likely to be in vain. In situations in which researchers cannot obtain the power they need for a specific research question (e.g., perhaps researchers are studying a limited-access population), we recommend revising the alpha level (e.g., using an alpha threshold of .10 instead of .05) for the significance test so that the power is not compromised.

Many researchers are uncomfortable with adjusting alpha to balance the theoretical Type I and Type II error rates of a research design, claiming that if researchers were free to choose their own alpha levels, everyone would be publishing "significant findings." We have two rejoinders to this argument. First, we believe that it only makes sense to adjust alpha *before* the data are collected. If alpha is adjusted after the data are collected to make a finding "significant," then, yes, the process of adjusting alpha would be biased. Second, and more important, allowing researchers to choose their alpha levels a priori is no more subjective than allowing researchers to choose their own sample sizes a priori. Current convention dictates that alpha be set to .05, but also allows researchers the freedom to choose any sample size they desire. As a consequence, some researchers simply run research subjects until they get the effects they are seeking. If *any* conventions are warranted, we argue that it would be better for the field if researchers were expected to design studies with .80 power rather than holding researchers to an alpha of .05 while allowing power to vary whimsically. Such a convention would lower

the Type II error rate of research in our field which, according to the estimates in Table 9.2, is fairly high for effects in the small to medium range. In short, we recommend that researchers design studies with .80 power to detect the effects hypothesized and select their sample sizes (or alpha rates, when N is beyond the researcher's control for logistic or financial reasons) accordingly. Such a practice would help to improve the quality of research design in personality psychology without making it impossible for researchers to study populations to which they have limited access.

Perhaps the real fear that psychologists have is that by allowing researchers to choose their own alpha levels to decrease the Type II error rate in psychological research, a number of Type I errors (i.e., findings that are statistically significant when in actuality the null hypothesis is true) would be published. Type I errors are made when researchers obtain a significant result but, in fact, the true effect is zero. Are Type I errors worth worrying about in personality psychology? It depends on how likely it is that the null hypothesis is credible in personality research, a topic we turn to in the next section.

We close this section with a final thought, one that we have not seen articulated before. The impetus for using NHST is the recognition that sampling error makes it difficult to evaluate the meaning of empirical results. Sampling error is most problematic when sample sizes are small, and thus when statistical power is low. When statistical power is high and sample sizes are large, however, sampling error is less a problem. The irony is that researchers use significance tests in precisely the conditions under which they are most likely to lead to inferential errors (namely, Type II errors). When the Type II error rate is reduced by increasing sample size, sampling error is no longer a big problem. Defenders of NHST often claim that significance tests should not be faulted simply because the researchers who use them fail to appreciate the limitations of low power studies. What defenders of NHST fail to recognize, however, is that there would be little need for significance tests if power were taken seriously.

The Null Hypothesis Is Almost Always False in Psychological Research

Recall that the primary reason for conducting a significance test is to test the null hypothesis— to determine how likely the data would be under the assumption that the effect does not really exist. Thus, in principle, the test is necessary only if the null hypothesis has a priori credibility. Given the prevalence of significance testing in personality research, a disinterested observer might conclude that the null hypothesis is a serious contender in many domains in our field.

But is the null hypothesis really a credible explanation for the data we collect? According to Lykken (1991) and Meehl (1990), everything is correlated with everything else to some non-zero degree in the real world. If this is the case, then, technically, the null hypothesis is unlikely to be true in virtually every research situation in personality psychology. Because significance tests are used to test the hypothesis of zero difference or zero association, any test conducted will produce a significant result so long as its statistical power is sufficiently high. Of course, because power is typically modest in personality research (see the previous section), not all tests will lead to significant results, thereby fostering the illusion that the null hypothesis might be correct most of the time.

To provide a less speculative analysis of the credibility of the null hypothesis in personality research, we again turned to our sample of coefficients from the 2004 volumes of the *JPSP* and *JP*. We recorded all correlations that were intended to represent associations between distinct variables (i.e., cases in which two variables were thought to load on the same factor were not recorded). A summary of these correlations is reported in Table 9.2. According to these data, the average correlation in personal-

ity research is .24 (SD = .17; Mdn = .21). Indeed, if we break down the effects into discrete ranges (e.g., .00 to .05, .06 to .10, .11 to .15), the proportion of correlations that fall between .00 and .05 is only 14%. (The proportion of correlations that are 0.00, as implied by the null hypothesis, is 1%.) In summary, a study of a broad cross section of the effects reported in the leading journals in the field of personality suggests that correlations are rarely so small as to suggest that the null hypothesis offers a credible explanation in any area of personality research. It really does seem that, in personality psychology, everything is correlated with everything else (at least 99% of the time).

It could be argued that this conclusion is premature because our analysis highlights only studies that "worked"—studies in which the null hypothesis was rejected. Our first response to this point is that, yes, the sample is a biased one. However, the reason it is biased is not that we drew a biased sample from the literature, but that the empirical literature itself is biased. We view this as an enormous problem for the field and discuss it—and the role that NHST has played in creating it—in more depth in the sections that follow. Our second response is that only some of the correlations we studied were focal ones (i.e., correlations relevant to a favored prediction on the part of the authors). Some of the correlations were auxiliary ones (i.e., relevant to the issues at hand, but the value of which was not of interest to the investigators) or discriminant validity correlations (i.e., correlations that, in the mind of the investigators, should have been small). Although this is unlikely to solve any biasing problems, it does make the results less biased than might be assumed otherwise.

Assuming for now that our conclusions are sound, why is it the case that most variables studied in personality psychology are correlated with one another? According to Lykken (1991), many of these associations exist owing to indirect causal effects. For example, two seemingly unrelated variables, such as political affiliation and a preference for the color blue, may be weakly correlated because members of a certain political group may be more likely to wear red, white, and blue ties, which, in turn, leads those colors to become more familiar and, hence, preferable. There is no causal effect of political orientation and color preferences, obviously, but the variety of complex, indirect, and, ultimately uninteresting pathways are sufficient to produce a non-zero correlation between the variables.[4]

In summary, the null hypothesis of zero correlation is unlikely to be true in personality research. Thus, personality researchers who use significance tests should relax their concerns about Type I errors, which can occur only if the null hypothesis is true, and focus more on minimizing Type II errors. Better yet, a case could be made for ceasing significance testing altogether. If the null hypothesis is unlikely to be true, testing it is unlikely to advance our knowledge.

The Paradox of Using NHST as a "Hypothesis Test"

Textbook authors often write about significance tests as if they are "hypothesis tests." This terminology is unfortunate because it leads researchers to believe that significance tests provide a way to test *theoretical*, as opposed to *statistical*, hypotheses. As we mentioned previously, the link between theoretical hypotheses, statistical hypotheses, and data, however, does not receive much attention in psychology (Link 1 in Figure 9.1, see Meehl, 1990). In fact, explicit training on translating theoretical hypotheses into statistical ones is absent in most graduate programs. The only mathematical training that students typically receive is concerned with the relation between statistical hypotheses and data (Link 2 in Figure 9.1)—the most trivial part of the equation, from a scientific and philosophical perspective (Meehl, 1990).

One limitation of significance tests is that the null hypothesis will always be rejected as sample size approaches infinity, because no statistical model (including the null model) is accurate to a large number of decimal places. This fact leads to an interesting paradox, originally articulated by Meehl (1967): In cases in which the null hypothesis is the hypothesis of interest (e.g., in some domains of physics or in psychological applications of structural equation models), the theory is subjected to a more stringent test as sample size and measurement precision increase. In cases in which the null hypothesis is the straw man (e.g., in most personality research), the theory is subjected to a weaker test as sample size and precision increase.

According to Meehl, a theoretical model that is good, but not perfect, should have a greater chance of being rejected as the research design becomes more rigorous (i.e., as more observa-

tions are collected and with greater fidelity). As precision increases, researchers are able to ignore the problem of how sample values relate to population values (i.e., the right-hand side of Figure 9.1) and focus more on the implication of those values for the theoretical predictions under consideration (i.e., the left-hand side of Figure 9.1). Because psychologists equate the significance test with the test of the theoretical hypothesis, however, the process flows in the opposite direction in psychology. Our studies bode well for the research hypothesis, whether it is right or not, as our sample sizes increase because the probability of rejecting the null approaches 1.00.

NHST Has Distorted the Scientific Nature of Our Literature

Although any single study in personality psychology is likely to meet the key criteria for being scientific (i.e., based on *systematic* empirical observation), the literature is unlikely to do so. Because researchers are selective in which studies they choose to submit for publication, the research published in the leading journals represents a biased sample of the data actually collected by psychologists.

Research by Cooper, DeNeve, and Charlton (1997) indicates that this bias creeps into the scientific publication process at multiple levels. For example, based on a survey of researchers who submitted studies for review to the Internal Review Board (IRB) at the University of Missouri, Cooper and his colleagues found that, of the 155 studies that were approved and started, only 121 were carried forward to the data analysis stage. Among those studies, only 105 led to a written document and only 55 of those were submitted as articles or book chapters. The reasons investigators cited for not drafting written reports included design problems, uninteresting findings, and the lack of significant results. It is important to note that 74% of studies with significant results were submitted for publication, whereas only 4% of studies with nonsignificant results were submitted, indicating a strong reporting bias due to the use of significance tests (see also Sterling, Rosenbaum, & Weinkam, 1995).

Many researchers are aware of the publication bias problem in the literature. Nonetheless, they operate as if the bias is unidirectional: The bias works against decent studies that do not get published, but what does get published is valid. However, one of the artifacts of the NHST publication bias is that the published findings can be inaccurate too. Schmidt (1996) has illustrated this problem nicely. Assume that a researcher is interested in the effect of a specific treatment on an outcome and that the true effect size is equal to a standardized mean difference of .50. Using a sample size of 15 per cell, the researcher conducts a significance test to determine whether the observed difference allows him or her to reject the null hypothesis. Because the null hypothesis is false in this scenario, the Type I error rate is undefined. As a consequence, the only error that can be made is a Type II error (the failure to reject the null when it is false). In Schmidt's example, the power to do so is 37%, indicating that the researcher has only a 37% chance of coming to the correct conclusion. The point of this example, however, is not to revisit the problems of low power in psychological research. The crucial point is that, because of power problems, the researcher must observe a standardized mean difference of .62 to obtain a significant result—a difference that is larger than the actual effect size. Thus, the only way for the researcher to correctly reject the null hypothesis it to make an error in the direction of overestimating the effect by capitalizing on sampling variability. More troubling, if multiple studies were conducted and only the significant effects were published, the published literature would lead to a meta-analytic estimate of .89—a value that is 78% higher than the true difference of .50 (Schmidt, 1996).

Let us assume for a moment that some of the nonsignificant results were published and that a psychologist were to peruse the empirical literature. The reviewer would notice that the treatment worked in some studies, but failed to work in others. This raises the question: Why? The most common answer to this question would be that there is a moderator that explains why the effect emerges in some cases but not in others. However, as Schmidt (1996) notes, the variation in effect size estimates across the studies in this example is due entirely to sampling errors. According to Schmidt, it is probably the case that many of the moderator variables that have been proposed in the literature are based on false leads. That is, given the current statistical power problems in psychological research, the most plausible explanation for why an effect emerges in one study but not in the next is low power, not the existence of moderators.

We share one final observation on how significance testing can distort the answers psychologists obtain. Because power considerations are rare, many researchers, instead of designing a study and including a predetermined number of participants, continue the study until they get significant results (or until they run out of patience). This leads to two problems. First, if the null hypothesis is true, this practice leads to an inflated Type I error rate. We do not elaborate on this point here because we do not think Type I errors are a real problem in personality research, although we suspect they are a problem in experimental social psychology (see Greenwald, 1975). Second, and related to Schmidt's (1996) point, this practice leads to overestimates of effect sizes because, for a study to produce a significant result, the association that is required may be larger than the true association. Thus, when sampling variability produces a deviation from the true value that favors a significant result, it will always be in the direction of overestimating the association rather than underestimating it (Berger & Berry, 1988). Indeed, in the coefficients we studied in our literature review, the correlation between the magnitude of correlations and the sample size from which they came was −.24. In other words, studies with smaller Ns tended to produce larger effects or, more accurately, larger effects were necessary in order to detect significant differences with small sample sizes.

In summary, one of the criticisms of the use of NHST, especially when coupled with inattention to power considerations, is that it can lead to the wrong answers. Specifically, the habits and traditions that govern the use of NHST can result in (1) a biased literature and (2) inflated effect sizes. In the rare case in which the null hypothesis is true, these same traditions lead to inflated Type I error rates.

What Are the Alternatives to Significance Testing?: Recommendations and Considerations

In this final section we make some recommendations on what researchers can do to break NHST habits. We emphasize at the outset that there are no magical alternatives to NHST. From our point of view, the best solution is to simply stop using significance tests. We realize, however, that this solution is too radical to lead to constructive change in the field. Thus, in the meantime, we advocate that if significance tests are used, they be used in an educated and judicious way. We believe the first step in this process is to follow Meehl's (1990) recommendation: Always ask yourself, If there was no sampling error present (i.e., if the sample statistics *were* the population values), what would these data mean and does the general method provide a strong test of my theory? If one feels uncomfortable confronting this question, then one is probably relying on significance testing for the wrong reasons. If one can answer this question confidently, then the use of significance tests will probably do little harm.

Distinguish Parameter Estimation from Theory Testing

Our first recommendation is that researchers make a sharper distinction between two distinct functions of empirical research: to describe the world and to test theoretical models. In our opinion, most of the research that is conducted in social and personality psychology is best construed as descriptive, parameter-estimation research. Just about any research question posed in psychology can be spun as one of parameter estimation. For example, an article that states that the research was conducted to "test the hypothesis" that two variables are related in a specific manner can just as easily be framed as being conducted to "determine the correlation" between those variables because the value of that correlation has important implications for the theory or theories under consideration.

Once researchers recognize that most of their research questions are really ones of parameter estimation, the appeal of statistical tests will wane. Specifically, researchers will find it much more important to report estimates of parameters and effect sizes, to report error bands associated with those estimates (e.g., standard errors or confidence intervals), and to discuss in greater detail the sampling process (e.g., whether a convenience sample was used, how attrition might impact estimates, how the reliability of measures might compromise the estimate of the population parameter).

We also think that once researchers begin to equate inferential statistics with estimation, they will be less inclined to confuse "hypothesis testing," as it is discussed in the philosophy of science, with "significance testing." Specifically, without NHST, hypothesis testing will become much more rigorous and informative because researchers will need to find creative ways to test hypotheses without relying on *p*-values.

Don't Test the Null Hypothesis When It Is Known to Be False

One of the absurdities of significance testing is that it encourages researchers to test the hypothesis of "no difference" or "zero correlation" even in situations in which previous research has shown the null hypothesis to be false. In our experience in reviewing manuscripts, we have repeatedly seen cases in which a specific association is examined across a handful of samples and the association was significant in one sample but not significant in the other. Even when the effect sizes are identical in the two studies, researchers speculate on possible moderator effects that may have led to the effect in one situation and not the next.

In such cases, does it make sense to test the null hypothesis of 0.00 in the second study? We do not see a reason to do so. In fact, it may be best to combine the different estimates to create a single estimate that takes into account the information gleaned from the two samples. Regardless of how researchers choose to handle this kind of situation, we recommend against concluding that there is an effect in one sample and not in the other when the effect sizes are in the same general ballpark. Without considering issues of power, sampling variability, and effect sizes, there are little grounds for assuming that a nonsignificant result in one study is incompatible with a significant result from a previous study.

Take Steps to Remove the Bias in the Literature

One of the key points we made previously was that the existing literature in psychology is not as scientific as it could be. If researchers and editors are deciding on which data to publish based primarily on study outcome rather than study design, they are ensuring that significant effects will be overrepresented in the literature. How can this problem be fixed? One solution is to make the publishing process more similar to that used by granting agencies. In other words, manuscripts should be evaluated and accepted based solely on the potential importance of the questions being addressed and the soundness of the methods proposed to answer those questions. If reviewers appreciate the significance of the questions and have confidence in the methods used to address them, then the research will, by definition, make a contribution to knowledge—even if that contribution is the documentation of a so-called null effect.

Another potential advantage of such a publishing system is that it would encourage researchers to focus on strengthening their research designs. The current publishing system appears to reward significant findings at the expense of the quality of research design. For example, it is possible for a researcher with a carefully designed longitudinal study to have a manuscript rejected because his or her key results fail to reach statistical significance, whereas a researcher with a cross-sectional study and a significant result may have his or her manuscript accepted. If researchers were competing for journal space on the basis of research design rather than the statistical significance of findings, researchers would likely pay more attention to measurement and design issues and their role in advancing knowledge.

Perhaps the take-home message here is that "knowledge" is more than just knowing what variables are associated with one another; knowledge also entails knowing which variables are *not* associated with one another. Our publication system currently encourages investigators to function like detectives who devote their time to poking around for clues to indict any suspect, while never attempting to gather the kind of information needed to rule out suspects.

Do Not Fall into the Trap of Assuming That the Bigger the Effect, the Better the Theory

In many research circles (although not necessarily in personality psychology), the concept of effect size is relatively new. For example, in experimental social psychology, researchers have traditionally omitted standard deviations from their empirical reports, thereby giving readers nothing to judge *except* the *p*-value associated with an effect. Fortunately, psychologists are now starting to emphasize effect sizes and parameter estimates more in their research (Wilkinson & the Task Force on Statistical Inference, 1999). The recent emphasis on the reporting of effect sizes, however, has raised a second and equally precarious problem. Namely, there appears to be a "bigger the

better" heuristic that has evolved in psychology, such that larger effect sizes are treated as being more important than smaller ones.

Why are researchers impressed with large effect sizes—even when those effects are estimated with little precision? The answer may have to do with limitations in the way in which psychologists derive predictions from theories, coupled with a dash of insecurity. Specifically, many quantitative predictions in personality psychology are *ordinal* ones, making claims about the directions of effects (e.g., positive or negative) rather than the specific values of parameters or the ratios between them. When an ordinal prediction is made, testing it without NHST is fairly straightforward: The correlation is either the right sign (i.e., positive or negative) or it is not. There is simply no way to impose a stiffer hurdle on a directional prediction other than by demanding larger effects.

Emphasizing the *size* of effects is not a wise strategy if one is genuinely interested in understanding the *true* relationships between variables in the natural world. Without an accurate map of how the psychological world is organized, there is no foundation for theory construction and theory testing. For example, if a researcher is interested in knowing the relationship between neuroticism and mortality (e.g., Mroczek & Spiro, 2005), there are good reasons for wanting to get the answer right, at least for the neurotic among us. If the true relationship is equal to a coefficient of .15, an empirical result is "better" if it estimates this particular quantity with precision rather than overestimating it as .30.

We should make it clear that the tendency to equate bigger with better does not typically emerge when researchers make point predictions instead of ordinal predictions. A *point prediction* is a specific quantitative value or ratio implied by a theory. For example, according to the commonly used additive genetic (*ACE*) model in behavior genetics, the correlation between phenotypes for DZ twins is expected to be half that of the MZ correlation. Thus, if the DZ correlation is much higher than the predicted value (i.e., and even more statistically significant), such a finding would be problematic for researchers testing hypotheses concerning additive genetic effects.

We mentioned previously that part of the "bigger = better" mentality might stem from insecurity. The field of personality psychology has often been accused of concerning itself with small effects. Should personality psychologists harbor these insecurities? There are two points that researchers should bear in mind when considering this matter. First, one should never expect the association between any two variables in the natural world to be too large due to the phenomenon of multiple causation (see Ahadi & Diener, 1989). To the extent to which multiple factors play a role in shaping individual differences in a domain, the association between any one factor and that outcome will necessarily be limited. For example, if 80% of the variance in an outcome is due to eight independent variables with identical weights, the maximum value of the correlation between any one of those variables and the outcome will be .32. One should expect high correlations only in situations in which a researcher is trying to assess the same variable in distinct ways or in cases in which variation in the outcome of interest is, in reality, affected by only a small number of variables.

The second critical point is that the "small" associations typically observed in personality research are on par with those observed in other areas of scientific inquiry. Several decades ago personality psychology got a bad rep because the correlations reported in the literature rarely peaked above .30, a value that came to be known as the "personality coefficient" (Mischel, 1968). What critics of the field failed to appreciate, however, is that most effects, when expressed in a standard effect size metric, such as the correlation coefficient, rarely cross the .30 barrier. As Funder and Ozer (1983) cogently observed, the classic studies in experimental social psychology, when expressed in a standard effect size metric, are no larger than those commonly observed in personality research. In an extraordinarily valuable article, Meyer and his colleagues (2001) summarized via meta-analysis the effect sizes associated with various treatments and tests. We have summarized some of their findings in Table 9.4, and highlight a few noteworthy ones here. For example, the effect of chemotherapy on surviving breast cancer is equivalent to a correlation of .03, whereas the effect of psychotherapy on well-being is equal to a correlation of .30.

In closing this section, we make a final point. Namely, psychologists in general do not have a well-honed intuition for judging effect sizes. In other words, researchers often label correlations in the .10 range as "small" because, implicitly, they are comparing the value of the correlation against its theoretical maximum— 1.00. To see why this can be a problem, consider a concrete example. No one would doubt that shooting someone in the knee caps would severely impair that person's ability to walk without a limp. In fact, when asked what the phi correlation should be between (1) being shot in the kneecaps and (2) walking with a limp, most people we have queried have indicated that it is likely .80 or higher. For the sake of discussion, let us throw some hypothetical numbers at the problem and see how they pan out. Let us imagine that we have a sample of 20 people who were shot in the kneecaps, 18 of whom were walking with a limp shortly after the incident. Let us also assume that 3,000 people in our sample have not been shot in the kneecaps and 500 of these 3,000 are walking with a limp. In this scenario, the phi correlation between being shot in the knee and walking with a limp is only .16. Nonetheless, there is certainly a powerful effect underlying these data. Consider the fact that 90% of people who were shot in the kneecaps exhibited a limp. (Some did not, simply because they were too busy running away from the shooter.) This intuitively powerful effect appears weak in a correlational metric for two reasons. Most important, the base rate of being shot in the kneecaps is low, occurring in less than 1% of the population. Second, there is a lot of variability in gait among those who were not shot in the kneecaps. Some are walking briskly, but some are limping for a variety of reasons (e.g., they suffer from arthritis, they pulled a leg muscle during a soccer game, they have a ball and chain attached to the left ankle). Because the correlation takes into account the relative rates of gait across the two situations, the natural variability that exists in one situation works to diminish the overall comparison. In order for the effect to emerge as a strong one in a correlational metric, it would not only have to be the case that being shot in the knees impairs gait, but that people who have not been shot are able to walk briskly. In short, sometimes powerful effects appear small when expressed in correlational metrics. Thus, researchers should avoid rushing to judgment too quickly.

In summary, we caution psychologists to avoid the trap of assuming that bigger effect sizes are better. The size of an effect is often contingent not only on the relationship between the two variables in question, but on *all* of the variables involved in the causal system in which they exist. Without understanding the broader system, there is no context in which to evaluate the size of an effect. It is also important to note that personality psychologists should not feel insecure about so-called small correlations. The effects typically observed in personality psychology are no smaller than those observed in other sciences, including other domains of psychology as well as medicine (Meyer et al., 2001) and the physical sciences (Hedges, 1987). Indeed, by some standards, personality psychologists are accomplishing many of their goals (e.g., predicting job performance) with better success than other scientific disciplines (Meyer et al., 2001).

Generating Point Predictions and Model-Data Bootstrapping

It is our belief that the use of NHST has impeded the development of more sophisticated models in personality psychology—models that either make point predictions or place severe constraints on the range of plausible empirical values. But how can researchers move beyond directional predictions? In this section we make some modest recommendations on steps that researchers can take to derive more precise predictions from their theoretical assumptions.

Our first recommendation is that researchers move beyond bivariate associations and focus instead on multivariate patterns. For example, in path analysis, the focus is typically on explaining the *pattern of associations* between variables rather than the specific value of any one association. Indeed, in path analysis the model-implied correlation or covariance matrix is tested, not necessarily the value of any one path. To illustrate, take a simple theoretical model in which certain kinds of appraisals lead to the experience of negative emotions which, in turn, lead people to behave in a less supportive way toward their romantic partners (see Figure 9.2). It is important to note that the theory that inspired this model makes no assumptions about the specific values of causal paths a and b; nonetheless, the range of possible correlations matrices among the three variables is tightly constrained. Using covariance algebra, it can be shown that the correlation between appraisals and affect is equal to a, the correla-

tion between appraisals and support is equal to $a \times b$, and the correlation between affect and support is equal to b. Thus, although the model is fairly vague in the predictions it makes about the precise value of specific causal paths, it is specific in the predictions it makes about the *pattern* of associations between variables.

This point leads to our second recommendation: Researchers should use model-data bootstrapping to derive quantitative predictions. Once a model (such as the one articulated above) is specified—and once certain parameters are estimated—severe constraints are placed on kinds of empirical values that should be observed if the model is correct. In the previous example, if researchers already had data on (1) the correlation between appraisals and negative affect and (2) the correlation between negative affect and supportive behavior, it would be possible to estimate paths a and b and then derive the expected correlation between appraisals and supportive behavior—a correlation that has yet to be empirically observed. If a and b are estimated as .50, then the expected correlation between appraisals and supportive behavior is $a \times b$ or .25. It would now be possible for researchers to collect empirical data on the correlation between appraisals and supportive behavior to test this prediction. Without model-data bootstrapping, researchers could only predict a positive association between these two variables. With model-data bootstrapping, however, it is possible to specify a specific value (i.e., $r = .25$) that should be observed if the theory is correct.

We offer one more example of this process from our own work as a means of driving the point home. There have been debates in recent years about the stability of individual differences in basic personality traits, such as neuroticism, attachment security, and subjective well-being. Although the debate has focused largely on the mechanisms of stability and change, the predictions that are tested are fairly vague. One camp might argue that the test–retest correlation over a long span of time will be small, whereas the others might argue that the correlation should be large. To illustrate how it is

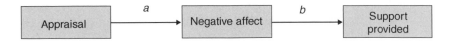

FIGURE 9.2. A model of the causal relations among three variables that constrains the patterns of correlations expected among the measured variables.

possible to go beyond vague directional predictions in this situation, let us consider a simple autoregressive model of stability and change. According to this model, a person's trait score at time T will be a function of his or her trait score at time $T - 1$ plus any other factors that lead to trait change (see Fraley & Roberts, 2005). When this model is formalized, it predicts that the test–retest correlation over interval T will equal a^T, where a is the path leading from the trait at time T to time $T + 1$. If we knew, on the basis of previous research, that the test–retest coefficient for a personality trait over 1 week was .90, then it would be possible to substitute that parameter into the model to generate point predictions about other values that might be observed. Substituting .90 in to the previous equation leads to the prediction that, over 5 weeks, the test–retest correlation will be .59 and that, over 10 weeks, the correlation will be .35. The bottom line is that if one has a theoretical model of the process in question, estimating one or two parameters can sometimes be sufficient to squeeze more precise predictions from the model. Those point predictions, in turn, can then be tested in a more rigorous fashion.[5] We should note that in the absence of such bootstrapping, researchers would simply predict a positive correlation between measurements of a trait across different occasions, a prediction that is not only loose, but, as Fraley and Roberts (2005) explained, perfectly compatible with theoretical perspectives that are incompatible with one another.

Our final recommendation is that researchers experiment with "thinking backward" regarding the relationship between theory and data. When researchers study complex causal models, they often begin by collecting data and then attempt to fit those data to one or more theoretical models. In other words, researchers often treat modeling as a "data analysis" strategy rather than a theoretical exercise, as is revealed in the use of phrases such as "running a model" or "fitting the data." There is a lot to be learned by moving in the other direction. By beginning with several theoretical models, formalizing them, and exploring their unique implications for the data, it is possible to understand the constraints of a model better and to identify exactly which kinds of data are necessary to test alternative theoretical assumptions (see Roberts & Pashler, 2000). In our own theoretical work on stability and change, we have sometimes discovered that by simply formalizing a set of assumptions and exploring their im-

plications mathematically, the predictions implied by the model can be surprisingly different from what might be expected otherwise (Fraley, 2002). There is a lot that can be learned by exploring formal models without actually doing any data analyses. Such explorations can help clarify the predictions of theories, as well as the precise points of convergence and divergence between theoretical models, and, most important, can point the way to the crucial tests that are needed to allow two theoretical models to be distinguished.

Use Confidence Intervals, but Not as Replacements for NHST

It is sometimes suggested that researchers abandon significance tests in favor of confidence intervals. Those who favor this proposal often diverge in exactly how it should be implemented. Some researchers recommend the use of confidence intervals as a useful way to quantify the amount of sampling variability that is associated with a sample estimate. Others argue that confidence intervals should be used because, in addition to providing a more straightforward means for quantifying sampling variability, they can be used for significance testing if desired. For example, if a 95% confidence interval around a correlation overlaps with 0.00, then, conceptually, one might argue that 0.00 offers a plausible account of the data. (This claim, however, is debatable without the use of Bayesian confidence or "credible" intervals. See Salsburg, 2001, for further discussion.) We strongly encourage researchers who wish to use confidence intervals not to fall into the trap of using them as if they were significance tests. Granted, using them as such would still be more informative than using p-values, but replacing NHST with another kind of significance test does not solve the problems that accompany the field's reliance on NHST.

Adopt a Do-It-Yourself Attitude

There tends to be a generational lag in the scientific process (Sulloway 1996). Thus, although the significance-testing war has been waged for some time, it will probably take another generation until researchers can confront the issues in a less contentious way and evaluate the pros and cons of significance testing rationally. In the meantime, it will be necessary for researchers who want to think outside the

NHST box to adopt a do-it-yourself attitude. If you think you would benefit from learning more about formalizing theoretical models (i.e., the left-hand side of Figure 9.1), you will have to start reading more books on philosophy and mathematics, "sitting in" on courses in other areas of science, and looking for good examples of non-NHST research to emulate. Unless there is a revolution on the horizon, this kind of training will not come to you; you will have to hunt it down—or, if you are a graduate student, demand it from your graduate program.

To facilitate this process, we recommend that you start learning how to use mathematical software packages other than *SPSS*. There is an increasing trend toward "click and point" data analysis in mainstream statistical packages. This trend will constrain, not liberate, your ability to explore new approaches to theory testing and data analysis. *R*, *S-Plus*, *Mathematica*, *Matlab*, and other packages exist that allow you to do things your own way. We strongly encourage you to explore these packages. The learning curve is a bit steep at first, but keep in mind, most people do not master *SPSS* in a day either.

Nature does not present itself as an ANOVA problem. If you chose to explore theoretical modeling techniques, chances are that the models you develop for psychological phenomena will not conform to those available in the *SPSS* tool chest. You will need to be able to build, explore, and test these models via alternative means.

Conclusions

Cohen (1994) opened his well-cited article on the significance-testing debate by stating, "I make no pretense of the originality of my remarks in this article. . . . If [the criticism] was hardly original in 1966, it can hardly be original now" (p. 997). Many of the points we have made in this chapter overlap considerably with those that have been made in the past. Yet it seems prudent to revisit the key ideas behind the significance debate again, given that a new generation of researchers have come of age since the debate was last waged. In this chapter we have summarized some of the core ideas, but we have also tried to contextualize the discussion to make it clear how significance testing may impact the study of personality and

how we might be able to move beyond significance tests. It is our hope that this chapter will help stimulate discussion of these matters and encourage some personality psychologists to reconsider the role of significance testing in their research.

Notes

1. Einstein's theory predicted an angular deflection of 1.75, whereas Newton's theory predicted an angular deflection of 0.875. If observation site is used as the unit of analysis, the Eddington data do not differ from 0.875 ($t[1] = 7.13$, $p = .09$), but they do differ from 0 ($t[1] = 14.417$, $p = .04$).
2. When the values of σ^2 are unknown, as they often are in applied research, they can be estimated by the sample variance, using well-known corrections.
3. When there are multiple hypotheses, the term $P(D|H_1)$ is expanded accordingly. In this example, we assume that the research hypothesis, H_1, is inclusive of all values other than 0.00 (i.e., a nondirectional prediction).
4. This problem is less severe in experimental research because when people are randomly assigned to conditions, the correlations between nuisance variables and the independent variable approaches zero as the sample size increases.
5. For the record, a simple autoregressive model of continuity and change in personality traits does not fare well in empirical tests (Fraley & Roberts, 2005).

Recommended Readings

Meehl, P. E. (1978). Theoretical risks and tabular asterisks: Sir Karl, Sir Ronald, and the slow progress of soft psychology. *Journal of Consulting and Clinical Psychology, 46*, 806–834.

Meehl, P. E. (1990). Appraising and amending theories: The strategy of Lakatosian defense and two principles that warrant it. *Psychological Inquiry, 1*, 108–141.

Meyer, G. J., Finn, S. E., Eyde, L., Kay, G. G., Moreland, K. L., Dies, R. R., et al. (2001). Psychological testing and psychological assessment: A review of evidence and issues. *American Psychologist, 56*, 128–165.

Oakes, M. (1986). *Statistical inference: A commentary for the social and behavioral sciences.* New York: Wiley.

Schmidt, F. L., & Hunter, J. E. (1997). Eight common but false objections to the discontinuation of significance testing in the analysis of research data. In L. A. Harlow, S. A. Mulaik, & J. H. Steiger (Eds.), *What if there were no significance tests?* (pp. 37–64). Mahwah, NJ: Erlbaum.

References

Ahadi, S., & Diener, E. (1989). Multiple determinants and effect size. *Journal of Personality and Social Psychology*, 56, 398–406.

Berger, J. O., & Berry, D. A. (1988). Statistical analysis and illusion of objectivity. *American Scientist*, 76, 159–165.

Cohen, J. (1962). The statistical power of abnormal-social psychological research: A review. *Journal of Abnormal and Social Psychology*, 65, 145–153.

Cohen, J. (1992). A power primer. *Psychological Bulletin*, 112, 155–159.

Cohen, J. (1994). The earth is round (*p* < .05). *American Psychologist*, 49, 997–1003.

Cooper, H., DeNeve, K., & Charlton, K. (1997). Finding the missing science: The fate of studies submitted for review by a human subjects committee. *Psychological Methods*, 2, 447–452.

Fraley, R. C. (2002). Attachment stability from infancy to adulthood: Meta-analysis and dynamic modeling of developmental mechanisms. *Personality and Social Psychology Review*, 6, 123–151.

Fraley, R. C., & Roberts, B. W. (2005). Patterns of continuity: A dynamic model for conceptualizing the stability of individual differences in psychological constructs across the life course. *Psychological Review*, 112, 60–74.

Funder, D. C., & Ozer, D. J. (1983) Behavior as a function of the situation. *Journal of Personality and Social Psychology*, 44, 107–112.

Gigerenzer, G. (1993). The superego, the ego, and the id in statistical reasoning. In G. Keren & C. Lewis (Eds.), *A handbook for data analysis in the behavioral sciences: Methodological issues* (pp. 311–339). Hillsdale, NJ: Erlbaum.

Greenwald, A. G. (1975). Consequences of prejudice against the null hypothesis. *Psychological Bulletin*, 82, 1–20.

Greenwald, A. G., Gonzalez, R., Harris, R. J., & Guthrie, D. (1996). Effect sizes and *p* values: What should be reported and what should be replicated? *Psychophysiology*, 33, 175–183.

Harris, R. J. (1997). Significance tests have their place. *Psychological Science*, 8, 8–11.

Hedges, L. V. (1987). How hard is hard science, how soft is soft science?: The empirical cumulativeness of research. *American Psychologist*, 42, 443–455.

Kaku, M. (2004). *Einstein's cosmos*. New York: Atlas Books.

Krueger, J. (2001). Null hypothesis significance testing: On the survival of a flawed method. *American Psychologist*, 56, 16–26.

Lykken, D. L. (1991). What's wrong with psychology? In D. Cicchetti & W. M. Grove (Eds.), *Thinking clearly about psychology: Vol. 1. Matters of public interest: Essays in honor of Paul E. Meehl* (pp. 3—39). Minneapolis: University of Minnesota Press.

Meehl, P. E. (1967). Theory-testing in psychology and physics: A methodological paradox. *Philosophy of Science*, 34, 103–115.

Meehl, P. E. (1978). Theoretical risks and tabular asterisks: Sir Karl, Sir Ronald, and the slow progress of soft psychology. *Journal of Consulting and Clinical Psychology*, 46, 806–834.

Meehl, P. E. (1990). Appraising and amending theories: The strategy of Lakatosian defense and two principles that warrant it. *Psychological Inquiry*, 1, 108–141.

Meyer, G. J., Finn, S. E., Eyde, L., Kay, G. G., Moreland, K. L., Dies, R. R., et al. (2001). Psychological testing and psychological assessment: A review of evidence and issues. *American Psychologist*, 56, 128–165.

Mischel, W. (1968). *Personality and assessment*. New York: Wiley.

Mroczek, D. K., & Spiro, A., III. (2005). *Personality change influences mortality in older men*. Manuscript submitted for publication.

Oakes, M. (1986). *Statistical inference: A commentary for the social and behavioral sciences*. New York: Wiley.

Roberts, S., & Pashler, H. (2000). How persuasive is a good fit? A comment on theory testing. *Psychological Review*, 107, 358–367.

Rozeboom, W. W. (1960). The fallacy of the null hypothesis significance test. *Psychological Bulletin*, 57, 416–428.

Salsburg, D. (2001). *The lady tasting tea: How statistics revolutionized science in the twentieth century*. New York: Freeman.

Scarr, S. (1997). Rules of evidence: A larger context for the statistical debate. *Psychological Science*, 8, 16–17.

Schmidt, F. L. (1996). Statistical significance testing and cumulative knowledge in psychology: Implications for training of researchers. *Psychological Methods*, 1, 115–129.

Sedlmeier, P., & Gigerenzer, G. (1989). Do studies of statistical power have an effect on the power of studies? *Psychological Bulletin*, 105, 309–316.

Sohn, D. (1998). Statistical significance and replicability: Why the former does not presage the latter. *Theory and Psychology*, 8, 291–311.

Sterling, T. D., Rosenbaum, W. L., & Weinkam, J. J. (1995). Publication decisions revisited: The effect of the outcome of statistical tests on the decision to publish and vice versa. *American Statistician*, 49, 108–112.

Sulloway, F. J. (1996). *Born to rebel: Birth order, family dynamics, and creative lives*. New York: Pantheon.

Wilkinson, L., & the Task Force on Statistical Inference. (1999). Statistical methods in psychology journals: Guidelines and explanations. *American Psychologist*, 54, 594–604.

## CHAPTER 10

Cross-Cultural Personality Research

Conceptual and Methodological Issues

Verónica Benet-Martínez

Personality is shaped by both genetic and environmental factors; among the most important of the latter are cultural influences. Culture consists of shared meaning systems that provide the standards for perceiving, believing, evaluating, communicating, and acting among those who share a language, a historic period, and a geographic location (Triandis, 1996). More recently Chiu and Chen (2004) have defined culture as "a network of knowledge that is produced, distributed, and reproduced among a collection of interconnected people" (p. 173). Culture is transmitted through language, media messages, cultural practices and institutions, and through the modeling of behavior. Cultural influences on personhood were a prevalent concern in early personality psychology (e.g., Allport, 1954; Kluckhohn & Murray, 1948; McClelland, 1961), but largely ignored in modern personality theory and research until the early 1990s. However, many cultural studies conducted during the last de-cade on issues such as self-processes, emotion, and personality traits have firmly established the following: Culture is a key determinant of what it means to be a person (see reviews by Church, 2000; Diener, Oishi, & Lucas, 2003; Triandis & Suh, 2002).[1] Furthermore, our personality—the affective, motivational, and cognitive dispositions that influence our evaluations and reactions to the environment—cannot be separated from the broad social and cultural context where it develops and is expressed. In fact, as Markus and Kitayama (1998) eloquently say:

> A cultural psychology approach assumes that personality . . . is completely interdependent with the meanings and practices of particular sociocultural contexts. People develop their personalities over time through their active participation in the various social worlds in which they engage. A cultural psychological perspective implies that *there is no personality without culture*; there is only a biological entity. (p. 67; emphasis added)

Most personality psychologists would agree that the systematic study of how culture influences social and intrapersonality behavior should be an essential part of our discipline. Yet cultural studies continue to be somewhat underrepresented in personality psychology. Why is this? One reason may be historical. Because of the serious methodological, theoretical, and ethical limitations of several cultural anthropological studies conducted in the middle decades of the 20th century (e.g., "culture and personality" or "national character" studies), some psychologists may still view cultural studies of personality with skepticism (LeVine, 2001). In addition, cultural psychological studies pose unique methodological challenges (concerning the conditions and parameters of research) to traditional personality psychology. Comparisons across cultural groups are often challenging and expensive; many cultural studies require painstaking translations, new hypotheses and instruments, expensive overseas trips, and networking with foreign researchers who are familiar with the cultures under study. Furthermore, several factors may limit the interpretation of results, including problems in translation, the presence of response biases, and the unfamiliarity of respondents in some cultures with the use of rating scales.

Despite the aforementioned challenges, cultural research offers scientists exciting and interesting benefits and opportunities not available with traditional research approaches (Matsumoto, 2000). Cultural personality studies help elucidate how macrocontextual factors mediate and moderate personality outcomes (e.g., McCrae, 2001; Schimmak, Radhakrishnan, Oishi, Dzokoto, & Ahadi, 2002), help dispel shaky cultural stereotypes (e.g., Terracciáno et al., 2005), and test the generalizability of our theories (e.g., Benet-Martínez & John, 1998). Cultural studies, which often rely on multiple languages and samples, also offer researchers a way of dealing with classic methodological issues regarding construct validity and generalizability (e.g., need to control for possible confounding variables such as socioeconomic status (SES) or language proficiency; use of multisample, multitrait, multimethod designs, etc.).

Early cultural research in psychology was problematic in that it was often based on three implicit or explicit faulty assumptions (Padilla & Lindholm, 1995), as in the following: (1) the use of White college samples as the standard against which other groups should be compared; (2) assuming that psychological instruments and theories are universally applicable across cultural groups or can be used with small adjustments; and (3) neglect of possible confounding variables such as social class, education, gender, or English proficiency. This chapter challenges these assumptions and offers suggestions for conducting valid cross-cultural personality research.

Theoretical Issues

Most cultural studies in personality are concerned with one or both of the following (interrelated) two questions: As people of varying cultures and ethnicities, how are we different and how are we alike? How do culture and ethnicity shape our identities and personalities? Notice that the first question deals with the issue of *differences/universality* in personality, and the second question is concerned with the origin of and *processes* behind these differences. Regardless of the questions at hand, any personality psychologists doing cultural work should be familiar with the following conceptual and definitional issues: (1) differences between culture ethnicity, race, and social class; (2) interdependence between culture and personality; (3) the emic versus etic debate; and (4) differences between cultural and cross-cultural approaches.

Awareness of these issues can help cultural personality researchers frame their questions properly. Furthermore, these issues inform the methodological considerations reviewed in the following sections of this chapter.

Culture, Ethnicity, and Race

Culture, ethnicity, and race are three different constructs, yet researchers often used them interchangeably. Confusion or oversights with regard to these categories result in research findings that are difficult to compare and inappropriate hypotheses and discussions. *Culture* is the broadest construct of the three, as defined earlier in this chapter. *Ethnicity* is a central component of culture. Ethnicity is neither simple nor clear-cut, but it entails one or more of the following: common background or social origins; shared culture and traditions that are distinctive, maintained between generations, and result in a sense of identity and group membership; and shared language or religious tradition (Senior & Bhopal, 1994). *Race* refers to shared genetic heritage, expressed by common external physical characteristics such as facial features, skin color, and hair texture. Because the construct of race was developed as a social classification system in which certain populations were categorized, race as an explanatory variable (at least in psychology) has been and continues to be controversial and dangerous. Accordingly, most social scientists use the more inclusive concept of ethnicity, which encompasses elements of race (for some groups only) and culture (Phinney, 1996).

A common mistake is to use the terms *ethnicity* and *race* interchangeably, but as said earlier, ethnicity usually implies shared identity and cultural ancestry, and race does not. Take the ethnic label "Hispanic" or "Latino," for instance. Racially speaking, Hispanic individuals can be White (e.g., Spaniards or Argentineans), Black (e.g., individuals from Cuba or the Dominican Republic), or Native American (e.g., many Mexicans and Guatemalans). Still, Hispanics define a univocal (yet admittedly very broad) distinct ethnic group because of their shared linguistic, religious, and historical traditions (i.e., predominance of the Spanish language and the Catholic religion, and being colonized by Spain).

Because of their shared elements, *ethnicity* and *culture* are also confused. Culture encompasses macrolevel processes and deals specifically with the values and norms that govern and organize a group of people (e.g., capitalistic culture), defining characteristics and behaviors that are deemed appropriate or inappropriate for an organized group (e.g., American business customs). Culture also specifies the context and environment (i.e., specific place, time, and stimuli) in which ethnicity exists. Obviously, not all individuals sharing a common "cultural space" (e.g., the United States) have the same ethnicity (e.g., Hispanic, Asian American, African American, etc.).

The above definitional issues translate into some specific methodological recommendations. First, ironically, culture is rarely measured in most cultural studies (i.e., nationality is instead used as a proxy for culture). However, the inclusion of measures of cultural identification and/or culture-specific values and behaviors provides researchers with a tool to conduct possible mediational analyses of their effects (or lack of thereof). Second, when dealing with ethnicity as an explanatory variable, it is important to measure each of its three components (Phinney, 1996): (1) cultural values, attitudes, and behaviors associated with it; (2) strength of ethnic identification or group membership; and (3) minority status experience (e.g., discrimination, prejudice). Finally, given the growing numbers of individuals who are multiracial and/or multicultural, researchers should be careful not exclude these individuals from participation.

Mutual Constitution of Culture and Personality

Although many studies have established that cultural forces influence the expression of personality (i.e., culture → personality effects), almost no attention has been given to the processes by which personality may in turn influence culture (personality → culture effects). Evidence from recent studies shows that our personalities shape the cultural contexts in which we live by influencing both micro- (e.g., personal spaces, music preferences, content and style of personal webpages, etc.; Gosling, Ko, Mannarelli, & Morris, 2002; Rentfrow & Gosling, 2003; Vazire & Gosling, 2004) and macro- (e.g., political orientation, social activism, etc.; Cole & Stewart, 1996; Jost, Glaser, Kruglanski, & Sulloway, 2003) cultural elements. Thus, future cultural work in personality may benefit from using designs in which researchers also explore personality effects on culture.

A related limitation of many cultural personality studies is their conceptualization of culture and personality influences as unrelated forces that shape people's lives in a largely independent fashion. Even in those few studies where personality and cultural variables have been considered simultaneously (e.g., Kwan, Bond, & Singelis, 1997; Schimmack et al., 2002), the possible links between these two kinds of variables are not explicitly acknowledged. One factor contributing to this tendency to treat culture and personality as separate effects is researchers' preference for designs in which culture is operationalized exclusively as an "objective," exogenous variable (e.g., country of birth, race, ethnicity) that influences (i.e., moderates) the phenomenon of interest (e.g., link between personality and well-being). However, this traditional separation of cultural and personality influences is at odds with recent cultural psychology views that emphasize the inseparability and mutual constitution of psyche and culture (Aaker, Benet-Martínez, & Garolera, 2001; Markus & Kitayama, 1998; see also Church, 2000, for a review).

An example of a study examining the joint influence of culture on personality is Benet-Martínez and Karakitapoglu-Aygun's (2003) cultural study on well-being. This study explored the following two questions: Do cultural syndromes, such as individualism and collectivism (Triandis, 1996), predict variations in broad personality dispositions, which in turn predict well-being? (i.e., personality as a mediator of the relationship between culture and well-being). Or, rather, do personality traits drive the internalization of individualism and collectivism, which in turn relate to different levels of well-being? (i.e., cultural values as mediators of the relationship between personality traits and well-being).[2] Results from this study supported the first model (personality as a mediator between cultural values and well-being).

Emic versus Etic Debate

A key notion in cultural research is the distinction between *imposed-etic* (imported) and *emic* (indigenous) approaches to data collection (Berry, 1980). The imposed-etic approach (the most commonly used until recently) involves the use of instruments that are either imported in their original form or translated into the local language. This approach is economical and appropriate when the researcher's only goal is to examine how the psychometric properties of a particular "measure" (notice that I do not say "theory" or "construct") generalize to other cultures. However, the imposed-etic approach has a key limitation: It precludes researchers from making valid conclusions about the cross-cultural status of the construct of interest—that is, its definition, nomological network, and prevalence in the other culture. The main problem with the imposed-etic approach is that it assumes that the construct under study (e.g., personality structure) is defined in the culture-of-interest culture in exactly the same way as it is in the culture where the construct and measure were developed (e.g., in terms of five dimensions similar to those captured by the Five-Factor Model [FFM]); thus, the culture-specific elements of the construct (i.e., its *emic* meaning) are likely to be lost when using translated instruments.

Emic approaches, however, explore a particular psychological construct from within the cultural system. With the emic approach, the instruments and theories indigenous to the target culture are developed by relying on a systematic process (through focus groups, interviews, content analyses of popular media, or culturally informed traditional scale development methods) that generates a set of indigenous attributes and stimuli.

The advantages of the imposed-etic strategy is that it is cheap and makes cross-cultural comparisons statistically feasible (given that quantitative judgments of similarity require stimuli that are equivalent); however, as said earlier, the imposed-etic strategy may distort the meaning of constructs in some cultures or overlook their culture-specific (emic) aspects, and thus results from cross-cultural studies that rely on this method are not fully interpretable. Conversely, an emic strategy, in which the construct is identified and measured from scratch, is well suited to identify culture-specific aspects of a construct (i.e., it is ecologically valid), but it is expensive and renders empirical comparisons across cultures very difficult (see Church, 2001, for an excellent review of all the issues to consider in deciding between imposed-etic and emic measures).

One solution to the emic–etic debate has been to pool both approaches in what is known as a *combined emic–etic* approach (see Benet-Martínez, 1999; Yang & Bond, 1990, for illustrations of this approach). The application of a combined emic–etic approach involves the following steps: (1) identifying the emic (indigenous) elements of the construct (again, through focus groups, interviews, etc.) in the target culture, and developing and administering measures that adequately tap these constructs; (2) administering translated measures of the construct (i.e., imposed-etic tests) in addition to the emic measures; and (3) statistically assessing the specificity and overlap between the imported and indigenous measures. This last step is key in that it allows researchers to quantify how well imported and indigenous constructs overlap/differ, and to clarify the meaning of the nonoverlapping indigenous elements (e.g., see Benet-Martínez, 1999, Table 2 and Fig. 1).

Jahoda (1995) has argued that both emic and imposed-etic strategies are needed for the advancement of knowledge. In the same way that "a person is in some ways similar to all other people, in some ways to some other people, and in some ways to no other people" (Kluckhohn & Murray, 1948), some elements of social behaviors are universal (e.g., ways in which societies regulate group sharing and power; Fiske, 1991), others are common to a group or type of cultures (e.g., such as Western cultures' emphasis on the self), and some aspects are unique to a culture (e.g., the Latin trait *simpatía*).

Cultural versus Cross-Cultural Psychology

Researchers are often confused with the distinction between cross-cultural and cultural psychology. It may seem as if the main difference between these two approaches is that the first involves cultural comparisons whereas the second does not; however, the distinction is not so simple. These two approaches have relatively distinct conceptual, methodological, and historical elements (Greenfield, 2000), although at times the differences between these two camps have been overemphasized. Undoubtedly, both approaches share an overarching concern with the understanding of how cultural factors affect behavior.

Church's (2001) recent review of these two traditions clarifies their differences while providing ideas for possible synergy. He notes that cross-cultural studies typically have the following features: (1) a focus on individual differences (particularly personality traits); (2) comparisons of multiple cultures in the search for cultural universals, or culture-specifics along with universals; (3) conceptualization of culture as a variable "outside" the individual (e.g., ecology, economic structure, value system) that influences personality and behavior; (4) use of traditional, standardized (i.e., context-free) psychometric scales and questionnaires; and (5) concern with the cross-cultural equivalence of constructs and measures. The majority of studies examining cultural influences on personality fit within the cross-cultural perspective. Many of these studies share an explicit or implicit optimism regarding the universality of personality dispositions and processes, particularly the Big Five (e.g., McCrae & Costa, 1997).

According to Church (2001), studies within cultural psychology, conversely, are often characterized by (1) a concern with psychological processes (vs. individual differences); (2) a focus on highly contextual descriptions of psychological phenomenon in one or more cul-

tures, with little expectation of finding cultural universals; (3) a conceptualization of culture and psychological functioning as mutually constitutive; and (4) an emphasis on experimental methodology, coupled with qualitative or interpretive approaches. Most studies examining cultural influences on self-processes (e.g., self-enhancement, self-concept) and social behavior (e.g., attribution, dissonance, etc.) fit within the cultural perspective. Cultural psychology also speaks to the socially constructed nature of the construct of personality (e.g., how the notions of traits and personality consistency are particularly meaningful in the West).

I believe that the boundaries between the two disciplines will become less significant as the old debates between social and personality psychology about the meaning and status of the construct of personality finally die out, as new generations of culturally savvy psychological researchers are trained, and as the processes by which culture influences behavior become more understood. In fact, many studies are starting to combine features from both approaches, focusing on individual differences while supporting a view of culture and personality as mutually constituted (e.g., Aaker et al., 2000; Lu & Gilmour, 2004; Oishi & Diener, 2001). Implicit in these recent personality studies is the view that personality variables (e.g., self- and other-ascribed traits, self-concept, well-being, goals) are often inseparable from cultural processes, in that the ways that situations are framed and experienced and the factors a person brings to a situation (e.g., expectations, values, etc.) are cultural products themselves.

Finally, in my view, the future of both cultural and cross-cultural psychology does not rest only in the integration of these camps, but also in their ability to respond to the theoretical and methodological challenges posed by the growing phenomenon of multiculturalism. Both cultural and cross-cultural psychologists often assume that culture is a stable, uniform influence and that nations and individuals are culturally homogeneous. But rapid globalization, continued massive migration, and the resulting demographic changes have resulted in social spaces (schools, homes, work settings) that are culturally diverse and in growing numbers of individuals who identify with, and live in, more than one culture (Hermans & Kempen, 1998; Hong, Morris, Chiu, & Benet-Martínez, 2000). Current and future cultural studies need to develop theoretical models and methodologies that are sensitive to the multiplicity and malleability of cultural meanings *within* and between individuals.

Types of Research Questions

A personality researcher interested in how culture influences self-esteem may ask him- or herself the following questions: Is self-esteem a meaningful psychological variable in non-Western societies, and if so, does it mean the same? Do individuals in Western cultures report higher levels of self-esteem than individuals in so-called collectivist societies, and if so, why? Do traditional measures of self-esteem replicate well in other cultures? Is the link between self-esteem and happiness universal? Do adolescent girls in every society suffer from lower levels of self-esteem as compared with boys, and is the drop in girls' self-esteem around adolescence universal? Notice that five these questions, although interrelated, deal with different issues (i.e., they ask questions about cultural differences in meaning, prevalence, nomological network, and processes in self-esteem, respectively) and thus call for different methodologies.

According to Van de Vijver and Leung (1997), most types of studies and designs in cultural research can be described in terms of three relatively independent dimensions or concerns: (1) level-oriented versus structure-oriented studies (the most basic dimension); (2) hypothesis-driven versus exploratory studies; and (3) contextualized versus noncontextualized studies (as Van de Vijver and Leung note, this taxonomy describes prototypes, and most cultural studies fit into more than one category). Level-oriented studies are mainly concerned with questions of universality versus difference with regard to a certain personality dimension. Early cross-cultural research relied heavily on this approach; these studies found robust cultural differences in key personality variables such as locus of control (Smith, Trompenaars, & Dugan, 1995), self-concept (Bond & Cheung, 1983), and personality traits (Eysenck & Long, 1986). In structure-oriented studies, however, the emphasis is on examining cultural differences with regard to associations among variables (i.e., examining the cultural invariance of correlational patterns, regression functions, factor structures, and causal rela-

tionships). Studies using this approach have examined issues such as whether locus of control has the same correlates in different cultures (Hui & Triandis, 1983), whether the FFM is generalizable to all cultures (McCrae, Yik, Trapnell, Bond, & Paulhus, 1998), whether self-esteem and relational esteem are related to life satisfaction in the same way in Hong Kong and in the United States (Kwan, Bond, & Singelis, 1997), and whether experimental manipulations of success versus criticism produce similar increases/decreases in self-esteem in Japan and the United States (Kitayama, Markus, Matsumoto, & Norasakkunkit, 1997).

Cultural studies can also be organized along two additional dimensions: whether the purpose of the study is mainly hypothesis testing or exploratory, and whether or not contextual factors are measured. Contextual factors are variables that can be used to validate the interpretation of cross-cultural differences and can be either individual related (e.g., gender, generation status, or psychological characteristics such as values or personality) or, more commonly, culture related (e.g., gross national product [GNP], type of religious or economic structure, or country-level scores on individualism–collectivism). Variability in the aforementioned two dimensions (exploration vs. hypothesis testing and inclusion of contextual variables) leads to four different types of studies: psychological difference, generalizability, ecological linkage, and contextual theory studies (see Van de Vijver & Leung, 1997, Table 1; note that both structure- and level-oriented studies are possible in each of these four types of research).

Psychological difference studies are mainly exploratory and do not include contextual variables. Many early comparative personality studies fit within this category (e.g., Benet & Waller, 1995; Eysenck & Long, 1986; McCrae & Costa, 1997). Generalizability studies specify and test hypotheses concerning cultural differences/similarities in the absence of contextual variables (see, e.g., Tafarodi & Swann, 1996). As pointed out by Van de Vijver & Leung (1997), a commendable feature of most psychological difference and generalizability studies is their psychometric rigor, but they are also limited because of their neglect of contextual variables and overreliance on imposed-etic designs.

Ecological linkage studies explore possible explanatory variables for cultural similarities and differences reported in the literature. Such studies are usually conducted at the culture level (i.e., work with aggregate country scores) and include a large number of contextual variables. Examples of ecological-linkage personality studies are McCrae's (2001) study seeking associations between aggregate FFM personality traits and cultural variables (e.g., GNP, country scores on Individualism and Power Distance values); and Van Hemert, Van de Vijver, Poortinga, and Georgas's (2002) study exploring the links between depression and subjective well-being and various relevant country characteristics (e.g., objective and relative living conditions, beliefs and values concerning happiness). Finally, studies with the most theory-building potential, according to Van de Vijver & Leung (1997), are contextual theory studies, which are hypothesis driven and include contextual variables. For instance, Tsai and Levenson's (1997) study tested several hypotheses regarding possible cultural differences in emotional responding during conflict between Chinese Americans and European Americans, while also examining the role of acculturation status in explaining these differences.

Van de Vijver and Leung's (1997) taxonomy of cultural studies provides a useful and long-needed conceptual organization of *traditional* comparative cross-cultural and cultural studies (i.e., studies comparing two or more cultural groups). However, this taxonomy is limited in that it does not include process-oriented studies, that is, studies concerned with cultural processes and dynamics within single groups or within individuals (e.g., acculturation and biculturalism studies). And yet process-oriented studies, particularly those relying on longitudinal designs, are instrumental in elucidating the dynamic interaction of cultural and personality factors in individuals' lives. For instance, recent process-oriented studies have examined the influence of personality traits in the adjustment and identity structure of acculturating individuals (e.g., Benet-Martínez & Haritatos, 2005) and the personality changes that result from immigration (e.g., McRae et al., 1998).

Sampling Issues

Sampling of Cultures

Very commonly, psychologists rely on samples of *convenience* for their cultural studies. This choice is typically driven by considerations of cost, logistics, and collaborator availability (Church & Ortiz, 2005). In studies using samples of convenience, the choice of culture is not theory driven and the questions and conclusions are often haphazard. Samples of convenience are often found in psychological differences studies. Unfortunately, this practice has led to an overrepresentation in mainstream cultural research of modernized societies (e.g., United States, Canada, Japan, Korea) and cultures that are relatively similar to each other (i.e., cultures where researchers live or can access easily).

A *systematic* selection of cultures is the optimal approach. Selection of cultures is purposeful (i.e., theory driven) in that the cultures vary as to the construct of primary interest (e.g., high vs. low emphasis on individual choice) or the construct expected to mediate the cultural difference of interest (e.g., interdependence vs. independence), while attempting to control for extraneous variables (e.g., literacy levels, GNP, religion, climate) (Church & Ortiz, 2005).[3] But when selecting cultures systematically, how many cultures should be included? Because observed differences between cultural groups can rarely be explained in terms of a single explanatory construct, Aaker and colleagues (2001) and Norenzayan and Heine (2005) propose a triangulation method whereby at least three cultural groups, each representing variations on two possible explanatory constructs, are used. For instance, in their study of cultural differences in "brand personality" (the abstract and instrumental qualities ascribed to a commercial brand), Aaker and colleagues selected the United States, Japan, and Spain; the rationale behind this selection was twofold: (1) these three cultural groups vary on the sociocultural dimensions of individualism (United States vs. Spain and Japan) and affective autonomy/expressiveness (Spain and the United States vs. Japan), two value orientations relevant to the perception of commercial brands; (2) at the same time, the United States, Japan, and Spain are similar in their approach to, and resources devoted for, advertising (a possible confound).[4]

Finally, some cautionary words: Researchers should be careful with the common practice of setting Western cultural groups as control groups or standards of comparison against which other cultural groups' results will be interpreted. The problem does not lie in using Western samples—which is both useful and understandable, given that most cultural research is conducted in Western universities—but in the interpretation of differences. Most of the world's population lives in collectivistic rather than individualistic societies, and thus behaviors and values such as self-effacement, filial piety, or interdependence do in fact represent the norm. Furthermore, discussions of difference should be wary of language implying the "othering" or "exoticization" of non-Western individuals.

Sampling of Participants

Within-culture diversity with respect to ethnicity, language, religion, and social class is very common. Unfortunately, however, cultural researchers often simply assume that the study participants are univocally representative of the cultures of interest, and when differences are found, they interpret these differences as "cultural." There is often a tradeoff between representativeness of samples *within* cultures and equivalence of samples *between* cultures (Church & Ortiz, 2005). For instance, researchers often rely on college students to facilitate between-culture comparisons, despite the fact that college students in most cultures are more similar than they are different with regard to preferences (e.g., valuing self-expression and independence) and level of affluence. A systematic approach to the sampling of participants can be used to tease apart these issues. For example, by including both high and low SES subgroups within each culture, researchers will be able to interpret between-cultural group differences as cultural—versus class or education differences (Church & Ortiz, 2005). Using this approach, Haidt and colleagues (Haidt, Koller, & Dias, 1993) found larger differences in morality reasoning between different SES groups than between cultures (Brazil and the United States). Systematic participant sampling can also be used to rule out other powerful confounds such as linguistic ability, generation status, immigrant versus colonized groups, acculturation level, and so forth. However, as Matsumoto (2000) points out, "noncultural" variables (e.g., demographic characteristics) are often intricately blended with culture and cannot be eliminated or controlled in a study. In these cases, researchers should conduct statistical tests to examine the contribution of these characteristics to their variables of interest and temper their interpretations accordingly.

Choice and Adaptation of Instruments

Item Generation and Translation Issues

As introduced earlier, when faced with the task of measuring a particular psychological construct in another culture, researchers can use one of three strategies: (1) rely on translations of already existing measures of the construct of interest (imposed-etic approach); (2) use locally derived instruments capturing the indigenous conceptualization of the construct (emic approach); or (3) use a combination of both types of measures (combined emic–etic approach). The emic approach is, of course, more labor-intensive and involves a first step in which the local meaning, expressions, and behavioral correlates attached to the construct of interest are identified, and a second step in which the researcher and his or her team write items that adequately measure these issues. Some techniques successfully used for the first step are (1) examining how the local media and the popular and academic literature define the construct; (2) polling local psychologists and experts; (3) conducting focus-group discussions and in-depth interviews with relevant samples; and (4) sampling, partially or completely, the local language (in the case of taxonomic personality studies). Ideally, two or more of these strategies should be used in combination (see, e.g., Kim, Atkinson, & Yang, 1999). Furthermore, in the item-writing phase, researchers should exert particular effort in writing statements that are clear and can potentially be translated into other languages. The latter is particularly important if the researcher plans to later compare the predictive validity of two different measures tapping different culture-specific definitions of a construct (e.g., American and Chinese notions of "agency") by administrating both instruments to participants in both cultures. Brislin (1986) developed a set of guidelines for writing new items and modifying existing ones. These guidelines are summarized in Table 10.1.

When translations of already existing instruments are necessary, researchers should use the translation-back-translation procedure (Brislin, 1986). In this iterative method (see Figure 10.1), one or two bilingual individuals (ideally, experts on the construct of interest) undertake the translation of the instrument from the original language into the new language. Using the

TABLE 10.1. Guidelines for Writing New Items and Editing Existing Ones

1. Use short, simple sentences of fewer than 16 words.
2. Employ the active rather than the passive voice, because the former is easier to comprehend.
3. Repeat nouns instead of using pronouns, because the latter may have vague referents; in English, for example, *you* can refer to any number of persons.
4. Avoid metaphors and colloquialisms.
5. Avoid the subjunctive form, with words like *could* and *would*. Many languages express this meaning in different ways, thereby putting a burden on the translator.
6. Add sentences to provide context for key ideas. Redundancy is not harmful for communicating key aspects of the instrument.
7. Avoid verbs and prepositions telling "where" and "when" that do not have a definite meaning. How many times a week do you have to see someone in order to say that you see him "often"?
8. Avoid possessive forms where possible, because it may be difficult to determine the ownership. The ownership such as "his" in "his dog" has to be derived from the context of the sentence, and languages do not have similar rules for expressing this ownership.
9. Use specific rather than general terms. Who is included in "members of your family" strongly differs across cultures; more precise terms are less likely to run into this problem.

Note. From Van de Vijver and Leung (1997). Copyright 1997 by Sage Publications, Inc. Reprinted by permission.

same dictionaries, a second set of bilingual experts independently translate these materials back into the original language. The combination of (1) examining the back translated versions, (2) discussions between translators, and (3) back-and-forth new translations should lead to a final set of translated items that are symmetrically translatable to the original language counterparts.

After the translation-back-translation procedure, the researcher may wish to conduct a small bilingual study to pilot test the translation accuracy of the new instrument. In this bilingual design, bilingual participants complete both language versions of a questionnaire simultaneously (see Benet-Martínez & John, 1998; for a detailed illustration of this method). Dissimilar item statistics between the two versions are usually indicative of poor translations (although, see Ramírez-Esparza, Gosling, Benet-Martínez, Potter, & Pennebaker, 2006). Bilingual designs have important advantages over monolingual designs because they can help unconfound the effects of language and sample differences. Notice that the bilingual design is an extension of the multitrait–multimethod approach (Campbell & Fiske, 1959), because different kinds of "method" (i.e., language) and "trait" (i.e., construct) effects can be tested (see Benet-Martínez & John, 1998, Fig. 1). Most recently, a set of psychometric techniques known as item response theory (IRT) has become a popular and effective tool for examining cross-linguistic equivalence (e.g., Ellis, 1989).

As the preceding discussion attests, the cultural and linguistic challenges involved in the choice and adaptation of instruments for cultural research are not trivial; these challenges, however, can be greatly alleviated by including members of the community or culture of interest in the research team. This strategy seems to be particularly advantageous when these individuals are included as true research partners,

Step	Description
A	Two simultaneous independent translations are made from source to target language by two bilingual experts.
B	Each target language version is blindly back-translated to the source language by two new bilingual experts.
C	The four bilingual experts involved meet with the investigators to review the back-translations, identify differences in meaning, and adapt the target language version to achieve the most accurate culturally equivalent meaning.
D	The new version is independently back-translated by two more bilingual experts.
E	A second meeting of the bilingual experts is held to review the new back-translations. If necessary, the process continues until the team agrees on the culturally equivalent meaning in the srouce- and target-language versions of the instrument.
F	Validation of the back-translated instrument is done by testing for reliablility and equivalence using a sample of bilingual subjects.

FIGURE 10.1. Translation–back-translation model. *Note.* From Jones, Lee, Phillips, Zhang, and Jaceldo (2001). Copyright 2001 by Lippincott Williams & Wilkins. Adapted by permission.

not just as translators or interviewers (Matsumoto, 2000).

Measurement and Conceptual Equivalence

Perhaps the most crucial methodological issue in cultural research is demonstrating the equivalence of the conceptual meaning and methodological operationalization of variables across the cultures under study. This equivalence is an indispensable requirement for valid cross-cultural comparisons. Cultural differences in either the conceptual definitions of variables or their measurement are very common, and researchers need to be aware of these biases' origins and consequences and the available methods to control them (see Van de Vijver & Leung, 1997, for an excellent review of these issues). The notions of "equivalence" and "bias" are, of course, interrelated; equivalence can be seen as the absence of conceptual and measurement biases.

Van de Vijver and Leung (1997) describe three kinds of bias in cross-cultural research: construct bias, method bias, and item bias. Possible sources for each of these types of biases are summarized in Table 10.2. Because these biases are discussed in great detail in Van de Vijver and Leung's book, I provide only short definitions and some examples for them. *Construct bias* exists when the definitions or behavioral markers of the construct being measured do not fully overlap across cultures. For instance, the concept of "good student" is likely to be defined very differently across cultures because notions such as what constitutes good grades, sustained academic effort, appropriate amount of daily homework, and good classroom behavior vary widely across nations (Stevenson et al., 1990). Researchers should be particularly wary of the fact that, even when the constructs are defined similarly, construct bias may exist owing to "construct underrepresentation" (i.e., insufficient sampling of a behavioral domain).

Even if a construct is well represented in the instrument, *method biases* may arise from particular features of the instrument or administration. Method bias comes in three forms: (1) sample bias (e.g., samples are not comparable in terms of SES, age, or familiarity with the construct of interest); (2) instrument bias (e.g., presence of differential response styles, such as acquiescence and extremity)[5]; and (3) administration bias (e.g., miscommunications between researcher and participants, doing individual administration in one culture and group ad-

---

TABLE 10.2. Overview of Types of Bias and Their Most Common Causes

Type of Bias	Source
Construct	• Incomplete overlap of definitions of the construct across cultures. • Differential appropriateness of (sub)test content (e.g., skills do not belong to the repertoire of one of the cultural groups). • Poor sampling of all relevant behaviors (e.g., short instruments). • Incomplete coverage of the construct (e.g., not all relevant domains are sampled).
Method	• Differential social desirability. • Differential response styles such as extremity scoring and acquiescence. • Differential stimulus familiarity. • Lack of comparability of samples (e.g., differences in educational background, age, or gender composition). • Differences in physical conditions of administration. • Differential familiarity with response procedures. • Tester/interviewer effects. • Communication problems between respondent and tester/interviewer in either cultural group.
Item	• Poor item translation. • Inadequate item formulation (e.g., complex wording). • Item(s) may invoke additional traits or abilities. • Incidental differences in appropriateness of the item content (e.g., topic of item of educational test not in curriculum in one cultural group).

Note. From Van de Vijver and Leung (1997). Copyright 1997 by Sage Publications, Inc. Reprinted by permission.

ministration in the other). Finally, *item bias* (also known as differential item functioning; DIF) can result from such factors as complex wording or translation nonequivalence for particular items (e.g., the English and Spanish trait terms *assertive* and *assertivo* do not mean the same, despite being linguistic cognates). The best way to reduce item bias is to ensure a good translation of the instrument items. Available methods for investigating translation equivalence include bilinguals studies (see page 178) and cross-language studies of differential item functioning (e.g., Huang, Church, & Katigbak, 1997).

Relatedly, Van de Vijer and Leung (1997) also describe three levels of equivalence: construct (or structural), measurement unit, and scalar. *Construct or structural equivalence* is present when a construct's definition and behavioral markers are cross-culturally equivalent. This type of equivalence is usually established by showing cross-cultural similarity in factorial structure and nomological networks by means of multigroup confirmatory factor analyses and path analyses (see, e.g., Benet-Martínez & Karakitapoglu-Aygun, 2003; Katigbak, Church, & Akamine, 1996). *Measurement unit equivalence* is present when the measure has the same unit of measurement across cultures (but perhaps different origins). *Scalar equivalence*, however, is present when the measure has the same measurement unit *and* origin across cultures. These last two types of equivalence are the hardest to establish, and researchers often erroneously claim scalar equivalence after establishing construct equivalence. The presence of item bias makes scalar or full-score comparability questionable.

In conclusion, researchers should be aware that comparisons of means across cultures without demonstration of conceptual and measurement equivalence can be misleading and lead to erroneous cultural stereotypes. Furthermore, even after establishing equivalence, researchers can have more confidence in the cultural mean differences they find when the following two conditions are met (Church, 2001): (1) the cultural differences are replicated with different samples and procedures and (2) the cultural differences are predicted and theory driven. Alternatively, researchers may choose to rely on emic, culture-specific measures if the study is exploratory and notions of universality or cross-cultural comparability are not as important, or when the likeli-

hood of obtaining measurement equivalence across cultures is small (Church, 2001).

Other Procedural Issues

Experimenter's Characteristics

A couple of interrelated procedural issues that often emerge during the administration of instruments in a cross-cultural context also need to be considered—namely, the cultural background of the experimenter and the nature of the interaction between experimenter and participant (see Van de Vijver & Leung, 1997, for a review). Specifically, the mere presence of a culturally different person can strongly affect respondents' behavior by eliciting distrust, timidity, or a display of certain demand characteristics. Misunderstandings between experimenter and participants can also give rise to administration problems, and, as said earlier, unambiguous communication is a prerequisite for adequate instrument use across cultures. Because of these two issues—the experimenter's cultural and linguistic background—cultural studies often rely on local individuals as experimenters or test administrators (notice that this recommendation does not imply that cultural groups should be studied only by researchers who belong to the same cultural/ethnic group).

Ethical and Political Concerns

The ethical and political issues involved in the treatment and counseling of cultural, ethnic, and linguistic minority populations have been discussed quite extensively (see, e.g., the American Psychological Association's (APA) 1993 "Guidelines for Providers of Psychological Services to Ethnic, Linguistic, and Culturally Diverse Populations"), yet the role of these issues in cultural research has received much less attention, perhaps because non-U.S. and non-White cultural groups have only recently begun to be studied by mainstream psychology. For instance, many new cultural researchers may not be aware that most American research institutions stipulate that research conducted in foreign countries remains under the institution's purview and guidelines. Typically, cross-cultural research projects must have been approved by the foreign equivalent of an Internal Review Board (IRB) before they can be approved by the investigator's local IRB. Where there is no equivalent board or group, investigators must rely on local experts or community leaders to provide approval. These principles allow for the fact that, although the investigator's institution cannot impose its standards for written documentation on the cultures under study, the standards for ethical conduct of research (e.g., consent process) should be applied.

Furthermore, ethical considerations in doing cultural research call for a careful consideration and respect of the social (e.g., SES), cultural (e.g., intragroup differences in language and values), and political (e.g., immigrant status) contexts of the cultural groups under study. Overlooking these issues may not only be unethical but may compromise the quality of the data and their interpretation. For instance, participants who are unfamiliar with research practices, and/or have different cultural expectations about what these entail, may be reluctant to disclose information about risky or highly personal behaviors because of their standards of decorum or concern that such disclosure may harm their own or their family's reputation and legal status. Furthermore, because of these possible differences in expectations and beliefs, some participants may mistakenly believe that the researcher can actively assist them in obtaining help for personal and communal issues revealed during the course the project (Fisher et al., 2002).

As in the case of dealing with potential linguistic bias (see page 178), it is important when dealing with these ethical and political issues to include the opinions of individuals with knowledge of and experience with the culture and behaviors that are the target of investigation. Respectful and successful community and participant consultation often depends on establishing a relationship of trust early in the research design phase and relying on this expertise continuously through the data interpretation, implementation, and dissemination phases (Fisher et al., 2002).

Priming Effects

Cultural researchers must also be aware of potential priming effects in their procedures. Specifically, the order and wording of certain questions and stimuli may move participants' responses in a direction that facilitates or makes more difficult the hypothesized behavior or differences (see also Note 5). For instance,

merely asking people to think for 2 minutes about what they have in common with their families and friends often functions as a prime that shifts people toward collectivism, whereas asking them to think of what makes them different from family and friends shifts them toward individualism (Trafimow, Triandis, & Goto, 1991). This cultural "frame switching" is even more pronounced among bicultural individuals (Hong et al., 2000).

Do the preceding findings mean that many reported cultural differences are superficial or not meaningful? No. Recent cultural studies suggest that, at least at the level of basic social values and schemas (or what Bond calls "social axioms"; Bond et al., 2004), all individuals, regardless of their cultural background, possess both "individualist" and "collectivist" cognitive structures (i.e., schemas about agency and uniqueness, and schemas about interrelatedness and obligation), and yet the *chronic accessibility* to these structures differs greatly cross-culturally because of national differences in institutions, discourse, and practices (e.g., prevalence of the Protestant ethic, value of free agency and competition, capitalism; Kitayama et al., 1997). Still, as mentioned earlier, researchers should be aware that the presence of certain stimuli (e.g., images or words associated with a particular cultural worldview) may make certain value schemas or mindsets *temporarily accessible* and thus influence participants' responses.

Reference-Group Issue

Several cultural researchers (Heine, Lehman, Peng, & Greenholtz, 2002; Peng, Nisbett, & Wong, 1997) have argued that some of the null results obtained from cross-cultural comparisons of means from attitude, trait, and value measures (e.g., Oyserman, Coon, & Kemmelmeir, 2001) are problematic and noninterpretable because of cultural differences in participants' choice of a comparison standard, or what is known as the "reference-group" effect; that is, those in one culture may compare themselves with different others and standards than do those in another culture, thus potentially confounding cross-cultural comparisons. These researchers argue that reliable and coherent cultural group differences are more likely to be observed when cultural differences are made salient by placing contrastive cultural paradigms in juxtaposition, such as when Japanese and Canadians are asked to use each other as a reference group to calibrate their self-ratings (Heine et al. 2002), when individualism scores and collectivism scores are pitted against each other (Schimmack et al. 2002), or when using scenarios understood by people from both target cultures (Peng et al., 1997). Oishi and colleagues (2004) provide an excellent conceptual and empirical analysis of this issue and the advantages and disadvantages of each of these aforementioned methods.

Data Analyses and Interpretation of Results

Data analysis in cultural research, as in any other types of research, involves a strategic choice of statistical techniques made on the basis of substantive considerations such as the research questions or hypotheses, sample size, data type, and so forth. Analysis and interpretation of cultural data, however, often involves the additional task of demonstrating measurement and conceptual equivalence (see the section, "Choice and Adaptation of Instruments").

Preliminary Analyses: Cultural Response Sets and Item Biases

A careful examination of the psychometric characteristics of instruments is an important first step in the analysis of cultural data. A preliminary (but incomplete) method of examining possible biases is to compare the instruments' reliabilities across the cultures under study (Van de Vijver & Leung, 1997). If significant differences are observed, which is common, their source should be explored (e.g., examine item–total correlations for each scale and sample). Of course, such differences can be produced by item bias due to bad translation, administration problems (e.g., experimenter effects or low interjudge reliability), sample characteristics (e.g., cultural differences in test familiarity or education levels), and differential response styles (e.g., acquiescence or social desirability).

Cultural response sets are tendencies for members of a given culture to use certain parts of a scale when responding (e.g., social desirability biases, extreme responding, acquiescence). For instance, individuals from collectivistic cultures may be reluctant to use the extreme endpoints of a scale, consistent with a cultural resistance to "stick out." Alternatively, individuals less familiar with Likert scales may be more inclined to use the endpoints to signal yes/no or true/false responses. Overall, work on this topic seems to suggest that persons who are older, less educated, or come from lower socioeconomic strata are more likely to display response styles (Van de Vijver & Leung, 1997). Cultural response sets cloud the interpretation of results, because any differences found among cultures may reflect these response tendencies rather than actual cultural differences on the items and constructs of interest. However, correction for the biases does not always reduce these differences (Grimm & Church, 1999).

Prior to any statistical analysis, the researcher also has to decide if the data should be *standardized* within each cultural group, and if so, which standardization procedure is to be used (Leung & Bond, 1989). Generally, standardization is defined as the computation of z scores: ($z = [X - M]/S$), where X is the score to be standardized, M is the mean of the cultural group, and S is its standard deviation. Typically, researchers use standardization to reduce or eliminate unwanted cultural differences due to response sets. However, when scores are standardized per cultural group, all (true and biased) cultural differences in means, standard deviations, or both are eliminated. Thus, it is appropriate to use this method prior to factor analyses (e.g., as when the goal is to compare factor structures; Benet-Martínez & Waller, 1997; Yang & Bond, 1990) but not for cross-cultural mean score comparisons.

When the demonstration of lack of *item bias* is important, differential item functioning statistical techniques such as analyses of variance, IRT, or Mantel–Haenszel statistic (see Van de Vijer & Leung, 1997, for a review of these procedures) provide much more rigorous tests than classical item statistics. Ramirez-Esparza and colleagues (2005), for instance, used these kinds of item-bias analyses to rule out translation anomalies before interpreting differences in responses to Big Five questionnaires in English and Spanish in bilingual subjects. But when item biases are detected, how should the researcher deal with them? Item biases can be seen as an indication that an instrument, or a particular item, is not inadequate for cross-cultural comparison. Such an approach is prudent but sometimes too restrictive, because item biases are likely in any study of highly dissimilar cultural groups (Van de Vijver & Leung, 1997). Alternatively, item-biases can be seen as providing clues to possible meaningful cultural idiosyncrasies, although the appropriateness of this approach is contingent on successfully finding reasons for the presence and absence of bias, possibly aided by one or more local experts.

It is important to note that the use of item-bias statistics is not free of limitations (Van de Vijver & Leung, 1997). First, it is often very difficult to identify reasons why an item is biased. Second, different procedures for identifying bias often do not yield the same results. Third, the stability of item-bias statistics is often poor. Still, the value of item-bias analyses should not be underestimated.

Structure- and Level-Oriented Studies

In structure-oriented studies, in which the main goal is to examine construct equivalence across cultures, a relatively large set of statistical techniques is available. The most frequently used is exploratory factor analysis, followed by target rotations and the computation of an index of factorial agreement across cultural groups (see, e.g., McCrae, Terracciano, et al., 2005). A key complication in factor comparison is the "rotation problem": The spatial orientation of factors in factor analysis is arbitrary. Factor solutions obtained in different cultural groups may be rotated with regard to each other (without this rotation factor, similarity will be underestimated). The problem is that one cultural group needs to be arbitrarily designated as the target factor structure, and, unfortunately, most studies set the imported structure (e.g., the English NEO structure obtained with U.S. participants) as the target toward which the other group structures will be shifted (see discussion on pages 176–177).

A more sophisticated method to test construct equivalence is to use multigroup confirmatory factor analysis (MCFA), which allows researchers to test the fit of a series of hypothesized factorial structures in two or more cultural groups simultaneously (e.g., Benet-Martínez & John, 1998). Joint confirmatory factor analysis (JCFA), in which the common underlying structure of two or more instruments is examined, is also particularly useful in structure-level cultural studies, particularly in those using a combined emic–etic approach (see Figure 10.2). Recall that a key goal of this approach is to examine the degree of overlap/difference between indigenous and imported (i.e., translated) constructs. As Figure 10.2 shows, JCFA techniques are optimal at revealing which (and to what extent) identified indigenous personality dimensions have cultural-specific versus common meaning, and thus how much imported definitions of a particular construct leave out meaning that is unique to the culture under study. When the goal is to examine the cross-cultural invariance of a particular nomological network, pattern of variable associations, or causal model, multigroup path analyses are also quite advisable (see, e.g., Benet-Martínez & Karakitapoglu-Aygun, 2002; Kwan et al., 1997). This technique (another variant of structural equation modeling techniques) allows for the examining of multiple dependent variables and direct and indirect effects.

Cross-validation is key in determining the plausibility of postulated structural and causal models within or across cultures. When a replication study is not feasible, split-sample cross-validation techniques are recommended, assuming that the sample size is large enough. In this technique, the (new or hypothesized) factor structure is identified using one random half of the sample, and the second half is used to examine how well the identified structure replicates with a different sample (see, e.g., Benet-Martínez, 1999).

In level-oriented studies, the most frequently used statistical tests are the t-test and analysis of variance (ANOVA). As emphasized earlier, unless the presence of bias cannot be ruled out, the interpretation of significant difference found through these tests may be ambiguous. Also often used in cultural research are the more complex so-called factorial designs, where in addition to cultural group, one or more independent variables such as gender, age, SES, or generation or acculturation status (i.e., key possible confounds or covariates) are included. These tests can also be achieved with multiple regression techniques, in which culture is entered as a dummy-coded variable. Multiple regression analyses are particularly useful when the goal is to examine whether the relative importance (i.e., beta weights) of a specific set of independent variables varies across two cultural groups.

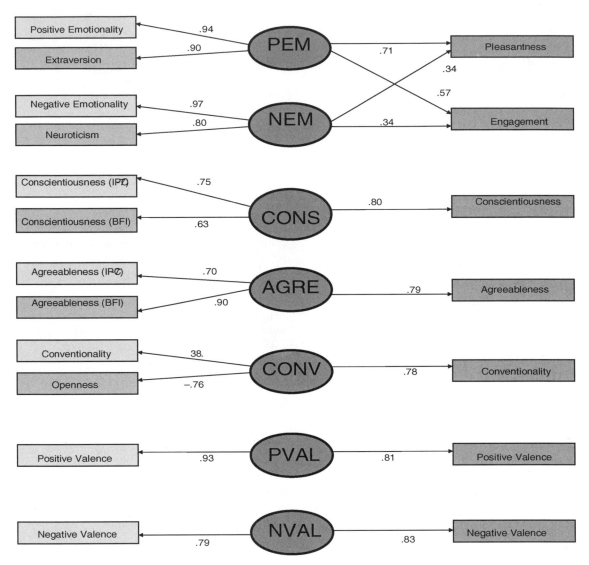

FIGURE 10.2. Example of analyses and results from a combined emic–etic approach in cultural personality research. $N = 894$ Spanish college students. Seven latent personality factors (PEM = Positive Emotionality; NEM = Negative Emotionality; CONS, Conscientiousness; AGRE, Agreeableness; CONV, Conventionality; PVAL, Positive Valence; NVAL, Negative Valence). CFI = .945 and χ^2/df = 2.3. From Benet-Martínez (1999). Copyright 1999 by Swets and Zeitlinger. Reprinted by permission.

Interpretation of Results: Individual versus Cultural Level

At least two levels of analysis are possible in cultural research (Leung & Bond, 1989). In the *culture-level* approach, culture or nation is the unit of analysis and the results inform the characterization of cultures but not of individuals. Hofstede's (1980) classic study of cultural values across 50+ cultures was based on this approach (see these dimensions in Table 10.4). In the *individual-level* approach, the individual is the unit of analysis (see Table 10.3). Dimensions and results obtained at the individual level may not replicate at the cultural level, and vice versa. For instance, notice that the names of the value dimensions reported in Tables 10.3 (individual level) and 10.4 (cultural level), as well as their personality, well-being, and income correlates, are different. This indicates that both the meaning of and dynamics among these variables vary across the psychological and ecological levels. Subjective well-being, for instance, is positively associated with GNP at the cultural level (i.e., richer countries report higher levels of well-being), but at the individual level, happiness and income do not seem to be related (Myers & Diener, 1995).

Two data analysis techniques with great potential value in cultural research and capable of handling the aforementioned complexities are multilevel modeling (see, e.g., Bryk & Raudenbush, 1992; Van de Vijver & Leung, 1997) and latent class analysis (see, e.g., Eid & Diener, 2001). These techniques allow researchers to compare and link findings at the individual and cultural levels and are particularly useful for identifying within-culture heterogeneity as well as between-culture differences. I believe these

underused techniques have the potential of fostering a fruitful synergy between the field of personality psychology—which has provided a wealth of information regarding individual-level psychological characteristics (e.g., traits and values)—and the fields of and anthropology and sociology, which are very informative regarding culture-level phenomena (e.g., economy, religion, and many other key demographic factors).

Conclusions

As this chapter attests, cultural research offers scientists unique benefits and opportunities (e.g., to elucidate links between individual and ecological influences on personality, dispel cultural stereotypes, test theory generalizability). Cultural studies, in fact, may make us better at "seeing" personality. Supporting this idea, anthropologist Margaret Mead observed, "The individual's inclination to respond in a certain way is relatively stable when the cultural context is understood" (as cited in Friedman & Schustack, 2003). In other words, by understanding the cultural backdrop of a particular behavior or script, culturally informed personality researchers may correctly

TABLE 10.3. Correlations between Big Five and Cultural and Economic Variables (Individual Level)

	N	E	O	A	C
Singelis value dimensions[a]					
Individualism	−.34	.52	.52	.11	.17
Collectivism	−.02	.01	−.23	.33	.09
Schwartz value dimensions[b]					
Benevolence	−.02	.01	−.06	.45	.04
Universalism	−.02	−.07	.47	.15	−.17
Self-Direction	−.10	.10	.48	−.25	−.01
Stimulation	−.07	.26	.33	−.26	−.24
Hedonism	−.01	.18	.07	−.34	−.05
Achievement	−.21	.31	−.06	−.41	.22
Power	.08	.13	−.38	−.45	.05
Security	.02	−.11	−.29	.06	.22
Conformity	.02	−.13	−.34	.20	.16
Tradition	.12	−.29	−.29	.36	−.10
Conscientiousness	−.04	−.18	−.26	−.04	.40
Life Satisfaction[a]	−.47	.34	.18	.26	.26
Salary[c]	−.03	.22	−.01	.01	.09

Note. N, Neuroticism; E, Extraversion; O, Openness; A, Agreeableness; C, Conscientiousness. Correlations in bold are significant.
[a] N = 122 U.S. college students from Benet-Martínez and Karakitapoglu-Aygun's (2002) study.
[b] N = 246 Israelis from Roccas, Sagiv, Schwartz, and Knafo's (2002) study.
[c] N = 163 U.S. men from Soldz and Vaillant's (1999) study.

TABLE 10.4. Correlations between Big Five and Cultural and Economic Variables (Culture Level)

	N	E	O	A	C
Hofstede value dimensions					
Power Distance	.20	−.46	−.41	−.31	.11
Uncertainty Avoidance	.30	.07	−.03	−.02	.20
Individualism	.05	.51	.33	.37	−.14
Masculinity	−.14	.00	.10	.04	.03
Schwartz value dimensions					
Conservatism	−.20	−.02	−.70	−.51	.15
Affective Autonomy	.13	.24	.55	.61	−.03
Intellectual Autonomy	.37	−.15	.51	.44	.07
Hierarchy	−.24	−.12	−.32	−.23	−.10
Mastery	−.27	−.31	.10	−.09	−.15
Egalitarian Commitment	.25	.20	.55	.44	−.09
Harmony	.08	.09	.26	.09	.15
Life Satisfaction	.01	.63	.35	.48	−.02
GDP	.04	.44	.47	.46	.02

Note. N = 22–49 different cultures. GDP, per capita gross domestic product. Other abbreviations as in Table 10.3. Correlations in bold are significant. From McCrae et al. (2005). Copyright 2005 by the American Psychological Association. Adapted by permission.

see consistency and coherence in individual differences and patterns of personality where other researchers would see only situational or random variability (Oishi, 2004).

Finally, let's not forget the important societal and applied benefits of cultural personality studies. Cultural personality research offers scientists, managers, policymakers, and the public ways to understand, manage, and benefit from the omnipresent cultural diversity that characterizes our society (Fowers & Richardson, 1996).

Notes

1. The terms *cross-cultural psychology* and *cultural psychology* refer to two different research traditions with somewhat distinct theoretical approaches, goals, and methodologies (see pages 174–175 for a discussion of these issues). However, for the sake of simplicity, throughout the chapter I use the broader term *cultural* (e.g., cultural psychology, cultural research, cultural methods) to refer to both kinds of traditions and their theories and methodologies.

2. Note that these two questions deal, if not directly, with a basic disagreement within personality psychology—namely, the opposing views that see the Big Five as largely representing either (1) endogenous and inherited basic tendencies that are independent from culture (genotypic view; McCrae & Costa, 1997) or (2) observable behavioral regularities that reflect characteristic adaptations to the sociocultural context (phenotypic view; Saucier & Goldberg, 1996).

3. In choosing systematically the cultures for study, researchers often rely on Hofstede's (1980) rankings of more than 50 cultures along the dimensions of Individualism–Collectivism, Power Distance, Uncertainty Avoidance, and Masculinity–Femininity. Other useful rankings of cultures along meaningful sociocultural dimensions (e.g., values) can be found in Schwartz (1994) and Smith, Trompenaars, and Dugan (1996).

4. Note that *random* sampling of cultures is often not feasible or desirable, but in some large-scale exploratory studies this has been an ideal approach (e.g., Buss, 1989; Diener, Diener, & Diener, 1995).

5. Instrument biases are complex and deserve special attention, although their cultural reliability is still being debated (Grimm & Church, 1999). Moreover, in multilingual persons, there is evidence suggesting that the language of assessment may be a potential source of method bias because of either *cultural frame-switching* (i.e., each language primes different aspects of the self; Ramírez-Esparza et al. (2006) or *cultural accommodation* effects (i.e., the respondent answers the questionnaire in a manner that accommodates or favors the culture associated with the language being used; Ralston, Cunniff, & Gustafson, 1995; Yang & Bond, 1990).

Recommended Readings

Church, A. T. (2001). Personality measurement in cross-cultural perspective. *Journal of Personality, 69,* 979–1006.

Church, A. T., & Ortiz, F. A. (2005). Culture and personality. In V. J. Derlaga, B. A. Winstead, &

W. H. Jones (Eds.), *Personality: Contemporary theory and research* (3rd ed., pp. 420–456). Belmont, CA: Wadsworth.

Heine, S. J., Lehman, D. R., Peng, K., & Greenholtz, J. (2002). What's wrong with cross-cultural comparisons of subjective Likert scales?: The reference-group effect. *Journal of Personality and Social Psychology, 82*, 903–918.

Leung, K., & Bond, M. H. (1989). On the empirical identification of dimensions for cross-cultural comparisons. *Journal of Cross-Cultural Psychology, 20*, 133–151.

Matsumoto, D. R. (2000). *Culture and psychology: People around the world*. Delmar, CA: Wadsworth Thomson Learning.

Van de Vijver, F., & Leung, K. (1997). *Methods and data analysis for cross-cultural research*. London: Sage.

References

Aaker, J., Benet-Martínez, V., & Garolera, J. (2001). Consumption symbols as carriers of culture: A study of Japanese and Spanish brand personality constructs. *Journal of Personality and Social Psychology, 81*, 249–264.

Allport, G. W. (1954). *The nature of prejudice*. Cambridge, MA: Addison-Wesley.

American Psychological Association Office of Ethnic Minority Affairs. (1993). Guidelines for providers of psychological services to ethnic, linguistic, and culturally diverse populations. *American Psychologist, 48*, 45–48.

Benet, V., & Waller, N. G. (1995). The "Big Seven" model of personality description: Evidence for its cross-cultural generality in a Spanish sample. *Journal of Personality and Social Psychology, 69*, 701–718.

Benet-Martínez, V. (1999). Exploring indigenous Spanish personality constructs with a combined emic-etic approach. In J. C. Lasry, J. G. Adair, & K. L. Dion (Eds.), *Latest contributions to cross-cultural psychology* (pp. 151–175). Lisse, The Netherlands: Swets and Zeitlinger.

Benet-Martínez, V., & Haritatos, J. (2005). Bicultural identity integration (BII): Components and socio-personality antecedents. *Journal of Personality, 73*, 1015–1050.

Benet-Martínez, V., & John, O. (1998). Los Cinco Grandes across cultures and ethnic groups: Multitrait multimethod analyses of the Big Five in Spanish and English. *Journal of Personality and Social Psychology, 75*, 729–750.

Benet-Martínez, V., & Karakitapoglu-Aygun, Z. (2003). The interplay of cultural values and personality in predicting life-satisfaction: Comparing Asian- and European-Americans. *Journal of Cross-Cultural Psychology, 34*, 38–61.

Benet-Martínez, V., & Waller, N. G. (1997). Further evidence for the cross-cultural generality of the Big Seven Factor model: Indigenous and imported Spanish personality constructs. *Journal of Personality, 65*, 567–598.

Berry, J. W. (1980). Introduction to methodology. In H. C. Triandis & J. W. Berry (Eds.), *Handbook of cross-cultural psychology: Methodology* (Vol. 2, pp. 1–28). Boston: Allyn & Bacon.

Bond, M. H., Leung, K., Au, A., Tong, K. K., Reimel de Carrasquel, S., Murakami, F., et al. (2004). Culture-level dimensions of social axioms and their correlates across 41 cultures. *Journal of Cross-Cultural Psychology, 35*, 548–570.

Brislin, R. W. (1986). The wording and translation of research instruments. In W. J. Lonner & J. W. Berry (Eds.), *Field methods in cross-cultural psychology* (pp. 137–164). Beverly Hills, CA: Sage.

Bryk, A. S., & Raudenbush, S. W. (1992). *Hierarchical linear models: Applications and data analysis methods*. Thousand Oaks, CA: Sage.

Buss, D. M. (1989). Sex differences in human mate preferences: Evolutionary hypotheses tested in 37 cultures. *Behavioral and Brain Sciences, 12*, 1–49.

Campbell, D. T., & Fiske, D. W. (1959). Convergent and discriminant validation by the multitrait–multimethod matrix. *Psychological Bulletin, 56*, 81–105.

Chiu, C. Y., & Chen, J. (2004). Symbols and interactions: Application of the CCC Model to culture, language, and social identity. In S. H. Ng, C. N. Candlin, & C. Y. Chiu (Eds.), *Language matters: Communication, culture, and identity* (pp. 155–182). Hong Kong: City University of Hong Kong Press.

Church, A. T. (2000). Culture and personality: Toward an integrated cultural trait psychology. *Journal of Personality, 68*, 651–703.

Church, A. T. (2001). Personality measurement in cross-cultural perspective. *Journal of Personality, 69*, 979–1006.

Church, A. T., & Ortiz, F. A. (2005). Culture and personality. In V. J. Derlaga, B. A. Winstead, & W. H. Jones (Eds.), *Personality: Contemporary theory and research* (3rd ed., pp. 420–456). Belmont, CA: Wadsworth.

Cole, E. R., & Stewart, A. J. (1996). Meanings of political participation among Black and White women: Political identity and social responsibility. *Journal of Personality and Social Psychology, 71*, 130–140.

Diener, E., Diener, M., & Diener, C. (1995). Factors predicting the subjective well-being of nations. *Journal of Personality and Social Psychology, 69*, 851–864.

Diener, E., Oishi, S., & Lucas, R. E. (2003). Personality, culture, and subjective well-being: Emotional and cognitive evaluations of life. *Annual Review of Psychology, 54*, 403–425.

Eid, M., & Diener, E. (2001). Norms for experiencing emotions in different cultures: Inter- and intranational differences. *Journal of Personality and Social Psychology, 81*, 869–885.

Ellis, B. B. (1989). Differential item functioning: Implications for test translations. *Journal of Applied Psychology, 74*, 912–921.

Eysenck, S. B. G., & Long, F. Y. (1986). A cross-cultural comparison of personality in adults and children:

Singapore and England. *Journal of Personality and Social Psychology, 50,* 124–130.

Fisher, C. B., Hoagwood, K., Boyce, C., Duster, T., Frank, D. A., Grisso, T., et al. (2002). Research ethics for mental health science involving ethnic minority children and youths. *American Psychologist, 57,* 1024–1040.

Fiske, A. P. (1991). *Structures of social life: The four elementary forms of human relations.* New York: Free Press.

Fowers, B. J., & Richardson, F. C. (1996). Why is multiculturalism good? *American Psychologist, 51,* 609–621.

Friedman, H., & Schustack, M. W. (2003). *Personality: Classic theories and modern research* (2nd ed.). Boston: Allyn & Bacon.

Gosling, S. D., Ko, S. J., Mannarelli, T., & Morris, M. E. (2002). A room with a cue: Judgments of personality based on offices and bedrooms. *Journal of Personality and Social Psychology, 82,* 379–398.

Greenfield, P. M. (2000). Three approaches to the psychology of culture: Where do they come from? Where can they go? *Asian Journal of Social Psychology, 3,* 223–240.

Grimm, S. D., & Church, A. T. (1999). A cross-cultural study of response biases in personality measures. *Journal of Research in Personality, 33,* 415–441.

Haidt, J., Koller, S., & Dias, M. (1993). Affect, culture, and morality, or is it wrong to eat your dog? *Journal of Personality and Social Psychology, 65,* 613–628.

Heine, S. J., Lehman, D. R., Peng, K., & Greenholtz, J. (2002). What's wrong with cross-cultural comparisons of subjective Likert scales? The reference-group effect. *Journal of Personality and Social Psychology, 82,* 903–918.

Hermans, H., & Kempen, H. (1998). Moving cultures: The perilous problem of cultural dichotomies in a globalizing society. *American Psychologist, 53,* 1111–1120.

Hofstede, G. (1980). *Culture's consequences.* Beverly Hills, CA: Sage.

Hong, Y. Y., Morris, M., Chiu, C. Y., & Benet-Martínez, V. (2000). Multicultural minds: A dynamic constructivist approach to culture and cognition. *American Psychologist, 55,* 709–720.

Huang, C. D., Church, A. T., & Katigbak, M. S. (1997). Identifying cultural differences in items and traits: Differential item functioning in the NEO Personality Inventory. *Journal of Cross-Cultural Psychology, 28,* 192–218.

Hui, C. H., & Triandis, H. C. (1983). Multistrategy approach to cross-cultural research: The case of locus of control. *Journal of Cross-Cultural Psychology, 14,* 65–83.

Jahoda, G. (1995). In pursuit of the emic–etic distinction: Can we ever capture it? In N. R. Goldberger & J. B. Veroff (Eds.), *The culture and psychology reader* (pp. 128–138). New York: New York University Press.

Jones, P. S., Lee, J. W., Phillips, L. R., Zhang, X. E., & Jaceldo, K. B. (2001). An adaptation of Brislin's translation model for cross-cultural research. *Nursing Research, 50,* 300–304.

Jost, J. T., Glaser, J., Kruglanski, A. W., & Sulloway, F. (2003). Political conservatism as motivated social cognition. *Psychological Bulletin, 129,* 339–375.

Katigbak, M. S., Church, A. T., & Akamine, T. X. (1996). Cross-cultural generalizability of personality dimensions: Relating indigenous and imported dimensions in two cultures. *Journal of Personality and Social Psychology, 70,* 99–114.

Kim, B. S. K., Atkinson, D. R., & Yang, P. H. (1999). The Asian Values Scale: Development, factor analysis, validation, and reliability. *Journal of Counseling Psychology, 46,* 342–352.

Kitayama, S., Markus, H. R., Matsumoto, H., & Norasakkunkit, V. (1997). Individual and collective processes in the construction of the self: Self-enhancement in the United States and self-criticism in Japan. *Journal of Personality and Social Psychology, 72,* 1245–1267.

Kluckhohn, C., & Murray, H. E. (1948). *Personality in nature, society, and culture.* New York: Knopf.

Kwan, V. S. Y., Bond, M. H., & Singelis, T. M. (1997). Pancultural explanations for life-satisfaction: Adding relationship harmony to self-esteem. *Journal of Personality and Social Psychology, 73,* 1038–1051.

Leung, K., & Bond, M. H. (1989). On the empirical identification of dimensions for crosscultural comparisons. *Journal of Cross-Cultural Psychology, 20,* 133–151.

LeVine, R. A. (2001). Culture and personality studies, 1918–1960: Myth and history. *Journal of Personality, 69,* 803–818.

Lou, L., & Gilmour, R. (2004). Culture and conceptions of happiness: Individual oriented and social oriented subjective wellbeing. *Journal of Happiness Studies, 5,* 269–291.

Markus, H. R., & Kitayama, S. (1998). The cultural psychology of personality. *Journal of Cross-Cultural Psychology, 29,* 63–87.

Matsumoto, D. R. (2000). *Culture and psychology: People around the world.* Delmar, CA: Wadsworth Thomson Learning.

McClelland, D. C. (1961). *The achieving society.* Princeton, NJ: Van Nostrand.

McCrae, R. R. (2001). Trait psychology and culture: Exploring intercultural comparisons. *Journal of Personality, 69,* 819–846.

McCrae, R. R., & Costa, P. T., Jr. (1997). Personality trait structure as a human universal. *American Psychologist, 52,* 509–516.

McCrae, R. R., Terracciano, A., & 79 members of the Personality Profiles of Cultures Project. (2005). Universal features of personality traits from the observer's perspective: Data from 50 cultures. *Journal of Personality and Social Psychology, 88,* 547–561.

McCrae, R. R., Yik, M. S. M., Trapnell, P. D., Bond, M. H., & Paulhus, D. L. (1998). Interpreting personality profiles across cultures: Bilingual, acculturation, and peer rating studies of Chinese undergraduates. *Jour-*

nal of Personality and Social Psychology, 74, 1041–1055.

Myers, D. G., & Diener, E. (1995). Who is happy? *Psychological Science, 1,* 10–19.

Norenzayan, A., & Heine, S.J. (2005). Psychological universals: What are they and how can we know? *Psychological Bulletin, 131,* 763–784.

Oishi, S. (2004). Personality in culture: A neo-Allportian view. *Journal of Research in Personality, 38,* 68–74.

Oishi, S., & Diener, E. (2001). Goals, culture, and subjective well-being. *Personality and Social Psychology Bulletin, 27,* 1674–1682.

Oishi, S., Hahn, J., Schimmack, U., Radhakrishan, P., Dzokoto, V., & Ahadi, S. (2004). The measurement of values across cultures. *Journal of Research in Personality, 39,* 299–305.

Oyserman, D., Coon, H. M., & Kemmelmeier, M. (2002). Rethinking individualism and collectivism: Evaluation of theoretical assumptions and meta-analyses. *Psychological Bulletin, 128,* 3–72.

Padilla, A. M., & Lindholm, K. J. (1995). Quantitative educational research with ethnic minorities. In J. Banks & C. A. McGee Banks (Eds.), *Handbook of research on multicultural education* (pp. 97–113). New York: Macmillan.

Peng, K., Nisbett, R. E., & Wong, N. Y. C. (1997). Validity problems comparing values across cultures and possible solutions. *Psychological Methods, 2,* 329–344.

Phinney, J. S. (1996). When we talk about American ethnic groups, what do we mean? *American Psychologist, 51,* 918–927.

Ralston, D. A., Cunniff, M. K., & Gustafson, D. A. (1995). Cultural accommodation: The effect of language on the responses of bilingual Hong Kong Chinese managers. *Journal of Cross-Cultural Psychology, 26,* 714–727.

Ramírez-Esparza, N., Gosling, S. D., Benet-Martínez, V., Potter, J., & Pennebaker, J. W. (2006). Do bilinguals have two personalities?: A special case of frame switching. *Journal of Research in Personality, 40,* 99–120.

Rentfrow, P. J., & Gosling, S. D. (2003). The do re mi's of everyday life: The structure and personality correlates of music preferences. *Journal of Personality and Social Psychology, 84,* 1236–1256.

Roccas, S., Sagiv, L., Schwartz, S. H., & Knafo, A. (2002). The Big Five personality factors and personal values. *Personality and Social Psychology Bulletin, 28,* 789–801.

Saucier, G., & Goldberg, L. R. (1996). The language of personality: Lexical perspectives on the five-factor model. In J. S. Wiggins (Ed.), *The five-factor model of personality: Theoretical perspectives* (pp. 21–50). New York: Guilford Press.

Schimmack, U., Radhakrishnan, P., Oishi, S., Dzokoto, V., & Ahadi, S. (2002). Culture, personality, and subjective well-being: Integrating process models of life-satisfaction. *Journal of Personality and Social Psychology, 82,* 582–593.

Schwartz, S. H. (1994). Beyond individualism-collectivism: New dimensions of values. In U. Kim, H. C. Triandis, C. Kagitcibasi, S. C. Choi, & G. Yoon (Eds.), *Individualism and collectivism: Theory, method and application* (pp. 85–119). Newbury Park, CA: Sage.

Senior, P. A, & Bhopal, R. (1994). Ethnicity as a variable in epidemiological research. *Briths Medical Journal, 309,* 327–330.

Smith, P. B., Trompenaars, F., & Dugan, S. (1995). The Rotter locus of control scale in 43 countries: A test of cultural relativity. *International Journal of Psychology, 30,* 377–400.

Soldz, S., & Vaillant, G. E. (1999). The Big Five personality traits and the life course: A 45-year longitudinal study. *Journal of Research in Personality, 33,* 208–232.

Stevenson, H. W., Lee, S. Y., Chen, C., Lummis, M., Stigler, J., Fan, L., et al. (1990). Mathematics achievement of children in China and the United States. *Child Development, 61,* 1053–1066.

Tafarodi, R. W., & Swann, W. B., Jr. (1996). Individualism–collectivism and global self-esteem: Evidence for a cultural trade-off. *Journal of Cross-Cultural Psychology, 27,* 651–672.

Terracciano, A., Abdel-Khalek, A. M., Adam, N., Adamovova, L., Ahn, C. K., Ahn, H. N., et al. (2005). National character does not reflect mean personality trait levels in 49 cultures. *Science, 310,* 96–100.

Trafimow, D., Triandis, H. C., & Goto, S. G. (1991). Some tests of the distinction between the private self and the collective self. *Journal of Personality and Social Psychology, 60,* 649–655.

Triandis, H. C. (1996). The psychological measurement of cultural syndromes. *American Psychologist, 51,* 407–415.

Triandis, H. C., & Suh, E. M. (2002). Cultural influences on personality. *Annual Review of Psychology, 53,* 133–160.

Tsai, J. L., & Levenson, R. W. (1997). Cultural influences on emotional responding: Chinese and European American dating couples during interpersonal conflict. *Journal of Cross-Cultural Psychology, 28,* 600–625.

Van de Vijver, F., & Leung, K. (1997). *Methods and data analysis for cross-cultural research.* London: Sage.

Van Hemert, D. A., Van de Vijver, F. J. R., Poortinga, Y. H., & Georgas, J. (2002). Structural and functional equivalence of the Eysenck Personality Questionnaire within and between countries. *Personality and Individual Differences, 33,* 1229–1249.

Vazire, S., & Gosling, S. D. (2004). E-perceptions: Personality impressions based on personal websites. *Journal of Personality and Social Psychology, 87,* 123–132.

Yang, K., & Bond, M. H. (1990). Exploring implicit personality theories with indigenous and imported constructs: The Chinese case. *Journal of Personality and Social Psychology, 58,* 1087–1095.

## CHAPTER 11

Measuring Personality in Nonhuman Animals

Simine Vazire
Samuel D. Gosling
Audrey S. Dickey
Steven J. Schapiro

Animal research has the potential to help address many fundamental questions about personality. The experimental control and wide range of methods associated with animal studies means that they provide unique opportunities to examine the biological, genetic, and environmental bases of personality and to study personality change, personality–health links, and personality perception. However, the field of animal personality research is relatively young; it has yet to establish the measurement foundations on which research on substantive topics must be based. Most fundamentally, questions remain about how best to assess personality in nonhuman subjects. In this chapter, we examine and evaluate the methods currently used to assess personality in animals, demonstrate how these methods are used, and offer some suggestions for improvement.

The Appeal of Animal Personality Research

Animal studies have contributed to many areas of psychology because they afford numerous methodological advantages (Domjan & Purdy, 1995; Vazire & Gosling, 2003). First, animal studies allow greater experimental control and facilitate more extensive experimental manipulations than is possible in studies of humans. Animal studies can be used to test specific hypotheses that, with humans, must often rely on suboptimal designs. For example, one study manipulated animals' social environments in order to examine the links between the stability of social environments and physical health (Capitanio, Mendoza, & Baroncelli, 1999). The findings showed that monkeys' sociability predicted both behavioral responses to social manipulations (stable versus unstable conditions) and antibody response to simian immunodeficiency virus (SIV) inoculation, both of which, in turn, predicted length of survival. Such a controlled and comprehensive study could not have been conducted with humans for practical as well as ethical reasons. Cross-fostering studies use another powerful design that cannot be used in humans. For example, researchers have used cross-fostering studies to examine the role of genetics in personality traits such as anxiety and reactivity (see, e.g., Gordon & Hen, 2004; Suomi, 1987). Of course, cross-fostering studies can also highlight the effects of environmental factors; studies of rats have emphasized the role of maternal care, rather than genetics, in the transmittal of some traits (Francis, Diorio, Liu, & Meaney, 1999).

The second advantage conferred by animal studies is that observations of animals can be made in far greater detail and for more extensive periods than is possible with humans. For example, Virgin and Sapolsky (1997) drew on 5 years' worth of behavioral observation of baboons to illuminate the links between male social behavior and endocrine responses.

Third, animal studies permit the use of a wide range of physiological interventions and the measurement of a wide range of physiological parameters, providing the type of data that are necessary to identify the biological mechanisms underlying psychological processes (Mehta & Gosling, 2006). For example, Zuckerman (1996) drew on animal studies involving measures of neurotransmitters, enzymes, and hormones to develop a psychobiological model for sensation seeking.

Fourth, the short lifespan of many species allows researchers to conduct longitudinal studies in shorter periods than is possible with humans. For example, in a period of only 4 years, Fahlke and colleagues (2000) examined how rhesus macaques' rearing experiences and stress responses in infancy predicted alcohol consumption in young adulthood.

Fifth, detailed quantitative and molecular genetic information is available for some species (see, e.g., Blake, Eppig, Richardson, Davidson, et al., 2000), and animal research permits transgenic, knock-out, and cloning studies that can provide novel opportunities to further understand the genetic influences on psychology and biology (Flint, 2002; Gosling & Mollaghan, 2006). For example, Dulawa, Grandy, Low, Paulus, and Geyer (1999) used knock-out mice to examine the links between the dopamine receptor (D4R) gene and novelty-seeking behavior.

In addition, using new genomic techniques, it is now possible to investigate directly the relationship between gene expression and behavior in the brains of animal models. For example, with gene-expression profiling, it is possible to monitor the activity of thousands of genes simultaneously in a particular tissue or brain area immediately following test subjects' exposure to a particular stimulus.

Three Concerns about the Validity of Personality Assessments in Animals

Despite the many advantages of studying animals, their use in research on these issues is still somewhat unconventional and many researchers have concerns about the validity of personality assessments in animals. Generally, these concerns fall into three categories:

- Concern 1: Personality cannot be measured reliably in animals.
- Concern 2: Assessments of animal personality are overly subjective.
- Concern 3: The methods required to obtain valid personality assessments of animals are not practical.

Interestingly, these three concerns have also been addressed in the context of human personality research (see, e.g., Block, 1977; Mischel, 1968). Thus, establishing the validity of personality assessment methods is a goal shared by both human and animal personality researchers. This chapter addresses these concerns in the context of animal personality assessment, but the implications have relevance for both human and animal studies.

Methods of Assessing Personality in Animals

Several methods have been used in researchers' attempts to assess personality in animals. In the dog literature, which reflects the variety of methods used across all species, Jones and Gosling (2006) identified four main assessment methods: test batteries, observational tests, ratings of individual animals, and expert ratings of breed prototypes. The first two categories are based on observers' codings of dog behaviors in response to test situations (e.g., exposing the subject to a novel stimulus) or in naturally occurring settings (e.g., while on a walk in the park). The last two categories rely on humans to intuitively aggregate and interpret dogs' behaviors and provide ratings on personality traits. Thus, at a broad level, two main approaches to assessing animal personality can be distinguished: behavior codings and observer trait ratings.

Behavior codings and trait ratings reflect different solutions to the apparent tradeoff between quantifying personality in terms of objective behaviors and using humans to record and interpret information more subjectively (Block, 1961; Stevenson-Hinde, 1983; Stevenson-Hinde, Stillwell-Barnes, & Zunz, 1980). Some researchers have tried to take an objective stance by coding narrowly defined behaviors and assessing individual animals over a series of behavioral tests, such as by coding an animal's response to a new environment (e.g., Hinde, Leighton-Shapiro, & McGinnis, 1978; Mather & Anderson, 1993; Spencer-Booth & Hinde, 1969). Other researchers have chosen to sacrifice the objectivity supposedly gained from such detailed behavior codings in favor of obtaining ratings by people who are familiar with individual animals on traits such as confident, curious, and playful (e.g., Bolig, Price, O'Neill, & Suomi, 1992; Buirski, Plutchik, & Kellerman, 1978; Gosling, 1998; Gosling, Kwan, & John, 2003; Stevenson-Hinde et al., 1980).

Although both methods have been used for assessing personality, many animal behavior researchers regard behavior codings as intrinsically superior to global personality ratings. Historically, rating data obtained from observers have been derided as subjective and inappropriate for the objective requirements of scientific measurement. Although he provided no data, Donald Hebb alluded to the appeal of coding methods in his classic 1946 article, and described a system implemented to assess chimpanzees:

> A thoroughgoing attempt to avoid anthropomorphic description in the study of temperament was made over a two-year period at the Yerkes Laboratory. A formal experiment was set up to provide records of the actual behavior of adult chimpanzees, and from these records to get an objective statement of the differences from animal to animal. (p. 88)

In contrast, many human researchers argue that behavior codings actually deserve the closest scrutiny. They point to research on human personality, where consensual observer ratings are often considered to be the *sine qua non* of personality traits. The relative merits of the two methods are also being debated in the child psychology literature (Stevenson-Hinde, 2005), where both sides have their adherents. Surprisingly, this question has never been addressed directly in the animal personality literature. Some validation studies have simultaneously utilized the two methods (e.g., Capitanio, 1999; Pederson, King, & Landau, 2005), but in these studies it is always the behavior codings that are used to validate the trait ratings. This makes reasonable conceptual sense because trait ratings are ultimately meant to reflect behavior, yet it again illustrates the widespread assumption that behavior codings are superior to trait ratings, even though there is, as yet, no empirical data directly supporting this view. To provide a background for our empirical comparison of the two methods, we next describe the procedures typical of each method.

Behavior Codings

Behavior codings have been used widely in animal personality studies, although only rarely with noncaptive animals. In a comprehensive review, Gosling (2001) found that 74% (137) of the animal personality studies to that date had used behavior codings to assess personality. Behavior codings typically require repeated observations of individuals and so can be performed only with animals whose behavior is easily visible or recorded. It is surprisingly difficult to summarize the specific methods and procedures used in the typical behavior-coding study because researchers often neglect to report vital details. We suspect this is because behavior codings are often assumed to be objective reflections of behavior, and so the methods used are not considered essential. For example, researchers seldom report how many observers coded each animal, who the observers were (e.g., experts or undergraduate research assistants), how the observers were trained, or even how many hours of observation were collected for each animal. In fact, researchers often do not even report the reliabilities of the codings, making it impossible to judge whether the method used was sufficiently reliable.

In the typical study, trained observers record

the behavior of one animal at a time in "focal-animal samples." The number of observers for each animal varies across studies, but is usually as low as one or two. The focal samples can vary in duration from study to study (e.g., from 10 seconds to 30 minutes), and the number of times each animal is sampled (from 6 to more than 100) also varies.

The choice of which behaviors to code is largely driven by the goals of the study. Once the behaviors have been chosen, the observers must be trained to recognize and record these behaviors. This can be done with basic paper-and-pencil techniques or with more sophisticated computer-based techniques (e.g., Noldus Observer). To facilitate the process of deciding which behaviors to code, many researchers refer to published ethograms, which are lists of species-typical behaviors.

Trait Ratings

Trait ratings are used less commonly than behavior codings in animal personality studies. In Gosling's (2001) review, only 34%[1] (62) of the studies used trait ratings to measure animal personality. Typically, researchers have quantified impressions by asking observers who were familiar with the animals to rate each one on a number of personality traits. Usually these ratings were made by more than one observer, and occasionally they were made at several points in time.

To demonstrate and evaluate the two methods, we draw on an illustrative study of chimpanzees that implemented both methods. First, we describe how the two methods were carried out. Next, we present new data from this study and examine the reliability, subjectivity, and practicality of the two methods, drawing also on the lessons learned in past research on human personality. In addition to this empirical analysis, we also provide a conceptual analysis of the two methods. Finally, we offer some conclusions about the validity of the two methods and recommendations for future research.

Illustrative Study: Behavior Codings and Trait Ratings of Chimpanzees

Few researchers have empirically examined the advantages and limitations of behavior codings and trait ratings. In the human literature, researchers' overreliance on self-reports has led to a dearth of empirical evidence on the validity of these alternative methods. Despite the wider use of these methods in the animal literature, to our knowledge there has not been a direct empirical comparison of the two methods. The illustrative study we present here allows us to provide a description of behavior codings and trait ratings, as well as a direct comparison of the two methods in assessing the personalities of 52 captive chimpanzees. Specifically, we examine the levels of agreement between trait ratings and codings of those behaviors theoretically associated with each trait. To understand the points of divergence between the two methods, we take a close look at the item content, implementation, and reliability of the two methods.

The subjects were 21 male and 31 female chimpanzees (*Pan troglodytes*) housed in groups of 9–14 at the Department of Veterinary Sciences of the University of Texas, M. D. Anderson Cancer Center, in Bastrop, Texas. The chimpanzees ranged in age from 2 to 40 years. Each social group lived in a large (75-foot diameter) outdoor compound connected to indoor quarters. Each compound contained several play objects and structures, including poles, ladders, ropes, tires, and plastic barrels.

Behavior Codings

A single observer collected behavior codings from all 52 chimpanzees using a focal-sampling method. Subjects were observed for 15-minute focal animal samples as they freely interacted within their social groups. More than 135 hours of data were collected across morning and afternoon sessions between September 2001 and March 2002. To capture samples of behavior at different points in the animals' circadian cycles (e.g., immediately after feeding or during the afternoon resting period), the sessions were deliberately conducted at a variety of times of day. Based on previous research on rhesus macaques (Nystrom, Schapiro, & Hau, 2001), which suggested a stabilized average for meaningful analyses of behavioral data can be obtained with between 6 and 12 observations per subject, we collected a minimum of 8 and a maximum of 12 focal animal samples for each chimpanzee.

The Noldus Observer observational software package (Noldus, 1991) was used to record (1) subjects' behaviors, (2) subjects' social locations, and (3) the social direction of the subjects' behaviors. Each behavior was defined, along with examples of how the behavior might be manifested in the present context. For example, the behavior "social groom given" is defined as "picking through the hair or skin of another chimpanzee and removing debris with hands and/or mouth. Does not include pulling hair" (a full description of the behavioral definitions is available from the authors). For the purpose of data analysis, the behaviors were grouped into categories based on published chimpanzee ethograms.

The ethogram used, along with the operational definitions and categories in the ethogram, was derived from several published chimpanzee ethograms. Most of the operational definitions in the ethogram were adapted from earlier ethograms, and many of the categories formed from specific behaviors are very similar to categories from earlier studies. In the interest of observational accuracy, and consistent with standard coding procedures (see, e.g., Schapiro, 2002; Schapiro & Bloomsmith, 1995), the behaviors were coded using mutually exclusive categories. Of course, chimpanzees may perform several behaviors at once (e.g., walking, looking, and chewing). Thus, in accord with standard coding procedures, we used three criteria to determine which behavior should be recorded. First, we gave highest priority to behaviors that were socially directed. This was our most important criterion and superseded the other two. For example, an animal that was eating while it was being groomed was recorded as receiving grooming. Second, we gave the next level of priority to behaviors that required the most calories to perform. For example, an animal that was eating and looking was recorded as eating. Third, we gave the next level of priority to behaviors that occupied more of the animal's attention.

Trait Ratings

Four observers, each of whom knew the animals well (mean acquaintance = 7.4 years), rated all 52 individuals using a list of 34 adjectives. These adjectives were a subset of those used by Gosling (1998) and Capitanio (1999) and selected by two chimpanzee experts on the basis of their relevance to chimpanzee behaviors in the context of their particular housing situation. Each trait was defined by a behavioral description of how that trait might be manifested. For example, the trait "curious" was defined by "readily explores new situations" (a full description of the trait definitions is available from the authors).

Before rating the chimpanzees, the observers clarified their understanding of the traits as defined in the present research. The observers made their ratings independently and were instructed not to discuss their ratings or the personality characteristics of the animals for the duration of the study. They were asked to base their ratings on the full length of their acquaintance with the chimpanzees. Observers were instructed to focus on chimpanzee-to-chimpanzee interactions, not chimpanzee-to-human interactions. All ratings were completed over a 5-week period. Ratings were made on a 7-point scale, ranging from extremely uncharacteristic (1) to extremely characteristic (7). Observers were encouraged to use the full range of the scale where such a range could be meaningfully applied to the animals.

Convergence between Codings and Ratings

Both rating and coding methods are designed to assess personality. If they both work, rating and coding measures of the same traits should converge. To test this, we selected a subset of behaviors and traits designed to assess similar constructs. For example, five behaviors were classified in the ethogram as indicators of aggression: attack, charge, threat, display, and displace. We next selected three traits also designed to assess aggression: aggressive, belligerent, and irritable. Selection was based on the definition of the traits. For example, belligerent was defined as "unprovoked aggression or aggressive gestures directed at another animal; e.g., one female grabbing or hurting through intention another female's baby," and irritable was defined as "reacts negatively with little provocation; an aggressive response to mild or inadvertent provocation." In a similar fashion, we selected behaviors and traits indicative of submissiveness, abnormal behavior, affiliation, solitariness, activity, and playfulness. We then correlated the behavioral measures with the trait measures. The resulting correlations are shown in Table 11.1, with the convergent correlations, which are predicted to be strong, shown in bold.

TABLE 11.1. Correlations between Trait Ratings and Behavioral Codings

Behavior category / Behavior label[a]	Aggression			Submissiveness				Abnormal		Affiliation		Solitariness		Activity	Playfulness
	Aggr.	Bell.	Irrit.	Subm.	Domi.	Assr.	Effe.	Ecce.	Depr.	Frie.	Soci.	Soli.	Sull.	Acti.	Play.
Aggressive behaviors															
Attack	.13	**.21**	**.21**	−.24	.28*	.25	.33*	.10	−.12	.07	.13	−.14	−.11	−.02	.15
Charge	.12	**.20**	**.17**	.01	.07	.00	.08	−.08	−.04	−.14	.04	−.03	−.04	.16	.09
Threat	.35*	**.52**	**.41**	−.24	.22	.26	.24	−.13	−.16	.00	−.13	−.11	−.01	−.08	.08
Display	.36*	**.28***	.24	−.19	.20	.18	.20	−.22	.04	−.04	−.15	.04	.18	−.01	.04
Displace	.17	**.09**	.10	−.16	.16	.14	.14	−.02	−.07	.05	.06	−.03	−.14	−.06	−.06
Submissive behaviors															
Flee	−.09	.21	.08	**.15**	**−.13**	**−.16**	**−.04**	.18	−.23	.24	.22	−.38**	−.17	.29*	.43**
Crouch	−.02	.20	.05	**.10**	**−.08**	**−.08**	**.00**	−.06	−.17	.14	.18	−.25	−.10	.28*	.31*
Avoid	−.17	.12	−.03	**.24**	**−.24**	**−.17**	**.11**	−.03	−.20	.27	.31*	−.33*	−.20	.33*	.41**
Scream	.06	.04	.09	**.05**	**.10**	**.04**	**.06**	.00	.12	.02	.09	−.09	−.07	−.15	−.03
Abnormal behavior															
Ingestion	−.01	.03	.04	.07	.02	−.13	−.07	**.20**	**−.01**	−.28*	−.04	.08	.08	−.08	−.25
Pace	−.15	−.13	−.17	.14	−.10	−.10	−.16	**.25**	**.05**	−.04	−.16	.28*	.07	−.03	−.23
Repetitive	−.01	.02	.13	.01	.07	−.02	.01	**.48**	**−.05**	.05	−.01	−.05	−.07	−.04	.07
Other abnor.	−.18	−.05	.16	.12	−.13	−.13	−.16	−.07	−.04	.03	−.01	.09	.05	−.11	−.06
Affiliatory behavior															
Social play	−.22	.17	−.07	.08	−.31*	−.09	−.08	−.05	−.36**	**.48**	**.38**	−.51**	−.38**	.34*	**.59**
Groom given	.09	.06	.04	−.10	.23	.13	.14	.04	.18	**.02**	**−.03**	.10	.09	−.27	−.28*
Groom received	.20	.30*	.09	−.08	.20	.31*	.18	.06	−.03	**−.24**	**−.17**	.04	.02	−.43**	−.23
Hold infant	−.27	−.16	−.13	.25	−.28*	−.24	−.26	.07	−.03	**.03**	**.10**	−.04	−.06	.07	.18
Contact—infant	−.43**	−.29*	−.35*	.14	−.41**	−.21	−.12	−.14	−.32*	**.46**	**.49**	−.41**	−.43**	.44**	.48**
Solitary behaviors															
Solitary play	−.40**	−.16	−.33*	.07	−.40**	−.16	−.17	−.17	−.38**	**.56**	**.44**	**−.52**	**−.41**	.37*	**.54**
Obj. manip.	−.16	.19	.00	.17	−.36**	−.27	−.12	.10	−.38**	**.31***	**.32***	**−.48**	**−.39**	.48**	**.58**
Nestbuild	−.13	.04	.00	.02	−.09	−.02	.04	.05	−.10	.16	.25	**−.32***	−.14	.06	.33*
Self-groom	.28*	.08	.32*	−.26	.36**	.33*	.30*	−.11	.27	−.22	−.11	**.24**	.19	−.31*	−.28*
Scratch	.23	.10	.15	−.12	.24	.22	.21	−.06	.13	−.08	.01	−.05	.00	−.14	−.06
Locomotor															
Locomotion	−.28*	−.08	−.25	.22	−.20	−.23	−.20	−.06	−.25	.26	.30*	−.21	−.17	**.33***	.44**

Trait label[b]

Note. N = 52. Correlations that are predicted to be strong are printed in **bold**.
[a] Abbreviated labels used; see Table 11.2 for full labels.
[b] Abbreviated labels used; see Table 11.3 for full labels.
* p < .05, two-tailed; ** p < .01, two-tailed.

195

As shown in Table 11.1, the level of agreement between trait ratings and theoretically associated behavior codings varied greatly, even within categories. For example, the aggression-related trait ratings converged strongly with some behavior codings (threat and display) but weakly with others (attack, charge, and displace). In general, the strongest convergent correlations were found for affiliation, activity, and playfulness. The convergent correlations for submissiveness, abnormal behavior, and solitariness were much weaker, and in some cases were even in the opposite direction than predicted. In addition, there were several strong correlations where no correlations were predicted.

What message should be drawn from this pattern of findings? On one hand, the numerous strong convergent correlations offer some encouragement, suggesting that the two methods are indeed assessing the same constructs. It is reassuring that personality ratings of animals predict relevant behaviors coded in a little more than 2 hours of observations. These predicted convergences make sense and require little further discussion. On the other hand, the weak correlations along the diagonal and strong correlations in unexpected places provide cause for concern. If two measures of a trait do not converge, then at least one of them is not working. What could explain the disagreement? Which method is better? The remaining sections of this chapter seek to address these potentially troubling questions.

Criteria for Evaluating Methods

We evaluate behavior-coding methods and trait-rating methods with respect to the reliability, subjectivity, and practicality of the two methods.

The first concern expressed by researchers is that trait ratings cannot be assessed reliably. Clearly, if a method is not reliable, it cannot be valid. The same criticism is less commonly directed at behavior-coding methods. Therefore, the first question we address is, Are trait-rating methods less reliable than behavior-coding methods?

The second concern held by some researchers is that trait-rating methods are too subjective to have any external validity. Behavior-coding methods, however, are typically viewed as immune to subjectivity. Therefore, the second question we address is, Are trait-rating

methods more subjective than behavior-coding methods?

Finally, researchers are concerned with the practicality of the methods. Behavior-coding methods are typically viewed as labor-intensive and difficult to implement rigorously. Trait-rating methods are usually considered more practical. Therefore, the third question we address is, Are behavior-coding methods less practical than trait-rating methods?

Question 1: Are Trait-Rating Methods Less Reliable Than Behavior-Coding Methods?

To evaluate the reliability of the behavior codings, reliabilities were computed for each behavior across the 50 chimpanzees for which we had at least 9 focal samples, treating the 9 focal samples as independent observations. The reliabilities of their composites are shown in Table 11.2. The mean intraclass correlation (ICC [1, k]) was .42, ranging from a high of .93 for solitary play to a low of .00 for twelve of the behaviors, including crouch and copulate.[2] The mean of the pairwise ICCs [1,1] was .11. We also computed composites of the behaviors within the eight categories to which they had been assigned a priori; the mean ICC [2, k] for the eight categories was only .17.

To evaluate the reliability of the trait ratings, we computed reliabilities for each trait across the 52 chimpanzees, treating the four observers as independent observations. The reliabilities of their composite are shown in Table 11.3. The mean intraclass correlation (ICC [2, k]) was .61, ranging from a high of .87 for submissive to a low of .03 for opportunistic. These values, equivalent to Cronbach's coefficient alphas, are at least as high as those found by John and Robins (1993) for single-item ratings of humans, where the mean alpha was .55.

The magnitude of alpha is affected by the number of observers. Therefore, to provide estimates of internal consistency that are unbiased by the number of observers, we also report the mean pairwise interjudge agreement. The mean of the pairwise ICCs [2,1], which are similar to pairwise correlations, was .30, as compared with a mean pairwise r of .24 in the John and Robins (1993) study.

As demonstrated in these tables, the reliabilities of the trait ratings were substantially higher on average than the reliabilities of the behavior codings. These findings are consistent with those of human studies, which have re-

TABLE 11.2. Reliability of Behavior Codings and Categories and Interitem Agreement

Behavioral category Behavior label[a]	Reliability (ICC [1, k])[a]	Interitem agreement (ICC [1, 1])	Reliability of composite (ICC[2, k])[b]
Aggressive behaviors			.16
Attack (aggressive interaction involving physical contact)	.61	.15	
Charge (locomotion toward another, often at full speed with piloerection)	.32	.06	
Threat (includes head tip, arm-raise threat, lunging)	.00	−.02	
Display (includes vocal [e.g., drumming] and nonvocal displays)	.45	.08	
Displace (where dominant animal physically supplants another)	.00	−.02	
Submissive behaviors			.59
Flee (animal moves away from another at full speed)	.28	.06	
Crouch (includes lowering of body and submissive presentation)	.00	−.01	
Avoid (animal moves away or out of the path of another)	.39	.07	
Fear grimace/bared-teeth scream	.05	.01	
Reconciliatory behaviors			n/a[c]
(includes embrace, extending hand to other, mouth-to-mouth contact)	.00	−.02	
Abnormal behavior			.22
Abnormal ingestion (e.g., of feces, hair)	.00	−.00	
Pace (repeated slow locomotion)	.44	.17	
Repetitive movements (includes rocking, head shaking)	.81	.31	
Other abnormal behavior (includes abnormal posturing, self-slapping)	.00	−.01	
Sexual behavior			.08
Copulate	.00	−.02	
Social explore (visual, oral, or manual inspection of ano-genital area)	.35	.06	
Masturbation (animal stimulates own genitals)	.60	.23	
Self-explore (animal manually inspects own genitals)	.34	.05	
Affiliatory behavior			.08
Social play (includes chasing, leaping, object manipulation with others)	.88	.45	
Social groom given (picking through hair or skin of another)	.11	.01	
Social groom received (having hair or skin picked through by another)	.00	−.01	
Embrace/hold infant (subject holds an infant)	.66	.17	
Social contact–infant (includes tandem walking, riding, nursing)	.80	.36	
Solitary behaviors			−.22
Solitary play (includes swinging, dangling, object manipulation alone)	.93	.61	
Manipulate object/environment (not included as part of play activity)	.68	.19	
Nestbuild (use of objects to form a place of retreat)	.31	.05	

(continued)

TABLE 11.2. *(continued)*

Behavioral category Behavior label[a]	Reliability (ICC [1, k])[a]	Interitem agreement (ICC [1, 1])	Reliability of composite (ICC[2, k])[b]
Solitary behaviors *(continued)*			
Self-groom (picking through own hair or skin)	.17	.02	
Scratch (scaping of fingernails across the skin)	.00	−.01	
Feeding behaviors			.13
Forage in (gathering of food in a substrate or puzzle)	.44	.08	
Feed on (taking food into the mouth)	.02	.00	
Drink (taking liquid into the mouth)	.38	.06	
Locomotor			−.02
Locomotion (includes running, climbing, walking)	.66	.18	
Sway (shifting weight from one side back to the other)	.14	.02	
Vocalizations and other behaviors			n/a[c]
Agonistic vocalization	.00	−.01	
Food call	.36	.06	
Cry/whimper	—[c]	—[d]	
Interact with contraspecific (focus is directed to non-chimpanzee individual)	.45	.08	
Inactive (any nonactive behavior not encompassed by the other scan codes)	.39	.07	
Other (any behavior not included in the rest of ethogram)	.00	.00	
Out of view (animal cannot be seen to record the behavior)	.29	.04	
Social location			n/a[c]
Nonsocial location (more than 3 feet from another chimpanzee)	.59	.14	
Contact (touching another chimpanzee)	.77	.27	
Near (less than 3 feet but not touching another chimpanzee)	.71	.22	
Social direction of behavior			n/a[c]
Self-directed (all behaviors not directed at another chimpanzee)	.80	.30	
Directed toward adult female	.28	.04	
Directed toward adult male	.44	.08	
Directed toward subadult female	.35	.06	
Directed toward subadult male	.83	.35	
Directed toward infant	.77	.27	
Directed toward multiple animals	.00	−.01	

Note. The *N* for these analyses is 50 because there were at least nine focal samples for these animals.

[a] A reliability less than zero does not make sense so ICCs less than zero are reported as zero.

[b] These values are equivalent to alphas.

[c] Reliabilities are not reported for categories that include only one item, include mutually exclusive items, or consist of items that were not intended to be theoretically related.

[d] Only one cry or whimper was recorded during the course of the study.

TABLE 11.3. Reliability of Composite Ratings and Pairwise Interobserver Agreement

Trait label	Reliability (ICC [2, k])[a]	Interobserver agreement r	Interobserver agreement (ICC [2,1])
Active	.49	.25	.19
Aggressive	.61	.27	.28
Anxious	.78	.47	.47
Assertive	.75	.43	.43
Belligerent	.54	.22	.23
Cautious	.53	.21	.22
Confident	.65	.30	.31
Consistent	.34	.10	.12
Curious	.64	.30	.30
Depressed	.50	.20	.20
Dominant	.85	.57	.58
Eccentric	.49	.18	.20
Effective	.80	.50	.50
Equable	.20	.04	.06
Excitable	.51	.18	.20
Fearful	.73	.39	.41
Friendly	.39	.15	.14
Gentle	.54	.25	.22
Impulsive	.50	.20	.20
Insecure	.75	.43	.43
Irritable	.68	.35	.35
Jealous	.49	.19	.20
Opportunistic	.03	.02	.01
Permissive	.55	.23	.23
Playful	.79	.49	.48
Protective	.36	.11	.12
Sensitive	.54	.24	.23
Slow	.68	.35	.35
Sociable	.61	.29	.28
Solitary	.69	.37	.36
Submissive	.87	.64	.63
Sullen	.71	.38	.38
Tense	.68	.35	.35
Vigilant	.64	.34	.31
Mean	.61	.30	.30

[a] These values are equivalent to alphas.

peatedly shown that codings of behavior yield unstable estimates (Borkenau, 1992) and can be difficult to assess reliably (Gosling, John, Craik, & Robins, 1998). Only 8 out of 34 traits (23%) had reliabilities below .50, whereas 35 out of 50 behaviors (70%) had reliabilities below .50. Note that among the convergent correlations in Table 11.1 (in bold), convergence between trait ratings and behavior codings occurred only for behaviors that were coded reliably. This makes conceptual sense (because if the behavior codings are not reliable, they are essentially meaningless as measures of personality traits) and suggests that the extent to which the two methods did not converge can be attributed to the unreliability of the behavior codings.

WHY ARE TRAIT RATINGS MORE RELIABLE THAN BEHAVIOR CODINGS?

Behavior varies in many ways. For example, variation in behavior can be due to seasonal effects, daily fluctuations, or changes in the social or physical environment (e.g., presence of a predator). For researchers trying to assess the consistent aspects of behavior (i.e., personality traits), this variance represents noise. Trait ratings successfully reduce this variability in two ways.

First, some of the variability in behavior is due to changes in the animal's situation or environment. For example, an individual may be active at one moment but inactive at another, but the variability in activity level may be due to situational factors (e.g., feeding time). One way to reduce the effects of this kind of variability is to take the situation into account when assessing personality. Observers making trait ratings can discount situational influences on behavior when making their ratings. In contrast, an observer making behavior codings would treat all instances of a behavior the same way, regardless of the situation. As Martin and Bateson (1993) wrote: "The human rater has played an active role in filtering, accumulating, weighting, and integrating information over a considerable period of time" (p. 81).

Second, another large portion of variability in behavior can be attributed to random variance. One way to reduce the effects of random variance is to aggregate those measures across time so that nonsystematic sources of variance will tend to cancel out one another. Trait ratings inherently benefit from this kind of aggregation because when observers rate an animal, they implicitly summarize that animal's behavior across all the years they have known it. Thus, data collected from trait ratings are essentially already aggregated across all the times the observer has observed the target animal. This quality of trait ratings drastically improves their reliability.

Behavior codings, in contrast, are at a disadvantage because they can be aggregated only across a shorter amount of the time (the amount of time each animal was observed). This results in a greater sensitivity to the situational variation in animals' behavior over time. Although this aspect of behavior codings may be an advantage in some research contexts (e.g., detecting the effects of experimental manipulations), it is problematic for personality trait research because the situational variance obscures the reliable cross-situational component of behavior that is a result of stable personality characteristics. If cross-situational variation in behavior is in part responsible for the low reliability of behavior codings, we would expect interobserver reliability (based on the same observation) to be higher than the interobservation reliability (across multiple observations) we report in this chapter. Indeed, previous animal research (Schapiro & Bloomsmith, 1995; Schapiro, Bloomsmith, Porter, & Suarez, 1996) has shown that the reliability of codings across multiple observers at the same time (interobserver reliability) is substantially higher than the reliability of codings across multiple observations across time (interobservation reliability). This pattern of findings supports the interpretation that low reliability in behavior codings is due, in part, to their sensitivity to situational variance (and not just to measurement error).

The variance in behaviors across situations and time can sometimes be extreme, thus producing behaviors that occur only in very rare circumstances. For example, in the 135 hours of behavior codings in this study, only a single whimper was ever recorded. In such extreme cases, behavior codings are not likely to be reliable; indeed they may fail to detect the behavior at all. Trait ratings, in contrast, are better able to detect low base-rate behaviors because of their greater aggregation across time. For example, a dog owner can accurately report whether or not her dog tends to bite humans, whereas even months of detailed observation may not be enough to detect such behavior if it is infrequent.

Another form of aggregation that improves reliability is aggregation across observers. In theory, both coding and rating methods could reap the benefits of this tactic, but, as they are currently practiced, only trait-rating methods do so. Aggregating ratings (or codings) across multiple observers enhances reliability by reducing measurement error due to the systematic idiosyncrasies of an observer (Block, 1961). For example, one observer may consistently interpret submissive behavior as playful, but this source of error will be minimized when ratings are aggregated across multiple observers.

Researchers may worry that aggregating across multiple observers leads to an artificial boost in reliability because of observers communicating with each other about the animals they are rating. However, even when observers are told not to communicate with each other about the animals (as in this study), interobserver reliabilities remain high. Of course, it must be acknowledged that in practice it is often impossible to completely eliminate sharing of information among raters (e.g., raters may have communicated with each other about the animals' personalities before the study began).

In summary, trait-rating methods capitalize on the benefits of aggregation on two levels—

by aggregating across time within each individual observer, and by aggregating across multiple observers. In contrast, the amount of aggregation necessary to obtain reliable behavior codings is often impossible to achieve. Trait-rating methods also have the advantage that observers can take context into account when interpreting a behavior, whereas behavior codings treat all instances of a behavior as identical, regardless of context. The reliabilities obtained in our study suggest that even when considerable effort is made to aggregate behavior codings, trait ratings still provide substantially more reliable estimates of personality than behavior codings across a variety of situations. With the psychometric odds stacked in favor of global ratings, substantial effort and resources are typically required to code behaviors as reliably as trait ratings (Moskowitz & Schwarz, 1982).

Given all of the apparent benefits of trait-rating methods with respect to reliability, why have they not been adopted more widely? One concern among researchers seems to be that trait ratings are compromised by their subjectivity. Specifically, researchers may worry that trait ratings are corrupted by rater bias or anthropomorphism. We address this possibility in the next section.

Question 2: Are Trait-Rating Methods More Subjective Than Behavior-Coding Methods?

For a method to be valid, it must be relatively free of subjective interpretation. A major appeal of behavior codings is their apparent objectivity because they do not seem to require much interpretation on the part of the human coders. In contrast, rating methods are often seen as idiosyncratic and subjective. Is this characterization fair?

In principle, measuring personality-relevant behavior directly is an appealing approach. However, as anyone who has actually coded behavior knows very well, behavior codings can quickly become quite complex. Subjectivity is introduced in the decisions that need to be made during both the development of the coding system and its implementation. We address each of these in turn.

When developing a coding system, researchers must first decide which behaviors to include. This decision involves determining which behaviors are indicators of which traits. For example, researchers dictate the meaning

of a category, such as "abnormal behavior," by deciding which behaviors should be included in the category and which ones should not. Selecting behaviors that are psychologically meaningful and categorizing them is a process that is subjective and susceptible to error.

In our illustrative study, the results suggest that some of the behaviors were indeed miscategorized. For example, the behavior "flee" was included in the category "submissive behaviors," when in fact it does not correlate with trait ratings of submissiveness. In fact, "flee" correlated better with the trait terms "active" and "playful" than with the submissive traits. In hindsight, this can be understood because the act of "mov[ing] away from another at full speed" could be a marker of playfulness (as running and chasing characterizes much rough-and-tumble chimpanzee play behavior). But without the trait-rating data, there is a danger that this interpretation of "flee" would not have come to light and the behavior would have continued to be categorized in the submissiveness category.

An alternative explanation for this pattern of results is that fleeing is, in fact, a marker of submissiveness and that raters were incorrectly interpreting it as a marker of playfulness and activity level. This explanation, however, is unlikely to be true, because the observers' ratings were based on their global impressions of the chimpanzees and so were not likely to be influenced greatly by a single behavior such as fleeing.

This type of categorization error occurred for many behaviors in our own study and, we suspect, is common in other studies as well. The validity of behavior codings can easily be compromised if researchers do not interpret the behaviors of animals correctly, if they attribute the behaviors to incorrect traits, or, more likely, if they simply neglect to account for the fact that a single behavior can be indicative of several different traits. Indeed, the results presented in Table 11.2 show that our ethogram-based classification of behavior was not borne out by the data—our behavior categories generally did not form reliable composites. If researchers do not verify the reliabilities of their behavior-coding categories, they may aggregate across behaviors that in reality do not co-occur and may be reporting meaningless results.

Next, researchers must decide at what level to code the behaviors. The most micro level of analysis might involve recording specific muscle movements. This has the advantage of being precise and objective, but makes subsequent steps of collecting and interpreting data much more difficult. As Martin and Bateson (1993) wrote, "The cost of gaining detail can be that higher-level patterns, which may be the most important or relevant features, are lost from view" (p. 9). In contrast, researchers could choose to measure behavior at the most global level, such as coding psychologically meaningful acts (e.g., fighting). As we discuss later, this introduces problems in the implementation stage.

Finally, to make the coding system easier to implement, researchers often make categories of behavior mutually exclusive, as we did in our illustrative study. This can impair the accuracy of behavior codings because, in reality, behaviors may reflect more than one trait. For example, playing may be underreported if sexual play is coded only as sexual behavior and not as playing behavior. Obviously, such decisions can have a big impact on animals' scores and are not necessarily supported by empirical research.

In addition to the subjectivity of decisions that are made in designing the coding system, subjectivity is also introduced when the behavior-coding system is implemented. For example, observers may apply the behavioral definitions strictly or loosely. As Block (1989) has noted in the context of assessing human behaviors, if the behavioral definitions are applied strictly—which presumably they must if the feared subjectivity is to be avoided—then relevant behaviors can easily be missed and irrelevant behaviors captured. For example, a behavior from the aggressive category, "charge," is defined as "locomotion during which an animal moves toward another at full speed often with piloerection (often as a component of a display). Can be male or female exhibiting this." Thus, an animal that locomotes aggressively toward another, but does so at three-fourths (vs. full) speed, would be classified as nonaggressive. Conversely, an animal that moves at full speed toward another should get a check in the aggression box even if it is doing so incidentally, in the service of escaping from another animal or in the service of play.

Another reason that the implementation of behavior-coding systems can be subjective is that many behaviors are ambiguous. This is particularly true if the behaviors are defined at the psychologically meaningful macrolevel. Even carefully defined behaviors are not immune from interpretational issues. For example, locomotion seems like a very simple, easy-to-define behavior, but what counts as locomotion? One step? Two?

The normal response to questions of this kind is to loosen the standards a bit, allowing the observer to use his or her knowledge of the species and to take contextual factors into account to determine whether a behavior really was an aggressive behavior. This is reasonable, but it immediately blurs the distinction between behavior codings and trait ratings. We suggest that, in practice, there is little difference between allowing the observer some slack in interpreting behaviors and simply asking the observer to rate how aggressively the animal behaves (a global trait rating).

In sum, it may seem that behavior codings do not deserve their reputation for being unconditionally objective. How do trait ratings compare?

The major concerns of researchers about the subjectivity of trait ratings can be summarized in two questions. First, are trait ratings fraught with the idiosyncratic biases of the individual observers? Second, are trait ratings simply anthropomorphic projections of human traits onto animals? We address each of these questions in turn.

Humans are not perfect information filters, and it is reasonable to question whether human observers introduce more bias than validity into the assessment process. If each observer is simply providing his or her own unique interpretation of an animal's behavior, this can greatly impede the objectivity of trait ratings. However, as Block (1961) has argued, aggregating across multiple observers essentially eliminates the idiosyncratic biases of each observer and the resulting average is not subjective. Indeed, our study shows that even as few as four observers per animal can provide reliable and consensual ratings for almost all traits.

The strong agreement among observers ensures that ratings are not purely idiosyncratic interpretations or biases. Nevertheless, the possibility remains that trait ratings reflect shared anthropomorphic projections. This concern, however, has been largely discredited (Gosling, 2001; Gosling & Vazire, 2002). Specifically, trait ratings have been validated against real-world behaviors and outcomes, they exhibit high levels of interobserver agreement, and they yield a factor structure similar to the factor structure of behavior codings. These findings suggest that trait ratings are measuring real attributes of the individuals being assessed and do not merely reflect anthropomorphic projections or lay theories about how traits covary in animals.

We have presented arguments and evidence suggesting that, contrary to widespread belief, behavior-coding methods are less objective than they might seem, and trait-rating methods less subjective. If researchers make their decisions about which methods to employ based on these unsubstantiated beliefs, they may foreclose on methods that would be useful. Obviously, researchers would be best served by basing their decisions on the validity of the methods, not their preconceptions about which method is more objective. Hebb (1946) expressed a similar sentiment: "A rigid refusal to 'anthropomorphize' may have its scientific disadvantages. . . . In spite of its mentalistic flavor and connotation of reference to conscious processes, the anthropomorphic terminology in this field may have another and more valuable significance as a classification of overt behavior" (p. 88).

Question 3: Are Trait-Rating Methods More Practical Than Behavior-Coding Methods?

Although practicality is not a central threat to the validity of a method, it can impact how well the method is carried out and therefore the quality of the results obtained. It is also a major consideration for researchers when deciding which method to use. It probably will not surprise researchers familiar with the two methods that comparing their practicality is a very simple matter: Trait-rating methods are usually more practical than behavior-coding methods.

The major advantage of trait-rating methods is that because researchers rely on the expertise of the observers, data collection is relatively effortless if sufficient observers are available. For example, in our study trait ratings were obtained by observers who each spent about 13 hours completing all 52 ratings. In contrast, the collection of the behavior-coding data required 135 hours of coding (not including training) over 7 months. The relative ease of obtaining trait ratings reduces the likelihood of errors

due to lack of training, misunderstandings, or fatigue on the part of the observer.

One practical limitation of trait-rating methods is that it may be difficult to identify multiple observers who are sufficiently familiar with the target animals to provide expert ratings. However, researchers wanting to use behavior-coding methods are faced with the equally (if not more) difficult problem of identifying multiple individuals who are willing and able to spend the hundreds of hours necessary to undergo training and to code behavior.

Conclusion

Now that we have examined the three main concerns related to behavior codings and trait ratings, we can return to the central question of this chapter: Which method is a better way to measure personality in animals, trait rating or behavior coding? Based on our analysis of the advantages and limitations of the two methods, we conclude that trait-rating methods are more reliable and practical than behavior-coding methods and are not as subjective as many researchers believe. Our empirical analyses demonstrated that trait ratings are reliable and hence well suited for detecting consistencies in animals' behavior, the very foundation of personality. Behavior codings, in contrast, are notoriously difficult to measure reliably, particularly when observations are made across different times of day or under varying conditions. Even when behaviors are measured at the same time of day or under the same conditions, they may reflect other characteristics of the environment (e.g., situational influences), not personality. We emphasize that we are not saying behavior codings are poor measures of *behavior*, but that they are poor measures of *personality*. Behavior-coding methods may be better suited for experimental manipulations, where researchers are concerned with detecting the effects of situational variables on behavior.

Our findings with respect to reliability indicate that researchers cannot assume that behavior codings are reliable, and should compute and report reliabilities for behavior codings as has been the practice for trait ratings. In addition, we recommend that researchers using either method take steps to improve the reliability of their measures. For example, behavior codings can probably be made more reliable by increasing the number of observers, increasing the number and length of observations, providing specific definitions of the behaviors to be coded, and training observers extensively. Trait ratings can also be made more reliable by increasing the number of observers, ensuring that all observers are well acquainted with the animals they are rating, and providing specific definitions of the traits being rated.

Our conceptual analyses of the potential threats to objectivity in the two methods revealed that, contrary to widespread belief, behavior codings are not immune to bias and subjectivity. In fact, the lack of standard systematic procedures for behavior codings raises concerns about the validity of results based on behavior codings. Our analyses suggest several important steps researchers can take to improve the objectivity of behavior codings. Specifically, researchers' decisions regarding which behaviors to code (e.g., "threat" vs. "displace" as an indicator of aggressiveness), the level at which behaviors are coded (e.g., "arm-waving and lunging toward another animal" vs. "threatening another animal"), and how to implement the coding procedures should be based on previous empirical research whenever possible, including research based on trait ratings.

Although the threats to objectivity in trait ratings are more familiar to researchers, we want to reiterate that researchers using trait ratings should continue to take precautions against anthropomorphism. Although the accumulated evidence presented here and elsewhere (Gosling, Lilienfeld, & Marino, 2003; Gosling & Vazire, 2002) suggests that anthropomorphism cannot fully account for the covariation among ratings, it is incumbent on investigators to demonstrate that ratings exhibit meaningful external correlates.

In order to estimate and reduce the effects of observer biases in both trait-rating and behavior-coding methods, we recommend that researchers perform variance partitioning analyses such as intraclass correlations or the Social Relations Model (Kenny, 1994). These analyses allow researchers to measure and statistically control for "perceiver effects," which are systematic idiosyncrasies in observers' ratings.

Our study also illustrated the practical advantages of trait-rating methods. Indeed, the efficiency with which ratings can be applied suggests that studies of personality could be carried out in many contexts where researchers

are perhaps discouraged by the efforts they associate with coding methods. These findings suggest that rating studies of personality can piggyback on animal studies already underway.

In many ways, our conclusions are consistent with the current consensus in the field of human personality research. That is, after facing many of the same issues that currently face animal researchers, human researchers concluded that trait ratings are in many respects better than behavior codings for describing personality and predicting future behavior. Nevertheless, human researchers frequently fail to take advantage of some of the most significant benefits of trait-rating methods we have illustrated here, such as aggregating across observers. Instead of relying on a single self-rating, researchers should also incorporate informant trait ratings (e.g., by the targets' friends, coworkers, spouses, etc.) as a powerful tool for personality assessment (Vazire, 2006).

Our conclusion that trait ratings are generally more valid than behavior codings is consistent with almost all empirical data on animal personality so far. This conclusion was anticipated in Hebb's reflections on his own study more than half a century ago:

> All that resulted [of behavior codings] was an almost endless series of specific acts in which no order or meaning could be found. On the other hand, by the use of frankly anthropomorphic concepts of emotion and attitude one could quickly and easily describe the peculiarities of the individual animals, and with this information a newcomer to the staff could handle the animals as he could not safely otherwise. Whatever the anthropomorphic terminology may seem to imply about conscious states in the chimpanzee, it provides an *intelligible and practical guide to behavior.* (Hebb, 1946, p. 88; original emphasis).

Of course, this does not mean that researchers should abandon behavior codings. Several studies, including our own, have found evidence for convergence between ratings and behavior codings. As in all assessments, the strongest evidence is obtained from converging sources of data. Therefore, where resources permit, we recommend using both rating and coding methods. Where resources are limited, however, our analyses suggest that rating methods, performed with care and rigor by observers who know the targets well, provide the most valid and efficient means of assessing personality in animals.

Notes

1. The proportion of coding and rating studies adds up to more than 100% because some studies (8%) used both methods to assess personality.
2. ICCs less than zero were set at zero because a reliability of less than zero does not make sense.

Recommended Readings

Capitanio, J. P. (1999). Personality dimensions in adult male rhesus macaques: Prediction of behaviors across time and situation. *American Journal of Primatology*, 47, 299–320.

Gosling, S. D. (2001). From mice to men: What can we learn about personality from animal research? *Psychological Bulletin*, 127, 45–86.

Gosling, S. D., Kwan, V. S. Y., & John, O. P. (2003). A dog's got personality: A cross-species comparative approach to evaluating personality judgments. *Journal of Personality and Social Psychology*, 85, 1161–1169.

Gosling, S. D., & Vazire, S. (2002). Are we barking up the right tree? Evaluating a comparative approach to personality. *Journal of Research in Personality*, 36, 607–614.

Hebb, D. O. (1946). Emotions in man and animal: An analysis of the intuitive process of recognition. *Psychological Review*, 53, 88–106.

Martin, P., & Bateson, P. (1993). *Measuring behavior: An introductory guide* (2nd ed.). Cambridge, UK: Cambridge University Press.

References

Blake, J. A., Eppig, J. T., Richardson, J. E., Davisson, M. T., & the Mouse Genome Database Group (2000). The Mouse Genome Database (MGD): Expanding genetic and genomic resources for the laboratory mouse. *Nucleic Acids Research*, 28, 108–111.

Block, J. (1961). *The Q-sort method in personality assessment and psychiatric research*. Springfield, IL: Charles C. Thomas.

Block, J. (1977). Advancing the psychology of personality: Paradigmatic shift or improving the quality of research? In D. Magnusson & N. S. Endler (Eds.), *Personality at the crossroads: Current issues in interactional psychology* (pp. 37–63). Hillsdale, NJ: Erlbaum.

Block, J. (1989). Critique of the act frequency approach to personality. *Journal of Personality and Social Psychology*, 56, 234–245.

Bolig, R., Price, C. S., O'Neill, P. L., & Suomi, S. J. (1992). Subjective assessment of reactivity level and personality traits of rhesus monkeys. *International Journal of Primatology*, 13, 287–306.

Borkenau, P. (1992). Implicit personality theory and the five-factor model. *Journal of Personality*, 60, 295–327.

Buirski, P., Plutchik, R., & Kellerman, H. (1978). Sex differences, dominance, and personality in the chimpanzee. *Animal Behaviour*, 26, 123–129.

Capitanio, J. P. (1999). Personality dimensions in adult male rhesus macaques: Prediction of behaviors across time and situation. *American Journal of Primatology*, 47, 299–320.

Capitanio, J. P., Mendoza, S. P., & Baroncelli, S. (1999). The relationship of personality dimensions in adult male rhesus macaques to progression of simian immunodeficiency virus disease. *Brain, Behavior, and Immunity*, 13, 138–154.

Domjan, M., & Purdy, J. E. (1995). Animal research in psychology: More than meets the eye of the general psychology student. *American Psychologist*, 50, 496–503.

Dulawa, S. C., Grandy, D. K., Low, M. J., Paulus, M. P., & Geyer, M. A. (1999). Dopamine D4 receptor-knock-out mice exhibit reduced exploration of novel stimuli. *Journal of Neuroscience*, 19, 9550–9556.

Fahlke, C., Lorenz, J. G., Long, J., Champoux, M., Suomi, S. J., Higley, J. D. (2000). Rearing experiences and stress-induced plasma cortisol as early risk factors for excessive alcohol consumption in nonhuman primates. *Alcoholism: Clinical and Experimental Research*, 24, 644–650.

Flint, J. (2002). Animal models of personality. In J. Benjamin & R. P. Ebstein (Eds.), *Molecular genetics and the human personality* (pp. 63–90). Washington, DC: American Psychiatric Press.

Francis, D., Diorio, J., Liu, D., & Meaney, M. J. (1999). Nongenomic transmission across generations of maternal behavior and stress responses in the rat. *Science*, 286, 1155–1158.

Gordon, J. A., & Hen, R. (2004). Genetic approaches to the study of anxiety. *Annual Review of Neuroscience*, 27, 193–222.

Gosling, S. D. (1998). Personality dimensions in spotted hyenas (*Crocuta crocuta*). *Journal of Comparative Psychology*, 112, 107–118.

Gosling, S. D. (2001). From mice to men: What can we learn about personality from animal research? *Psychological Bulletin*, 127, 45–86.

Gosling, S. D., John, O. P., Craik, K. H., & Robins, R. W. (1998). Do people know how they behave? Self-reported act frequencies compared with on-line codings by observers. *Journal of Personality and Social Psychology*, 74, 1337–1349.

Gosling, S. D., Kwan, V. S. Y., & John, O. P. (2003). A dog's got personality: A cross-species comparative approach to evaluating personality judgments. *Journal of Personality and Social Psychology*, 85, 1161–1169.

Gosling, S. D., Lilienfeld, S. O., & Marino, L. (2003). Personality. In D. Maestripieri (Ed.), *Primate psychology: The mind and behavior of human and nonhuman primates* (pp. 254–288). Cambridge, MA: Harvard University Press.

Gosling, S. D., & Mollaghan, D. M. (2006). Animal research in social psychology: A bridge to functional genomics and other unique research opportunities. In P. A. M. van Lange (Ed.), *Bridging social psychology: Benefits of trans-disciplinary approaches* (pp. 123–128). Mahwah, NJ: Erlbaum.

Gosling, S. D., & Vazire, S. (2002). Are we barking up the right tree? Evaluating a comparative approach to personality. *Journal of Research in Personality, 36*, 607–614.

Hebb, D. O. (1946). Emotions in man and animal: An analysis of the intuitive process of recognition. *Psychological Review, 53*, 88–106.

Hinde, R. A., Leighton-Shapiro, M. E., & McGinnis, L. (1978). Effects of various types of separation experience on rhesus monkeys 5 months later. *Journal of Child Psychology and Psychiatry and Allied Disciplines, 19*, 199–211.

John, O. P., & Robins, R. W. (1993). Determinants of interjudge agreement on personality traits: The big five domains, observability, evaluativeness, and the unique perspective of the self. *Journal of Personality, 61*, 521–551.

Jones, A. C., & Gosling, S. D. (2006). Temperament and personality in dogs (*Canis familiaris*): A review and evaluation of past research. *Applied Animal Behavior Science, 95*, 1–53.

Kenny, D. A. (1994). *Interpersonal perception: A social relations analysis.* New York: Guilford Press.

Martin, P., & Bateson, P. (1993). *Measuring behavior: An introductory guide* (2nd ed.). Cambridge, UK: Cambridge University Press.

Mather, J. A., & Anderson, R. C. (1993). Personalities of octopuses (*Octopus rubescens*). *Journal of Comparative Psychology, 107*, 336–340.

Mehta, P. H., & Gosling, S. D. (2006). How can animal studies contribute to research on the biological bases of personality? In T. Canli (Ed.), *Biology of personality and individual differences* (pp. 427–448). New York: Guilford Press.

Mischel, W. (1968). *Personality and assessment.* New York: Wiley.

Moskowitz, D. S., & Schwarz, J. C. (1982). Validity comparison of behavior counts and ratings by knowledgeable informants. *Journal of Personality and Social Psychology, 42*, 518–528.

Noldus L. P. (1991). The Observer: S software system for collection and analysis of observational data. *Behavior Research Methods, Instruments and Computers, 23*, 415–429.

Nystrom, P., Schapiro, S. J., & Hau, J. (2001). Accumulated means analysis: A novel method to determine reliability of behavioral studies using continuous focal sampling. *In Vivo, 15*, 29–34.

Pederson, A. K., King, J. E., & Landau, V. I. (2005). Chimpanzee (*Pan troglodytes*) personality predicts behavior. *Journal of Research in Personality, 39*, 534–549.

Schapiro, S. J. (2002). Effects of social manipulations and environmental enrichment on behavior and cell-mediated immune responses in rhesus macaques. *Pharmocology, Biochemistry and Behavior* [Special Issue: Environmental manipulations in rodents and primates: Insights into pharmacology, biochemistry and behavior], *73*, 271–278.

Schapiro, S. J., & Bloomsmith, M. A. (1995). Behavioral effects of enrichment on singly-housed, yearling rhesus monkeys: An analysis including three enrichment conditions and a control group. *American Journal of Primatology, 35*, 89–101.

Schapiro, S. J., Bloomsmith, M. A., Porter, L. M., & Suarez, S.A. (1996). Enrichment effects on rhesus monkeys successively housed singly, in pairs, and in groups. *Applied Animal Behaviour Science, 48*, 159–172.

Spencer-Booth, Y., & Hinde, R. A. (1969). Tests of behavioural characteristics for rhesus monkeys. *Behaviour, 33*, 180–211.

Stevenson-Hinde, J. (1983). Individual characteristics and the social situation. In R. A. Hinde (Ed.), *Primate social relationships: An integrated approach* (pp. 28–35). Sunderland, MA: Sinauer.

Stevenson-Hinde, J. (2005). The interplay between attachment, temperament, and maternal style: A madingley perspective. In K. E. Grossmann, K. Grossmann, & E. Waters (Eds.), *Attachment from infancy to adulthood: The major longitudinal studies* (pp. 198–222). New York: Guilford Press.

Stevenson-Hinde, J., Stillwell-Barnes, R., & Zunz, M. (1980). Subjective assessment of rhesus monkeys over four successive years. *Primates, 21*, 66–82.

Suomi, S. J. (1987). Genetic and maternal contributions to individual differences in rhesus monkey biobehavioral development. In N. Krasnegor, E. Blass, M. Hofer, & W. Smotherman (Eds.), *Perinatal development: A psychobiological perspective* (pp. 397–420). New York: Academic Press.

Vazire, S. (2006). Informant reports: A cheap, fast, and easy method for personality assessment. *Journal of Research in Personality, 40*, 472–481.

Vazire, S., & Gosling, S. D. (2003). Bridging psychology and biology with animal research. *American Psychologist, 5*, 407–408.

Virgin, C. E., Jr., & Sapolsky, R. M. (1997). Styles of male social behavior and endocrine correlates among low-ranking baboons. *American Journal of Primatology, 42*, 25–39.

Zuckerman, M. (1996). The psychobiological model for impulsive unsocialized sensation seeking: A comparative approach. *Neuropsychobiology, 34*, 125–129.

PART II

Methods for Assessing Personality at Different Levels of Analysis

## CHAPTER 12

Taxonomies, Trends, and Integrations

Kenneth H. Craik

From day to day, from year to year, from birth to death, every individual generates a steady and diverse flow of information about the kind of person that individual is.

In its most generic sense, our knowledge of persons derives from a rich variety of sources of information about them, including (1) their everyday conduct, (2) their reputations in their communities, (3) the impressions they make on others, (4) their self-characterizations, (5) their imaginative and interpretive productions, (6) their behavior in standardized test situations, and (7) their life histories and fate in society.

The field of personality psychology seeks to marshall such information to address an array of questions: How does that person compare with other persons? How has the person developed and changed over the life course? And what impact has the person made on the individual's own environment, community and society, and on other persons?

In retrospect, the historical development of personality research methods can be viewed as a rather unsystematic effort to identify more or less comprehensively the kinds of information a person generates and to devise means of monitoring or recording these various ways of knowing a person (Craik, 2000b).

A historical perspective on research methods suggests that as personality psychology initially achieved its identity as a distinct field of scientific inquiry, researchers devoted some attention to each domain of knowing persons (Craik, 1986). Over the first half century of the field's development, however, scientific attention granted to these methods fluctuated. Some methods displayed continued, sustained development and others arrested or interrupted development. Nevertheless, this discipline has been guided by the recognition that scientific investigation of personality requires multiple and diverse forms of inquiry. Indeed, in recent decades, the full breadth of coverage has again been demonstrated, whereas attention to specific techniques within each method category has waxed and waned.

This chapter reviews a taxonomy of seven ways of knowing a person that is rooted in the historical development of personality research methods. Each taxonomic category subsumes a set of methodological issues and a variety of specific research tools.

Taxonomy of Personality Research Methods as Types of Information Sources about Persons

Persons Are Known through Their Everyday Conduct and Experiences

Persons are known by the kinds of actions they take throughout everyday life. For example, one meaning of personality trait constructs, such as *dominant*, is that over a period of observation, a person so described tends to display a relatively high frequency of prototypically dominant acts, such as "taking charge of the situation after the accident" (Buss & Craik, 1983). Thus, one way in which personality is revealed is through the situated, daily actions of individuals.

Historically, field studies of personality have shown a pattern of interrupted development (Craik, 1986). Early uses can be found in the period when personality psychology emerged as a distinct field of scientific inquiry (Craik, Hogan, & Wolfe, 1993). They include Newcomb's (1929) studies of extraversion among children at a summer camp and the naturalistic experiments of the Character Education Inquiry (Hartshorne & May, 1928, 1929; Hartshorne, May, & Shuttleworth, 1930). Perhaps the most thorough monitoring of everyday conduct was Barker and Wright's *One Boy's Day* (1951), which reported the full text of one behavior specimen record, giving the continuous and detailed descriptions by a relay team of monitors working from breakfast to bedtime and tracking the ongoing conduct of 7-year-old Raymond.

Following a decline in interest during the 1950s and 1960s, attention to monitoring the flow of experience and conduct *in situ* has continued steadily since the mid-1970s (Hormuth, 1986). Technical developments in field methods have assisted in depicting everyday manifestations of personality from the inside agent's

perspective and from the outside observers' perspective (Craik, 1994).

For time-sampling reports of situated experience and conduct, portable computer programmed beeper devices provide prompts and permit the person to record coded reports of emotions, behaviors, and settings (Conner, Feldman Barrett, Tugade, & Tennen, Chapter 5, this volume; Mehl, Gosling, & Pennebaker, 2006). In contrast, video recordings of the lived days of persons focus on the observer's point of view. In this approach, video-recording teams generate more or less continuous recordings of situated conduct over extended periods of observation within the person's own ecological niches (Craik, 2000a).

The goal of field studies is to enhance the ecological validity of personality research by moving investigations out of the laboratory, clinic, or assessment center and into the often mundane environments in which personality develops and lives are lived.

Methodological research issues in the use of these methods include gauging the influence of reactivity in the reports of persons taking part in time-sampling beeper studies and the possible adjustment of behavior in response to being video recorded in lived day analyses. Systematic research can delineate the impact of such reactivity. A second issue is the importance of developing coding systems appropriate to personality field studies. For example, video recordings of daily conduct can be categorized into several alternative systems, such as behavior setting categories, trait construct categories, and goal–task categories (Craik, 2000a). Attention must also be paid to the potential bias toward overemphasizing either the mundane, quotidian aspects of everyday life or its relatively infrequent but accentuating and revealing episodes (Caspi & Moffett, 1993; Craik, 1993). Finally, note must be taken of trait-relevant behavioral residues that offer multiple cues to personality within an individual's environment, such as those from prototypical conscientious acts that leave behind an alphabetized CD collection (Gosling, Ko, Mannarelli, & Morris, 2002)

Persons Are Known by Their Reputations in Their Lifelong Idiographic Communities

Persons are known through their reputations, that is, how they are collectively viewed by those who know them in their communities and in society at large. How persons have become represented throughout their particular reputational networks is a product of ongoing community observation and communication. Thus, a person's prevailing reputation is an inescapable part of social reality for the individual as well as a source of information about that person.

Throughout the life course, each person is discussed and represented by the unique and evolving network of other individuals who have come to know the person. At any given moment, information about the person may be flowing across certain segments of the reputational network. What is being said about the person, the overt communication and discussion, can be considered the discursive facet of the person's reputation. In addition, each and every reputational network member forms and maintains some more or less extensive representation of the person; these dispersed beliefs, evaluations, and impressions can be considered the distributive facet of the person's reputation. The research approach appropriate for analysis of the discursive facet of reputation requires a different set of techniques than the analysis of the distributive facet of a person's reputation (Craik, 2006). The former enlists expertise in social linguistics and communication analysis, and the latter bears more on sampling methods in survey research.

Seven decades after the emergence of the scientific field of personality psychology, the analysis of reputation remains largely in an arrested stage of development. Mark A. May (1932) had unsuccessfully attempted to foster a dual conception of personality, balancing the notion of the person as an agent of integrative action with the notion of the person as a social stimulus, and thus directing attention to how the person is viewed by others. Alas, in his pioneering textbook on personality, Gordon W. Allport (1937) explicitly and decisively dismissed the study of reputation or social stimulus value from the domain of personality, associating it with the realm of mere gossip and rumor.

Thus, reputational analysis remains the category of research methods most in need of attention, and it is beginning to receive it. Hogan (1996) has advocated this conception, treating reputation as the outer view of personality and agentic dynamics as the inner view. Bromley (1993) has contributed a broad and multidisci-plinary review of the topic, and Emler (1990) has taken a social-psychological approach that includes the serious scientific analysis of the functions and processes of gossip.

In his sketch of a dual conception of personality, May had failed to incorporate a network perspective with regard to the views and impressions that others form of a person (Craik, 2006). Yet the evidence is ubiquitous in everyday social life that people share and discuss their impressions of a person with other individuals. Social networks can be interpreted as one component of reputational networks, consisting of those individuals with whom the person has a mutual acquaintance, in contrast to those others who know the person but whom the person does not know. A network interpretation of reputation is facilitated by a program of empirical study of social networks (Pool, I. de Sola, & Kochen, 1978) and by more general recent advances in network theory (Watts, 2003).

The goal of reputational analysis in personality research is to make use of the formidable amount of both systematic and incidental surveillance and interactions that generate reputation, as well as the distillation of ongoing communication and commentary that they afford.

Several methodological issues are posed by reputational analysis and many still wait to be addressed thoroughly. The matter of bias, either toward denigration or bolstering, is a tendentious influence that must be recognized and understood. The impact of false negative assertions on reputation is sufficiently potent that the common law affords individuals actions for libel and slander as a protection against false defamation.

From a research point of view, truth in reputation focuses on two lines of inquiry. One issue deals with appraising the accuracy of the reputational analysis of network structure and content. Network structure entails accuracy in determining size and membership, the density or interrelatedness among network members, delineation of clusters or cliques among members, and so forth. The reputational content encompasses the kinds of information circulating and stored within the network. For example, content can refer to (1) social facts (e.g., "was born on March 28, 1970"), (2) anecdotes and act descriptions regarding the person (e.g., "a woman poured a bowl of sugar on his head during a party"), and (3) personality attributes (e.g., "she is dominant, curious").

A second mission deals with appraising the validity of reputational content claims. Whatever the reputed birth date and age might be, the validity of this reputational content claim requires detective work in checking official birth certificates. Similarly, information concerning the prevailing belief about the sugar bowl incident requires inquiry with reputational network members, but validation of the story itself entails interviews with on-the-scene witnesses to the goings on at that party. Finally, samples of network members might provide personality trait ratings, but the validation of these claims encounters the complex arena of construct validity and the marshaling of such evidence as degree of consensus among the raters, relation to monitored trends in everyday conduct, self-ratings, and other candidates for status as validational criteria (Furr & Funder, Chapter 16, this volume; McCrae & Weiss, Chapter 15, this volume).

Persons Are Known through the Impressions They Make on Others

Persons are known by their impressions on others and the descriptions others render of them. Human observers are sensitive instruments for monitoring and interpreting information about the personality of others. Furthermore, ordinary language is rich in descriptive and evaluative terms that are available to observers for portraying and communicating their impressions of other persons.

From the beginning years of personality research, investigators have had frequent recourse to personality ratings as a primary form of data in their empirical studies to assess and examine individual differences in personality characteristics (Hollingworth, 1922; Roback, 1927). This immediate mobilization of personality judgments and ratings is understandable because the format closely mimics the use of trait adjectives and related terms in describing persons in everyday social life. Indeed, Allport and Odbert (1936) and other early researchers systematically examined dictionaries to delineate the broad domain of ordinary language personality descriptors (Bromley, 1977; John & Srivastava, 1999). In addition, techniques such as Q-sort procedures and adjective checklists were introduced to aid in standardizing personality descriptions in research and applied contexts (Block, 1978; Gough & Heilbrun, 1983).

The identification of a recurrent five-factor structure (i.e., the "Big Five") in ordinary language personality ratings has gained wide attention. This development has focused research on the functions of these broad dimensions and the specific descriptors that are subsumed by each bipolar dimension (Goldberg, 1992; John & Srivastava, 1999).

The goal of this method of study in personality is to employ the nuanced interpretive and integrative skills of observers to organize and convey the information to be found in the impressions a person has made on them.

The reader will note that the impressions of a person formed by network members constitutes one—though only one—component of reputational content. However, some authorities draw firm distinctions between personality judgments and interpersonal perception, on one hand, and facets of reputation, on the other. For example, in his influential reviews and analytic models, Kenny (1994) has explicitly restricted his examination of interpersonal perception to processes that occur online during social interactions (p. 148) and excludes the role of third-party communications that are, of course, a ubiquitous and pervasive feature of reputational processes.

Similarly, in his comprehensive analysis of personality judgments, Funder (1999) acknowledges the nature and importance of reputation but sets sharp Allportian boundaries between the study of personality judgments and the study of reputation. He argues that although reputation can be examined in its own right, with regard to personality ratings, reputation enters this picture only to "the degree to which one's reputation might be among the indicators of what a person is *really* like" (p. 6). Within reputational analysis, we have referred to this issue as that of determining the validity of the personality component of reputational content claims.

Among the methodological issues in the use of this method of personality study is the recognition that gauging the reliability or reproducibility of observer-based assessments of personality requires the use of aggregated ratings from a panel of observers recording their impressions independently. Other parameters that warrant attention are the individual variations among persons in the amount of agreement to be found in observer descriptions of them and the various contextual attributes of assessments, such as prior acquaintance and the particular domain of personality constructs being rated (John & Robins, 1993a).

Persons Are Known through Their Self-Reflexive Assertions about Themselves

Persons are known through their claims about themselves. Thus, the self-descriptions individuals render about their own actions, beliefs, emotions, habits, interests, and other characteristics offer an important form of information about the personality of individuals.

One mode for this self-report method of study in personality research is to treat the person as simply another observer and to tap the impressions the person has made on him- or herself. However, it is commonly acknowledged that the person has certain forms of privileged, or at least distinctive, access to information about experiences, intentions, and motives that is less readily available to acquaintances and other individuals.

Recently, the question has been raised about whether self-reports of this kind have themselves been granted an unduly privileged status in personality research (Hofstee, 1994). Self-ratings of personality, in general, appear to be used much more frequently in published studies than informant ratings (Vazire, 2006). Furthermore, in appraising the accuracy of personality judgments, self-reports seem to be more often employed as a criterion, in comparison to informant reports (Funder, 1999).

Empirical studies have focused on delineating and understanding certain biases in self-reports, such as self-enhancement (John & Robins, 1994), which can then be taken into account in the use of this source of information about persons. Furthermore, nuanced conceptual analyses can tease out the relative validational pertinence of self versus other personality ratings, according to the specific personality construct being studied (Ozer, 1989).

A second mode for using self-reports is found in personality scales and inventories. The development of these techniques followed from the early discovery that self-assertions endorsing widely varied statements about one's attitudes, interests, beliefs, and conduct turned out to have value in assessing individual differences in personality.

Pioneering personality inventories included the Woodworth Personal Data Sheet (1917), the Strong Vocational Interest Blank (1927),

the Allport–Vernon Study of Values (1933) and the Minnesota Multiphasic Personality Inventory (1943) (Goldberg, 1971).

Current comprehensive personality inventories have been derived through several different approaches and methods of scale construction, often within the development of the same inventory. The construction of the Myers–Briggs Type Indicator (MBTI) (Myers & McCaulley, 1985) was guided by constructs drawn from C. G. Jung's theory of psychological types (Jung, 1923); indeed, the initial item pool was closely derived from Jung's detailed descriptive text.

Guiding the development of the original individual scales of the California Psychological Inventory (CPI) (Gough, 1957) was the choice of folk concepts, such as dominance and tolerance, that differentiate persons within societies and possess predictive implications for how a person is viewed by others and for forecasting important life outcomes. Subsequent statistical and conceptual analysis revealed a higher-order internal structure derived from orientations toward interpersonal life (externality–internality), toward societal imperatives (norm-favoring–norm questioning), and toward self-realization. In a resulting typological model, the first pair of these orthogonal vectors depicts four styles of living, each with seven levels of integration calibrated along the third vector (Gough, 2002; Gough & Bradley, 2002).

The empirical identification of a Big Five structure in the domain of observer-based personality trait ratings has generated efforts to conceptualize and examine a more general theoretical five-factor model of personality structure (John & Robins, 1993b; McCrae & Weiss, Chapter 15, this volume). This research program has fostered the development of self-report personality instruments seeking to assess these dimensions of extraversion, agreeableness, conscientiousness, neuroticism, and openness. They include the NEO Personality Inventory—Revised (NEO-PI-R) (Costa & McCrae, 1992), the Trait Descriptive Adjectives (TDA) (Goldberg, 1992), and the Big Five Inventory (BFI)(John & Srivastava, 1999).

From the post–World War II era and across four or more decades, the program of research using personality scales to predict theoretically and practically important nontest criteria and life outcomes was a dominant feature of personality research and continues to be strong (Wiggins, 1973, 2003). This methodological tradition has contributed an impressive array of self-critical and clarifying concepts and techniques, such as construct validation, conceptual analysis of scale scores, and heterotrait–heteromethod analysis. Special scales have been developed within some inventories to identify test-taking intentions to create favorable or unfavorable impressions. Major personality inventories are accompanied by manuals that provide an abundant amount of empirical research findings that help to delineate the psychological meaning and implications of personality scale scores and categories.

Persons Are Known by Expressions of Their Imaginations and How They Construe Their Experiences

Persons are known through their imaginative productions and the ways they construe their life experiences. Thus, the distinctive products that persons generate through their apperceptions, fantasies, stories, and other imaginative and constructive formats yield information about their personalities.

This method has been a long-standing, and at times almost dominant, force in personality research. In 1910, Jung reported on his investigations with the word association method in the *American Journal of Psychology*. Rorschach introduced his inkblot test in 1922, and Morgan and Murray presented the first report on the Thematic Apperception Test (TAT) in 1935.

In his discussion of projective techniques, L. K. Frank (1939) offered an organizing term and perspective on this early set of procedures, emphasizing the challenge to persons to perceive, apperceive and impose meaning upon the inkblots, pictures, and so forth.

Subsequently, the scope of this method has been expanded in several ways. First, the techniques of thematic analysis within the framework of Murray's (1938) need–motive system have been applied to assess motives such as achievement, affiliation, intimacy, and power in personal documents, letters, speeches, and archival materials (Winter, 1991) Second, adapting a procedure first used in the 1920s, Loevinger (1979) devised the Sentence Completion Test of Ego Development (SCT) with a coding manual for assessing six sequential stages: impulsive, protective, conformist, conscientious, autonomous, and integrated.

Third, Kelly (1955) introduced the Role Construct Repertory Test (REP Test) to analyze

how a person construes the interpersonal world. Finally, in his analysis of identity and personal myth in an individual's own life stories, McAdams (1996) examined the autobiographical materials generated by a person. His model encompasses affects (reflected in the tone of the personal life story), imagery (e.g., residues of childhood make-believe), motivation (expressed in themes), beliefs (e.g., ideology), memories (e.g., of key life episodes), and imagoes (e.g., central characters).

Between the two major pioneering techniques within this category of research methods, a shift in research standing seems to be occurring. Although predominant in the post–World War II era, the Rorschach technique in recent years remains persistently controversial with regard to its scientific validation (Wood, Nezworski, Lilienfeld, & Garb, 2003). In the meantime, TAT spin-off methods have earned a notable place in mainstream personality research; these include the thematic analysis of personal life stories (McAdams, 1996) and the TAT-based content analyses of motives (Winter, 1991).

The goal of procedures within this method of personality study is to evoke the apperceptive and interpretive styles of a person. Within the historical development of each procedure, a route is often apparent, beginning with its use by sometimes talented individual interpreters and progressing to more standard instruments, accompanied by more or less successful efforts to advance evidence of reproducibility and validity. For these purposes, coding systems and teaching materials for coders have been devised, as well as efforts to identify and correct for various potential biases, such as verbal fluency and productivity.

Persons Are Known by How They React to Certain Kinds of Challenges and Tasks

Persons are known by how they react to specific kinds of challenges and perform in certain kinds of tasks. Thus, how persons conduct themselves in standard test situations provides an important source of information about their personalities. In addition, systematic examination of sources of influence on behavior in such controlled settings can generate knowledge about the dynamics of affect, thought, and action.

The well-established resort to laboratory methods in the study of personality dynamics can be traced to such pioneering efforts as those conducted in the 1920s and 1930s in Berlin by Kurt Lewin (1935), whose research team studied such topics as level of aspiration and selective memory for uncompleted tasks. In the 1930s, German military psychologists reported on use of the leaderless group discussion (LGD) to assess individual differences in initiative and leadership (Bass, 1954). Subsequently, British and American wartime assessment programs also employed the technique (Eysenck, 1953; Office of Strategic Services Assessment Staff, 1948), and the procedure continues to be employed in both managerial and personality assessment centers (Craik et al., 2002).

Subsequent exemplars of this method include Lazarus's (1986) use of films of industrial accidents as elicitors of psychological stress in studies of individual differences in coping. In addition, coding techniques initiated by Ekman and Friesen (1978) were developed to assess emotions based on facial expressions. These two lines of inquiry have fostered research programs on emotional communication and control, for example, in the context of aging (Levenson, 2000; Diamond & Otter-Henderson, Chapter 22, this volume).

Research on the delay of gratification and the development of self-control has employed standard situations in which children's capacity to delay the consumption of candies or the use of toys is assessed (Bem & Funder, 1978; Block, 1977; Mischel, 1966). Individual differences in delay of gratification among children have been related to concurrent descriptions of them as planful and reflective and to ratings later in adolescence as being self-controlled (Shoda, Mischel, & Peake, 1990).

The use of standard tasks to assess individual differences can be contrasted with employing the same tasks in experimental research examining the impact of various situational variables on aspects of task performance. For example, Asch (1952) devised the conformity situation to examine the influence of group pressure in opinion on the judgments of an individual, for example, comparing a partial majority to a unanimous majority. Taking the same standard task and situation, Crutchfield (1956) adapted it to assess individual differences in independence of judgment or resistance to pressure. Variations in resisting majority views were related positively to independent assessment staff descriptions of the same par-

ticipants on such personality descriptors as (1) Is persuasive; tends to win other people over to his point of view and (2) Is self-reliant; independent in judgment; able to think for him- or herself, and negatively related to (1) Is conforming; tends to do what is prescribed and (2) Is unable to make decisions without vacillation or delay (Crutchfield, 1956, pp. 194–195).

The goal of standard tasks and situations is to assess individual differences in aspects of personality that bear upon the underpinnings and dynamics of thought and action (Beer & Lombardo, Chapter 21, this volume; Ebstein, Bachner-Melman, Israel, Nemanov, & Gritsenko, Chapter 23, this volume; Robinson, Chapter 20, this volume). An important methodological issue in the use of this method is the role of aggregation of responses in ensuring reliable and reproducible findings (Epstein, 1983). Psychometric standards apply in this context, just as in the use of multiple observers and multiple scale items with other methods of personality study.

Persons Are Known by the Kinds of Lives They Have Lived

Persons are known by the nature of their own life histories. Although the amount of information available about their specific pasts may vary among persons, it is nevertheless an important source of our understanding of their personalities.

In this method of personality study, as Runyan (1982) has emphasized, the life history is the subject matter, that is, "the sequence of events and experiences in a life from birth until death" (p. 6). In this sense, all the information afforded by all of the other methods of study in personality is grist for the mill in conducting a life history analysis of a person.

The goal or aspiration for objectivity in historical representations rests upon an openness to continuing scrutiny and revision and a sensitivity to such factors as the partial survival of records and evidence (Elms, Chapter 6, this volume; Lowenthal, 1996; Novick, 1988; Pompa, 1990).

Of course, life history analysis of a person constitutes a special kind of historical research and draws aid from the craft of biography and such fields of inquiry as psychobiography and lifespan developmental psychology. At the beginning era of personality psychology, psychobiographical reports were a common feature of the journal *Character and Personality* (later to become the *Journal of Personality*). Efforts to promote systematic inquiry included Dollard's (1935) criteria for compiling life histories and Allport's (1942) guidelines for the use of personal documents. Even these modest initiatives were accompanied by backstage opposition within academic psychology (Barenbaum & Winter, 2003).

Despite notable contributions (e.g., Erikson, 1958, 1963), attention to this endeavor waned during the post–World War II years. The interrupted development of life history analysis ended in the 1980s. A turning point was Runyan's (1982) *Life Histories and Psychobiography*, which presented a comprehensive argument for the field and a compelling vision of its prospects. Procedural advice for undertaking projects in this domain appeared (Alexander, 1990; Elms, 1994, and Chapter 6, this volume; Runyan, 2005), as well as treatments of the diversity and organization of case study materials (Bromley, 1986).

A strategic issue for this method of personality study is whether a particular project in life history analysis is to attempt a comprehensive representation of the entire life of a person or whether it is to pursue an equally valuable detailed focus on a particular question or notable episode in the person's life (Elms, 1994). Thus, an account might be rendered of the early life and career of Gordon W. Allport through the 1930s (Nicholson, 2003), or the implications of Allport's meeting in Vienna with Sigmund Freud might be examined (Elms, Chapter 6, this volume).

Detailed examination of specific puzzles or episodes, such as the import of Woodrow Wilson's neurological illness (George & George, 1981–82; Weinstein, Anderson, & Link, 1978–79) or the psychological meaning of Dodge Morgan's solo circumnavigation (Nasby & Read, 1997) can be considered a form of basic research within life history analysis.

Finally, useful distinctions can be drawn among life histories, personal life stories, and collective life stories of a person. As indicated earlier, a life history of a person is rendered by means of an objectivity-aspiring combination of historical and psychological research. Personal life stories constitute the representations of the same life by that person (McAdams, 1996), which have been reviewed in the earlier discussion of the method analyzing interpretive and imaginative expressions. Collective life sto-

ries are found in the social representations of the same life (Craik, 1996), which can readily be seen to form a component of the content claims within a person's reputational network, and thus a topic for the method of reputational analysis.

Integrative Methodological Pluralism

When the field of personality psychology first emerged, a full range of methods was represented, tapping each of our seven sources of information for knowing a person. By the mid-1980s, a promise of return to full coverage once again seemed possible, even though two method categories had shown interrupted development, namely, field studies of everyday conduct and life history analysis. This period of relative neglect occurred during the post–World War II era, when personality inventories and projective techniques were dominant. One method—reputational analysis—had suffered arrested development, despite some hints at attention in the 1930s.

Since the 1980s, the promising trends toward a comprehensive array of methods have continued. Field studies of one kind or another are now fairly routine (e.g., Moskowitz & Cote, 1995). Life history analysis has matured since the 1980s; a handbook has been published (Schultz, 2005), and relevant journals emerged between 1978 and 1991. And since the 1980s, with regard to the severely neglected method of reputational analysis, valuable overviews have appeared from Bromley (1993) and Emler (1990), as well as from researchers in organizational behavior (Rein, Kotler, & Stoller, 1997).

Thus, from its outset as a distinct field of inquiry until the present time, personality psychology has recognized that persons are complex, multifaceted entities whose understanding will require a wide array of methods of study. One challenge facing personality psychologists is to advance our grasp of the mutual relevance of our diverse methods and sources of knowledge about persons.

Method Guilds

A continuing barrier to more integrative use of these methods of study is the influence of method guilds (Craik, 1986). The development of particular methods and associated specific instruments, procedures, and analytic techniques has often been accompanied by special workshops, regularly scheduled conferences, societies, and journals.

Method guilds serve constructive scientific functions in fostering sophisticated technical aspects of specific methods. A certain degree of method specialization follows readily from this process. An expert in multivariate scale construction (Angleitner & Wiggins, 1986) is not necessarily savvy in disentangling the alternative meanings of a life history incident, such as van Gogh's cutting off his ear (Runyan, 1981).

At least two downside effects can be discerned regarding method guilds. The first is that the social institutional apparatus and its inertia result in some methods or specific procedures persisting in use well beyond any adequate claims to validity. This possibility has been raised, for example, concerning the Rorschach technique (Meyer, 2000; Wood, Nezworski, Stejskal, & Garven, 2001).

More central to our concern here is the inadvertent effect of method guilds in promoting isolated use of methods in research programs on substantive topics. To address this danger, countervailing forces toward integrated methodological pluralism must be generated in research projects and in research training programs.

The Challenge

A general impression to be gained from the current journals and research literature is at least a small trend toward the use of multiple methods. Overwhelmingly, the goal of multiple-method usage is a generic form of comprehensive coverage of variables relevant to the particular project at hand. Less frequently, the explicit aim is to examine the prospects and nature of integrative understandings yielded by the conjoint use of different methods and forms of knowledge about persons. Yet such cumulative understandings derived from integrative methodological pluralism are essential for progress in personality psychology.

Case Studies in Integrative Methodological Pluralism

This endeavor poses both a conceptual challenge that must be addressed by personality theorists and a methodological challenge to personality assessors, to gather, organize, and examine the interrelationships among the varied forms of information about persons. A brief review of the following three studies will serve to illustrate the kinds of conceptual and methodological issues that are encountered in efforts toward integrative methodological pluralism in personality research.

Traits and Personal Life Stories: Personality Scales, Imaginative Productions, and Life History Analysis

In 1997 an entire special issue of the *Journal of Personality* was devoted to a multimethod case study of an exemplary sailor, Dodge Morgan (Craik, 1997; Nasby & Read, 1997; Wiggins, 1997). In 1985–86, Morgan had completed a solo circumnavigation in what was then a record-setting 150 days. Morgan had also been the strong self-financed leader-client of the team that designed and built his ship and plotted the strategy for the successful and challenging voyage.

With Morgan's participation, Nasby and Read mobilized an impressive array of research methods covering at least four of our ways of knowing a person. For field study methods, Morgan completed reports of affect and motive in a pre-arranged schedule throughout his voyage. For imaginative and interpretive methods, Nasby and Read (1997) gathered life story reports and Thematic Apperception Test (TAT) protocols. For self-report methods, they administered the Personality Research Form (PRF; Jackson, 1984) before and after the voyage. And for life history analysis, they gathered early memories and an array of biographical materials.

As one component of this ambitious project, Nasby and Read (1997) deployed this exercise in methodological pluralism to examine conceptual implications of particular methods of personality study. Specifically, they arranged a conceptual encounter between the five-factor model of personality dispositions (John & Srivastava, 1999) and the personal life story approach (McAdams, 1996).

The dispositional portrait of Morgan and the thematic thrust of his life story appeared to cohere. His central traits included autonomy, exhibition, achievement, and endurance and dominance, and his thematic life story mode emerged as a set of tales of heroic adventure.

Nevertheless, the psychological issue is the potential relations between various formulations of disposition (Craik, 1997), on one hand, and the specific purposive-cognitive model entailed in the personal life story approach (McAdams, 1996). Do dispositional constructs simply offer one taxonomic system for the categorization of narrative accounts from personal life stories? Do dispositions, as strong causes, more or less directly generate the particular conduct and content of personal life stories? Or do dispositions and purposive-cognitive structures, such as identity, personal myth, and the like, serve as reciprocal causes in generating personal life stories?

Traits and Motives:
Personality Scales, Imaginative Productions,
and Life History Analysis

In their multimethod project, Winter, John, Stewart, Klohnen, and Duncan (1998) argue that self-report personality scales yield a psychologically different kind of information from that of imaginative productions. Even when the concept is the same, such as assessed motives, self-report measures of motives will intercorrelate more highly with self-report measures of traits than they will with measures of motives based on imaginative productions (such as the TAT). This cross-method barrier applies as well, of course, to the relations between self-report measures of traits (such as the CPI) and motives assessed by the TAT. These various relationships have been demonstrated empirically many times and suggest that the two methods provide distinctive kinds of information about persons.

The researchers provide an extensive analysis of the distinctive characteristics of self-report inventories and imaginative productions such as the TAT. The basic contrasts include the explicit responses to a menu of specific behaviors, interests, and attitudes in the case of the personality scales, and the implicit, tacit, and sometimes covert themes generated within the TAT stories.

In their effort to attain some kind of integration of these two seemingly isolated traditions of personality research, Winter and his colleagues drew upon data from two longitudinal studies of talented women, which both began when their participants were college age and include life history outcomes gathered during their 40s. A major personality trait, that of extraversion–introversion, was assessed by the CPI, and the two major social motives of affiliation and power were assessed by means of TAT stories.

As anticipated, the trait measure was empirically independent of the two measures of social motives. One implication might be that in forecasting life history outcomes, the trait measures and social motive measures could each account for nonoverlapping facets of the outcome criteria. Winter and colleagues (1998) go beyond that consideration of incremental validity and hypothesize an interactive model of the relationships between the two types of predictors and the outcome criteria. These moderated effects are illustrated by the result that extraverts were more engaged than introverts with multiple roles (e.g., work and family), but especially among those extraverts scoring high on the social motive of affiliation. And in a second result, relationships at work were more important for extraverts than for introverts, but especially for those extraverts scoring high on the power motive. Thus, as they conclude, "traits channel the behavioral expression of motives throughout the life course" (p. 230).

Combining Managerial
and Personality Assessment Programs

From its outset in the 1930s, personality psychology has featured multimethod personality assessment programs, in which diverse methods are employed to assess the same sample of persons. Their origins can be traced to the Harvard Psychological Clinic (1938) and the World War II assessment programs of the U.S. Office of Strategic Services (OSS, 1948) and the British War Office Selection Boards (Eysenck, 1953).

Yet even within this tradition, one explicitly and demonstratively committed to multimethod programs, distinct meta-method guilds have emerged (Craik et al., 2002; Lifton, 1983; Wiggins, 1973, 2003).

One assessment center guild has focused on comprehensive assessment of personality, often for basic research purposes (MacKinnon, 1962, 1975). This type of assessment program combines personality staff descriptions of participants, based on observation of varied situations, procedures, and informal social contexts, with results from other methods, such as personality inventories.

A second assessment center guild has focused on the assessment and selection of managers within business and industry (Hough & Oswald, 2000; Thornton, 1992). This type of assessment program involves the use of specific situational exercises analyzed as simulated work conditions, and behavior-anchored observations made by assessment staff are categorized within an array of managerial performance dimensions, rather than traditional trait categories (Lifton, 1983; Sackett, 1987).

To heed the call for systematic research examining the relations between the managerial and personality approaches (Bray, & Howard, 1983), a combined assessment program was devised to study MBA students (Craik et al., 2002).

The 3-day program entailed two independently operating assessment teams. The managerial assessment team conducted such procedures as the In-Basket Exercise, the LGD, work and professional field interviews, and an integrative staff council meeting for each participant. The managerial assessors completed ratings on 14 managerial performance dimensions, which subsequent analyses showed reflected two underlying managerial styles: the Strategic Managerial Style (e.g., decision making, fact finding, and delegation) and the Interpersonal Managerial Style (e.g., oral communication, initiative, and leadership).

The personality assessment team hosted the participants at breakfast, lunch, and social hours (all informal contexts for interaction and observation) and conducted sessions entailing role improvisations, team charades, life history interviews, and administration of standard personality inventories and questionnaires. The personality assessors also observed the LGD. The managerial staff were kept isolated from any interaction with participants beyond the standard managerial assessment procedures. Following the program, the personality assessors recorded their personality descriptions of each participant in several ways, including use of the 300-item Adjective Check List (ACL; e.g., *alert*, *zany*) (Gough & Heilbrun, 1983).

The two managerial performance styles and an overall managerial potential measure rendered by the managerial staff were related to the personality staff descriptions recorded on the ACL. This analysis, joining the findings of both managerial and personality assessment programs, revealed that the Strategic Managerial Style was significantly related to adjectival trait descriptions drawn from five-factor model (FFM) (John & Srivastava, 1999) categories for Conscientiousness (e.g., clear-thinking) and Openness (e.g., insightful). The Interpersonal Managerial Style, in addition to those two themes, showed a substantial number of significant relations to adjectival trait descriptors from the Extraversion category (e.g., outgoing) and a smaller set of negative associations for the Agreeableness category (e.g., argumentative). The overall Managerial Potential measure demonstrated the associations with trait adjectival descriptions from the Extraversion, Conscientiousness, and Openness categories, but not those from the negative Agreeableness category.

Note that in these analyses, observer-based judgments in the construct language of managerial performance by one assessment staff were meaningfully associated with observer-based judgments in the construct language of personality traits made by an independent assessment staff.

Further research is required to advance our understanding of how elements of observed conduct are categorized by assessors within the categories of managerial dimensions, on one hand, and according to personality trait constructs, on the other. Are the same facets of conduct attended to but simply assigned within differing category systems, or do the two domains of managerial and personality constructs cognitively prime observers to attend to or interpret differing elements of conduct? In short, how do we come to know these associated individual differences between persons via managerial assessments and through personality assessments?

Conclusions

This review of methods available for the study of personality has been organized around an epistemological theme—the kinds of information available to us for knowing a person. We have seen that, historically, the various method categories have shown differing patterns of development. Although at least hints of each were evident at the outset of personality psychology, only some have displayed continued development while others experienced interrupted or arrested development. In the past few decades, the full pattern has become available once again.

In an analysis relevant to our epistemological theme, McAdams (1995) posed the question: What do we know when we know a person? His taxonomy identified three conceptual levels, comprising dispositional traits, personal concerns, and identity narratives. His purpose did not directly concern a taxonomy of methods of study but rather a set of construct criteria for achieving an adequate description of a person. The associated methods of study for his construct sets fall across different method categories. Trait assessment relates to several methods, whereas personal concern assessment and analysis of personal life stories are more method focused. Nevertheless, the aggregate of available specific tools within and across our proposed set of seven method categories does suggest a richer and more diverse array of opportunities and media for knowing a person.

With regard to our historical perspective on personality methods, attention must be drawn to Wiggins's (2003) contribution of a comprehensive and authoritative historical chart dealing with personality research. Its basic taxonomic elements include five research traditions (i.e., the psychodynamic, interpersonal, personological, multivariate, and empirical), organized by eight periods from the pre-1930s through the 1990s and illustrated by distinctive theoretical concepts, empirical research reports, or new research instruments.

In contrast, the present taxonomy derives from an earlier exercise in historical perspective taking that focused solely on research methods (Craik, 1986, 2000b) and has now evolved to deal with the broader categories of information about persons distinctively generated by particular kinds of methods for the study of personality.

Recommended Readings

Barenbaum, N. B., & Winter, D. G. (2003). Personality. In D. K. Freedheim (Ed.), *Handbook of psychology: Vol. 1. History of psychology* (pp. 177–204). New York: Wiley.

Craik, K. H. (1986). Personality research methods: An historical perspective. *Journal of Personality, 54,* 18–51.

Craik, K. H., Hogan, R., & Wolfe, R. W. (Eds.). (1993). *Fifty years of personality psychology.* New York: Plenum Press.

McAdams, D. P. (1995). What do we know when we know a person? *Journal of Personality, 64,* 365–396.

Wiggins, J. S. (2003). *Paradigms of personality assessment.* New York: Guilford Press.

References

Alexander, I. E. (1990). *Personology: Method and content in personality assessment and psychobiography.* Durham, NC: Duke University Press.

Allport, G. W. (1937). *Personality: A psychological interpretation.* New York: Holt.

Allport, G. W. (1942). *The use of personal documents in psychological science.* New York: Social Science Research Council.

Allport, G. W., & Odbert, H. S. (1936). Trait-names: A psycho-lexical study. *Psychological Monographs, 47,* 1–171.

Angleitner, A., & Wiggins, J. S. (Eds.). (1986). *Personality assessment via questionnaires: Current issues in theory and measurement.* New York: Springer-Verlag.

Asch, S. E. (1952). *Social psychology.* New York: Prentice-Hall.

Barenbaum, N. B., & Winter, D. G. (2003). Personality. In D. K. Freedheim (Ed.), *Handbook of psychology: Vol. 1. History of psychology* (pp. 177–204). New York: Wiley.

Barker, R. G., & Wright, H. F. (1951). *One boy's day: A specimen record of behavior.* New York: Harper & Row.

Bass, B. M. (1954). The leaderless group discussion. *Psychological Bulletin, 51,* 465–492.

Bem, D. J., & Funder, D. G. (1978). Predicting more of the people more of the time: Assessing the personality of situations. *Psychological Review, 85,* 485–501.

Block, J. (1977). Advancing the psychology of personality: Paradigmatic shift or improving the quality of research? In D. Magnusson & N. S. Endler (Eds.), *Personality at the crossroads: Current issues in interactional psychology* (pp. 37–63) . Hillsdale, NJ: Erlbaum.

Block, J. (1978). *The Q-sort method in personality assessment and psychiatric research.* Palo Alto, CA: Consulting Psychologists Press.

Bray, D. W., & Howard, A. (1983). Personality and the assessment center method. In C. D. Spielberger & J. N. Butcher (Eds.), *Advances in personality assessment* (pp. 1–34). Hillsdale, NJ: Erlbaum.

Bromley, D. B. (1977). *Personality description in ordinary language.* London: Wiley.

Bromley, D. B. (1986). *The case study method in psychology and related disciplines.* Chichester, UK: Wiley.

Bromley, D. P. (1993). *Reputation, image and impression management.* New York: Wiley.

Buss, D. M., & Craik, K. H. (1983). The act frequency approach to personality. *Psychological Review, 90,* 105–126.

Caspi, A., & Moffett, T. E. (1993). When do individual differences matter? A paradoxical theory of personality coherence. *Psychological Inquiry, 4,* 247–271.

Costa, P. T., & McCrae, R. R. (1992). *The NEO PI-R professional manual*. Odessa, FL: Psychological Assessment Resources.

Craik, K. H. (1986). Personality research methods: An historical perspective. *Journal of Personality, 54,* 18–51.

Craik, K. H. (1993). Accentuated, revealed and quotidian personalities. *Psychological Inquiry, 4,* 278–280.

Craik, K. H. (1994). Manifestations of individual differences in personality within everyday environments. In D. Bartussek & M. Amelang (Eds.), *Fortschritte der Differentiellen Psychologie und Psychologischen Diagnostik: Festschrift zum 60. Geburtstag von Kurt Pawlik* (pp. 19–25). Gottingen, Germany: Hogrefe.

Craik, K. H. (1996). The objectivity of persons and their lives: A noble dream for personality psychology? *Psychological Inquiry, 7,* 326–330.

Craik, K. H. (1997). Circumnavigating the personality as a whole: The challenge of integrative methodological pluralism. *Journal of Personality, 65,* 1087–1111.

Craik, K. H. (2000a). The lived day of an individual: A person–environment perspective. In W. B. Walsh, K. H. Craik, & R. H. Price (Eds.), *Person–environment psychology: New directions and perspectives* (pp. 233–266). Mahwah, NJ: Erlbaum.

Craik, K. H. (2000b). Personality psychology: Methods of study. *Encyclopedia of psychology* (Vol. 6, pp. 133–140). New York: American Psychological Association and Oxford University Press.

Craik, K. H. (2006). *Reputational networks*. Berkeley: Institute of Personality and Social Research, University of California.

Craik, K. H., Hogan, R., & Wolfe, R. N. (1993). *Fifty years of personality psychology: Celebrating the Allport and Stagner textbooks*. New York: Plenum Press.

Craik, K. H., Ware, A. P., Kamp, J., O'Reilly, C., III, Staw, B., & Zedeck, S. (2002). Explorations of construct validity in a combined managerial and personality assessment programme. *Journal of Occupational and Organizational Psychology, 75,* 171–193.

Crutchfield, R. S. (1956). Conformity and character. *American Psychologist, 10,* 191–198.

Dollard, J. (1935). *Criteria for the life history*. New Haven, CT: Yale University Press.

Ekman, P., & Friesen, W. V. (1978). Measuring facial movements. *Environmental Psychology and Nonverbal Behavior, 1,* 56–75.

Elms, A. C. (1994). *Discovering lives: The uneasy alliance of biography and psychology*. New York: Oxford University Press.

Emler, N. (1990). The social psychology of reputation. *European Review of Social Psychology, 1,* 171–193.

Epstein, S. (1983). Aggregation and beyond: Some basic issues on the prediction of behavior. *Journal of Personality, 51,* 360–392.

Erikson, E. H. (1958). *Young Martin Luther*. New York: Norton.

Erikson, E. H. (1963). *Childhood and society*. New York: Norton. (Original work published 1950)

Eysenck, H. J. (1953). Assessment of men. In H. J. Eysenck, *The uses and abuses of psychology* (pp. 138–159). Harmomdsworth, UK: Penguin Books.

Frank, L. K. (1939). Projective methods for the study of personality. *Journal of Psychology, 8,* 389–413.

Funder, D. C. (1999). *Personality judgment: A realistic approach to person perception*. New York: Academic Press.

George, A. L., & George, J. L. (1981–82). Woodrow Wilson and Colonel House: A reply to Weinstein, Anderson, and Link. *Political Science Quarterly, 96,* 641–655.

Goldberg, L. R. (1971). A historical survey of personality scales and inventories. In P. McReynolds (Ed.), *Advances in psychological assessment* (Vol. 2, pp. 293–336). Palo Alto, CA: Science and Behavior Books.

Goldberg, L. R. (1992). The development of markers for the Big Five factor structure. *Psychological Assessment, 4,* 26–42.

Gosling, S. D., Ko, S. J., Mannarelli, T., & Morris, M. E. (2002). A room with a cue: Judgments of personality based on offices and bedrooms. *Journal of Personality and Social Psychology, 82,* 379–398.

Gough, H. G. (1957). *Manual for the California Psychological Inventory*. Palo Alto, CA: Consulting Psychologists Press.

Gough, H. G. (2002). *Comprehensive bibliography of the CPI assessment, 1948–2002*. Mountain View, CA: Consulting Psychologists Press.

Gough, H. G., & Bradley, P. (2002). *California Psychological Inventory manual* (3rd ed.). Mountain View, CA: Consulting Psychologists Press.

Gough, H. G., & Heilbrun, A. B., Jr. (1983). *The Adjective Check List manual* (2nd ed.). Palo Alto, CA: Consulting Psychologists Press.

Hartshorne, H., & May, M. A. (1928). *Studies in the nature of character: Vol. 1. Studies in deceit*. New York: Macmillan.

Hartshorne, H., & May, M. A. (1929). *Studies in the nature of character: Vol. 2. Studies in service and self-control*. New York: Macmillan.

Hartshorne, H., May, M. A., & Shuttleworth, F. K. (1930). *Studies in the nature of character: Vol. 3. Studies in the organization of character*. New York: Macmillan.

Hofstee, W. K. B. (1994). Who should own the definition of personality? *European Journal of Personality, 48,* 149–162.

Hogan, R. (1996). A socioanalytic perspective on the Five-Factor Model. In J. S. Wiggins (Ed.), *The five-factor-model of personality* (pp. 163–179). New York: Guilford Press.

Hollingworth, H. L. (1922). *Judging human character*. New York: Appleton-Century.

Hormuth, S. E. (1986). The sampling of experience in situ. *Journal of Personality, 54,* 282–294.

Hough, L. B., & Oswald, F. L. (2000). Personnel selection: Looking toward the future—remembering the past. *Annual Review of Psychology, 51,* 631–664.

Jackson, D. N. (1984). *Personality Research Form manual.* Port Huron, MI: Research Psychologists Press.

John, O. P., & Robins, R. W. (1993a). Determinants of interjudge agreement on personality traits: The Big Five domains, observability, evaluativeness, and the unique perspective of the self. *Journal of Personality, 61,* 521–551.

John, O. P., & Robins, R. W. (1993b). Gordon Allport: Father and critic of the five factor model. In K. H. Craik, R. Hogan, & R. W. Wolfe (Eds.), *Fifty years of personality psychology* (pp. 215–236). New York: Plenum Press.

John, O. P., & Robins, R. W. (1994). Accuracy and bias in self-perception: Individual differences in self-enhancement and the role of narcissism. *Journal of Personality and Social Psychology, 66,* 206–219).

John, O. P., & Srivastava, S. (1999). The Big Five trait taxonomy: History, measurement and theoretical perspectives. In L. A. Pervin & O. P. John (Eds.), *Handbook of personality theory and research* (pp. 102–138). New York: Guilford Press.

Jung, C. G. (1910). The association method. *American Journal of Psychology, 21,* 219–269.

Jung, C. G. (1923). *Psychological types, or the psychology of individuation.* London: Routledge & Kegan Paul.

Kelly, G. A. (1955). *The psychology of personal constructs* (Vols. 1 & 2). New York: Norton.

Kenny, D. A. (1994). *Interpersonal perception: A social relations analysis.* New York: Guilford Press.

Lazarus, R. S. (1986). *Psychological stress and the coping process.* New York: McGraw-Hill.

Levenson, R. W. (2000). Expressive, physiological and subjective changes in emotion across adulthood. In S. H. Qualls & N. Abeles (Eds.), *Psychology and the aging revolution* (pp. 123–140). Washington, DC: American Psychological Association.

Lewin, K. (1935). *A dynamic theory of personality.* New York: McGraw-Hill.

Lifton, P. D. (1983). Assessment centers: The AT&T and IPAR methods. *Journal of Personality Assessment, 47,* 442–445.

Loevinger, J. (1979). Construct validity of the sentence completion test of ego development. *Applied Psychological Measurement, 3,* 281–311.

Lowenthal, D. (1996). *Possessed by the past: The heritage debate and the spoils of history.* New York: Free Press.

MacKinnon, D. W. (1962). The nature and nurture of creative talent. *American Psychologist, 17,* 484–496.

MacKinnon, D. W. (1975). IPAR's contribution to the conceptualization and study of creativity. In I. A. Taylor & J. W. Getzels (Eds.), *Perspectives in creativity* (pp. 60–89). Chicago: Aldine.

May, M. A. (1932). The foundations of personality. In P. S. Achilles (Ed.), *Psychology at work* (pp. 81–101). New York: McGraw-Hill.

McAdams, D. P. (1995). What do we know when we know a person? *Journal of Personality, 64,* 365–396.

McAdams, D. P. (1996). Personality, modernity, and the storied self: A contemporary framework for studying persons. *Psychological Inquiry, 7,* 295–321.

Mehl, M. R., Gosling, S. D., & Pennebaker, J. W. (2006). Personality in its natural habitat: Manifestations and implicit folk theories of personality in daily life. *Journal of Personality and Social Psychology, 90,* 862–877.

Meyer, G. J. (2000). The science of Rorschach research. *Journal of Personality Assessment, 75,* 46–81.

Mischel, W. (1966). Theory and research on the antecedents of self-imposed delay of reward. In B. A. Maher (Ed.), *Progress in experimental personality research* (Vol. 3, pp. 85–132). New York: McGraw-Hill.

Morgan, C. D., & Murray, H. A. (1935). A method for investigating fantasies. *Archives of Neurology and Psychiatry, 32,* 29–39.

Moskowitz, D. S., & Cote, S. (1995). Do interpersonal traits predict affect? A comparison of three models. *Journal of Personality and Social Psychology, 69,* 915–924.

Murray, H. A. (1938). *Explorations in personality.* New York: Oxford University Press.

Myers, I. B., & McCaulley, M. H. (1985). *Manual: A guide to the development and use of the Myers-Briggs Type Indicator.* Palo Alto, CA: Consulting Psychologists Press.

Nasby, W., & Read, N. W. (1997). The life voyage of a solo circumnavigator: Integrating theoretical and methodological perspectives. *Journal of Personality, 65,* 785–1068.

Newcomb, T. M. (1929). *Consistency of certain extravert–introvert behavior patterns in 51 problem boys.* New York: Columbia University Teachers College.

Nicholson, I. A. M. (2003). *Inventing personality: Gordon Allport and the science of selfhood.* Washington, DC: American Psychological Association.

Novick, P. (1988). *That noble dream: The "objectivity question" and the American historical profession.* Cambridge, UK: Cambridge University Press.

Office of Strategic Services Assessment Staff. (1948). *Assessment of men.* New York: Rinehart.

Ozer, D. J. (1989). Construct validity in personality assessment. In D. M. Buss & N. Cantor (Eds.), *Personality psychology: Recent trends and emerging directions* (pp. 224–236). New York: Springer-Verlag.

Pompa, L. (1990). Historical consciousness and historical knowledge. In L. Pompa (Ed.), *Human nature and historical knowledge: Hume, Hegel, and Vico* (pp. 192–225). Cambridge, UK: Cambridge University Press.

Pool, I. de Sola, & Kochen, M. (1978). Contacts and influence. *Social Networks, 1,* 1–51.

Rein, I., Kotler, P., & Stoller, M. (1997). *High visibility: The making and marketing of professionals into celebrities.* Chicago: NTC Business Books.

Roback, A. A. (1927). *A bibliography of character and personality*. Cambridge, MA: Sci-Art.

Rorschach, H. (1922). *Psychodiagnostics: A diagnostic test based on perception*. New York: Grune & Stratton.

Runyan, W. M. (1981). Why did Van Gogh cut off his ear?: The problem of alternative explanations in psychobiography. *Journal of Personality and Social Psychology, 40*, 1070–1077.

Runyan, W. M. (1982). *Life histories and psychobiography*. New York: Oxford University Press.

Runyan, W. M. (2005). Evolving conceptions of psychobiography and the study of life histories: Encounters with psychoanalysis, personality psychology, and historical science. In W. T. Schultz (Ed.), *Handbook of psychobiography* (pp. 19–41). New York: Oxford University Press.

Sackett, P. R. (1987). Assessment centers and content validity: Some neglected issues. *Personnel Psychology, 40*, 13–25.

Schultz, W. T. (Ed.). (2005). *Handbook of psychobiography*. New York: Oxford University Press.

Shoda, Y., Mischel, W., & Peake, P. K. (1990). Predicting adolescent cognitive and self-regulatory competencies from preschool delay of gratification: Identifying diagnostic conditions. *Developmental Psychology, 26*, 978–986.

Thornton, G. C. (1992). *Assessment centers in human resource management*. Reading, MA: Addison-Wesley.

Vazire, S. (2006). Informant reports: A cheap, fast, and easy method for personality assessment. *Journal of Research in Personality, 40*, 472–481.

Watts, D. J. (2003). *Six degrees: The science of a connected age*. New York: W. W. Norton.

Weinstein, E. A., Anderson, J. W., & Link, A. S. (1978–79). Woodrow Wilson's political personality: A reappraisal. *Political Science Quarterly, 93*, 586–594.

Wiggins, J. S. (1973). *Personality and prediction: Principles of personality assessment*. Reading, MA: Addison-Wesley.

Wiggins, J. S. (1997). Circumnavigating Dodge Morgan's interpersonal style. *Journal of Personality, 65*, 1069–1086.

Wiggins, J. S. (2003). *Paradigms of personality assessment*. New York: Guilford Press.

Winter, D. G. (1991). Measuring personality at a distance: Development of an integrated system for scoring motives in running texts. In A. J. Stewart, J. M. Healy, & D. Ozer (Eds.), *Perspectives in personality: Approaches to understanding lives* (pp. 59–89). London: Jessica Kingsley.

Winter, D. G., John, O. P., Stewart, A. J., Klohnen, E. C., & Duncan, L. E. (1998). Traits and motives: Towards an integration of two traditions in personality research. *Psychological Review, 105*, 230–250.

Wood, J. M., Nezworski, M. T., Lilienfeld, S. O., & Garb, H. N. (2003). *What's wrong with the Rorschach? Science confronts the controversial inkblot test*. San Francisco: Jossey-Bass.

Wood, J. M., Nezworski, M. T., Stejskal, W. J., & Garven, S. (2001). Advancing scientific discussion of the controversy surrounding the Comprehensive System for the Rorschach: A reply to Meyer (2000). *Journal of Personality Assessment, 76*, 369–378.

## CHAPTER 13

The Self-Report Method

Delroy L. Paulhus
Simine Vazire

If you want to know what Waldo is like, why not just ask him? Such is the commonsense logic behind the self-report method of personality assessment. It remains the field's most commonly used mode of assessment—by far (see Robins, Tracy, & Sherman, Chapter 37, this volume). Despite its popularity and demonstrated utility, the self-report method has been a frequent target of criticism from the early days of psychological assessment (Allport, 1927) right up to the present (Dunning, Heath, & Suls, 2005).

The psychological processes underlying an act of self-reporting are now understood to be exceedingly complex (e.g., Hogan & Nicholson, 1988; Johnson, 2004; Schwarz, 1999; Tourangeau, Rips, & Rasinksi, 2001). Examination of these processes requires burrowing deep into the affective and cognitive substrates of personality. Among the challenging issues are the role of motives in self-perception (Robins & John, 1997), the applicability of performative models (Johnson,

2004), the effectiveness of introspection (Wilson, 2002), the degree of automaticity (Mills & Hogan, 1978; Paulhus & Levitt, 1986), and the meaning of nonresponding (Tourangeau, 2004).

The goal of this chapter is more limited: to provide a brief guide to nonexpert researchers interested in using the self-report method to assess personality. We begin by delineating three categories of self-reports. We then review the advantages and the disadvantages of the self-report method. Next, we examine the convergence of self-reports with other methods of assessing personality. Finally, we provide a practical guide to choosing a self-report instrument.

Types of Self-Reports

Variants of the self-report method are numerous and could be organized in a number of ways. We restrict ourselves to cases in which respondents are aware that they are reporting on their personalities. Thereby ruled out are such methods as projective tests, handwriting analysis, conditional reasoning, and nonverbal coding techniques. As a result, we are left with three broad categories.

Direct Self-Ratings

In the simplest form of the self-report method, people are asked to report directly on their own personalities. In the case of a *global self-rating*, the respondent is furnished with a face-valid label of the construct and asked to give a summary self-appraisal. For some constructs, a single global rating can be surprisingly valid (Burisch, 1983). A recent example is the Single-Item Self-Esteem Scale (Robins, Hendin, & Trzeszniewski, 2001). Other successful examples are the Five-Item Personality Inventory (FIPI) (Gosling, Rentfrow, & Swann, 2003) and the Single-Item Measures of Personality (SIMP)(Woods & Hampson, 2005), which capture each of the Big Five factors with a single item.

The authors of these single-item measures took pains to ensure that the item supplied a clear description of the attribute being assessed. In short, they sought high *face validity*. Of course, the validity of a clear item depends on the respondent's willingness and ability to provide that information (see below). The point here is that earnest attempts to disclose one's personality are facilitated by a clear question.

As a general rule, however, single-item assessment is not recommended because its reliability is usually lower than that of multi-item composites.[1] The availability of multiple items also makes it easier to control for certain response styles such as acquiescence and extremity (see below). Because a variety of items are administered to assess each construct, it may be less obvious what the test is designed to assess. Nonetheless, respondents usually try to make sense of the test and their interpretation gets more confident as more items are presented (Knowles & Condon, 1999). To help clarify the construct to the respondent, items can be grouped and labeled (Goldberg, 1992).

Some constructs (e.g., openness to experience, ego-resiliency) are too complex to be directly rated and, even with multiple items, may never crystallize in the mind of the respondent. Nonetheless, the aggregation of items may yield a scientifically meaningful score.

To summarize, the key features in the direct-rating approach—especially the global self-rating—are clarity and simplicity. In many cases, a direct request for personality information will yield the most valid assessment.

Indirect Self-Reports

Like direct self-ratings, *indirect self-reports* pose questions about the respondent's personality. The primary difference is that indirect self-reports usually obscure the construct being measured: Respondents may even be intentionally misled about the purpose of the test.[2] For example, the Narcissistic Personality Inventory (NPI; Raskin & Hall, 1981) asks respondents about their competence, their leadership ability, their storytelling ability, and their physical attractiveness. In truth, the NPI is not actually targeting any of those traits. Instead, a respondent accumulates a high narcissism score by repeatedly choosing the grandiose option across that whole range of superlative qualities.

Note that a corresponding self-rating measure of narcissism would simply ask for degree of agreement with the item "I am narcissistic." Because narcissists are defensive and deluded, however, a direct measure would be pointless. Thus, the choice of the indirect approach was theoretically driven.

A similar logic applies to several measures of socially desirable responding (e.g., the Marlowe-Crowne scale or the Balanced Inventory of Desirable Responding). For example, one item on the latter instrument reads "My first impressions about people are always right" (Paulhus, 1991). Yet the test aims to measure not interpersonal perspicuity, but the tendency to ascribe desirable (yet highly unlikely) qualities to oneself. Rather than the specific content, a respondent's score is based on the total number of desirable but unlikely qualities claimed. Indirect approaches have also been tried in the measurement of defense mechanisms via self-report (but see Davidson & MacGregor, 1998).

Another type of indirect test involves the use of *subtle items*. Here, the purpose of the item is obscure. The 49-item version of the MMPI Alcoholism Scale, for example, is composed entirely of subtle items (e.g., "I have had periods when I carried out activities without knowing later what I had been doing" and "My hardest battles are with myself"). They do not directly mention, but are predictive of an alcoholic predisposition. The subtle approach has been subjected to substantial research, most of it indicating that subtle items are actually less valid than more obvious items (e.g., Holden, Fekken, & Jackson, 1985; Osberg, 1999).

In sum, indirect tests are designed to minimize face validity: The assessment of personality is based on the researcher's interpretation of the answers, not on the content of the respondent's intended message. The major advantage claimed for such measures is resistance to faking: If the respondent has no idea what the administrator is assessing, then faking is precluded.

Nonetheless, respondents do make inferences about what is being assessed. With an indirect test, however, the respondent's interpretation is likely to differ from the researcher's. Moreover, different respondents tend to make different inferences. For example, high scorers on anxiety scales assume that the test measures emotional honesty, whereas low scorers assume that it measures mental illness. High scorers on integrity tests assume that the assessor will hire people who admit no past misbehavior; low scorers take a more cynical stance in assuming that the assessor will take admissions of misbehavior as an indicator of honesty (Cunningham, Wong, & Barbee, 1994). The fact that such instruments show predictive validity may result from the finding that the differential interpretation is diagnostic by itself.

Note that the distinction between direct and indirect self-reports involves a continuum, rather than a strict dichotomy. Many measures are neither completely direct nor completely indirect. On most Big Five inventories, for example, the items are mixed up or rotated and, accordingly, only partly transparent. With enough repetition in the items, the respondent may eventually see the pattern.

Open-Ended Self-Descriptions

In this third general category, self-reports are derived from participants' free descriptions of their own personalities. Unlike structured measures (such as those described above), this open-ended form of self-report allows respondents to use any constructs they wish in describing themselves. The researcher may request a focus on certain trait domains, or be as loose as possible with an instruction such as "Describe your personality in the space provided." For example, the Twenty Statements

Test (TST; Kuhn & McPartland, 1954) asks respondents to complete 20 sentences, each beginning with the phrase "I am."

For such self-descriptions to be quantified, they must be content coded. A systematic coding system must be developed and its meaningfulness confirmed by establishing good interrater reliabilities (see Woike, Chapter 17, this volume, for an example). Although the codings involve some degree of subjectivity, high reliabilities can often be established. For example, narcissism might be assessed by coding for (1) self-focus on positive as opposed to negative qualities and (2) implicit derogation of others. Note that the coding process is often protracted and labor-intensive, and there is no guarantee that a reliable and valid coding scheme can ever be developed.

Objective elements can also be coded from free descriptions. For example, narcissism might be measured by the sheer volume of self-description or the proportion of pronouns that are in the first person singular (*I* or *me*). Trait-relevant words can be indexed using the computer program Linguistic Inquiry and Word Count (LIWC) developed by Pennebaker, Francis, and Booth (2001). Note that some subjectivity is involved in mapping language use onto traits: The researcher must rationally designate which categories of words are indicators of which traits (see Vazire, Gosling, Dickey, & Schapiro, Chapter 11, this volume).

In sum, all three categories involve self-reports in the sense that respondents are aware that they are being asked about their personalities. Although the methods vary with respect to the assumption that respondents are capable of reporting their own personalities, and with respect to the amount of structure provided, they all share the assumption that self-reports can tell us a great deal about personality. Except where otherwise indicated, the issues discussed in the rest of this chapter apply to all three types of self-reports.

Advantages of Self-Reports

The best criterion for a target's personality is his or her self-rating. . . . Otherwise, the whole enterprise of personality assessment seriously needs to rethink itself.

—Reviewer A

Like Reviewer A, many researchers take for granted that self-reports are the ultimate measure of personality. Although alternative methods have an equally long history, self-reports remain the most popular choice. Their popularity appears to be based on a number of persuasive advantages: These include easy interpretability, richness of information, motivation to report, causal force, and sheer practicality. A substantial body of research supports all of these claims (Lucas & Baird, 2006; Swann, Chang-Schneider, & McClarty, in press).

Interpretability. Self-reports are communicated in the language common to the assessor and the respondent. Although there may be some variation within a culture, the assessor's request to a literate adult for a rating of, say, anxiety, can reasonably be assumed to be understood. This feature is one shared with informant reports. But compare that verbal equivalence to the case of behavioral measures such as galvanic skin response, heart rate, and blood pressure. Such behavioral measures are always subject to multiple interpretations (Wiggins, 1973). Life data, although often objectively scored, entail even more ambiguity. Variables such as socioeconomic status, educational level, and longevity are most certainly multiply determined and impossible to equate with a single psychological construct (Loevinger, 1957).

Information Richness

The notion that people are the best-qualified witnesses to their own personalities is supported by the indisputable fact that no one else has access to more information. First, the self has an the opportunity to observe a wide range of behaviors covering a wide swath of time. These include behaviors that are typically performed in private—for example, masturbation, academic cheating, napping, and singing in the shower. In short, people have access to a great *quantity* and *breadth* of information. Second, the self has access to intrapsychic information—thoughts, feelings, and sensations that are unavailable to others (Robins, Norem, & Cheek, 1999). In this sense, people possess a better *quality* of information about themselves. For example, an observer witnessing the theft of a candy bar has no access to the underlying motivation: The thief may have been motivated by thrill seeking, hunger, or the desire to make a political statement against corporations. In

general, the self is better able to contextualize when reporting on personality-relevant information and, therefore, better able to provide a valid report.

Even when the same information is available to self and others, people are more likely to remember information that is self-relevant (Rogers, Kuiper, & Kirker, 1977). It is not surprising, then, that people's self-schemas are especially well developed. Although not necessarily improving the accuracy of self-perceptions, a well-developed schema certainly quickens the speed of trait-relevant information retrieval (Fekken & Holden, 1992).

Motivation to Report

Another advantage of the self-report method is that no one is more fascinated by the target of assessment than is the assessor. Up to a point, then, people are usually pleased to talk about themselves. Of course, the motivation to reflect on the self varies across individuals (Trapnell & Campbell, 1999).

Self-preoccupation may also lead people to answer more diligently when completing self-reports. Whereas ratings of others may be done carelessly or superficially, people tend to put in more time and effort when reporting on their own personalities. Greater validity should ensue. This argument applies all the more when respondents are completing questionnaires in order to get private feedback on their personalities.

Causal Force

Another advantage of the self-report method is that it engages the respondent's identity (Hogan & Smither, 2001). Accurate or not, self-perceptions have a strong influence on how people interact with the world. They affect behavior (Ickes, Snyder, & Garcia, 1997), self-presentation to others (Vazire & Gosling, 2004), and expectations about how one will be seen by others.

Although not synonymous with personality, identity is unquestionably a central aspect of personality (McAdams, 2000). A person's identity reflects the phenomenological experience of his or her personality: "What it feels like to be me." If someone thinks of him- or herself as neurotic, whether or not the objective evidence supports the person's self-view, that perception constitutes one aspect of his or her personality.

Although identifying oneself as shy may not be equivalent to being genetically shy, it does influence one's behavior (Cheek & Watson, 1989). In some cases, simply being asked to characterize oneself can influence one's future behavior (Greenwald, Carnot, Beach, & Young, 1987). In sum, the causal force of self-perceptions make them important to personality assessment in a rather different fashion from other indicators—reputation, for example (Hogan & Smither, 2001).

Practicality

Finally, a singular advantage of self-reports is their extraordinary practicality. They are both efficient and inexpensive. They require only the cooperation of the target person; in contrast, the collection of informant ratings, behavior assessment, or life data all require the involvement of less available parties. Self-reports are efficient because they can be administered in mass testing sessions (as opposed to one-on-one interviews, for example). Hundreds of variables can easily be collected in one sitting.

Self-reports also tend to be the least expensive data source. Although researchers may need to provide compensation for more effortful, intensive methods (e.g., diary studies), questionnaire administrations seldom require more incentive than the opportunity to express oneself. When an incentive is needed, provision of personality feedback will often suffice; for students, extra course credit will do. Indeed, self-reporters often volunteer and will sometimes pay to be assessed. Expenses for study materials seldom go beyond those for photocopying, and even these may be eliminated if the items are administered via the Internet. Data entry costs can be minimized by collecting responses on machine-scorable sheets.

In the case of some constructs, self-report is the only appropriate method (Ozer & Reise, 1994). For example, researchers interested in self-efficacy, a construct that is by nature a self-perception, must obtain self-reports. Self-esteem researchers often argue that methods other than self-report are simply inadequate (Robins et al., 2001). Other personality-related concepts best measured via self-report include well-being (Diener, Sandvik, Pavot, & Gallagher, 1991), values (Trapnell, 2006), personal projects (Little, 1998), and life goals (Roberts, O'Donnell, & Robins, 2004).

Beyond their virtues, self-reports are often a necessity: They may be the only available method. Survey research, for example, is entirely self-reported (Tourangeau, 2004). Internet studies of personality rely on self-reports: Responses are completed anonymously and, therefore, are not easily linked to other corroborative measures such as behavior or informant reports (Gosling, Vazire, Srivastava, & John, 2004).

Disadvantages of Self-Reports

Self-reports suffer from many of the same measurement artifacts as other assessment methods. These include anchoring effects, primacy and recency effects, time pressure, and consistency motivation. Such issues are beyond the scope of this chapter; instead, we focus on several problems that are unique to the self-report method.

An overarching issue is the credibility of self-reports. Why should we trust what people say about themselves? Clearly, accuracy is not the only motive shaping self-perceptions (Sedikides & Strube, 1995). Among the other powerful motives are consistency seeking, self-enhancement, and self-presentation (Robins and John, 1997; Swann et al., in press). Even when respondents are doing their best to be forthright and insightful, their self-reports are subject to various sources of inaccuracy. Of special interest, as discussed below, are limitations such as self-deception and memory.

Self-reports in the context of face-to-face interviews raise a host of other problems such as effects of self-consciousness, rapport, transference, and modeling. Unique issues are raised by computerized testing (Butcher, 2003) and Internet surveys (Gosling et al., 2004). Such issues go beyond the scope of our review, and we restrict our discussion to self-reports in the form of pencil-and-paper questionnaires.

Classic Response Sets and Styles

Some people show a tendency to respond to questions in a manner that, although systematic, interferes with the validity of the response (for a review, see Paulhus, 1991). Well-known examples are socially desirable responding (SDR), acquiescent responding (AR), and extreme responding (ER). When specific to the situation, these tendencies are termed *response* sets; when consistent across time and assessment context, they are termed *response styles*.

Self-Presentation

We use the term *self-presentation* to subsume all self-report propensities of an evaluative nature. It includes self-aware forms—*impression management*—as well as unconscious forms—*self-deception*. Impression management includes such variants as exaggeration, faking, and lying, whereas self-deception includes variants such as self-favoring bias, self-enhancement, defensiveness, and denial. Self-presentation can be negative, as in *malingering* (Morey & Lanier, 1998), but the more common concern in personality research has been with positive biases such as SDR (Paulhus, 2002).

A temporary SDR set can be induced when a situational press compels the individual to give an overly positive self-description. For example, a job applicant may have such motivation to land a specific job that she exaggerates her credentials only on that one assessment. More or less random events (e.g., a recent job loss due to downsizing) can create a press for self-presentation that is independent of personality and ability and is, perforce, unpredictable. This response set should pervade all the variables in the specific assessment context but should not generalize to other contexts.

When stable across time and different questionnaires, this trait-like form of SDR is considered to be a response style (Edwards, 1957). Instruments are available to capture several variants of this concept (e.g., impression management, self-deceptive enhancement, self-deceptive denial, malingering) . Eight popular instruments were reviewed in detail by Paulhus (1991).

Originally, response styles were assumed to be limited to the questionnaire context. The consistency of styles across time and settings, however, implicates underlying personality traits (see below). Nonetheless, unless otherwise noted, our subsequent discussion and recommendations apply to SDR sets as well as styles.

The nature of concern about SDR differs somewhat between survey and personality researchers. Survey researchers would worry about an overall bias even if all respondents engaged in SD to the same degree. In personality research, however, the primary concern is that respondents may *differ* in their tendency to engage in SDR because it creates a confounding between SDR and personality content scales.

CONTROL OF SD EFFECTS

The litany of methods aimed at controlling SD contamination can be organized into three categories: (1) rational techniques, (2) demand reduction, and (3) covariate techniques. They correspond to methods applied during test construction, during test administration, and during data analysis, respectively.

Rational techniques prevent the respondent from answering in an unduly desirable fashion. For example, the test constructor can restrict item choice to those neutral in social desirability. Forced-choice items can be equated for social desirability. Demand reduction includes maximizing anonymity and confidentiality. If feedback is to be provided, respondents can be reminded that the feedback will be useful only if responses are honest. Of course, all such instructions must be provided *before* the test administration in order for them to reduce demand for socially desirable responses. Covariate techniques involve the administration of an SDR scale along with the content measure of interest. Scores on SDR are then partialed out of the content measure in an attempt to create a purified measure of content. We do not recommend the use of covariate techniques because they typically remove valid variance and, if anything, reduce the validity of the content measure (Ones, Viswesvaran, & Reiss, 1996). We do recommend that assessors use rational methods and demand reduction.

Note that concern over SDR may be unwarranted in many research contexts. In research on student or volunteer samples, there is little reason to be concerned about contamination from this response bias (Piedmont, McCrae, Riemannn, & Angleitner, 2000). SDR observed under such low-demand conditions is likely to reflect substantive variance, that is, traits with desirability implications.

STYLES AS TRAITS

Because consistent styles are likely to have their own cognitive or motivational roots, they can be studied as personality traits in their own right. As such, their manifestations are likely to go well beyond test-taking behaviors. The classic example is the Marlowe-Crowne scale. Originally designed to measure socially desirable responding, the scale came to be interpreted in terms of need for approval (Crowne & Marlowe, 1964).

To further complicate the issue, repeated biases can eventually become honest self-reports: With enough repetition (Paulhus, 1993) or reinforcement (Jones, Davis, & Gergen, 1961), a self-presentation can be incorporated into the respondent's true self-image (Johnson & Hogan, 1981).

Acquiescent Responding (AR)

The label *acquiescent* is used for respondents who tend to agree with statements without regard to their content. Those with the opposite tendency, indiscriminant disagreement, are called *reactant*. Such tendencies are rarely absolute: Usually everyone agrees with some statements and disagrees with others. On dichotomous response formats (e.g., Yes–No, True–False, Agree–Disagree), the phenomenon is evident if respondents show dramatically high or low proportions of "Yes" answers across a wide range of items Another way of diagnosing either extreme is to index the tendency to agree with an affirmation and its exact negation (e.g., "happy" and "not happy").

The traditional concern is that acquiescence can be viewed as an individual difference variable in its own right—a personality trait with conceptual links to conformity and impulsiveness (see, e.g., Couch & Kenniston, 1960). If so, a problem arises when a self-report instrument measures acquiescence along with (or instead of) the construct it was designed to measure. For example, on most anxiety scales, the majority of items ask respondents to indicate which anxiety-related symptoms they have experienced. The respondent who agrees with all the symptoms may indeed be a very anxious person—or merely a yea-sayer. For this reason, some researchers have worried that acquiescence might be a serious confound in self-reports (Schuman & Presser, 1981). Other researchers have concluded that acquiescence effects are insignificant (Rorer, 1965).

In one sense, acquiescence is more problematic in attitude and survey research than in personality assessment (Krosnick, 1999). In survey research, the overall percentage agreement with an item (e.g., I favor capital punishment) is more critical than in personality items (e.g., I am friendly), where individual differences are the issue. Moreover, in many personality inventories, the items are simply trait adjectives, thereby simplifying the control of acquiescence. In sharp contrast, Schuman and Presser (1981) have shown that the complex statements required in much survey research are highly susceptible to acquiescence in agree–disagree, interrogative, or true–false formats.

Instead, the major problem for personality research is that acquiescence exaggerates the correlations among same-valenced items and decreases the correlations among opposite-valenced items. Moreover, acquiescence in one personality domain correlates with acquiescence in other personality domains (Knowles & Nathan, 1997). Consequently, correlations between scales with items keyed in the same direction may be inflated and, conversely, two scales may appear orthogonal because their items are scored in opposite directions (McCrae, Herbst, & Costa, 2001; Paulhus, 1984).

A recent example of the substantive import of acquiescence is the debate about the bipolarity of affect. Carroll, Yik, Russell, and Barrett (1999) argued that AR artifactually reduces the correlation between positive and negative affect. A complex structural model was required to show that, in fact, the correlation remains modest even after taking into account the effects of acquiescence and therefore positive and negative affect can be measured separately (McCrae et al., 2001; Tellegen, Watson, & Clark, 1999).

CONTROL OF AR EFFECTS

The standard control for AR bias at the test construction stage is simply to balance the scoring key. That is, half the items should be written as true-keyed (a high rating indicates possession of the trait) and half the items are false-keyed (a low rating indicates possession of the trait).

This simple precaution controls the classical form of acquiescence (agreement acquiescence) because, to get an overall high content score, the respondent must agree with some items and disagree with others. Any effects of an acquiescent tendency on the true-keyed items will be canceled out on the false-keyed items. In other words, one cannot get a high content score simply by yea-saying or nay-saying (Wiggins, 1973).

An imbalanced key can even be dealt with post hoc. If the correlations are high between true- and false-keyed subtotals and their correlations with other variables are comparable, one may safely combine the two. If not, one could differentially weight the two subtotals to simulate a balanced key.

Two unfortunate problems arise from attempts to control acquiescence by balancing the key. One is a reduction in the alpha reliability of the instrument (as compared to one with unidirectional keying). Second, factor analyses often yield two factors—one for the true-keyed items and one for the false-keyed items—even when the underlying construct is unidimensional. The reason for both problems is that items keyed in the same direction tend to have higher correlations than items keyed in opposite directions.

MEASUREMENT OF AR

Only a handful of instruments have been designed to measure individual differences in AR (e.g., Couch & Kenniston, 1960) but none is widely used. A number of the larger assessment batteries permit computation of an acquiescence index across all the items in the battery. Gough's (1983) Adjective Check List (ACL), for example, permits calculation of the "checking factor," that is, the total number of adjectives checked as true of the self. This score is often factored out of subsequent analyses (e.g., Tracey, Rounds, & Gurtman, 1996). Note that this procedure may eliminate measurement of some content variables unless one has administered the ACL in True–False format to ensure some response to each item. The most credible measure of AR bias is an overall sum of items on a large relatively balanced personality inventory such as the NEO-PI-R (McCrae et al., 2001).

Extreme Responding (ER)

ER is the tendency to use the extreme choices on a rating scale (e.g., 1's and 7's on a 7-point scale). Situational factors such as ambiguity, emotional arousal, and rapid responding induce temporary increases in extreme responding. The individual exhibiting this tendency across time and stimuli may be said to have an extreme response style. Low scorers on this variable may be said to show moderate responding, that is, the tendency to use the midpoint as often as possible.

Early reviews (e.g., Peabody, 1962) concluded that ER bias is a consistent individual difference, and more recent studies have sustained this conclusion. ER bias appears to be highly stable over time and a major source of individual differences in raters. There is little support, however, for a link between ER bias and any traditional personality dimensions (Schwartz & Sudman, 1996).

Contamination of a dataset with ER bias precludes the direct comparability of one respondent's scores to another's: One cannot ordinarily distinguish whether an extreme rating indicates a strong opinion or a tendency to use the extremities of rating scales. A second problem is that ER bias induces spurious correlations among otherwise unrelated constructs. A third source of problems is the interaction between ER bias and demographic variables such as gender, race, and education (Schuman & Presser, 1981).

CONTROL OF ER EFFECTS

ER bias cannot be corrected simply by balancing the key because extremity operates in both directions. Standardizing the within-subject variance equates subjects on extremity but subject variances are often inextricably confounded with subject means. In measuring self-esteem, for example, most responses are on the positive side of the rating scale, thus confounding high self-esteem and ER bias.

In some situations, ER bias can be controlled by rendering all items in a dichotomous format. After all, a "Yes" response is no more or no less extreme than a "No" response. The loss of reliability in moving from a multipoint to a dichotomous format can be compensated for by adding additional items.

Another approach is to require fixed distributions. For example, the respondent may be asked to give equal numbers of each response option. A more common forced distribution is a normal approximation: On a 5-point scale, for example, the required proportions of each rating would be 1(.05), 2(.10), 3(.70), 4(.10), 5(.05). Typing the item statements on small cards is often used to facilitate the adjustment of these proportions. This approach, called the *Q*-sort, capitalizes on the fact that it is much easier to judge the height of a stack of cards than it is to keep track of how many 5's one has used (Block, 1961).

MEASUREMENT OF ER BIAS

There are no standard instruments for assessing ER bias as a response style. In some applications, the variance of a subject's ratings across an inventory has been used as an index (e.g., Van der Kloot, Kroonenberg, & Bakker, 1985). Of course, this approach is inappropriate if the key for each dimension is not balanced or if the means depart substantially from the scale midpoint. Note that if only one dimension is being assessed, it is difficult to distinguish any index of ER bias from a measure of dimensional importance or salience for that topic.

Miscellaneous Response Sets

Other response biases—for example, pattern responding, random responding, and inconsistent responding—create less cause for concern. In pattern responding, participants simply mark their responses in a physical pattern (e.g., 1, 2, 3, 4, 5, 1, 2, 3, 4, 5, etc., or all 3's). This phenomenon is best recognized by human eye, although some researchers have developed computer programs to recognize the most common of these. Random responding is more difficult to detect even by eye (Baer, Kroll, Rinaldo, & Ballenger, 1999). Both of these sets can be detected instead by including a subset of rare items in the subject's inventory (e.g., "I was born in Pago-Pago"; "I recently had a liver transplant"). Although all are possible, an accumulation of "Yes" responses to such items suggests that none of the respondent's answers can be trusted. These miscellaneous response sets are reviewed in more detail by Paulhus (1991).

The MMPI includes measures of several miscellaneous response biases (e.g., F, F-K, FBS). They are less common in batteries aimed at normal-range personality. The most well-researched measures of inconsistent and infrequent responding are available in the Multivariate Personality Questionnaire (Patrick, Curtin, & Tellegen, 2002; Tellegen, in press) and Personality Assessment Index (Morey, 1991).

Other Limitations

Constraints on Self-Knowledge

It is often assumed that an honest self-disclosure is sufficient to yield an accurate self-description that can outperform informant consensus and predict future behavior. According to this view, only response biases stand in the way of accuracy. The assumption is that there is only one "truth" about an individual, a truth that is fully available to that individual.

In fact, there are good reasons to believe otherwise. For one thing, much information is unavailable to the earnest self-assessor. Dunning, Heath, and Suls (2005) distinguish between information unavailable to the self-assessor and information that tends to be ignored by the self-assessor. People do not have an infinite ability to recall all information relevant to a posed question. Conversely, they may be overwhelmed with a plethora of information, in which case the process of integration and simplification may be too challenging a task. A self-reporter may have to resort to a "press release" version of his or her personality just to get on with the task.

Of more concern than lack of access is the claim that introspection may actually diminish accuracy. Timothy Wilson has argued that any extended attempt to clarify one's self-descriptions can undermine their validity. This effect may be restricted to gross evaluations of unfamiliar targets (e.g., Wilson & LaFleur, 1995).

Further research is needed to determine the relevance of this work to personality assessment. To date, we know of no such research on the effects of introspection on the validity of self-reports of personality. We do know that, up to a point, speeding the administration of a personality test has little effect on its validity (Holden, Wood, & Tomashewski, 2001).

Cultural Limitations

Respondents from different cultures may not treat self-reports in the fashion we expect from those of European heritage (Hamamura, Heine, & Paulhus, 2006). Those with Asian heritage, for example, show more moderacy bias and ambivalence (Chen, Lee, & Stevenson, 1995). Such stylistic differences may create artifactual differences between groups. When expected cultural differences are *not* found, the failure may sometimes be traced to the *reference group effect* (Heine, Lehman, Peng, & Greenholtz, 2002): That is, respondents normally evaluate themselves relative to their own culture and not to some unspecified external group. In principle, then, mean group differences should vanish or, at least, diminish in size.

Research on cultural differences in self-report styles has just begun and will become more complex as other cultural groups are studied in detail. In the meantime, we recommend that readers treat with caution any claims for cultural differences based purely on survey data.

Convergence with Other Methods

Because there is no absolute criterion against which a personality self-report can be evaluated, evidence for its construct validity must be marshaled from a variety of sources in a cumulative process called *construct validation* (Loevinger, 1957). Necessary for this process is support for convergent and discriminant validity. Convergent validity is advanced by the confirmation of associations among available self-report measures of the construct. If our new measure of extraversion correlates highly with the Extraversion scales on Eysenck's Personality Inventory and the Big Five Inventory, then potential users of the new instrument will have more faith that it is capturing the intended construct.

An even more impressive demonstration is the convergence among different modes of measurement. To the degree that a self-report of extraversion correlates highly with informant ratings, behavioral, and life data measures, then its credibility is boosted considerably. Established measures of the Big Five personality traits, for example, have demonstrated substantial convergence (in the .40–.60 range) with aggregated ratings of knowledgeable informants (e.g., McCrae & Weiss, Chapter 15, this volume). Research on moderators of self–other agreement can also give us some insight into the conditions under which self-reports are more likely to be accurate. For example, self–other agreement is high when the respondents are self-consistent and certain about the trait, and when the trait being rated is important to the respondent, unambiguous, more observable, and evaluatively neutral (John & Robins, 1993). Self–other agreement is higher for personality traits than for affective traits (Watson, Hubbard, & Wiese, 2000). Overall, the correspondence between self-reports and informant reports is moderate in size, suggesting that the two methods provide

some overlapping and some complementary information (Vazire, 2006).

Convergence of self-reports with behavioral measures is more variable and depends on the degree of aggregation, the reliability, and the relevance of the behavioral measures. Research has found that self-behavior convergence is higher for affect-related traits (Spain, Eaton, & Funder, 2000) and for evaluatively neutral behaviors (Gosling, John, Craik, & Robins, 1998). Overall, the relation between self-reports and behavior tends to be modest (Meyer et al., 2001; Vazire, 2006). However, as Meyer and colleagues (2001) point out, those correlations are within the range of other well-established real-world effects (e.g., mammogram results predicting breast cancer).

Convergence with other modes of measurement can reduce concerns about *common method variance*. The term refers to possible contamination ensuing from the use of a single measurement method: It can exaggerate the apparent association between two constructs measured with the same method (Wiggins, 1973). These concerns are often justified because large datasets are often composed entirely of self-report measures. Response biases common to self-reports (see section above) may distort the intercorrelations. Associations among self-report measures of the Big Five, for example, may be exaggerated by the operation of self-favoring biases (McCrae & Costa, 1989) and acquiescence (McCrae et al., 2001). Spurious associations may result when self-reports are used to measure predictors such as coping, defensiveness, or self-enhancement as well as adjustment outcomes (Colvin, Block, & Funder, 1994; Cramer, 1998).

As noted earlier, in some assessment situations, the self-report mode of measurement is the most credible and is therefore used as the criterion method. The literature on so-called *zero acquaintance*, for example, examines the increases in the validity of observer ratings with increases in level of acquaintanceship. The size of the association with a corresponding self-report measure is used to index the validity of an observer judgment (Kenny, 1994).

Selecting a Self-Report Instrument

Having selected the construct to be measured and having concluded that self-report is the method of choice, the researcher still has a series of decisions to make.

Established or New Instrument?

As a general rule, the researcher should use an established instrument rather than one with less scientific credibility. An established measure is likely to have undergone an extensive program of construct validation. Normative data are also more likely to be available. A comparison of one's results with norms helps ensure that one hasn't miscored or misapplied the instrument.

If no credible instrument is available, one might have to construct a new one. This task requires a lengthy and often expensive program of construct validation (see Simms & Watson, Chapter 14, this volume). Without such validation, the use of an ad hoc measure is vulnerable to criticism. Any association (or nonassociation) found with the measure can be explained away as a faulty operationalization of the construct.

Which One?

The choice of an established instrument will require substantial homework and consultation with experts. If one seeks to cover the broad domain of personality, a number of well-researched inventories are available. Many of them have organized personality into the well-known Five-Factor Model alternatively known as the "Big Five."

Only a few instruments provide a multifaceted breakdown of the Big Five factors. One is the commercially available NEO Personality Inventory—Revised (NEO-PI-R; Costa & McCrae, 1989), the most widely used. Another is the International Personality Item Pool (IPIP) inventory, which can be freely downloaded from Lewis Goldberg's website (*www.ipip.ori.org/*; Goldberg et al., 2006). A sixth factor (Honesty-Humility) is included along with the Big Five factors in the HEXACO measure; facet scales are included for all six factors (Lee & Ashton, 2004). The Hogan Personality Inventory (HPI; Hogan & Hogan, 1992) comprises seven factors and was the first to subdivide major personality dimensions into meaningful facets. Finally, the Five Factor Inventory (Hofstee & de Raad, 2002) was developed in Dutch, but with easy translation into other languages in mind.

Several other instruments are much shorter, with the more modest goal of capturing the Big Five factors without the facets. These include John and Srivastava's (1999) Big Five Inventory (BFI), Costa and McCrae's (1989) NEO Five-Factor Inventory (NEO-FFI), and Goldberg's (1990) Trait Descriptive Adjective (TDA) markers. Saucier (1994) has developed an abbreviated set of adjective minimarkers.

Other comprehensive instruments organize the personality space using a variety of alternative schemes. These include Gough's (1957/1995) California Personality Inventory (CPI), Block's (1961) Q-Set, Cattell's (Cattell & Schuerger, 2003) 16PF, Jackson's (1984) Personality Research Form (PRF) and Tellegen's (in press) Multidimensional Personality Questionnaire (MPQ) (see Patrick, Curtin, & Tellegen, 2002).

Despite the availability of all the variables measured in those inventories, new constructs are proposed and measured on a regular basis. Instead of writing original items, researchers sometimes start with one of the comprehensive item sets cited above. These inventories contain a wide enough variety of items for use in developing new personality measures. For example, a set of experts might be asked to rate the 100 Q-Set items for prototypicality with regard to sanctimoniousness. The items with the highest mean ratings could then be assembled to form a new Sanctimone Scale. An advantage to this approach is that the new measure can be scored on archived datasets that include the full inventory (see Cramer, Chapter 7, this volume).[3]

The Eysenck Personality Questionnaire (EPQ) may well have been administered more often than any other inventory of normal personality, but only three variables can be scored (Extraversion, Neuroticism, Psychoticism). Several other broad instruments are organized in terms of temperament—for example, the Tridimensional Character Inventory (Cloninger, 1987) and the EAS (Buss & Plomin, 1984). Other narrower domain instruments include Block's (1965) ego-control and ego-resiliency scales. Several focus specifically on maladaptive personality traits: the Dark Triad (Paulhus & Williams, 2002) and the Hogan Personality Factors measure (Hogan & Hogan, 2001).

Single Variables

Although researchers are often interested in studying the role of a specific personality variable, we recommend that it be measured along with a careful selection of other variables—especially those that may provide an alternative interpretation of the findings. Inclusion of parallel measures addresses convergent validity, and competing measures can provide discriminant validity. Critics want to know the incremental validity of the focal instrument. What does it capture above and beyond well-established traits? For example, a researcher claiming to study the role of self-esteem or coping must show that self-reports of those variables cannot be fully explained by other traits (e.g., neuroticism). Common these days is the inclusion of an instrument capturing all of the Big Five factors. All of these procedures reduce the possibility of researchers "reinventing the wheel."

In short, single-variable research is not recommended in isolation. The obvious tradeoff is with the space and time it takes to administer corroborative measures. Without such corroboration, however, interpretation of results with the key variable may remain ambiguous.

There are literally hundreds of single-construct self-report personality measures. Less than 50, we estimate, have sufficiently documented construct validity to be taken seriously. Two popular collections of established personality tests are the handbook by Robinson, Shaver, and Wrightsman (1991) and the online Social-Personality Psychology Questionnaire Instrument Compendium compiled by Reifman (2006). Reviews of commercially available instruments are provided in the venerable series of *Mental Measurement Yearbooks* (Plake, Impara, & Spies, 2003).

Summary

There are several indisputable advantages to the self-report method. It opens a pipeline to prodigious amounts of unique information about the target of assessment. It directly taps his or her self-perceived personality, that is, identity. Clarity of communication and ease of administration are also clear advantages. More than other methods, self-reports allow for the collection of large numbers of personality-relevant variables in one administration.

The disadvantages of self-reports have been given much scrutiny, especially in regard to response styles such as socially desirable responding. It is only prudent to be skeptical about respondents' claims about their personality—especially on highly evaluative traits. Although self-reports of personality can be faked, it is rarely a serious problem in most research settings. In high-stakes testing such as job interviews, self-presentation remains an issue. As with the use of any method, self-reports should be corroborated with alternative assessment methods.

Nonspecialist researchers planning to use self-reports can profit from choosing a well-established instrument: The necessary but arduous accumulation of psychometric credibility has already been carried out for measures of many constructs. The use of such measures will allow researchers to build on a cumulative science.

Well-constructed self-report scales can predict a wide range of important outcomes with ease and efficiency. Although relentlessly criticized, they remain the most popular means of personality assessment. We conclude by borrowing Winston Churchill's comparison of democracy to other political systems: As a method for accurate personality assessment, self-report is dreadful—yet, overall, more effective than any alternative.

Notes

1. In fact, the alpha reliability cannot even be calculated with a single item. It must be estimated from previous research in which that item was included with similar others.
2. Funder (2004) describes this approach as collecting behavioral data via self-report data.
3. Note that inventories sold commercially usually place legal restrictions on what items can be used in new measures. Nonetheless, one learn from them what type of item taps the new construct and then devise similar but noncopyrighted items.

Recommended Readings

Dunning, D. (2005). *Self-insight: Roadblocks and detours on the path to knowing oneself.* New York: Psychology Press.

Lucas, R. E., & Baird, B. M. (2006) Global self-assessment. In M. Eid & E. Diener (Eds.), *Handbook of multimethod measurement in psychology* (pp. 29–42). Washington, DC: American Psychological Association.

Paulhus, D. L. (1991). Measurement and control of response bias. In J. P. Robinson, P. R. Shaver, & L. S. Wrightsman (Eds.), *Measures of personality and so-*

cial psychological attitudes (pp. 17–59). New York: Academic Press.

Schwarz, N., & Sudman, S. (Eds.). (1996). *Answering questions: Methodology for determining cognitive and communicative processes in survey research*. San Francisco: Jossey-Bass/Pfeiffer.

Tourangeau R., Rips, L. J., & Rasinski, K. (2001). *The psychology of survey response*. New York: Cambridge University Press.

Wilson, T. D. (2002). *Strangers to ourselves: Discovering the adaptive unconscious*. Cambridge, MA: Belknap Press/Harvard University Press.

References

Adams, D. P. (2000). *The person: An integrated introduction to personality psychology*. Fort Worth, TX: Harcourt.

Allport, F. H. (1927). Self-evaluation: a problem in personal development. *Mental Hygiene, 11*, 570–583.

Baer, R. A., Kroll, L. S., Rinaldo, J., & Ballenger, J. (1999). Detecting and discriminating between random responding and overreporting on the MMPI-A. *Journal of Personality Assessment, 72*, 308–320.

Block, J. (1961). *The Q-Sort method in personality assessment and psychiatric research*. Springfield, IL: Charles C. Thomas.

Block, J. (1965). *The challenge of response sets*. New York: Century.

Burisch, M. (1983). Approaches to personality inventory construction: A comparison of merits. *American Psychologist, 39*, 214–227.

Buss, A. H., & Plomin, R. (1984). *Temperament*. Boston: Allyn-Bacon.

Butcher, J. N. (2003). Computerized psychological assessment. In J. R. Graham & J. A. Naglieri (Eds.), *Handbook of psychology: Assessment psychology* (Vol. 10, pp. 141–163). Hoboken, NJ: Wiley.

Carroll, J. M., Yik, M. S. M., Russell, J. A., & Barrett, L. F. (1999). On the psychometric principles of affect. *Review of General Psychology, 3*, 14–22.

Cattell, H. E. P., & Schuerger, J. M. (2003). *Essentials of 16PF assessment*. New York: Wiley.

Cheek, J. M., & Watson, A. K. (1989). The definition of shyness: Psychological imperialism or construct validity? *Journal of Social Behavior and Personality, 4*, 85–95.

Chen, C., Lee, S. Y., & Stevenson, H. W. (1995). Response style and cross-cultural comparisons of rating scales among east Asian and North American students. *Psychological Science, 6*, 170–175.

Cloninger C. R. (1987). A systematic method for clinical description and classification of personality variants. *Archives of General Psychiatry, 44*, 573–580.

Colvin, C. R., Block, J., & Funder, D. C. (1995). Overly positive self-evaluations and personality: Negative implications for mental health. *Journal of Personality and Social Psychology, 68*, 1152–1162.

Costa, P. T., & McCrae, R. R. (1989). *Manual for the NEO Personality Inventory: Five Factor Inventory/NEO-FFI*. Odessa, FL: PAR.

Couch, A., & Kenniston, K. (1960). Yeasayers and naysayers: Agreeing response set as a personality variable. *Journal of Abnormal and Social Psychology, 60*, 151–174.

Cramer, P. (1998). Coping and defense mechanisms: What's the difference? *Journal of Personality, 66*, 919–931.

Crowne, D. P., & Marlowe, D. (1964). *The approval motive*. New York: Wiley.

Cunningham, M. R., Wong, D. T., & Barbee, A. P. (1994). Self-presentational dynamics on overt integrity tests: Experimental studies of the Reid Report. *Journal of Applied Psychology, 79*, 643–658.

Davidson, K., & MacGregor, M. W. (1998). A critical appraisal of self-report defense mechanism measures. *Journal of Personality, 66*, 965–992.

Diener, E., Sandvik, E., Pavot, W., & Gallagher, D. (1991). Response artifacts in the measurement of subjective well-being. *Social Indicators Research, 24*, 35–56.

Dunning, D., Heath, C., & Suls, J. M. (2005). Flawed self-assessment: Implications for education, and the workplace. *Psychological Science in the Public Interest, 5*, 69–106.

Edwards, A. L. (1957). *The social desirability variable in personality assessment and research*. New York: Dryden.

Fekken, G. C., & Holden, R. R. (1992). Response latency evidence for viewing personality traits as schema indicators. *Journal of Research in Personality, 26*, 103–120.

Funder, D. C. (2004). *The personality puzzle*. San Francisco: Norton.

Goldberg, L. R. (1990). The structure of phenotypic personality traits. *American Psychologist, 48*, 26–34.

Goldberg, L. R. (1992). The development of markers for the Big Five structure. *Psychological Assessment, 4*, 26–42.

Goldberg, L. R., Johnson, J. A., Eber, H. W., Hogan, R., Ashton, M. C., Cloninger, C. R., et al. (2006). The international personality item pool and the future of public-domain personality measures. *Journal of Research in Personality, 40*, 84–96.

Gosling, S. D., John, O. P., Craik, K. H., & Robins, R. W. (1998). Do people know how they behave? Self-reported act frequencies compared with on-line codings by observers. *Journal of Personality and Social Psychology, 74*, 1337–1349.

Gosling, S. D., Rentfrow, P. J., & Swann, W. B., Jr. (2003). A very brief measure of the Big Five personality domains. *Journal of Research in Personality, 37*, 504–528.

Gosling, S. D., Vazire, S., Srivastava, S., & John, O. P. (2004). Should we trust Web-based studies?: A comparative analysis of six preconceptions about Internet questionnaires. *American Psychologist, 59*, 93–104.

Gough, H. G. (1983). *The adjective check list*. Palo Alto, CA: Consulting Psychologists Press.

Gough, H. G. (1995). *Manual for the California Psychological Inventory* (3rd ed.). Palo Alto, CA: Consulting Psychologists Press. (Original work published 1957)

Greenwald, A. G., Carnot, C. G., Beach, R., & Young, B. (1987). Increasing voter behavior by asking people if they expect to vote. *Journal of Personality and Social Psychology, 72,* 315–318.

Hamamura, T., Heine, S. J., & Paulhus, D. L. (2006). *Cultural differences in response styles: The role of dialectical thinking.* Manuscript under review.

Heine, S. J., Lehman, D. R., Peng, K., & Greenholtz, J. (2002). What's wrong with cross-cultural comparisons of subjective Likert scales? The reference-group problem. *Journal of Personality and Social Psychology, 82,* 903–918.

Hofstee, W. K. B., & de Raad, B. (2002). The Five-Factor Personality Inventory: Assessing the Big Five by means of brief and concrete statements. In B. de Raad & M. Perugini (Eds.), *Big Five assessment* (pp. 79–100). Amsterdam: Hogrefe & Huber.

Hogan, R., & Hogan, J. (1992). *Hogan Personality Inventory manual.* Tulsa, OK: Hogan Assessment Systems.

Hogan, R., & Hogan, J. (2001). Assessing leadership: A view from the dark side. *International Journal of Selection and Assessment, 9,* 40–51.

Hogan, R., & Nicholson, R. A. (1988). The meaning of personality test scores. *American Psychologist, 43,* 621–626.

Hogan, R., & Smither, R. (2001). *Personality: Theory and applications.* Boulder, CO: Westview Press.

Holden, R. R., Fekken, G. C., & Jackson, D. N. (1985). Structured personality test item characteristics and validity. *Journal of Research in Personality, 19,* 386–394.

Holden, R. R., Wood, L. L., & Tomashewski, L. (2001). Do response time limitations counteract the effect of faking on personality inventory validity? *Journal of Personality and Social Psychology, 81,* 160–169.

Ickes, W., Snyder, M., & Garcia, S. (1997). Personality influences on the choice of situations. In R. Hogan, J. A. Johnson & S. R. Briggs (Eds.), *Handbook of personality psychology* (pp. 165–195). San Diego, CA: Academic Press.

Jackson, D. N. (1984). *Personality Research Form manual.* London, ON, Canada: Research Psychologists Press.

John, O. P., & Robins, R. W. (1993). Determinants of interjudge agreement on personality traits: The Big Five domains, observability, evaluativeness, and the unique perspective of the self. *Journal of Personality, 61,* 521–551.

John, O. P., & Srivastava, S. (1999). The Big Five trait taxonomy: History, measurement, and theoretical perspectives. In L. A. Pervin & O. P. John (Eds.), *Handbook of personality psychology* (pp. 102–139). New York: Guilford Press.

Johnson, J. A. (2004). Impact of item characteristics on item and scale validity. *Multivariate Behavioral Research, 39,* 273–302.

Johnson, J. A., & Hogan, R. (1981). Moral judgments and self-presentations. *Journal of Research in Personality, 15,* 57–63.

Jones, E. E., Davis, K. E., & Gergen, K. J. (1961). Some determinants of being approved or disapproved as a person. *Journal of Abnormal and Social Psychology, 63,* 302–310.

Kenny, D. A. (1994). *Interpersonal perception: A social relations analysis.* New York: Guilford Press.

Kolar, D. W., Funder, D. C., & Colvin, C. R. (1996). Comparing the accuracy of personality judgments by the self and knowledgeable others. *Journal of Personality, 64,* 311–337.

Knowles, E. S., & Condon, C. A. (1999). Why people say "yes": A dual process theory of acquiescence. *Journal of Personality and Social Psychology, 77,* 379–386.

Knowles, E. S., & Nathan, K. T. (1997). Acquiescent responding in self-reports: Cognitive style or social concern? *Journal of Research in Personality, 31,* 293–301.

Krosnick, J. A. (1999). Maximizing questionnaire quality. In J. P. Robinson, P. R. Shaver, & L. S. Wrightsman (Eds.), *Measures of political attitude* (pp. 37–57). San Diego, CA: Academic Press.

Kuhn, M. H., & McPartland, T. S. (1954). An empirical investigation of self-attitudes. *American Sociological Review, 19,* 68–76.

Lee, K., & Ashton, M. C. (2004). Psychometric properties of the HEXACO personality inventory. *Multivariate Behavioral Research, 39,* 329–358.

Little, B. R. (1998). Personal project pursuit: Dimensions and dynamics of personal meaning. In P. T. Wong & P. Fry (Eds.), *The human quest for meaning: A handbook of psychological research and clinical applications* (pp. 193–212). Hillsdale, NJ: Erlbaum.

Lucas, R. E., & Baird, B. M. (2006). Global self-assessment. In M. Eid & E. Diener (Eds.), *Handbook of multimethod measurement in psychology* (pp. 29–42). Washington, DC: American Psychological Association.

Loevinger, J. (1957). Objective tests as instruments of psychological theory. *Psychological Reports, 3*(Suppl. 9), 635–694.

McAdams, D. P. (2000). *The person. An integrated introduction to personality psychology.* Fort Worth, TX: Harcourt.

McCrae, R. R., & Costa, P. T. (1989). Different points of view: Self-reports and ratings in the assessment of personality. In J. P. Forgas & J. M. Innes (Eds.), *Recent advances in social psychology: An interactional perspective* (pp. 429–439). Amsterdam: Elsevier.

McCrae, R. R., Herbst, J. H., & Costa, P. T. (2001). Effects of acquiescence on personality factor structures. In R. Reimann, F. M. Spinath, & F. Ostendorf (Eds.), *Personality and temperament: Genetics, evolution, and structure* (pp. 216–231). Berlin: Pabst Science.

Meston, C. M., Heiman, J. R., Trapnell, P. D., & Paulhus, D. L. (1998). Socially desirable responding and sexuality self-reports. *Journal of Sex Research*, 35, 148–157.

Meyer, G. J., Finn, S. E., Eyde, L. D., Kay, G. G., Moreland, K. L., Dies, R. R., et al. (2001). Psychological testing and psychological assessment: A review of evidence and issues. *American Psychologist*, 56, 128–165.

Mills, C., & Hogan, R. (1978). A role theoretical interpretation of personality scale item responses. *Journal of Personality*, 46, 778–785.

Morey, L. C. (1991). *The Personality Assessment Inventory Professional manual*. Odessa, FL: Psychological Assessment Resources.

Morey, L. C., & Lanier, V. W. (1998). Operating characteristics of six response distortion indicators for the Personality Assessment Inventory. *Assessment*, 5, 203–214.

Ones, D. S., Viswesvaran, C., & Reiss, A. D. (1996). Role of social desirability in personality testing for personnel selection: The red herring. *Journal of Applied Psychology*, 81, 660–679.

Osberg, T. M. (1999). Comparative validity of the MMPI-2 Wiener–Harmon subtle–obvious scales in male prison inmates. *Journal of Personality Assessment*, 72, 36–48.

Ozer, D. J., & Reise, S. P. (1994). Personality assessment. *Annual Review of Psychology*, 45, 357–393.

Patrick, C. J., Curtin, J. J., & Tellegen, A. (2002). Development and validation of a brief form of the Multidimensional Personality Questionnaire. *Psychological Assessment*, 14, 150–163.

Paulhus, D. L. (1984). Two-component models of socially desirable responding. *Journal of Personality and Social Psychology*, 46, 598–609.

Paulhus, D. L. (1991). Measurement and control of response bias. In J. P. Robinson, P. R. Shaver, & L. S. Wrightsman (Eds.), *Measures of personality and social psychological attitudes* (pp. 17–59). New York: Academic Press.

Paulhus, D. L. (1993). Bypassing the will: The automatization of affirmations. In D. M. Wegner & J. W. Pennebaker (Eds.), *Handbook of mental control* (pp. 373–587). Englewood Cliffs, NJ: Prentice-Hall.

Paulhus, D. L. (2002). Socially desirable responding: The evolution of a construct. In H. Braun, D. N. Jackson, & D. E. Wiley (Eds.), *The role of constructs in psychological and educational measurement* (pp. 67–88). Hillsdale, NJ: Erlbaum.

Paulhus, D. L., & & Levitt, K. (1986). Desirable responding triggered by affect: Automatic egotism? *Journal of Personality and Social Psychology*, 52, 245–259.

Paulhus, D. L., & Williams, K. (2002). The dark triad of personality: Narcissism, Machiavellianism, and psychopathy. *Journal of Research in Personality*, 36, 341–350.

Peabody, D. (1962). Two components in bipolar scales: Direction and extremeness. *Psychological Review*, 69, 65–73.

Pennebaker, J. W., Francis, M. E., & Booth, R. J. (2001).

Linguistic inquiry and word count (LIWC 2001). Mahwah, NJ: Erlbaum.

Piedmont, R. L., McCrae, R. R., Riemann, R., & Angleitner, A. (2000). On the invalidity of validity scales: Evidence from self-reports and observer ratings in volunteer samples. *Journal of Personality and Social Psychology*, 78, 582–593.

Plake, B. S., Impara, M. C., & Spies, R. A. (Eds.). (2003). *The Fifteenth Mental Measurements Yearbook*. Lincoln, NE: Buros Institute of Mental Measurements.

Raskin, R. N., & Hall, C. S. (1981). The narcissistic personality inventory: Alternative form reliability and further evidence of construct validity. *Journal of Personality Assessment*, 45, 159–162.

Reifman, A. (2006). *Social-Personality Psychology Questionnaire Instrument Compendium*. El Paso: University of Texas at El Paso. Available at *www.hs.ttu.edu/research/reifman/qic.htm*.

Roberts, B. W., O'Donnell, M., & Robins, R. W. (2004). Goal and personality trait development in emerging adulthood. *Journal of Personality and Social Psychology*, 87, 541–550.

Robins, R. W., Hendin, H. M., & Trzesniewski, K. H. (2001). Measuring global self-esteem: Construct validation of a single-item measure and the Rosenberg Self-Esteem Scale. *Personality and Social Psychology Bulletin*, 27, 151–161.

Robins, R. W., & John, O. P. (1997). The quest for self-insight: Theory and research on accuracy and bias in self-perception. In R. Hogan, J. A. Johnson, & S. R. Briggs (Eds.), *Handbook of personality psychology* (pp. 649–679). San Diego, CA: Academic Press.

Robins, R. W., Norem, J. K., & Cheek, J. M. (1999). Naturalizing the self. In L. A. Pervin & O. P. John (Eds.), *Handbook of personality: Theory and research* (2nd ed., pp. 443–477). New York: Guilford Press.

Robinson, J. P., Shaver, P. R., & Wrightsman, L. S. (1991). *Measures of personality and social psychological attitudes*. San Diego, CA: Academic Press.

Rogers, T. B., Kuiper, N. A., & Kirker, W. S. (1977). Self-reference and the encoding of personal information. *Journal of Personality and Social Psychology*, 35, 677–688.

Rorer, L. G. (1965). The great response-style myth. *Psychological Bulletin*, 63, 129–156.

Saucier, G. (1994). Mini-markers: A brief version of Goldberg's unipolar Big-Five markers. *Journal of Personality Assessment*, 63, 506–516.

Schuman, H., & Presser, S. (1981). *Questions and answers in attitude surveys*. New York: Academic Press.

Schwartz, N., & Sudman, S. (1996). *Answering questions: Methodology for determining cognitive and communicative processes in survey research*. San Francisco: Jossey-Bass.

Sedikides, C., & Strube, M. J. (1995). The multiply motivated self. *Personality and Social Psychology Bulletin*, 21, 1330–1335.

Spain, J. S., & Eaton, L. G., & Funder, D. C. (2000).

Perspectives on personality: The relative accuracy of self versus others for the prediction of emotion and behavior. *Journal of Personality, 68,* 837–867.

Swann, W. B., Jr., Chang-Schneider, C., & McClarty, K. L. (in press). Do our self-views matter?: Self-concept and self-esteem in everyday life. *American Psychologist.*

Tellegen, A. (in press). *Multidimensional Personality Questionnaire.* Minneapolis: University of Minnesota Press.

Tellegen, A., Watson, D., & Clark, L. A. (1999). On the dimensional and hierarchical structure of affect. *Psychological Science, 10,* 297–303.

Tourangeau, R. (2004). Survey research and societal change. *Annual Review of Psychology, 55,* 775–801.

Tourangeau, R., Rips, L. J., & Rasinski, K. (2001). *The psychology of survey responses.* New York: Cambridge University Press.

Tracey, T. J., Rounds, J., & Gurtman, M. (1996). Examination of the general factor with the interpersonal circumplex structure: Application to the Inventory of Interpersonal Problems. *Multivariate Behavioral Research, 31,* 441–466.

Trapnell, P. D. (2006). *A new measure of agentic and communal values.* Manuscript under review.

Trapnell, P. D., & Campbell, J. D. (1999). Private self-consciousness and the five-factor model of personality: Distinguishing rumination from reflection. *Journal of Personality and Social Psychology, 76,* 284–304.

Van der Kloot, W. A., Kroonenberg, P. M., & Bakker, D. (1985). Implicit theories of personality: Further evidence of extreme response style. *Multivariate Behavioral Research, 20,* 369–387.

Vazire, S. (2006). Informant reports: A cheap, fast, easy method for personality assessment. *Journal of Research in Personality, 40,* 472–481.

Vazire, S., & Gosling, S. D. (2004). e-Perceptions: Personality impressions based on personal websites. *Journal of Personality and Social Psychology, 87,* 123–132.

Watson, D., Hubbard, B., & Wiese, D. (2000). Self-other agreement in personality and affectivity: The role of acquaintanceship, trait visibility, and assumed similarity. *Journal of Personality and Social Psychology, 78,* 546–558.

Wiggins J. S. (1973). *Personality and prediction: Principles of personality assessment.* Boston: Addison-Wesley.

Wilson, T. D. (2002). *Strangers to ourselves: Discovering the adaptive unconscious.* Cambridge, MA: Belknap Press/Harvard University Press.

Wilson, T. D., & LaFleur, S. J. (1995). Knowing what you'll do: Effects of analyzing reasons on self-prediction. *Journal of Personality and Social Psychology, 68,* 21–35.

Woods, S. A., & Hampson, S. E. (2005). Measuring the Big Five with single items using a bipolar response scale. *European Journal of Personality, 19,* 373–390.

## CHAPTER 14

The Construct Validation Approach to Personality Scale Construction

Leonard J. Simms
David Watson

Scale construction continues to be a popular activity among basic and applied personality researchers. We conducted a *PsycINFO* search of English-language journal articles published during the past 55 years that (1) included the keywords *test construction*, *scale development*, *scale construction*, or *measure development* and (2) also included the keyword *personality*. Using these criteria, our search revealed a total of 5,071 articles published since 1950, of which 3,609 (69.4%) have been published since 1985. Through the late 1980s and the 1990s, approximately 168 such articles, on average, were published each year, but this number has increased markedly in first half of this decade. Between the years 2000 and 2004, an average of 218 personality scale construction articles were published each year, representing a 30% increase as compared with the 15 years prior.

Several points are notable from these data. First, approximately two-thirds of all personal-

ity scale construction articles have been published over the past 20 years, likely reflecting both a resurgence of personality-based research and the proliferation of psychology journals in general. Second, although stable between 1985 and 1999, the pace of such publications appears to be increasing of late. Moreover, even the most recent articles have used a wide variety of approaches to construct and validate personality measures, with many reporting inadequate or outdated methodology, suggesting that the need for sound scale construction resources has never been greater (Clark & Watson, 1995; Watson, 2006). Thus, the primary goal of this chapter is to review basic principles of personality scale construction and describe an integrative method for constructing objective personality measures under the broad umbrella of construct validity.

The confusion often observed in the scale construction literature is not surprising when one considers the limited, and often outdated, guidance provided for such endeavors in many personality and assessment texts. In most texts, methods of personality scale construction are described through a discussion of various specific scale construction approaches or strategies. In particular, many texts organize these strategies into those based on (1) rational or theoretical justifications, (2) empirical criterion keying, and (3) factor analytic and internal consistency methods (e.g., Anastasi & Urbina, 1997; Kaplan & Saccuzzo, 2005)—which usually are described as mutually exclusive methods. As we discuss later, each approach carries clear strengths and limitations relative to the others. However, the combination of these approaches into a more integrative method of scale construction capitalizes on the unique strengths of each and makes it more likely that resultant measures will evidence adequate construct validity.

But what is "construct validity"? Often misunderstood and oversimplified, the concept of construct validity first was articulated in a seminal article by Cronbach and Meehl (1955), who argued that explicating the construct validity of a measure involves at least three steps: (1) describing a theoretical model—what Cronbach and Meehl called "the nomological net"—consisting of one or more hypothetical constructs and their relations to one another and to observable criteria, (2) building measures of the constructs identified by the theory, and (3) empirically testing the hypothesized relations between the constructs and observable criteria as specified by the theoretical model. Different scale construction approaches tend to favor some aspects of the construct validation process while ignoring others. For example, measures derived using purely rational-theoretical methods may have direct connections to a clear, well-defined theory of a construct, but often fail to yield a clean pattern of convergent and discriminant relations when compared with other measures and with observable, nontest criteria. In contrast, the empirical criterion-keying approach results in measures that may reliably predict observable criteria but are devoid of any connection to theory.

How is construct validity involved in the scale construction process? All too often, researchers consider construct validity only in a post hoc fashion, as something that one establishes after the test has been constructed. However, construct validation is more appropriately

considered a process, rather than an endpoint to which one aspires (Clark & Watson, 1995; Loevinger, 1957; Messick, 1995). To maximize the practical utility and theoretical meaningfulness of a measure, the concepts of construct validity articulated by Cronbach and Meehl (1955) should be consulted at all stages of the scale construction process, including initial conceptualization of the construct(s) to be measured, development of an initial item pool, creation of provisional scales, cross-validation and finalization of scales, and validation against other test and nontest indicators of the construct(s).

Moreover, construct validity is not a static quality of a test that can be "established" in a definitive way with a single study or even a series of studies. Rather, the process of construct validation is dynamic. As Cronbach and Meehl (1955) describe, "In one sense, it is naïve to inquire 'Is this test valid?' One does not validate a test, but only a principle for making inferences. If a test yields many different types of inferences, some of them can be valid and others invalid" (p. 297). Thus, as new scales begin to be examined against observable criteria, some aspects of the theory that guided its construction likely will be supported. However, other aspects of the theory may be refuted, and in such cases one must decide whether the fault lies with the test or the theory. This can be a tricky issue. Clearly, one cannot discard years of empirical work supporting a given theory because of a single study of a new measure. However, scales constructed rigorously, in accordance with the principles described in this chapter, have the potential to highlight problems with our understanding of theoretical constructs and lead to alternative hypotheses to be tested in future studies.

In addition to construct validity, researchers often speak of many other forms of validity—such as content validity, face validity, convergent validity, discriminant validity, concurrent validity, and predictive validity—that often are described as independent properties of a given measure. Recently, however, growing consensus has emerged that construct validity is best understood as a single overarching concept (American Psychological Association, 1999; Messick 1995; Watson, 2006). Indeed, as stated in the revised *Standards for Educational and Psychological Testing* (American Psychological Association, 1999), "Validity is a unitary concept. It is the degree to which all the accumulated evidence supports the intended interpretation of test scores for the proposed purpose" (p. 11). Thus, the concept of construct validity not only encompasses any form of validity that is relevant to the target construct, but also subsumes all of the major types of reliability. In sum, construct validity "has emerged as the central unifying concept in contemporary psychometrics" (Watson, 2006).

Loevinger (1957) was the first to systematically describe a theory-driven method of test construction firmly grounded in the concept of construct validity. In her monograph, Loevinger distinguished between three aspects of construct validity that she termed *substantive validity*, *structural validity*, and *external validity*. She argued that "these three aspects are mutually exclusive, exhaustive of the possible lines of evidence for construct validity, and mandatory" (pp. 653–654) and are "closely related to three stages in the test construction process: constitution of the pool of items, analysis of the internal structure of the pool of items and consequent selection of items to form a scoring key, and correlation of test scores with criteria and other variables" (p. 654). Modern application of Loevinger's test construction principles has been described in detail elsewhere (e.g., Clark & Watson, 1995; Watson, 2006). In this chapter, our goals are to (1) summarize the basic features of substantive, structural, and external validity in the test construction process, (2) discuss a number of personality-relevant examples, and (3) propose ways to integrate principles of modern measurement theory (e.g., item response theory) in the development of construct valid personality scales.

To illustrate key aspects of the scale construction process, we draw on a number of relevant examples, including a personality measure currently being constructed by one of us (L. J. S.). This new measure, provisionally called the Evaluative Person Descriptors Questionnaire (EPDQ), was conceived and developed to provide an enhanced understanding of the Positive Valence and Negative Valence factors of the Big Seven model of personality (e.g., Benet-Martínez & Waller, 2002; Saucier, 1997; Tellegen & Waller, 1987; Waller, 1999). Briefly, the Big Seven model builds on the lexical tradition in personality research, which generally has suggested that five broad factors underlie much of the variation in human personality (i.e., the Big Five, or five-factor model of personality).

However, Tellegen and Waller (1987; Waller, 1999) argued that restrictions historically imposed on the dictionary descriptors used to identify the Big Five model ignored potentially important aspects of personality, such as stable individual differences in mood states and self-evaluation. Their less restrictive lexical studies resulted in seven broad factors: the familiar Big Five dimensions, plus two evaluative factors—*Positive Valence* (PV) and *Negative Valence* (NV)—reflecting extremely positive (e.g., describing oneself as exceptional, important, smart) and negative (e.g., describing oneself as evil, immoral, disgusting) self-evaluations, respectively. To date, only one measure of the Big Seven exists in the literature, the Inventory of Personal Characteristics #7 (IPC-7; Tellegen, Grove, & Waller, 1991), and this measure includes only global indices of PV and NV. Thus, the EPDQ is being developed to (1) provide an alternative measure of PV and NV to be used in structural personality studies, and (2) explore the lower-order facet structure of these dimensions.

The Substantive Validity Phase: Construct Conceptualization and Item Pool Development

A flowchart depicting the scale construction process appears in Figure 14.1. In it, we divide the process into three general phases, corresponding to the three aspects of construct validation originally articulated by Loevinger (1957) and reiterated by Clark and Watson (1995). The first phase—substantive validity—is centered on the tasks of construct conceptualization and development of the initial item pool.

Review of Literature

The substantive phase begins with a thorough review of the literature to discover all previous attempts to measure and conceptualize the construct(s) under investigation. This step is important for a number of reasons. First, if this review reveals that we already have good, psychometrically sound measures of the construct, then the scale developer must ask him- or herself whether a new measure is, in fact, necessary and, if so, why. With the proliferation of scales designed to measure nearly every conceivable personality attribute, the justifica-

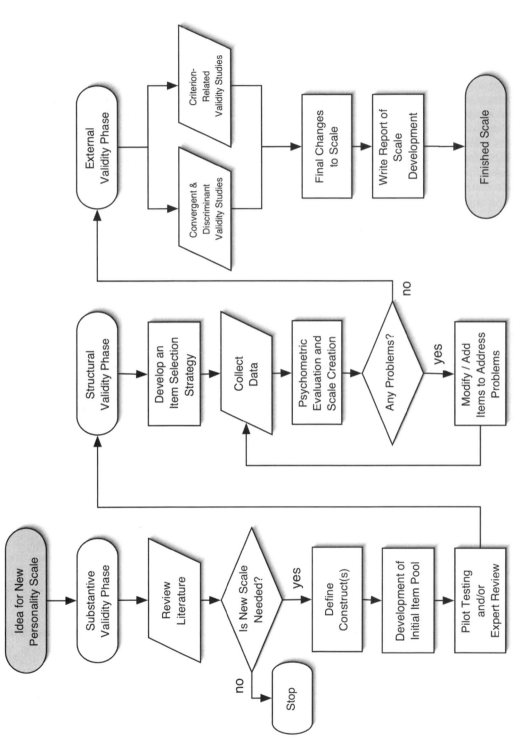

FIGURE 14.1. Flowchart depicting the substantive, structural, and external validity phases of construct valid personality scale development.

tion for a new measure should be very carefully considered.

However, the existence of psychometrically sound measures of the construct does not necessarily preclude the development of a new instrument. Are the existing measures perhaps based on a very different definition of the construct? Are the existing measures perhaps too narrow or too broad in scope as compared with one's own conceptualization of the construct? Or are new measures perhaps needed to help advance theory or to cross-validate the findings achieved using the established measure of the construct? In the early stages of EPDQ development, the literature review revealed several important justifications for a new measure. First, as described above, the single available measure of PV and NV included only broad scales of these constructs, with too few items to identify meaningful lower-order facets. Second, factor analytic studies seeking to clarify personality structure require more than single exemplars of the constructs under investigation to yield theoretically meaningful solutions. Thus, despite the existence of the IPC-7 to tap PV and NV, the decision to develop the EPDQ appeared justified, and formal development of the measure was undertaken.

Construct Conceptualization

The second important function of a thorough literature review is to develop a clear conceptualization of the target construct. Although one often has a general sense of the construct before starting the project, the literature review likely will reveal alternative conceptualizations of the construct, related constructs that potentially are important, and potential pitfalls to consider in the scale development process. Clark and Watson (1995) recommend writing out a formal definition of the target construct in order to finalize one's model of the construct and clarify its breadth and scope. For the EPDQ, formal definitions were developed for PV and NV that included not only the broad aspects of extremely positive and negative self-evaluations, respectively, but also potential lower-order components of each identified in the literature. For example, the concept of PV was refined by Benet-Martínez and Waller (2002) to include a number of subcomponents, such as self-evaluations of distinction, intelligence, and self-worth. Therefore, the conceptualization of PV was expanded for the EPDQ to include these potentially important facets.

Development of the Initial Item Pool

Once the justification for the new measure has been established and the construct formally defined, it is time to create the initial pool of items from which provisional scales eventually will be drawn. This is a critical step in the scale construction process. As Clark and Watson (1995) described, "No existing data-analytic technique can remedy serious deficiencies in an item pool" (p. 311). Thus, great care must be taken to avoid problems that cannot be easily rectified later in the process. The primary consideration during this step is to generate items sampling all content that potentially is relevant to the target construct. Loevinger (1957) provided a particularly clear description of this principle, saying that "the items of the pool should be chosen so as to sample all possible contents which might comprise the putative trait according to all known alternative theories of the of the trait" (p. 659).

Thus, *overinclusiveness* should characterize the initial item pool in at least two ways. First, the pool should be broader and more comprehensive than one's theoretical model of the target construct. Second, the pool should include some items that may ultimately be shown to be tangential or perhaps even unrelated to the target construct. Overinclusiveness of the initial pool can be particularly important later in the scale construction process when one is trying to establish the conceptual and empirical boundaries of the target construct(s). As Clark and Watson (1995) put it, "Subsequent psychometric analyses can identify weak, unrelated items that should be dropped from the emerging scale but are powerless to detect content that should have been included but was not" (p. 311).

Central to substantive validity is the concept of content validity. Haynes, Richard, and Kubany (1995) defined content validity as "the degree to which elements of an assessment instrument are relevant to and representative of the targeted construct for a particular assessment purpose" (p. 238). Within this definition, *relevance* refers to the appropriateness of a measure's items for the target construct. When applied to the scale construction process, this principle suggests that all items in the finished measure should fall within the boundaries of the target construct. Thus, although the principle of overinclusiveness suggests that some items be included in the initial item pool that fall outside the boundaries of the target construct, the principle of content validity suggests that final decisions regarding scale composition should take the relevance of items into account (Haynes et al., 1995; Watson, 2006).

A second important principle highlighted by Haynes and colleagues' (1995) definition is the concept of *representativeness*, which refers to the degree to which the item pool adequately samples content from all important aspects of the target construct. Representativeness includes at least two important considerations. First, the item pool should contain items reflecting all content areas relevant to the target construct. To ensure adequate coverage, many psychometricians recommend creating formal subscales to tap each important content area within a domain. In the development of the EPDQ, for example, an initial sample of 120 items was written to assess all areas of content deemed important to PV and NV, given the various empirical and theoretical considerations revealed by the literature review. More specifically, the pool contained "homogeneous item composites" (HICs; Hogan, 1983; Hogan & Hogan, 1992), tapping a variety of relevant content highlighted by the literature review, including depravity, distinction, self-worth, perceived stupidity/intelligence, perceived attractiveness, and unconventionality/peculiarity (see, e.g., Benet-Martínez & Waller, 2002; Saucier, 1997).

A second aspect of the representativeness principle is that the initial pool should include items reflecting all levels of the trait that need to be assessed. This principle is most commonly discussed with regard to ability tests, wherein a range of item difficulties are included so that the instrument can yield equally precise scores along the entire ability continuum. In personality measurement, this principle often is ignored for a variety of reasons. Items with extreme endorsement probabilities (e.g., items with which nearly all individuals will either agree or disagree) often are removed from consideration because they offer relatively little information relevant to most people's standing on the dimension, especially for traits with normal or nearly normal distributions in the general population. However, many personality measures are used across a diverse array of respondents—including college students, community-dwelling adults, psychiatric patients, and incarcerated individuals—who may differ substantially in their average trait levels. Thus, the item pool should reflect the entire range of trait levels along which reliable measurement is

desired. Notably, psychometric methods based on *classical test theory*—which currently inform most personality scale construction projects—usually favor selection of items with moderate endorsement probabilities. However, as we will discuss in greater detail later, *item response theory* (IRT; see, e.g., Embretson & Reise, 2000; Hambleton, Swaminathan, & Rogers, 1991) offers valuable tools for quantifying the "trait level" of the items in the pool.

Haynes and colleagues (1995) recommend that the relevance and representativeness of the item pool be formally assessed during the scale construction process, rather than in a post hoc manner. A number of approaches can be adopted to assess content validity, but most involve some form of consultation with experts who have special knowledge of the target construct. For example, in the early stages of development of a new measure of posttraumatic symptoms, one of us (L. J. S.) and his colleagues are in the process of surveying practicing psychologists in order to gauge the relevance of a broad range of items. We expect that these expert ratings will highlight the full range of item content deemed relevant to the experience of trauma and will inform all later stages of item writing and scale development.

Writing Clear Items

Basic principles of item writing have been detailed elsewhere (e.g., Clark & Watson, 1995; Comrey, 1988). However, here we briefly discuss two broad aspects of item writing: item clarity and response format. Unclear items can lead to confusion among respondents, which ultimately results in less reliable and valid measurement. Thus, items should be written using simple and straightforward language that is appropriate for the reading level of the measure's target population. Likewise, it is best to avoid using slang and trendy or colloquial expressions that may quickly become obsolete, as they will limit the long-term usefulness of the measure. Similarly, one should avoid writing complex or convoluted items that are difficult to read and understand. For example, "double-barreled" items—such as the true–false item "I would like the work of a librarian because of my generally aloof nature"—should be avoided, because they confound two different characteristics: (1) enjoyment of library work and (2) perceptions of aloofness or introversion. How are individuals to answer if they agree with one aspect of the item but not the other? Such dilemmas infuse unneeded error into the measure and ultimately reduce reliability and validity.

The particular phrasing of items also can influence responses and should be considered carefully. For example, Clark and Watson (1995) suggested that writing items with stems such as "I worry about . . . " or "I am troubled by . . . " will build a substantial neuroticism/negative affectivity component into a scale. In addition, many writers (e.g., Anastasi & Urbina, 1997; Comrey, 1988; Kaplan & Saccuzzo, 2005) recommend writing a mix of positively and negatively keyed items to guard against response sets characterized by acquiescence (i.e., yea-saying) or denial (i.e., nay-saying). In practice, however, this can be quite difficult for some constructs, especially when the low end of the dimension is not well understood.

It also is important to phrase items so that all targeted respondents can provide a reasonably appropriate response (Comrey, 1988). For example, items such as "I get especially tired after playing basketball" or "My current romantic relationship is very good" assume contexts or situations that may not be relevant to all respondents. Rewriting the items to be more context-neutral—for example, "I get especially tired after I exercise" and "I've been generally happy with the quality of my romantic relationships"—increases the applicability of the resulting measure. A related aspect of this principle is that items should be phrased to maximize the likelihood that individuals will be willing to provide a forthright answer. As Comrey (1988) put it, "Do not exceed the willingness of the respondent to respond. Asking a subject a question that he or she does not wish to answer can result in several possible outcomes, most of them bad" (p. 757). However, when the nature of the target construct requires asking about sensitive topics, it is best to phrase such items using straightforward, matter-of-fact, and nonpejorative language.

Choice of Response Format

The two most common response formats used in personality measures are dichotomous (e.g., true–false or yes–no) and polytomous (e.g., Likert-type rating scales) (see Clark & Watson, 1995, for an analysis of alternative but less frequently used response formats, such as checklists, forced-choice items, and visual analog scales). Dichotomous and polytomous formats each come with certain strengths and limitations to be considered. Dichotomously scored items often are less reliable than their polytomous counterparts, and scales composed of such items generally must be longer in order to achieve comparable scale reliabilities (e.g., Comrey, 1988). Historically, many personality researchers adopted dichotomous formats for easier scoring and analyses. However, the power of modern computers and the extension of many psychometric models to polytomous formats have made these advantages less important. Nevertheless, all other things being equal, dichotomous items take less time to complete than polytomous items; thus, given limited time, a dichotomous item format may yield more information (Clark & Watson, 1995).

Polytomous item formats can vary considerably across measures. Two key decisions to make are (1) choosing the number of response options to offer and (2) deciding how to label these options. Opinions vary widely on the optimal number of response options to offer. Some argue that items with more response options yield more reliable scales (e.g., Comrey, 1988). However, there is little consensus on the "best" number of options to offer, as the answer likely depends on the fineness of discriminations that participants are able to make for a given construct (Kaplan & Saccuzzo, 2005). Clark and Watson (1995) add, "Increasing the number of alternatives actually may reduce validity if respondents are unable to make the more subtle distinctions that are required" (p. 313). Opinions also differ on whether to offer an even or odd number of response options. An odd number of response options may entice some individuals to avoid giving careful consideration to some items by responding neutrally with the middle option. For that reason, some investigators prefer using an even number of options to force respondents to provide a nonneutral response.

Response options can be labeled using one of several anchoring schemes, including those based on agreement (e.g., *strongly disagree* to *strongly agree*), degree (e.g., *very little* to *quite a bit*), perceived similarity (e.g., *uncharacteristic of me* to *characteristic of me*), and frequency (e.g., *never* to *always*). Which anchoring scheme to use depends on the nature of the construct and the phrasing of items. In this regard, the phrasing of items must be compatible with the response format that has been chosen. For example, frequency modifiers may be quite useful for items using agreement-based Likert scales, but will be quite confusing when used with a frequency-based Likert scale. Consider the item "I frequently drink to excess." As a true–false or agreement-based Likert item, the addition of "frequently" clarifies the meaning of the item and likely increases its ability to discriminate between individuals high and low on the trait in question. However, using the same item with a frequency-based Likert scale (e.g., 1 = *never*, 2 = *infrequently*, 3 = *sometimes*, 4 = *often*, 5 = *almost always*) is confusing to individuals because the frequency of the sample behavior is sampled twice.

Pilot Testing

Once the initial item pool and all other scale features (e.g., response formats, instructions) have been developed, pilot testing in a small sample of convenience (e.g., 100 undergraduates) and/or expert review of the stimuli can be quite helpful. Such procedures can help identify potential problems—such as confusing items or instructions, objectionable content, or the lack of items in an important content area—before a great deal of time and money are expended to collect the initial round of formal scale development data.

The Structural Validity Phase: Psychometric Evaluation of Items and Provisional Scale Development

Loevinger (1957) defined the structural component of construct validity as "the extent to which structural relations between test items parallel the structural relations of other manifestations of the trait being measured" (p. 661). In the context of personality scale development, this definition suggests that the structural relations between test and nontest manifestations of the target construct should be parallel to the extent possible—what Loevinger called "structural fidelity"—and, ideally, this structure should match that of the theoretical model underlying the construct. According to this principle, for example, the nature and magnitude of relations between behavioral manifestations of extraversion (e.g., sociability, talkativeness, gregariousness) should match the structural relations between comparable test items designed to tap these same aspects of the construct. Thus, the first step is to develop an

item selection strategy that is most likely to yield a measure with structural fidelity.

Rational–Theoretical Item Selection

Historically, item selection strategies have taken a number of forms. The simplest of these to implement is the rational–theoretical approach. Using this approach, the scale developer simply writes items that *appear* consistent with his or her particular theoretical understanding of the target construct, assuming, of course, that this understanding is completely correct. The simplicity of this method is quite appealing, and some have argued that scales produced on solely rational grounds yield equivalent validity as compared with scales produced with more rigorous methods (e.g., Burisch, 1984). However, such arguments fail to account for other potential pitfalls associated with this approach. For example, although the convergent validity of purely rational scales can be quite good, the discriminant validity of such scales often is poor. Moreover, assuming that one's theoretical model of the construct is entirely correct is unrealistic and likely will result in a suboptimal measure.

For these reasons, psychometricians argue against adopting a purely rational item selection strategy. However, some test developers have attempted to make the rational–theoretical approach more rigorous through additional procedures designed to guard against some of the problems described above. For example, having experts evaluate the relevance and representativeness of the items (i.e., content validity) can help identify problematic aspects of the item pool, so that changes can be made prior to finalizing the measure (Haynes et al., 1995). In another application, Harkness, McNulty, and Ben-Porath (1995) described the use of *replicated rational selection* (RRS) in the development of the PSY-5 scales of the second edition of the Minnesota Multiphasic Personality Inventory (MMPI-2; Butcher, Dahlstrom, Graham, Tellegen, & Kaemmer, 1989). RRS involves asking many trained raters—who are given a detailed definition of the target construct—to select items from a pool that most clearly tap the construct, given their interpretations of the definition and the items. Then, only items that achieve a high degree of consensus make the final cut. Such techniques are welcome advances over purely rational methods, but problems with discriminant validity often still emerge unless additional psychometric procedures are employed.

Criterion-Keyed Item Selection

Another historically popular item selection strategy is the empirical criterion-keying approach, which was used in the development of a number of widely used personality measures, most notably the MMPI-2 and the California Psychological Inventory (CPI; Gough, 1987). In this approach, items are selected for a scale based solely on their ability to discriminate between individuals from a "normal" group and those from a prespecified criterion group (i.e., those who exhibit the characteristic that the test developer wishes to measure). In the purest form of this approach, item content is irrelevant. Rather, responses to items are considered samples of verbal behavior, the meanings of which are to be determined empirically (Meehl, 1945). Thus, if one wishes to create a measure of extraversion, one simply identifies groups of extraverts and introverts, administers a range of items to each, and identifies items, regardless of content, that extraverts reliably endorse but introverts do not. The ease of this technique made it quite popular, and tests constructed using this approach often show reasonable validity.

However, empirically keyed measures have a number of problems that limit their usefulness in many settings. An important limitation is that empirically keyed measures are entirely atheoretical and fail to help advance psychological theory in a meaningful way (Loevinger, 1957). Furthermore, scales constructed using this approach often are highly heterogeneous, making the proper interpretation of scores quite difficult. For example, tables in the manuals for both the MMPI-2 (Butcher et al., 1989) and CPI (Gough, 1987) reveal a large number of internal consistency reliability estimates below .60, with some as low as .35, demonstrating a pronounced lack of internal coherence for many of the scales. Similarly problematic are the high correlations often observed among scales within empirically keyed measures, reflecting poor discriminant validity (e.g., Simms, Casillas, Clark, Watson, & Doebbeling, 2005). Thus, for these reasons, psychometricians recommend against adopting a purely empirical item selection strategy. However, some limitations of the empirical approach may reflect problems in the way the approach was implemented, rather than inherent deficiencies in the approach itself. Thus, combining this approach with other psychometric item selection procedures—such as those focusing on internal consistency and content validity considerations—offers a potentially powerful way to create measures with structural fidelity.

Internal Consistency Approaches to Item Selection

The internal consistency approach actually represents a variety of psychometric techniques drawing from classical reliability theory, factor analysis, and more modern techniques such as IRT. At the most general level, the goal of this approach is to identify relatively homogenous scales that demonstrate good discriminant validity. This usually is accomplished with some variant of factor or component analysis, often combined with classical and modern psychometric approaches to hone the factor-based scales. In developing the EPDQ, for example, the initial pool of 120 items was administered to a large sample and then factor analyzed to determine the most viable factor structure underlying the item responses. Provisional scales were then created based on the factor analytic results as well as reliability considerations. The primary strength of this approach is that it usually results in homogeneous and differentiable dimensions. However, nothing in the statistical program helps to label the dimensions that emerge from the analyses. Therefore, it is important to note that the use of factor analysis does not obviate the need for sound theory in the scale construction process.

Data Collection

Once an item selection strategy has been developed, the first round of data collection can begin. Of course, the nature of this data collection will depend somewhat on the item selection strategy chosen. In a purely rational–theoretical approach to scale construction, the scale developer might choose to collect expert ratings of the relevance and representativeness of each candidate item and then choose items based primarily on these ratings. If developing an empirically keyed measure, the developer likely would collect self-ratings on all candidate items from groups that differ on the target construct (e.g., those high and low in PV) and then choose the items that reliably discriminate between the groups.

Finally, in an internal consistency approach, the typical goal of data collection is to obtain self-ratings for all candidate items in a large sample representative of the population(s) for which the measure ultimately will be used. For measures with broad relevance to many populations, data collection may involve several specific samples chosen to represent an optimal range of individuals. For example, if one wishes to develop a measure of personality pathology, sole reliance on undergraduate samples would not be appropriate: Although undergraduate samples can be important and helpful in the scale construction process, data also should be collected from psychiatric and criminal samples in which personality pathology is more prevalent.

As depicted in Figure 14.1, several rounds of data collection may be necessary before provisional scales are ready for the external validity phase. Between each round, psychometric analyses should be conducted to identify problematic items, gaps in content, or any other difficulties that need to be addressed before moving forward.

Psychometric Evaluation of Items

Because the internal consistency approach is the most common method used in contemporary scale construction (see Clark & Watson, 1995), in this section we focus on psychometric techniques from this tradition. However, a full review of internal consistency techniques is beyond the scope of this chapter. Thus, here we briefly summarize a number of important principles of factor analysis and reliability theory, as well as more modern approaches such as IRT, and provide references for more detailed discussions of these principles.

Factor Analysis

The basic goal of any exploratory factor analysis is to extract a manageable number of latent dimensions that explain the covariations among the larger set of manifest variables (see, e.g., Comrey, 1988; Fabrigar, Wegener, MacCallum, & Strahan, 1999; Floyd & Widaman, 1995; Preacher & MacCallum, 2003). As applied to the scale construction process, factor analysis involves reducing the matrix of interitem correlations to a set of factors or components that can be used to form provisional scales. Unfortunately, there is a daunting array of choices awaiting the prospective factor analyst—such as choice of rotation, method of

factor extraction, the number of factors to extract, and whether to adopt an exploratory or confirmatory approach—and many avoid the technique altogether for this reason. However, with a little knowledge and guidance, factor analysis can be used wisely as a valuable tool in the scale construction process. Interested readers are referred to detailed discussions of factor analysis by Fabrigar and colleagues (1999), Floyd and Widaman (1995), and Preacher and MacCallum (2003).

Regardless of the specifics of the analysis, exploratory factor analysis is extremely useful to the scale developer who wishes to create homogeneous scales (i.e., scales that measure one thing) that exhibit good discriminant validity. For demonstration purposes, abridged results from exploratory factor analyses of the initial pool of EPDQ items are presented in Table 14.1. In this particular analysis, all 120 items were included, and five oblique (i.e., correlated) factors were extracted. We should note here that there is no gold standard for deciding how many factors to extract in an exploratory analysis. Rather, a number of techniques—such as the scree test, parallel analyses of eigenvalues, and fit indices accompanying maximum likelihood extraction methods—provide some guidance as to a range of viable factor solutions, which should then be studied carefully (for discussions of the relative merits of these approaches, see Fabrigar et al., 1999; Floyd & Widaman, 1995; Preacher & MacCallum, 2003). Ultimately, however, the most important criterion for choosing a factor structure is the psychological and theoretical meaningfulness of the resultant factors. In this case, five factors—tentatively labeled Distinction, Worthlessness, NV/Evil Character, Oddity, and Perceived Stupidity—were extracted from the initial EPDQ data because (1) the five-factor solution was among those suggested by preliminary analyses and (2) this solution yielded the most compelling factors from a psychological standpoint.

In the abridged EPDQ output, six markers are presented for each factor in order to demonstrate a number of points (note that these are not simply the best six markers of each factor). The first point is that the goal of such an analysis is not necessarily to form scales using the top markers of each factor. Doing so might seem intuitively appealing, because using only the best markers will result in a highly reliable scale. However, high reliability often is gained at the expense of construct validity. This phenomenon is known as the *attenuation paradox* (Loevinger, 1954, 1957), and it reminds us that the ultimate goal of scale construction is validity. Reliability of measurement certainly is important, but excessively high correlations within a scale will result in a very narrow scale that may show reduced connections with other test and nontest exemplars of the same construct. Thus, the goal of factor analysis in scale construction is to identify a range of items within each factor to serve as candidates for scale membership. Table 14.1 includes a number of candidate items for each EPDQ factor, some good and some bad.

Good candidate items are those that load at least moderately (at least |.35|; see Clark & Watson, 1995) on the primary factor and only minimally on other factors. Thus, of the 30 candidate items listed, only 18 meet this criterion, with the remaining items loading moderately on at least one other factor. Bad items, in contrast, are those that either load weakly on the hypothesized factor or cross-load on one or more factors. However, poorly performing items should be carefully examined before they are removed completely from consideration, especially when an item was predicted a priori to be a strong marker of a given factor. A number of considerations can influence the performance of an individual item. One's theory can be wrong; the item may be poorly worded or have extreme endorsement properties (i.e., nearly all or none of the participants endorsed the item); or perhaps sample-specific factors are to blame.

TABLE 14.1. Abridged Factor Analytic Results Used to Construct the Evaluative Traits Questionnaire

Line	Item	Abbreviated item text	I	II	III	IV	V
1	52	People admire things I've done.	.74				
2	83	I have many special aptitudes.	.71				
3	69	I am the best at what I do.	.68				
4	48	Others consider me valuable.	.64	−.29			
5	106	I receive many awards.	.61				
6	66	I am needed and important.	.55	−.40			
7	118	No one would care if I died.		.69			
8	28	I am an unimportant person.		.67			
9	15	I would describe myself as stupid.		.55			.29
10	64	I'm relatively insignificant.		.55			
11	113	I have little to offer the world.	−.29	.50			
12	11	I would describe myself as depraved.		.34	.24		
13	84	I enjoy seeing others suffer.			.75		
14	90	I engage in evil activities.			.67		
15	41	I am evil.			.63		
16	100	I lie, cheat, and steal.			.63		
17	95	When I die, I'll go to a bad place.		.23	.36		
18	1	I am a good person.	.26	−.23	−.26		
19	14	I am odd.				.78	
20	88	My behavior is strange.				.75	
21	9	Others describe me as unusual.				.73	
22	29	I have unusual beliefs.				.64	
23	93	I think differently from everybody.	.33			.49	
24	98	I consider myself normal.	.29			−.66	
25	45	Most people are smarter than me.					.55
26	94	It's hard for me to learn new things.					.54
27	110	My IQ score would be low.		.22			.48
28	80	I have very few talents.		.27			.41
29	104	I have trouble solving problems.					.41
30	30	Others consider me foolish.		.25		.31	.32

Note. Loadings < |.20| have been removed.

For example, Item 110 of the EPDQ (line 27 of Table 14.1: "If I took an IQ test, my score would be low") loaded as expected on the Perceived Stupidity factor, but also loaded secondarily on the Worthlessness factor. Because of its face valid connection with the Perceived Stupidity factor, this item was tentatively retained in the item pool pending its performance in future rounds of data collection. However, if the same pattern emerges in future data, the item likely will be dropped. Another problematic item was Item 11 (line 12 of Table 14.1; "I would describe myself as depraved"), which loaded predictably but weakly on the NV/Evil Character factor, but also cross-loaded (more strongly) on the Worthlessness factor. In this case, the item will be reworded in order to amplify the "depraved" aspect of the item and eliminate whatever nonspecific aspects contributed to its cross-loading on the Worthlessness factor.

Internal Consistency and Homogeneity

Once a reduced pool of candidate items has been identified through factor analysis, additional item-level analyses should be conducted to hone the scale(s). In the service of structural fidelity, the goal at this stage is to identify a set of items whose intercorrelations match the internal organization of the target construct (Watson, 2006). Thus, for personality constructs—which typically are hypothesized to be homogeneous and internally coherent—this principle suggests that items tapping personality constructs also should be homogenous and internally coherent. The goal of most personality scales, then, is to measure a single construct as precisely as possible. Unfortunately, many scale developers and users confuse two related but differentiable aspects of internal coherence—(1) *internal consistency*, as measured by indices such as coefficient alpha (Cronbach, 1951), and (2) *homogeneity* or *unidimensionality*—often using the former to establish the latter. However, internal consistency is not the same as homogeneity (see, e.g., Clark & Watson, 1995; Schmitt, 1996). Whereas internal consistency indexes the overall degree of interrelation among a set of items, homogeneity (or unidimensionality) refers to the extent to which all of the items on a given scale tap a single factor. Thus, although internal consistency is a necessary condition for homogeneity, it clearly is not sufficient (Watson, 2006).

Internal consistency estimators such as coefficient alpha are functions of two parameters: (1) the average interitem correlation and (2) the number of items on the scale. Because such estimates confound internal coherence with scale length, scale developers often use a variety of alternative approaches—including examination of interitem correlations (Clark & Watson, 1995) and conducting confirmatory factor analyses to test the fit of a single-factor model (Schmitt, 1996)—to assess the homogeneity of an item pool. Here, we focus on interitem correlations. To establish homogeneity, one must examine both the mean and the distribution of the interitem correlations. The magnitude of the mean correlation generally should fall somewhere between .15 and .50. This range is wide to account for traits of varying bandwidths. That is, relatively narrow traits—such as those in the provisional Perceived Stupidity scale from the EPDQ—should yield higher average interitem correlations than broader traits such as those in the overall PV composite scale of the EPDQ (which is composed of a number of narrow but related facets, including reversed-keyed Perceived Stupidity). Interestingly, the provisional Perceived Stupidity and PV scales yielded average interitem correlations of .45 and .36, respectively, which was only somewhat consistent with expectations. The narrow trait indeed yielded a higher average interitem correlation than the broader trait, but the difference was not large, suggesting either that (1) the PV item pool is not sufficiently broad or (2) the theory underlying PV as a broad dimension of personality requires some modification.

The distribution of the interitem correlations also should be inspected to ensure that all cluster narrowly around the average, inasmuch as wide variation among the interitem correlations suggests a number of potential problems. Excessively high interitem correlations suggest unnecessary redundancy in the scale, which can be eliminated by dropping one item from each pair of highly correlated items. Moreover, significant variability in the interitem correlations may be due to multidimensionality within the scale, which must be explored.

Although coefficient alpha is not a perfect index of internal consistency, it continues to provide a reasonable estimate of one source of scale reliability. Thus, alpha should be computed and evaluated in the scale development process. However, given our earlier discussion of the attenuation paradox, higher alphas are not necessarily better. Accordingly, some psychometricians recommend striving for an alpha of at least .80 and then stopping, as adding items for the sole purpose of increasing alpha beyond this point may result in a narrower scale with more limited validity (see, e.g., Clark & Watson, 1995). Additional aspects of scale reliability—such as test–retest reliability (see, e.g., Watson, 2006) and transient error (see, e.g., Schmidt, Le, & Ilies, 2003)—also should be evaluated in this phase of scale construction to the extent that they are relevant to the structural fidelity of the new personality scale.

Item Response Theory

IRT refers to a range of modern psychometric models that describe the relations between item responses and the underlying latent trait they purport to measure. IRT can be an extremely useful adjunct to other scale development methods already discussed. Although originally developed and applied primarily in the ability testing domain, the use of IRT in the personality literature recently has become more common (e.g., Reise & Waller, 2003; Simms & Clark, 2005). Within the IRT literature, a variety of one-, two-, and three-parameter models have been proposed to explain both dichotomous and polytomous response data (for an accessible review of IRT, see Embretson & Reise, 2000, or Morizot, Ainsworth, & Reise, Chapter 24, this volume). Of these, a two-parameter model—with parameters for *item difficulty* and *item discrimination*—has been applied most consistently to personality data. Item difficulty (also known as "threshold" or "location") refers to the point along the trait continuum at which a given item has a 50% probability of being endorsed in the keyed direction. High difficulty values are associated with items that have low endorsement probabilities (i.e., that reflect higher levels of the trait). Discrimination reflects the degree of psychometric precision, or *information*, that an item provides at its difficulty level.

The concept of *information* is particularly useful in the scale development process. In contrast to classical test theory—in which a constant level of precision typically is assumed across the entire range of a measure—the IRT concept of information permits the scale developer to calculate conditional estimates of measurement precision and generate item and test information curves that more accurately reflect reliability of measurement across all levels of the underlying trait. In IRT, the standard error of measurement of a scale is equal to the inverse square root of information at every point along the trait continuum:

$$SE(\theta) = \frac{1}{\sqrt{I(\theta)}}$$

where $SE(\theta)$ and $I(\theta)$ are the standard error of measurement and test information, respectively, evaluated at a given level of the underlying trait, θ. Thus, scales that generate more information yield lower standard errors of measurement, which translates directly into more reliable measurement. For example, Figure 14.2 contains the test information and standard error curves for the provisional Distinction scale of the EPDQ. In this figure, the trait level, θ, is plotted on a *z*-score metric, which is customary for IRT, and the standard error axis is on the same metric as θ. Test information is not on a standard metric; rather the maximum amount of test information increases as a function of the number of items in the test and the precision associated with each item. These curves indicate that this scale, as currently constituted, provides most of its information, or measurement precision, at the low and moderate levels of the underlying trait dimension. In concrete terms, this means that the strongest markers of the underlying trait were relatively "easy" for individuals to endorse; that is, they had higher endorsement probabilities.

This may or may not present a problem, depending on the ultimate goal of the scale developer. If, for instance, the goal is to discriminate between individuals who are moderate or high on this dimension—which likely would be the case in clinical settings—or if the goal is to measure the construct equally precisely across the all levels of the trait—which would be desirable for computerized adaptive testing—then items would need to be added to the scale that provide more information at trait levels greater than 1.0 (i.e., items reflecting the same construct but with lower response base rates). If, however, one wishes only to discriminate between individuals who are low or moderate on the trait, then the current items may be adequate.

IRT also can be useful for examining the performance of individual items on a scale. Item information curves for five representative items

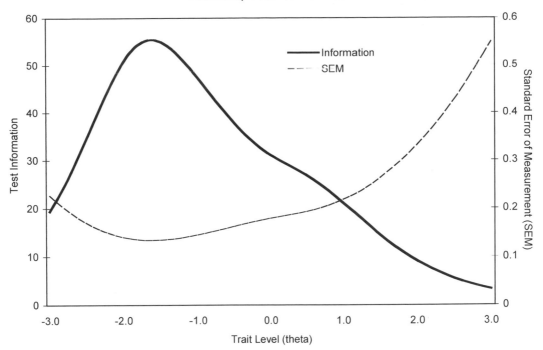

FIGURE 14.2. Test information and standard error curves for the provisional EPDQ Distinction scale. Test information represents the sum of all item information curves, and standard error of measurement is equal to the inverse square root of information at all levels of theta. The standard error axis is on the same metric as theta. This figure shows that measurement precision for this scale is greatest between theta values of –2.0 and +1.0.

of the EPDQ Distinction scale are presented in Figure 14.3. These curves illustrate several notable points. First, not all items are created equal. Item 63 ("I would describe myself as a successful person"), for example, yielded excellent measurement precision along much of the trait dimension (range = –2.0 to +1.0), whereas Item 103 ("I think outside the box") produced an extremely flat information curve, suggesting that it is not a good marker of the underlying dimension. This is particularly interesting, given that the structural analyses that guided construction of this provisional scale identified Item 103 as a moderately strong marker of the Distinction factor. In light of these IRT analyses, this item likely will be removed from the provisional scale. Item 86 ("Among the people around me, I am one of the best"), however, also yielded a relatively flat information curve but provided incremental information at the very high end of the dimension. Therefore, this item was tentatively retained, pending the results from future data collection.

IRT methods also have been used to study item bias, or *differential item functioning*

(DIF). Although DIF analyses originally were developed for ability testing applications, these methods have begun to appear more often in the personality testing literature to identify DIF related to gender (e.g., Smith & Reise, 1998), age cohort (e.g., Mackinnon et al., 1995), and culture (e.g., Huang, Church, & Katigbak, 1997). Briefly, the basic goal of DIF analyses is to identify items that yield significantly different difficulty or discrimination parameters across groups of interest, after equating the groups with respect to the trait being measured. Unfortunately, most such investigations are done in a post hoc fashion, after the measure has been finalized and published. Ideally, however, DIF analyses would be more useful during the structural phase of construct validation to identify and fix potentially problematic items before the scale is finalized.

A final application of IRT potentially relevant to personality is Computerized Adaptive Testing (CAT), in which items are individually tailored to the trait level of the respondent. A typical CAT selects and administers only those items that provide the most "psychometric in-

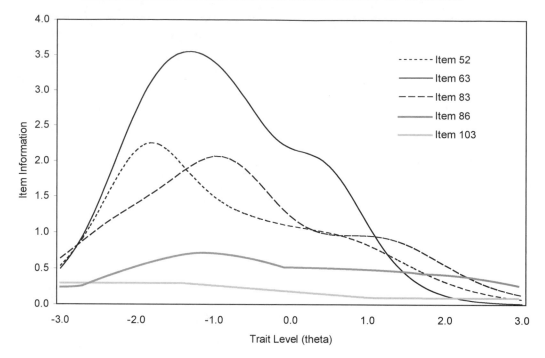

FIGURE 14.3. Item information curves associated with five example items of the provisional EPDQ Distinction scale.

formation" at a given ability or trait level, eliminating the need to present items that have a very low or very high likelihood of being endorsed or answered correctly, given a particular respondent's trait or ability level. For example, in a CAT version of a general arithmetic test, the computer would not administer easy items (e.g., simple addition) once it was clear from an individual's responses that his or her ability level was far greater (e.g., he or she was correctly answering calculus or matrix algebra items). CAT methods have been shown to yield substantial time savings with little or no loss of reliability or validity in both the ability (Sands, Waters, & McBride, 1997) and personality (e.g., Simms & Clark, 2005) literatures.

For example, Simms and Clark (2005) developed a prototype CAT version of the Schedule for Nonadaptive and Adaptive Personality (SNAP; Clark, 1993) that yielded time savings of approximately 35% and 60%, as compared with full-scale versions of the SNAP completed via computer or paper-and-pencil, respectively. Interestingly, these data suggest that CAT, and nonadaptive computerized administration of questionnaires, offer potentially significant efficiency gains for personality researchers. Thus,

CAT and computerization of measures may be attractive options for the personality scale developer that should be explored further.

The External Validity Phase: Validation against Test and Nontest Criteria

The final piece of scale development depicted in Figure 14.1 is the external validity phase, which is concerned with two basic aspects of construct validation: (1) convergent and discriminant validity and (2) criterion-related validity. Whereas the structural phase primarily involves analyses of the items *within* the new measure, the goal of the external phase is to examine whether the relations between the new measure and important test and nontest criteria are congruent with one's theoretical understanding of the target construct and its place in the nomological net (Cronbach & Meehl, 1955). Data consistent with theory supports the construct validity of the new measure. However, discrepancies between observed data and theory suggest one of several conclusions—(1) the measure does not adequately measure the target construct, (2) the theory requires modification, or (3) some of both—that must be addressed.

Convergent and Discriminant Validity

Convergent validity is the extent to which a measure correlates with other measures of the same construct, whereas *discriminant validity* is supported to the extent that a measure does not correlate with measures of other constructs that are theoretically or empirically distinct. Campbell and Fiske (1959) first described these aspects of construct validity and recommended that they be assessed using a multitrait–multimethod (MTMM) matrix. In such a matrix, multiple measures of at least two constructs are correlated and arranged to highlight several important aspects of convergent and discriminant validity.

A simple example—in which self-ratings and peer ratings of preliminary PV, NV, Extraversion, and Agreeableness scales are compared—is shown in Table 14.2. We must, however, exercise some caution in drawing strong inferences from these data, because the measures are not yet in their final forms. Nevertheless, these preliminary data help demonstrate several important aspects of an MTMM matrix. First, the underlined values in the lower-left block are convergent validity coefficients comparing self-ratings on all four traits with their respective peer ratings. These should be positive and at least moderate in size. Campbell and Fiske (1959) summarized: "The entries in the validity diagonal should be significantly

different from zero and sufficiently large to encourage further examination of validity" (p. 82). However, the absolute magnitude of convergent correlations will depend on specific aspects of the measures being correlated. For example, the concept of *method variance* suggests that self-ratings of the same construct generally will correlate more strongly than will self-ratings and peer ratings. In our example, the convergent correlations reflect different methods of assessing the constructs, which is a stronger test of convergent validity.

Ultimately, the power of an MTMM matrix lies in the comparisons of convergent correlations with other parts of the table. The ideal matrix would include convergent correlations that are greater than all other correlations in the table, thereby establishing discriminant validity, but three specific comparisons typically are made to explicate this issue more fully. First, each convergent correlation should be higher than other correlations in the same row and column in same box. Campbell and Fiske (1959) labeled the correlations above and below the convergent correlations *heterotrait–heteromethod triangles*, noting that convergent validity correlations "should be higher than the correlations obtained between that variable and any other variable having neither trait nor method in common" (p. 82). In Table 14.2, this rule was satisfied for Extraversion and, to a lesser extent, Agreeableness, but PV and NV clearly have failed this test of discriminant validity. The data are particularly striking for PV, revealing that peer ratings of PV actually correlate more strongly with self-ratings of NV and

TABLE 14.2. Example of Multitrait–Multimethod Matrix

Method	Scale	Self-ratings				Peer ratings			
		PV	NV	E	A	PV	NV	E	A
Self-ratings	PV	(.90)							
	NV	−.38	(.87)						
	E	.48	−.20	(.88)					
	A	−.03	−.51	.01	(.84)				
Peer ratings	PV	*.15*	−.29	.09	.26	(.91)			
	NV	−.09	*.39*	.00	−.41	−.64	(.86)		
	E	.19	−.05	*.42*	−.05	.37	−.06	(.90)	
	A	−.01	−.35	.05	*.50*	.54	−.66	.06	(.92)

Note. N = 165. Correlations above |.20| are significant, *p* < .01. Alpha coefficients are presented in parentheses along the diagonal. Convergent correlations are underlined. PV = positive valence; E = Extraversion; NV = negative valence; A = Agreeableness.

Agreeableness than with self-ratings of PV. Such findings highlight problems with either the scale itself or our theoretical understanding of the construct, which must be addressed before the scale is finalized.

Second, the convergent correlations generally should be higher than the correlations in the *heterotrait–monomethod triangles* that appear above and to the right of the heteromethod block just described. Campbell and Fiske (1959) described this principle by saying that a variable should "correlate higher with an independent effort to measure the same trait than with measures designed to get at different traits which happen to employ the same method" (p. 83). Again, the data presented in Table 14.2 provide a mixed picture with respect to this aspect of discriminant validity. In both the self-rating and peer-rating triangles, four of six correlations were significant and similar to or greater than the convergent validity correlations. In the self-rating triangle, PV and NV correlated –.38 with each other, PV correlated .48 with Extraversion, and NV correlated –.51 with Agreeableness, again suggesting poor discriminant validity for PV and NV. A similar, but more amplified, pattern emerged in the peer-rating triangle. Extraversion and Agreeableness, however, were uncorrelated with each other in both triangles, which is consistent with the theoretical assumption of the relative independence of these constructs.

Finally, Campbell and Fiske (1959) recommended that "the same pattern of trait interrelationship [should] be shown in all of the heterotrait triangles" (p. 83). The purpose of these comparisons is to determine whether the correlational pattern among the traits is due more to true covariation among the traits or to method-specific factors. If the same correlational pattern emerges regardless of method, then the former conclusion is plausible, whereas if significant differences emerge across the heteromethod triangles, then the influence of method variance must be evaluated. The four heterotrait triangles in Table 14.2 show a fairly similar pattern, with at least one key exception involving PV and Agreeableness: Whereas self-ratings of PV were uncorrelated with self-ratings and peer ratings of Agreeableness (*r*s = –.03 and –.01, respectively), peer ratings of PV correlated moderately to strongly with self-ratings and peer ratings of Agreeableness (*r*s = .26 and .54, respectively). Such findings suggest a significant role for method variance within the peer ratings of PV. It should be

noted that this particular form of test of discriminant validity is particularly well suited to confirmatory factor analytic methods in which observed variables are permitted to load on both trait and method factors, thereby allowing for the relative influence of each to be quantified.

Criterion-Related Validity

A final source of validity evidence is criterion-related validity, which involves relating a measure to nontest variables deemed relevant to the target construct, given its nomological net. Most texts (e.g., Anastasi & Urbina, 1997; Kaplan & Saccuzzo, 2005) divide criterion-related validity into two subtypes based on the temporal relationship between the administration of the measure and the assessment of the criterion of interest. *Concurrent validity* involves relating a measure to criterion evidence collected at the same time as the measure itself, whereas *predictive validity* involves associations with criteria that are assessed at some point in the future. In either case, the primary goals of criterion-related validity are to (1) confirm the new measure's place in the nomological net and (2) provide an empirical basis for making inferences from test scores.

To that end, criterion-related validity evidence can take a number of forms. In the EPDQ development project, self-reported behavior data are being collected to clarify the behavioral correlates of PV and NV, as well as the facets of each. For example, to assess the concurrent validity of the provisional Perceived Stupidity facet scale, undergraduate participants in one study are being asked to report their current grade point averages. Pending these results, future studies may involve other related criteria, such as official grade point average data provided by the university, results from standardized achievement/aptitude test scores, or perhaps even individually administered intelligence test scores. Likewise, to examine the concurrent validity of the provisional Distinction facet scale, the same participants are being asked to report whether they have recently received any special honors, awards, or merit-based scholarships, or whether they hold any leadership positions at the university.

Finally, as depicted in Figure 14.1, once sufficient reliability and validity data have been collected to support the initial construct validity of the new measure, the provisional scales should be finalized and the data published in a research article or test manual that thoroughly describes the methods used to construct the measure, appropriate administration and scoring procedures, and interpretive guidelines (American Psychological Association, 1999).

Summary and Conclusions

In this chapter we provide an overview of the personality scale development process in the context of construct validity (Cronbach & Meehl, 1955; Loevinger, 1957). Construct validity is not a static quality of a measure that can be established in any definitive sense. Rather, construct validation is a dynamic process in which (1) theory and empirical work inform the scale development process at all phases and (2) data emerging from the new measure have the potential to modify our theoretical understanding of the target construct. Such an approach also can serve to integrate different conceptualizations of the same construct, especially to the extent that all possible manifestations of the target construct are sampled in the initial item pool. Indeed, this underscores the importance of conducting a thorough literature review prior to writing items and of creating an initial item pool that is strategically overinclusive. Loevinger's (1957) classic three-part discussion of the construct validation process continues to serve as a solid foundation on which to build new personality measures, and modern psychometric approaches can be easily integrated into this framework.

For example, we discussed the use of IRT to help evaluate and select items in the structural phase of scale development. Although sparingly used in the personality literature until recently, IRT offers the personality scale developer a number of tools—such as detection of differential item functioning across groups, evaluation of measurement precision along the entire trait continuum, and administration of personality items through modern and efficient approaches such as CAT—which are becoming more accessible to the average psychometrician or personality scale developer. Indeed, most assessment texts include sections devoted to IRT and modern measurement principles, and many universities now offer specialized IRT courses or seminars. Moreover, a number of Windows-based software packages have emerged in recent years to conduct IRT analyses (see Embretson & Reise, 2000). Thus, IRT can and should play a much more prominent role in personality scale development in the future.

Recommended Readings

Clark, L. A., & Watson, D. (1995). Constructing validity: Basic issues in objective scale development. *Psychological Assessment*, 7, 309–319.

Embretson, S. E., & Reise, S. P. (2000). *Item response theory for psychologists*. Mahwah, NJ: Erlbaum.

Floyd, F. J., & Widaman, K. F. (1995). Factor analysis in the development and refinement of clinical assessment instruments. *Psychological Assessment*, 7, 286–299.

Haynes, S. N., Richard, D. C. S., & Kubany, E. S. (1995). Content validity in psychological assessment: A functional approach to concepts and methods. *Psychological Assessment*, 7, 238–247.

Simms, L. J., & Clark, L. A. (2005). Validation of a computerized adaptive version of the Schedule for Nonadaptive and Adaptive Personality. *Psychological Assessment*, 17, 28–43.

Smith, L. L., & Reise, S. P. (1998). Gender differences in negative affectivity: An IRT study of differential item functioning on the Multidimensional Personality Questionnaire Stress Reaction Scale. *Journal of Personality and Social Psychology*, 75, 1350–1362.

References

American Psychological Association. (1999). *Standards for educational and psychological testing*. Washington, DC: Author.

Anastasi, A., & Urbina, S. (1997). *Psychological testing* (7th ed.). New York: Macmillan.

Benet-Martínez, V., & Waller, N. G. (2002). From adorable to worthless: Implicit and self-report structure of highly evaluative personality descriptors. *European Journal of Personality*, 16, 1–41.

Burisch, M. (1984). Approaches to personality inventory construction: A comparison of merits. *American Psychologist*, 39, 214–227.

Butcher, J. N., Dahlstrom, W. G., Graham, J. R., Tellegen, A., & Kaemmer, B. (1989). *Minnesota Multiphasic Personality Inventory (MMPI-2): Manual for administration and scoring*. Minneapolis: University of Minnesota Press.

Campbell, D. T., & Fiske, D. W. (1959). Convergent and discriminant validation by the multitrait–multimethod matrix. *Psychological Bulletin*, 56, 81–105.

Clark, L. A. (1993). *Schedule for nonadaptive and adaptive personality (SNAP): Manual for administration, scoring, and interpretation*. Minneapolis: University of Minnesota Press.

Clark, L. A., & Watson, D. (1995). Constructing validity: Basic issues in objective scale development. *Psychological Assessment*, 7, 309–319.

Comrey, A. L. (1988). Factor-analytic methods of scale development in personality and clinical psychology. *Journal of Consulting and Clinical Psychology, 56,* 754–761.

Cronbach, L. J. (1951). Coefficient alpha and the internal structure of tests. *Psychometrika, 16,* 297–334.

Cronbach, L. J., & Meehl, P. E. (1955). Construct validity in psychological tests. *Psychological Bulletin, 52,* 281–302.

Embretson, S. E., & Reise, S. P. (2000). *Item response theory for psychologists.* Mahwah, NJ: Erlbaum.

Fabrigar, L. R., Wegener, D. T., MacCallum, R. C., & Strahan, E. J. (1999). Evaluating the use of exploratory factor analysis in psychological research. *Psychological Methods, 4,* 272–299.

Floyd, F. J., & Widaman, K. F. (1995). Factor analysis in the development and refinement of clinical assessment instruments. *Psychological Assessment, 7,* 286–299.

Gough, H. G. (1987). *California Psychological Inventory administrator's guide.* Palo Alto, CA: Consulting Psychologists Press.

Hambleton, R., Swaminathan, H., & Rogers, H. (1991). *Fundamentals of item response theory.* Newbury Park, CA: Sage.

Harkness, A. R., McNulty, J. L., & Ben-Porath, Y. S. (1995). The Personality Psychopathology-5 (PSY-5): Constructs and MMPI-2 scales. *Psychological Assessment, 7,* 104–114.

Haynes, S. N., Richard, D. C. S., & Kubany, E. S. (1995). Content validity in psychological assessment: A functional approach to concepts and methods. *Psychological Assessment, 7,* 238–247.

Hogan, R. T. (1983). A socioanalytic theory of personality. In M. Page (Ed.), *1982 Nebraska Symposium on Motivation* (pp. 55–89). Lincoln: University of Nebraska Press.

Hogan, R. T., & Hogan, J. (1992). *Hogan Personality Inventory manual.* Tulsa, OK: Hogan Assessment Systems.

Huang, C., Church, A., & Katigbak, M. (1997). Identifying cultural differences in items and traits: Differential item functioning in the NEO Personality Inventory. *Journal of Cross-Cultural Psychology, 28,* 192–218.

Kaplan, R. M., & Saccuzzo, D. P. (2005). *Psychological testing: Principles, applications, and issues* (6th ed.). Belmont, CA: Thomson Wadsworth.

Loevinger, J. (1954). The attenuation paradox in test theory. *Psychological Bulletin, 51,* 493–504.

Loevinger, J. (1957). Objective tests as instruments of psychological theory. *Psychological Reports, 3,* 635–694.

Mackinnon, A., Jorm, A. F., Christensen, H., Scott, L. R., Henderson, A. S., & Korten, A. E. (1995). A latent trait analysis of the Eysenck Personality Questionnaire in an elderly community sample. *Personality and Individual Differences, 18,* 739–747.

Meehl, P. E. (1945). The dynamics of structured personality tests. *Journal of Clinical Psychology, 1,* 296–303.

Messick, S. (1995). Validity of psychological assessment: Validation of inferences from persons' responses and performances as scientific inquiry into score meaning. *American Psychologist, 50,* 741–749.

Preacher, K. J., & MacCallum, R. C. (2003). Repairing Tom Swift's electric factor analysis machine. *Understanding Statistics, 2,* 13–43.

Reise, S. P., & Waller, N. G. (2003). How many IRT parameters does it take to model psychopathology items? *Psychological Methods, 8,* 164–184.

Sands, W. A., Waters, B. K., & McBride, J. R. (1997). *Computerized adaptive testing: From inquiry to operation.* Washington, DC: American Psychological Association.

Saucier, G. (1997). Effect of variable selection on the factor structure of person descriptors. *Journal of Personality and Social Psychology, 73,* 1296–1312.

Schmidt, F. L., Le, H., & Ilies, R. (2003). Beyond alpha: An empirical examination of the effects of different sources of measurement error on reliability estimates for measures of individual differences constructs. *Psychological Methods, 8,* 206–224.

Schmitt, N. (1996). Uses and abuses of coefficient alpha. *Psychological Assessment, 8,* 350–353.

Simms, L. J., Casillas, A., Clark, L. A., Watson, D., & Doebbeling, B. N. (2005). Psychometric evaluation of the restructured clinical scales of the MMPI-2. *Psychological Assessment, 17,* 345–358.

Simms, L. J., & Clark, L. A. (2005). Validation of a computerized adaptive version of the Schedule for Nonadaptive and Adaptive Personality. *Psychological Assessment, 17,* 28–43.

Smith, L. L., & Reise, S. P. (1998). Gender differences in negative affectivity: An IRT study of differential item functioning on the Multidimensional Personality Questionnaire Stress Reaction Scale. *Journal of Personality and Social Psychology, 75,* 1350–1362.

Tellegen, A., Grove, W., & Waller, N. G. (1991). *Inventory of personal characteristics #7.* Unpublished manuscript, University of Minnesota.

Tellegen, A., & Waller, N. G. (1987). *Reexamining basic dimensions of natural language trait descriptors.* Paper presented at the 95th annual meeting of the American Psychological Association, New York.

Waller, N. G. (1999). Evaluating the structure of personality. In C. R. Cloninger (Ed.), *Personality and psychopathology* (pp. 155–197). Washington, DC: American Psychiatric Press.

Watson, D. (2006). In search of construct validity: Using basic concepts and principles of psychological measurement to define child maltreatment. In M. Feerick, J. Knutson, P. Trickett, & S. Flanzer (Eds.), *Child abuse and neglect: Definitions, classifications, and a framework for research.* Baltimore: Brookes.

## CHAPTER 15

Observer Ratings of Personality

Robert R. McCrae
Alexander Weiss

Long before self-report personality scales were invented—as long ago as Theophrastus's *Characters*, 319 B.C.E.—observers described personality traits in other people. Psychoanalysts and psychiatrists developed formal languages for the description of personality traits in patients, which Block (1961) distilled into a common language in a set of Q-sort items. In psychology, perhaps the first important use of observer ratings was Webb's 1915 study of trait ratings of teacher trainees (Deary, 1996), and the discovery of the five-factor model (FFM) of personality was made through the analysis of eight observer rating studies (Tupes & Christal, 1961/1992). Yet despite their historical importance, observer ratings are used far less often than self-reports in personality assessment. This is unfortunate, because self-reports have well-known limitations, and observer ratings can complement and supplement them. There is now a solid body of evidence that ratings by informants well acquainted with a target pro-

vide reliable, stable, and valid assessments of personality traits (e.g., Funder, Kolar, & Blackman, 1995; Riemann, Angleitner, & Strelau, 1997).

There are several methods of obtaining observer rating data. When members of a group are asked to assess each other, a ranking technique is sometimes used, in which each group member ranks every other member. Alternately, group members may nominate the single individual who shows the highest level of a trait. Expert raters can be asked to complete a Q-sort to describe targets (see, e.g., Lanning, 1994). However, in recent years most informant ratings have been obtained by the use of questionnaires that parallel familiar self-report instruments. The Big Five Inventory (BFI; Benet-Martínez & John, 1998) uses a format that can be applied to either self-reports or observer ratings; the Revised NEO Personality Inventory (NEO-PI-R; Costa & McCrae, 1992) has parallel forms, with "I . . . ," "He . . . ," and "She . . . " phrasings. The first-person version is called Form S, the third-person version Form R.

Observer ratings can be used in almost every context in which self-reports are normally used, but they are particularly valuable when (1) targets are not available to make self-reports; (2) self-reports are untrustworthy; or (3) researchers wish to evaluate and improve the accuracy of assessments by aggregating multiple raters (Hofstee, 1994). In this chapter we focus on ratings of personality (including traits, motives, temperaments, and so on), but the method can also be used to assess psychopathology, moods, social attitudes, and many other psychological constructs.

A Step-by-Step Guide

Selecting or Developing the Scale

A researcher or practitioner who wishes to assess a personality construct needs some assessment instrument. For personality traits, standardized and validated instruments should be the first choice. The BFI provides a quick assessment of the five major personality factors, as does the short version of the NEO-PI-R, the NEO Five-Factor Inventory (NEO-FFI; Costa & McCrae, 1992). The full, 240-item NEO-PI-R provides more reliable measures of the factors, together with scores for 30 specific traits, or facets, that define the factors. Goldberg's (1990) adjective scales have been used for observer ratings (see, e.g., Rubenzer, Faschingbauer, & Ones, 2000). The California Adult Q-Set (CAQ; Block, 1961) was originally intended for quantifying expert ratings, but it has been adapted for lay use (Bem & Funder, 1978) and can be scored in terms of the FFM (McCrae, Costa, & Busch, 1986).

There are several considerations in selecting among these instruments. The CAQ requires the rater to sort items from least to most characteristic according to a fixed distribution. This procedure eliminates certain response biases, but it is a lengthy and cognitively challenging task relative to completing standard questionnaires. The full NEO-PI-R gives much more detailed information than the NEO-FFI, but takes correspondingly longer to complete. The Goldberg adjectives and the BFI are chiefly useful for research, because they do not offer normative information. The NEO-FFI and NEO-PI-R have norms for observer ratings, and thus

can be used in assessing individual cases as well as in research.

Observer ratings have generally been the preferred method of assessing temperament and personality in children. Among the validated measures available are the EASI-III Temperament Survey (Buss & Plomin, 1975), the Hierarchical Personality Inventory for Children (Mervielde & De Fruyt, 1999), and the California Child Q-Set (Block, 1971), which can be scored for FFM factors (John, Caspi, Robins, Moffitt, & Stouthamer-Loeber, 1994).

Because the FFM is a comprehensive model of personality traits, scales from these instruments will be relevant in most applications. In some instances, however, the construct of interest will be highly specialized (e.g., expectancy of occupational success) or only weakly related to FFM dimensions (e.g., religiosity). In these cases, researchers have two options. The first is to adapt an existing self-report scale for use by observers; the second is to develop a scale *de novo*. The first option is clearly preferable; it saves time and effort, and there is now considerable experience suggesting that observer rating adaptations of self-report instruments maintain most of the psychometric properties of the original (see, e.g., McCrae, Terracciano, et al., 2005). Research employing a newly adapted observer rating scale should ideally include established measures that can be used to provide validity evidence for the new scale.

If no established self-report measure is available, researchers can develop a new scale, following the same procedures and standards that are used in the development of self-report scales: writing relevant items, piloting the scale, examining internal consistency and factor structure, and gathering evidence of retest reliability and convergent and discriminant validity. Observer rating scales are subject to biases and response sets much as self-report scales are, and these biases must be considered in creating new scales. Acquiescent responding (McCrae, Herbst, & Costa, 2001) is effectively neutralized by including approximately equal numbers of positively and negatively keyed items. Evaluative bias in observer ratings is usually called a *halo effect*, a tendency to attribute desirable or undesirable characteristics indiscriminately to a target. Such biases can be controlled to some extent by phrasing items in objective terms, by instructing raters to give a careful and honest description of the target, and by choosing raters who are unbiased, or whose biases cancel each other out: One's true personality probably lies somewhere between the descriptions given by one's best friend and one's worst enemy.

Selecting Raters

The targets in an observer rating study are usually dictated by the research question: If one wants to look for personality predictors of heart disease, the targets will be coronary patients and controls. But there are several possibilities for selecting the raters. Researchers who are interested in impression formation normally choose unacquainted individuals and provide them with a controlled exposure to the target. For example, raters may be shown a videotape of the target in a social interaction and asked to provide ratings (Funder & Sneed, 1993). More commonly, researchers are interested in obtaining accurate assessments of the target's personality and choose raters who are already well acquainted with the target: spouses, coworkers, roommates, or friends.

There is some controversy about the effect of length of acquaintance on the accuracy of ratings. Kenny (2004) goes so far as to say that "acquaintance is not as important in person perception as generally thought" (p. 265). His conclusions are based chiefly on laboratory studies, however, where short adjective scales are typically used and correlations across raters are generally small (*Mdn r* = .15; Kenny, 2004, Table 1) and remain so after further exposure to the target. Real-life settings and questionnaire measures yield more evidence of an acquaintance effect. For example, Kurtz and Sherker (2003) used the NEO-FFI on samples of college roommates tested after 2 weeks and 15 weeks and found that median self–other agreement rose from .27 to .43 across the five scales. It is likely, however, that a ceiling is reached fairly soon in such settings, because self–peer agreement in a study that involved raters who had been acquainted with the target for up to 70 years showed a median correlation of only .41 (Costa & McCrae, 1992).

These correlations are substantially higher than the ".3 barrier" once thought to characterize the upper limit of personality scale validities, but they are also substantially less than 1.0, which would indicate perfect concordance. Researchers who want higher correlations have two choices: They can select intimate informants instead of merely well-acquainted informants, or they can aggregate judgments from multiple raters. There is evidence from American (Costa & McCrae, 1992) and Russian (McCrae et al., 2004) samples that spouse ratings agree with self-reports more highly than do other informants' ratings (*Mdn*s = .58 vs. .40), presumably because people share more personal thoughts and feelings with spouses. In a Czech study (McCrae et al., 2004), high self–other agreement (*Mdn* = .57) was found for ratings by siblings, other relatives, and friends as well as spouses. Perhaps Czechs are generally more self-disclosing than Americans and Russians.

Gathering data from multiple raters of each target has two advantages. First, one can assess interrater agreement, which gives a sense of the amount of confidence to be placed in the ratings; it is particularly useful as evidence for the validity of new scales. Second, one can aggregate (that is, average) across raters to improve the accuracy of the assessment. Agreement between raters is called *consensus* in the literature on person perception, and it can in principle arise from inaccurate shared stereotypes. But correlations between aggregated observer ratings and self-reports are less likely to be due to stereotypes, and studies show that increasing the number of raters increases self–other agreement and thus, presumably, validity. Four raters per target appears to be the practical maximum, although there are diminishing returns from any more than two raters (McCrae & Costa, 1989). There has been no systematic research on the optimal combination of raters; however, it seems that the fullest portrait would be obtained by combining reports from raters acquainted with the target in different ways—for example, a family member and a coworker, or a same-sex friend and an opposite-sex friend.

Implementing the Study

To this day, the bulk of personality research is conducted by collecting self-report data from college students. The reason for this is simply convenience: College students are at hand, and they can give informed consent and complete a questionnaire in a single sitting. It is perfectly possible to conduct observer rating studies in the same way, as long as anonymous targets are used. For example, if one wished to know whether the association between Openness to

Experience and political preferences varied across the lifespan, one could randomly assign students to think of a young, middle-aged, or old man or woman and provide ratings of their personalities and political beliefs (cf. McCrae et al., 2005).

More commonly, however, the researcher wants to know about particular targets: psychotherapy patients (see Bagby et al., 1998), job applicants, dating couples. In these situations, the design is a bit more involved. It is first necessary to identify raters, who are usually nominated by the target, and then in most cases it will be necessary to get informed consent from both target and rater. In obtaining consent, it would be important to specify what information from the observer rating, if any, would be divulged to the target: Some targets might want to participate only if they will receive feedback; some raters might want to participate only if their ratings are strictly confidential. In preparing instructions, it would be essential to make it clear to the rater who the intended target is, and to include some check on this—for example, by requiring the rater to provide the name and age of the target being rated. Beyond that, little special attention is needed in the instructions: Raters are simply asked to describe the target by judging the accuracy of personality items. People have very little difficulty with such a task. Vazire (2006) advocated and illustrated the use of informant reports in Internet assessments.

In clinical practice, a psychotherapy patient may be asked to name a significant other who could provide ratings of him or her; that person would then be contacted (perhaps by mail) and asked to provide the ratings. (Written informed consent would not be required if the data were used exclusively for clinical purposes, but mutual agreement among clinician, patient, and rater would probably be needed in order to obtain valid and clinically useful ratings.)

In the 1980s, cross-observer agreement on personality traits was offered as evidence that traits were veridical, and skeptics sometimes argued that the rater and target may have conspired to give similar ratings. Usually, instructions to avoid discussing the questionnaire with the target are sufficient; if this is a serious concern, it may be necessary to gather data in a controlled setting, with the rater physically separated from the target.

Research using couples often gathers self-reports and partner ratings from both partners. This is a rich experimental design, because it allows the researcher to study such issues as assortative mating (whether the two have similar personalities) and assumed similarity (whether people tend to see others as they themselves are). But it also requires particular care in creating a data file that clearly distinguishes the different method and target data, and that accurately matches data from the two partners. Variable labels should reflect both the source and target of the rating.

Examples of Observer Rating Research

Observer ratings can be used in almost any assessment of personality, but there are several research circumstances in which they are particularly valuable. In some of these, their value comes from their use in conjunction with self-reports. We provide three examples of these applications, in personality research, in the interpretation of an individual case, and in latent trait modeling. For other research problems, self-reports are not feasible, or even possible, and we illustrate the use of observer ratings for assessing cognitively impaired adults, historical figures, and chimpanzees. The use of observer ratings for the assessment of personality in children is already widely practiced (see, e.g., Mervielde & De Fruyt, 1999).

Personality Research in the Augmented Baltimore Longitudinal Study of Aging

Some of the research that led to the prominence of the FFM was conducted in the 1980s on members of the Augmented Baltimore Longitudinal Study of Aging (ABLSA). The BLSA (Baltimore Longitudinal Study of Aging) itself was begun in 1958 as a study of aging men; in 1978 women were added to the study, but at a rather modest rate. Participants visited the Gerontology Research Center every 1–2 years to complete a battery of biomedical and psychosocial tests. To increase the number of women in the study, we augmented the BLSA by inviting the spouses of then current BLSA members to complete questionnaires at home (McCrae, 1982). Among the first data gathered from the ABLSA in 1980 were self-reports on the NEO Inventory, a three-factor precursor of the NEO-PI-R, and, a few months later, spouse ratings on a third-person version of the NEO Inventory. As new versions of the instrument were developed that included scales for Agreeableness and Conscientiousness, both Form S and Form R were readministered. Beginning in 1983, ABLSA participants were asked to nominate peer raters, and these individuals in turn were asked to complete Form R to describe the participants. The NEO-PI-R was administered to peer raters in 1990.

These data, in combination with the other psychological data collected in the BLSA and ABLSA, led to several key findings:

• Different observers agreed with each other and with self-reports at a level that was both statistically significant and socially important, and the differences in method made it unlikely that this was the result of artifacts. Personality traits could be consensually validated, and thus the claim, prevalent in the 1970s, that traits were mere cognitive fictions could be dismissed (McCrae, 1982).

• When a self-report scale is correlated with a measure of social desirability, it may mean that the scale is contaminated by the desire of the individual to present him- or herself in a flattering light, or it may mean that the social desirability measure is actually assessing genuine aspects of personality. Researchers routinely presumed that the former interpretation was correct, and the dispute could not be resolved if only self-reports were available. But significant correlations between self-reported social desirability scales and observer ratings of personality could not plausibly be attributed to a shared bias, and thus demonstrated that social desirability scales assess more substance than style (McCrae & Costa, 1983).

• Longitudinal studies of self-reports had consistently shown that individual differences in personality traits are extremely stable in adults, with uncorrected retest correlations near .80 over 6–10-year intervals. But perhaps that simply reflected the effects of a crystallized self-concept; people might be blind to changes in their basic personality traits. If personality changed with age whereas self-concept did not, self-reports should become increasingly inaccurate, and self–other agreement should be lower for old than for young targets. Observer rating data showed that was not the case (McCrae & Costa, 1982), and longitudinal stability coefficients in observer rating data were as high as in self-reports (Costa & McCrae, 1988).

• In principle, NEO-PI-R facet scale scores contain variance common to the five factors, variance that is specific to the facet, and error. But unless there is substantial specific variance, there is no need to assess facets; all personality traits would simply be combinations of the five factors. It was possible to separate the specific variance from the common variance by partialling out the factor scores, but against what criteria could one validate the residuals? Residuals from observer ratings of the same facets were the natural choice, and correlations of the residuals from the two methods in fact demonstrated the consensual validation of specific variance in NEO-PI-R facet scales (McCrae & Costa, 1992).

• The wish that we could "see oursels as others see us" (in Burns's language) is based on the widespread belief that there are noticeably different public and private selves. Hogan and Hogan (1992) referred to the former as *reputation* and believed that the private self, available to introspection, must show a different structure of personality. But the same FFM is found in self-reports and observer ratings (Ostendorf & Angleitner, 2004), and agreement among different observers is not systematically higher than agreement between self and other (McCrae & Costa, 1989). The distinction between public and private selves is thus in some sense an illusion; there is no perfect consensus on our public self that we could hope to see, and our self-reports are not based on some direct intuition of our inner nature, but on self-observations that substantially overlap with what others observe.

• The essence of good science is replication, and multimethod replications are powerful because they reduce the possibility that findings are due to some artifact of a particular method. In ABLSA studies, we showed that self-reports on the NEO-PI-R were related to psychological well-being, interpersonal traits, Jungian types, and ways of coping. All of these findings were replicated when spouse or peer ratings were used as the measure of personality (Costa & McCrae, 1992).

Interpreting a Case Study: Madeline G

Costa and Piedmont (2003) reported a study of Madeline G, a flamboyant Native American lawyer who volunteered to be a case study for a variety of personality assessors (Wiggins, 2003). She completed Form S of the NEO-PI-R, and her common-law husband completed Form R to describe her.

Consistent with the general impression that she was a volatile and forceful character,

Madeline G's responses consisted almost exclusively of *strongly disagree* (33.8%) or *strongly agree* (48.8%), and the resulting profile was correspondingly extreme: Four of the five domains and 25 of the 30 facets were in the "Very Low" or "Very High" range. Such a profile is statistically very unusual, and in isolation it would have been difficult to know whether it was meaningful or merely an artifact of extreme responding. A comparison with Form R was therefore more than usually informative in this case. Although not as extreme, her husband's descriptions agreed in direction with her self-reports for three factors and 19 facets, suggesting that her self-reports were exaggerated but not meaningless.

It is possible to assess the degree of agreement between two personality profiles (for example, Madeline G's self-report and her husband's rating of her), although all the currently used metrics have limitations. As Cattell pointed out in 1949, simple Pearson correlations are problematic because they reflect only the similarity of shape of the profile, not similarity of level. Cattell's proposed alternative, r_p, takes into account the difference between profile elements, but not the extremeness of the trait. When Madeline G scores $T = 16$ on Agreeableness, whereas her husband places her at $T = 4$ (where T-scores have a mean of 50 and standard deviation of 10), there is more than a standard deviation difference between the scores—yet both depict her as profoundly antagonistic (recall that she was a lawyer). McCrae (1993) proposed a different metric, the coefficient of profile agreement, r_{pa}, that is sensitive to both the difference between corresponding profile elements and the extremeness of the average score.

The computer-generated Interpretive Report (Costa & McCrae, 1992; Costa, McCrae, & PAR Staff, 1994) for the NEO-PI-R calculates this quantity and shows in the case of Madeline G that agreement is .95, which is very good as compared with agreement between most married couples. The high value is found in spite of major disagreements between the two sources on some factors and facets, because r_{pa} takes extremeness of scores into account, and Madeline G has a very extreme profile. In such cases, r_{pa} probably overestimates agreement; this is one of its limitations. But empirical tests (McCrae, 1993) have shown that it is generally superior to Cattell's r_p as a measure of overall profile agreement.

The Interpretive Report also uses r_{pa} statistics to pinpoint agreement or disagreement on specific factors and facets. Madeline and her husband disagreed on 12 facets and on two factors, Neuroticism and Conscientiousness. Madeline regarded herself as very low in Neuroticism and high in Conscientiousness, whereas her husband saw her as high in Neuroticism and low in Conscientiousness. Within the six Conscientiousness facets, there was both agreement and disagreement: Both believed that she was high in C4: Achievement Striving and very low in C6: Deliberation, but she saw herself as high in C3: Dutifulness, whereas he saw her as very low. Here is a woman with lofty goals who sets out to achieve them without much thought about the ramifications of her actions. Perhaps she focused on the ends and viewed herself as highly principled; perhaps he focused on the means and saw her as unscrupulous.

How should observer rating data be integrated with self-report data in the interpretation of individual cases? First, they can be used to evaluate the quality of the self-report. Many validity scales have been devised to assess the trustworthiness of self-reports, but evidence suggests that they are of limited value (Piedmont, McCrae, Riemann, & Angleitner, 2000). An independent source of information is preferable. A comparison with her husband's ratings suggests that, overall, Madeline's self-report is valid, but that there are some particular trait assessments (such as C3: Dutifulness) that are questionable.

Second, the two sources can be combined to provide an optimal estimate of personality trait levels. It is probable that Madeline is neither as dutiful as she says nor as unethical as her husband claims; averaging them should give a better estimate of the true level. (In fact, the Interpretive Report provides an average with a slight adjustment to account for the fact that the variance of means is reduced; see McCrae, Stone, Fagan, & Costa, 1998.)

But there is a third possibility, of particular importance in clinical settings, where the psychologist expects to interact with the client on repeated occasions. It is not necessary to stop the assessment after the questionnaires have been scored. Instead, discrepancies between two sources ought to be explored with the client, the observer, or both. On the one hand, that should yield a better assessment of the disputed trait; on the other hand, it may offer insights into the nature of their relationship. It does not bode well for a marriage when one partner thinks the other is unethical, and in this case, Madeline G's relationship ended shortly after the assessments.

The Estimation of Latent Traits

Riemann and colleagues (1997) provided an elegant example of the integrative use of data from multiple observers and self-reports. They assessed personality using self-reports and ratings from two informants on the NEO-FFI in a sample of mono- and dizygotic twins. Typically, behavior genetic studies use only self-reports and partition the variance into genetic, shared environmental, and nonshared environmental effects. Most behavior genetic studies of personality have shown that the shared environment (experiences shared by children living in the same family) accounts for little or no variance; instead, personality is about equally determined by genetic influences and the nonshared environment (Bouchard & Loehlin, 2001). When Riemann and colleagues analyzed self-reports, they reported heritabilities, a measure of the proportion of variance that arises from genetic differences, of .42–.56.

In these analyses, however, the *nonshared environment* term is somewhat mysterious: It includes real effects on personality that are due to unique experiences of different children in the same family (such as the fact that one took piano lessons whereas the other studied the flute), but it also includes measurement error. It is possible to eliminate random measurement error by correcting for test unreliability; this typically increases the estimate of genetic effects modestly.

But reliability estimates only deal with random error, not systematic bias. For example, a rater may think that a target is more extraverted than the target actually is, but because the rater maintains this view consistently, the misperception does not introduce unreliability. Riemann and colleagues (1997) used data from two raters to estimate heritability using latent trait analyses, in which both random error and systematic biases of the two raters were statistically controlled. In this design, the heritabilities were higher (.57–.81); and when the latent traits (the "true scores") were estimated from a combination of self-reports and the two informant ratings, heritabilities were generally even higher, .66–.79. This study suggests that the

heritability of personality traits has been systematically and substantially underestimated by monomethod studies.

Monomethod studies may also have been misleading with respect to factor intercorrelations. Digman (1997) proposed that the Big Five factors were themselves intercorrelated, yielding two factors he called α, Personal Growth, and β, Socialization. Markon, Krueger, and Watson (2005) elaborated on this scheme, using data from a meta-analysis of self-report studies. However, using multitrait–multimethod confirmatory factor analyses of self-reports and peer and parent ratings, Biesanz and West (2004) found that "none of the Big Five latent factors were significantly correlated" (p. 865), and suggested that within-method evaluative biases were probably responsible for the apparent higher-order structure of FFM factors.

Personality and Its Changes in Alzheimer's Disease

Although geriatricians have often observed that there seem to be personality changes in patients with Alzheimer's disease, there was very little research on the topic until the 1990s. One of the major reasons for that was, of course, that the self-report instruments typically used to assess personality were of dubious applicability. Would dementing patients have insight into their own personality, or indeed, would they be able to complete a questionnaire at all? Certainly not in the later stages of the disease.

Siegler and her colleagues realized that observer ratings provided a feasible alternative (Siegler et al., 1991). They asked caregivers to rate 35 patients with memory impairment on an older version of the NEO-PI-R in two conditions: as they were now, and as they had been before onset of the disease (the premorbid ratings). The premorbid profiles were generally in the normal range, but there were dramatic differences for the current descriptions: Patients were seen as high in Neuroticism, low in Extraversion, and very low in Conscientiousness. The increase in Neuroticism was not surprising, because Alzheimer's disease had often been linked to depression. But no one had anticipated changes in Conscientiousness, although they seem obvious in hindsight: People who have difficulty concentrating and remembering show behavior that is poorly organized and not goal directed.

That groundbreaking study, subsequently replicated by several teams of investigators, was imperfect in a few respects. First, it was not clear whether the premorbid ratings were accurate, because they depended on the memory of the caregiver and might be distorted by contrast with current traits. For example, premorbid Conscientiousness might have been overestimated because it was so much higher than current levels. Strauss, Pasupathi, and Chatterjee (1993) recruited two independent raters—the caregiver and another friend or relative—and asked for premorbid and current ratings of the patient. The two raters generally agreed on both ratings, suggesting that both were accurate reflections of the patient's personality at different times.

In a later study, Strauss and Pasupathi (1994) obtained observer ratings of Alzheimer's patients on two occasions, 1 year apart. They showed continuing changes in the direction of higher Neuroticism and lower Conscientiousness over the course of the year, suggesting that observer ratings are sensitive to relatively small changes.

Observer ratings have also been used to study other psychiatric disorders in which self-reports from patients were suspect, including Parkinson's disease and traumatic brain injury. In addition, Duberstein, Conwell, and Caine (1994) gathered informant reports about suicide completers as part of a "psychological autopsy," which suggested that suicide completers are more likely to be closed than open to experience.

Portraits of Historical Figures

Was Abe really honest? Was Washington cold? We cannot ask these men to complete self-report questionnaires, and it is not clear how much we would learn from reading the many biographies that have been written about each of them, because the data would not be standardized in a way that could make meaningful comparisons possible. Rubenzer and colleagues (2000) solved this problem by inviting biographers of U.S. presidents to describe their subjects using observer rating forms of the NEO-PI-R, the California Adult Q-Set (Block, 1961), and a set of adjective scales (Goldberg, 1990). (See Song and Simonton, Chapter 18, this volume, for another approach to the assessment of historical figures.)

It is one thing to ask caregivers to rate the personality of an Alzheimer's patient as he or she was 5 years ago; it is another to ask historians to rate the personality of an individual who has been dead for two centuries. How would they respond to items like "[George Washington] really loves the excitement of roller coasters" or "[Abraham Lincoln] believes that the 'new morality' of permissiveness is no morality at all," when these are clearly anachronistic? Fortunately, Rubenzer and colleagues (2000) identified only three such items in the NEO-PI-R, and even those could probably be meaningfully rated: Does anyone really think that Washington would have loved roller coaster rides if he had been given the opportunity to try one?

Rubenzer and colleagues argued that their assessments were valid because they were internally consistent and showed cross-rater agreement (using the r_{pa} measure) comparable to that seen in contemporary peer rating studies. Based on descriptions by 10 experts, George Washington was average in Neuroticism, low in Extraversion, Openness, and Agreeableness, and very high in Conscientiousness—a portrait that seems to aptly characterize his steadfast but formal personality. Lincoln was rather more interesting, scoring high on Neuroticism, Extraversion, Agreeableness, and Conscientiousness, and very high on Openness. The high Neuroticism scores are consistent with his well-known episodes of depression, and the high Openness is seen in his legendary love of books. Curiously, although he was generally agreeable, he was ranked very low in Straightforwardness, being a far shrewder politician than he pretended to be.

McCrae (1996) reported a case study of the French-Swiss philosopher, composer, and novelist, Jean-Jacques Rousseau. Figure 15.1 shows his profile, based on ratings by a political scientist who had written a book on his political ideology. In this figure, the five factor scores are given on the left, and the 30 facet scales are grouped by factor toward the right. Because only one rater was available, interrater agreement could not be assessed, but this profile is consistent with the writings of Rousseau's contemporaries, who described both his paranoia and his genius. Like Madeline G, Rousseau shows an extreme profile, with scores literally off the chart for several facets (e.g., N4: Self-Consciousness, O1: Fantasy). Perhaps this reflects the rater's use of extreme response options, but it must be recalled that Rousseau was one of the most extraordinary figures in history, and these ratings may be completely accu-

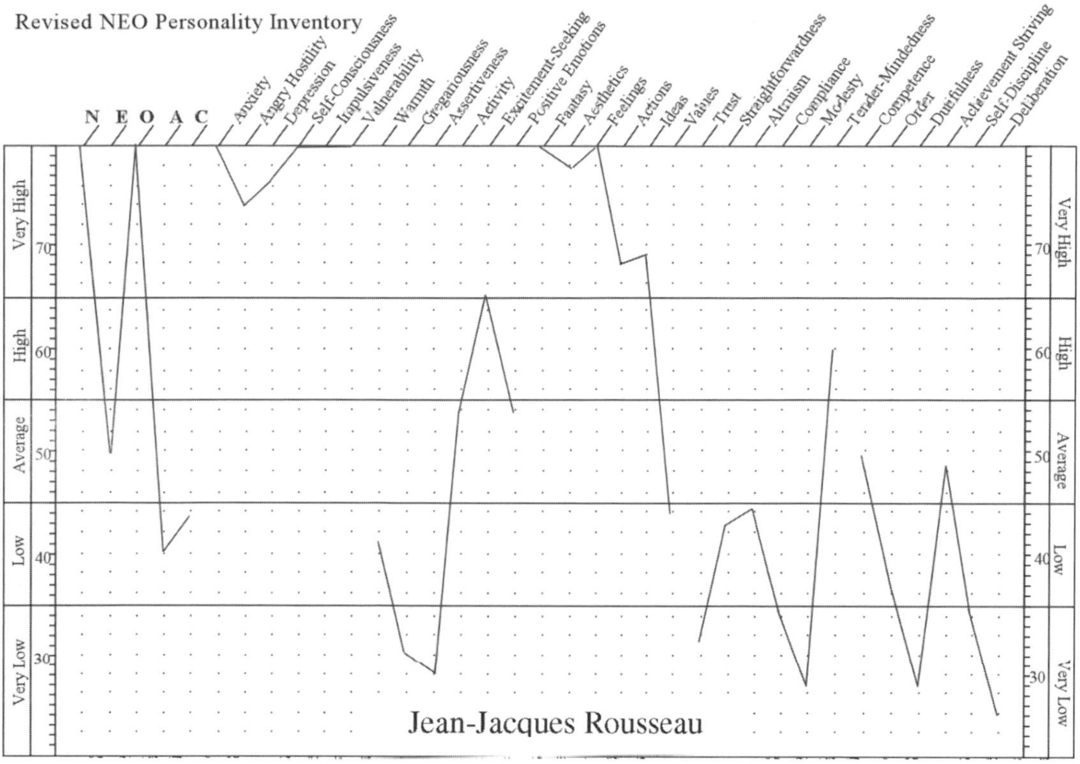

FIGURE 15.1. Revised NEO Personality Inventory profile for J.-J. Rousseau, as rated by A. M. Melzer. Adapted from McCrae (1996). Profile form reproduced by special permission of the publisher, Psychological Assessment Resources, Inc., 16204 North Florida Avenue, Lutz, Florida 33549, from the Revised NEO Personality Inventory by Paul T. Costa, Jr., and Robert R. McCrae. Copyright 1978, 1985, 1989, 1992 by PAR, Inc. Further reproduction is prohibited without permission of PAR, Inc.

rate. If the reader still feels the need for a second opinion on Rousseau—good. Personality psychologists, clinicians, and historians should all cultivate a taste for multiple assessments of personality (McCrae, 1994).

Personality Assessment in Chimpanzees

Another chapter (Vazire, Gosling, Dickey, & Schapiro, Chapter 11, this volume) discusses the use of observer ratings to assess personality in other species, but we feel it is worth focusing on some issues in observer ratings of the personality of our closest nonhuman relatives, chimpanzees (*Pan troglodytes*). King and Figueredo (1997) asked zoo workers to rate individual chimpanzees on a 43-item questionnaire that was based on adjective measures of the FFM. Each adjective was accompanied by a short description to clarify the intended construct. Factor analysis of the 43 items suggested

six factors. The first factor, Dominance, was a large chimpanzee-specific factor that was indicative of competitive prowess. The remaining five factors were analogous to the domains of the FFM.

Because the validity of observer ratings of chimpanzee personality cannot be assessed by comparing them with self-reports, King and Figueredo (1997) had multiple raters assess each target and used intraclass correlations to show that individual $[ICC(3, 1)]$ and mean $[ICC(3, k)]$ ratings were consistent across raters (Shrout & Fleiss, 1979). The interrater reliability of individual ratings can be used to compare reliabilities of similar factors across different species even if the number of raters differs. The interrater reliability of mean ratings is typically used to describe the reliability of scores based on multiple raters. Because using a mean of several ratings will reduce measurement error, it should be no surprise that the reliability of mean ratings will be higher.

A recent study (King, Weiss, & Farmer, 2005) on the personality of chimpanzees in zoos and in a sanctuary in the Republic of Congo (Brazzaville) challenged Kenny's (2004) conclusion that length of acquaintance has little effect on the reliability of ratings. Raters at zoos knew their charges for an average of 6.5 years, and there were a mean of 3.7 raters per zoo chimpanzee. Raters at the sanctuary knew their charges for a mean of only 6.9 months, but each chimpanzee in this habitat was rated by an average of 16.2 raters (King et al., 2005). Interrater reliabilities of individual ratings were considerably higher (*Mdn* = .46) for ratings of chimpanzees in zoos than for ratings at the sanctuary (*Mdn* = .26), suggesting that length of acquaintance does affect accuracy, and that one should be skeptical of any conclusions drawn from single ratings of chimpanzees based on limited acquaintance. However, the same study showed that the reliabilities of the mean ratings of the chimpanzees in the African sanctuary (*Mdn* = .87) were comparable to or greater than those of chimpanzees living in zoos (*Mdn* = .77). In short, the use of more raters per chimpanzee all but eliminated any disparity between the reliabilities of ratings that arose due to differences in the length of acquaintance.

Observer ratings of chimpanzee personality traits can also be validated by a pattern of correlations with external criteria. Supporting evidence has been found in two studies that have related each of the chimpanzee factors to frequencies of relevant behaviors (Pederson, King, & Landau, 2005), and Dominance, Extraversion, and Dependability (analogous to Conscientiousness) to ratings of subjective well-being (King & Landau, 2003).

Cautions in the Use of Observer Ratings

We advocate multimethod approaches to personality assessment because no method, including observer ratings, is perfect. Some of the potential problems with observer ratings are familiar to readers of the self-report literature. Acquiescence, extreme responding, and random responding are threats to the validity of observer ratings, much as they are to the validity of self-reports. Efforts to identify or correct invalid protocols have so far met with limited success (Piedmont et al., 2000), in part because

even carelessly completed inventories typically have some useful information: The validity of most assessments is a matter of degree (Carter et al., 2001). Users of both Form S and Form R of the NEO-PI-R are thus given four rather conservative rules for discarding protocols as invalid: (1) more than 40 missing items; (2) a response of *disagree* or *strongly disagree* to the validity check item "I have tried to answer all these questions honestly and accurately;" (3) a *no* response to the validity check item "Have you entered your responses in the correct areas?;" or (4) random responding, as evidenced by strings of repetitive responses (e.g., more than six consecutive *strongly disagree*s). Even in these instances, however, clinicians are advised to retain the responses, discuss the potential problems with the respondent, and interpret the profile cautiously. For research purposes, the optimal solution is to score all protocols (replacing missing items with *neutral* or the group mean) and report analyses with and without the exclusion of nominally invalid protocols.

McCrae and colleagues (2005) extended the assessment of protocol validity to entire samples in their cross-cultural study of observer-rated personality. Personality questionnaires are familiar to American and European college students, but they are less widely used in Asia and Africa, so there is reason to believe that the quality of personality data might be better in some cultures than in others. McCrae and colleagues created a Quality Index that took into account random responding, acquiescence, missing data, the fluency of the sample in the language of the questionnaire, the quality of the translation, and miscellaneous problems reported by the test administrator. This index was not used to exclude samples, but to help interpret the data. For example, the factor structure of NEO-PI-R Form R was less well replicated in African cultures. Was that because African cultures have a personality structure that is different from that of Americans, or was it simply due to error of measurement? The fact that the Quality Index was low in most of the African cultures suggested the latter interpretation, and when noise was reduced by pooling responses from the five African cultures, the FFM structure was clearly replicated.

Judging by the attention it has been given by psychometricians, the major concern with self-reports is social desirability, individual differences in the tendency to exaggerate one's strengths and minimize one's failings. One of the chief merits of observer ratings is that they do not share this bias: Mary Jones may be particularly prone to socially desirable responding, but there is usually no reason to think that her raters will also feel a need to paint a rosy picture of her.

Although the assessment and control of individual differences in socially desirable responding is problematic (Piedmont et al., 2000), this does not mean that there are no evaluative biases in self-reports and observer ratings. Individuals who are applying for a job typically score higher on self-reports of all desirable traits than disinterested volunteers, and their scores must be interpreted in terms of job applicant norms, not volunteer norms. Similar biases might well be found in observer ratings if the observer has an interest in the outcome. For example, spouse ratings of job applicants might also be unrealistically favorable, because the whole family would benefit from the job offer.

A striking instance of negative bias in observer ratings was reported by Langer (2004), who administered Form S and Form R of the NEO-PI-R to 20 couples being evaluated for child custody litigation. Their mean self-reports for the five factors all fell within the normal range, although they tended toward higher-than-average Extraversion, Agreeableness, and Conscientiousness, and lower-than-average Neuroticism scores. Their mean ratings of their spouses, however, were dramatically different: They described their spouses as high in Neuroticism, low in Openness, and very low (mean T-scores = 26.3 and 25.2) in Agreeableness and Conscientiousness. The moral is that in interpreting observer rating data in groups or individuals, one must take into account normative biases attributable to the situation. (Among chimpanzees, situational biases to consider in rater reports may include whether the individuals live in the wild, in sanctuaries, or in research labs.) Ideally, this would mean the use of relevant norms (e.g., from a large sample of spouse ratings of custody litigants); otherwise, clinical judgment must be used to discount suspicious data. It is of considerable interest that Langer reported Form S/Form R correlations ranging from .18 to .46 for the five factors, with significant agreement for Extraversion and Openness. This suggests that some validity in individual differences is retained even when the mean levels are dramatically distorted.

Future Directions

Research on Ratings

A number of researchers have been interested in the factors that affect agreement between judges (Funder et al., 1995; John & Robins, 1993). Differences in observability and evaluation appear to influence cross-observer agreement, and Extraversion is usually found to be the most consensually rated factor (Borkenau & Liebler, 1995). In a cross-cultural extension of that work, McCrae and colleagues (2004) reported similar findings for American and European samples, but not for Chinese data. Perhaps agreement across raters depends on the salience of the trait in the raters' culture.

There is ample evidence that ratings from observers who are well acquainted with the target provide reliable and valid assessments of the full range of personality traits, but many questions remain about how to optimize observer rating assessments. Is some particular combination of raters (e.g., a spouse and a friend) preferable, and should these sources be differentially weighted? Should special instructions be given, perhaps asking raters to focus on the person in a particular context (at work, at home), or emphasizing that they should report both strengths and weaknesses? We know already that observer rating methods and instruments work well in translation and across a variety of cultures (McCrae et al., 2005); are any special problems posed by the use of informant ratings of personality gathered via the Internet (e.g., "flaming")?

In most cases, research using observer ratings replicates findings based on self-reports, but in a few instances, substantive findings differ across these methods. For example, cross-sectional ratings of Agreeableness consistently increase across the adult lifespan when self-reports are examined, but not when observer ratings are analyzed (McCrae et al., 2005). How do we account for such discrepancies, and which set of findings should we believe?

In the assessment of chimpanzee personality, continued work is needed on assessment instruments. One important question about chimpanzee personality is whether deviations from the FFM structure previously reported are an artifact of the specific measure. The questionnaire King and Figueredo (1997) used was based on the human FFM, but it was not a standard measure, and it was modified for use with chimpanzees. Thus, we do not know whether the Dominance factor and a unipolar Agreeableness factor found in chimpanzees reflect unique characteristics of chimpanzees' personality trait structure, or whether these are attributable to the particular set of adjectives chosen. Observer rating studies need to be conducted in which human targets are rated on the chimpanzee personality questionnaire and a well-validated measure of the FFM. Factor analysis of the chimpanzee items in this human sample would indicate whether the human or chimpanzee structure would be found using this instrument (cf. Gosling, Kwan, & John, 2003). Correlations with the FFM measure would aid in the interpretation of the chimpanzee items and factors.

Wider Applications

Observer ratings provide a simple, valid, and still underutilized source of personality data. If researchers want to evaluate the correlation of Scale A with Scale B, they typically administer them to college students. There is no reason why the students should not be asked to provide observer ratings rather than (or in addition to) self-reports. With some thought, researchers may be able to obtain more generalizable findings in this way, by requiring that raters select targets of specified age, gender, or socioeconomic status (SES).

Informant ratings can also be used effectively on hypothetical targets. The Personality Profiles of Cultures Project (Terracciano et al., 2005) included informant reports on the traits of the "typical" member of each culture, allowing a comparison of national stereotypes (e.g., the typical Canadian is thought to be more compliant than the typical American). Informants can rate ideal romantic partners (Figueredo et al., 2005) or preferred roommates. Strictly speaking, these are not observer ratings, because the hypothetical targets have not been observed. They do, however, provide useful psychological information using the observer rating methodology.

Observer ratings have one more important feature that makes them especially valuable for survey research: They require minimal involvement of the target. Survey researchers often complain that their interviews do not leave enough time to administer a full personality inventory, and if they assess personality at all, it is likely to be with a handful of questions of limited reliability. But most survey respondents can easily identify a significant other or friend who could be asked to make ratings of the respondent's personality and return them to the interviewer, either in person or by mail (cf. Achenbach, Krukowski, Dumenci, & Ivanova, 2005). Although those data might not meet the stringent sampling requirements of the study, they would provide important auxiliary information that could confirm or extend results of the interview assessment and validate the abbreviated self-report personality assessments. Obviously, the same advantage should make observer ratings attractive to clinicians or researchers whose current test batteries already tax the patience of their clients or research participants.

Acknowledgment

This research was supported by the Intramural Research Program of the National Institutes of Health, National Institute on Aging.

Recommended Readings

Benet-Martínez, V., & John, O. P. (1998). *Los Cinco Grandes* across cultures and ethnic groups: Multitrait multimethod analyses of the Big Five in Spanish and English. *Journal of Personality and Social Psychology, 75,* 729–750.

Costa, P. T., Jr., & Piedmont, R. L. (2003). Multivariate assessment: NEO-PI-R profiles of Madeline G. In J. S. Wiggins (Ed.), *Paradigms of personality assessment* (pp. 262–280). New York: Guilford Press.

Funder, D. C., Kolar, D. C., & Blackman, M. C. (1995). Agreement among judges of personality: Interpersonal relations, similarity, and acquaintanceship. *Journal of Personality and Social Psychology, 69,* 656–672.

Kenny, D. A. (2004). PERSON: A general model of interpersonal perception. *Personality and Social Psychology Review, 8,* 265–280.

McCrae, R. R. (1994). The counterpoint of personality assessment: Self-reports and observer ratings. *Assessment, 1,* 159–172.

McCrae, R. R., Stone, S. V., Fagan, P. J., & Costa, P. T., Jr. (1998). Identifying causes of disagreement between self-reports and spouse ratings of personality. *Journal of Personality, 66,* 285–313.

References

Achenbach, T. M., Krukowski, R. A., Dumenci, L., & Ivanova, M. Y. (2005). Assessment of adult psychopathology: Meta-analyses and implications of cross-informant correlations. *Psychological Bulletin, 131,* 361–382.

Bagby, R. M., Rector, N. A., Bindseil, K., Dickens, S. E.,

Levitan, R. D., & Kennedy, S. H. (1998). Self-report ratings and informant ratings of personalities of depressed outpatients. *American Journal of Psychiatry, 155,* 437–438.

Bem, D. J., & Funder, D. C. (1978). Predicting more of the people more of the time: Assessing the personality of situations. *Psychological Review, 85,* 485–501.

Benet-Martínez, V., & John, O. P. (1998). Los Cinco Grandes across cultures and ethnic groups: Multitrait multimethod analyses of the Big Five in Spanish and English. *Journal of Personality and Social Psychology, 75,* 729–750.

Biesanz, J. C., & West, S. G. (2004). Towards understanding assessments of the Big Five: Multitrait-multimethod analyses of convergent and discriminant validity across measurement occasion and type of observer. *Journal of Personality, 72,* 845–876.

Block, J. (1961). *The Q-sort method in personality assessment and psychiatric research.* Springfield, IL: Charles C. Thomas.

Block, J. (1971). *Lives through time.* Berkeley, CA: Bancroft Books.

Borkenau, P., & Liebler, A. (1995). Observable attributes as manifestations and cues of personality and intelligence. *Journal of Personality, 63,* 1–25.

Bouchard, T. J., & Loehlin, J. C. (2001). Genes, evolution, and personality. *Behavior Genetics, 31,* 243–273.

Buss, A. H., & Plomin, R. (1975). *A temperament theory of personality development.* New York: Wiley.

Carter, J. A., Herbst, J. H., Stoller, K. B., King, V. L., Kidorf, M. S., Costa, P. T., Jr., et al. (2001). Short-term stability of NEO-PI-R personality trait scores in opioid-dependent outpatients. *Psychology of Addictive Behaviors, 15,* 255–260.

Cattell, R. B. (1949). r_p and other coefficients of pattern similarity. *Psychometrica, 14,* 279–298.

Costa, P. T., Jr., & McCrae, R. R. (1988). Personality in adulthood: A six-year longitudinal study of self-reports and spouse ratings on the NEO Personality Inventory. *Journal of Personality and Social Psychology, 54,* 853–863.

Costa, P. T., Jr., & McCrae, R. R. (1992). *Revised NEO Personality Inventory (NEO-PI-R) and NEO Five-Factor Inventory (NEO-FFI) professional manual.* Odessa, FL: Psychological Assessment Resources.

Costa, P. T., Jr., McCrae, R. R., & PAR Staff. (1994). NEO Software System [Computer software]. Odessa, FL: Psychological Assessment Resources.

Costa, P. T., Jr., & Piedmont, R. L. (2003). Multivariate assessment: NEO PI-R profiles of Madeline G. In J. S. Wiggins (Ed.), *Paradigms of personality assessment* (pp. 262–280). New York: Guilford Press.

Deary, I. J. (1996). A (latent) Big Five personality model in 1915? A reanalysis of Webb's data. *Journal of Personality and Social Psychology, 71,* 992–1005.

Digman, J. M. (1997). Higher-order factors of the Big Five. *Journal of Personality and Social Psychology, 73,* 1246–1256.

Duberstein, P. R., Conwell, Y., & Caine, E. D. (1994). Age differences in the personality characteristics of suicide completers: Preliminary findings from a psy-chological autopsy study. *Psychiatry: Interpersonal and Biological Processes, 57,* 213–224.

Figueredo, A. J., Sefcek, J., Vasquez, G., Brumbach, B. H., King, J. E., & Jacobs, W. J. (2005). Evolutionary personality psychology. In D. M. Buss (Ed.), *Handbook of evolutionary psychology* (pp. 851–877). Hoboken, NJ: Wiley.

Funder, D. C., Kolar, D. C., & Blackman, M. C. (1995). Agreement among judges of personality: Interpersonal relations, similarity, and acquaintanceship. *Journal of Personality and Social Psychology, 69,* 656–672.

Funder, D. C., & Sneed, C. D. (1993). Behavioral manifestations of personality: An ecological approach to judgmental accuracy. *Journal of Personality and Social Psychology, 64,* 479–490.

Goldberg, L. R. (1990). An alternative "description of personality": The Big-Five factor structure. *Journal of Personality and Social Psychology, 59,* 1216–1229.

Gosling, S. D., Kwan, V. S. Y., & John, O. P. (2003). A dog's got personality: A cross-species comparative approach to personality judgments in dogs and humans. *Journal of Personality and Social Psychology, 85,* 1161–1169.

Hofstee, W. K. B. (1994). Who should own the definition of personality? *European Journal of Personality, 8,* 149–162.

Hogan, R., & Hogan, J. (1992). *Hogan Personality Inventory manual.* Tulsa, OK: Hogan Assessment Systems.

John, O. P., Caspi, A., Robins, R. W., Moffitt, T. E., & Stouthamer-Loeber, M. (1994). The "little five": Exploring the five-factor model of personality in adolescent boys. *Child Development, 65,* 160–178.

John, O. P., & Robins, R. W. (1993). Determinants of interjudge agreement on personality traits: The Big Five domains, observability, evaluativeness, and the unique perspective of the self. *Journal of Personality, 61,* 521–551.

Kenny, D. A. (2004). PERSON: A general model of interpersonal perception. *Personality and Social Psychology Review, 8,* 265–280.

King, J. E., & Figueredo, A. J. (1997). The Five-Factor Model plus Dominance in chimpanzee personality. *Journal of Research in Personality, 31,* 257–271.

King, J. E., & Landau, V. I. (2003). Can chimpanzee (*Pan troglodytes*) happiness be estimated by human raters? *Journal of Research in Personality, 37,* 1–15.

King, J. E., Weiss, A., & Farmer, K. H. (2005). A chimpanzee (*Pan troglodytes*) analogue of cross-national generalization of personality structure: Zoological parks and an African sanctuary. *Journal of Personality, 73,* 389–410.

Kurtz, J. E., & Sherker, J. L. (2003). Relationship quality, trait similarity, and self–other agreement on personality traits in college roommates. *Journal of Personality, 71,* 21–48.

Langer, F. (2004). Pairs, reflections, and the EgoI: Exploration of a perceptual hypothesis. *Journal of Personality Assessment, 82,* 114–126.

Lanning, K. (1994). Dimensionality of observer ratings

on the California Adult *Q*-Set. *Journal of Personality and Social Psychology, 67*, 151–160.

Markon, K. E., Krueger, R. F., & Watson, D. (2005). Delineating the structure of normal and abnormal personality: An integrative hierarchical approach. *Journal of Personality and Social Psychology, 88*, 139–157.

McCrae, R. R. (1982). Consensual validation of personality traits: Evidence from self-reports and ratings. *Journal of Personality and Social Psychology, 43*, 293–303.

McCrae, R. R. (1993). Agreement of personality profiles across observers. *Multivariate Behavioral Research, 28*, 13–28.

McCrae, R. R. (1994). The counterpoint of personality assessment: Self-reports and observer ratings. *Assessment, 1*, 159–172.

McCrae, R. R. (1996). Social consequences of experiential openness. *Psychological Bulletin, 120*, 323–337.

McCrae, R. R., & Costa, P. T., Jr. (1982). Self-concept and the stability of personality: Cross-sectional comparisons of self-reports and ratings. *Journal of Personality and Social Psychology, 43*, 1282–1292.

McCrae, R. R., & Costa, P. T., Jr. (1983). Social desirability scales: More substance than style. *Journal of Consulting and Clinical Psychology, 51*, 882–888.

McCrae, R. R., & Costa, P. T., Jr. (1989). Different points of view: Self-reports and ratings in the assessment of personality. In J. P. Forgas & M. J. Innes (Eds.), *Recent advances in social psychology: An international perspective* (pp. 429–439). Amsterdam: Elsevier Science.

McCrae, R. R., & Costa, P. T., Jr. (1992). Discriminant validity of NEO-PI-R facets. *Educational and Psychological Measurement, 52*, 229–237.

McCrae, R. R., Costa, P. T., Jr., & Busch, C. M. (1986). Evaluating comprehensiveness in personality systems: The California *Q*-Set and the five-factor model. *Journal of Personality, 54*, 430–446.

McCrae, R. R., Costa, P. T., Jr., Martin, T. A., Oryol, V. E., Rukavishnikov, A. A., Senin, I. G., et al. (2004). Consensual validation of personality traits across cultures. *Journal of Research in Personality, 38*, 179–201.

McCrae, R. R., Herbst, J. H., & Costa, P. T., Jr. (2001). Effects of acquiescence on personality factor structures. In R. Riemann, F. Ostendorf, & F. Spinath (Eds.), *Personality and temperament: Genetics, evolution, and structure* (pp. 217–231). Berlin: Pabst Science.

McCrae, R. R., Stone, S. V., Fagan, P. J., & Costa, P. T., Jr. (1998). Identifying causes of disagreement between self-reports and spouse ratings of personality. *Journal of Personality, 66*, 285–313.

McCrae, R. R., Terracciano, A., & 78 Members of the Personality Profiles of Cultures Project. (2005). Universal features of personality traits from the observer's perspective: Data from 50 cultures. *Journal of Personality and Social Psychology, 88*, 547–561.

Mervielde, I., & De Fruyt, F. (1999). Construction of the Hierarchical Personality Inventory for Children. In I. Mervielde, I. Deary, F. De Fruyt, & F. Ostendorf (Eds.), *Personality psychology in Europe: Proceedings of the Eighth European Conference on Personality Psychology* (pp. 107–127). Tilburg, The Netherlands: Tilburg University Press.

Ostendorf, F., & Angleitner, A. (2004). *NEO-Persönlichkeitsinventar, revidierte Form, NEO-PI-R nach Costa und McCrae* [Revised NEO Personality Inventory, NEO-PI-R of Costa and McCrae]. Göttingen, Germany: Hogrefe.

Pederson, A. K., King, J. E., & Landau, V. I. (2005). Chimpanzee (*Pan troglodytes*) personality predicts behavior. *Journal of Research in Personality, 39*, 534–549.

Piedmont, R. L., McCrae, R. R., Riemann, R., & Angleitner, A. (2000). On the invalidity of validity scales in volunteer samples: Evidence from self-reports and observer ratings in volunteer samples. *Journal of Personality and Social Psychology, 78*, 582–593.

Riemann, R., Angleitner, A., & Strelau, J. (1997). Genetic and environmental influences on personality: A study of twins reared together using the self- and peer report NEO-FFI scales. *Journal of Personality, 65*, 449–475.

Rubenzer, S. J., Faschingbauer, T. R., & Ones, D. S. (2000). Assessing the U.S. presidents using the Revised NEO Personality Inventory. *Assessment, 7*, 403–420.

Shrout, P. E., & Fleiss, J. L. (1979). Intraclass correlations: Uses in assessing rater reliability. *Psychological Bulletin, 86*, 420–428.

Siegler, I. C., Welsh, K. A., Dawson, D. V., Fillenbaum, G. G., Earl, N. L., Kaplan, E. B., et al. (1991). Ratings of personality change in patients being evaluated for memory disorders. *Alzheimer Disease and Associated Disorders, 5*, 240–250.

Strauss, M. E., & Pasupathi, M. (1994). Primary caregivers' descriptions of Alzheimer patients' personality traits: Temporal stability and sensitivity to change. *Alzheimer Disease and Associated Disorders, 8*, 166–176.

Strauss, M. E., Pasupathi, M., & Chatterjee, A. (1993). Concordance between observers in descriptions of personality change in Alzheimer's disease. *Psychology and Aging, 8*, 475–480.

Terracciano, A., Abdel-Khalak, A. M., Ádám, N., Adamovová, L., Ahn, C.-k., Ahn, H.-n., et al. (2005). National character does not reflect mean personality trait levels in 49 cultures. *Science, 310*, 96–100.

Tupes, E. C., & Christal, R. E. (1992). Recurrent personality factors based on trait ratings. *Journal of Personality, 60*, 225–251. (Original work published 1961)

Vazire, S. (2006). Informant reports: A cheap, fast, and easy method for personality assessment. *Journal of Research in Personality, 40*, 472–481.

Wiggins, J. S. (2003). *Paradigms of personality assessment.* New York: Guilford Press.

## CHAPTER 16

Behavioral Observation

R. Michael Furr
David C. Funder

How can we tell which of two people is more extraverted? According to the most widely used method of assessment in personality psychology, the answer is, "Give them both an extraversion questionnaire, and their answers will tell you." The only issue that remains is which inventory to use (and whether you want to measure extraversion or extroversion). The reliance on self-report measures has a long and productive history in personality psychology, and they have become the default assessment method in the field.

How can we tell which of two people is more extraverted? If you ask this question of a student who has not yet been initiated into the rituals of personality psychology, you may well receive a different but quite reasonable answer. The student may advise you to "see how they act" or offer the slightly more sophisticated recommendation to "put them both in a room with other people and see which one is more outgoing."

As reasonable and even obvious as it might be to "see how they act," personality psychology has historically paid surprisingly scant attention to how people actually behave. Yet among the most interesting and important tasks for the field is an understanding of the links between who people are and what they do. The measurement of behavior is a fundamental part of the task of addressing this issue.

The measurement of behavior entails many difficulties. However, a well-conceived and well-executed plan of behavioral observation can offer valuable insights into many of the issues that personality psychologists find fascinating. In this chapter, we primarily consider behavioral observation in the context of interpersonal behavior in laboratory settings. We discuss some of the core underlying conceptual issues and practical considerations in the assessment of directly observed behavior. Specifically, we consider the costs and benefits of behavioral observation, discuss the process of selecting and designing a behavioral coding system, and examine some basic issues in conducting research using behavioral observation. In addition, we present a basic introduction to and illustration of generalizability theory (Cronbach, Gleser, Nanda, & Rajaratnam, 1972), as a useful framework for evaluating the quality of data derived from behavioral observations. Careful consideration and negotiation of these issues can result in observational research that provides a wealth of rare and important information.

In a move to correct the historical neglect of behavior in the study of personality, some researchers have recently made increasing use of behavioral assessment (e.g., Asendorpf, Banse, & Mücke, 2002; Borkenau, Mauer, Riemann, Spinath, & Angleitner, 2004; Furr & Funder, 1998, 2004; Markey, Markey, & Tinsley, 2004; Mast & Hall, 2003; Mehl & Pennebaker, 2003). In part, this movement is due to an increasing recognition of the importance of behavior and partly due to an increasing availability of manageable and nonintrusive technologies. The increasing examination of actual behavior is an exciting trend that reflects shifts in the perceived balance of costs and benefits associated with behavioral observation.

The Challenges and the Importance of Behavioral Observation

Compared to questionnaires, behavioral observation is difficult, expensive, and can also be limited in scope. Therefore, the first step in behavioral assessment should be a careful consideration of the costs and benefits of the method in the relevant research context.

The Costs of Behavioral Observation

There are at least three reasons why extensive behavioral observations are relatively rare. One reason is that other, easier methods have been sufficient to yield interesting and important advances. The use of self-report questionnaires is ubiquitous in the field, for conceptually and practically important reasons. At relatively low cost, a good deal of data can be quickly gathered on almost any topic, using questionnaires. It is obvious that practical and ethical considerations prevent (or even prohibit) the direct observation of many of people's important behaviors in many of the important contexts of their lives. In a questionnaire, by contrast, it is possible to ask about virtually anything (though whether the participant will answer honestly, or at all, is another matter). Indeed, much of what we currently know about personality traits, personality change, and culture and personality is derived from the analysis of self-report data. Because of its efficiency and potential range, it is possible to build a productive and valuable career on self-report data alone.

A second reason why extensive behavioral observations are relatively rare is that few behavioral coding systems have been extensively developed, refined, and psychometrically evaluated. At a molecular level of analysis, the Facial Action Coding System (FACS; Ekman, Friesen, & Hager, 2002) is the most widely used coding system in the analysis of facial displays of emotion (Rosenberg, 1997). At a broader level of analysis, the 64-item Riverside Behavioral Q-Sort (RBQ; Funder, Furr, & Colvin, 2000) was developed to capture a range of important interpersonal behaviors such as "Initiates humor," "Expresses criticism," and "Acts playful." The RBQ has been translated from English into German (Spinath, Spinath, & Funder, 2000) and Dutch (De Corte & Buysse, n.d.), and it has been adapted for use with children (Markey et al., 2004).[1] Aside from these measures, most historical examples of behavioral observation in personality psychology—as well as other areas of psychology—are based on ad hoc sets of behaviors narrowly relevant to specific theoretical or applied issues. Researchers who do not want to spend time developing and validating a behavioral observation system thus might shy away from the process.

The third and perhaps most powerful reason that behavioral observations are relatively rare is that the process can be expensive in terms of time, money, and effort. Aside from developing the observation system itself, the process of actually using such a system can be overwhelmingly demanding. The technique begins to draw heavily on time and resources in the training phase. For example, Ekman and colleagues (2002) indicate that training six experts in the FACS required about 100 hours of learning and practice. In addition, the greatest demand might be in the actual data collection and coding phase. In one use of the RBQ (see, e.g., Furr & Funder, 2004) 116 participants were observed in six dyadic interactions, and each participant in each interaction was coded by at least four judges using the 64 items of the RBQ. Because of theoretically based practical constraints on the number of times that a given judge could contribute codings, the process of accumulating reliable codings for all participants in all situations required literally years of work, *after* the conclusion of the last experimental session. The prospect of spending years to collect and code behavioral observations might not appear to fit well with researchers' desires to publish frequently and with editors' preferences for multiple-study articles.

The Benefits of Behavioral Observation

Given the potential practical difficulties and expense of behavioral observation and the relative simplicity and ease of alternative methods, one might wonder whether it would be worth the trouble. The answer is yes, it can be. Behavioral data are fundamental to personality psychology, for two reasons.

The first reason emerges from the fact that behavior may be considered the defining characteristic of scientific psychology, including, of course, personality psychology. In fact, personality has been defined as "a pattern of relatively permanent traits, dispositions, or characteristics that give some measure of consistency to a person's behavior" (Feist & Feist, 2002, p. 4) and as "those characteristics of the person that account for consistent patterns of feeling, thinking, and behaving" (Pervin & John, 2001, p. 4). Despite the centrality of behavior, personality psychology has been accused of a relative lack of attention to it. The study of personality psychology involves the understanding of persons, situations, and behaviors, as well as the links within this triad (Funder, 2006). But Funder (2001) observed that the field's understanding of the elements in this triad has been severely skewed in favor of the person and away from both situations and behaviors. As a result, although we know much about how to classify traits, we know relatively little about how to classify behaviors or the situations in which they occur.

This lack of understanding of behavior and of the links between personality characteristics and the situational manifestation of behavior reflects an empirical and theoretical soft spot in the field. Throughout the late 1960s and until the late 1980s the field grappled with the fact that little evidence was available to support the assumption that personality traits had any meaningful association with actual behaviors in actual situations. Putting aside the potential theoretical explanation for this lack of evidence for a moment (i.e., that traits are in fact not meaningfully associated with actual behaviors in actual situations), one simple fact was that there was just not much information about how personality characteristics were associated with actual behavior in actual situations. The stack of articles that even attempted to examine the personality–behavior links was embarrassingly short. The stack has grown, but not as much as it should have—the soft spot remains (Funder, 2001). The recently emerging interest in behavioral observation (e.g., Borkenau et al., 2004; Mehl & Pennebaker, 2003) is an encouraging sign that the field is recognizing and addressing the importance of behavior.

The second reason behavioral data are fundamental to personality psychology is that, in the final analysis, behavior is the source of all psychological information. We have no direct access to anyone's thoughts, emotions, motivations, interests, or attitudes. Any clue to a person's psychology emerges from what that person *does*—what the person says, what the person writes, how the person responds to a questionnaire, how the person's heart rate changes, which choices the person makes, what kind of intonations are present in his or her voice, or how the person reacts with others. All sources of information about personality derive from some kind of observation and measurement of a physical act—intentional or unintentional, subtle or obvious, verbal or nonverbal, internal or external, rapid or slow.

For both of these reasons, behavioral observation is a ubiquitous and important part of comprehensive frameworks that have been developed to categorize the kinds of data that are relevant to personality psychology (see, e.g., Cattell, 1965; Mayer, 2004). No single type of information offers a perfectly clear window on personality; each type—including self-reports, informant reports, and observations of social behavior—has advantages and disadvantages. The primary disadvantage of behavioral observations as a means of personality assessment is that the link between a specific behavior and a specific personality characteristic may not be direct. Imagine that we observe a new acquaintance being talkative and friendly in a social situation. Do these two behavioral observations (i.e., a high level of talkativeness and a high level of friendliness) indicate that the individual has a high level of extraversion? Perhaps so. But perhaps the person is nervous and deals with anxiety through constant chatter. Or perhaps the person is in an unusually good mood and would not ordinarily act this way, so our observations do not reflect a more stable facet of the person. Or perhaps the observation that the individual is "friendly" has nothing to do with whether the person is extraverted— friendliness might be a behavior that is more closely tied to another trait, such as agreeableness or even manipulativeness. In sum, we need to be careful when drawing psychological inferences from observations of specific behaviors in specific situations.

Even though behavioral observations are not perfect indicators of personality, their advantages can complement the advantages offered by different sources of personality-relevant information. One advantage of behavioral observations in laboratory situations is that very specific kinds of psychological situations and behavioral interactions can be created. For example, Downey, Freitas, Michaelis, and Khouri (1998, Study 2) examined the role of rejection sensitivity in romantic interactions. To observe the behavioral styles that were exhibited during arguments between romantic partners, the researchers used procedures to elicit discussion of conflictual issues that were specific to each participant couple. A second advantage is that behavioral observations are not as strongly affected by some response biases that affect other forms of personality assessment. When relying on self-reports, researchers may be concerned about random responding, psychological defensiveness, social desirability biases, and acquiescence biases. When relying on informant reports, researchers may be concerned about similar biases, along with the possibility that informants have limited information relevant to the personality characteristics of interest. With behavioral observations, we do not have to rely on anyone to tell us how talkative, friendly, timid, argumentative, or dominant our target participants are or might be in specific situations. We see for ourselves how talkative, friendly, timid, argumentative, and dominant they are, and we can quantify this directly.

Recent research by Borkenau and his colleagues (Borkenau et al., 2004; Borkenau, Riemann, Angleitner, & Spinath, 2001) provides compelling examples of the use of behavioral observation as a source of personality trait information. In their research, observers watched videotapes of target participants engaging in one of a series of behavioral tasks (e.g., introducing themselves, telling stories, telling a joke, reading aloud newspaper headlines), and they rated their impressions of the targets along a set of personality trait dimensions. In addition, targets provided self-report ratings, and acquaintances of the targets provided informant report ratings on the personality trait dimensions. Results revealed wide-ranging correlations between these sources of trait information, and even evidence of genetic heritability, which underscores the utility of behavioral observations as a complement to the more traditional methods of assessing personality.

Behavioral observation provides data that are essential for the theoretical and empirical well-being of personality psychology. Although the field has often been hesitant to collect such data, recent years provide encouraging signs that the need for observational data is being filled. Greater familiarity with some of the basic issues in collecting behavioral observation data can help this to happen.

Selecting or Designing a Coding System for Behavioral Observation

Once a researcher decides to conduct a study using behavioral observation, he or she faces a number of important decisions. Our discussion focuses on issues that we have found most compelling in the context of personality and social psychology. There are several sources that provide other perspectives on behavioral observation across several areas of psychology (e.g., Bakeman, 2000; Bakeman & Gottman, 1997; Margolin et al., 1998; Thompson, Symons, & Felce, 2000). When making decisions concerning the preparation of a behavioral coding system, an overarching consideration is that they should be made on the basis of both practical and theoretical considerations. If the system used in a behavioral observation study turns out to be practically or theoretically flawed in any important way, then all the time and money that have been invested in designing, using, and analyzing the behavioral data might well be for naught. Figure 16.1 summarizes several key considerations in the design,

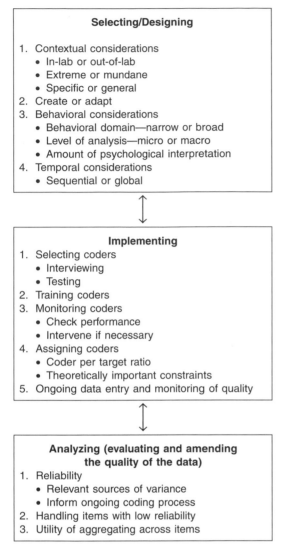

Selecting/Designing

1. Contextual considerations
   - In-lab or out-of-lab
   - Extreme or mundane
   - Specific or general
2. Create or adapt
3. Behavioral considerations
   - Behavioral domain—narrow or broad
   - Level of analysis—micro or macro
   - Amount of psychological interpretation
4. Temporal considerations
   - Sequential or global

Implementing

1. Selecting coders
   - Interviewing
   - Testing
2. Training coders
3. Monitoring coders
   - Check performance
   - Intervene if necessary
4. Assigning coders
   - Coder per target ratio
   - Theoretically important constraints
5. Ongoing data entry and monitoring of quality

Analyzing (evaluating and amending the quality of the data)

1. Reliability
   - Relevant sources of variance
   - Inform ongoing coding process
2. Handling items with low reliability
3. Utility of aggregating across items

FIGURE 16.1. Considerations in designing, implementing, and analyzing a behavioral coding system.

implementation, and analysis of behavioral coding systems.

Observational Context

The first consideration in the use of a behavioral coding system is the context within which it will be used (Rosenblum, 1978). The situation in which behavior will be observed has implications for both the content and complexity of the coding system. When preparing to adapt or develop a behavioral coding system, researchers must consider several basic contextual facets that are relevant to many kinds of personal-

ity research. For example, are the observations going to be conducted in naturalistic "real world" settings, or will they be conducted in a laboratory? Are observations intended to capture behavior in a common or mundane kind of situation, or are they intended to capture behavior in an unusual or extreme situation? Are observations going to be conducted in a specific situation or should the coding system be applicable to a wide range of situations?

Behavioral observations to be conducted in a real-world setting may require novel developments in content and technology. One interesting new development is the electronically activated recorder (EAR), which has been developed to monitor the sounds of participants' daily lives (Mehl & Pennebaker, 2003). The EAR is a small digital recording device that is worn by a participant, and it activates every 12 minutes to record whatever the participant may be saying or hearing. As with many observational technologies, the EAR generates a great deal of raw information to be transcribed and coded. In one study, Mehl and Pennebaker (2003) used the Social Environment Coding of Sound Inventory to code each segment recorded by the EAR. This coding system was designed to categorize the raw data in terms of the nature of each segment's interaction, activity, and location. By taking advantage of recent developments in technology, the EAR and its associated coding systems expand researchers' ability to capture real-world behavior.

As with any kind of research, observational research conducted in unusual situations has benefits and costs. For example, the study of topics such as altruism or obedience may require the creation of unusual situations that afford participants an opportunity to manifest (or fail to manifest) helping behavior or obedience. Similarly, researchers may tailor situations in order to evaluate behavior at the extremes. For example, a personality psychologist who is interested in anxiety may desire to observe participants in an extremely stressful situation. Despite the potential theoretical and practical value of observations in novel situations, they do have a downside. Ethical considerations limit the degree to which situations can be designed to be demanding, embarrassing, or otherwise stressful for participants. Extreme situations may be difficult to construct in ways that truly involve participants; for example, if deception is involved (such as telling participants that important outcomes ride on their performance), the deception may not be believed. Finally, participants' behaviors in a strange or unusual situation may not tell us much about what people do under more ordinary real-life circumstances.

An additional contextual consideration regarding the selection or development of a behavioral coding system is situational specificity versus generality. A researcher may desire a coding system that would be applicable to a very specific kind of situation. This researcher will likely choose or develop a system focused on those behaviors that are expected to be relevant in that situation. Alternatively, a researcher may wish to examine a set of behaviors that are applicable across a range of situations. This researcher will likely choose or develop a coding system that includes a set of behaviors that pertain to many different kinds of social contexts. For example, the RBQ (Funder et al., 2000) was developed to be applicable to a wide range of interpersonal situations. Reflecting this generality, the RBQ has been used to code unstructured, competitive, and cooperative dyadic interactions in college students (e.g., Furr & Funder, 1998, 2004), it has been adapted and used to code parent–child interactions (Markey et al., 2004), and it has been used to code communications situations in a German sample (Spinath & Spinath, 2004). Recently, the RBQ has been revised to be even more applicable to social settings in general. The newest version—along with a program enabling Q-sorts to be completed and recorded via computer—is available at *www.rap.ucr.edu/qsorter.*

Adapting or Developing a Coding System?

A second issue regarding the use of a coding system is whether one can be adapted or whether one must be fully designed and developed. Bakeman (2000) points out that researchers may be tempted to plunge headlong into developing a new system for coding behavioral observations, but this "makes as much sense as each student of heat developing his or her own thermometer"(p. 141). At this point in the research process, some time invested in searching for existing coding systems may pay off handsomely in terms of avoiding investments in developing a new system and in terms of being able to tie into existing literatures. Even if no existing coding system fits exactly with a researcher's requirements, the researcher

might find one that can be adapted without much difficulty. Even though using an existing coding system may initially feel like "wearing someone else's underwear" (Bakeman & Gottman, 1997, p. 15), a little work can make it feel quite comfortable. If the only coding systems that are available are too far removed from a researcher's new research questions (or if they are all three sizes too small), then he or she will have to develop a new coding system. Developing a new coding system for behavioral observation involves decisions about the nature of the behaviors to be observed and the temporal units in which observations will be made.

Behaviors in the Coding System

The process of designing a new coding system involves a number of important decisions about the nature of the behaviors to be included. One of the primary design decisions concerns the content domain of behaviors to be included. Of course, this is a decision based on theory and the larger purpose of a coding system. Some coding systems may be focused on a single behavioral domain. For example, Asendorpf and colleagues (2002) recently examined behavioral expression of shyness, and they videotaped participants engaging in a dyadic shyness-inducing 5-minute conversation. Observers watched the videotapes and coded six behaviors that were hypothesized as manifestations of shyness—speech duration, illustrator duration (i.e., movements illustrating speech), facial adaptor duration (touching one's face or neck), body adaptor duration (touching other parts of one's body), gaze aversion, and bodily tension. Focused coding systems such as this may include only a few behaviors chosen to pinpoint a particular issue of direct theoretical relevance. Other coding systems are more wide-ranging, covering many different domains of behavior. The RBQ (Funder et al., 2000) is an example of a coding system that was developed to assess a wide variety of behaviors. In our analyses, we have typically used the RBQ as 64 separate and potentially important behavioral items that provide a rich portrait of participants' overall behavioral style (e.g., Furr & Funder, 1998).

Although wide-ranging coding systems such as the RBQ can be reduced through principal components analysis (e.g., Funder et al., 2000), researchers who use such a system should consider carefully the pros and cons of such decisions. Certainly some items within most coding systems will appear to share some meaning, but the meaning of any particular item may change in subtle but important ways from situation to situation. Factorial combination of items could present problems for generalizing across situations and/or studies—both in terms of the psychological meaning of behaviors and in a potential lack of invariance of the factor structure across situations. Consider the RBQ item "Smiles frequently." At first glance, this item may seem to reflect an underlying friendliness. But many students of psychology quickly recognize that frequent smiling may also reflect an attempt to cope with or cover up anxiety. Furthermore, frequent smiling in an interaction with an opposite-sex stranger may have different meaning than frequent smiling in an interview situation or in an argument with a significant other. Such potentially important differences would be masked if "frequent" smiling were combined with other behaviors that might show different patterns of meaning across situations. In sum, although compositing behaviors in a system may have some psychometric and statistical advantages for reliability and in the number of significant tests to be conducted, it risks losing information of potential psychological importance and raising other psychometric problems. At the very least, researchers using a wide-ranging coding system might opt to analyze the data at the item level before moving to a composite or factor level—to evaluate the degree to which important psychological meaning is lost by presenting only composite-level results.

A second important issue in designing a coding system is its specificity versus generality. Some "molecular" systems focus on very specific physical behaviors such as occurrence of eyeblinks, the occurrence of eyewinks, and the amount of "backward lean" (Ekman et al., 2002; Ellgring, 1989; Kalbaugh & Haviland, 1994). In contrast, some observational studies have focused on more general-level analysis, oriented toward more "molar" behavioral styles such as *managerial-autocratic, blunt-aggressive,* or *cold and socially avoidant* (e.g., Alden & Phillips, 1990; Hokanson, Lowenstein, Hedeen, & Howes, 1986). A coding system could be designed at any level of specificity within this continuum.

The specificity of the behavioral observation system selected or designed by a researcher should match his or her research questions. For example, the RBQ was designed at a mid-level of specificity, with items such as "Behaves in a cheerful manner," "Seeks advice," and "Initiates humor." The decision to focus the RBQ at this level was driven by several considerations. First, the RBQ was designed in part to be used in research addressing the links between personality and behavior. In designing the RBQ, we wanted to include behavioral items that would have clear and direct links to many of the personality characteristics described by the California Adult Q-set (CAQ; Block, 1978). For instance, the RBQ behavioral item "Is talkative (as observed in this situation)" was included as a cognate for the CAQ item "Is a talkative individual." Thus, the generality of the RBQ items was motivated in part by the desire for convergence with the CAQ. Second, items at this level of generality were assumed to fit the phenomenology of people engaged in everyday types of social interactions more closely than items at a more molecular level. Although the molecular movements that comprise facial displays might affect perceptions of emotional states, we assumed that the degree to which an actor "Behaves in a cheerful manner" is more salient to other people and has a more direct impact on their overall perceptions and behavioral responses to the actor. Third, items at this level of generality can be combined into more general composites reflecting behavioral styles (see the discussion of compositing above), but items coded at a broader level cannot subsequently be broken into their components. Reflecting this point, Bakeman and Gottman (1997) suggest that researchers consider using a coding system that is focused at a level of analysis that is slightly more molecular than the level at which the research questions are framed. Among other rationales, they point out that more specific behaviors can be empirically "lumped" together to form more general categories of behavior (pp. 24–26).

A third consideration in the design of a coding system is the amount of interpretation to be required of observers. Some coding systems, and even the behaviors within a given coding system, restrict observers to recording the occurrence of well-defined events. Others require observers to make inferences about the psychological meaning of the events. Cairns and Green (1979) make this distinction in terms of behavioral observations (recording of actual activities) and behavioral ratings (social judgments that observers make, regarding the target's standing on a psychological dimension). This issue is also closely tied to the behavioral specificity versus generality issue and to what Bakeman and Gottman (1997) describe as a distinction between physical and social behaviors (pp. 17–22). The detection of a particular muscle movement, as coded by the FACS, requires no inference about the psychological meaning of the event. The coding might be subjective in terms of whether the movement occurred or not, but it does not seem to require subjectivity in terms of the meaning of the event. Moving up in generality, a coding of the RBQ item "Smiles frequently" might be subjective in terms of what constitutes a smile and what constitutes "frequently," but it again does not require inferences about the meaning of the smile. Observers are simply asked about the occurrence of the behavior, they are not asked to judge whether the actor is expressing true friendliness, faux friendliness, anxiety, or happiness. Moving up in generality even more, observers making judgments of behavioral styles such as *managerial-autocratic*, *blunt-aggressive*, or *cold and socially avoidant* (see, e.g., Alden & Phillips, 1990; Hokanson et al., 1986) are being asked to make much more inferential judgments about the overall psychological message being communicated through an actor's behavior.

Temporal Units in the Coding System

In addition to making a decision regarding the nature of the behaviors to be included in the coding system, researchers must also consider the temporal units of observation. Again, decisions regarding this issue will be driven by the research questions to be addressed.

A crucial issue is whether the observed interaction will be taken as a whole or be divided into discrete temporal units. Consider a coding system designed for observing paternal behavior within a game-playing interaction between fathers and their children. For some research questions, a global, overall judgment about the talkativeness, punitiveness, or encouragement that a father expresses during the interaction will be sufficient. For example, the researcher may hypothesize that paternal encouragement will be positively correlated with child self-esteem. In this case, overall judgments about differences between fathers in the degree of encouragement they express will provide adequate information for

the research question, and there is no need for a more fine-grained (and vastly more expensive) analysis of the stream of behavior as it unfolded. In contrast, some research questions may require a sequential analysis that focuses on recording behavior as it unfolds. For example, the researcher studying father–child interactions may be interested in the speed with which fathers might transition from a positive to a negative behavioral style. Alternatively, the researcher may be interested in the temporal locations or sequences of specific behavioral events—when a punitive behavior is emitted by the father, is it followed by attempts to soften the potential emotional distress experienced by the child? For such questions, the researcher would carefully code the sequence of behaviors, recording behavior as it occurs during the interaction instead of providing a summary of the overall behavioral style. Bakeman and his colleagues (Bakeman & Gottman, 1997; Bakeman & Quera, 1995) provide a wealth of information regarding the design and statistical analysis of sequential observations.

Clearly, a coding system's complexity, in terms of its temporal units, has implications for the ease and expense with which it can be used. The theoretical relevance of a coding system is a crucial issue to consider, but, as a practical matter, researchers should also consider carefully whether the information potentially obtained from a more complex coding strategy will be worth the time, effort, and money that will be invested. This issue is important not just because everyone wishes to save time and money, but also because research resources invested needlessly in fine-grained behavioral recording become unavailable for other empirical and theoretical efforts that may prove more fruitful.

Collecting Behavioral Observation Data

Alongside the issues involved with adapting and designing a behavioral coding system are many important practical issues involved with actually collecting the observational data and evaluating its quality. In addition to the technological options involved with behavioral coding (for which readers can refer to Thompson, Felce, & Symons, 2000, Chaps. 3–7), important considerations include the selection, training, and monitoring of observers and the assignment of observers to tasks.

Selecting, Training, and Monitoring Observers

As in any research project, researchers conducting a behavioral observation study will benefit by working with assistants who are likely to perform well. The opportunity to maximize the performance of coders is enhanced by efficient selection, training, and monitoring procedures.

Given the amount of training that can be required for some coding procedures, researchers will be interested in selecting coders who are most likely to develop into good, reliable observers. Some selection procedures are exactly what may be used in many "hiring" processes. One of our colleagues conducts ongoing research in parent–child interactions. In his lab, all potential research assistants went through a rigorous application and interview process. This process included gathering information about academic performance, interest in psychology, interest in parent–child interactions, and other questions intended to gauge the potential observers' level of potential conscientiousness and motivation. Bishop and DiLalla (1998) reported a small-sample study in which reliable coders and nonreliable coders scored differently on reasoning and rule consciousness. These results suggest that reliable coders were more abstract reasoners and less rule conscious, which the authors interpreted as indicating that reliable coders were "able to interpret the coding rules more broadly" (p. 166). Given the limited sample size in this study ($n = 27$), we should interpret these results with care—but the idea of developing personality-based predictors of coding reliability is a potentially useful contribution.

At the Riverside Accuracy Project (RAP), the selection process has asked potential observers to demonstrate an ability to understand the coding procedure and achieve a criterion level of proficiency. After an initial training meeting, potential observers engage in the coding process, independently observing a videotape of a specific target participant and using the RBQ to code the participant's behavior. The specified target participant had been coded previously by several senior lab personnel, providing a set of "criteria" codes. Potential observers whose coding agreed highly with the criteria codes were invited to continue within the training process.

Although selection procedures, such as those discussed here, do not guarantee that the final pool of observers will be perfect, we encourage researchers to consider carefully a rigorous evaluation process for potential observers. A great deal of time and energy can be invested in training and employing observers, and it is worthwhile to minimize the risk of these investments.

Potential observers need to learn the nuts and bolts of the coding system. Depending on the research application, training includes issues such as accessing the target stimuli (e.g., where, when, how to obtain video or audio recordings of target participants), learning the coding system itself (e.g., learning to identify the different muscular movements in the FACS), and learning the procedures for recording the codes (e.g., paper-and-pencil, computerized entry, etc.). Coding systems can vary dramatically in the time required to train reliable observers. For example, the training of observers to use the RBQ for the RAP (e.g., Furr & Funder, 1998) usually required 2–4 hours. The RBQ was intended to be a relatively intuitive coding system, and the RBQ was applied as a global system in the RAP. Therefore, observers did not need to be trained to perform codings of highly specialized behaviors in a sequence of discrete temporal units. In contrast, other types of observer training are much more time intensive; Bishop and DiLalla (1998) report that their process required approximately 7 weeks of training, and the FACS manual states that the training of six experts in the FACS required about 100 hours of learning and practice (Ekman et al., 2002). Ideally, investing time in the training process will pay off in high-quality observational data.

After observers are trained and begin the coding process, it is wise to regularly monitor the observational data. Even observers who have passed selection criteria and have completed a rigorous training process can decline in accuracy over time. A regular monitoring process can catch such declines early and allow intervention. A coding process that goes unchecked will produce data, but it may produce data with problems that become apparent only after data collection is supposedly completed. At best, this state of affairs could be remedied by recoding some portion of the data. At worst, it may require a complete recoding of the entire dataset. In the RAP, we checked interrater agreement approximately every 2 weeks. When we found an observer who exhibited a trend of low agreement with other observers, we contacted the observer in an attempt to identify and ameliorate the problem or confusion.

Assigning Observers

Assuming that observers are selected carefully, trained well, and monitored regularly, careful thought needs to be given to the ways in which observers are assigned to coding tasks. Some considerations are purely practical, whereas others are more conceptually tied to the research questions being addressed. The practical considerations are basic issues such as ensuring that every target participant is observed by a some minimal number of coders and ensuring that every target participant is coded on every behavior.

Conceptual considerations are those with implications for the researcher's ability to make inferences about the theoretical questions driving the research. A researcher conducting a behavioral observation study may need to think carefully about the way in which the coding process will affect the strength of his or her theoretical conclusions. For example, we (Furr & Funder, 2004, Study 2) were interested in factors affecting cross-situational behavioral consistency—the degree to which participants' behavior is stable from one situation to another. For this, we analyzed data from the RAP, in which participants were observed in six dyadic interactions. An important consideration in this research was that correlations between participants' behavior in one situation and their behavior in another would reflect only their actual behavioral consistency. To be able to make clear inferences about behavioral consistency, the research question required that the participants' *behavioral consistency* across situations was not confounded with the *consistency of observers* across situations.

Several assignment strategies could have been used for this observational study. In some strategies, assignments may have been made without regard to which observers were coding which participants in which situations—an observer may have been assigned to code a participant in more than one situation. For example, observer Rick may have been assigned to target Chris in situation 1 and in situation 2. But if Chris's behavioral profile was then found to ex-

hibit a high correlation between the two situations, we would wonder whether the consistency in Chris's data reflected either a true consistency of Chris's behavior or a consistent bias in Rick's perception of Chris. In the assignment strategies actually used in Furr and Funder's (2004) data, great care was taken to ensure that an observer coded a particular target participant in only one situation. For example, observer Rick coded target Chris's behavior in situation 1, and observer Bob coded Chris's behavior in situation 2. With this assignment strategy, a high correlation between Chris's two behavioral profiles could not be due to consistency in a single observer's perceptions. Although it is possible that the two observers might have a common bias in their perceptions of Chris, the semirandom assignment of multiple coders across multiple targets across multiple situations would seem to minimize such a problem. The bottom line is that both practical and conceptual matters should be considered in a strategy for assigning observers to targets.

Evaluating Behavioral Observation Data: An Example of Judgments of Extraversion Based on Observation of Nonverbal Behavior

Any kind of behavioral data need to be evaluated in terms of their psychometric quality. With behavioral observations, a primary psychometric consideration is typically the degree to which the observers agree on the behavioral codes assigned to target participants. Several issues arise in evaluating interrater reliability, with the statistical alternatives having related strengths and weaknesses (see, e.g., Bakeman & Gottman, 1997, Chap. 4). Generalizability theory (G theory; Cronbach et al., 1972) is a psychometric perspective that offers some advantages over many alternatives. Perhaps the most practical advantage offered by G theory is the ability to explore the effects that multiple facets of the measurement design have on the psychometric quality of the data.

To describe and illustrate the use and interpretation of G theory for behavioral data, we return to our initial question—how can we tell which of two people is more extraverted? Using behavioral observation to make inferences about underlying personality characteristics is a key application of the techniques discussed in this chapter (see, e.g., Borkenau et al., 2004). We present an example of this application, with observers of nonverbal behavior making judgments about target participants' extraversion. For this example, observers watched videotapes of participants in the RAP, and they rated each target participant along a set of dimensions. Two of these dimensions were intended to be indicators of extraversion.

We present these analyses for three reasons. First, we hope that this presentation provides a useful example of the application and interpretation of the statistical procedures at the heart of G theory. Analyses based on G theory can be highly technical, and they are often presented in ways that seem accessible only to those with deep interest in the technical issues and the patience to grapple with them. We hope that our presentation helps to illustrate and explain the concepts and procedures in a way that can facilitate others' use of the techniques. Second, we hope that this presentation is conceptually interesting to personality psychologists. Third, we hope that the presentation provides useful psychometric information for future researchers. The results of these analyses can be used to plan future research procedures, in terms of maximizing the efficiency of behavioral observations. G theory can afford insight into the reliability of such data, based on various numbers of items and various numbers of observers. Such insight can be used to plan new research procedures, balancing theoretical interests, practical constraints, and desired psychometric qualities of the data.

Selecting the Indicators

Each observer watched 60 or 61 target participants and rated each participant on two items reflecting extraversion. Using Goldberg's (1992) markers, we asked the observers to rate each target on Talkativeness and Shyness (reverse scored). These two items were selected because of their strong extraversion loadings in Goldberg's factor analysis.

Assigning Targets to Raters

Fourteen observers and 121 targets were divided into two "panels"—with each observer rating approximately one-half of the target participants. Within each panel, each of the seven observers watched videotapes of each of the approximately 60 participants in each of two 5-minute situations. The first situation was an unstructured dyadic interaction with an opposite-sex stranger, and the second situation was an unstructured dyadic interaction with a same-sex acquaintance.[2] Each observer rated only one of the two target participants from each of the pairs in the dyadic interactions. Observers independently focused on an assigned target, watched the interaction with the sound completely muted, and then provided ratings of the target on both of the extraversion items.

Quality of the Data

Reliability

The first psychometric concern is the reliability of the data—do observers use the two items in a way that provides a consistent measure of the differences between the target participants? That is, to what degree does the rank order of the target participants generalize across the two items and across the seven raters?

G theory offers a distinct advantage over classical test theory (CTT) in its ability to provide information regarding the impact of multiple factors on the reliability of a measurement. Variability in observed scores may be created by many different facets of the assessment context, and these assessment facets may in turn affect the measure's reliability. For example, we may be concerned about the impact that the number of items has on reliability, the impact that number of raters has on reliability, and the way in which these two facets combine to affect reliability. According to CTT, total variance in a measure's observed scores is decomposed into either true score variance or error variance, and error variance is viewed as undifferentiated, amorphous, and monolithic (Brennan, 2001; Cronbach et al., 1972). Therefore, CTT cannot differentiate the effects of items and observers—they are all pooled into a single "measurement error." In contrast to CTT, G theory allows us to distinguish and understand observers and items as separable but potentially synergistic sources of measurement error.

G theory views "error" variance as potentially differentiated, which is the basis of a two-step procedure for evaluating and improving measurement. In the first step, the various facets that affect observed score variance (and thus that affect reliability) can be identified and their effects can be estimated. For example, we can estimate the degree to which observers' ratings of targets' extraversion are affected by a set of facets—differences between target participants, differences between items, differences between observers, and the ways in which these facets interact with each other (e.g., the degree to which the observers use the items differently). In the second step of an analysis based on G theory, the results of the first step can be used to estimate the reliability of various combinations of the facets. For example, we can estimate the number of items and observers that would be needed to obtain a reliability of .80 for judgments of extraversion based on observations of behavior. For a given research protocol, it may be difficult or expensive to increase the number of observers that can contribute ratings. Therefore, we may be quite interested in estimating the number of items that would be required to obtain a particular reliability, based on a design with a small number of observers.

The core results of a G theory analysis are variance components, and several sources provide technical discussions of the statistical methods for obtaining estimates of variance components (Brennan, 2001; Cronbach et al., 1972). Variance components are often obtained from the results of an analysis of variance (ANOVA) that is specified to partition the rating data into the desired set of effects. In our data, we are interested in the degree to which ratings are affected by three facets (differences between target participants, differences between observers, and differences between items) and the interactions between those facets. So, for each of the two panels' data for each of the two situations, we conducted a three-way ANOVA. From this, we obtained three main effects, three two-way interactions, and a residual term that combined the three-way interaction and error variance. Table 16.1 presents the relevant results of the ANOVA for panel 1's ratings in the Stranger situation, and Table 16.2 presents the equations for estimating the variance components in the model. At least two popular statistical packages (SAS, SPSS) offer options for directly estimating variance components (e.g., SAS "proc varcomp"), which relieves the researcher of the burden of computing these estimates from the results of ANOVA "by hand." For the current analyses, the three facets are treated as random effects.

TABLE 16.1. ANOVA Results for Panel 1, Stranger Interaction

Effect	df	SS	MS
Target	60	573.246	9.554
Observer	6	167.897	27.983
Item	1	172.665	172.665
Target × Observer	360	781.246	2.170
Target × Item	60	101.906	1.698
Observer × Item	6	49.532	8.255
Residual	360	293.897	.816

Table 16.3 presents the estimates of the variance components and the proportion of variance for each variance component (the variance component divided by the sum of the variance components). The results reveal the degree to which each of the facets affected the ratings of extraversion that were derived from observations of nonverbal behavior, and Table 16.4 presents interpretations and examples to illustrate the meaning of these effects. In evaluating the reliability of the coding procedures as a measure of individual differences in the Targets' extraversion, four of the effects are of interest.

The primary effect of interest is the *main effect of Target*. As mentioned in Table 16.4, this effect reflects the degree to which the Targets

TABLE 16.2. Equations for Estimating Variance Components in the Target × Observer × Item Model

Effect	Equation
Target	$\sigma_t^2 = \dfrac{MS_t - MS_{to} - MS_{ti} + MS_{Res}}{n_o n_i}$
Observer	$\sigma_o^2 = \dfrac{MS_o - MS_{to} - MS_{oi} + MS_{Res}}{n_t n_i}$
Item	$\sigma_i^2 = \dfrac{MS_i - MS_{ti} - MS_{oi} + MS_{Res}}{n_t n_i}$
Target × Observer	$\sigma_{to}^2 = \dfrac{MS_{to} - MS_{Res}}{n_i}$
Target × Item	$\sigma_{ti}^2 = \dfrac{MS_{ti} - MS_{Res}}{n_o}$
Observer × Item	$\sigma_{oi}^2 = \dfrac{MS_{oi} - MS_{Res}}{n_t}$
Residual	$\sigma_{Res}^2 = MS_{Res}$

TABLE 16.3. Results of Generalizability Analysis

Effect	Variance component				Proportion of variance			
	StrP1	StrP2	AcqP1	AcqP2	StrP1	StrP2	AcqP1	AcqP2
Target	.464	.382	.605	.497	.170	.156	.227	.189
Observer	.151	.000	.072	.000	.055	.000	.027	.000
Item	.383	.078	.201	.078	.140	.032	.075	.030
T × O	.677	.736	.667	.769	.247	.302	.250	.293
T × I	.126	.113	.090	.080	.046	.046	.034	.030
O × I	.122	.094	.116	.122	.045	.038	.044	.046
Residual	.816	1.038	.912	1.081	.298	.425	.342	.411

elicited different mean ratings, averaged across Observers and Items. Across the two situations and the two panels, differences between Targets accounts for 15–23% of the variance in observed ratings. The reliability estimates to be computed will reveal the degree to which these differences are generalizable—the degree to which the rank order of the Target participants is consistent across Observers and across Items.

In terms of our ability to detect differences between the Target participants, measurement error includes three effects. The *Target × Observer interaction* reflects the degree to which the Observers provided different rank orderings of the Targets. Again, the primary goal of our measurement process is to obtain a clear and consistent measure of the relative ordering of Target participants on extraversion scores (i.e., to obtain a generalizeable measure of individual differences in extraversion). The Target × Observer effect is considered to be a reflect error because a large effect would indicate that the relative ordering of the Target participants is *not* consistent across the Observers. As

TABLE 16.4. Substantive Interpretations and Examples of the Effects in Generalizability Theory Analysis

Effect	Interpretation (the degree to which . . .)	Example
Target	Targets elicited different mean ratings, averaged across the 7 Observers and the 2 Items.	Target *X* gets higher average rating than Target *Y*.
Observer	Observers provided different mean ratings, averaged across the 60 Targets and the 2 Items.	Observer *A* gives higher average ratings than Observer *B*.
Item	Items elicited different mean ratings, averaged across the 60 Targets and the 7 Observers.	Item 1 has a higher average rating than Item 2.
T × O*	Targets were rank ordered differently across Observers, in terms of their ratings averaged across the 2 items.	Observer *A* rates target *X* higher than Target *Y*, but Observer *B* rates Target *X* as lower than Target *Y*.
T × I*	Targets were rank ordered differently across Items, in terms of their ratings averaged across the Observers.	On Item 1 Target *X* was rated higher than Target *Y*, but on Item 2 Target *X* was rated lower than Target *Y*.
O × I	Items were rank ordered differently by the Observers, in terms of the ratings averaged across Targets.	Observer *A* tends to rate Item 1 higher than Item 2, but Observer *B* tends to rate Item 1 lower than Item 2.
Residual*	Variance in ratings is not associated with any of the above effects.	

* These terms are considered as contributing to "error" in the relative generalizability of the Target effect.

shown in Table 16.3, the Target × Observer interaction is relatively large in our ratings (25–30% of the variance). The *Target* × Item *interaction* reflects the degree to which the Targets were rank ordered differently across the items. This suggests that the Items were operating somewhat inconsistently across the Targets, thus potentially clouding the differences between the Targets. That is, the difference between Targets is not consistent across the Items. As shown in Table 16.3, the Target × Item interaction is relatively small in our ratings (3–5% of the variance). Finally, the *Residual* term is composed of two components that are considered error. Because our Observers provided only one rating of each Target on each Item (in each situation), we cannot separate the three-way interaction between Targets, Observers, and Items from pure "error" variance. Both of these components would be considered measurement error, because they would contribute to ambiguity/inconsistency in terms of the rank ordering of Targets across Observers and Items. As Table 16.3 indicates, the Residual accounts for 30–43% of the variance in our ratings.

For the sake of clarity, a brief discussion of the three remaining effects may be useful. These effects are *not* considered to be measurement error because they do not compromise the rank ordering of the Targets. A large *main effect of Observer* would indicate that some Observers provided higher mean ratings than other Observers. The fact the some Observers consistently made higher ratings of extraversion in general than did others has no effect on the consistency of the relative ordering of the Targets within a panel. Similarly, a large *main effect of Item* would indicate that some Items elicited higher mean ratings than did other Items. These mean differences are independent of the relative ordering of the Targets. Note that the Target × Item interaction, discussed above, indicates the degree to which Item differences are inconsistent across Targets (which would be considered measurement error), but this is statistically and conceptually separate from the possibility that some Items are rated higher than other Items, in general, across all Targets. Finally, the *Observer* × *Item* interaction indicates the degree to which Observers differed in their average rank orderings of the Items, with this difference being consistent across Targets. This consistency ensures that the Observers' differences in Item usage cancel each other out and do not obscure differences between Targets. Therefore, the Observer × Item interaction is not considered to be measurement error, in terms of our ability to detect a clear and consistent rank ordering of the Targets.

G theory's differentiation of measure error allows us to understand the degree of impact and the nature of the impact that each facet has on the reliability of the ratings, as a measure of individual differences in extraversion. We can then use the variance components in Table 16.3 to inform decisions about the number of observers and the number of items that may be used in future research.

The extrapolation to future research designs for behavioral observation involves computing "coefficients of generalizability" for combinations of numbers of observers and items. Because we are interested in obtaining a measure of individual differences between the target participants, we are interested in a "relative" generalizability coefficient.[3] Thus, the coefficient of generalizability is analogous to reliability as defined by CTT. Conceptually, it is the ratio of the variance component of the measured effect (Targets) and the variance components of that effect plus its error variance components. More specifically, to obtain an estimate of the coefficient of generalizability (ρ^2), we obtain a ratio of the appropriate variance components weighted by the numbers of observers and items that we are considering:

$$\rho^2 = \frac{\sigma_t^2}{\sigma_t^2 + \frac{\sigma_{to}^2}{n_o'} + \frac{\sigma_{ti}^2}{n_i'} + \frac{\sigma_{Res}^2}{n_o' n_i'}} \qquad (1)$$

where ρ^2 is the generalizability coefficient for the differences between Targets, σ_t^2 is the estimated variance component for the Target effect, σ_{to}^2 is the estimated variance component for the Target × Observer effect, σ_{ti}^2 is the estimated variance component for the Target × Item effect, σ_{Res}^2 is the estimated variance component for the Residual term, n_o' is the number of Observers being considered, and n_i' is the number of Items being considered. For example, we can use the variance components from panel 1's data in the opposite-sex stranger interaction to estimate the reliability for a design in which two observers each rated the targets on only one item:

$$\rho^2 = \frac{.464}{.464 + \frac{.677}{2} + \frac{.126}{1} + \frac{.816}{2 \times 1}} = \frac{.464}{1.3365} = .35$$

This indicates that we would obtain an unacceptably low reliability, and that we should consider increasing the number of observers and/or the number of items. In our data, with seven observers in a panel, and two items, the generalizability coefficient is .68.

Equation 1 reveals the core advantage of a generalizability approach over a CTT approach to measurement. From the CTT perspective, in which error is undifferentiated, there is no ability to separately estimate the effect of different combinations of Observers and Items. However, based on the G Theory perspective, researchers can use Equation 1 along with variance components in Table 16.3 to estimate reliability for various combinations of observers and items. By systematically testing various combinations of numbers of observers and numbers of items as separate facets, a researcher can estimate the reliability that would likely be obtained from a particular measurement strategy. This information, considered along with the practical costs and benefits of adding observers and/or items, can help optimize the efficiency and quality of the researcher's measurement methods.

Table 16.5 and Figure 16.2 provide reliability estimates for various combinations of observers and items. These estimates are derived from Equation 1, using the variance components from panel 1's data in the opposite-sex stranger interaction. The estimates illustrate two important points. First, we can find the combinations of observers and items that would be estimated to produce a specific reliability. For example, a reliability of .75 is estimated to be obtained through several combinations of observers and items. Specifically, 12 observers using 2 items, 9 observers using 3 items, 7 observers using 4 items, and 6 observers using 5 items would all be estimated to provide reliability of approximately .75. So, if a researcher desires a minimum reliability of .75, then he or she could weigh the costs and benefits of each of these four combinations. Second, we can see the points at which adding more ob-

servers and/or items produces minimal increments in reliability. For example, consider the increment in reliability associated with using 8 items instead of 4. Figure 16.2 indicates that this increment is relatively small, particularly considering the possible "cost" of doubling the number of items that each observer rates for each target. Similarly, the benefits of adding more observers appear to diminish about 6–8 observers, and they appear to flatten out almost completely by about 17 or 18 observers. Again, this kind of information may be useful in planning an efficient strategy for collecting behavioral observations.

Two caveats should be mentioned regarding the estimated variance components and generalizability coefficients presented in these analyses. First, the stability of the estimates of the variance components is affected by the number of observations for each component. For example, the effects that include the Item facet (i.e., the I, TI, OI, and Residual effects) may be less stable than the others because they are estimated from data that include only two items. Second, the generalizability coefficients that are presented in Table 16.5 and Figure 16.2 are derived from the variance component estimates for panel 1's ratings in the opposite-sex stranger interaction. It should be noted that the variance components from the other panel and the other interaction vary somewhat in their sizes, which produces some variation in the reliability estimates that would be obtained.

Behavioral data face some unique psychometric challenges. Without question, the psychometric properties of any measurement device are a fundamental concern, and behavioral observation is no exception. However, when interpreting the reliability of behavioral codings, it may be worth considering the nature of the behaviors in relation to the interaction in which they are observed, and the analytic use of the behavioral data. Some behaviors may be relatively difficult to code in particular interactions. For example, the RBQ

TABLE 16.5. Generalizability Coefficients Estimated Using Variance Components from Panel 1's Ratings in the Opposite-Sex Stranger Interaction

Observers (n'_o)	1	2	7	20	1	2	7	20	1	2	7	20	1	2	7	20
Items (n'_i)	1	1	1	1	2	2	2	2	3	3	3	3	5	5	5	5
ρ^2	.22	.35	.58	.70	.29	.43	.68	.80	.32	.47	.72	.84	.35	.51	.76	.87

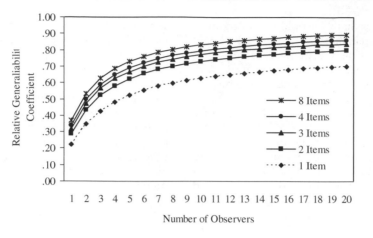

FIGURE 16.2. Relative generalizability coefficients as a function of number of observers and number of items.

includes the behavior "Competes with partner" (Funder et al., 2000, item #56), and this behavior exhibited dramatically different reliability in the two interactions reported by Funder and colleagues (2000). The behavior was coded with a reliability of .20 in the "unstructured" interaction, in which pairs of participants engaged in a 5-minute open-ended conversation with an opposite-sex stranger. Conversely, the behavior was coded with a reliability of .62 in the "competitive" situation, in which pairs of participants played a memory game (for a small cash prize) against each other for 5 minutes. So, even within a given coding system, a given behavior can vary in its reliability, depending on the degree to which the behavior may be relevant to various situations. In the unstructured interaction, participants did not differ from each other much in the degree to which they exhibited competitive behavior, and the reliability of the behavioral observation codings of that behavior was therefore relatively low. But in the competitive interaction, participants differed quite dramatically in the degree to which they seemed to compete against each other, and the reliability of the codings was therefore noticeably higher. The second consideration regarding the reliability of individual behaviors is the intended use of the data. For example, Furr and Funder (2004) used the RBQ to examine behavioral consistency across pairs of situations, and consistency was approached from two conceptual and analytic perspectives. One approach was

variable centered, with each behavior examined separately—indicating the degree to which individual differences in a behavior are consistent across two situations. The second approach was person centered, with each person's profile of behaviors examined separately—indicating the degree to which a person's profile of behaviors in one situation is similar to his or her profile of behaviors in a second situation. The reliability of any single behavior will have a large effect on the results of the variable-centered approach but a smaller effect on the results of the person-centered approach.

Validity

Validity is the next concern regarding the quality of the data derived from this example of behavioral observation. We may expect that ratings of extraversion derived from observations of nonverbal behavior will be moderately positively correlated with extraversion scores from personality inventories. Self-report, informant report, and behavioral observation each have different strengths and weaknesses as sources of information about a target's personality. They may capture different facets of personality (e.g., Borkenau et al., 2004).

In the RAP data, self-report and informant report data are available for the targets' extraversion. The target participants completed self-report versions of the NEO Personality Inventory (NEO-PI) (Costa & McCrae, 1985). In addition, each target participant was asked to recruit both parents, two hometown acquaintances, and two college acquaintances to provide informant report descriptions of the target's extraversion, using the NEO-PI. We computed composite scores within each informant domain (e.g., averaged the scores provided by the two hometown acquaintances) to obtain three composite informant report scores. In addition, we computed an overall informant report composite by averaging across all available informants.

To evaluate the validity of the data obtained from the behavioral observations, we examined the correlations between the behavioral observation data and the self-report and informant report inventory data. Table 16.6 presents these correlations and shows generally small to moderate positive correlations, providing evidence of convergent validity. The correlations were somewhat stronger for the ratings obtained through the observation of nonverbal behavior of targets in the opposite-sex stranger interaction, as compared with the ratings from the same-sex acquaintance interaction. To evaluate the discriminant validity of the ratings, we examined the correlations between the extraversion ratings obtained from the behavioral observations and the inventory scores on the other four factor scores from the NEO-PI. These correlations were not consistently different from zero, providing support for the discriminant validity of the behavioral observation extraversion ratings.

Summary and Conclusion

After a long history of neglect, direct behavioral observation is beginning to take its rightful place as a key method of personality psychology. Although behavioral observation is more difficult than gathering self-reports, does not include very many well-developed coding systems, and is time-consuming and expensive, behavioral data remain fundamental to personality psychology because behavior is a key psychological phenomenon in its own right and is the only route to deeper psychological knowledge. Researchers who decide to use behavioral observations need to consider the observational context they will use, such as laboratory versus real-world settings, whether to develop their own coding system or adapt one already developed by others, which behaviors to code, and the temporal units to be employed. Each of these considerations raises important issues, and the "right" choice, as always, depends on the theoretical aims of the investigation.

Once a behavioral observation study is begun, important practical issues include the selection and training of observers, the method of assigning them to particular interactions to code, and tracking reliability over the course of the coding process (as well as assessing it once the process is completed). Analyses based on G theory can be helpful not just for assessing validity and reliability, but also for making operational choices such as the number of coders to employ.

The direct assessment of behavior presents numerous practical and conceptual difficulties. But if psychology is to progress, there is no avoiding the need to develop and employ new methods for capturing what people actually are seen to do. The continued status of psychology as a science requires that we directly confront, rather than avoid, the difficulties of measuring the key phenomena in our field.

TABLE 16.6. Correlations between "Nonverbal" Extraversion and Extraversion Inventory Scores

Inventory source	Beh. Obs. from OSS situation		Beh. Obs. from SSA situation	
	Panel 1	Panel 2	Panel 1	Panel 2
Self	.32*	.27*	.13	.28*
Par. Comp.	.29*	.24	.03	.20
HT Comp.	.26*	.53***	.11	.31*
Coll. Comp.	.20	.11	.16	.10
Inf. Composite	.37**	.31*	.10	.23†

Note. N ranges between 42 and 64 across inventories and panels.
* $p < .05$; ** $p < .01$; *** $p < .001$; † $p < .10$; OSS, opposite-sex stranger; SSA, same-sex acquaintance.

Notes

1. All versions of the RBQ are available online at *www.faculty.ucr.edu/~funder/lab/supplemental.htm*.
2. The analyses that we present are part of a larger set of behavioral codings. Observers rated each target on 18 characteristics, but we focus only on the 2 characteristics relevant to extraversion. These ratings are based on observations of videotaped interactions that have been used with the RBQ in previously published research (e.g., Furr & Funder, 1998, 2004). The data based on *nonverbal* ratings have never been reported.
3. Other coefficients can be obtained as well. An "index of dependability" reflects the quality of the estimate of Targets' absolute scores, not the relative ordering of Target scores (Brennan, 2001). This index is appropriate when the test is used to make inferences about Targets' absolute scores (e.g., deciding whether a student's score meets a specific criterion to place her in a particular classroom). This index will probably not be directly relevant as a measure of reliability for most research in personality psychology.

Recommended Readings

Bakeman, R. (2000). Behavioral observations and coding. In H. T. Reis & C. K. Judd (Eds.), *Handbook of research methods in social psychology* (pp. 138–159). New York: Cambridge University Press.

Bakeman, R., & Gottman, J. M. (1997). *Observing interaction: An introduction to sequential analysis* (2nd ed.). New York: Cambridge University Press.

Brennan, R. L. (2001). *Generalizability theory.* New York: Springer-Verlag.

Cairns, R. B. (Ed.). (1979). *The analysis of social interactions: Methods, issues and illustrations.* Hillsdale, NJ: Erlbaum.

Funder, D. C., Furr, R. M., & Colvin, C. R. (2000). The Riverside Behavioral Q-Sort: A tool for the description of social behavior. *Journal of Personality, 68,* 451–489.

Margolin, G., Oliver, P. H., Gordis, E. B., O'Hearn, H. G., Medina, A. M., Ghosh, C. M., et al. (1998). The nuts and bolts of behavioral observation of marital and family interaction. *Clinical Child and Family Psychology Review, 4,* 195–213.

References

Alden, L. E., & Phillips, N. (1990). An interpersonal analysis of social anxiety and depression. *Cognitive Therapy and Research, 14,* 499–513.

Asendorpf, J. B., Banse, R., & Mücke, D. (2002). Double dissociation between implicit and explicit personality self-concept: The case of shy behavior. *Journal of Personality and Social Psychology, , 83,* 380–393.

Bakeman, R. (2000). Behavioral observations and coding. In H. T. Reis & C. K. Judd (Eds.), *Handbook of research methods in social psychology* (pp. 138–159). New York: Cambridge University Press.

Bakeman, R., & Gottman, J. M. (1997). *Observing interaction: An introduction to sequential analysis* (2nd ed.). New York: Cambridge University Press.

Bakeman, R., & Quera, V. (1995). *Analyzing interaction: Sequential analysis with SDIS and GSEQ.* New York: Cambridge University Press.

Bishop, E. G., & DiLalla, L. F. (1998). A method for predicting behavioral rating success. *Infant Behavior and Development, 21,* 163–166.

Block, J. (1978). *The Q-sort method in personality assessment and psychiatric research.* Palo Alto, CA: Consulting Psychologists Press. (Original work published 1961)

Borkenau, P., Mauer, N., Riemann, R., Spinath, F. M., & Angleitner, A. (2004). Thin slices of behavior as cues of personality and intelligence. *Journal of Personality and Social Psychology, 86,* 599–614.

Borkenau, P., Riemann, R., Angleitner, A., & Spinath, F. M. (2001). Genetic and environmental influences on observed personality: Evidence from the German Observational Study of Adult Twins. *Journal of Personality and Social Psychology, 80,* 655–668.

Brennan, R. L. (2001). *Generalizability theory.* New York: Springer-Verlag.

Cairns, R. B., & Green, J. A. (1979). How to assess personality and social patterns: Observations or ratings? In R. B. Cairns (Ed.), *The analysis of social interactions: Methods, issues and illustrations* (pp. 209–226). Hillsdale, NJ: Erlbaum.

Cattell, R. B. (1965). *The scientific analysis of personality.* Baltimore: Penguin Press.

Costa, P. T., & McCrae, R. R. (1985). *The NEO Personality Inventory manual.* Odessa, FL: Psychological Assessment Resources.

Cronbach, L. J., Gleser, G., C., Nanda, H., & Rajaratnam, N. (1972). *The dependability of behavioral measurements: Theory of generalizability for scores and profiles.* New York: Wiley.

De Corte, C. K., & Buysse, A. (n.d.) *The Riverside Behavioral Q-sort: Dutch translation.* Retrieved June 28, 2005, from *www.faculty.ucr.edu/%7Efunder/lab/DutchRBQ.htm*

Downey, G., Freitas, A. L., Michaelis, B., & Khouri, H. (1998). The self-fulfilling prophecy in close relationships: Rejection sensitivity and rejection by romantic partners. *Journal of Personality and Social Psychology, 75,* 545–560.

Ekman, P., Friesen, W. V., & Hager, J. C. (2002). *The facial action coding system* (2nd ed.). Salt Lake City, UT: Research Nexus eBook. Retrieved May 20, 2005, from *face-and-emotion.com/dataface/facs/description.jsp*

Ellgring, H. (1989). *Nonverbal communication in de-*

pression. Cambridge, UK: Cambridge University Press.

Feist, J., & Feist, G. J. (2002). *Theories of personality* (5th cd.). Boston: McGraw-Hill.

Funder, D. C. (2001). Personality. *Annual Review of Psychology, 52,* 197–221.

Funder, D. C. (2006). Towards a resolution of the personality triad: Persons, situations and behaviors. *Journal of Research in Personality, 40,* 21–34.

Funder, D. C., Furr, R. M., & Colvin, C. R. (2000). The Riverside Behavioral Q-Sort: A tool for the description of social behavior. *Journal of Personality, 68,* 451–489.

Furr, R. M., & Funder, D. C. (1998). A multi-modal analysis of personal negativity. *Journal of Personality and Social Psychology, 74,* 1580–1591.

Furr, R. M., & Funder, D. C. (2004). Situational similarity and behavioral consistency: Subjective, objective, variable-centered, and person-centered approaches. *Journal of Research in Personality, 38,* 421–447.

Goldberg, L. R. (1992). The development of markers for the Big-Five factor structure. *Psychological Assessment, 4,* 26–42.

Hokanson, J. E., Lowenstein, D. A., Hedeen, C., & Howes, M. J. (1986). Dysphoric college students and roommates: A study of social behaviors over a three-month period. *Personality and Social Psychology Bulletin, 12,* 311–324.

Kalbaugh, P. E., & Haviland, J. M. (1994). Nonverbal communication between parents and adolescents: A study of approach and avoidance behaviors. *Journal of Nonverbal Behavior, 18,* 91–113.

Margolin, G., Oliver, P. H., Gordis, E. B., O'Hearn, H. G., Medina, A. M., Ghosh, C. M., et al. (1998). The nuts and bolts of behavioral observation of marital and family interaction. *Clinical Child and Family Psychology Review, 4,* 195–213.

Markey, P. M., Markey, C. N., & Tinsley, B. (2004). Children's behavioral manifestations of the five-factor model of personality. *Personality and Social Psychology Bulletin, 30,* 423–432.

Mast, M. S., & Hall, J. A. (2003). Anybody can be a boss but only certain people make good subordinates: Behavioral impacts of striving for dominance and dominance aversion. *Journal of Personality, 71,* 871–892.

Mayer, J. D. (2004). A classification system for the data of personality psychology and adjoining fields. *Review of General Psychology, 8,* 208–219.

Mehl, M. R., & Pennebaker, J. W. (2003). The sounds of social life: A psychometric analysis of students' daily social environments and natural conversations. *Journal of Personality and Social Psychology, 84,* 857–870.

Pervin, L. A., & John, O. P. (2001). *Personality: Theory and research* (8th ed.). New York: Wiley.

Rosenberg, E. L. (1997). Introduction: The study of spontaneous facial expressions in psychology. In P. Ekman & E. L. Rosenberg (Eds.), *What the face reveals: Basic and applied studies of spontaneous expression using the Facial Action Coding System (FACS)* (pp. 3–17). London: Oxford University Press.

Rosenblum, L. (1978). The creation of a behavioral taxonomy. In G. P. Sackett (Ed.), *Observing behavior: Vol. 2. Data collection and analysis methods* (pp. 15–24). Baltimore: University Park Press.

Spinath, B., & Spinath, F. M. (2004). Verhaltensbeobachtungen in dyadischen Interaktionssituationen: Die deutsche Form des Riverside Behavioral Q-Sort (RBQ-D). *Zeitschrift für Differentielle und Diagnostische Psychologie, 25,* 105–115.

Spinath, B., Spinath, F. M. & Funder, D. C. (2000). *Die deutsche Form des Riverside Behavioral Q-Sort (RBQ-D): Ein Instrument zur Beschreibung von Verhalten in sozialen Interaktionssituationen.* Unveröffentlichtes Testmaterial, Universität Bielefeld.

Thompson, T., Felce, D., & Symons, F. J. (Eds.). (2000). *Behavioral observation: Technology and applications in developmental disabilities.* Baltimore: Brookes.

Thompson, T., Symons, F. J., & Felce, D. (2000). Principles of behavioral observation: Assumptions and strategies. In T. Thompson, D. Felce, & F. J. Symons (Eds.), *Behavioral observation: Technology and applications in developmental disabilities* (pp. 3–16). Baltimore: Brookes.

## CHAPTER 17

Content Coding
of Open-Ended Responses

Barbara A. Woike

This chapter deals with the content coding of written or verbal responses to open-ended questions. Responses to open-ended questions can range from the completion of sentences to extended narratives. The content may be derived from the respondent's imagination, opinions on various topics, or autobiographical memory. The amount of and variability in the material generated about thoughts, feelings, and behavior in response to an open-ended question can be staggering. Yet this material may arguably be the richest information available to personality psychologists. As more and more researchers turn to these techniques to investigate complex personality processes, it is important for the field to establish a set of guidelines for conducting content coding of open-ended responses. This chapter attempts to bring to light the unique advantages and challenges of this method. It also seeks to stimulate the reader's imagination about the possible uses of content coding in research. Moreover, it warns against treating data yielded by content scoring techniques as though they were data derived from questionnaires and argues for a specific set of rules governing issues of reliability and validity of content-coded data that can maintain both methodological rigor and the richness of the material. Thus, the chapter presents (1) information on the history and development of open-ended scoring techniques, followed by (2) a review of the basic types of scoring systems, (3) a step-by-step guide to using these scoring techniques, and (4) a case example of developing a hypothesis-driven content scoring system. The final section discusses briefly the complexities involved in determining reliability and validity of data collected with open-ended scoring techniques.

History and Development of Open-Ended Scoring Methods

Throughout the history of psychology, open-ended-style questions have been a common choice for researchers interested in complex, subjective experiences, including intentions, patterns of reasoning, and attempts to find meaning in personal experiences. In the late 19th century and early 20th century, the most influential psychologists of the day, including Galton, William James, Wundt, Freud, G. Stanley Hall, and Piaget, made extensive use of narrative accounts of personal experiences in their early explorations of the inner workings of the mind (Smith, 2000). These researchers were concerned with the broad issues of how people think, reason, and make use of their experiences to understand themselves and the world around them. Even as the behaviorists rejected the subjective, introspective, and mentalistic aspects of the person and limited their psychological investigations to observable behavior, some personologically and clinically oriented psychologists, such as Murray and Allport, continued to explore the inner life of the person using a variety of open-ended techniques.

When interest in cognition and affect returned to mainstream psychology during the 1950s and 1960s, a foundation had been laid to explore these topics with increased experimental rigor (Smith, 2000). For some researchers this meant developing reliable measures in the form of fixed-response instruments such as inventories and questionnaires. Some investigators found that these methods did not capture the complexity of human thought, feelings, and behavior, and they turned to content and narrative analysis as an alternative that provided less structure and greater insight into the richness of the subjective experience of the individual. The research programs that attempted to assess personality motives via storytelling techniques, such as the work on the achievement motive (McClelland, Atkinson, Clark, & Lowell, 1958), put forth the notion that indirect, open-ended measures of personality can be highly revealing of a person's preferences and enduring concerns (see Schultheiss & Pang, Chapter 19, this volume).

Since the mid-1980s, there has been a burgeoning of interest in open-ended responses that involve content-analytic techniques. Notably, McAdams (1985) put forth a model of identity as being rooted in one's personal life story. According to this view, an individual's life story is an internalized and evolving narrative of the self that serves to integrate disparate roles and to bring together the reconstructed past, perceived present, and anticipated future. Moreover, the groundbreaking work of Pennebaker (1997; Pennebaker, Mehl, & Niederhoffer, 2003) demonstrated the importance of narratives in making meaning of traumatic and difficult personal experiences. Thus, personal narratives have been shown to provide a person's life with some degree of unity, purpose, and meaning.

Interest in open-ended responses reached a new height when Smith (1992) devoted an entire book to issues of thematic content analysis that included 14 different scoring systems for open-ended responses for motives, attributions and cognitive orientations, and psychosocial orientations. The topics investigated by the various content scoring systems in the book included personality change and development, stress and coping, goal setting, physical health and illness, and societal trends. This book provided practical information on using content-analytic methods and helped to make the techniques more accessible to researchers interested in open-ended responses.

Nowadays, it is quite common for personality psychologists interested in complex psychological processes to employ open-ended response techniques. Many researchers have found that by asking people to write or to express orally their thoughts and reactions, it is possible to discover unique patterns of expression that would be extremely difficult to capture in the form of fixed-response questionnaires. Thus, despite its labor-intensiveness and complications involving reliability and validity (discussed below), many researchers find content coding of open-ended responses to be an invaluable tool.

A unique, and perhaps most important aspect of open-ended responses is that they offer individuals freedom of expression. Some personality psychologists have argued that individual differences are most easily detected in situations that are loosely structured so that the person cannot rely on external social cues on how to act, think, and feel. Open-ended techniques can create such ambiguity. Participants may find that the open-ended format gives them more freedom to explore their thoughts, feelings, and reactions in ways that they had not done previously. So the qualitative material generated from open-ended questions may reveal innermost thoughts, frames of reference, emotional reactions, and cultural assumptions that may or may not be accessible by other methods.

In contrast, when developing a fixed-response format, researchers use their expertise to come up with typically four or fewer alternatives from which the participant must select one that best represents his or her thoughts, feelings, and reactions to the question. The procedure obviously limits the participants' choices and restricts their options to what the researcher views as most probable or relevant. Participants may endorse responses that do not at all represent their true reactions—even if they are the most representative ones available. It may be that a question is simply irrelevant to the individual. For example, if a researcher is interested in the characteristic of "zaniness" and develops a zaniness questionnaire, it may have utility only with people who have the characteristic of zaniness and offer no predictive utility for those who lack this characteristic (cf. Baumeister & Tice, 1988).

Open-ended responses are more likely to be personally relevant and important to the individual because they are generated by the individual—often spontaneously. Because responses to open-ended questions are generated without a great deal of prompting, they may be more likely to reveal the individual's most candid and least self-critical thoughts, feelings, and reactions. For this reason, response biases such as social desirability effects, which often plague questionnaire methods (see Paulhus & Vazire, Chapter 13, this volume), should be of less concern for responses to open-ended questions. The content of open-ended responses may reveal more about people than they want to disclose, or even more than they know about themselves.

Another related advantage of open-ended responses is that they can often bring to light issues that the researcher did not think to inquire about directly. There may be aspects of the phenomenon in question that are extremely important to the participant but go undetected owing to preconceived ideas or lack of awareness of the researcher. For instance, in a pilot study that my colleagues and I conducted (Wang, 2004) on how young women balance their commitments to work and relationships, we asked fixed-response questions about the number of mentors and how much social support the participants received from the mentors. We found that the participants generally reported few mentors and very little social support. It was later discovered via the responses to open-ended items, such as "Describe someone in

your life who is helpful to you," that the words *mentor* and *social support* had very negative connotations. For the young women in the sample, these words implied subordinate relationships and lack of ability to cope. By asking them open-ended questions about helpful people in their lives, the participants were able and quite willing to express their experiences with mentors and social support, but in their own words. If we had not asked the questions in an open-ended way, we would never have known about these supportive relationships that were central to the study. Open-ended responses may help lessen unknown researcher biases. Thus, the open-ended response method offers a unique set of advantages and challenges.

Types of Open-Ended Responses

It is beyond the scope of this chapter to inventory every established content scoring system created to analyze open-ended response data (see Smith, 1992, 2000, for a more extensive list). Three major types of open-ended responses are discussed here: (1) sentence completion, (2) verbal material from essays or archives, and (3) personal narratives, stories, and diaries. It is intended that the examples of each type be given in enough detail for the reader to appreciate the breadth of content that can be studied with these methods.

Sentence Completion Tests

Sentence completion tests generally involve providing participants with a set of sentence stems each from which they must complete to form a complete thought. Participants are usually instructed to respond quickly or to go with their initial reactions to the stem. Sentence completion tests are often employed to measure motivation, as well as to assess moral and cognitive reasoning. The idea is to obtain a sample of the participants' thoughts, reasoned opinions, and/or preoccupations in response to a minimal prompt, such as "I feel good when . . . ," "It is important to . . . ," "I am trying to . . . ," and "Most people are. . . . "

Three examples of sentence completion scoring systems are discussed below. The first two coding systems are excellent examples of the operationalization of complex psychological characteristics derived from well-known theories of personality development. The final example is a very successful attempt to measure and to classify personal goals. In examining the responses to the sentence stems, one often finds that no two responses are alike. Yet these classification systems can reliably identify the common characteristics of complex psychological processes. Numerous studies have validated the utility of these tests.

The first example of a sentence completion test measures human motivation based on Maslow's (1954) hierarchy of needs. Aronoff (Aronoff & Wilson, 1985) developed the sentence completion test to measure three of the needs from Maslow's well-known hierarchy. On the basis of his knowledge of Maslow's theory, Aronoff developed scoring categories that were articulated in enough detail for independent coders to reliably identify the responses. For instance, sentence completions such as "I feel good when *I have enough money*" and "Most people are *rude*" demonstrate a desire for safety, whereas responses like "Most people are *potential friends*" and "I feel good when *I am loved*" indicate a need for affiliation. Responses like "I feel good when *I am doing my best*" and "It is important to *make a lasting contribution*" represent the need for esteem. Individuals complete a series of sentence stems that are then scored for these motives by independent judges. Aronoff conducted a series of studies both cross-culturally and with college students in the United States that offered convincing evidence for the validity of the scoring system. Research on developmental antecedents and group behavior validated the system's power in distinguishing individuals concerned with safety and esteem needs (Aronoff & Wilson, 1985).

Loevinger's model of ego development (1976) has been especially influential in personality psychology because it allows the ego stages to be measured via a standardized sentence completion test, called the Washington University Sentence Completion Test for Ego Development (WUSCTED; Loevinger & Wessler, 1970). The work is theoretically grounded in a cognitive-developmental paradigm, influenced by Piaget and concepts from the psychoanalytic tradition. The WUSCTED is used to study how people make sense of and synthesize experiences as they move across the lifespan. As in Maslow's theory, development is viewed as a progression through hierarchical stages. Earlier stages must be mastered before subsequent stages can be approached. In general, moving from lower to higher stages, one becomes less governed by immediate impulses and more flexible, operating according to internalized standards of conduct. Interpersonally, the person moves from egocentrism through conformity to relative autonomy and mutual interdependence. The WUSCTED is composed of a series of sentence stems, such as "The thing I like about myself . . . " and "I am . . . " For each stem, the person writes an ending to the sentence. Each response is classified into one of Loevinger's stages, ranging from impulsive to integrated, according to carefully designed scoring manuals. The scores are then tabulated, and a final ego-state score is derived according to a numerical formula. The test has generated a considerable amount of research that, to a great extent, has shown the validity of this classification system. For instance, researchers interested in personality development over time have used this system to develop a tripartite typology of personality characteristics and have demonstrated coherent patterns over time (e.g., John, Pals, & Westenberg, 1998; York & John, 1992).

A sentence completion format can also be used to classify the content of personal goals. Notably, Emmons (1986,1992) developed the concept of personal strivings, defined as "characteristic, recurring goals that a person is trying to accomplish" (Emmons, 1992, p. 292). The participant is asked to list 10–15 different personal strivings, or what he or she is "currently trying to do." Examples used to complete the stem "Trying to:" include "avoid anything that upsets me," "be a kinder person," "attain positions of leadership," and "not eat between meals." Emmons (1992) developed a 12-category coding system to capture the idiographic nature of these strivings and demonstrated that they are related to other important motivational constructs, as well as quality-of-life measures. For example, strivings related to intimacy, generativity, and spirituality are correlated with well-being, whereas avoidance and power strivings are negatively correlated with life satisfaction (Emmons, 1992). It has also been possible to examine the interrelationship between and among different strivings (Emmons & King , 1988) and how these goals may be related to different levels of motivation that can predict action (Emmons & McAdams, 1991).

Paragraphs from Essays, Archives, and Other Verbal Material

Content-analytic methods have also been used to identify patterns of content and structure in essays written in response to specific questions, as well as in archival material such as letters, diaries, and speeches, which may provide a rich source of information about a person's inner life. Archives may be the only source of information about persons who are deceased, unavailable, or uncooperative. Written or oral records may provide the only feasible way of studying individuals in depth, and at the same time take into account historical periods, cohort, and social/cultural influences on the individual (see Cramer, Chapter 7, this volume, for a more detailed discussion).

The length of such material can range from a paragraph to many pages of text. Therefore, to analyze this type of material, the researcher must first decide on a meaningful unit of analysis. This may be the whole response, regardless of length, or the unit may be arbitrarily decided by using some factor, such as the number of words or paragraphs, that is unrelated to the content of the material. Another strategy is to develop a criterion for meaningful passages that lend themselves to further analysis and discard the other material that does not meet the criterion. Once the unit of analysis is identified, a scoring system may be created to quantify the characteristics of interest. Below are two examples of such scoring systems.

One well-known scoring system used with lengthy material of this sort is the Content Analysis of Verbatim Explanations (CAVE; Peterson, Schulman, Castellon, & Seligman, 1992), which measures the explanatory style that individuals use to make sense of events. The CAVE technique involves extracting casual explanations from verbal material and then rating these explanations on 7-point scales according to their internality, stability, and globality. The system was developed to approximate the Attributional Style Questionnaire (ASQ; Peterson et al., 1982), and make it possible to research "all manner of interesting subjects, including those inaccessible with the ASQ—the quick, dead, famous, belligerent, sensitive or remote" (Peterson et al., 1992, p. 380). The CAVE technique has been used reliably by independent judges unaware of the research hypotheses. There is a good deal of validation data supporting the CAVE technique as a measure of explanatory style. Studies show that highly internal, stable, and global causes preceded increased depression and that highly external, unstable, and specific causes preceded decreased depression in psychotherapy transcripts coded with the use of CAVE. Peterson, Seligman, and Vaillant (1988) used the CAVE technique to analyze data from a 35-year longitudinal study of the psychological precursors of physical illness. They found that a pessimistic explanatory style found in the written responses around age 25 predicted poor health from ages 45 through 60, even when initial mental and physical health were held constant, thereby lending a good deal of support for the powerful influence of explanatory style.

A second scoring system used extensively to analyze text is the Integrative Complexity Coding Manual (Baker-Brown et al., 1992). This system has been developed from successive versions of theory that focus on the complexity of information processing and decision making. Complexity includes two components: differentiation and integration. *Differentiation* refers to the perception of different dimensions within a stimulus domain, and to the taking of different perspectives when considering the domain. In this scoring system, differentiation is a necessary but not sufficient prerequisite for *integration*, which is the development of conceptual connections between differentiated dimensions or perspectives. Examples of such connections include references to tradeoffs between alternatives, a synthesis between them, and a reference to a higher-order concept that subsumes them. Integrative complexity is scored on a 1–7 scale, where 1 indicates no evidence of either differentiation or integration, 3 indicates moderate to high differentiation but no integration, 5 indicates moderate to high differentiation and moderate integration, and 7 indicates both high differentiation and high integration. A great deal of research has demonstrated the utility of the system. Nonarchival research has been directed toward the general topics of social perception, attitude and attitude change, and attribution; preparation of speeches, organization problems, attitudes concerning social policy decisions, and moral dilemmas. Archival work has addressed the prediction of international crises and their outcomes, the effects of social and political roles, the succession and duration of leader careers, and the relation between political ideology and political climate (Suedfeld, Tetlock, &

Streufert, 1992). It also has been possible to examine the interplay of archival, case study, and experimental research, deriving hypotheses from one that can be tested by the others. For instance, this convergent approach had been used to study complexity, value conflict, and political ideology and the effects of accountability on complexity (Tetlock, 1983; Tetlock & Kim, 1987; Tetlock, Skitka, & Boettger, 1989).

Personal Narratives, Stories, and Diaries

In recent years, personality psychologists have become increasingly interested in the stories people tell about their own lives (e.g., Pillemer, 1998; Singer & Salovey, 1993; Thorne, 2000). Autobiographical essays and stories may hold special significance because they provide valuable information about a person's self-perceptions, including self-identity, life scripts, and beliefs in how the world works pertaining to the person's destiny. Moreover, research suggests that personal narratives promote healing from personal traumas and other difficult life experiences and can aid in integrating life experiences into a stable sense of identity (McAdams, 1985). The telling of personal stories allows individuals to make sense of difficult or discordant events and to integrate these experiences with the self.

Most notably, the work of Pennebaker (1997) suggests that translating personal traumas into words has long-term health benefits. This basic writing paradigm, used in a large number of these studies, involves having participants write about assigned topics for 3–5 consecutive days, 15–30 minutes each day. The writing is generally done in the laboratory with no feedback given. Participants assigned to the control condition are typically asked to write about superficial topics, whereas participants in the experimental condition are asked to "[Write about the] very deepest thoughts and feelings about an extremely important emotional issue that has affected you and your life" (Pennebaker, 1997, p. 162). Common themes found in these emotional essays include lost loves, deaths, incidents of sexual and physical abuse, and tragic failures. In order to study the cognitive changes associated with writing about traumatic experiences, Pennebaker and Francis (1996) created the Linguistic Inquiry and Word Count (LIWC), a computer program

that analyzes essays in text format. The LIWC was developed by having judges evaluate the degree to which more than 2,000 words were related to several different categories. These categories included negative emotion words (*sad*, *angry*), positive emotion words (*happy*, *laugh*), causal words (*because*, *reason*), and insight words (*understand*, *realize*). The LIWC program allows for the quick computation of the percentage of the total words that are represented in each of these categories.

Three linguistic factors have been found to reliably predict improved physical health. First, the more positive words people used, the better their subsequent health. Second, moderate use of negative emotion words was associated with better health, whereas the use of very high or very low numbers of negative emotion words correlated with poorer health. And perhaps most important, an increase in both causal and insight words over the course of the writing was strongly associated with improved health (Pennebaker, Mayne, & Francis, 1997). That is, people who benefited most from writing began with poorly organized descriptions and progressed to a coherent story by the end of the writing assignment.

The life story model of personality is another highly influential narrative approach (McAdams, 1985). According to this model, identity itself is the life story that an individual begins constructing in late adolescence and young adulthood. McAdams created a life story interview in which participants divide their lives into chapters and provide a plot summary for each. They are then asked to describe eight key episodes (e.g., low and high points, turning point, earliest memory). Participants then identify and describe their greatest life challenges, the most influential people in their lives as the main characters, future plot, personal ideology, and life theme.

Obviously, much information is gleamed from these extensive life narrative interviews. McAdams has developed two different scoring techniques to capture the variability and common themes among these highly idiographic accounts. First, by examining the thematic lines of the stories, it was found that many characters strive for love or power or both. Love and power reflect Bakan's (1966) themes of agency and communion, which he argues are the two fundamental modalities of experience. *Agency* refers to the individual's efforts to expand, assert, perfect, and protect the self, to separate the self from others, and to master the environment. *Communion* refers to the individual's efforts to merge with other individuals, to join together with others in bonds of love, intimacy, friendship, and community. McAdams, Hoffman, Mansfield, and Day (1996) developed and validated a system that breaks down agency and communion into four main subthemes that can be reliably coded in narrative accounts of key episodes in a life story, such as high points or turning points. For agency, life story episodes can be reliably coded for the subthemes of self-mastery, status/victory, achievement/responsibility, and empowerment. For communion, life story episodes can be reliably coded for subthemes of friendship/love, dialogue, care/help, and unity/togetherness. Research suggests that these themes are consistently related to people's motivational tendencies (McAdams et al., 1996; Woike, 1994, 1995; Woike, Gershkovich, Piorkowski, & Polo, 1999; Woike & Polo, 2001).

Second, McAdams' more recent work looks at the life stories of midlife adults. A general theme from these life narratives is the commitment story, similar to Tomkins's (1987) notion of a commitment script. In the commitment story, the protagonist (1) enjoys an early family blessing or advantage, (2) is sensitized to the suffering of others at an early age, (3) is guided by a clear and compelling personal ideology that remains relatively stable over time, (4) transforms or redeems bad events into good outcomes, and (5) sets goals for the future to benefit society and its institutions. Commitment life stories are common among adults committed to promoting the well-being of youth and the next generation, or what Erikson referred to as *generativity*. For both midlife adults and students, the tendency to construct life stories in which bad events are ultimately redeemed into good outcomes is associated with greater psychological well-being (McAdams & de St. Aubin, 1992; McAdams, de St. Aubin, & Logan, 1993).

Many of the aforementioned scoring techniques can be applied to smaller snippets of data, such as short diary entries and data gathered from experience sampling techniques (see Conner, Feldman Barrett, Tugade, & Tennen, Chapter 5, this volume). For instance, Mehl, Pennebaker, Crow, Dabbs, and Price (2001) developed the Electronically Activated Recorder (EAR), a device for sampling naturalistic daily activities and conversations. The EAR tape-

records for 30 seconds once and every 12 minutes for 2–4 days. It is also possible to examine daily diary entries by adapting the scoring criteria to smaller units of analysis. For instance, Woike (1995; Woike & Polo, 2001) converted McAdams's agentic and communal scoring criteria to score narratives of significant life events into a scoring system for daily diary entries.

Thus, content-analytic methods are used to measure a wide range of personological phenomena. By giving people simple guidelines for open-ended questions, it is possible to tap into their most important aspirations, hopes, and fears—as well as their unique capacity of understanding themselves and the world around them. Evidence shows that these systems can be used reliably, by independent judges, to discern and to categorize a wide array of responses. A large body of validation data demonstrates that these techniques reveal complex personality processes, including motivations, beliefs, and even probable courses of action.

A Step-by-Step Guide to Using Content Coding Techniques

The basic steps involved in content coding of open-ended responses have been identified (Smith, 2000). Each of these steps is discussed here in terms of general issues and decisions that must be made at each respective point in the research process.

• *Step 1: What is the research question? What is to be identified, described, or measured?* In personality psychology, open-ended response data may be used to test three basic types of hypotheses, which are not necessarily mutually exclusive. First, the method may be employed to identify a personality characteristic that is assumed to be relatively stable over time, such as explanatory style or achievement motivation. Second, open-ended responses may be used to assess a person's understanding of a certain event, such as in Pennebaker's (1997) technique for retelling traumatic experiences. This allows the researcher to ask questions pertaining to how a person reasons or makes sense of particular events and issues. There is the potential to uncover numerous patterns from these data. The technique may also allow researchers to uncover how describing the experience itself influences the individual—for example, how writing about an event many times changes the person's understanding of that event over time. Finally, coding techniques for open-ended responses may be employed as outcome or dependent measures—for instance, studies that show that experimental manipulations such as accountability (Tetlock, 1983) influence the complexity of a person's narrative opinion of various issues. In addition, open-ended scoring procedures may valuable in post hoc explorations and as unobtrusive manipulation checks.

• *Step 2: Decide whether content analysis will provide the needed information, either by itself or in conjunction with another method.* It is often preferable to employ some other measure for cross-validation of the scoring system for open-ended responses, particularly if it is a newly developed system. However, it is often the case that the reason a content-analytic technique is employed is that the phenomena under investigation cannot be properly studied via other methods. It is also important to be mindful of the associations, or lack thereof, between self-report questionnaires and data coded from open-ended responses, inasmuch as lack of association may be due to method variance.

If the open-ended response system is used to assess a stable personality characteristic, such as the need for achievement, the results of the study itself may verify the validity of the open-ended measure. If open-ended responses are to be used as dependent variables, it may be especially desirable to obtain multiple measures derived from more than one assessment technique. Demonstrating an effect with converging methods offers convincing evidence for the hypotheses and validates the open-ended scoring technique at the same time.

• *Step 3: Decide what type of qualitative material will best provide the information needed and how to obtain it.* There are some important issues for consideration at this step in the research process. First, what questions should be asked? The task is to create enough structure to make meaningful comparisons and for meaningful differences to be detected, if they do in fact exist. A researcher would probably not want to approach an elderly participant and simply say, "Tell me the story of your life." Insufficient structure would probably introduce too much variability. However, the questions should not be so structured that they resemble those of a self-report questionnaire.

Should similar questions be asked more than once as a way to obtain a more stable measure? This technique works well in the scoring systems of measures such as sentence completion tests, in which many stems are provided, each response is scored, and then the total scores are examined to derive the participant's score. Other methods, such as interviews, do not provide a way to obtain repeated measures, but asking questions in sequence provides continuity and some degree of structure across participants.

Should response time or number of words be limited in order to create some degree of standardization? How might this influence the responses? It may not be practical to allow participants an unlimited amount of time to tell their personal accounts. Yet imposing a time or word limit can create demand characteristics and limit spontaneity. Should the questions be asked via computer, written format, or orally? A computer format may be most efficient if the data will be analyzed using a computer-assisted scoring procedure. However, it is necessary that participants know how to use a computer and feel comfortable in responding this way. The written format may be the most common form of collecting open-response data, as it is easy for the participant to see the question or stem and then construct an answer in a standard format created by the researcher. Oral responding may be more appropriate for participants less familiar with a writing format, such as children, elderly individuals, and persons with learning disabilities.

Should responses be anonymous or given in face-to-face interviews? Anonymity is often preferable, as it believed to increase honesty and candidness. However, it may be necessary to conduct face-to-face interviews if participants are unfamiliar with the procedure or need more guidance to maintain their interest and increase the appropriateness of their responses, such as with children, elderly people, individuals with learning disabilities, or those who speak a different native language. Of course, if the researcher is analyzing archival data, he or she must take what is available in the format in which it is found. It may still be worthwhile to consider how the format may have influenced the responses—as some open-ended methods may be more susceptible to context effects than questionnaires.

• *Step 4: Determine the unit of analysis to be coded.* Depending on the decisions made in the previous steps, the length of open-ended response material can range from a phrase, to a sentence, a paragraph, or many pages of text. Whatever the amount, a central task is deciding on a meaningful unit of analysis. Coding units used in prior research include (1) the entire text unit, such as an essay, (2) linguistically defined segments, such as meaningful words, clauses, or sentences, (3) response segments, such as a response to an interview question, (4) physically defined segments, such as a set number of words, and (5) temporal segments, such as number of minutes of a verbal response (Smith, 2000). Once the unit of analysis has been identified, a scoring system may be created to quantify the characteristics of interest.

- *Step 5: Select or develop a content coding system.* A number of scoring systems for open-ended responses have been developed in prior research. Therefore, reviewing the literature relevant to the research question is an important task. An example of how to develop a new scoring system for open-ended responses is presented in a case study in the next section of this chapter. In deciding on a scoring system, it is important to consider what types of scores are most desirable for understanding the data. There are three kinds of scores that may be generated from the content coding of open-ended responses: categories, ratings, and frequencies.

A categorization system is typically used to describe and identify broad orientations that are assumed to be related to personality structures and processes. The researcher develops a description of the characteristics that must be present for the responses to be categorized. The description must be general enough to apply to the various responses generated from the open-ended questions, as well as specific enough that coders can use the system reliably.

Ratings systems are similar to categories, except that they are incremental, and therefore it is not possible to score a unit of analysis for more than one rating. The psychosocial phenomenon being rated necessarily has a valenced quality. For example, the scale may range from positive to negative or from simple to complex. As with a categorization system, the researcher develops a description of the characteristics that must be present for the responses to be given a certain rating. The description must be general enough to apply to the various responses but specific enough to be used reliably. As in the integrative complexity scoring system (Baker-Brown et al., 1992) and Loevinger and Wessler's (1970) ego development coding system, the response to each open-ended question is given a rating. In this way, an average rating can be computed from each category. A potential problem with ratings is that there must be enough open-ended response questions so that when the ratings are used as a dependent measure they are relatively stable—that is, not based on one data point. This issue may be particularly problematic if specific meaningful units are being selected and certain cases contain only a smaller number of these units. Another problem can be obtaining enough variability among scores in the sample.

Frequency coding involves developing criteria for meaningful units of the response and recording the number of instances of these units in the data. Frequency coding can be quite labor-intensive, especially if responses are dense and lengthy. However, frequencies are a good choice for data in which the meaningful units occur rather infrequently and the researcher has multiple scoring criteria that can be discerned reliably from the data.

Another issue is whether it is most efficient to score the data using trained coders or whether the data can be scored via computer. There are obvious advantages to computer scoring in terms of efficiency and consistency. However, computers may miss important variability and nuances in the data that trained judges can detect easily. Computer-assisted scoring may be most useful for voluminous text in which simple sentences and phrases are to be counted, such as in the LIWC. But complex sentence structures and themes that may have an infinite number of semantic manifestations in open-ended responses do not lend themselves easily to computer-assisted techniques.

- *Step 6: Obtain pilot data to test and to refine the coding system.* An important consideration is whether the coding system will be (or has been) developed using an a priori approach, in which the criteria are specified before the material is examined, or an empirical approach, in which the criteria emerge from material to be analyzed (Smith, 2000). If the system is developed a priori, the researcher must compare the coding criteria with the pilot data and consider whether the phenomena of interest are meaningfully represented in the data. If not, then the researcher must consider whether the criteria can be modified to better suit the data or whether a different set of a priori criteria should be used. If the a priori criteria are in fact found in the pilot data, then the researcher must decide if the definitions of the coding system are specific enough for independent judges, unaware of the hypotheses, to detect this content using the specified criteria.

If the empirical approach is employed, researchers can provide independent judges, unaware of the hypotheses, with broad definitions of the phenomena of interest and see what they find. Alternatively, researchers can examine the pilot data themselves and come up with scoring criteria based on the patterns in the pilot data. Then the researcher must develop the definitions of the coding system to be specific enough for a new set of independent judges, unaware of the hypotheses, to reliably detect the content of interest.

• *Step 7: Train coders and ensure that intercoder agreement is satisfactory.* Essential requirements for training coders are a clear coding manual, ample practice material, and an opportunity to discuss coding decisions with an expert scorer (Smith, 2000). The rules and procedures for the coding system must be explicitly defined in a scoring manual. These manuals typically include a general orientation to the phenomena of interest, then specific definitions of the content to be identified, as well as how it is to be identified, (e.g., categories, ratings, or frequencies). Many established scoring systems also include practice exercises for coders to hone their scoring skills. The practice exercises can be used to help coders achieve interrater agreement and to give researchers a good estimate of how accurately each coder is able to score the data. In general, it is a good idea for an expert coder to meet regularly with the group of coders to discuss their progress in learning the scoring criteria and to discuss any difficulties or ambiguities in the scoring system. It is most desirable for all data to be scored by at least two coders who are unaware of the hypotheses. In some cases, it may be acceptable for the data to be scored by one expert scorer and one naive coder. The scoring systems mentioned in this chapter should be appropriate for advanced undergraduates or graduate students. It may be desirable to train more coders than needed and use only those coders who demonstrate the highest aptitude on practice or pilot data (Smith, 2000).

Intercoder agreement is computed differently, depending on whether the data are scores or categories. When coding systems yield scores, a correlation coefficient can be used to assess agreement. Assessing intercoder reliability with categories can be more complex. The simplest and most frequently reported category index is the percentage of agreement between two or more coders in classifying materials into two or more categories. For example, two coders may agree 75% of the time. There are two problems with this measure. First, it is affected by the frequency with which the category is present. Second, it does not take into account chance agreement. The first problem is most evident with low or high frequency of occurrences—for example, if achievement imagery is present in 2 out of 100 imaginative stories. If a coder misses the two instances and codes achievement imagery as being absent in 100 out of 100 stories, then the coder's agreement with the practice exercises would be 98%. To correct the percentage of agreement for the frequency with which the category occurs, the following index was developed by McClelland and colleagues (1958):

$$\frac{2 \ (\text{# of agreements between coders on presence of category})}{(\text{# scored present by coder 1}) + (\text{# scored present by coder 2})}$$

If the scoring system involves several categories, it may be useful to compute the index for each category, both to assess agreement and to discover categories that may need to be eliminated or revised.

To correct for chance agreement, Cohen's (1960) kappa is often employed when the coding categories are independent and mutually exclusive. A weighted kappa may be used to evaluate agreement with ordinal categorical data. Kappa is an index that characterizes agreement in applying a coding scheme that varies from 0 (indicating no agreement) to 1 (indicating perfect agreement). It is a summary statistic derived from a matrix of the proportion of agreement actually observed and the proportion of agreement expected. For more details concerning computation and available programs, see Bakeman (2000).

What should be considered an acceptable level of intercoder reliability? Published research has tended to regard 85% agreement, or an interscorer correlation of .85 or more, as acceptable (Smith, Feld, & Franz, 1992), although a kappa score of .80 or more can be viewed as satisfactory, depending on the data (see McDowell & Acklin, 1996). Once agreement is calculated and an acceptable level of intercoder reliability is achieved, coders can discuss their disagreements. In the final analyses, disagreements can be resolved through a consensus discussion or the disparate scores can be averaged.

• *Step 8: Obtain final material to be analyzed.* The final material should be collected by researchers unaware of the hypotheses. Ideally, the data should be collected by a group of researchers different from those who will score the open-ended response data. As in all data collections, it is important that all participants receive the same instructions and are tested in the same context under the same conditions. Open-ended responses can have a good deal of variability, and the experimenter needs to be careful to not inadvertently introduce more while collecting the responses.

• *Step 9: Code the material with identifying characteristics removed, and determine interrater reliability; or perform computer-assisted content analysis.* Ideally, handwritten data should be transcribed. Coders who have achieved an acceptable level of reliability on practice materials or pilot data, and who are unaware of the hypotheses, should work independently to score the data. The scores should then be compared; the data must meet acceptable levels of reliability, as discussed in Step 7, before any data analysis or interpretation is performed on the data.

• *Step 10: Analyze the data; carry out cross-validation if appropriate.* An exhaustive discussion of data analytic strategies is beyond the scope of the chapter. However, some important issues for consideration when using categories, ratings, and frequencies are discussed here. First, if responses may be classified into a fixed number of mutually exclusive categories, then they must be treated as categories in the analyses. If hypotheses are to be tested with inferential statistics, it is essential that there is a large enough sample size for each category. If the other variables in the study are also categorical, then the chi-square statistic may be most appropriate. For instance, Woike, Candela, and Osier (1996) investigated the relationship between college men's attachment styles (secure, avoidant, anxious) and the violent imagery they used to write imaginative stories about relationships. Criteria for scoring violent imagery developed by Pollack and Gilligan (1982) were adopted, and the discrete categories of violent imagery (e.g., verbal threats, murder) were combined into one violent imagery category because the individual categories occurred in low frequency. A chi-square analysis was conducted using the three attachment categories and the presence or absence of violent imagery. The frequency of anxious men who wrote stories with the presence of violent imagery was significantly greater than expected by chance.

If the other variables in the study are continuous, it is possible to compare the means of these variables between categories using parametric statistics. For instance, Woike, Mcleod, and Goggin (2003) asked people to describe two memories, which were then categorized as either agentic or communal following McAdams's (1985) scoring criteria. The prediction was that people would be more likely to recall a memory that was congruent with their motivation (either achievement/power or intimacy). To test the prediction, *t*-tests were performed on the motive scores, which were continuous variables between the presence and absence of the categories. For instance, the investigators compared the average of the achievement/power motives scores for participants who recalled a memory categorized as agentic with the scores of those who recalled memories that were not categorized as agentic. It was found that those who recalled an agentic memory had higher achievement motivation scores than those who did not recall an agentic memory, and the same pattern was found for intimacy motivation and communal memories.

Second, the data yielded from scoring open-ended responses may be ratings on a continuum. In this case, it is important to first examine the descriptive properties of the data. Is there a normal distribution? In many cases, rating systems for variables reflecting psychological or intellectual maturity, such as the scoring systems for ego development and integrative complexity, tend to be skewed or restricted in range on the lower end of the scale, particularly in college populations (Woike, 1994). Thus, it is important to obtain a sufficient sample size and ratings that represent a number of responses per participant. It may be useful to correct for range restriction. If there is a broad range of skewed scores, it may be useful to convert ratings to standard scores. After taking these issues into consideration, the ratings can be used to test a range of hypotheses with most inferential statistics.

Finally, the scoring of open-ended responses may yield frequency data. As with ratings, it is important to examine the distribution of frequency data. Another very important consideration is how the frequencies relate to the size of the response, that is, how do frequencies relate to the number of words used in the response? Many researchers argue that all frequency data should be corrected for word count (see Schultheiss & Pang, Chapter 19, this volume, for more details about correction techniques). However, it may behoove the researcher to consider alternatives. If we are scoring for specific themes that by necessity need words to be presented, it is the mere presence of these themes—not the number per number of words—that is important. For instance, if an individual's written recollection of a traumatic event reflects a greater insight and understanding based on the frequency of certain specified words, the actual written recollection may be longer than one that does not reflect such insight and understanding. It would be an inaccurate representation of the response to calculate the "insight per word" ratio, as it would lose all external validity.

• *Step 11: Interpret results. Compare your findings with norms, if available.* The interpretation and generalizability of the findings depends largely on the research questions. Open-ended response data will provide some corroboration of past findings and current hypotheses and add new information to the psychological phenomena under question.

Case Example: Using and Developing Hypothesis-Driven Content-Analytic Scoring Systems

My research deals with how personality motivation influences social perceptual-cognitive processes, most specifically autobiographical memory. In doing this work, my colleagues and I have used several open-ended response scoring systems. Therefore, the work seems suitable for a case demonstration of the development and use of open-ended response scoring techniques. The steps outlined above are used to organize the case study, and in some instances the methods of multiple studies (e.g., Woike, 1994, 1995; Woike & Aronoff, 1992; Woike et al., 1999; Woike, Mcleod, & Goggin, 2003; Woike & Polo, 2001) are combined for ease of presentation.

• *Step 1: What is the research question? What is to be identified, described, or measured?* The empirical question was, How

does personality motivation influence autobiographical memory—specifically, what is remembered and how is it remembered? To conduct the study, we needed a measure of personality motivation, a measure of memory content (what) and a measure of memory of process or structure (how). In considering how to measure two broad and contrasting types of personality motivation (achievement/power and intimacy), we decided to use a version of the Thematic Apperception Test (TAT; see Chapter 19, this volume). For gathering the memory data, open-ended questions were useful to test the hypothesis involving *what*, that is, What are people's most important memories about? Specifically, we predicted that the content of people's most important memories would be thematically related to their motivations. Therefore, we needed to identify memory content related to these two broad motivational categories, agency (or task-related concerns) and communion (or socially related concerns). Because we were also interested in *how*—that is, How does one explain an autobiographical memory?—open-ended data were used to examine patterns in the written recollections of these experiences. It was predicted that the structure of the memories would be related to motivations as well. We predicted that achievement/power-motivated individuals would focus on differences as a way to gauge their performance, whereas intimacy-motivated individuals would focus on similarities as a way to relate to others (for a more thorough discussion of this reasoning, see Woike, 1994). Thus, we needed a way to identify the perception of differences and similarities in the memory data.

• *Step 2: Decide whether content analysis will provide the needed information, either by itself or in conjunction with another method.* In order to test the hypotheses, we needed separate measures of personality motivation and autobiographical memories. To obtain a measure of autobiographical memory, we determined that asking an open-ended question or series of questions would be the best way to gather information on the variability in content and in structure of autobiographical material. Because our research question did not hinge on accuracy or corroboration of the events, we determined that an autobiographical memory written by each participant from his or her own point of view would be an appropriate and sufficient measure of autobiographical memory. In considering how to measure personality motivation, we decided to use an open-ended scoring technique, a version of the TAT, that was already well established in the literature. These measures do not correlate with self-report measures of motivation (see Woike, 1995), so no other personality measures were employed for cross-validation. Thus, we assessed motive and memory variables independently—but because both assessment procedures involved open-ended responses that were content scored, the measures were at the same level of analysis and therefore did not introduce unnecessary method variance.

• *Step 3. Decide what type of qualitative material will best provide the information needed and how to obtain it.* For the measure of autobiographical memory, we thought that one memory of an important or significant event in the participant's life would suffice. Participants were instructed to think for a few moments about their life experiences and then chose *one* experience that they felt was significant and important. They were told that they had about 10 minutes to write out their memory. This allowed them time to write about an experience without being rushed, but did not provide extended time for deliberation or to edit or revise their writing, thus increasing the spontaneity of their responses. In these ways, we attempted to control for unnecessary method variance. It was also decided that participants would write their memories by hand on paper that could be transcribed into typewritten text. In doing so, we were able to test a large group of participants at a time. Participants' personal identification information was removed from their materials in an effort to reduce their social desirability concerns. However, it was likely that, given free choice to write about any important experience, participants would chose one that they would enjoy recalling (rather than a painful or negative experience that was also significant), which was consistent with our motivation hypothesis, that people are more likely to recall experiences related to their motives.

• *Step 4: Determine the unit of analysis to be coded.* Because each memory pertained to a specific event, the whole memory was used as the unit of analysis for the content scoring procedure. To score the memories for differences and similarities, it seemed most reasonable to identify meaningful phrases within the memories that had these respective qualities.

• *Step 5: Select or develop a content coding system.* In a review of the literature on motivation and personal narratives, we found McAdams's (1985) life experiences scoring system, in which each personal narrative could be sorted into agency, communion, both, or neither, based on broad thematic scoring criteria, to be suitable to measure of task (agency) versus social (communion) themes.

In a review of the literature on social perception and cognitive complexity, we found that the Conceptual/Integrative Complexity System (Baker-Brown et al., 1992) was the best system to measure differences and similarities in the text of the memories because it had operational definitions for both differentiation and integration. However, because this system is based on ratings, it did not provide a way to measure differentiation and integration independently—which was essential for our hypotheses. Therefore, we decided to develop a scoring system for the two components of complexity, differentiation and integration (Woike, 1994, 1997; Woike & Aronoff, 1992), to measure the frequencies of two forms of complexity found in open-ended responses. This system allowed for the separate assessment of the components of differentiation and integration.

• *Step 6: Obtain pilot data to test and to refine the coding system.* In developing the system for cognitive complexity, we consulted different systems in the literature (see Woike & Aronoff, 1992, for a complete list). We then wrote out descriptions of the characteristics that pertained to differentiation and integration for a group of naive coders to find in pilot data of autobiographical memories. From these initial scorings, the system was further developed; in some cases categories were eliminated because they could not be found reliably in the pilot data. In other cases, categories were too broad and were divided into subcategories that could be identified reliably. The system went through several revisions; each revision in the scoring definitions was tested with pilot data until each subcategory would be identified reliably, based on the definition in the scoring manual. In the end, we had four subcategories for differentiation and four for integration.

• *Step 7: Train coders and ensure that intercoder agreement is satisfactory.* A scoring manual was developed that included clear definitions and examples for each of the subcategories. We used the pilot data to create sets of practice exercises to allow the coders to learn the system and to assess their reliability. Reliability was determined using the formula for establishing reliabilities with frequency data discussed earlier. Each coder needed to achieve 90% agreement with the expert scoring key before he or she could begin scoring the data.

• *Step 8: Obtain final material to be analyzed.* Participants were pretested for agentic and communal motives as described above. Those who scored high on one motive and low on the other were called back to participate in a follow-up study by research assistants unaware of the hypotheses. In a neutral classroom setting, all participants received the same written and verbal instructions for completion of the memory writing task. Their names did not appear on the materials.

• *Step 9: Code the material with identifying characteristics removed, and determine interrater; or perform computer-assisted content analysis.* Two coders categorized the memories for agency and communal themes, and another group of coders scored the frequencies of the categories of complexity in the memory data. Their reliabilities were determined, using Cohen's kappa for the category data, and the formula for determining the reliability of frequency data for the complexity data, as discussed above.

• *Step 10: Analyze the data; carry out cross-validation if appropriate.* To test the hypotheses, we first conducted a chi-square comparing the number of agentic versus communal individuals who had memories categorized as agentic versus communal. As predicted, we found that more agentic participants wrote about a significant memory that was categorized as agentic, whereas the more communal individuals wrote about memories categorized as communal. Next, we looked at the complexity of the memories within a 2(motive) × 2(theme) multiple analysis of variance (MANOVA) with differentiation and integration as the dependent variables. An interaction was found between motive, theme, and type of complexity, in which agency-motivated individuals whose memories had agentic themes organized their memories using more differentiation and communal-motivated individuals whose memories had communal themes organized their memories using more integration.

• *Step 11: Interpret results. Compare your findings with norms, if available.* From these findings it appeared that personality motivation did indeed influence what and how autobiographical memories were recalled. Multiple tests of the content hypothesis (Woike, 1994, 1995; Woike et al., 1999, 2003; Woike & Polo, 2001) have replicated the same thematic patterns under different conditions. The influence of these motives on the complexity with which personal experiences are recalled in written recollections has also been replicated (Woike, 1994; Woike et al., 1999; Woike & Polo, 2001). Further studies have shown evidence that the organizational patterns found in written narratives reflect the influence of motivation on the patterns of encoding, processing, and retrieval of the memory of personal experiences. Computer-based encoding and retrieval studies have found that these motives serve a selective and organizing function for incoming information, and then influence the retrieval of this information as well (Woike, Lavezzary, & Barsky, 2001; Woike, Mcleod, & Salzberg, 2007). This work has led to the development of a model of the influence of personality motivation on memory processes beyond written recollections (Woike, 2007). Without the initial open-ended response data from which the scoring system for differentiation and integration was derived, it would not have been possible to make this discovery.

Complexities: Determining Reliability and Validity with Open-Ended Response Data

This final section deals with some considerations for determining the psychometric properties of open-ended data. Open-ended data differ from questionnaire data in several ways. Therefore, it is important not to subject data derived from coding open-ended responses to statistical techniques that have been designed to test reliability and validity of questionnaire data.

Questionnaires have different properties. In using questionnaires, it is assumed that each item is discrete and can be presented in any order to the participant and that this will not affect the participant's score. Data from open-ended responses are typically a coherent set of verbal responses that form a specific rather than a random pattern. Open-ended responses typically have a beginning, middle, and end. If the sentence were to be scrambled (as is possible with questionnaire items), the response would lose its meaning. Therefore, a technique like factor analysis, which is based on having a fixed number of responses to a number of discrete questions, would not be an appropriate technique to use to examine the internal properties of open-ended responses. Other techniques, such as split half reliability, are also not appropriate for the same reasons.

Test–retest reliability may also be difficult to achieve with open-ended data using standard procedures. Even if the participants are asked the same questions, at different points in time, there are an infinite number of ways they can respond to an open-ended question, whereas questionnaires have a limited number of choices. Test–retest reliability may also be lower with open-ended data if questions involve creativity or storytelling, as the participant may make efforts to not repeat the same response. As open-ended responses may have more problems with reliability than questionnaires, the validity of open-ended response instruments may arguably be easier to establish. By asking people directly what they think and feel, we know about their cognitive representations of their thoughts and feelings and what sorts of information are important to them, rather than those of the researcher.

Recommended Readings

Aronoff, J. (1967). *Psychological needs and cultural systems: A case study.* Princeton, NJ: Van Nostrand.

McAdams, D. P. (1985). *Power, intimacy, and the life story: Personological inquiries into identity.* Chicago: Dorsey Press.

Pennebaker, J. W. (1997). *Opening up: The healing power of expressing emotions.* New York: Guilford Press.

Singer, J. A., & Salovey, P. (1993). *The remembered self.* New York: Free Press.

References

Aronoff, J., & Wilson, J. P. (1985). *Personality in the social process.* Hillsdale, NJ: Erlbaum.

Bakan, D. (1966). *The duality of human existence.* Chicago: Rand McNally.

Bakeman, R. (2000). Behavioral observation and coding. In H. T. Reis & C. M. Judd (Eds.), *Handbook of research methods in social and personality psychology* (pp. 138–159). New York: Cambridge University Press.

Baker-Brown, G., Ballard, E. J., Bluck, S., deVries, B., Suedfeld, P., & Tetlock, P. (1992). The integrative complexity coding manual. In C. Smith (Ed.), *Handbook of thematic analysis* (pp. 605–611). Cambridge, UK: Cambridge University Press.

Baumeister, R. F., & Tice, D. M. (1988). Metatraits. *Journal of Personality, 56,* 571–598.

Cohen, J. A. (1960). A coefficient of agreement for nom-

inal scales. *Educational and Psychological Measurement, 20,* 37–46.

Emmons, R. A. (1986). Personal strivings: An approach to personality and subjective well-being. *Journal of Personality and Social Psychology, 51,* 1058–1068.

Emmons, R. A. (1992). Abstract versus concrete goals: Personal striving level, physical illness, and psychological well-being. *Journal of Personality and Social Psychology, 62,* 292–300.

Emmons, R. A., & King, L. A. (1988). Conflict among personal strivings: Immediate and long-term implications for psychological and physical well-being. *Journal of Personality and Social Psychology, 54,* 1040–1048.

Emmons, R. A., & McAdams, D. P. (1991). Personal strivings and motive dispositions: Exploring the links. *Personality and Social Psychology Bulletin, 17,* 648–654.

John, O. P., Pals, J. L., & Westenberg, P. M. (1998). Personality prototypes and ego development: Conceptual similarities and relations in adult women. *Journal of Personality and Social Psychology, 74,* 1093–1108.

Loevinger, J. (1976). *Ego development.* San Francisco: Jossey-Bass.

Loevinger, J., & Wessler, R. (1970). *Measuring ego development: Volume I. Construction and use of a sentence completion test.* San Francisco: Jossey-Bass.

Maslow, A. (1954). *Motivation and personality.* New York: Harper & Row.

McAdams, D. P. (1985). *Power, intimacy, and the life story: Personological inquiries into identity.* Chicago: Dorsey Press.

McAdams, D. P., & de St. Aubin, E. (1992). A theory of generativity and its assessment through self-report, behavioral acts, and narrative themes in autobiography. *Journal of Personality and Social Psychology, 62,* 1003–1015.

McAdams, D. P., de St. Aubin, E., & Logan, R. L. (1993). Generativity among young, midlife, and older adults. *Psychology and Aging, 8,* 221–230.

McAdams, D. P., Hoffman, B. J., Mansfield, E. D., & Day, R. (1996). Themes of agency and communion in significant autobiographical scenes. *Journal of Personality, 64,* 339–377.

McClelland, D. C., Atkinson, J. W., Clark, R. A., & Lowell, E. L. (1958). A scoring manual for the achievement motive. In J. W. Atkinson (Ed.), *Motive in fantasy, action, and society* (pp. 179–204). Princeton, NJ: Van Nostrand.

McDowell, C., & Acklin, M. W. (1996). Standardizing procedures for calculating Rorschach inter-rater reliability: Conceptual and empirical foundations. *Journal of Personality Assessment, 66,* 308–320.

Mehl, M. R., Pennebaker, J. W., Crow, D. M., Dabbs, J., & Price, J. H. (2001). The Electronically Activated Recorder (EAR): A device for sampling naturalistic daily activities and conversations. *Behavior Research Methods, Instruments, and Computers, 33*(1), 517–523.

Pennebaker, J. W. (1997). Writing about emotional experiences as a therapeutic process. *Psychological Science*, 8, 162–166.

Pennebaker, J. W., & Francis, M. E. (1996). Cognitive, emotional, and language processes. *Cognition and Emotion*, 10, 601–626.

Pennebaker, J. W., Mayne, T. J., & Francis, M. E. (1997). Linguistic predictors of adaptive bereavement. *Journal of Personality and Social Psychology*, 72, 863–871.

Pennebaker, J. W., Mehl, M. R., & Niederhoffer, K. G. (2003). Psychological aspects of natural language use: Our words, ourselves. *Annual Review of Psychology*, 54, 547–577.

Peterson, C., Schulman, P., Castellon, C., & Seligman, M. E. P. (1992). CAVE: Content analysis of verbatim explanations. In C. P. Smith (Ed.), *Motivation and personality: Handbook of thematic content analysis* (pp. 383–392). New York: Cambridge University Press.

Peterson, C., Seligman, M. E. P., & Vaillant, G. E. (1988). Pessimistic explanatory style is a risk factor for physical illness: A thirty-five year longitudinal study. *Journal of Personality and Social Psychology*, 55, 23–27.

Peterson, C., Semmel, A., von Baeyer, C., Abramson, L. Y., Metalsky, G. I., & Seligman, M. E. P. (1982). The attributional style questionnaire. *Cognitive Therapy and Research*, 6, 287–300.

Pillemer, D. B. (1998). *Momentous events, vivid memories*. Cambridge, MA: Harvard University Press.

Pollack, S., & Gilligan, C. (1982). Images of violence in TAT test stories, *Journal of Personality and Social Psychology*, 42, 159–167.

Singer, J. A., & Salovey, P. (1993). *The remembered self*. New York: Free Press.

Smith, C. P. (1992). (Ed.). *Handbook of thematic analysis*. Cambridge, UK: Cambridge University Press.

Smith, C. P. (2000). Content analysis and narrative analysis. In H. T. Reis & C. M. Judd (Eds.), *Handbook of research methods in social and personality psychology* (pp. 313–335). New York: Cambridge University Press.

Smith, C. P., Feld, S. C., & Franz, C. E. (1992). Methodological considerations: Steps in research employing content analysis systems. In C. P. Smith (Ed.), *Motivation and personality: Handbook of thematic content analysis* (pp. 515–536). New York: Cambridge University Press.

Suedfeld, P., Tetlock, P. E., & Streufert, S. (1992). Conceptual-integrative complexity. In C. Smith (Ed.), *Handbook of thematic analysis* (pp. 401–418). Cambridge, UK: Cambridge University Press.

Tetlock, P. E. (1983). Accountability and complexity of thought. *Journal of Personality and Social Psychology*, 45, 74–83.

Tetlock, P. E., & Kim, J. (1987). Accountability and judgment in a personality prediction task. *Journal of Personality and Social Psychology*, 52, 700–709.

Tetlock, P. E., Skitka, L., & Boettger, R. (1989). Social and cognitive strategies of coping with accountability: Conformity, complexity and bolstering. *Journal of Personality and Social Psychology*, 57, 632–641.

Thorne, A. (2000). Personal memory telling and personality development. *Personality and Social Psychology Review*, 4, 45–56.

Tomkins, S. S. (1987). Script theory. In J. Aronoff, A. I. Rabin, & R.A. Zucker (Eds.), *The emergence of personality* (pp. 147–216). New York: Springer.

Wang, S. W. (2004). *The relations of perceptions of work–love tensions to personality characteristics and well-being*. Unpublished senior thesis, Department of Psychology, Barnard College, New York.

Woike, B. A. (1994). The use of differentiation and integration processes: Empirical studies of "separate" and "connected" ways of thinking. *Journal of Personality and Social Psychology*, 67, 142–150

Woike, B. A. (1995). Most memorable experiences: Evidence for a link between implicit and explicit motives and social cognitive processes in everyday life. *Journal of Personality and Social Psychology*, 68, 1081–1091.

Woike, B. A. (1997). *Cognitive complexity: Theory and method* [Technical document]. New York: Department of Psychology, Barnard College, Columbia University.

Woike, B. A. (2007). *The influence of implicit and explicit motives on autobiographical memory: A review*. Manuscript under review.

Woike, B. A., & Aronoff, J. (1992). Antecedents of complex social cognitions. *Journal of Personality and Social Psychology*, 63, 97–104.

Woike, B. A., Candela, K., & Osier, T. (1996). Attachment style and violent imagery in thematic stories about relationships. *Personality and Social Psychology Bulletin*, 22, 1030–1034.

Woike, B. A., Gershkovich, I., Piorkowski, R., & Polo, M. (1999). The role of personality motives in the content and structure of autobiographical memories. *Journal of Personality and Social Psychology*, 76, 600–612.

Woike, B. A., Lavezzary, E., & Barsky, J. (2001). The influence of implicit motives on memory processes. *Journal of Personality and Social Psychology*, 81, 935–945.

Woike, B., Mcleod, S., & Goggin, M. (2003). Implicit and explicit motives influence accessibility to different autobiographical memories. *Personality and Social Psychology Bulletin*, 29, 1046–1055.

Woike, B., Mcleod, S., & Salzberg, A. (2007). *The role of organizational structure in the link between implicit motives and autobiographical memory*. Manuscript under review.

Woike, B. A., & Polo, M. (2001). Motive-related memories: Content, structure, and affect. *Journal of Personality*, 69, 391–415.

York, K. L., & John, O. P. (1992). The four faces of Eve: A typological analysis of women's personality at midlife. *Journal of Personality and Social Psychology*, 63, 494–508.

## CHAPTER 18

Personality Assessment at a Distance

Anna V. Song
Dean Keith Simonton

Most personality research is conducted using undergraduates as participants. Yet occasionally personality psychologists turn to other research samples to study the extent and nature of individual differences. Of particular interest are those occasions when investigators study individuals who have made a name for themselves as exceptional creators, leaders, geniuses, or talents. These research subjects have been called "significant samples" (Simonton, 1999). Such significant samples serve two main purposes in the field of personality psychology. First, samples of famous persons can be used to demonstrate the generalizability of findings derived from traditional methods and samples. For example, a major goal in political psychology is to show that psychological principles that have been firmly established using mainstream methods can be applied to political leaders and thereby can help us understand the politicians that affect our everyday lives. Second, significant samples are used because they are representative of a particular class of human beings—people who represent the extreme upper tail of the distribution of human traits. Such individuals can be said to constitute pure exemplars of an important attribute, such as creativity or leadership. The hope is to isolate the psychological characteristics that enable these persons to attain such a unique position in the general population of humanity.

Although significant samples provide an opportunity to study the extent of generality and individuality, they also present a unique quandary: Because the subjects are frequently too famous, are averse to psychological inquiry, or are deceased, traditional assessment methods are not applicable. For instance, an investigator who wishes to examine the relationship between personality traits and political leadership may choose to study those individuals who have served as president of the United States. Yet it is clear that most living presidents would not be inclined to expose themselves to direct psychological inquiry by filling out a researcher's personality inventories or questionnaires. Worse yet, the vast majority of U.S. presidents are now deceased and therefore incapable of serving as research participants even if they may have been positively inclined to do so. As a result, this specific significant sample is not amenable to mainstream forms of personality assessment.

To overcome these difficulties, personality psychologists have devised ingenious methods to study subjects "at a distance." These methods range from qualitative to quantitative techniques and also encompass an array of theoretical perspectives. Our goal in this chapter is to provide an overview of such methods through examples of techniques used to measure personality at a distance.

General Approaches

Research methods using significant samples usually take one of two approaches: qualitative or quantitative. In qualitative methods, the data are in the form of biographical and historical information and the analysis is expressed in terms of descriptive narratives or interpretations (Simonton, 2003). Alternatively, in quantitative approaches, variables are given operational definitions, measured numerically, and analyzed using statistical techniques. In the following sections, we discuss examples of both qualitative and quantitative approaches.

Qualitative Approaches: Psychobiographical Analyses

In general psychology, qualitative research is usually conducted as naturalistic observations or case studies. In the study of significant samples, qualitative research is represented by psychohistory or psychobiography. The practice of psychohistory involves the use of psychological concepts to explain historically significant events. Psychobiography is considered a subset of psychohistory; instead of focusing on historical events, psychobiography focuses on lives of historically significant people. Subsequently, psychobiography is the application of psychological theory to biographical data.

Usually, the psychological theory that is applied in psychobiography is psychodynamic in orientation. The dominance of psychoanalysis in this area is most likely due to the fact that

Sigmund Freud (1910/1964) conducted the first psychobiography—a psychoanalysis of Leonardo da Vinci (Elms, 1994). Midway through his career, Freud proclaimed his desire to take psychoanalysis into the realm of biography in order to extend psychoanalysis beyond those on the couch to consider eminent individuals previously unreachable. Although Freud's work on da Vinci is considered the most influential psychobiography (Elms, 1994; Runyan, 1982), it was far from perfect. Indeed, much of its influence is due to the fact that it was theoretically and methodologically flawed (Elms 1994). Even though subsequent psychobiographers have tried to avoid the mistakes Freud made, the major criticisms aimed at the first psychobiography are also aimed at the whole field, in past as well as the present.

One of the criticisms that personality psychologists make regarding psychobiography is that it is inherently subjective. This subjectivity creates major chinks in psychobiography's scientific façade. For example, psychologists often choose to conduct a psychobiographical study on a subject for whom they feel some emotion, positive or negative. Elms (1994) showed that Freud's objectivity was clouded by identification with his subject. Freud not only admired da Vinci, but also began to see himself in his subject's life and work. Moreover, feelings toward the subject are not always positive. Sometimes psychobiographers dislike their subjects, which makes their work prone to pathography or inaccuracy. For instance, many psychobiographical works on politicians are clouded by the psychobiographer's political bias. Freud again provides a prime example: his hatred for U.S. president Woodrow Wilson motivated his collaboration with William Bullitt (1966) to publish the scathing psychobiographical work *Thomas Woodrow Wilson: A Psychological Study*. Because of the pervasive biases apparent in the work and the criticisms leveled by leading psychobiographers and presidential historians (Elms, 1994; George & George, 1964), the work continues to be the classic example of how a psychobiography can go wrong.

Quantitative Approaches: Content Analysis, Historiometry, and Expert Surveys

The problems of psychobiography have led personality psychologists who wish to study personality at a distance to search for alternative approaches. Simonton (1990, 2003) presents several quantitative methodologies that avoid the pitfalls common to qualitative approaches. Unlike descriptive narratives and qualitative interpretations, quantification removes subjectivity by utilizing measurement and statistics to establish testable, falsifiable arguments (Simonton, 2003). Although many psychologists credit psychophysicist Gustav Fechner (1860/1912) for bringing quantification into psychology, Belgian social scientist Adolphe Quételet (1835/1968) demonstrated quantification of psychological characteristics a quarter of a century earlier. In particular, he used data on historical individuals to conduct a longitudinal study of the relationship between creative productivity and age. Since Quételet, at-a-distance methods have advanced to include three types of quantitative strategies. These include content analysis, historiometry, and expert surveys.[1] In the following discussion, we briefly present the history behind these three methods.

Content Analysis

Content analysis most often involves the systematic examination of verbal text for words or themes associated with psychological constructs. Verbal text includes a wide range of materials, such as speeches (Winter, 1987, 1988), spontaneous political remarks (Hermann, 1980), letters (Suedfeld, Corteen, & McCormick, 1986), diaries, writing assignments, and journal abstracts (Pennebaker & King, 1999). Content analysis has also expanded beyond the bounds of words and into nonverbal text, such as musical pieces and works of art (see Simonton, 2003, for a review).

The genesis of content analysis in personality psychology can be traced to work by Morgan and Murray (1935) on the Thematic Apperception Test (TAT). The scoring for this projective test involves showing participants ambiguous images and asking them to write stories about the pictures. The stories are then analyzed for themes and imagery associated with specific motives and needs. David McClelland furthered this work by developing a content-analytical scoring system using experimental manipulation of motives (McClelland & Atkinson, 1948). Subsequently, Winter (1973) and his colleagues continued McClelland & Atkinson's (1948) work by adapting their scor-

ing scheme to verbal text—the coding scheme yields an imagery score per 1,000 words of any oral or written text. This technique allowed researchers to measure motives from virtually any historical document about a subject.

For example, in their analysis of President Nixon, Winter and Carlson (1988) quantitatively measured Nixon on three personality motives: the need for power, achievement, and affiliation. Winter and Carlson content analyzed Nixon's inaugural addresses using Winter's (1973) at-a-distance scoring scheme for each motive. From these speeches, Winter and Carlson determined a personality profile for Nixon: high in the achievement and in affiliation motives, but moderate in the power motive. They also found that his paradoxical behavior in office, such as in the Watergate scandal, corresponded to this personality profile, thus providing a psychological explanation for one of the most perplexing U.S. presidents in history.

The technique used by Winter and Carlson (1988) is not limited to the measurement of personality motives. Suedfeld, Tetlock, and Streufert (1992) devised an at-a-distance scoring technique for integrative complexity—the degree to which people differentiate and integrate alternative perspectives. To assess how political figures might differentiate or integrate complex information, researchers can now quantitatively measure levels of integrative complexity by scoring written materials such as letters, speeches, and interviews. For example, Suedfeld and colleagues (1986) measured General Robert E. Lee's level of integrative complexity during six major battles. They scored dispatches, orders, and private letters written by Lee and his opposing generals. They found that, with the sole exception of the battle at Gettysburg, when Lee was higher in integrative complexity than his opposing commanders, he would win the battles. Only General Ulysses Grant was higher in complexity, and Lee lost both battles to Grant.

Historiometry

As mentioned earlier, one of the first instances of quantitative methods in psychology was Quételet's (1835) longitudinal study on age and creative productivity. This obscure study is also the first example of historiometry—the testing of nomothetic psychological hypotheses using quantitative methods on historical data

(Simonton, 1999). Some 30 years later, Galton (1869) left his own mark on the field with *Hereditary Genius*. This historiometric work, unlike that of Quételet, led directly to other historiometric endeavors, including those of Woods (1909), Cattell (1903), and Thorndike (1950).

Indeed, not only did Woods demonstrate historiometric methods through several studies on individual differences in morality and virtue in European monarchs, he was the first to use the term *historiometrics* in his 1909 paper in *Science*. At the time, the editor was J. M. Cattell, who offered his own contribution to historiometry through his work "A Statistical Study of Eminent Men" (1903). The influence of these early historiometricians can be seen in the works of subsequent psychologists. For instance, Cattell's student E. L. Thorndike, better known for his experimental work on learning, also published studies on personality traits of eminent individuals (Thorndike, 1950).

Perhaps one of the best examples of historiometric research in personality psychology emerged from Lewis Terman's studies of intelligence. After developing the Stanford-Binet Test, Terman (1917) showed that IQs could be measured at a distance by using the case of Sir Francis Galton, whose IQ was estimated to be 200. This work continued through his graduate student, Catharine Cox, who wrote her dissertation on the relationship between IQ and eminence. Her magnum opus, the 842-page book *The Early Mental Traits of Three Hundred Geniuses* (1926), included IQ scores and personality profiles for highly eminent individuals—all measured at a distance. Based on Cattell's (1903) earlier work on eminent geniuses, Cox chose leaders and creators born after 1450, eliminated those who inherited their positions (monarchs), and imposed a cutoff in eminence rating. For the remaining 301 individuals, she compiled biographical abstracts containing key developmental markers, such as the age at which each person learned to read, learned mathematics, and produced his or her first domain-specific accomplishment (e.g., novel, concerto, military battle). Because IQ scores are a ratio between mental and chronological age, she distributed biographical abstracts to raters (including Terman), who provided estimated IQ scores.

In addition, Cox (1926) devised methods for assessing a subset of her geniuses ($n = 100$) on 67 personality characteristics. This pioneering effort also influenced subsequent research on the personal characteristics of highly eminent individuals. Simonton's (1986) study on presidential personalities is an example. Simonton collected biographical data of all the presidents, removing all identifying information. Independent raters, using the Gough Adjective Check List, then evaluated the presidents on 300 descriptors, 110 of which could be assessed to an acceptable degree of reliability. A factor analysis of these traits produced 14 factors, including moderation, friendliness, intellectual brilliance, and Machiavellianism. A personality profile based on these 14 trait dimensions was computed for each president and then subjected to hierarchical cluster analysis. This analysis allowed Simonton to group presidents according to personality profile and to assess whether they exhibited similar leadership styles while in office. For example, John Adams and his son John Quincy Adams were very similar to each other. In addition, these two were very similar to Tyler, Cleveland, and Wilson, all of whom experienced some type of moralistic impasse with their political opposition (e.g., Wilson and the League of Nations).

Expert Surveys

The use of expert surveys is the least common of the three at-a-distance measures discussed thus far, but it has increasingly found utility among researchers. Some of the best examples of expert survey assessments are political psychological studies of the characteristics of politicians, especially U.S. presidents. An example is Arthur Schlesinger Sr.'s (1948) study of presidential performance. He sent surveys to 55 experts (mostly presidential historians) and asked them to rank presidential leadership on a 5-point scale: Great, Near Great, Average, Below Average, and Failure. The top six presidents in order of greatness were Lincoln, Washington, FDR, Wilson, and Jackson.

Since Schlesinger (1948), several social scientists have continued the tradition of expert surveys to measure characteristics at a distance. For instance, Murray and Blessing (1983) had 846 experts evaluate presidential greatness, but also determined the extent to which the expert evaluations were influenced by ideology and other possible contaminants. Even more interesting from a personality perspective is a study by Maranell (1970), who had 571 American historians assess the presidents on idealism, flexibility, activeness, strength, prestige, and accomplishment. Simonton's (1986, 1988) research on presidential greatness has shown that these expert-based assessments agree with his own historiometrically derived personality traits. For instance, Maranell's idealism trait correlates negatively with Machiavellianism but positively with intellectual brilliance. Two recent applications of expert survey methodology deserve special mention.

First is Sulloway's (1996) study of the relationship between personality and birth order. Sulloway was specifically interested in the question, "Why do some people have the genius to reject the conventional wisdom of their day and to revolutionize the way we think?" (p. xi). To address this question, Sulloway gathered a sample of 6,566 subjects involved as either advocates or opponents in 121 major movements toward innovation. He then had historians rate the individuals on several traits, including their social attitudes and the stance each took on the historic event. The interrater reliability coefficients were exceptionally high, ranging from .76 to .93. Using these data, Sulloway showed that scientists who were firstborns tended to support mainstream, status quo theories. Conversely, later-born scientists were more likely to engage in revolutionary thinking that significantly changed their respective fields.

The second example is Rubenzer, Faschingbauer, and Ones's (2000) study of the personality structure of presidential leadership. Rubenzer and colleagues asked experts and biographers of specific presidents to score their subjects on all five personality factors represented in Costa and McCrae's (1992) NEO Personality Inventory (NEO-PI). Subsequently, neuroticism, extraversion, openness, conscientiousness, and agreeableness scores were used to predict greatness, as measured by Murray and Blessing (1983). Rubenzer and colleagues' findings were congruent with Simonton's (1988) findings on presidential success: Openness (or intellectual brilliance) is one of the most important personality predictors of greatness. Rubenzer and Faschingbauer's (2004) subsequent work using expert surveys to measure presidential personalities not only reiterated the importance of openness in presidential leadership, but also presented eight personality types: dominators (e.g., LBJ and Nixon), introverts (e.g., both John and John Quincy Adams), extroverts (e.g., FDR and JFK), good guys (e.g., Washington, Eisenhower, and Ford), innocents (e.g., Grant and Harding), actors (e.g., Reagan and Clinton), maintainers (e.g., Truman and George H. W. Bush), and philosophers (e.g., Jefferson, Lincoln, and Carter).

From Eminent Creators to Musical Stanzas: Choosing Your Sample

As in most psychological research, the first consideration to be discussed in personality research is sampling. Very often, the sample of interest is immediately apparent. Political leadership studies call for a sample of politicians; creativity investigations sample scientists, artists, writers, or musicians. In addition, it is often the case that the specific individuals making up the samples are evident because the target population is finite and data on this group are accessible. Examples include U.S. presidents (Simonton, 1986, 1988; Winter, 1987), literary figures (Porter & Suedfeld, 1981), creators (Cassandro, 1998; Martindale, 1973, 1990), and military figures (Suedfeld et al., 1986). At other times, sampling choices are much more difficult. The potential sample could be too large, making it nearly impossible to include all members of the group in the study. Moreover, membership in groups such as geniuses or great leaders may be ambiguous (Simonton, 1999, 2003).

Another sampling issue that is less likely to be addressed in traditional personality research methods is one of unit definition. As Simonton (2003) frames it, "When a study consists of a sample of size N, what is being counted when determining N? What is the unit on which the variables are to be assessed?" (p. 625). Unlike most psychological research that is based on individuals (or animals), at-a-distance research sometimes uses "micro-units" consisting of creative products (Martindale, 1973, 1990), leader actions or decisions (Song, 2005; Suedfeld et al., 1986), or some other cross-sectional unit smaller than a single human being. Conversely, at-a-distance research psychologists may use "macro-units" such as whole nations (Winter, 1987). Furthermore, longitudinal designs can add an additional level of analysis in terms of specific time units, such as months, years, or even decades (Simonton, 1998). A personality psychologist can thus study a micro-unit (e.g., music, literature, decisions) within individuals (e.g., leaders, writers, artists), within a macro-unit (e.g., artistic medium, literature genre, partisan-controlled legislature, nations), or across time (Martindale, 1990; Porter & Suedfeld, 1981; Simonton, 1998). This method also lends itself to creative combinations: Units can take the form of distinctive combinations, such as individual–generational analysis that combines individual-level data with generational-level data (Simonton, 1976).

The second consideration is the type or source of data to be used in assessing personality. In this case, data sources fall in two categories, primary and secondary (Simonton, 2003; Song, 2005). Primary sources, usually in written form, may be public, such as campaign speeches, inaugural addresses, diplomatic communiqués, court decisions, poems, short stories, publication titles, and journal abstracts (e.g., Winter, 1987), whereas others may be private, such as correspondence and diaries (e.g., Porter & Suedfeld, 1981). Nonverbal materials provide another useful primary source, including artworks, musical compositions, architectural monuments, and various cultural artifacts. Secondary sources are written by historians and scholars and are in the form of biographies, histories, encyclopedias, biographical dictionaries, bibliographies, and obituaries.

Assessment Techniques

Techniques for assessing individuals at a distance fall into two major categories: (1) those that entail the adaptation of already established measures and (2) those that require the invention of new measures without obvious connections to standard methods.

Adapting Standard Instruments

Often, there are preexisting scales or techniques that can be used to measure the personality construct of interest, but their use necessitates contact with the person to be measured. Thus, researchers hoping to measure personality constructs from afar adapt established measurement instruments for at-a-distance applications. For instance, McCrae (1996) investigated behaviors and correlates of the five-factor model dimension of Openness in one historically relevant individual: Jean-Jacques

Rousseau. In this study, McCrae identified several behaviors and thoughts akin to Openness. He also expanded the scope of the construct by linking it with other established personality characteristics, such as authoritarianism, attitude formation, and political affiliation. Using these characteristics of Openness as his construct identifiers, he content analyzed Rousseau's biography to show how the French philosopher could serve as an exemplar of a person particularly high in Openness.

Numerous examples can be drawn from the extensive literature on integrative complexity. The majority of studies on stress and well-being focus on short-term effects (or at least measure effects as if they were finite). These studies also focus on outcome variables such as physical health, emotions, or instances of psychopathology. Porter and Suedfeld (1981) deviated from tradition by focusing on long-term, cumulative effects of stress on individuals' lives. Specifically, they focused on how stressful life events might impact individuals' cognitive functioning, or integrative complexity, throughout their lives.[2] Ordinarily, to study such a phenomenon, scientists would have to engage in a monumental data collection effort on par with Terman's *Genetic Studies of Genius*. That is, Porter and Suedfeld would have to follow individuals throughout their lives, recording life events, the stress incurred as a result of these events, and changes in each person's cognitive abilities.

Bypassing the difficulties of traditional longitudinal methods, the researchers adapted preexisting measures of integrative complexity to study personalities of historical literary figures. Originally, integrative complexity was measured with the Paragraph Completion Task (PCT), which is given to participants in person. Participants are asked to respond to stem sentences such as "What I think about rules . . . " Responses are scored on a 1–7 scale for complexity (i.e., 1 = inflexible; 7 = cognitively complex). The 1–7 scale used to code PCT samples was adapted to include levels of differentiation (scores of 1–3) and integration (scores of 5–7), and subsequent measures of integrative complexity have employed this scoring technique (see Suedfeld et al., 1992).

Porter and Suedfeld (1981) describe their use of the integrative complexity coding technique in three stages. First, a third party, who was blind to the hypothesis and focus of the study, collected personal letters of five British novelists that spanned across the writers' lives. In addition, the researchers documented any historical events that occurred during the writers' lives. These events included wars, civil unrest, and economic hardships. Second, all identifying information was removed from the letters in order to limit possible scorer biases. Third, Suedfeld scored the segments of the unidentifiable letters for integrative complexity, using the adapted version of the measure. Once the letters were scored, Porter and Suedfeld conducted a multiple regression to see what environmental events might affect integrative complexity. Specifically, they found that war negatively impacted cognitive functioning, but civil unrest increased integrative complexity. Moreover, they unexpectedly found that, excluding personal illnesses, personal stressors did not affect integrative complexity. Finally, Porter and Suedfeld showed that cognitive functioning significantly dropped a few years before the writers died.

Devising New Instruments

Occasionally, personality psychologists want to measure characteristics at a distance but find that there are no existing instruments for the construct. In this case, researchers must start from scratch and devise their own instruments, as Hermann (1980) did for her study on Soviet politicians. The primary goal of the study was to devise at-a-distance measures of foreign leaders in regard to six characteristics thought to influence decision-making processes. The six characteristics Hermann chose were nationalism (ethnocentrism), self-confidence, cynicism, conceptual complexity (not integrative complexity), need for power, and need for affiliation.[3] As an illustration, we consider Hermann's measure of nationalism. Hermann first operationally defined nationalism as "the view of the world in which one's own group holds center stage; strong emotional ties to one's own group with emphasis on group honor and group identity" (p. 338). To measure nationalism, a reference was scored if (1) nouns or phrases about the person's group were modified with positive adjectives or (2) nouns or phrases about an out-group were modified by negative descriptors. Finally, the nationalistic references were tallied and that number was divided by the total number of nouns and phrases within a 250-word segment.

In addition to their work in political psychology, researchers in the field of creativity have also provided groundbreaking techniques to measure psychological constructs at a distance. The preeminent example of such procedures is Martindale's (1973, 1990) work on primordial cognition and primary processing. Martindale observed that primary process imagery increases as competition to create original work increases. He theorized that part of the appeal of a great work of art is that it is original, exciting, and captures the attention of audiences in the midst of other artists trying to accomplish the same goal. Therefore, the drive to produce "the next big thing" also drives the artist to test boundaries and regress into primordial cognition, a type of primary processing. Martindale (1973) found empirical evidence of primordial regression during artistic constraints in the laboratory and recorded changes in stylistic patterns in primary processing. In conjunction with patterns seen in the laboratory, Martindale (1990) devised a Regressive Imagery Dictionary (RID)—a bank of words, images, and codes that indicate primary and secondary process thinking. This dictionary is the basis for his content-analytical software that can measure primordial cognition in literary texts. This measure has been usefully applied to problems as diverse as the aesthetic impact of Shakespeare's sonnets and the scientific influence of eminent American psychologists (Simonton, 1999, 2003).

Statistical Issues

To get a better appreciation of the methodology, we must now deal with two statistical issues: measure reliability and data analysis.

Measure Reliability

Although methods used in measuring the personalities of inaccessible subjects seem so different from traditional self-report methods, there is one common issue that unites them: reliability. Traditional self-report techniques rely on Cronbach's alpha to indicate agreement between items on a questionnaire. The logic behind this type of analysis is that if several questions are supposed to be measuring the same construct, they should correlate. This is also true for at-a-distance personality measures, except that instead of agreement between items, the issue is agreement between scorers. Moreover, acceptable levels of reliability extend to both methodologies. A respectable alpha in psychometrics is .70–.80, and different raters measuring personality from archival documents should correlate in the same range, if not more highly (Suedfeld et al., 1992).

A unique consideration in measuring personality from a distance is how many raters researchers should employ to create a reliable measure. On this point, there is some divergence. On one hand, researchers may use only one rater to code written text (e.g., McCrae, 1996; Porter & Suedfeld, 1981). In such cases, the coder is an expert in the field or has been trained extensively and generally correlates with expert scorers at the .85 level on other documents. On the other hand, some researchers recognize that just as researchers increase the number of items to increase reliability, the number of raters should increase as well. In these cases, researchers employ anywhere from 2 to 11 coders to score documents (e.g., Simonton, 1998). When a researcher decides to use multiple raters, there are several additional issues to consider. First, the number of coders is inversely related to the difficulty of the scoring measure. Scoring schemes for some constructs, such as integrative complexity or the power motive, require the recognition of subtle themes or arguments. Therefore, studies of this type usually require one or two scorers, each of whom is extensively trained. Scoring schemes

for other constructs, such as nationalism or the Big Five traits, are easier to recognize or require only word counts. In this case, training coders is not as arduous and it is possible to utilize a larger number of scorers.

Data Analysis

As is apparent from the preceding discussion, quantitative at-a-distance methodology encompasses a diverse array of techniques that lend themselves to a variety of statistical analyses. Once variables have been measured, those measurements can be subjected to the same analytical tools used in more traditional personality research, such as factor analysis (Simonton, 1986), cluster analysis (Simonton 1986, 1988), multiple regression (Cassandro, 1998), and other forms of statistical modeling.

Pulling It All Together: Procedures in Measuring Personality from a Distance

Thus far, we have described several different components of research studies of personality from a distance. In this section we use Simonton's (1998) study on King George III to illustrate how these steps come together to measure the personalities of inaccessible people (see Figure 18.1).

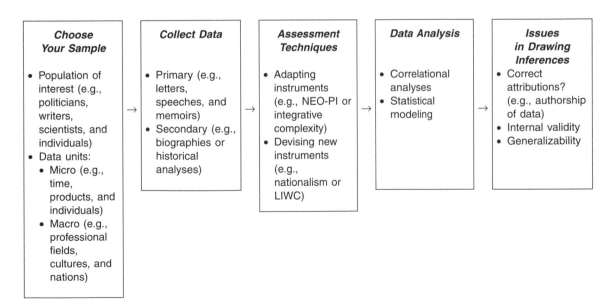

FIGURE 18.1. The process of studying personality from a distance.

Choosing the Sample

King George III was the British monarch who reigned during the American Revolution. His time on the throne was marked not only by political instability and the succession of one of England's colonies, but also by bouts of mental and physical breakdowns that led him to be branded as Mad King George. His symptoms included talking for days at a time, hearing voices he claimed to be angels, greeting a tree as a dignitary, and severe depression. He was frequently restrained in a straightjacket or chair and was bled on numerous occasions. Academics have posited various theories for his breakdown, including arsenic poisoning and a blood disease called porphyria (see Runyan, 1982, for a review).

Although a plethora of theories were already in existence, Simonton (1998) noted that no one had ever tested the simple possibility that King George was at times subjected to severe stress. Previous work had already established that stress negatively affects physical and cognitive well-being (Porter & Suedfeld, 1981). Subsequently, Simonton (1998) tested the hypothesis that personal and political stress caused King George's breakdowns. In this case, Simonton's sample was apparent—because his interest was the madness of King George III, his only choice was to collect documents pertaining to King George.

Collecting Documents

Simonton collected several biographies on King George, totaling five full-length works. These biographies were condensed into two mutually exclusive full-life chronologies that were compiled by two groups of research assistants who worked in independent teams. These biographical timelines documented two aspects of King George's life: personal and political events and all references to his physical and mental well-being. The teams pored through biographies and extracted all references to stress or physical/mental health. The teams then compiled verbatim quotes or amalgamations of different quotes to form chronologies. Although quotes were used in order to reduce any selection biases, the research assistants were inevitably required to provide some editing, but usually for clarification or to provide context (e.g., approximate conversion from 18th-century English currency to American dollars). In all, both chronologies contained a total of 71,400 words, or 124 pages (10-point font), and spanned King George's complete life.

Time Units

With the biographical information collected and organized, the next step was to decide the unit of analysis, or in this case, the unit of time. Occasionally, the type and amount of data limit this choice. If the amount of data is meager or if the data lack detail, the researcher may consider aggregation across large time increments. However, the opposite was true in Simonton's study. Because there was a vast amount of information on King George's life, Simonton could choose months, years, or even decades as his time unit. Simonton considered at least two issues in his decision. First, the time span had to be long enough to encompass the events related to the psychological construct. In terms of stress and health, events would most likely span across days and weeks. Therefore, it would make more sense to consider larger time units such as months or years. The second issue was that the magnitude of correlations would be related to the time unit's span. Specifically, because larger time increments encompass more events, they will most likely yield larger correlations than smaller time spans. Simonton decided to use a conservative approach and minimized the magnitude of correlations by examining King George's life in months. By using this approach, Simonton tested whether the relationship between health and stress would surface, using the most stringent statistical condition.

In addition to deciding on which unit of time to use, Simonton had to consider what portion of his subject's life to examine. Although data were compiled for the whole lifespan, Simonton confined the data to 624 months of King George's adult years, beginning with his ascension to the throne and ending with his abdication to his son King George IV (1760–1811). Simonton explains that most of the health and stress ratings occurred during these years, and data before and after this time period were less complete. In addition, the truncation did not affect the reliabilities of the measures.

Assessment Technique

Simonton's hypothesis focused on two main variables: stress and health. Using both chronologies, he was able to create three measures for stress (political, personal, and total stress) and three for health (physical, mental, and general health).

Eleven coders were asked to read the 624-month chronology of stress-related events experienced by King George. For each month, student raters who served as "judges" were asked to give a score between 0 and 100 for (1) total stress level, (2) stress from political events, and (3) stress arising from personal events. For the purposes of a reference point, Simonton provided the judges with a copy of Holmes and Rahe's (1967) Social Readjustment Rating Scale. Raters were instructed to use the scale to help them notice pertinent events and to gauge associated levels of stress. He cautioned them against applying the scale too strictly. Instead, he encouraged them to empathize with the subject's situation and reflect how they themselves would feel if they were King George. The same procedure was used to obtain physical, mental, and general health ratings.

Assessing the Assessment Technique

The scores from 11 judges were averaged to compute a composite score for six variables. To measure the reliability of each measure, Simonton assessed both interrater reliability and reliability coefficients for each measure. Interrater reliability was exceptionally high, reaching .92 in the stress ratings and .94 in the health assessments. Internal consistency reliabilities were computed by treating individual judges as items, and individual months within the 980-month chronology as cases. The resulting reliability coefficients were .94, .89, and .95 for total, personal, and political stress, respectively. Health scores were extremely reliable as well, with coefficients of .97, .97, and .96 for general, physical, and mental health, respectively.

Analyzing the Data

Simonton conducted time-series analyses to examine the relationship between stress and health. He reported three different sets of analyses: one analysis using raw scores and two analyses correcting for high autocorrelations between ratings from adjacent months. In addition to these analyses, Simonton also accounted for the possibility that the relationship

between stress and health does not operate instantaneously. It was more likely that the effects of stress would manifest themselves after a period of time. To examine this possibility, Simonton examined cross-correlations between stress and health time series and found a negative correlation at 9-month lags (e.g., $r = -.17$, $p < .001$). This finding was important because it represented the first quantitative evidence that King George's episodes could be at least partially attributed to stressful events that occurred 9 months before mental and physical breakdowns.

Issues

The use of historical data to measure personality characteristics at a distance raises several issues regarding authenticity. Historical data, particularly documents supposedly written by the subject in question, are criticized as being heavily shaped by impression management. Personal letters, for example, are shaped by how the authors want others to see them. In addition, Schafer (2000) points out that data derived from public rhetoric, including speeches, interviews, and press conferences, may contain significant biases that do not reflect the individual's true personality characteristics. This is especially true of at-a-distance research in political psychology. The use of political speechwriters has created a great deal of uncertainty as to whose personality is being measured. On one hand, the words most likely belong to the speechwriter him- or herself. Therefore, content-analytical techniques would measure personality characteristics of the writer, and not the intended subject. On the other hand, politicians rarely give speeches without editing or approving the pieces themselves. Extensive review of presidential archives reveals significant revisions of speeches and letters—mostly at the behest of the president himself (Song, 2005). Furthermore, politicians choose speechwriters who can express the political ideas and imagery they, the politicians, wish to promote (Winter, 1987). Some researchers have advocated the use of spontaneous materials to bypass the influence of impression management or ghostwriters. Dillie (2000) found that at-a-distance measures for cognition-related personality constructs (e.g., cognitive complexity, operational code) are susceptible to impression management and that these differences were more apparent in comparing prepared statements with spontaneous interviews. He argued that the difference between speeches and interviews is that politicians invest a considerable amount of time in preparing speeches and, consequently, are able to utilize impression management strategies. Conversely, interviews and press conferences force politicians to respond quickly, leaving little room for public-image maintenance. Therefore, researchers should seriously consider the use of spontaneous materials when measuring cognitively based personality variables.

Moreover, if we consider Campbell's (1957) definition of internal validity—the degree to which a chosen design can infer causality between variables x and y—research using at-a-distance methods may seem specious. Studies of this type are invariably correlational and lack the advantages of random assignment to conditions in establishing cause–effect relationships. Although researchers are increasingly using multivariate techniques, quasi-experimental designs, and time-series analyses to reduce spuriousness, possible threats to internal validity are never completely obliterated. In other words, at-a-distance researchers can infer causal relationships only with extreme care.

Evaluation

Although correlational studies are frequently criticized for lacking internal validity, they often compensate by possessing higher external validity—offering the ability to generalize observed effects beyond the studied sample (Campbell, 1957). Laboratory experiments are often criticized for having low external validity because they introduce sterile situations and artificial manipulations that evoke unrepresentative responses. "Guinea pig" effects, expectancy effects, acquiescence, satisficing, and demand characteristics are but several laboratory-induced responses (Krosnick, Narayan, & Smith, 1996). In addition, as Sears (1986) points out, most laboratory experiments use unrepresentative research participants, particularly college students taking introductory psychology courses. At-a-distance methods are necessarily "unobtrusive" and "nonreactive" and thus cannot be contaminated with experimenter effects (Simonton, 1999; Winter, 1987). Moreover, because historical data come from the "real world," there can be no doubt that

the results are applicable to the world beyond the research laboratory.

Even if experimental results seem prima facie applicable to the world outside the laboratory, there persists a profound gap between merely extrapolating those findings to the outside world and actually demonstrating that those findings can be so generalized. An outright empirical demonstration removes the intrinsically speculative nature of the extrapolation. In this case, at-a-distance methods provide an opportunity to test hypotheses under empirically rigorous settings, while maintaining aspects of the environment that have a bearing on how psychological phenomena play out in the real world.

Take, for instance, Cassandro's (1998) study on premature mortality rate of creative writers. Empirical data support the popular notion that in comparison to geniuses in nonartistic fields, creative writers and artists lead short, tumultuous lives (Jamison, 1993). In addition, research in clinical psychology provides evidence that mentally ill persons have increased risk of premature mortality. Both findings had been tested within more traditional settings but had yet to be tested under the strain of "real-world" settings. It also seems intuitive that these two lines of research have a bearing on each other, but the dynamics of how they relate had not been empirically tested. Combining the two lines of research, Cassandro found historiometric support for the "mad genius" phenomenon, and that premature mortality in creative writers could be explained by the high incidence of psychopathology. Hence, Cassandro demonstrates that not only can at-a-distance methods support research with inherent external validity, but that they can also provide the means to establish the generality of results obtained from more conventional research methods.

Future Directions

Where do we see at-a-distance research in 10, 20, or even 30 years from now? If psychology's embrace of technology is any indication of future directions, there is a good chance that studies will increasingly employ computer programs to measure personality constructs in verbal text and historical data. In fact, examples of such technological advances are already abundant in personality research. Simonton (1999, 2003) summarizes several studies of his

CHAPTER 19

Measuring Implicit Motives

Oliver C. Schultheiss
Joyce S. Pang

Over the past 10 years, the field of personality psychology has seen a resurgence of interest in implicit motives, nonconscious motivational needs that orient, select, and energize behavior (McClelland, 1987). This renewed interest has led to significant advances in our understanding of the biological, cognitive, emotional, social, and cultural manifestations of implicit motivational needs (e.g., Brunstein, Schultheiss, & Grässmann, 1998; Hofer & Chasiotis, 2003; Langner & Winter, 2001; Schultheiss, Pang, Torges, Wirth, & Treynor, 2005; Schultheiss, Wirth, & Stanton, 2004; Schultheiss, Wirth, et al., 2005; Woike, 1995; Zurbriggen, 2000). Some strides have also been made toward conceptual refinements of the implicit motive construct (e.g., Brunstein & Maier, 2005; Schultheiss, 2001a; Schultheiss & Brunstein, 2005).

However, as Schultheiss and Brunstein (2001) and Pang and Schultheiss (2005) recently pointed out, considerably less effort has

gone into the description, evaluation, and refinement of the implicit motive measures commonly used in research. As a result, the thematic content coding method of motive assessment has remained an enigma to researchers not familiar with the field, and the threshold for using these methods may therefore be higher than for other, more frequently used assessment tools in personality psychology. This chapter is intended to lower this threshold by (1) discussing the differential validity of implicit motive measures, as contrasted with measures of individuals' explicit, self-attributed motivational needs and goals, (2) reviewing the reliability of implicit motive measures, (3) providing a step-by-step guide for the assessment of implicit motives and the use of motive scores in analytic designs, (4) illustrating the use of implicit motive measures in research with case examples, and (5) pointing out some future directions for the development of better motive measures.

---

own that utilized computerized content analysis on verbal and nonverbal text. Hermann's (1980) coding scheme has been streamlined into a software program called Profiler+ (Young, n.d.). Martindale's Regressive Imagery Dictionary is also available as software. In addition, Pennebaker and colleagues have developed the Linguistic Inquiry and Word Count (LIWC) program to measure various personality constructs, such as emotional and cognitive processes (Pennebaker & King, 1999).

In addition to the ease afforded by computer programs, a further benefit for at-a-distance methods is the availability of data on the Internet. Take, for instance, the papers of President George Washington. During the adolescent years of at-a-distance research, scientists had to correspond with archivists to obtain just a small sample of documents written by the subject. The researcher would also have to travel to archives, libraries, or collection facilities to view a document in person. Now, a researcher need only go to the Library of Congress website to discover hundreds of pages from Washington's diary, letters written to various people, his exercise schedule, and his presidential papers. Indeed, there is so much data available that the researcher is left with the coveted quandary of choosing which samples of data to analyze! These advances in methods and technology have expanded the scope of at-a-distance methods, thereby making the technique more attractive and useful to researchers in personality psychology.

Notes

1. For suggested readings on these topics, see Table 18.1.
2. Integrative complexity is a style of information processing. Specifically, it is the degree to which people (a) differentiate ideas and perspectives and (b) integrate these perspectives in a general outlook on a situation.

3. Although there were preexisting measurement instruments for several constructs (e.g., self-confidence, need for power, and need for affiliation), Hermann used different conceptualizations of these constructs and thereby created new at-a-distance measurements for all six constructs.

Recommended Readings

Cox, C. (1926). *The early mental traits of three hundred geniuses.* Stanford, CA: Stanford University Press.

Rubenzer, S. J., Faschingbauer, T., & Ones, D. S. (2000). Assessing the U.S. presidents using the Revised NEO Personality Inventory. *Assessment, 7*(4), 403–420.

Simonton, D. K. (1986). Presidential personality: Biographical use of the Gough Adjective Check List. *Journal of Personality and Social Psychology, 51,* 149–160.

Simonton, D. K. (1990). *Psychology, science, and history: An introduction to historiometry.* New Haven, CT: Yale University Press.

Smith, C. P. (Ed.). (1992). *Motivation and personality: Handbook of thematic content analysis.* New York: Cambridge University Press.

Sulloway, F. (1996). *Born to rebel: Birth order, family dynamics, and creative lives.* New York: Pantheon.

Winter, D. G. (1987). Leader appeal, leader performance, and the motive profiles of leaders and followers: A study of American presidents and elections. *Journal of Personality and Social Psychology, 52,* 196–202.

References

Campbell, D. T. (1957). Factors relevant to the validity of experiments in social settings. *Psychological Bulletin, 54,* 297–312.

Cassandro, V. J. (1998). Explaining premature mortality across fields of creative endeavor. *Journal of Personality, 66,* 805–833.

Cattell, J. M. (1903). A statistical study of eminent men. *Popular Science Monthly, 62,* 359–377.

Costa, P. T., Jr., & McCrae, R. (1972). *The Revised NEO Personality Inventory professional manual.* Odessa, FL: Psychological Assessment Resources.

Cox, C. (1926). *The early mental traits of three hundred geniuses.* Stanford, CA: Stanford University Press.

TABLE 18.1. Essential Readings on Quantitative at-a-Distance Methods

	Quantitative techniques		
	Content analysis	Historiometry	Expert survey
Methodological writings	Smith (1992)	Simonton (1990)	Sulloway (1996)
Empirical examples	Winter (1987)	Cox (1926) Simonton (1986)	Rubenzer, Faschingbauer, & Ones (2000)

Dillie, B. (2000). The prepared and spontaneous remarks of Presidents Reagan and Bush: A validity comparison for at-a-distance measurements. *Political Psychology, 21*, 572–585.

Elms, A. E. (1994). *Uncovering lives: The uneasy alliance of biography and psychology.* New York: Oxford University Press.

Fechner, G. T. (1860/1912). Elemente der Psychophysik [Elements of psychophysics] (H. Langfield, Trans.). In B. Rand (Ed.), *The classical psychologists* (pp. 562–572). Boston: Houghton Mifflin.

Freud, S. (1910/1964). *Leonardo da Vinci and a memory of his childhood.* Oxford, UK: Norton.

Freud, S., & Bullitt, W. (1966). *Thomas Woodrow Wilson: A psychological study.* London: Weidenfeld & Nicolson.

Galton, F. (1869). *Hereditary genius: An inquiry into its laws and consequences.* London: Macmillan.

George, A. L., & George, J. L. (1964). *Woodrow Wilson and Colonel House.* New York: Dover.

Hermann, M. G. (1980). Assessing the personalities of Soviet Politburo members. *Personality and Social Psychology Bulletin, 6*, 332–352.

Holmes, R., & Rahe, R. (1967). The Social Adjustment Rating Scale. *Journal of Psychosomatic Research, 11*, 213–218.

Jamison, K. R. (1993). *Touched with fire: Manic–depressive illness and the artistic temperament.* New York: Free Press.

Krosnick, J. A., Narayan, S. S., & Smith, W. R. (1996). Satisficing in surveys: Initial evidence. In M. T. Braverman & J. K. Slater (Eds.), *Advances in survey research* (pp. 29–44). San Francisco: Jossey-Bass.

Maranell, G. M. (1970). The evaluation of presidents: An extension of the Schlesinger Polls. *Journal of American History, 57*, 104–113.

Martindale, C. (1973). An experimental simulation of literary change. *Journal of Personality and Social Psychology, 25*, 319–326.

Martindale, C. (1990). *The clockwork muse: The predictability of artistic styles.* New York: Basic Books.

McClelland, D. C., & Atkinson, J. W. (1948). The projective expression of needs: I. The effect of different intensities of the hunger drive on perception. *Journal of Psychology: Interdisciplinary and Applied, 25*, 205–222.

McCrae, R. R. (1996). Social consequences of experiential openness. *Psychological Bulletin, 120*, 323–337.

Morgan, C. D., & Murray, H. H. (1935). A method for investigating fantasies: The thematic Appercention Test. *Archives of Neurology and Psychiatry, 34*, 289–306.

Murray, R. K., & Blessing, T. H. (1983). The presidential performance study: A progress report. *Journal of American History, 70*, 535–555.

Pennebaker, J. W., & King, L. A. (1999). Linguistic styles: Language use as an individual difference. *Journal of Personality and Social Psychology, 77*, 1296–1312.

Porter, C. A., & Suedfeld, P. (1981). Integrative complexity in the correspondence of literary figures: Effects of personal and societal stress. *Journal of Personality and Social Psychology, 40*, 321–330.

Quételet, A. (1968). *A treatise on man and the development of his faculties.* New York: Franklin. (Original work published 1835; 1842 Edinburgh translation).

Rubenzer, S. J., & Faschingbauer, T. R. (2004). *Personality, character, and leadership in the White House: Psychologists assess the presidents.* Washington, DC: Brassey's.

Rubenzer, S. J., Faschingbauer, T., & Ones, D. S. (2000). Assessing the U.S. presidents using the Revised NEO Personality Inventory. *Assessment, 7*(4), 403–420.

Runyan, W. M. (1982). *Life histories and psychobiography: Explorations in theory and method.* London: Oxford University Press.

Schafer, M. (2000). Issues in assessing psychological characteristics at a distance: An introduction to the symposium. *Political Psychology, 21*, 511–527.

Schlesinger, A. M. (1948, November). Historians rate U.S. presidents. *Life*, pp. 65–66, 68, 73–74.

Sears, D. O. (1986). College sophomores in the laboratory: Influences of a narrow data base on social psychology's view of human nature. *Journal of Personality and Social Psychology, 51*, 515–530.

Simonton, D. K. (1976). Do Sorokin's data support his theory?: A study of generational fluctuations in philosophical beliefs. *Journal for the Scientific Study of Religion, 15*, 187–198.

Simonton, D. K. (1986). Presidential personality: Biographical use of the Gough Adjective Check List. *Journal of Personality and Social Psychology, 51*, 149–160.

Simonton, D. K. (1988). Presidential style: Personality, biography, and performance. *Journal of Personality and Social Psychology, 55*, 928–936.

Simonton, D. K. (1990). *Psychology, science, and history: An introduction to historiometry.* New Haven, CT: Yale University Press.

Simonton, D. K. (1998). Mad King George: The impact of personal and political stress on mental and physical health. *Journal of Personality, 66*, 443–466.

Simonton, D. K. (1999). Significant samples: The psychological study of eminent individuals. *Psychological Methods, 4*, 425–451.

Simonton, D. K. (2003). Qualitative and quantitative analyses of historical data. *Annual Review of Psychology, 54*, 617–640.

Smith, C. P. (Ed.). (1992). *Motivation and personality: Handbook of thematic content analysis.* New York: Cambridge University Press.

Song, A. V. (2005). Hiding the snark: Methodological considerations in studying elusive politicians. In W. Schultz (Ed.), *Handbook of psychobiography* (pp. 365–397). New York: Oxford University Press.

Suedfeld, P., Corteen, R., & McCormick, C. (1986). The role of integrative complexity in military leadership: Robert E. Lee and his opponents. *Journal of Applied Social Psychology, 16*, 498–507.

Suedfeld, P., Tetlock, P., & Streufert, S. (1992). Conceptual/integrative complexity. In C. P. Smith (Ed.), *Motivation and personality: Handbook of thematic content analysis* (pp. 393–400). New York: Cambridge University Press.

Sulloway, F. (1996) *Born to rebel: Birth order, family dynamics, and creative lives.* New York: Pantheon.

Terman, L. M. (1917). The intelligence quotient of Francis Galton in childhood. *American Journal of Psychology, 28*, 209–215.

Thorndike, E. L. (1950). Traits of personality and their intercorrelations as shown in biographies. *Journal of Educational Psychology, 41*, 193–216.

Winter, D. G. (1973). *The*[ ] Free Press.

Winter, D. G. (1987). Lead[ ]mance, and the motive pro[ ]ers: A study of American[ ] *Journal of Personality an*[ ] 196–202.

Winter, D. G., & Carlson, D.[ ] scores in the psychobiograph[ ] ual: The case of Richard Nix[ ] *ity, 56*, 75–103.

Woods, F. A. (1909, November[ ] new science. *Science, 30*, 70[ ]

Young, M. (n.d.). *Profiler softu*[ ] OH: Social Science Automat[ ]

Differential Validity of Implicit Motive Measures

Research on implicit motive constructs originated in the assumption that people do not have introspective access to many of the wellsprings of their behavior (McClelland, Atkinson, Clark, & Lowell, 1953; see also Gazzaniga, 1985; Kagan, 2002; Nisbett & Wilson, 1977). McClelland, Atkinson, and their colleagues therefore used motivation arousal studies to develop content coding measures of imaginative stories that research participants write in response to picture cues, a technique called the Picture Story Exercise (PSE; cf. McClelland, Koestner, & Weinberger, 1989; see Winter, 1999, for key differences between the PSE and Murray's, 1943, Thematic Apperception Test, TAT). These content coding measures were designed to capture individuals' implicit needs for power (or n Power; a concern for having impact on others), achievement (or n Achievement; a concern for doing well according to a standard of excellence), affiliation (or n Affiliation; a concern for establishing, maintaining, or restoring close, friendly relationships), and intimacy (or n Intimacy; a preference for experiences of warm, close, and communicative interactions with others) (for a compilation of these and other scoring systems, see Smith, 1992a). Of course, it is also possible to ask people directly to what extent they view themselves as being motivated to have power, achieve, or affiliate with and be close to others, and over time many carefully constructed instruments were developed for this purpose, such as Jackson's (1984) Personality Research Form (PRF) and, more recently, goal inventories that assess people's commitments to specific power, achievement, affiliation, and intimacy goals in their daily lives (e.g., Brunstein et al., 1998).

The parallel development of thematic-content and self-report measures of motivation revealed a pervasive lack of variance overlap between the two types of assessment, which soon instigated a fight over which type of measure was the more valid one (e.g., Atkinson, 1981; Entwisle, 1972; Fineman, 1977; McClelland, 1987). Eventually, this quarrel prompted researchers to delineate more carefully the differential validity of thematic-content measures of motivation (cf. McClelland et al., 1989; Schultheiss, 2001a; Spangler, 1992). Summarizing the main conceptual and empirical outcomes of this endeavor, Schultheiss (2001a, in press; Schultheiss & Brunstein, 2005) characterized the key characteristics of implicit motives as follows:

Implicit motives are more likely to become aroused by and respond to *nonverbal cues* than verbal stimuli (Schultheiss, 2001a). Klinger (1967) observed that individuals responded with increases in affiliation or achievement motivation expressed in imaginative stories, to watching an affiliation-oriented or achievement-oriented experimenter, even if they could not hear his verbal instructions. In a similar vein, Schultheiss and Brunstein (1999, 2002) demonstrated that experimenters who assigned and described a power-related goal verbally to their participants failed to arouse the participants' power motive. Only after participants had had an opportunity to translate the verbally assigned goal into an experiential format through a goal imagery exercise did their power motive predict goal commitment and task performance. Finally, recent research indicates that facial expressions of emotion are particularly salient nonverbal cues for implicit motives. Facial signals of friendliness and hostility interact with individuals' implicit affiliation motive, and facial signals of dominance and submission interact with individuals' implicit power motive, to shape attentional orienting and instrumental learning (Schultheiss & Hale, in press; Schultheiss, Pang, et al., 2005).

Consistent with motive bias toward responding to stimuli that are not verbally encoded, implicit motives are particularly likely to show an effect on behavior if *nondeclarative measures* (e.g., measures of behaviors and processes that are neither controlled by a person's conscious intentions nor the self-concept) are employed, but have very limited or no effects on declarative measures of motivation (i.e., measures that tap into a person's conscious sense of self and the beliefs, judgments, decisions, and attitudes associated with it). The differential effect of implicit motives on declarative and nondeclarative measures was first documented by deCharms, Morrison, Reitman, and McClelland (1955), who found that n Achievement predicted performance on a scrambled-word test (a nondeclarative measure), but not participants' attribution of achievement-related traits to themselves or others (declarative measures of motivation). Later, Biernat (1989) showed that the implicit achievement motive predicted performance on a math task (nondeclarative measure), but not subjects' decision to serve as a group leader on another task (declarative measure). In a similar vein, Brunstein and Hoyer (2002) found that high-achievement individuals showed superior performance on a vigilance task (nondeclarative measure), but were not more likely than low-achievement individuals to continue on the task if given the choice (declarative measure). Finally, Schultheiss and Brunstein (2002) found that the implicit power motive predicts nonverbal (e.g., gesturing, facial expressions) and paraverbal (e.g., speech fluency) behaviors on a persuasion task, but not the actual content of the arguments presented, which can be conceived of as a declarative measure.

To summarize, implicit motives are not accessible to introspection and self-report, respond preferentially to nonverbal stimuli, and predict nondeclarative measures of motivation and behavior better than declarative measures. In addition, it is important to keep in mind that individual motives respond specifically to certain types of incentives, but not others. For instance, power-motivated individuals respond to opportunities to have impact on others, but not to situations that allow relaxed, friendly contact with others, whereas the reverse is true of affiliation-motivated individuals.

Reliability of Implicit Motive Measures

The reliability of implicit motive measures has most frequently been estimated through (1) their internal consistency, (2) interscorer agreement, and (3) their test–retest reliability. PSE motive measures appear to have low reliability when their internal consistency is assessed, that is, when motive scores derived from stories written in response to different picture cues are correlated with each other. Typically, these correlations tend to be low, resulting in internal consistency coefficients (e.g., Cronbach's alpha) in the .20–.50 range.

However, as Atkinson (1981; Atkinson & Birch, 1970) has pointed out in the context of his dynamics-of-action theory, estimates of internal consistency may not be applicable to the assessment of implicit motives in the first place. Atkinson essentially argued that internal consistency estimates are suitable for assessment

tools, such as trait inventories, that tap *declarative, self-related memories and beliefs*. These frequently capitalize on a person's long-term memory of his or her past behavior and on his or her short-term memory of answers given to earlier items on the same test; in conjunction with the compelling need to maintain a consistent self-concept, people are likely to provide answers on subsequent items that are consistent with earlier ones (cf. Gazzaniga, 1985). But internal consistency measures are *not* suitable for the assessment of a *motivational process*, which by its very nature is not constant but characterized by a dynamic waxing and waning of need states, depending on environmental incentive cues and opportunities for need satisfaction. According to Atkinson, the PSE picks up such a motivational process and thereby indirectly taps the strength of an underlying motive disposition. The stronger the motive, the easier it is to arouse and show up in participants' stories and actual behavior. And then, by the very act of being expressed in imaginative thought (or actual behavior), the motive becomes consummated and drops for some time from the surface of participants' stories (or behavior). Atkinson, Bongort, and Price (1977) showed in computer simulations that individuals with a strong underlying motive disposition cycle more quickly back and forth between motive expression and satiation than individuals with a weak motive, and predicted that, given equal PSE length, a motive therefore can be more validly assessed in the former than in the latter. Reuman (1982) empirically confirmed this prediction of Atkinson's motivational theory by demonstrating that PSE motive scores with high variability, resulting in *negative* Cronbach alpha coefficients (!), have better predictive validity than motive scores with low variability and positive alphas.

A second source of interstory variability of motive scores may be found in the *dissimilarity* of PSE picture cues. Whereas Atkinson's dynamics-of-action model assumes a picture pool with similar, constant cue characteristics for a given motive, PSE picture sets used in research frequently consist of pictures showing a wide variety of situations (cf. Table 19.1). McClelland and colleagues (1953) have speculated that a motive's strength is reflected not only in the intensity of individuals' responses to the same type of cue, but also in the *extensity*

TABLE 19.1. Raw Motive Scores and Word Counts across Picture Cues

Picture	N Power		N Achievement		N Affiliation		Words	
	M	SD	M	SD	M	SD	M	SD
Women in laboratory								
U.S.[a]	<u>0.77</u>	<u>0.85</u>	<u>1.08</u>	<u>0.93</u>	0.19	0.50	93.38	26.09
German[b]	<u>0.80</u>	<u>0.84</u>	<u>0.66</u>	<u>0.77</u>	0.19	0.48	82.85	21.15
Ship captain								
U.S.[a]	<u>1.01</u>	<u>0.88</u>	0.14	0.47	0.21	0.53	98.24	27.46
German[b]	<u>1.16</u>	<u>0.92</u>	0.11	0.37	0.20	0.53	85.68	21.08
Couple by river								
U.S.[a]	0.23	0.54	0.00	0.21	<u>2.06</u>	<u>1.07</u>	99.42	25.73
German[b]	0.43	0.72	0.03	0.17	<u>1.84</u>	<u>1.05</u>	91.53	22.01
Trapeze artists								
U.S.[a]	<u>0.70</u>	<u>0.79</u>	<u>0.76</u>	<u>0.83</u>	0.49	0.80	97.00	26.96
German[b]	<u>0.79</u>	<u>0.85</u>	<u>0.78</u>	<u>0.84</u>	0.43	0.71	86.04	21.64
Nightclub scene								
U.S.[a]	<u>0.75</u>	<u>0.82</u>	0.01	0.30	<u>1.32</u>	<u>1.10</u>	99.53	28.09
German[b]	<u>0.86</u>	<u>0.83</u>	0.09	0.31	<u>1.29</u>	<u>1.08</u>	89.44	22.77
Boxer[c]								
U.S.[a]	<u>0.79</u>	<u>0.90</u>	<u>1.14</u>	<u>1.06</u>	0.17	0.51	97.60	29.09
Architect at desk[c]								
German[b]	0.22	0.46	0.29	0.55	<u>1.16</u>	<u>0.84</u>	90.75	22.73
Bicycle race								
U.S.[c]	<u>0.95</u>	<u>0.95</u>	<u>1.65</u>	<u>1.08</u>	0.16	0.41	109.61	27.27
Woman and man arguing								
U.S.[c]	<u>1.70</u>	<u>0.94</u>	0.31	0.66	0.18	0.53	102.46	27.23
Hooligan attack								
U.S.[c]	<u>2.26</u>	<u>0.95</u>	0.01	0.14	0.15	0.43	109.36	27.86
Lacrosse duel								
U.S.[c]	0.69	0.84	<u>1.22</u>	<u>0.96</u>	0.16	0.50	102.77	27.08
Men on ship deck								
U.S.[d]	<u>1.82</u>	<u>1.26</u>	0.48	0.63	0.20	0.51	110.52	24.71
German[e]	<u>1.14</u>	<u>0.95</u>	0.47	0.73	0.29	0.63	77.49	18.61
Soldier								
German[e]	<u>0.94</u>	<u>1.01</u>	0.35	0.64	0.17	0.36	81.52	21.81
Soccer duel								
German[e]	<u>0.74</u>	<u>0.77</u>	<u>1.79</u>	<u>0.81</u>	0.07	0.27	80.47	18.28
Couple sitting opposite a woman								
U.S.[f]	<u>1.05</u>	<u>0.98</u>	0.40	0.79	<u>0.73</u>	<u>0.90</u>	104.45	23.84
Girlfriends in café with male approaching								
U.S.[f]	0.53	0.65	0.38	0.76	<u>1.62</u>	<u>1.43</u>	105.45	22.42

Note. Underlined motive scores indicate that more than 50% of participants have responded with at least one instance of codable motive imagery to the picture cue. Motive imagery was scored using Winter's (1994) coding system.
[a]From Pang and Schultheiss (2005); N = 323.
[b]From Schultheiss and Brunstein (2001); N = 428.
[c]From Wirth, Welsh, and Schultheiss, Study 2 (2006); N = 109.
[d]From Schultheiss, Campbell, and McClelland (1999); N = 42 (male participants only).
[e]From Schultheiss and Rohde (2002); N = 66 (male participants only).
[f]From Schultheiss, Wirth, and Stanton (2004); N = 60.

of the cues that elicit a motivational response, that is, how many different contexts and situations a person has learned to associate with need satisfaction. According to this view, individuals who, for instance, inject power imagery into stories written in response to pictures showing couples, but not into stories about pictures showing competitive situations, may have learned to express their need for power only in close relationships, but not in competitive situations, whereas someone writing power-related stories about both types of pictures would have a more extensive power motive, because he or she responds to a greater variety of situations with power imagery. To our knowledge, there has been no systematic research on the extensity postulate. But if the postulate is correct, then lower internal consistency on the PSE would be due, at least in part, to a bandwidth-fidelity problem, according to which a PSE that samples motive imagery in response to highly dissimilar picture cues would by necessity have lower internal consistency, but broader validity, than a PSE with highly similar picture cues. We return to this issue when we discuss picture selection.

Motive score reliability is high when examined from the perspective of coding agreements between two or more independent coders of the same PSE stories. Usually, high coding reliability is ensured from the outset, because most coding systems require the coder to train on practice stories prescored by an expert until the coder reaches a criterion of .85 percentage agreement or better. A coder who has reached this criterion and follows further steps to ensure high coding reliability (as detailed below) typically also achieves good to excellent agreement with other coders who independently code the same PSE stories (cf. Pang & Schultheiss, 2005; Smith, 1992b).

Motive score reliability is also satisfactory when viewed from the perspective of retest stability. To illustrate this point, we conducted a meta-analysis that included a comprehensive set of retest reliability studies, both published and unpublished, with the requirement that they employed motive scoring systems that were developed empirically in the McClelland–Atkinson tradition and used standard PSE administration conditions. The regression function we obtained for retest coefficients from these studies is 0.71–0.13 × base-10 log (retest interval in days; cf. Figure 19.1). According to this formula, the average stability coefficient is

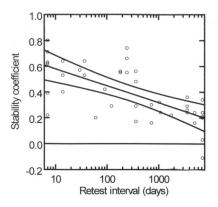

FIGURE 19.1. Regression line (plus 95% confidence interval) for motive stability coefficients as a function of test–retest time interval (log-transformed).

.71 if the retest interval is 1 day, .60 if the retest interval is 1 week, .52 if the retest interval is 1 month, .37 if the retest interval is 1 year, .29 if the retest interval is 5 years, and .25 if the retest interval is 10 years. Average retest stability did not differ across the motive domains power, achievement, and affiliation/intimacy (collapsed into one category), and neither was motive stability differentially affected by motive domain across retest intervals (i.e., the slope was the same for all motive domains). Factors that also influence retest stability, but which we did not control for, include test–retest instructions (e.g., allowing participants at the retest session to write stories that are similar to those they wrote at the first session increases stability; Lundy, 1985; Winter & Stewart, 1977), number and suitability of picture cues (longer tests and higher cue-strength pictures typically provide more stable or comprehensive estimates of an individual's true score; cf. Reumann, 1982), whether different pictures or the same pictures were used at both assessments (same pictures yield higher stability coefficients; cf. Lundy, 1985; Winter & Stewart, 1977), and the occurrence of motive-arousing or stressful life events during the test interval (critical life events can have a profound impact on motive scores and lower retest stability; cf. Smith, 1992b). Overall, our findings suggest that implicit motive scores are moderately stable over time and that stability decreases with increasing retest intervals at a rate similar to that observed for questionnaire trait measures (e.g., Schuerger, Zarrella, & Hotz, 1989).

Step-by-Step Guide

In the following discussion, we provide detailed instructions for the assessment of implicit motives and the use of motive scores derived from the combined use of the PSE and implicit motive coding systems developed in the McClelland–Atkinson research tradition. Although verbal cues are sometimes used instead of picture cues to elicit stories, we focus on the PSE as the primary means of story collection, because it is the most widely used and best studied assessment tool for implicit motive measurement. In our recommendations, we build on both the excellent chapter by Smith, Feld, and Franz (1992; see also the other chapters in Smith, 1992a, for recommendations for the assessment of specific motives) and our lab's own best practices, which we developed across dozens of studies and thousands of PSE stories (cf. Pang & Schultheiss, 2005; Schultheiss & Brunstein, 2001). Our goal is to provide the uninitiated reader with robust guidelines for the collection of valid and reliable motive scores.

Which Motives to Assess?

The first question that needs to be answered in the planning of motive research is whether a single motive should be assessed—and if so, which—or whether several motives should be measured. The answer to this question depends on the nature and focus of the research and will determine not only the choice of coding system(s), but also the number and kinds of pictures that will be used.

Therefore, we start with brief descriptions of the most commonly used coding systems for *n* Achievement, *n* Affiliation, *n* Intimacy, and *n* Power (detailed versions of these coding systems can be found in Smith, 1992a; see also Schultheiss, 2001b; Winter, 1994). These coding systems have two common characteristics.

First, they were constructed either by examining the effects on story themes of experimental manipulation of the target motive, or by examining the differences in stories written by members of theoretically relevant, naturally occurring groups that differ in the strength of that motive. Second, each scoring system typically follows a general theoretical framework of the sequence for motivated behavior. The motivated behavioral sequence is often initiated when the person feels a need or a motive

(*Need*). The person may either anticipate successful attainment of this goal or may become frustrated and anticipate nonattainment (*Goal Anticipation*). In order to accomplish his or her goal, the person engages in instrumental activity that is either successful or not (*Instrumental Activity*). He or she may experience positive or negative affect in response to the goal-directed activity and its consequences (*Affect*).

Achievement-Related Coding Systems

McClelland and colleagues' (1953) scoring system for the achievement motive provided the blueprint for many other subsequent motive scoring systems. They introduced the technique of using experimental arousal to manipulate and examine the effects of a motive and applied the general behavioral sequence outlined above to provide an organizing framework for their scoring system. The *n* Achievement scoring system also provided a guideline for making scoring decisions that would be adopted by many other authors—the scorer must first determine whether a story contains any reference to the motive goal before going on to score the motive-related subcategories. With respect to achievement, the scorer must determine whether the story contains any reference to an achievement-related goal in order to justify scoring achievement-related subcategories. For the *n* Achievement scoring system and other scoring systems described here, a scoring decision is made for the absence or presence (given a value of +1) of each scoring category and subcategory. Each category and subcategory can be scored only once per story. The motive score for each story is calculated by adding the category and subcategory scores for that picture, and the motive score for each individual is computed by adding the motive scores for all pictures.

According to McClelland and colleagues (1953), stories are scored for achievement-related imagery if there is mention of *competition with a standard of excellence*. Having determined that a story contains achievement imagery, a coder then proceeds to score for seven possible subcategories: (1) stated need for achievement; (2) successful, doubtful, or unsuccessful instrumental activity; (3) positive and negative anticipatory goal states; (4) obstacles or blocks that can come either from within the person or from elements in the world at large; (5) nurturant press, which refers to forces that aid the story character in the goal pursuit; (6) positive or negative affective states associated with goal attainment or nonattainment; and (7) achievement thema, which is a weighting category scored whenever achievement imagery is elaborated in such a way that it becomes the central plot of the story.

The latent distinction between a success-approaching and a failure-avoiding component of *n* Achievement inherent in McClelland and colleagues' (1953) scoring system was later made explicit in Heckhausen's (1963) scoring system, which yields separate scores for hope of success and fear of failure. This scoring system, which was extensively validated with German samples (cf. Heckhausen, 1991), is now available in an English translation, which also includes extensive training materials (Schultheiss, 2001b).

Affiliation-Related Coding Systems

There are two main approaches to measuring affiliative tendencies—the *n* Affiliation scoring system (Heyns, Veroff, & Atkinson, 1958), which was developed to assess concerns about establishing, maintaining, or restoring relationships, and the *n* Intimacy scoring system (McAdams, 1980), which assesses a preference for warm, close, and communicative social interactions. While *n* Affiliation is related to an active striving to attain and maintain social relationships, *n* Intimacy is focused on the quality of these relationships. In other words, intimacy involves a focus on the experience of "being" in a relationship, whereas affiliation emphasizes the act of "doing" or "getting" a relationship.

A story is scored for affiliation only if there is evidence of a concern about establishing, maintaining, or restoring a positive affective relationship with another person or persons. If a story meets this criterion, the scorer goes on to code for subcategories that are similar to those featured in McClelland and colleagues' (1953) *n* Achievement scoring system. These include (1) stated need for affiliation; (2) instrumental activity; (3) anticipatory goal states; (4) obstacles or blocks; (5) affective states; and (6) affiliation thema.

The scoring system for *n* Intimacy comprises two "prime tests" and eight subcategories. The scorer first determines whether a relationship produces positive affect or whether there is dialogue or any verbal or nonverbal exchange between (or among) characters in a story. If either or both of these criteria are met, the scorer goes on to code for the subcategories: (1) psychological growth and coping; (2) commitment or concern by a story character for others; (3) time- or space-transcending quality of a relationship; (4) physical or figurative union of people who have been apart; (5) harmony; (6) surrender or acquiescence by a story character to uncontrollable outside forces that control interpersonal relationships; (7) escape to intimacy, which is when a story character escapes to a situation that affords greater interpersonal growth; (8) connections with the outside world, which is scored when at least one of the story characters experiences a metaphoric interaction with aspects of the nonhuman world (e.g., "communion with nature") or a direct interaction that has a demonstrable effect on the character's thought, behavior, or feelings (e.g., "the heat sapped his energy").

Power-Related Coding Systems

The original coding system for *n* Power (Veroff, 1957) was conceived of as a concern for controlling the means of influence. However, motive scores derived from this coding system were related to assertive behavior in some conditions (e.g., Veroff, 1957) but not in others (e.g., Berlew, 1961). These results were interpreted as indicating a *fear of weakness*, rather than a positive desire for power. In other words, people who received high scores on Veroff's (1957) measure of *n* Power were interested in controlling the means of influence only to ensure that they would not become victims of others' influence. In order to address the approach aspects of power, Winter (1973) constructed a revised scoring system for *n* Power, which incorporates aspects of Veroff's coding system, as well as aspects of a more approach-oriented need for influence measure developed by Uleman (1972), but which goes beyond both in developing a broader view of the power motive as a concern for having impact on others. We therefore present a brief summary of Winter's revised coding system here and refer interested readers to Veroff and Ulemann for more information about earlier measures of power motivation.

According to Winter (1973), power imagery is scored when a story character is concerned about having an impact on or influence over another person, persons, or the world at large.

If power imagery is scored, a coder then goes on to check for the following subcategories: (1) prestige of actor; (2) stated need for power; (3) instrumental activity; (4) external blocks to power goal; (5) goal anticipation; (6) affective goal states; (7) effect, which refers to physical, mental, or emotional responses to the power attempts of a story character.

Winter's Integrated Scoring System

The scoring system outlined in Winter's (1994) *Manual for Scoring Motive Imagery in Running Text* was based on the systems developed by McAdams (1980) for *n* Intimacy, Heyns and colleagues (1958) for *n* Affiliation, McClelland and colleagues (1953) for *n* Achievement, and Winter (1973) for *n* Power. Each subscale of the running text system is an abbreviated version of the original coding system on which it is based. In other words, only the basic imagery of each motive is scored; the subcategories are not used. The running text system also combines *n* Affiliation and *n* Intimacy into one conjoint category because of the theoretical and empirical overlap between the two constructs.

The running text scoring system has been psychometrically validated (Winter, 1991) and demonstrates good predictive validity in a variety of applications ranging from studies of political leaders (Winter, 1980; Winter & Carlson, 1988) to the effects of motives–goal congruence on emotional well-being (Brunstein et al., 1998). Thus, it provides a viable alternative to the original coding systems while substantially decreasing the amount of time and energy required of coders for training and research purposes. It was also developed to be used with other imaginative verbal material besides the PSE and has been successfully used with, for instance, political speeches, literary documents, and spoken interviews (e.g., Winter, 1991; Winter & Carlson, 1988). Its versatility and ease of use make the Winter (1994) running text system a good choice for researchers who require a valid, albeit less differentiated, measure of intimacy/affiliation, achievement, and power motives.

What Pictures to Use?

We now consider several issues in using pictures in PSE motive research, such as the optimum number of picture cues to be presented, the influence of order of presentation on motive scores, and the selection of appropriate pictures for single- or multimotive measurement.

• *Use a sufficient number of picture cues (at least four or five).* The two key issues concerning the number of pictures to include in a final PSE battery are validity and variance. Researchers should use batteries of eight pictures or fewer, because later stories tend to produce less valid scores than earlier pictures in a battery (Reitman & Atkinson, 1958). This decline in validity as test length increases is probably due to fatigue. The key is to use as few or as many pictures about which the participant will cooperate in producing stories in one session, while not sacrificing validity of scores. Conversely, having too few pictures is not optimal either, because variance of scores is affected as the number of pictures used in the PSE approaches zero. Logically, the degree of dispersion of scores within a population should increase proportionally with the number of items used in a test.

To illustrate this point, we have aggregated the motive scores from a dataset using a multimotive PSE and encompassing five different studies (for details on this dataset, cf. Pang & Schultheiss, 2005), and expressed the distribution of motive scores as a function of number of picture cues. Figure 19.2 shows the distribution of total motive imagery resulting from PSEs with as few as one and as many as six picture cues. As shown, the likelihood of detecting any motive imagery in a PSE protocol based on just one picture is less than 40%, and scores are Poisson-distributed, allowing the researcher to derive only a very crude dichotomy between the absence and presence of motive imagery, which is clearly too coarse and not adequate for most assessment and research purposes. Although the situation becomes slightly better in the case of two-, three-, and four-picture sets, the distribution of scores is nonetheless still considerably skewed to the left and, because too many individuals still show zero motive imagery, a normal distribution remains almost impossible to obtain, even if scores are subjected to square root or log transformations. Motive scores start to approximate a normal distribution once a five-story picture set is used.

Thus, to the extent that one wants to, first, use motive scores in regression analyses, which require normally distributed predictor and cri-

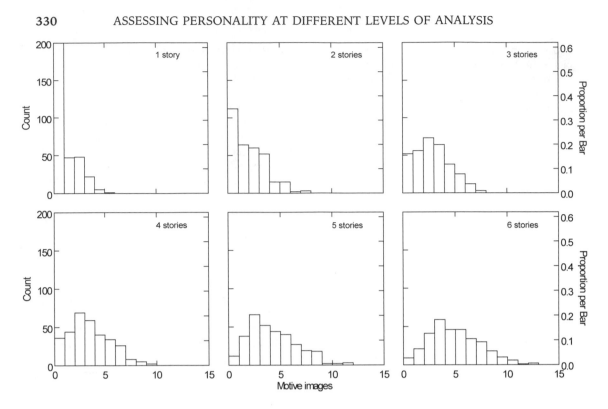

FIGURE 19.2. Distribution of motive images as a function of number of pictures in a picture set.

terion variables, and, second, make sufficiently fine-grained distinctions of motive strength among research participants, we recommend that a PSE include at least five pictures. Note, however, that this recommendation is based on a dataset using a multimotive picture set (i.e., a PSE with pictures aiming at several different motives) and that the minimum number of pictures to use may be slightly lower (i.e., four) if a PSE is employed whose pictures all have a strong pull for one single motive.

• *Use pictures that have sufficiently high cue strength for the motive(s) of interest.* Pictures can differ quite dramatically in their capacity to elicit motive imagery. Some pictures have a good "pull" for one kind of imagery (e.g., power), whereas others are suitable for assessing two or more motives, and yet others have very little pull for any motive. Moreover, some pictures suggest a motivational theme so explicitly that respondents will almost uniformly infuse their stories with a specific kind of motivational imagery; such a picture is therefore not suitable to differentiate between individuals low and high in the motive in question. For instance, a picture that shows a boxer punching another boxer in the face is certain to

elicit a great amount of power imagery from almost every respondent, because nearly everyone will write a story that describes the fight and the exchange of blows. Yet a picture showing a boxer staring absentmindedly into space may prompt some individuals to write about a fight ending in a knockout (e.g., high-power individuals), but others may write about a boxer taking a break from practicing (e.g., low-power individuals) or about a boxer looking forward to spending the evening with his sweetheart (e.g., high-affiliation individuals). Thus, the former picture would be less suitable for discriminating high- from low-power individuals than the latter.

Clearly, therefore, what a researcher needs are picture cues that elicit a sufficient amount of motive imagery in respondents' stories, but that are sufficiently ambiguous or also provide some cues for other motives so that story content can also revolve around other themes than the motive in question. To facilitate the task of compiling suitable picture sets for the assessment of one or several motives, we have started to examine picture profiles, that is, to describe frequently used and new PSE pictures in terms of how much power, achievement, and affiliation/intimacy imagery they elicit on average in respondents' stories (Pang & Schultheiss, 2005; Schultheiss & Brunstein, 2001). We have compiled this information, which comes from U.S. American (Pang & Schultheiss, 2005) and German samples (Schultheiss & Brunstein, 2001), in Table 19.1 and complemented it with picture profiles from other studies conducted in our lab that employed novel picture cues taken from newsmagazines. The stories these data are based on were all scored using Winter's (1994) integrated scoring system. Pictures that elicited at least one scoreable instance of imagery for a given motive in more than 50% of participants were considered high-pull pictures for that motive. Thus, for instance, *women in laboratory* has high pull for both power and achievement imagery, whereas *ship captain* pulls primarily for power imagery and *couple by river* pulls primarily for affiliation imagery.

Usage of this information is straightforward: if you are interested in assessing one specific motive, select the four to six pictures that have the highest pull for that motive. For instance, a researcher interested in assessing only power could compile a set using the *ship captain, woman and man arguing, hooligan attack,* and *men on ship deck*. Based on the mean levels of power imagery given for each of these pictures in Table 19.1, the average sum score for power motive imagery will be close to 7, which is high enough to ensure a good spread of individual scores ranging from the low end (i.e., close to 0) to the high end (i.e., 14 and higher) and thus to harvest a sufficient amount of variance representing interindividual differences in power motivation. More generally, for assessment of a single motive we recommend that at least four pictures be used that have high pull for that motive and for which a total score of 5 or more can be expected on average. For the simultaneous assessment of two motives, we recommend that at least five pictures be used that have high pull for either or both motives and for which total motive scores of 4 or more can be expected on average for each motive. And for the simultaneous assessment of all three major motives, we recommend that at least six pictures be used, with each picture ideally having high pull for at least two motives, and with total motive scores being at 3 or higher for each motive. For this case, we (Pang & Schultheiss, 2005) specifically recommended the use of the following set of pictures, which have been used and validated extensively in our lab: *couple by*

river, nightclub scene, women in laboratory, ship captain, trapeze artists, and *boxer*. If the picture sequence cannot be randomized, we recommend presenting them in the sequence indicated here.

- *Use pictures that are similar to the situation in which you assess your dependent variables.* An issue that has received very little attention in the research literature is the relationship between the picture cues and the situational context in which dependent measures are being assessed. How similar to that situational context should the picture cues be to yield optimally valid motive scores? In lieu of systematic empirical investigations of this issue, we recommend that, to the extent that emotions, cognitions, or behaviors are assessed as dependent variables in a specific situational context, the selected picture cues should be reasonably similar to, but not actual depictions of, the targeted situation. This recommendation is borne out by some observations in our lab. For instance, in a study on the effect of power motivation on persuasive communication (Schultheiss & Brunstein, 2001), the power motive score that best predicted participants' persuasiveness stemmed from the picture *ship captain*, which depicts a captain who seems to argue with another person, whereas the power motive score derived from the picture *trapeze artists*, which shows two trapeze artists in midflight, was a less valid predictor of persuasiveness, although when aggregated with the power motive scores from other pictures it contributed somewhat to the predictive validity of the overall power motive score. Conversely, power motive scores derived from cues that depicted individuals giving a presentation in front of a group of people held virtually no predictive validity in, and were therefore eliminated from, a set of studies in which the effects of power motivation on hormonal and behavioral responses to competition were assessed, whereas power motive scores stemming from pictures showing people in various aggressive or competitive situations had good predictive validity (Schultheiss et al., 2005b; Wirth, Wesh, & Schultheiss, 2006).

If implicit motives are assessed in studies that do not focus on specific thoughts, feelings, or behaviors in circumscribed situations but aim at revealing the relationship of motives to more global measures (e.g., emotional well-being over time or life outcome variables; cf. Brunstein et al., 1998; Jenkins, 1994), it may be more useful to employ picture sets that represent a broad spectrum of everyday situations and thus capture the extensity of a person's motives, that is, the range of contexts and situations in which the person's motives become engaged and may ultimately influence the outcome measures of interest (cf. our previous discussion of motive intensity and extensity). The picture set described by Pang and Schultheiss (2005) represents a good example of a PSE with a broad range of validity.

Finally, keep in mind that researchers are not restricted to the traditionally used PSE pictures, like those described in Table 19.1 or contained in Smith (1992a). If a particular study requires the fine-tailoring of picture cues to a particular assessment situation or social context, new picture cues can be introduced, for instance by using pictures from ads and reports in newspapers and magazines, as has frequently been done in the past (the picture *nightclub scene* is actually a beer ad from the 1960s). However, we recommend that new pictures be pretested with a small sample of participants (20–30) to ensure that they have sufficient pull for the motive(s) in question. We also recommend that, if new pictures are used, they be complemented with a suitable selection of PSE cues whose validity is already established to minimize the risk of obtaining null findings due to possible low validity of the new cues.

• *Picture order has little influence on scores.* Picture order has negligible effects on motive scores. As a general rule, picture profiles (i.e., how much power, affiliation, and achievement imagery they elicit) do not change differentially as a function of their position in the PSE set (Pang & Schultheiss, 2005). Pang and Schultheiss (2005) found some evidence, however, that some pictures are more likely to elicit overall more motive imagery in some serial positions than others. The practical significance of such findings is probably negligible, as they were obtained for only two out of six pictures and the size of the effect was small. In general, picture order effects are of little concern if picture sequence can be randomized across participants by, for instance, administering the PSE on a computer. If picture order is fixed because, for instance, the PSE is administered as a printed leaflet, Smith and colleagues (1992) have recommended that pictures with low and high pull for a given motive should be alternated. If several high-pull pictures for the assessment of one motive only are administered,

we recommend that similar pictures (e.g., pictures showing competitive situations) are not presented back-to-back, but interspersed with high-pull pictures with dissimilar content.

Test Administration

The PSE can be administered individually, with picture presentation and timing of stories being controlled either by an experimenter or by a computer, or in small groups, with picture presentation and timing of stories typically being controlled by the experimenter. Each picture is presented for about 10 to 15 seconds, after which participants are told to write a story on a sheet of paper or to type it directly into the computer. During the writing of the story, participants should no longer be able to see the picture so that their stories do not become confined to a mere description of the picture. After 4 minutes and 30 seconds have elapsed since picture presentation onset, participants are told to finish their stories, and when 5 minutes have elapsed since picture presentation onset, the next picture is presented. Thus, each picture presentation and story writing episode should last about 5 minutes. However, this is only a rough guideline. Inevitably, some participants will go overboard on a story and take more than the total allotted 5 minutes to write a story, and others will be done even before the 5 minutes are up. If assessment time is limited, but the researchers still would like to use a PSE with a large number of pictures, it is also possible to limit the total time allotted to each picture story to 4 minutes.

If the PSE is administered by an experimenter, we recommend that he or she exert as little pressure as possible and move on to the next picture presentation only when all participants are finished with a given story and make eye contact with the experimenter. If the PSE should not take longer than a specific amount of time in the overall data collection session, the experimenter can hold total PSE time constant by providing less time (or more time, in case participants finish early on a preceding picture) on subsequent pictures.

For computer administration of the PSE we recommend that the participants be reminded with a detectable, but low-key message (e.g., the words "Please finish your story and press a key to move on to the next picture" blinking on the screen, with a short beep repeating every 10 seconds) once time is up on a given story.

Moreover, to ensure that participants do not just skim through the PSE and produce insufficient story material in order to be finished early, we recommend that the software allow participants to move on to the next picture story only after some minimum time (e.g., 4 minutes) since picture onset has elapsed.

The overarching goal of PSE administration should be to exert *as little pressure as possible* on participants, because social pressure and demands can interact with participants' motives in ways that renders the motive scores harvested from PSEs invalid (cf. Lundy, 1988). For this reason, we actually recommend computer administration of the PSE over administration by an experimenter, whose very presence and nonverbal signals may already impact on participants' implicit motives (cf. Klinger, 1967). A viable, low-tech alternative is to use leaflets that contain all instructions and, in alternating order, picture cues and story writing sheets, and let participants work through the materials at their own pace, either in the lab or at home. Other measures that can decrease the pressure exerted on participants include (1) not referring to the PSE as a "test" of any kind, (2) not exerting time pressure on participants by requiring them to "write quickly," or making ostensible use of a stopwatch or other time-tracking device (stopwatches should be used only covertly), (3) keeping the interaction between experimenter and participant relaxed and friendly but professional, and (4) administering the PSE at the beginning of an experiment, because other tests and tasks administered during data collection may have unintended, but systematic motive-arousing effects on participants (cf. Lundy, 1988).

Instructions

In our lab, we have worked with PSE instructions adapted from Lundy (1988), who obtained good motive score validity coefficients with them. These instructions are in turn based on earlier standard instructions given in Atkinson (1958) and Smith and colleagues (1992). The instructions we present are as follows:

PICTURE STORY EXERCISE

In the Picture Story Exercise, your task is to write a complete story about each of a series of [number of pictures] pictures—an imaginative story with a beginning, a middle, and an end. Try to portray who the people in each picture are, what they are feeling, thinking, and wishing for. Try to tell what led to the situation depicted in each picture and how everything will turn out in the end.

On your desk are [number of pictures] sheets of paper for you to write your stories on. They are labeled PSE 1 through PSE [number of pictures] in the upper right-hand corner. In the upper left-hand corner there are some guiding questions—these should be used only as guides to writing your story. You do NOT need to answer them specifically.

[For computer administration:]

Each picture will be presented for 10 seconds. After it has disappeared, write whatever story comes to your mind. Don't worry about grammar, spelling, or punctuation—they are of no concern here. If you need more space, use the back of the sheet. You will have about 5 minutes for each story; the computer will then let you know when you have 20 seconds left. If you take less than the entire 5 minutes, the computer will be ready to move on after 4 minutes.

[For administration by experimenter:]

I will show you each picture for 10 seconds. After that, write whatever story comes to your mind. Don't worry about grammar, spelling, or punctuation—they are of no concern here. If you need more space, use the back of the sheet. You will have about 5 minutes for each story; I will let you know when you have 20 seconds left and when it's time to move on to the next picture.

At this point, let us emphasize again that instructions should be conveyed as suggestions, not commandments. If an experimenter is presenting the instructions orally, he or she should be able to present their gist by heart rather than formally reading them from a sheet.

In addition to the preceding instructions, a series of guiding questions are usually printed at the top of each writing page. These questions are adapted from Atkinson (1958):

What is happening? Who are the people?
What happened before?
What are the people thinking about and feeling?
What do they want?
What will happen next?

Although some investigators have spaced these questions apart evenly on the writing page in order to elicit specific responses to each question, we recommend against imposing this degree of structure to participants' responses, because it limits the free flow of the story narrative and may thus interfere with the expression of motivational impulses.

Sometimes participants are exposed to the same picture cues in two or more testing sessions. In these cases a sentence should be included in the instructions of the later session(s) that makes it explicit to participants that they are not expected to produce stories that are different from those they wrote before (Lundy, 1988; Winter & Stewart, 1977):

> You may remember seeing some of these pictures before. If you do, feel free to react to them as you did before, or differently, depending on how you feel now. In other words, tell the story the picture makes you think of now, whether or not it is the same as you told last time.

Format of Data Collection

Usually, participants write their stories on designated sheets containing the guiding questions in the upper left-hand corner and the PSE story number in the upper right-hand corner to allow for easy matching of a given story to the eliciting picture cue later on. A relatively unexplored issue is the effect of having participants type their responses using a computer. Blankenship and Zoota (1998) compared power imagery in PSEs written by hand and on a computer, and found no differences in n Power in participants' stories between these conditions. This is good news, because using a computer decreases the time required of human coders for transcription and word-counting tasks and makes data storage, organization, and sharing more convenient. Although stories typed in an untimed condition were longer than those that were typed in a timed condition, there were no significant differences in the motive scores. Thus, Blankenship and Zoota recommend that researchers use the untimed condition, because participants vary in their typing abilities.

Coding and Preparation for Coding

Coder Training

In order to move on from practice coding materials to actual protocols, scorers have to establish a percentage agreement of 85% or better with materials prescored by an expert, which are typically available with the training and practice materials of a coding system. Training materials for most scoring systems are reprinted in either Atkinson (1958) or Smith (1992a). If that is not the case, they can usually

be requested from the author. Smith and colleagues (1992) have provided an excellent section on recommendations for training scorers to achieve adequate reliability with expert materials. A number of key points deserve to be highlighted:

1. Read the coding manual several times before scoring practice materials until a sufficient level of reliability is obtained.
2. During training, review any errors before going on to the next set of practice stories.
3. Novice scorers should undergo at least 12 hours of training with practice materials when learning a coding system for the first time.
4. Construct, customize, and refer liberally to a "crib sheet" that contains the main points and definitions of each category and subcategory, important coding rules-of-thumb, and special coding considerations.
5. Justify every coding decision by noting the category or subcategory that the image falls under; if a specific coding category cannot be identified, do not score the image no matter how relevant it seems; when in doubt, it is better to err on the side of caution and not score a statement for imagery.
6. Do not make physical markings on the original practice or research materials, in case there is a need to return to these materials later for rescoring or retraining purposes; sets of photocopies should be made for each coder, and these may be marked up instead.

To these recommendations we add that if a novice coder does not achieve adequate reliability on the training materials on the first pass, he or she should score all training materials again, using a fresh set of unmarked copies, and as often as necessary until the 85% criterion is reached. We do not see a problem in the fact that the coder will be better at the subsequent scoring passes simply because the coder remembers his or her own correct and incorrect scores on the first pass. Rather, this is exactly what a good coder should rely on: explicit memory for specific instances in which an image should or should not be scored. For the same reason, we also recommend that even a coder who has already passed the 85% hurdle, and is starting to score stories from a research project, should keep the crib sheet or the original coding manual handy and refer to it *whenever even the slightest doubt arises* in the process of scoring. This will ensure that over time the coder will attain a full, explicit representation of the coding rules in all their complexity and be able to apply them with sufficient specificity and rigor.

An important statistic for coder training is the index of scoring reliability, which is the degree of scoring agreement between coders. Traditionally, there are two means of calculating interscorer reliability: (1) Spearman's rank order correlation between total motive scores and (2) percentage agreement, also known as index of concordance. Percentage agreement should be calculated for each motive, using the following formula: [2*(agreements on presence of motive imagery in story)]/[number of times coder 1 scored motive imagery in story + number of times coder 2 scored motive imagery in story]. This formula is conservative because it does not take into account agreements on the absence of imagery.

The use of intraclass correlation coefficients (ICCs) is an increasingly endorsed way of assessing interrater reliability. The ICC is a "chance-corrected reliability coefficient suitable to continuous data and equivalent to kappa under appropriate conditions" (Meyer et al., 2002). The one-way random effects ICC is a form of analysis of variance that is calculated by the following formula: [MS (between raters) − MS (within raters)]/[MS (between raters) + MS (within raters)]. It is especially meaningful for calculating interrater reliability because it calculates correlations between observations that do not have an obvious order. In other words, in a study with two coders, the assignment of who is "rater 1" or "rater 2" is assumed to be random.

Coding

There are a couple of tasks and decisions involved in the preparation for coding. First, regardless of how long it has been since coders have mastered a coding system, they should reacquaint themselves with it by rereading the training manual before scoring any research materials. Doing so will improve subsequent coding accuracy and interrater reliability because individual scorers are likely to have developed idiosyncratic coding rules based on their previous coding experiences—a rereading of the coding manual helps to alleviate the effects of this "scorer drift." We recommend that after long breaks from scoring, coders reestab-

lish reliability with practice materials before beginning to score research protocols.

Second, all materials for coding should be stripped of any identifying information such as participant biographical data and experiment condition. The only information to appear on the protocols should be participant identification number and picture cue number. If the identification numbers disclose demographic information such as gender, race, or any other group identity, new identification numbers should be assigned. Careful blinding of protocols also prevents the "halo effect." Occasionally, through scoring or being involved in other aspects of an experiment, a coder may form an impression of a participant that may influence his or her scoring of ambiguous responses by that participant. Smith and colleagues (1992) argue that one source of such a halo effect may simply be the coder's knowledge of previous stories written by a participant, which may then influence the coder's scoring of subsequent stories. They therefore recommend coding stories by picture cue as opposed to scoring them by participant. However, in our experience, careful application of the scoring rules usually prevents any carryover from the scoring of previous stories to subsequent stories of a given participant. Moreover, scoring stories by cue instead of by participant may introduce error variance due to scorer drift across picture cues and may also lead to more stereotypical scoring of stories because of similar story material. We therefore suggest that scoring by participant instead of picture cue is defensible, too.

Finally, a tedious but necessary task, in addition to scoring for motive imagery, is the determination of each story's word count. Participants' motive scores correlate with word count more than with the time participants have available to write each story or the time they actually take from the first word to the last, and word count is therefore the single most important variable to control for in participants' overall motive scores.

One Coder or Two?

A critical decision about coding concerns the number of coders to employ. We suggest that this decision should depend on coder experience. If a coder already has extensive coding experience (e.g., more than 1,000 stories coded) with a given scoring system in actual research, *not* counting the training materials he or she completed, it is, in our experience, sufficient to have this one coder score stories from a new study if the same scoring system and similar picture cues are used and the coder follows the recommendations we made in the section "Coder Training." In addition, we suggest that after the coding of all materials is completed, the coder should review all of his or her scores by reading through the coded stories again and use this opportunity to eliminate scores that, at second glance, do not hold up according to the coding rules, and to detect images that may have been overlooked during coding and should be scored. This second reading is critical for maintaining high coding accuracy even if the coder is already experienced. Moreover, it may sometimes be necessary for the single coder to recode a subset of fresh, unmarked copies of 50–100 stories from the same sample to establish intrarater reliability and demonstrate that coder drift has no substantial effect on the motive scores used in the data analysis.

If no experienced coder is available for coding, we recommend that two newly trained coders be used for independent coding of all stories. In our experience, interrater reliability can be substantially enhanced by first having both coders independently score 40 to 60 stories collected with the same picture cues as the ones that have been used in the study for which they are about to do coding. These stories can come from either a subset (5 to 10 participants) of the actual sample or, better yet, from pilot participants whose data will not be used in testing the research hypotheses. After scoring of this initial story pool, the coders should meet, compare their stories, discuss all coding discrepancies, and try to develop further coding guidelines to deal with coding issues and problems that are idiosyncratic to the specific picture cues and samples from which they obtained their stories. Of course, these specific guidelines should be consistent with the more general ones of the scoring manual employed by the coders. Then each coder independently works on a full set of copies of the PSE stories collected from the total research sample.

Once all coding is finished, each story's total motive score can be averaged between scorers for further analyses, or coders can get together for a final session in which coding discrepancies are discussed and resolved based on rigorous application of the rules contained in the scoring system. Although the latter option is more labor-intensive, it usually provides more accurate and rationally derived final scores and has the added pedagogical benefit of providing further training for the coders. Whether the averaging or the discrepancy-resolution approach is chosen, interrater reliability should be determined on the basis of each coder's original scores, before any changes are made to them owing to averaging or the coders' discussion of their scores. If intercoder reliability is determined by using correlation or ICC coefficients, it should be done on the basis of each participant's total score across all pictures, and not by picture.

A final comment on the effort invested in coding stories for motive imagery: On average, an experienced scorer needs 2–5 minutes to score one PSE story, not counting the time needed to determine word count (this task can be assigned to a research assistant). Thus, for a typical research sample of 80 participants who are administered a six-picture PSE, an experienced coder will need between 16 and 40 hours to code all materials, plus some additional time to review the assigned scores. This is certainly a large time investment, but it is necessary to obtain valid motive scores, and the investment is very likely to pay off, as we have found again and again in our own research. We realize that, as compared with the effort other sciences invest in their measurements, personality psychology often has an unfortunate tendency to sacrifice validity for economy. The PSE does not cater to this propensity, but neither is it excessively labor-intensive when compared with, for example, the assessment of hormones in psychoendocrinology or brain activation patterns in the cognitive and affective neurosciences.

Data Entry and Processing

We finish the step-by-step guide for implicit motive assessment by describing some data entry and processing strategies that we have found useful in our research. In the following discussion, we give recommendations about data entry, data aggregation and distribution issues, procedures for correcting for word count, and some basic approaches to data analysis using implicit motive scores.

• *Enter motive scores and word counts in as fine-grained a format as possible.* At a minimum, motive and word count scores should be entered into a spreadsheet for each picture separately to enable the researcher to later examine the contribution of each picture to the PSE's criterion validity. In some cases, it may even be useful to enter subscores for each imagery category separately for each picture. This may be useful in cases in which, for instance, the researcher would like to compare the specific validity contributions of each coding category to the test's predictive power or separate the approach and avoidance components of a given motive, which are often represented as separate coding categories within the overall coding system (e.g., in McClelland et al.'s 1953 coding system for *n* Achievement, negative instrumental activity, negative goal anticipation, negative goal affect, and the block categories may be used to assess the fear of failure aspect of achievement motivation; cf. Schultheiss & Brunstein, 2005, for further discussion).

As outlined in our previous discussion of reliability issues, researchers should not expect scores of the same motive derived from different picture cues to be correlated strongly. However, they can examine the differential validity of each picture's motive score by entering all pictures' motive scores, plus a word count variable representing the aggregated word count scores for each picture, into simultaneous regression equations with the dependent variables of interest. Not every picture score's regression weight will be significant, and sometimes even the signs of the picture scores may differ. However, before a specific picture's motive score is eliminated from a final total score, it should be firmly established that the picture's motive score differs from other pictures' scores because it (1) predicts a dependent variable with a different sign that is, moreover, (2) significant and (3) replicable for at least two critical criterion variables.

• *Examine score distributions after creating total motive and word count scores.* After summing motive and word count scores across pictures, examine the total scores for each motive and the word count using histograms and scatterplots. If deviations from a normal distribution are detected or total scores feature outliers, use a square root or log transformation to correct the problem of the offending score. Keep in mind that outliers can substantially influence the results of later analyses that test the actual research hypothesis.

• *If motive scores and word counts correlate, correct motive scores for word count.* Cal-culate Pearson correlations for all total motive scores with the total word count score. If a given motive score does not significantly correlate with the total word count score, do not correct it for word count; use the raw total motive score in all further analyses. If a total motive score does significantly correlate with the word count score (usually in the positive direction and even up to .50), there are two strategies to remove the influence of participants' verbal fluency from the motive score.

The first option is to use regression analysis to residualize motive scores for word count and use the residual scores in all subsequent analyses. This option has the advantage that it makes the resulting motive score exactly 0-correlated with the word count score and thus completely removes the influence of verbal fluency from the motive measure. But there are also two disadvantages to this correction. First, because regression analysis is used, it depends on the entire sample's motive and word count scores to calculate predicted and residualized motive scores for each participant. Thus, a given residualized motive score's meaning is always sample dependent. Second, the residualized scores lose the intuitive meaning of the raw score (an experienced researcher may easily classify a raw score of 5 as high, but may be stumped by a residual score of 0.89) and require subsequent transformations (e.g., into *z*-scores) to make them more meaningful again. Note, however, that the meaning of a *z*-score is, of course, entirely sample dependent.

The second option is to correct motive scores for word count by multiplying the total motive score by 1,000 and dividing the result by the total word count for each participant. The resulting score can be readily interpreted as motive images per 1,000 words. Owing to the nature of the correction, the resulting score does not depend on the specific sample in which the data were collected and can easily be compared to average images-per-1,000-word scores obtained in other samples. In other words, this transformation yields a readily interpretable metric that allows between-sample comparisons of motive scores. A major drawback of this correction is that the resulting scores are not necessarily 0-correlated with total word count. At worst, they can create serious biases and artifacts due to persisting significant overlap with the word count. Thus, the corrected motive score should always be checked for variance overlap with the total word count.

The correlation will rarely be 0; however, we recommend that it should not exceed |.15|. If this criterion is not fulfilled, we recommend using the regression approach to word count correction.

Finally, check the word-count-corrected motive score for distribution abnormalities using a histogram. If the corrected score is not normally distributed, but the raw total motive score and word count scores were, use square root or log transformations to make the corrected score conform to a normal distribution. If the raw total motive score or the raw word count score, or both, were not normally distributed to begin with, transform these first (or try a different transformation) so that the word-count-corrected motive score will more closely approximate a normal distribution.

• *Use continuous word-count-corrected motive scores in all statistical analyses.* If total motive scores were carefully examined and corrected for either distribution violations, the influence of verbal fluency, or both, they will provide the researcher with a good quantitative measure of motive strength. Thus, word-count/distribution-corrected motive scores should be entered as quantitative variables into all correlation and regression analyses testing the research hypotheses and should *not* be subjected to a median split or any other method of partitioning a quantitative measure into groups. This would only result in a rather dramatic reduction of test power, increase Type I error, and make it more difficult to test a research hypothesis. Usually, any kind of analysis that can be done with partitioned scores can also be done with quantitative scores when general regression methods are used. We highlight this issue with a couple of case examples in the following section and refer the reader to the excellent article on the use of quantitative personality predictors in analytical designs by West, Aiken, and Krull (1996) for a more systematic treatment of this topic.

Case Examples

In the following discussion, we showcase the use of PSE motive scores in a variety of research designs. Specifically, we briefly highlight the use of the PSE in studies on motivational arousal, longitudinal changes in motive levels, and motive × situation interactions in between-subject designs.

Using the PSE to Measure Motivational Arousal

Schultheiss and colleagues (2004) were interested in studying the effects of affiliation motivation arousal on progesterone release. To do so, they had one group of participants view an affiliation-arousing movie, another one a neutral control movie, and a third group a power-arousing movie to differentiate the specific effects of the affiliation-arousing movie from general effects due to the presentation of movies with social content. To verify that the different arousal conditions actually had the intended effect on participants' motivational state, they administered one three-picture PSE before, and one after the movie, in a counterbalanced design, with one-half of participants working on picture set A before and picture set B after the movie, and the other half working on the PSE in the reverse sequence. All PSE stories were scored for power and affiliation imagery using Winter's (1994) running text scoring system, and motive scores were residualized for total word count on each set. Motive data were analyzed using a multiple regression analysis with post-movie motive scores as dependent variable, pre-movie motive scores as covariate, and experimental condition (control, affiliation arousal, power arousal) as dummy-coded predictor. The results verified that experimental conditions aroused implicit motives differentially: After the movie, affiliation-arousal participants had increased affiliation and decreased power motive scores, whereas power-arousal participants showed the reverse pattern, and control-group participants registered virtually no changes in their motive levels. Eventually, the affiliation-arousal group was the only group that also had elevated progesterone levels after the movie. In essence, Schultheiss and colleagues used the assessment of motive changes on the PSE as a manipulation check, which allowed them to verify that the movie in the affiliation-arousal condition had the intended specific motivational effect. They therefore argued that the subsequent increase in progesterone observed in this condition reflected an affiliation-driven endocrine effect. Hormone assessments notwithstanding, their research design also represented a well-crafted study of the effects of motive arousal on changes in motivational content expressed in PSE stories and, in this aspect, is very similar to many motive arousal studies originally conducted to derive coding systems (e.g., Winter, 1973).

Assessing Longitudinal Changes in Implicit Motives

Schultheiss, Dargel, and Rohde (2003) examined the effects of menstrual cycle stage on longitudinal changes in implicit power and affiliation motivation. Their sample consisted of one group of normally cycling (NC) women, one group of women who were using oral contraceptives (OC), which prevent the hormonal changes typically associated with the various phases of the menstrual cycle from occurring, and one group of men. Three different sets of four-picture PSEs were carefully compiled to ensure that each set featured picture cues that, although not identical to those in the other sets, depicted similar situations and had similar and balanced pulls for the implicit needs for power and affiliation. These sets were administered at three phases of the menstrual cycle, corresponding to the follicular (T1), periovulatory (T2), and luteal phase (T3) of the female cycle (participants in the male group were scheduled on the basis of a pseudocycle). To prevent a confoundation between picture set and assessment phase, Schultheiss and colleagues systematically varied the sequence in which the sets A, B, and C were administered to participants across T1, T2, and T3, resulting in the six sequence permutations, ABC, ACB, BAC, BCA, CAB, and CBA. PSE stories were coded for power and affiliation imagery using Winter's (1994) integrated scoring system. All scores were converted to motive images per 1,000 words to adjust for differences in word count. Although the three sets did not differ in the length of the stories written in response to them, set B elicited significantly more power imagery and significantly less affiliation imagery than the other two sets. To correct for these differences, participants' corrected motive scores were converted to z-scores within each picture set. The influence of picture set on participants' motive scores in any given cycle phase was thus removed from the scores' variance. Repeated-measures regression analysis with motive (power, affiliation) and cycle phase (follicular, periovulatory, luteal) as within-subject factors and contraceptive use (OC, NC) as between-subject factors revealed that women had higher levels of affiliation motivation around ovulation than in the follicular phase and lower

power motivation in the periovulatory phase than in the luteal phase of the menstrual cycle, regardless of oral contraceptive use.

It is conceivable that the variance due to differences between picture sets may have obscured more fine-grained differences between groups and cycle phases. But Schultheiss and colleagues (2003) decided against administering the same PSE three times to participants, because they were concerned that this procedure might introduce even more error variance owing to participants' getting bored with writing stories about the same pictures again and again. Thus, although this study illustrates that the PSE measure of implicit motives can also be used in longitudinal research, it also illustrates some of the problems associated with devising PSEs suitable for this task.

Examining Motive × Situation Effects in an Experimental Study

A recent example of a study that examines the interplay between individuals' implicit motives and experimentally manipulated situations was provided by Schultheiss, Wirth, and colleagues (2005). Two studies, the first with male, the second with female participants, dealt with the effects of power-relevant situational outcomes, namely, experimentally varied victory and defeat in a one-on-one competition based on an implicit sequence learning task. At the start of each data collection session, participants' implicit power motive was assessed with a five-picture PSE. To optimize motive score validity for the prediction of physiological and behavioral changes associated with the competition situation created for this study, only picture cues that showed people in competitive or aggression-related contexts were used. The stories were coded for power imagery using Winter's (1973) revised power motive scoring system. Scores were corrected for word count by regression, and the distribution of the z-transformed residuals were checked for normality. In Study 2 (women), a square-root transformation was used to make the z-scores conform to a normal distribution. Before participants began the task, they listened to a tape-recorded guided imagery exercise that described the ensuing contest in rich contextual detail from the winner's perspective. The inclusion of this imagery exercise was based on earlier research indicating that mere verbal priming for and instructions about a potentially motive-relevant experimental task may not be sufficient to adequately engage participants' implicit motives in the typically language-heavy context of laboratory experiments (cf. our introduction and Schultheiss, 2001a, for further discussion of this issue). Dependent variables were changes in salivary testosterone as measured before and after the contest and postcontest learning gains on the serial response task used during the competition. The analytical design was based on multiple regressions with power motive scores as a quantitative personality variable, contest outcome as a dummy-coded experimental variable, and the multiplicative interaction term of these variables as predictors, and postcontest testosterone (residualized for precontest testosterone) and implicit learning gains as dependent variables.

The power motive × contest outcome effect was significant for implicit learning gains in both studies. Among contest winners, power motives scores significantly and positively predicted implicit learning gains, whereas they were a significant negative predictor of learning among losers in both studies. In Study 1 (men), the power motive × contest outcome effect was also significant for testosterone 15 minutes postcontest, controlling for precontest testosterone levels. Among contest winners, higher power motives scores predicted, with marginal significance, greater testosterone increases; among contest losers, higher power motives scores significantly predicted greater testosterone decreases. Notably, as in an earlier study (Schultheiss & Rohde, 2002), postcontest testosterone increases were positively related to implicit learning gains, and mediation analyses revealed that the negative effect of power motivation on learning gains among losers was mediated by the effect of power motivation on testosterone changes. In Study 2 (women), power motivation had a strong main effect on postcontest testosterone changes, with higher motive scores predicting greater hormone increases.

Ironically, although participants' self-reported mood was strongly influenced by contest outcome, with winners in both studies being much happier after the contest than losers, these changes in mood were neither predicted by participants' implicit power motivation nor associated with hormone changes or learning gains. These findings underscore the point we were making previously, namely, that nondeclarative measures of motivation, such as im-

plicit motive scores, implicit learning gains, or hormonal changes, are more closely associated with each other than with declarative measures, such as self-reported satisfaction or dissatisfaction with a situational outcome.

Conclusion and Some Future Directions

We hope that this chapter has made the procedures of measuring implicit motives with the PSE more transparent to potential users. To achieve this aim, we have relied on excellent earlier introductions to implicit motive assessment, which we recommend to anyone interested in motive assessment (e.g., Smith, 1992a; Smith et al., 1992), added recommendations based on our own experiences with PSE-based motive assessment (particularly in regard to the use of computers in the administration of the PSE), and compiled here for the first time crucial information on the motivational pull of traditionally used and more recent PSE picture cues. As we have emphasized throughout the chapter, valid assessment of implicit motives requires care, attention to detail, a thorough understanding of motivation in general and implicit motive dispositions in particular, and, of course, effort and time.

In regard to the last point, we should add that we think it is possible to develop faster, and possibly also better, measures of implicit motives, as long as these reside in the nondeclarative domain and assess motives by examining processes over which the individual has little conscious control and that tap some specific, crucial aspect of a given motive. An important step in this direction has recently been presented by Brunstein and Schmitt (2004), who adapted the Implicit Association Test (IAT; Greenwald, McGhee, & Schwartz, 1998) to assess implicit achievement motivation. Consistent with the idea that implicit motives influence nondeclarative, but not declarative indicators of motivation, these authors found that the IAT achievement motive measure was (1) uncorrelated with a self-report measure of achievement motivation based on the same stimulus material on which the IAT measure was based and (2) predicted participants' response times on a vigilance task when performance feedback was provided, but not participants' self-reported satisfaction with their performance. Although the convergent validity of the IAT measure of achievement motivation with PSE measures of this motive still needs to be established, we think that Brunstein and Schmitt's (2004) findings are very promising and could mark the beginning of a new era of implicit motive assessment.

Still, even if latency-based or other procedural measures of implicit motives will be developed more intensively in the future, we are certain that there will always be a place for PSE-type motive measures for two important reasons. First, the content-coding systems developed for the PSE can also be applied to many other forms of verbal material and therefore enable the researcher to assess at a distance the personality of individuals who are either dead or in other ways inaccessible (cf. Winter, 1991). This simply cannot be done with computerized, procedural motive measures, which always require the respondent to be present for the assessment. Second, those studies that use PSE-type methods to collect verbal material represent an immensely valuable resource, because stories can always be recoded once other or better content-coding measures are developed and become available to the researcher. Many old longitudinal studies that have employed the TAT for clinical or psychodynamic assessment purposes today represent a gold mine for motive researchers who code the TAT stories for implicit motive imagery to examine the impact of motives on life trajectories. Had the original authors of these studies used tests with a fixed response format instead of the open-ended collection of picture stories, later researchers would always be stuck with the necessarily more limited conceptual framework of the study authors and the dataset would therefore be of much more limited value.

For these reasons, we believe that for a long time to come, the development and refinement of content-coding methods for motive assessment, including the PSE technique, will remain an important task for researchers who are interested in the nonconscious sources of motivation and personality. Some important ways in which the content-coding approach to the assessment of motivation could be furthered include the development of scoring systems for neglected, but fundamental motivational needs, such as sex or curiosity, the refinement of existing motive scoring systems, and the development of coding systems that, based on experimental arousal studies, systematically differentiate between approach and avoidance components of each motive (cf. Schultheiss, in press; Schultheiss & Brunstein, 2005). Ultimately, such efforts toward better assessment of implicit motives are likely to pay off in the form of more meaningful findings, more sophisticated theories of implicit motivational processes, and a more prominent role of the implicit motive construct for personality psychology and neighboring disciplines, such as clinical psychology and affective neuroscience.

Author Note

All picture stimuli described in this chapter are available upon request from the authors.

Recommended Readings

Atkinson, J. W. (1981). Studying personality in the context of an advanced motivational psychology. *American Psychologist, 36,* 117–128.

Lundy, A. (1985). The reliability of the Thematic Apperception Test. *Journal of Personality Assessment, 49,* 141–145.

Lundy, A. (1988). Instructional set and Thematic Apperception Test validity. *Journal of Personality Assessment, 52,* 309–320.

Reuman, D. A. (1982). Ipsative behavioral variability and the quality of thematic apperceptive measurement of the achievement motive. *Journal of Personality and Social Psychology, 43*(5), 1098–1110.

Smith, C. P. (Ed.). (1992). *Motivation and personality: Handbook of thematic content analysis.* New York: Cambridge University Press.

Smith, C. P., Feld, S. C., & Franz, C. E. (1992). Methodological considerations: Steps in research employing content analysis systems. In C. P. Smith (Ed.), *Motivation and personality: Handbook of thematic content analysis* (pp. 515–536). New York: Cambridge University Press.

Winter, D. G. (1991). Measuring personality at a distance: Development of an integrated system for scoring motives in running text. In D. J. Ozer, J. M. Healy, & A. J. Stewart (Eds.), *Perspectives in personality* (Vol. 3, pp. 59–89). London: Jessica Kingsley.

References

Atkinson, J. W. (Ed.). (1958). *Motives in fantasy, action, and society.* Princeton, NJ: Van Nostrand.

Atkinson, J. W. (1981). Studying personality in the context of an advanced motivational psychology. *American Psychologist, 36,* 117–128.

Atkinson, J. W., & Birch, D. (1970). *The dynamics of action.* New York: Wiley.

Atkinson, J. W., Bongort, K., & Price, L. H. (1977). Explorations using computer simulation to comprehend thematic apperceptive measurement of motivation. *Motivation and Emotion, 1,* 1–27.

Berlew, D. E. (1961). Interpersonal sensitivity and motive strength. *Journal of Abnormal and Social Psychology, 63,* 390–394.

Biernat, M. (1989). Motives and values to achieve: Different constructs with different effects. *Journal of Personality, 57,* 69–95.

Blankenship, V., & Zoota, A. L. (1998). Comparing power imagery in TATs written by hand or on the computer. *Behavior Research Methods, Instruments, and Computers, 30*(3), 441–448.

Brunstein, J. C., & Hoyer, S. (2002). Implizites und explizites Leistungsstreben: Befunde zur Unabhängigkeit zweier Motivationssysteme [Implicit versus explicit achievement strivings: Empirical evidence of the independence of two motivational systems]. *Zeitschrift für Pädagogische Psychologie, 16,* 51–62.

Brunstein, J. C., & Maier, G. W. (2005). Implicit and self-attributed motives to achieve: Two separate but interacting needs. *Journal of Personality and Social Psychology, 89*(2), 205–222.

Brunstein, J. C., & Schmitt, C. H. (2004). Assessing individual differences in achievement motivation with the Implicit Association Test. *Journal of Research in Personality, 38,* 536–555.

Brunstein, J. C., Schultheiss, O. C., & Grässmann, R. (1998). Personal goals and emotional well-being: The moderating role of motive dispositions. *Journal of Personality and Social Psychology, 75,* 494–508.

deCharms, R., Morrison, H. W., Reitman, W., & McClelland, D. C. (1955). Behavioral correlates of directly and indirectly measured achievement motivation. In D. C. McClelland (Ed.), *Studies in motivation* (pp. 414–423). New York: Appleton-Century-Crofts.

Entwisle, D. R. (1972). To dispel fantasies about fantasy-based measures of achievement motivation. *Psychological Bulletin, 77,* 377–391.

Fineman, S. (1977). The achievement motive construct and its measurement: Where are we now? *British Journal of Psychology, 68,* 1–22.

Gazzaniga, M. S. (1985). *The social brain: Discovering the networks of the mind.* New York: Basic Books.

Greenwald, A. G., McGhee, D. E., & Schwartz, J. L. K. (1998). Measuring individual differences in implicit cognition: The Implicit Association Test. *Journal of Personality and Social Psychology, 74,* 1464–1480.

Heckhausen, H. (1963). *Hoffnung und Furcht in der Leistungsmotivation* [Hope and fear components of achievement motivation]. Meisenheim am Glan: Anton Hain.

Heckhausen, H. (1991). *Motivation and action.* Berlin: Springer.

Heyns, R. W., Veroff, J., & Atkinson, J. W. (1958). A scoring manual for the affiliation motive. In J. W.

Atkinson (Ed.), *Motives in fantasy, action, and society* (pp. 205–218). Princeton, NJ: Van Nostrand.

Hofer, J., & Chasiotis, A. (2003). Congruence of life goals and implicit motives as predictors of life satisfaction: Cross-cultural implications of a study of Zambian male adolescents. *Motivation and Emotion, 27,* 251–272.

Jackson, D. N. (1984). *Personality research form* (3rd ed.). Port Huron, MI: Sigma Assessment Systems.

Jenkins, S. R. (1994). Need for power and women's careers over 14 years: Structural power, job satisfaction, and motive change. *Journal of Personality and Social Psychology, 66,* 155–165.

Kagan, J. (2002). *Surprise, uncertainty, and mental structures.* Cambridge, MA: Harvard University Press.

Klinger, E. (1967). Modeling effects on achievement imagery. *Journal of Personality and Social Psychology, 7,* 49–62.

Langner, C. A., & Winter, D. G. (2001). The motivational basis of concessions and compromise: Archival and laboratory studies. *Journal of Personality and Social Psychology, 81,* 711–727.

Lundy, A. (1985). The reliability of the Thematic Apperception Test. *Journal of Personality Assessment, 49,* 141–145.

Lundy, A. (1988). Instructional set and Thematic Apperception Test validity. *Journal of Personality Assessment, 52*(2), 309–320.

McAdams, D. P. (1980). A thematic coding system for the intimacy motive. *Journal of Research in Personality, 14,* 413–432.

McClelland, D. C. (1987). *Human motivation.* New York: Cambridge University Press.

McClelland, D. C., Atkinson, J. W., Clark, R. A., & Lowell, E. L. (1953). *The achievement motive.* New York: Appleton-Century-Crofts.

McClelland, D. C., Koestner, R., & Weinberger, J. (1989). How do self-attributed and implicit motives differ? *Psychological Review, 96,* 690–702.

Meyer, G. J., Hilsenroth, M. J., Baxter, D., Exner, J. E., Jr., Fowler, J. C., Piers, C. C., et al. (2002). An examination of interrater reliability for scoring the Rorschach Comprehensive System in eight data sets. *Journal of Personality Assessment, 78*(2), 219–274.

Murray, H. A. (1943). *Thematic Apperception Test manual.* Cambridge, MA: Harvard University Press.

Nisbett, R. E., & Wilson, T. D. (1977). Telling more than we can know: Verbal reports on mental processes. *Psychological Review, 84,* 231–259.

Pang, J. S., & Schultheiss, O. C. (2005). Assessing implicit motives in U. S. college students: Effects of picture type and position, gender and ethnicity, and cross-cultural comparisons. *Journal of Personality Assessment, 85*(3), 288–294.

Reitman, W. R., & Atkinson, J. W. (1958). Some methodological problems in the use of thematic apperceptive measures of human motives. In J. W.

Atkinson (Ed.), *Motives in fantasy, action, and society* (pp. 664–683). Princeton, NJ: Van Nostrand.

Reuman, D. A. (1982). Ipsative behavioral variability and the quality of thematic apperceptive measurement of the achievement motive. *Journal of Personality and Social Psychology, 43*(5), 1098–1110.

Schuerger, J. M., Zarrella, K. L., & Hotz, A. S. (1989). Factors that influence the temporal stability of personality by questionnaire. *Journal of Personality and Social Psychology, 56*, 777–783.

Schultheiss, O. C. (2001a). An information processing account of implicit motive arousal. In M. L. Maehr & P. Pintrich (Eds.), *Advances in motivation and achievement: Vol. 12. New directions in measures and methods* (pp. 1–41). Stamford, CT: JAI Press.

Schultheiss, O. C. (2001b). *Manual for the assessment of hope of success and fear of failure.* Unpublished manuscript. University of Michigan, Ann Arbor.

Schultheiss, O. C. (in press). A biobehavioral model of implicit power motivation arousal, reward and frustration. In E. Harmon-Jones & P. Winkielman (Eds.), *Fundamentals of social neuroscience.* New York: Guilford Press.

Schultheiss, O. C., & Brunstein, J. C. (1999). Goal imagery: Bridging the gap between implicit motives and explicit goals. *Journal of Personality, 67*, 1–38.

Schultheiss, O. C., & Brunstein, J. C. (2001). Assessing implicit motives with a research version of the TAT: Picture profiles, gender differences, and relations to other personality measures. *Journal of Personality Assessment, 77*(1), 71–86.

Schultheiss, O. C., & Brunstein, J. C. (2002). Inhibited power motivation and persuasive communication: A lens model analysis. *Journal of Personality, 70*, 553–582.

Schultheiss, O. C., & Brunstein, J. C. (2005). An implicit motive perspective on competence. In A. J. Elliot & C. S. Dweck (Eds.), *Handbook of competence and motivation* (pp. 31–51). New York: Guilford Press.

Schultheiss, O. C., Campbell, K. L., & McClelland, D. C. (1999). Implicit power motivation moderates men's testosterone responses to imagined and real dominance success. *Hormones and Behavior, 36*(3), 234–241.

Schultheiss, O. C., Dargel, A., & Rohde, W. (2003). Implicit motives and gonadal steroid hormones: Effects of menstrual cycle phase, oral contraceptive use, and relationship status. *Hormones and Behavior, 43*, 293–301.

Schultheiss, O. C., & Hale, J. A. (in press). Implicit motives modulate attentional orienting to perceived facial expressions of emotion. *Motivation and Emotion.*

Schultheiss, O. C., Pang, J. S., Torges, C. M., Wirth, M. M., & Treynor, W. (2005). Perceived facial expressions of emotion as motivational incentives: Evidence from a differential implicit learning paradigm. *Emotion, 5*(1), 41–54.

Schultheiss, O. C., & Rohde, W. (2002). Implicit power motivation predicts men's testosterone changes and implicit learning in a contest situation. *Hormones and Behavior, 41*, 195–202.

Schultheiss, O. C., Wirth, M. M., & Stanton, S. (2004). Effects of affiliation and power motivation arousal on salivary progesterone and testosterone. *Hormones and Behavior, 46*(5), 592–599.

Schultheiss, O. C., Wirth, M. M., Torges, C. M., Pang, J. S., Villacorta, M. A., & Welsh, K. M. (2005). Effects of implicit power motivation on men's and women's implicit learning and testosterone changes after social victory or defeat. *Journal of Personality and Social Psychology, 88*(1), 174–188.

Smith, C. P. (1992a). *Motivation and personality: Handbook of thematic content analysis.* New York: Cambridge University Press.

Smith, C. P. (1992b). Reliability issues. In C. P. Smith (Ed.), *Motivation and personality: Handbook of thematic content analysis* (pp. 126–139). New York: Cambridge University Press.

Smith, C. P., Feld, S. C., & Franz, C. E. (1992). Methodological considerations: Steps in research employing content analysis systems. In C. P. Smith (Ed.), *Motivation and personality: Handbook of thematic content analysis* (pp. 515–536). New York: Cambridge University Press.

Spangler, W. D. (1992). Validity of questionnaire and TAT measures of need for achievement: Two meta-analyses. *Psychological Bulletin, 112*, 140–154.

Uleman, J. S. (1972). The need for influence: Development and validation of a measure, in comparison with need for power. *Genetic Psychology Monographs, 85*, 157–214.

Veroff, J. (1957). Development and validation of a projective measure of power motivation. *Journal of Abnormal and Social Psychology, 54*, 1–8.

West, S. G., Aiken, L. S., & Krull, J. L. (1996). Experimental personality designs: Analyzing categorical by continuous variable interactions. *Journal of Personality, 64*, 1–48.

Winter, D. G. (1973). *The power motive.* New York: Free Press.

Winter, D. G. (1980). Measuring the motives of southern African political leaders at a distance. *Political Psychology, 2*(2), 75–85.

Winter, D. G. (1991). Measuring personality at a distance: Development of an integrated system for scoring motives in running text. In D. J. Ozer, J. M. Healy, & A. J. Stewart (Eds.), *Perspectives in personality* (Vol. 3, pp. 59–89). London: Jessica Kingsley.

Winter, D. G. (1994). *Manual for scoring motive imagery in running text.* Unpublished manuscript, University of Michigan, Ann Arbor.

Winter, D. G. (1999). Linking personality and "scientific" psychology: The development of empirically derived Thematic Apperception Test measures. In L.

Gieser & M. I. Stein (Eds.), *Evocative images: The Thematic Apperception Test and the art of projection* (pp. 107–124). Washington, DC: American Psychological Association.

Winter, D. G., & Carlson, L. (1988). Using motive scores in the psychobiographical study of an individual: The case of Richard Nixon. *Journal of Personality, 56,* 75–103.

Winter, D. G., & Stewart, A. J. (1977). Power motive reliability as a function of test–retest instructions. *Journal of Consulting and Clinical Psychology, 45,* 436–440.

Wirth, M. M., Welsh, K. M., & Schultheiss, O. C. (2006). Salivary cortisol changes in humans after winning or losing a dominance contest depend on implicit power motivation. *Hormones and Behavior, 49*(3), 346–352.

Woike, B. A. (1995). Most-memorable experiences: Evidence for a link between implicit and explicit motives and social cognitive processes in everyday life. *Journal of Personality and Social Psychology, 68,* 1081–1091.

Zurbriggen, E. L. (2000). Social motives and cognitive power–sex associations: Predictors of aggressive sexual behavior. *Journal of Personality and Social Psychology, 78,* 559–581.

## CHAPTER 20

Lives Lived in Milliseconds

Using Cognitive Methods in Personality Research

Michael D. Robinson

Areas of psychology as diverse as those related to attention, consciousness, and religion frequently cite William James (1890), who offered important insights into these phenomena. In relation to the self, the same can be said. One particularly cogent insight contrasted the *I* versus the *me*. The *I* thinks; the *me* is thought about. The *I* lives in real time; the *me* does not. The *I* is the perceiver and cannot be perceived; the *me* can be perceived and in fact is the product of one's perceptions of the self. This distinction may capture some important differences between cognitive and self-report approaches to personality. Cognitive approaches seek to examine the processes, existing in real-time transactions with the environment, that are responsible for attention, perception, and interpretation. Self-report approaches, in contrast, seek to capture generalizations that the self makes about the self. These two aspects of personality may or may not correspond with each other.

There are other considerations favoring the development of cognitive approaches to personality. Cognitive processes can be measured in an objective fashion; in contrast, self-report approaches necessarily rely on some degree of subjectivity. Cognitive processes capture the self in its real-time interactions with the environment; in contrast, self-report approaches necessarily rely on abstraction and retrospection. Cognitive processes can provide an understanding of personality dynamics and flux; in contrast, self-report measures are often relatively silent on questions of personality process (Pervin, 1994). One could go on here. However, the important point is that cognitive processes, as slippery and fractionated as they may sometimes be, nonetheless allow the researcher to measure and manipulate objective, rather than subjective, personality processes.

Given that there are some important theoretical and methodological benefits to the cognitive assessment of individual differences, it is somewhat surprising that such methods are not used more frequently. The widespread availability of personal computers, along with a host of reliable experimental software packages, renders cognitive methods relatively easy to instantiate in the lab. Nonetheless, there are downsides to cognitive approaches as well, three of which are mentioned here. One, there is certainly an important learning curve in computer programming and data analysis. Indeed, budding cognitive psychologists are likely to view their early programming and analysis efforts as cumbersome at best and fatally flawed at worst. Two, cognitive approaches to personality are underdeveloped, both theoretically and methodologically, at present. For example, there are very few taxonomic efforts related to cognitive personality assessment. Data are promising, but in constant revision.

Three, it appears to be somewhat inevitably the case that cognitive measures of personality are less reliable than self-report measures of personality. This apparent fact can be attributed to at least two important sources. Cognitive measures are very much dependent on momentary states of mind. Such factors may be less important to trait self-report measures, which do not rely on state-related sources of information to the same extent. In addition, the reliability and stability of traits derive in part from the fact that people develop very stable beliefs about themselves. These beliefs, however, may provide a misleading picture of how much people's lives and personalities are actually changing (for a relevant review, see Robinson & Clore, 2002). The upshot of these two considerations leads to the suggestion that cognitive processing measures cannot, and should not, be as stable as self-reports of personality. Nevertheless, it is important to pay somewhat constant attention to the reliability of cognitive processing measures, as such measures may or may not in fact tap reliable and stable individual differences.

Why Use Cognitive Measures?

Given the aforementioned theoretical benefits and methodological costs of using cognitive measures in personality research, it may be useful to consider in greater depth the possible reasons to assess cognition in one's research. The first reason is that one is seeking to explain a trait–outcome relation. For example, it is plau-

sible and consistent with extant theory to propose that habitually anxious individuals are anxious in state-related terms in part because of cognitive processing tendencies favoring threatening information in the environment. Such an assumption has been validated in multiple ways within the clinical literature (for a review, see MacLeod, 1999). Anxious (versus nonanxious) individuals often appear to selectively attend to threatening information within spatial attention tasks. Moreover, attention to threat tendencies appear to mediate and cause state-related experiences of anxiety (MacLeod, 1999). In sum, an understanding of the cognitive processes underlying dispositional vulnerabilities answers important questions concerning the mechanisms involved in trait–state relations.

The second reason for assessing cognitive variables is that one hypothesizes that such variables should correlate with important individual difference outcomes, irrespective of possible correlations with self-reported traits. In the domain of emotional experience, MacLeod (1999) and Robinson (2004) present evidence for the predictive validity of cognitive processing measures. Often, such relations obtain despite the fact that the cognitive (or implicit) measures do not correlate with self-reported personality variables (Bornstein, 1999; Robinson, 2004). Thus, the use of cognitive measures often reveals important facts about individuals that cannot be assessed by self-report.

The third reason to assess cognitive variables is that one hypothesizes that such variables should moderate trait–outcome relations. For example, Matthews and Gilliland (1999) report that measures tapping cortical arousal, whether behavioral or brain related, often interact with the trait of extraversion in predicting relevant outcomes (e.g., speed of classical conditioning, memory recall performance). Such interactions tend to occur despite the fact that trait extraversion predicts cortical arousal variables to only a small extent (Matthews & Gilliland, 1999). Moderator effects have also been frequently observed in my program of research (e.g., Robinson, 2004).

In summary, trait–cognition correlations can help to provide a plausible basis for trait–outcome relations. Cognition–outcome relations are very useful in understanding the processes that lead to certain outcomes (e.g., such as aggression). Finally, trait–cognition interactions help to explain when and why traits are consequential for everyday experience and behavior. Overall, then, it seems apparent that a personality science embracing both self-reported traits and cognitive processing measures will necessarily be richer than one confined to either type of measure considered alone.

Types of Cognitive Measures: Overview and Guide

In seeking to add cognitive measures to one's repertoire, it must be recognized that cognition is not a unified process, but rather a diverse set of processes. Even seemingly very specific processes such as those associated with spatial attention, semantic priming, or executive control (all of which are reviewed below) can be further subdivided, depending on the specific cognitive paradigms used to measure the relevant constructs. From a personality-related perspective, it may be useful to focus on the larger effects reported in the cognitive literature. In this "molar" spirit, I present a broad taxonomy of cognitive processes rather than one that is paradigm specific.

To anticipate the subsequent taxonomy, it is helpful to refer to Table 20.1. As indicated in the table, the discussion includes five classes of cognitive measures, related to attention, accessibility, semantic priming, implicit self-attitudes, and executive control. Also as indicated there, all cognitive processes can be measured in ways that are more indirect or more direct. Indirect methods are those in which it is not at all obvious as to what is being measured, whereas direct methods are those in which it is potentially more obvious as to what is being measured. The table provides citations for direct and indirect measures of each cognitive process. As will be apparent in the discussion of specific cognitive processes, it may be that direct cognitive methods are typically more useful in personality research in sense that they are associated with effects that are more reliable and robust. For this reason, direct methods are favored in the following discussion.

Attention

In regard to either covert attention or eye movements, the mind's eye tends to select certain information for further processing. Such selective attention effects are apparent within 100 msec of stimulus exposure (Posner & Raichle, 1994). However, early selectivity effects are largely nonsemantic in nature, related to the prestimulus direction of attention as well as relatively crude features of stimuli such as bright colors or movement. Such early orienting operations are unlikely to be of great interest to personality psychologists. Admittedly,

TABLE 20.1 A Taxonomy of Cognitive Processes Linked to Individual Differences in Personality

Cognitive process	Method	Reference
Attentional disengagement	Indirect Direct	Fox et al. (2001) Wilkowski, Robinson, & Meier (2006)
Accessibility	Indirect Direct	Higgins & Brendl (1995) Meier & Robinson (2004)
Semantic priming	Indirect Direct	Mikulincer et al. (2000) Robinson & Kirkeby (2005)
Implicit self-attitudes	Indirect Direct	Koole, Dijksterhuis, & van Knippenberg (2001) Greenwald & Farnham (2000)
Executive control	Indirect Direct	Shah, Friedman, & Kruglanski (2002) von Hippel & Gonsalkorale (2005)

Note. Indirect procedures are those in which it is not obvious what is being measured. In direct procedures, it is somewhat more obvious what is being measured. The Reference column lists empirical studies using methods relevant to the particular combination of cognitive process and method (i.e., direct versus indirect).

this is a speculative suggestion. However, it is supported by recent studies suggesting that early aspects of attention are largely insensitive to the meaning of stimuli (e.g., Fox, Russo, Bowles, & Dutton, 2001).

Later attentional processes, such as those related to engagement and disengagement, are of far more interest to personality psychologists. Engagement operations are those associated with understanding a stimulus, whereas disengagement processes are those associated with inhibiting such elaborative processes in favor of a new stimulus (Posner & Raichle, 1994). In practice, it is difficult to distinguish engagement and disengagement processes, at least within behavioral paradigms. Accordingly, my colleagues and I make the general distinction between orienting and disengagement operations and suggest that the latter type of operation may be of more interest to personality psychologists (Fox et al., 2001).

The literature on anxiety and threat has typically examined one type of selective attention task, albeit with many variations. In the typical task, two words are simultaneously presented, one being threatening in nature (e.g., *snake*) and one being nonthreatening in nature (e.g., *chair*). Participants are told to attend to the words somewhat generally. After some delay (typically 500–700 msec, although often shorter or longer than this), the words disappear and a spatial probe almost immediately replaces one of the two words. Probe tasks can vary, but often require simple detection (e.g., "hit the space bar as soon as you detect the letter *x*") or discrimination (e.g., "press the letter key *q* or *p* as soon as you see the letter *q* or *p*"). If individuals are quicker to the spatial probe when it occurs in the location of threatening words, then the investigator makes the legitimate inference that the individual was preferentially attending to them. In this manner, one can index covert attention to threatening or nonthreatening words when both are presented simultaneously.

It is notable that traditional spatial probe tasks, in which two stimuli are simultaneously presented, cannot necessarily distinguish orienting processes from disengagement ones. Because there has been some suggestion that disengagement operations are of more interest to personality psychologists (e.g., Fox et al., 2001), my colleagues and I have developed a task designed to tap disengagement processes somewhat specifically (e.g., Wilkowski, Robin-son, & Meier, in press). In our modified version of the task, only one spatial cue is shown at one time. The cue is randomly assigned to either the left or right spatial location. To ensure that the meaning of the cue interacts with personality-related systems, participants are asked to categorize the word vocally (e.g., as "hurtful" or "helpful"; Wilkowski et al., in press). The vocal response removes the word. Almost immediately subsequent to the vocalization, the letter *q* or *p* appears in either the same location as the word or in the opposite location to the word. Participants then type *q* or *p*, depending on the letter shown.

In such studies, we have been interested in the question of whether participants are able to spatially disengage from word cues of a specific semantic category (e.g., "hurtful" words). In a recent study (Wilkowski et al., in press), we found that agreeable individuals were slow to spatially disengage from "helpful" primes, whereas disagreeable individuals were slow to spatially disengage from "hurtful" primes. It should be noted that these effects were in the neighborhood of 150 msec (for the Agreeableness × Cue Type interaction). This suggests to us that a spatial disengagement paradigm along these lines might be particularly useful in personality research. The task encourages meaning analysis and is specifically designed to measure spatial disengagement processes, which have been characterized as most sensitive to personality-related influences (Fox et al., 2001).

Category Accessibility

Bruner (1957) proposed that individuals are "prepared" to assign habitual categories to stimuli, a suggestion that has been confirmed in a large number of studies focusing on "chronic accessibility" measures of personality (for a review, see Robinson & Neighbors, 2006). Although such work has often focused on dependent measures such as those related to person perception, the basic ideas have considerable implications for personality functioning. For example, Kelly's (1963) theory of personality was primarily based on habitual semantic categories used to interpret events.

In a number of recent studies, my colleagues and I have sought to measure individual differences in category accessibility (for a review, see Robinson, 2004). We did so by using choice reaction time tasks. For example, assume that individuals differ in the accessibility of blame, defined as a tendency to assign blame to relevant events as they occur. We (Meier & Robinson, 2004) were interested in whether such tendencies to assign blame might predict anger and aggression in everyday life. To examine this question, we designed a blame categorization task that required individuals to classify relevant words as blameworthy (e.g., *malpractice*, *sin*) or not blameworthy (e.g., *mildew*, *baldness*) as quickly and accurately as possible. We measured the time taken to categorize such words within a choice reaction time task. We also controlled for individual differences in construct-irrelevant categorization speed, a point covered below. For now, note that we were able to order individuals along a fast (i.e., accessible) to slow (i.e., nonaccessible) dimension related to blame accessibility.

In the same study, we (Meier & Robinson, 2004) also assessed the trait of agreeableness, which has specific relevance to predicting anger and aggression. Finally, we measured tendencies to experience anger and engage in arguments in daily life, specifically within an experience-sampling protocol. We expected agreeable individuals to be less angry and aggressive in daily life. We also expected blame-accessible individuals to be more angry and aggressive in daily life. Such considerations may suggest that the two individual difference variables—that is, agreeableness and blame accessibility—would be significantly correlated. They were not in fact correlated, consistent with the general idea that implicit and explicit measures of personality are typically independent of each other (Robinson & Neighbors, 2006).

Of perhaps more importance, both blame accessibility and agreeableness predicted anger and aggression in daily life, but only in their interaction (Meier & Robinson, 2004). First, in regard to the effects pertaining to agreeableness, they were not significant if blame accessibility was low. This suggests that no one is particularly angry or aggressive, given low blame accessibility. Second, in regard to the effects pertaining to blame accessibility, it was a significant predictor of anger and aggression, but only at low levels of agreeableness. This suggests that accessible blame contributes to anger and aggression only among some people. Third, in regard to the interaction in total, it suggests that agreeable individuals are capable

of inhibiting implicit blaming tendencies, whereas disagreeable individuals are not capable and/or inclined to do so. This is consistent with other results from our lab, as reported below. In sum, recent investigations suggest that one can measure habitual categories in terms of choice reaction time performance (Robinson, 2004).

Semantic Priming

As people go about their lives, they learn to organize and structure related items of information together. For example, people learn that supermarkets are places where bread, meat, fruit, and other edibles are available for purchase. In contrast, they learn that zoos are places where tigers, zebras, monkeys, and other animals can be viewed by the modern city dweller. Such covariations in experience and knowledge are invaluable in organizing mental life. First, they allow for an organization of concepts rather than a willy-nilly configuration of facts. Second, they allow one to predict what will happen next. For example, the supermarket shopper is prepared to see bread, fruit, and meat rather than tigers, zebras, and monkeys. Integrated semantic memory networks therefore facilitate the encoding and retrieval of related facts in a manner that is typically adaptive to the individual.

Individuals are likely to organize mental life in a similar manner in some respects. For example, everybody learns that supermarkets contain food, whereas zoos contain live animals in cages. However, individuals would also be expected to differ in such semantic memory networks. This general notion has received a good deal of attention. Along these lines, Bargh, Raymond, Pryor, and Strack (1995) proposed that individuals differ in associations between power and sexual attraction. For the power-motivated individual, but not for others, dominance over opposite-sex others would be expected to "prime" sexual attraction (Bargh et al., 1995). Many other citations could be offered. The important point here is that there are a large number of theories assuming that semantic priming effects should vary across individuals.

Semantic memory networks are invisible and unconscious. They organize memory material, but cannot be directly observed. Within the cognitive literature, it is typical to examine such semantic memory networks in lexical decision or pronunciation tasks (Neely, 1991). Perhaps the most common task is the primed lexical decision task. The participant is told to categorize letter strings as words (e.g., *nurse*, *grape*: 9 key button press) or nonwords (e.g., *narsd*, *grite*: 1 key button press). Shortly before the presentation of target letter strings, participants are briefly flashed (typically for 200 msec) with a "prime" word that they are told is irrelevant to the target task. When primes and targets are related (e.g., *doctor–nurse*, *fruit– grape*), versus unrelated (e.g., *doctor–grape*, *fruit–nurse*), lexical decisions are some 10–20 msec faster (Neely, 1991). This is a small but robust effect. The nature of the effect suggests that (1) related words are clustered together within semantic memory and (2) word reading and recognition processes involve semantic meaning to some extent.

The primed lexical decision task has been profitably used in several studies of personality. For example, Mikulincer, Birnbaum, Woddis, and Nachmias (2000) used this task to show that stress-related primes (e.g., the word *death*) activate proximity-seeking thoughts (e.g., the word *love*) among secure and anxious, but not avoidant, individuals. Mikulincer et al. argued that avoidant individuals have learned to suppress the attachment system in part because they do not believe that others can be trusted to provide comfort during times of stress. The results are fascinating and supportive of the psychodynamic attachment theory that guided the investigation.

Nevertheless, from a psychometric perspective, it may be that the primed lexical decision task is not an ideal one to probe individual differences in semantic memory networks. There are a number of issues here. Here, I highlight two related ones. One, there is evidence that many lexical decisions can be made without reference to semantic factors (Joordens & Becker, 1997). Two, people can strategically ignore irrelevant sources of information when they are told to ignore them (Besner, 2001). In other words, it may often be the case that neither primes nor targets activate semantic memory networks within the primed lexical decision task (Joordens & Becker, 1997). Thus, it is generally concluded that the primed lexical decision task is useful for examining the automaticity of semantic processes (Neely, 1991). However, it is a somewhat poor task for examining the structure of semantic memory networks in that such networks often do not

contribute to task performance (Joordens & Becker, 1997).

Fortunately, there are alternatives to the primed lexical decision task. My colleagues and I have used variations of what we term the "continuous semantic priming task" (CSPT). Relative to the primed lexical decision task, there are at least two important differences. One, individuals categorize prime stimuli according to semantic categories. For example, they may classify picture primes as "gay" or "neutral," depending on whether the picture depicts gay sexual activity or not (Meier, Robinson, Gaither, & Heinert, 2006). This categorization task ensures that primes activate semantic meaning. Two, targets, like primes, are also categorized in terms of semantic meaning. For example, target stimuli may be categorized as "positive" or "negative" (Meier et al., 2006).

Because both primes and targets involve semantic distinctions, one can therefore examine priming effects across prime and target trials somewhat secure in the knowledge that both tasks involved semantic memory structures (Joordens & Becker, 1997). Therefore, facilitation or lack of facilitation can be more directly interpreted in terms of semantic memory networks. In the Meier and colleagues (2006) study discussed above, we found that gay prime pictures facilitated negative target evaluations only among a group that was high in both self-deception and homophobia. We concluded that aversive associations to gay sexual activity are potentiated by both self-deception and homophobia, but particularly in their combination.

Our CSPT procedures can be altered in a number of ways. Semantic tasks can be the same across prime and target trials (e.g., Meier, Robinson, & Wilkowski, 2006) or different across trials (e.g., Meier et al., 2006). Semantic tasks can involve dichotomous classifications (e.g., Meier, Robinson, & Wilkowski, 2006) or rating procedures (e.g., Wilkowski & Robinson, 2006). Prime and target judgments can involve the same response modality (e.g., both button presses; Meier, Robinson, & Wilkowski, 2006) or different response modalities (e.g., pronunciations followed by button presses; Meier et al., 2006). In short, the CSPT is flexible, but based on the fundamental assumption that individual differences in semantic priming are best examined within the context of semantic (rather than merely lexical) decisions.

Implicit Self-Attitudes

The emerging consensus is that there are two apparently reliable and valid procedures for measuring implicit self-attitudes, otherwise referred to as implicit self-esteem (e.g., Bosson, Swann, & Pennebaker, 2000). The first sort of measure is based on evaluations of letters of the alphabet, with the idea that positive attitudes toward the self will result in a preference for the letters in one's name. There are a number of very interesting developments along these lines, and a review article by Pelham, Carvallo, and Jones (2005) is recommended. Because of space limitations, however, we concentrate on the second assessment technique below.

The Implicit Association Test (IAT; Greenwald, McGhee, & Schwartz, 1998) has generated a great deal of interest since it was first introduced. Greenwald and Farnham (2000) subsequently introduced an IAT measure specific to self-esteem. The IAT self-esteem task involves two choice reaction time distinctions, one pertaining to the distinction between self (e.g., the word *me*) and other (e.g., the word *them*) and one pertaining to the distinction between pleasant (e.g., the word *sunshine*) and unpleasant (e.g., the word *vomit*). To measure IAT self-esteem, participants are asked to perform two "combined" blocks. In one of these blocks, self and pleasant words are associated with one response (e.g., pressing the 1 key), whereas other and unpleasant words are associated with a different response (e.g., pressing the 9 key). In a second combined block, such mappings are reversed (e.g., self or unpleasant = 1 key; other or pleasant = 9 key). IAT self-esteem is defined by subtracting speed in the self or pleasant block from speed in the self or unpleasant block, with higher scores indicating higher levels of implicit self-esteem (for further details, see Greenwald & Farnham, 2000).

There is an emerging consensus that IAT self-esteem may predict individual differences in emotional experience. Along these lines, two recent investigations sought to correlate IAT self-esteem with affective experiences in everyday life (Conner & Barrett, 2005; Robinson & Meier, 2005). Both studies found that individual differences in IAT self-esteem were associated with everyday experiences of negative affect, but not positive affect. In particular, both studies found that higher IAT self-esteem levels were associated with less negative affect in daily life. It therefore appears that high levels of IAT self-esteem buffer the individual from stress and distress (Conner & Barrett, 2005).

Why does IAT self-esteem buffer the individual from negative affect? Robinson, Mitchell, Kirkeby, and Meier (2006) proposed a theory related to spatial metaphor. Briefly, my colleagues and I viewed IAT self-esteem in terms of spatial compatibility principles and suggested that individual differences in IAT self-esteem tap tendencies to repel negative connotations from the self-concept. This general idea seems consistent with related themes involving introjection versus repulsion in the cognitive, psychodynamic, and linguistic literatures (Robinson, Mitchell, et al., 2006). In short, because of the spatial mapping properties of the IAT self-esteem measure, it may be tapping tendencies to introject versus repel negative connotations from the self-concept (Robinson, Mitchell, et al., 2006).

Consistent with another theme of this chapter, there is also good evidence for the idea that traits and IAT self-esteem tend to interact in the prediction of some outcome variables (Jordan, Spencer, Zanna, Hoshino-Browne, & Correll, 2003; Robinson & Wilkowski, in press). For example, Robinson and Wilkowski (2006) suggest that high levels of IAT self-esteem could be problematic at high levels of agreeableness because they would conflict with the more egalitarian style of agreeable individuals. Across three studies, the authors found that agreeableness and implicit self-esteem interacted to predict psychological distress such that high levels of agreeableness, combined with high levels of implicit self-esteem, were associated with higher levels of psychological distress. Although these findings were robust, we also suggest that a great deal of future research would be useful in this area.

Executive Control

Most cortical areas are involved in perception, memory, or attention. However, this is less obviously true in the case of the frontal cortex. Interestingly, the frontal cortex is also disproportionately large among human beings relative to other animals. What does the frontal cortex do? Some general answers are that it permits an individual to inhibit prior action tendencies, maintain goals within working memory, and alter behavior in the service of longtime (rather than short-term) goals. Such functions are often viewed in terms of self-regulation or executive control (Baddeley, 1996; Knight & Grabowecky, 2000).

Within the cognitive literature, executive control abilities are typically examined within cognitive ability tasks, such as those related to inhibiting prepotent responses or generating flexible responses over time (Baddeley, 1996). Such cognitive abilities appear to be important to personality-related outcomes. For example, damage to frontal lobes impairs a variety of abilities related to behavioral flexibility, behavioral inhibition, and perspective taking (Knight & Grabowecky, 2000). In addition, executive control deficits have been linked to a number of individual difference variables such as low IQ and behavioral impulsivity (Knight & Grabowecky, 2000).

Although the studies mentioned above did not assess the traits of the five-factor model, there is a recent suggestion that executive control abilities may be positively correlated with the trait of agreeableness. My colleagues and I have found such a suggestion to be supported in recent studies in our lab (e.g., Meier et al., 2006). Aside from the trait of agreeableness, however, other traits such as conscientiousness and neuroticism—seemingly somewhat related to executive control—have not tended to correlate with self-regulation abilities, at least in our studies. This said, we have found many cases in which neuroticism interacted with executive control abilities in predicting everyday experiences and displays of negative emotion (e.g., Robinson, Wilkowski, Kirkeby, & Meier, 2006; Robinson, Wilkowski, & Meier, 2006). Perhaps the most parsimonious conclusion to emerge from the latter research is that executive control abilities seem to be particularly important at high levels of neuroticism (Robinson et al., 2006).

The literature on executive control is clearly a growth industry. Therefore, there are likely to be important changes in conceptualizing and measuring such abilities in the future. For now, we note that we have found a simple color–word Stroop test to be useful in assessing a number of self-regulation processes (e.g., Robinson et al., 2006; Robinson, Wilkowski, & Meier, 2006). In the simplest version of this task, the words *green* and *red* could be presented in green or red font. Participants could be told to press one key for a green font color and another key for a red font color. Within this simplified choice reaction time task, there are two congruent conditions (i.e., *red* in red and *green* in green) and two incongruent responses (i.e., *red* in green and *green* in red). There are quite a few indications that greater difficulties with incongruent responses indicate some difficulties in executive control (MacLeod, 1991; von Hippel & Gonsalkorale, 2005). If so, one can operationalize executive control difficulties in terms of a larger incongruent RT minus congruent RT difference score.

In addition, the same Stroop task can be scored with respect to several other plausible self-regulation variables. First, average speed on the task should correlate negatively with IQ measures, which themselves are often viewed in terms of executive control abilities (Jensen, 1998). In addition to average speed, it is useful to quantify the standard deviation of performance. Higher standard deviations of performance across trials have been associated with frontal lobe damage, old age, and low IQ (Jensen, 1998). As there is typically some positive relation between average speed and the standard deviation of response speed, we suggest that researchers statistically control for average speed prior to examining the correlates of reaction time variability (Robinson, Wilkowski, & Meier, 2006).

Finally, there are theoretical reasons for examining reaction time performance as a function of the previous trial. I do not elaborate much here, given the other goals of this chapter. However, there are data suggesting that individual differences in self-regulation correlate positively with error control, defined as slower reaction times following errors and faster reaction times following correct responses. A recent study found that higher error-control tendencies predicted greater levels of subjective well-being (Robinson, in press). Additional studies have shown that difficulties associated with switching required responses across consecutive trials are associated with stronger trait–outcome relations, defined in terms of correlations between traits and relevant personality outcome measures (Robinson & Cervone, in press; Robinson et al., 2006).

Case Examples

Having somewhat briefly described implicit measures pertaining to attention, category accessibility, semantic priming, implicit self-attitudes, and executive control, the discussion now turns to two case studies using cognitive measures of personality. The first focuses on individual differences in category accessibility, and the second focuses on individual differences in semantic priming and self-regulation. In each case example, a greater amount of methodological detail is presented than in the brief overview above.

Case Example 1

Kelly (1963) proposed that individuals differ in their "personal constructs" or habitual categories and further suggested that such variations play a profound role in structuring everyday experience. For example, I met a woman who claimed that she never felt sad, angry, or guilty. The woman often dresses in pink or peach colors, has an extremely engaging personality, and rarely if ever expresses criticisms or complaints. I was intrigued and puzzled by this extremely cheerful person. How could someone go through life with such a cheerful disposition? The answer, from Kelly's point of view, is simple. It seems likely that this person rarely sees the glass as half empty; that is, she does not assign negative evaluations to events in her life. For this reason, very little in life can be distressing or disappointing to her.

Kelly's (1963) theory of personality is intriguing because it suggests that acts of meaning assignment do not follow from personality; rather, they *are* personality. My colleagues and I have sought to measure "personal constructs" in terms of acts of meaning assignment within choice reaction time tasks (Robinson, 2004). Here, one such investigation is reported. To examine the accessibility of negative evaluations, we asked participants to quickly and accurately categorize words in terms of whether they were neutral (e.g., *penny*; press 1 key) or negative (e.g., *decay*; press 9 key) in nature (Robinson, Vargas, Tamir, & Solberg, 2004). The "neutral" response pole is consistent with Kelly's theory in that Kelly assumed that personal constructs are dimensional in nature, necessarily including two poles such as "honest" versus "not honest." Of additional importance, choice reaction time tasks require a choice. The neutral alternative category seemed ideal because it was also an evaluative category, but not one that should elicit a good deal of either positive or negative affect.

Word stimuli were chosen from normed sources. Neutral words included *couch*, *jelly*, and *string*; negative words included *dirt*, *pimple*, and *trash*. Approximately 10 neutral and 10 negative words were chosen for each study.

There were 16 practice trials designed to give participants some familiarity with the words and response assignments. This practice block was followed by a 30-trial assessment-related block. The category "neutral" was presented to the left of the screen, and the category "negative" was presented to the right of the screen. The presentation of the categories was to help in the response mapping process (i.e., neutral = 1 key; negative = 9 key).

Words were randomly selected and presented in the center of the computer screen. We measured the amount of time needed to categorize each word. Correct responses were followed by a blank screen for 150 msec, which should allow sufficient time to prepare for the next trial. Incorrect responses were penalized by a 1,500 msec error message in order to ensure a relatively high accuracy rate. Reaction times are more informative if accuracy rates are high. Indeed, one typically penalizes inaccurate (but not slow) responses if speed is the desired unit of analysis. In contrast, one typically penalizes slow (but not inaccurate) responses if accuracy is the desired unit of analysis.

The most robust predictor of categorization speed (aside from death or coma) is practice. We therefore reasoned that faster performance within the negative categorization block would belie prior (i.e., preassessment) tendencies to assign negative evaluations to life events. However, one caveat here is that there are both general and task-specific contributions to choice reaction time performance. For example, individuals high in *g*, or fluid intelligence, are faster at every categorization task. Although this correlation is not large, it is robust (Jensen, 1998). Therefore, my colleagues and I sought to remove such general abilities through the use of a second categorization task that we believed was entirely neutral in nature. Trial procedures were parallel to those described above. However, within the control block, we asked participants to quickly and accurately categorize words in terms of whether they represented nonanimate (e.g., *chair*; press 1 key) or animate (e.g., *mouse*; press 9 key) objects.

As expected, accuracy rates for both blocks were high (*M* accuracy ~ 95%), which is desirable when examining reaction time. Inaccurate trials were deleted, as they may or may not reflect the processes of interest (Ratcliff, 1993). We were left with millisecond values for correct responses. Within most cognitive tasks, reaction time distributions are skewed. Therefore, it is desirable to reduce skew through one of several transformations (Ratcliff, 1993). Both log-transformed latencies (i.e., = log10[msec value]) and inverse latencies (i.e., = 1 / [msec value]) can be recommended, as they will reduce the positive skew of reaction time distributions (Ratcliff, 1993). We always log-transform reaction times in our studies.

Even after log-transforming reaction times, it is still the case that some of them are especially fast or slow. It is desirable to reduce the impact of outliers. This can be done by replacing or eliminating outlier latencies (Ratcliff, 1993). We define outlier latencies as those that are 2.5 standard deviations (SD's) faster or slower than the log-latency mean for the task and sample at hand. We then replace log-latencies faster or slower than these 2.5 SD cutoff scores with these cutoff scores. Alternate procedures for handling reaction time data are discussed by Ratcliff (1993). Suffice it to note that it seems desirable to develop an invariant set of procedures to prevent capitalizing on chance. Based on our experience, log-transformation followed by 2.5 SD replacements seems to produce desirable latency distributions.

To assess individual differences in the accessibility of negative evaluations, we then averaged trials within a given block (Robinson et al., 2004). To remove the general speed factor from consideration, we then performed a simple regression predicting negative block speed from animal block speed. The regression equation was used to remove the speed common to both blocks (typically ~ an r = .5 correlation). Residual negative evaluation scores were computed as follows: = (negative speed – [intercept + (slope * animal speed)]). Residual scores were necessarily highly correlated with speed in the negative evaluation block, but uncorrelated with speed in the animal control block. The residual variance left over is therefore specific to the negative evaluation block, as desired.

We then repeated the above procedures separately for odd and even trials of the two categorization tasks. We therefore obtained two estimates of negative evaluation speed (residualized), one of which was particular to odd trials and one of which was particular to even trials. To compute the split-half reliability of this measure of negative evaluation accessibility, we then correlated the two independent assessments of negative evaluation speed. The correlation was in the neighborhood of r = .70. This suggests that there are reliable individual differences in the accessibility of negative evaluations.

To examine the correlates of negative evaluation tendencies, we also assessed the traits of extraversion and neuroticism (Robinson et al., 2004). Neither of these traits correlated with negative evaluation tendencies. This suggests that implicit and explicit (i.e., trait-related) measures of personality are independent of each other, an observation consistent with a good deal of other data (Robinson & Neighbors, 2006). In the same three studies, we also assessed everyday tendencies toward negative affect and lower experiences of life satisfaction. As predicted, faster negative evaluations were associated with (1) more negative appraisals of daily life, (2) higher levels of negative emotional experience, and (3) lower levels of life satisfaction. These results remained significant when controlling for the traits of extraversion and neuroticism.

The results of the study support Kelly's (1963) theory of personality in that habitual negative evaluations, assessed by residual choice reaction time, predicted lower levels of subjective well-being within everyday life. These correlations remained significant when controlling for extraversion and neuroticism, the two traits most closely associated with subjective well-being. It therefore appears that habitual negative evaluations predispose individuals to lower levels of subjective well-being in their everyday transactions with the environment. We suspect, with no data, that our optimistic peach-colored individual, mentioned earlier, would exhibit particular difficulties with the negative evaluation task.

Case Example 2

Meier and Robinson (2004) found that blame categorization tendencies, measured in a manner parallel to that used in Case Example 1, did not correlate with the trait of agreeableness. This suggested to us that individuals low and high in agreeableness blame others with relatively equal frequency. However, Meier and Robinson also found that blame categorization speed interacted with levels of agreeableness in predicting everyday tendencies toward anger and aggression. Specifically, accessible blame predicted higher levels of anger and aggression among disagreeable, but not agreeable, individuals. This suggested to us that agreeable individuals are capable of self-regulating or inhibiting aggressive thoughts, in effect precluding their influence on subsequent affect and behavior.

To examine spontaneous tendencies to self-regulate (or inhibit) aggressive thoughts, we (Wilkowski & Robinson, 2006) designed two cognitive paradigms. The first paradigm used the continuous semantic priming task (CSPT) in combination with instructions to evaluate words (1 = extremely unpleasant; 8 = extremely pleasant) as they were presented. In Study 1 of this investigation, we compiled a list of 50 aggressive actions (e.g., *hit*, *punch*, *mutilate*) and 50 neutral actions (e.g., *lecture*, *converse*, *interact*). These words were randomly selected and presented one at a time within the center of the computer screen. Following the 100+ trials, we coded evaluations in terms of the nature of the target word (i.e., the word receiving the evaluation rating: neutral versus aggressive) as well as the nature of the prime word (i.e., the word presented in the immediately preceding trial: neutral versus aggressive). Evaluations were averaged across the four cells of the 2 (Prime) × 2 (Target) within-subject design. In addition, we measured trait anger with a common measure of this construct.

The design of Study 1 (of Wilkowski & Robinson, 2006), like most cognitive studies, is a factorial repeated-measures design. Almost any often used statistical software package will handle such designs. However, it is rare for cognitive studies to examine potential interactions between within-subject manipulations (e.g., neutral versus aggressive primes) and continuous between-subjects variables such as Trait Anger. In the past, such between-by-within designs have typically been handled by dichotomizing trait variables. However, such procedures have been heavily criticized (Aiken & West, 1991). It therefore seems desirable to examine interactions involving traits in a manner that preserves the continuous nature of such traits (Aiken & West, 1991). We have found that the general linear model (GLM) procedures of statistical analysis software (SAS) are quite flexible in handling such between-by-within designs.

With respect to the present predictions (Wilkowski & Robinson, 2006), we performed an analysis examining word evaluations as a function of the Prime × Target × Trait Anger design. Individuals low and high in trait anger rated aggressive targets equally negatively, and there was also no hint of a Prime × Target × Trait Anger interaction. However, there was a significant Prime × Trait Anger interaction. This interaction is not associated with cell means per se, as trait anger was a continuous rather than discrete variable within the analysis. We therefore sought to understand the interaction by performing two regressions. In one, we entered trait anger as a predictor of evaluations following neutral primes. In the other, we entered trait anger as a predictor of evaluations following aggressive primes. We used the regressions to estimate predicted means for those low (−1 SD) and high (+1 SD) in trait anger, for each of the prime conditions considered separately. Readers are encouraged to consult Aiken and West (1991) for further details concerning this procedure. As expected, the estimated means revealed that aggressive (versus neutral) primes had a larger effect on the evaluations of high trait anger individuals relative to low trait anger individuals. This result is consistent with the idea that low trait anger individuals self-regulate the negative affect induced by aggressive primes. This interaction was replicated in a second study.

Although the evaluation data reported by Wilkowski and Robinson (2006) are consistent with the idea that low anger individuals self-regulate (or inhibit) aggressive primes, we wanted to offer converging evidence for this hypothesis. To do so, we borrowed from theoretical frameworks suggesting that self-regulation is an effortful activity that takes time (e.g., Mischel & Ayduk, 2004). We further drew from the cognitive literature, which has shown that switching from one task to another involves effortful self-regulation processes (Posner & Raichle, 1994). Therefore, if we are correct that individuals low (but not high) in trait anger self-regulate aggressive primes, then such individuals should exhibit increased task-switching costs following aggressive primes.

To investigate such predictions, we designed a CSPT involving distinct prime and target tasks. In the priming phase of the task, individuals were asked to categorize words as hurtful (e.g., *hit*) or helpful (e.g., *hug*) in nature, specifically by pronouncing "hurtful" or "helpful" into a voice microphone. Sufficient sound pressure triggered the removal of the prime from the screen, which was somewhat immediately followed by the letter *q* or *p*. Participants were instructed to press the *p(q)* key on the keyboard in response to the *p(q)* letter.

If individuals low in trait anger spontaneously self-regulate aggressive primes, then they should exhibit task-switching difficulties following the "hurtful" (relative to the "helpful") primes. Indeed, this was the case in two studies (Wilkowski & Robinson, 2006). Specifically, there was a Prime (hurtful versus helpful) × Trait Anger interaction affecting q/p target categorizations. Estimated means for the interaction, along with follow-up analyses, revealed that prime type affected target performance among individuals low, but not high, in trait anger, suggesting an active self-regulation process triggered by aggressive primes.

In sum, the results of four studies involving two different CSPT tasks converged on the prediction that low anger individuals spontaneously self-regulate aggressive primes, whereas high anger individuals do not (Wilkowski & Robinson, 2006). Such results help to explain why low anger individuals are less reactive to aggressive primes and less vulnerable to outbursts of anger and aggression. The results are particularly noteworthy in that they illustrate the manner in which trait-related theories can be examined within relatively mundane cognitive processing tasks.

Complexities

Cognitive processing tasks tend to target rather specific sorts of abilities. For example, Stroop effects, although robust in general, interact with a variety of task variables such as performance instructions, visual angles, and procedural details (Besner, 2001; MacLeod, 1991). Cognitive psychology, in general, seems to favor the delineation of smaller and smaller contributions to performance over time. For this reason, it is useful for assessment-oriented researchers to distance themselves, to some extent, from the microanalytic contributions to performance that often characterize cognitive processes. That is, very specific reaction time processes are unlikely to provide much help in understanding individual differences, for two reasons. One, the reliability of very specific contributions to cognition is likely to be low. Two, very specific contributions to cognition are likely to predict a very narrow range of outcome variables. Therefore, our impression is that personality psychologists would be better served by focusing on the "big" rather than "small" effects within cognitive psychology.

Concerning the reliability and validity of cognitive measures, my colleagues and I find ourselves in sympathy with the literature on implicit motivation (e.g., Bornstein, 1999; McClelland, 1987). Over time, its researchers have had to deal with persistent criticisms concerning the reliability and face validity of their measures. Implicit measures of motivation are quite clearly less reliable than explicit measures of motivation (McClelland, 1987). Such reliability concerns are serious, and they should be. However, it is perhaps mistaken to assume that a given cognitive process should be as reliable as a given self-report variable. In particular, we suggest that cognition is, by its very nature, unstable. With respect to the predictive validity of implicit and explicit measures, we also agree with this prior literature that implicit measures of personality compete favorably with explicit measures of personality (Bornstein, 1999; McClelland, 1987). In sum, we suggest that the predictive validity of implicit cognitive measures is often as high as that of self-reported trait variables (Bornstein, 1999; Robinson & Neighbors, 2006).

We have suggested that cognitive and self-reported measures of personality often do not correlate with each other, even when it seems that they might do so (Robinson, 2004; Robinson & Neighbors, 2006). Therefore, studies limited to traits and cognitive measures may often produce null results—that is, no relation. Even when relations between traits and cognitive processing tendencies are found, it is often true that the relations are quite malleable in nature. For example, such relations appear to be affected by state arousal (Matthews & Gilliland, 1999), mood states (Tamir & Robinson, 2004), and a variety of procedural details (Matthews & Gilliland, 1999).

Researchers may be discouraged by the complexity of trait–cognition relations (Matthews & Gilliland, 1999; Robinson & Neighbors, 2006). Indeed, study after study examining trait–cognition relations has produced only incremental progress (Matthews & Gilliland, 1999; Rusting, 1998). In light of these complexities, we suggest that a "paradigm shift" may be useful. Specifically, the researcher need not be limited to examining trait–cognition relations. The assessment of third variables, related to everyday cognition, emotion, and behavior, permits a much wider consideration of the correlates of cognitive variables for a number of reasons. First, traits may correlate with cognitive processing tendencies, consistent with the "default" assumption in the literature (e.g., Wilkowski & Robinson, 2006). Second, cognitive processing tendencies may predict daily emotion and behavior even in the absence of correlations with traits (e.g., Robinson, in press). Third, trait–cognition relations may be moderated by transitory variables such as mood states (Rusting, 1998) or priming variables (Meier et al., 2006). Fourth, traits and cognitive processing tendencies may interact in predicting daily emotion and behavior (Meier & Robinson, 2004).

A research design limited to traits and cognitive processing tendencies can uncover evidence for only the first of the four patterns mentioned above. In contrast, a research design assessing traits, cognitive processing tendencies, and a third, state-related variable can uncover evidence for any of the four patterns mentioned above. Thus, it is necessarily true that our understanding of individual differences in cognition will advance to the extent that we, as personality researchers, are freed from the restrictive assumption that cognitive processing tendencies have to correlate with self-reported traits in order to predict meaningful outcomes.

An Emerging Integration of Personality and Cognition

Although early personality psychologists such as Eysenck (1947) emphasized both experimental and correlational methods in their research, the two sorts of methods have typically produced divergent, somewhat unrelated, bodies of knowledge. In the present view, both sorts of research traditions can benefit each other far more than is typically realized. Experimental cognitive psychology offers exciting tools that can be used to understand the inner workings of mind and their relevance to attention, self-regulation, and behavior (Posner & Raichle, 1994). Personality psychology forces one to consider critical issues related to construct and predictive validity. From this perspective, a cognitive effect should be more than just a 10 msec difference within a specific cognitive paradigm. It should also mean something with respect to people's everyday lives. That is, it should predict other construct-relevant outcomes.

In exploring the interface of personality and cognition, I suggest that investigators may be forced to relinquish some typically untested assumptions. On the cognitive side, correlational research necessarily challenges the assumption that a specific cognitive mechanism *matters*—

that is, has relevance to anything other than itself. On the personality side, experimental research necessarily challenges the assumption that personality traits can be easily understood in terms of cognitive processes. Correlations between these levels of analysis require intuition, persistence, and revision in the light of initial evidence. Nevertheless, the gains are worth such efforts, in that they necessarily enrich both levels of analysis.

In my view, there are signs pointing to a closer future relationship between experimental and correlational personality research. In the past several years, for example, cognitive researchers have become increasingly interested in variables related to temperament and personality. In addition, many personality psychologists seem ready to move beyond showing that personality predicts this or that amount of variance with respect to an outcome measure. Increasingly, personality psychologists seem to want to address questions of process and mechanism, a direction that must somewhat necessarily lead to a cognitive level of analysis.

Indeed, emerging research from several labs has sought to relate individual difference variables to the brain's reactions to stimuli in cognitive tasks. Canli's (2004) research program has found that extraversion and neuroticism predict specific sorts of brain processes in response to emotional stimuli. A key finding is that extraversion predicts the brain's reactions to positive stimuli, whereas neuroticism predicts the brain's reactions to negative stimuli (Canli, 2004). In other research, Luu, Collins, and Tucker (2000) found a relation between negative affectivity and activation of the anterior cingulate cortex following errors, and these findings begin to pave the way for understanding how neuroticism influences efforts after cognitive control.

Finally, Gray and colleagues (2005) found that a trait measure of approach motivation was associated with less brain activity in areas associated with cognitive control during a demanding working memory task. Interestingly, however, extraversion did not predict performance in the behavioral task. Thus, although personality and cognitive performance may often be unrelated, personality clearly predicts *how* people process affective and nonaffective stimuli (see Canli, 2004, for a review). Such insights are broadly consistent with the goals of this chapter, which involve highlighting the role of cognition for understanding individual differences in emotion and behavior.

A Final Note

It may be important to resist "reifying" cognitive measures, for example, by referring to a measure as one tapping "implicit neuroticism." Cognitive processes are necessarily dynamic in nature. Therefore, it is unlikely that any given measure of cognition can tap something as fixed and stable as a personality trait (Canli, 2004). However, cognitive processes can predict dispositional tendencies to experience certain emotional states (e.g., Robinson, in press; Robinson et al., 2004). But such relations, because they rely on correlations involving cognitive processing measures, must permit a greater latitude of change than is typical of personality traits. Personality processes, from the cognitive perspective, should be amenable to change.

Acknowledgment

I gratefully acknowledge support from the National Institute of Mental Health (Grant No. MH 068241).

Recommended Readings

Fox, E., Russo, R., Bowles, R., & Dutton, K. (2001). Do threatening stimuli draw or hold visual attention in subclinical anxiety? *Journal of Experimental Psychology: General, 130,* 681–700.

Joordens, S., & Becker, S. (1997). The long and short of semantic priming effects in lexical decision. *Journal of Experimental Psychology: Learning, Memory, and Cognition, 23,* 1083–1105.

Meier, B. P., & Robinson, M. D. (2004). Does quick to blame mean quick to anger?: The role of agreeableness in dissociating blame and anger. *Personality and Social Psychology Bulletin, 30,* 856–867.

Mikulincer, M., Birnbaum, G., Woddis, D., & Nachmias, O. (2000). Stress and accessibility of proximity-related thoughts: Exploring the normative and intraindividual components of attachment theory. *Journal of Personality and Social Psychology, 78,* 509–523.

Robinson, M. D., & Cervone, D. (in press). Riding a wave of self-esteem: Perseverative tendencies as dispositional forces. *Journal of Experimental Social Psychology, 42,* 103–111.

Tamir, M., & Robinson, M. D. (2004). Knowing good from bad: The paradox of neuroticism, negative affect, and evaluative processing. *Journal of Personality and Social Psychology, 87,* 913–925.

References

Aiken, L. S., & West, S. G. (1991). *Multiple regression:*
Testing and interpreting interactions. Thousand Oaks, CA: Sage.

Baddeley, A. (1996). Exploring the central executive. *Quarterly Journal of Experimental Psychology: Human Experimental Psychology, 49A,* 5–28.

Bargh, J. A., Raymond, P., Pryor, J. B., & Strack, F. (1995). Attractiveness of the underling: An automatic powersex association and its consequences for sexual harassment and aggression. *Journal of Personality and Social Psychology, 68,* 768–781.

Besner, D. (2001). The myth of ballistic processing: Evidence from Stroop's paradigm. *Psychonomic Bulletin and Review, 8,* 324–330.

Bornstein, R. F. (1999). Criterion validity of objective and projective dependency tests: A meta-analytic assessment of behavioral prediction. *Psychological Assessment, 11,* 48–57.

Bosson, J. K., Swann, W. B., & Pennebaker, J. W. (2000). Stalking the perfect measure of implicit self-esteem: The blind men and the elephant revisited? *Journal of Personality and Social Psychology, 79,* 631–643.

Bruner, J. S. (1957). On perceptual readiness. *Psychological Review, 64,* 123–152.

Canli, T. (2004). Functional brain mapping of extraversion and neuroticism: Learning from individual differences in emotional processing. *Journal of Personality, 72,* 1105–1132.

Conner, T., & Barrett, L. F. (2005). Implicit self-attitudes predict spontaneous affect in daily life. *Emotion, 5,* 476–488.

Eysenck, H. J. (1947). *Dimensions of personality.* Oxford, UK: Kegan Paul.

Gray, J. R., Burgess, G. C., Schaefer, A., Yarkoni, T., Larsen, R. J., & Braver, T. S. (2005). Affective personality differences in neural processing efficiency confirmed using fMRI. *Cognitive, Affective, and Behavioral Neuroscience, 5,* 182–190.

Greenwald, A. G., & Farnham, S. D. (2000). Using the Implicit Association Test to measure self-esteem and self-concept. *Journal of Personality and Social Psychology, 79,* 1022–1038.

Greenwald, A. G., McGhee, D. E., & Schwartz, J. L. K. (1998). Measuring individual differences in implicit cognition: The Implicit Association Test. *Journal of Personality and Social Psychology, 74,* 1464–1480.

Higgins, E. T., & Brendl, C. M. (1995). Accessibility and applicability: Some "activation rules" influencing judgment. *Journal of Experimental Social Psychology, 31,* 218–243.

James, W. (1890). *The principles of psychology.* New York: Holt.

Jensen, A. R. (1998). *The g factor: The science of mental ability.* Westport, CT: Praeger.

Jordan, C. H., Spencer, S. J., Zanna, M. P., Hoshino-Browne, E., & Correll, J. (2003). Secure and defensive high self-esteem. *Journal of Personality and Social Psychology, 85,* 969–978.

Kelly, G. A. (1963). *The psychology of personal constructs.* New York: Norton.

Knight, R. T., & Grabowecky, M. (2000). Prefrontal

cortex, time, and consciousness. In M. S. Gazzaniga (Ed.), *The new cognitive neurosciences* (2nd ed., pp. 1319–1339). Cambridge, MA: MIT Press.

Koole, S. L., Dijksterhuis, A., & van Knippenberg, A. (2001). What's in a name: Implicit self-esteem and the automatic self. *Journal of Personality and Social Psychology, 80,* 669–685.

Luu, P., Collins, P., & Tucker, D. M. (2000). Mood, personality, and self-monitoring: Negative affect and emotionality in relation to frontal lobe mechanisms of error monitoring. *Journal of Experimental Psychology: General, 129,* 43–60.

MacLeod, C. (1991). Half a century of research on the Stroop effect: An integrative review. *Psychological Bulletin, 109,* 163–203.

MacLeod, C. (1999). Anxiety and anxiety disorders. In T. Dalgleish & M. J. Power (Eds.), *Handbook of cognition and emotion* (pp. 447–477). New York: Wiley.

Matthews, G., & Gilliland, K. (1999). The personality theories of H. J. Eysenck and J. A. Gray: A comparative review. *Personality and Individual Differences, 26,* 583–626.

McClelland, D. C. (1987). *Human motivation.* New York: Cambridge University Press.

Meier, B. P., Robinson, M. D., Gaither, G. A., & Heinert, N. J. (2006). A secret attraction or defensive loathing?: Homophobia, defense, and implicit cognition. *Journal of Research in Personality, 40,* 377–394.

Meier, B. P., Robinson, M. D., & Wilkowski, B. M. (2006). Turning the other cheek: Agreeableness and the self-regulation of aggressive primes. *Psychological Science, 17,* 136–142.

Mischel, W., & Ayduk, O. (2004). Willpower in a cognitive–affective processing system: The dynamics of delay of gratification. In R. F. Baumeister & K. D. Vohs (Eds.), *Handbook of self-regulation: Research, theory, and applications* (pp. 99–129). New York: Guilford Press.

Neely, J. H. (1991). Semantic priming effects in visual word recognition: A selective review of current findings and theories. In D. Besner & G. W. Humphreys (Eds.), *Basic processes in reading: Visual word recognition* (pp. 264–336). Hillsdale, NJ: Erlbaum.

Pelham, B. W., Carvallo, M., & Jones, J. T. (2005). Implicit egotism. *Current Directions in Psychological Science, 14,* 106–110.

Pervin, L. A. (1994). A critical analysis of current trait theory. *Psychological Inquiry, 5,* 103–113.

Posner, M. I., & Raichle, M. E. (1994). *Images of mind.* New York: Scientific American Books.

Ratcliff, R. (1993). Methods for dealing with reaction time outliers. *Psychological Bulletin, 114,* 510–532.

Robinson, M. D. (2004). Personality as performance: Categorization tendencies and their correlates. *Current Directions in Psychological Science, 13,* 127–129.

Robinson, M. D. (in press). Gassing, braking, and self-regulating: Error self-regulation predicts subjective well-being. *Journal of Experimental Social Psychology.*

Robinson, M. D., & Clore, G. L. (2002). Belief and feeling: Evidence for an accessibility model of emotional self-report. *Psychological Bulletin, 128,* 934–960.

Robinson, M. D., & Kirkeby, B. S. (2005). Happiness as a belief system: Individual differences and priming in emotion judgments. *Personality and Social Psychology Bulletin, 135,* 78–91.

Robinson, M. D., & Meier, B. P. (2005). Rotten to the core: Neuroticism and implicit evaluations of the self. *Self and Identity, 4,* 361–372.

Robinson, M. D., Mitchell, K. A., Kirkeby, B. S., & Meier, B. P. (2006). The self as a container: Implications for implicit self-esteem and somatic symptoms. *Metaphor and Symbol, 21,* 147–167.

Robinson, M. D., & Neighbors, C. (2006). Catching the mind in action: Implicit methods in personality research and assessment. In M. Eid & E. Diener (Eds.), *Handbook of multimethod measurement in psychology* (pp. 115–125). Washington, DC: American Psychological Association.

Robinson, M. D., Vargas, P. T., Tamir, M., & Solberg, E. C. (2004). Using and being used by categories: The case of negative evaluations and daily well-being. *Psychological Science, 15,* 521–526.

Robinson, M. D., & Wilkowski, B. M. (2006). Loving, hating, vacillating: Agreeableness, implicit self-esteem, and neurotic conflict. *Journal of Personality, 74,* 935–978.

Robinson, M. D., Wilkowski, B. M., Kirkeby, B. S., & Meier, B. P. (2006). Stuck in a rut: Perseverative response tendencies and the neuroticism/distress relationship. *Journal of Experimental Psychology: General, 135,* 78–91.

Robinson, M. D., Wilkowski, B. M., & Meier, B. P. (2006). Unstable in more ways than one: Reaction time variability and the neuroticism/distress relationship. *Journal of Personality, 74,* 311–343.

Rusting, C. L. (1998). Personality, mood, and cognitive processing of emotional information: Three conceptual frameworks. *Psychological Bulletin, 124,* 165–196.

Shah, J. Y., Friedman, R., & Kruglanski, A. W. (2002). Forgetting all else: On the antecedents and consequences of goal shielding. *Journal of Personality and Social Psychology, 83,* 1261–1280.

von Hippel, W., & Gonsalkorale, K. (2005). "That is so bloody revolting!": Inhibitory control of thoughts better left unsaid. *Psychological Science, 16,* 497–500.

Wilkowski, B. M., & Robinson, M. D. (2006). *Catching anger control in the act: Trait anger and the spontaneous self-regulation of aggressive primes.* Manuscript submitted for publication.

Wilkowski, B. M., Robinson, M. D., & Meier, B. P. (in press). Agreeableness and the prolonged spatial processing of antisocial and prosocial information. *Journal of Research in Personality.*

CHAPTER 21

Patient and Neuroimaging Methodologies

Jennifer S. Beer
Michael V. Lombardo

Whedn you hear the phrase "lighting up," do you think of smoking, Christmas trees, or the brain? Personality psychologists have once again become interested in the brain and how its study may inform theories of personality processes. The most common complaint about this trend is that psychologists explain nothing by showing that a brain area has "lit up." This can be a fair criticism, but it is also important to remember that particular kinds of psychological functions have been associated with different brain networks. Modern phrenology can easily be avoided by well-designed research that is motivated by a psychological question. Generally, neuroscience methodologies can be useful (not exclusive) tools for comparing and contrasting personality processes or examining them in relation to a trait measurement. For example, a functional magnetic resonance imaging study has shown that Extraversion is correlated with increased amygdala activity in response to positive emotional stimuli (Canli et al., 2001; Canli, Sivers, Whitfield, Gotlib, & Gabrieli, 2002). This finding supports the theorized positive emotionality component of Extraversion at the neural level of analyses (e.g., John & Srivastava, 1999).

This chapter reviews some common neuroscience approaches in order to aid scientists interested in (1) conducting research with these methodologies and/or (2) becoming more informed consumers of this growing literature. Although it would be impossible for this chapter to replace training in these complicated methods, it provides a working knowledge of common neuroscience approaches. The chapter briefly introduces patient and imaging methodologies (functional magnetic resonance imaging and electroencephalographic/event-related potential recordings), provides examples of extant research, and reviews experimental design considerations. A comparison of the advantages and disadvantages of these approaches is presented in Table 21.1.

TABLE 21.1. Advantages and Disadvantages of Patient, fMRI, and ERP Approaches

Method	Advantages	Disadvantages
Patients with psychiatric or medical disorders	• Learn about changes	• Imprecise localization of function associated with disease • Generalization problematic
Patients with focal lesions	• Greater precision in localization of damage • Determine critical involvement • Wide range of experimental tasks possible	• Difficult to know if impairment is caused by damage or results from lack of communication to/from another structure • Lacks random assignment
fMRI	• Good spatial resolution • Event-related activity	• Poor temporal resolution • Tasks constrained by timing issues
EEG/ERP	• Good temporal resolution • Event-related activity	• Poor spatial resolution • Tasks constrained by timing issues

Patient Population Approaches

The study of patient populations is a classic methodology for understanding the relation between brain and behavior (Kolb & Whishaw, 2003; Rorden & Karnath, 2004). The patient methodology is deficit focused. Patients with brain damage are studied to determine how brain dysfunction impairs (or does not impair) specific behaviors. Patient studies usually include one of three broad population categories: patients with psychiatric disorders (e.g., depression, autism), patients with medical disorders (e.g., epilepsy, dementia, stroke), and patients with focal lesions (e.g., traumatic brain injury, tumor resection).

Studies of Psychiatric and Medical Disorders

Patients with psychiatric disorders and medical disorders are usually much more accessible but may be less informative for basic science questions. Patients who have psychiatric disorders or develop progressive medical disorders potentially have different developmental neural trajectories, are generally taking medications that affect brain function, and usually have diffuse areas of damage. Differential development and medication make it difficult to generalize findings from these populations to healthy populations. For example, Urbach–Wiethe is a rare disease that causes calcification of the amygdala in almost 50% of cases (e.g., Siebert, Markowitsch, & Bartel, 2003). Therefore, pa-

tients with this disease are natural models of amygdala damage. However, the lack of random assignment to the disease makes it unclear as to whether findings will generalize to normal populations with normal developmental trajectories. In addition, in some cases, the calcification spreads beyond the amygdala. Diffuse damage makes it difficult to isolate behavioral deficits in relation to a specific brain region. Generally, studying psychiatrically or medically disordered populations is most beneficial for understanding personality and social processing that change as a function of a particular disorder. These studies are also useful for understanding which kinds of dysfunction tend to cluster together. For example, autism spectrum disorders, Williams syndrome, and frontotemporal dementia are interesting examples of disorders that primarily affect social and personality processes (e.g., Bryson, Rogers, & Fombonne, 2003; Doyle, Bellugi, Korenberg, & Graham, 2004; Perry et al., 2001). The selective clustering of social or personality deficits in these disorders provides support for the conceptualization of traits as sets of abilities that are independent from basic cognitive processing.

Studies of Patients with Focal Lesions

Patients with focal lesions provide a better avenue for understanding how damage to specific brain regions affects personality and social processes. Focal lesions are most often the result of trauma from accidents, although other possible causes include tumor resection and stroke (e.g., Gazzaniga, Ivry, & Mangun, 1998; Kolb & Whishaw, 2003). If a behavioral deficit is observed in relation to damage to a specific brain region, then scientists consider that brain region to be critically involved (i.e., necessary) for that behavior. Although it is not the case that trauma is always limited to a specific brain region, some of the regions that are most likely to interest personality psychologists can be selectively damaged. For example, the jagged ridges that hold the eye orbits in place often selectively damage the orbitofrontal cortex. In high-speed collisions, the brain may bounce against the back of the skull and then shoot forward against the jagged ridges, causing damage to the orbitofrontal region.

For researchers interested in personality and social processes, lesion studies can be helpful for manipulating individual differences that are difficult to manipulate in the lab. For example, patients with orbitofrontal cortex damage have self-regulatory deficits in their interpersonal behavior (e.g., Beer, Heerey, Keltner, Scabini, & Knight, 2003; Beer, Shimamura, & Knight, 2004). Healthy adult participants often do not make social mistakes in a laboratory setting where they are highly concerned about their performance. By comparing patients who have experienced orbitofrontal damage with other patients and healthy controls, it is possible to examine the relation between individual differences in interpersonal self-regulatory ability and a personality trait or another personality process.

The method in which behavioral implications of brain lesions are examined has been underused by personality psychologists and has resulted in little extant work. However, some studies point out the potential of this method for researchers interested in personality and social processes. In one study, the relation between impaired reversal behavior with impulsivity and reward sensitivity was examined by comparing patients with orbitofrontal damage to patients with medial or dorsolateral frontal damage and healthy controls (Berlin, Rolls, & Kischka, 2004). The inclusion of both a healthy and patient control group ensures that effects are not generally associated with brain damage, but with damage in the area of interest. In addition, a large number of patients (23 with orbitofrontal damage, 20 without orbitofrontal damage) were included. The patients with orbitofrontal damage, in comparison to all other participants, failed reversal tasks of association. In the reversal task, participants were presented with a series of images and learned to respond to particular images to earn a reward. After they got nine trials correct, the associations would be reversed and response to other images would be rewarded. The patients with orbitofrontal damage performed poorly on this task in comparison to all other participants. These patients were unable to reverse their associations and kept responding to the originally rewarded images. Participants also completed questionnaire measurements of Impulsivity and Extraversion. In comparison to all other participants, patients with orbitofrontal damage were much more impulsive but did not differ in their Extraversion. The researchers interpreted these findings to mean that the impaired reversal of these patients was explained by their inability to stop themselves from responding (Impulsivity), rather than an insensitivity to reward (Extraversion). Although other researchers may have chosen a different measure of sensitivity to reward, this study is one example of how the "lesion approach" can be used to examine the relation between a personality process and a personality trait.

The lesion approach is less successful when patients with diffuse brain damage are studied. In one study, pretrauma and posttrauma measures of the five dimensions of personality (i.e., the NEO inventory) were compared between patients with head injuries and patients without head injuries (e.g., Lannoo, de Deyne, Colardyn, de Soete, & Jannes, 1997). This study also had a large sample of patients (68 patients with head injuries and 28 patients with non-head injuries). Peer reports from relatives were collected for almost all of the patients with head injuries. The patients were all at least 6 months posttrauma. This is important, as the impairment resulting from brain damage can be pronounced right after the injury because of hemorrhage or swelling. By 6 months, it is thought that impairment has stabilized. The researchers found that both groups reported significant changes in personality following their traumas but the magnitude of change did not differ across the two groups. Specifically, patients reported increased Neuroticism, decreased Extraversion, and decreased Conscientiousness after their traumas. In comparison to their relatives, patients with head injuries reported a smaller reduction in Extraversion and

Conscientiousness. However, it is difficult to draw any conclusions from this study because the area and extent of head injury for each patient are not reported. It may be that across a broad range of participants, personality changes are similar to those patients without head injuries. However, if patients could be sorted into area of brain damage, the results might suggest whether particular personality traits change more as a function of damage to areas associated with specific cognitive functions.

Although the study of focal lesions may be the most beneficial for basic science, there are still a number of things to consider when planning such a study. First, nonrandom assignment may be a particular concern for scientists interested in individual differences. If focal lesions result from trauma, it is important to consider whether patients with lesions prospectively differed on personality dimensions (e.g., risk taking), which may have made them more likely to incur brain damage.

Second, it is unlikely that there will be a one-to-one correspondence between the area damaged and the deficient behavior. Therefore, minor damage to a particular area may not yield a deficit at the behavioral level, but that does not rule out a possible relation between that area and a particular behavior. As in all research, null results should not be interpreted as evidence for a lack of effect.

Finally, it is impossible to know whether "critical involvement" means that an area is important for receiving or for sending a necessary signal. The damaged region may affect behavior because signals from the region directly affect the execution of that behavior. The damaged region may also affect behavior because fibers of passage have been damaged and a message cannot be relayed between two brain areas through the area of damage. Both of these possibilities should be acknowledged in the interpretation of experimental results.

An optimal patient study would compare patients with focal lesions in an area of interest, patients with focal lesions in an area of no interest, and healthy comparison subjects. Lesions should be homogeneous as to location and size within the patient group and depicted in the publication. Many personality studies may include 100 or more subjects; thus, it is important to consider time and size constraints when studying patient populations. In patient studies, sample size and testing time may be very limited. Therefore, it is wisest to focus that time on tasks that yield reliable and robust effects in small numbers of healthy comparison subjects. Patients may often come from different ethnic, educational, and economic backgrounds. This is particularly true if patients are referred from a Veterans Administration hospital or another nonrandom sample. It is important to match controls on these factors so that effects are not explained by demographic variables.

Brain Imaging Approaches

The study of healthy brain tissue is an important complement to approaches that study patients with brain lesions. Brain imaging approaches are activity focused. Brain activity is measured in various ways to explain differences in neural recruitment in specific tasks. In contrast to patient approaches, which are considered to test the critical involvement of a brain region for a specific task, imaging studies test whether a region may be recruited for a specific task. A wide range of brain imaging techniques exist, including functional magnetic resonance imaging (fMRI), electroencephalographic (EEG)/event-related potential (ERP) recordings, positron emission tomography (PET), transcranial magnetic stimulation (TMS), magnetoencephalogram (MEG), and intracranial recording in surgical patients (see, e.g., Gazzaniga et al., 1998; Kolb & Whishaw, 2003). This chapter focuses on two of the most commonly used methods: fMRI and EEG/ERPs.

Functional Magnetic Resonance Imaging

Functional magnetic resonance imaging (fMRI) is one of the most commonly used imaging techniques and is increasingly accessible to researchers (for further description, see Buxton, 2002; Gazzaniga et al., 1998; Huettal, Song, & McCarthy, 2004; Kolb & Whishaw, 2003). In order to understand fMRI, it is first important to understand nuclear magnetic resonance imaging (technically, NMRI, but more commonly known as MRI). Using MRI, an image of the brain's structure can be created by manipulating the orientation of hydrogen nuclei in the brain tissue (Horowitz, 1995). First, a participant is placed in a strong magnetic field (i.e., the MRI scanner) and the hydrogen nuclei align themselves to this field. The strength of the scanner is measured in Tesla (T), and scanners are often referred to by their strength (i.e., "3T" is a 3 Tesla magnet). A radio frequency pulse (RF pulse) is applied, which shifts the nuclei from their original positions. After the pulse stops, the nuclei shed the energy injected by the RF pulse and "relax" back into their original orientation to the external magnetic field. MRI images are derived through differences in relaxation rates. For example, the water molecules filled with hydrogen nuclei in blood relax at a different rate than water molecules in other tissues, making it possible to denote differences between blood and brain tissue.

When MRI is used to create images of brain activity rather than structural images of the brain, it is referred to as functional magnetic resonance imaging (fMRI). fMRI uses the blood oxygenation level dependent (BOLD) contrast effect in order to yield images of brain activity (Ogawa, Lee, Nayak, & Glynn, 1990; Ogawa et al., 1992). As a brain region becomes active, a hemodynamic response occurs in which oxygen is delivered to active regions via the blood. The proportion of deoxygenated blood to oxygenated blood creates a signal known as the BOLD contrast effect. Therefore, fMRI is not a direct measure of brain activity, but rather a measure of the aftermath of changes in blood flow associated with neural activity. The exact relation between neural activity and the BOLD signal is not currently known. It is also important to note that the temporal resolution of fMRI is not very precise. Once a change in brain activity occurs, it takes time for the hemodynamic response to unfold and create the BOLD signal, which is the basis of fMRI measurement.

In fMRI data analyses, images of activity from experimental and control conditions are statistically compared to determine significant activity. The images of activity are registered, or overlaid, on a structural image of the brain in order to identify where significant activity is generated. Therefore, it is not the case that significant areas "light up," that is, go from rest in the control condition to active in the experimental condition. Instead, activity in the experimental condition is statistically different from activity during the control condition. It is also important to remember that nonsignificance does not necessarily reflect a lack of activity. Nonsignificant differences may also arise in cases in which the brain region is similarly active in both the experimental and control conditions.

For researchers interested in personality and social processes, fMRI can be useful for understanding individual differences in information processing as well as their relation to traits. For example, a series of fMRI studies examined the cognitive processing underlying individual differences in self-regulation (Beer, Knight, & D'Esposito, 2006). In one study, participants were required to inhibit their attention to emotional stimuli while making risky gambles. In another study, participants were required to pay attention to emotional stimuli while making risky gambles. Specifically, participants were presented with an emotional or neutral picture and then placed a bet in a roulette game. In the condition in which participants were asked to pay attention to the emotional stimuli, they were told that negative stimuli predicted a bet that was unlikely to pay off. Individual differences in self-regulation of emotional influence on betting were related to orbitofrontal activity. Orbitofrontal activity was related to both inhibiting emotional influence in the "inhibit" study and to using emotional influence in the "attention" study. These findings suggest that individual differences in the ability to control emotional influence on decision making are related to recognizing the utility of the emotion for the decision, rather than the ability to control emotion per se.

Two other studies by Canli and colleagues have shown that Extraversion is associated with increased sensitivity to emotional stimuli at the neural level (Canli et al., 2001, 2002). In one study, participants completed trait questionnaires of Extraversion and then watched emotional pictures in the scanner (Canli et al., 2001). The results showed that individual differences in Extraversion predicted activity in brain regions associated with emotional processing including the frontal lobes, cingulate, amygdala, putamen, and caudate in response to positive emotional stimuli, as compared with neutral stimuli. Another study found that individual differences in Extraversion predicted increased amygdala activation in response to happy faces, in comparison to neutral faces (Canli et al., 2002). Together these studies suggest that individual differences in Extraversion are associated with differences in sensitivity to positive stimuli at the neural level and in distinct brain regions.

Electroencephalographic/Event-Related Potential Recordings

Another type of brain imaging is EEG and ERP recording. In comparison to fMRI, EEG/ERP recording is a direct and continuous measure of electrical brain activity (for further description, see Fabiani, Gratton, & Coles, 2000; Gazzaniga et al., 1998; Kolb & Whishaw, 2003). In order to understand ERPs, it is first important to understand EEG. In many EEG recordings, pairs of electrodes are connected to amplifiers and placed on the participant's scalp, and as a point of reference, on the ear. A greater number of amplifiers (and thus more scalp electrodes) are desirable, and researchers usually note this number in publications. The electrodes placed over various brain regions detect the summed electrical potentials from large bodies of neurons. Brain activity is considered significant when a wave's magnitude or rhythm statistically differs from the ear recording (where there are no electrical potentials). The output of this measurement is a wave for each electrode of continuous activity across time. Four major types of continuous rhythmic sinusoidal EEG waves are recognized (alpha, beta, delta, and theta). Typically, these waves have been examined in different states of consciousness (i.e., sleeping vs. awake) or across healthy and clinical populations. This recording is a general measure of brain activity and is not in relation to the presentation of a particular stimulus.

Changes in the EEG signal in response to a specific stimulus are known as event-related potentials (ERPS). These momentary changes in the EEG signal are difficult to detect among the other electrical responses in the brain. Therefore, reasonable ERP estimates require the averaging of EEG data over dozens to thousands of trials. The timing information provided by ERPs is far superior to that of fMRI. Timing information can be assessed by noting the length of time the change in magnitude occurs after the stimulus presentation. For scientists interested in psychological function, a number of ERPs have been identified and are theorized to reflect different cognitive functions. ERPs are usually named to indicate whether they are negative or positive (i.e., shift upward or downward from baseline, respectively), are assigned a number based on the time they are produced in relation to stimulus presentation, and are associated with a set of brain regions. For example, the P300 or P3 is one of the most commonly studied ERPs. The P300 is a positive ERP (P) that is produced 300 msec after a stimuli is presented (300) and is thought to indicate orientation or decoding of the meaning of the stimulus (e.g., Polich, 2004; Soltani & Knight, 2000). The P300 has been further split into the P3a and P3b because each has a distinct cognitive function and neural generator (e.g., Polich, 2004). The P3a is involved in automatic detection of novel stimuli and is associated with the frontal lobes and hippocampus. The P3b is involved with orienting toward a target and is associated with temporal and parietal areas. Another commonly studied ERP is the N400, which is thought to indicate error detection. Candidate generators include the sylvian fissure, orbitofrontal, dorsolateral prefrontal, superior temporal sulcus, and temporal pole (Halgren et al., 1994; McCarthy, Nobre, Bentin, & Spencer, 1995; Nobre, Allison, & McCarthy, 1994). The P600 is a later emerging ERP, which is involved in encoding as well as recognition. There is controversy over whether recognition reflects effort exerted for recognition or the success of recognition. Candidate brain generators for this wave include the hippocampus, parahippocampal gyrus, temporal pole, orbitofrontal cortex, fusiform, cingulate, medial temporal lobe, paralimbic areas, and inferior frontal gyrus (Guillem, Rougier, & Claverie, 1999; Halgren et al., 1994).

Both EEG and ERPs have been used to examine individual differences. For example, Davidson and colleagues have long claimed that individual differences in approach and avoidance are reflected in the resting level of brain activity in the frontal lobes. In one study, baseline measurements of resting EEG activity in the frontal lobes were assessed in participants (Sutton & Davidson, 1997). Participants also completed self-report measurements of approach and avoidance tendencies. The researchers computed an asymmetry score reflecting the difference in the alpha band of the frontal lobes in the left hemisphere as compared with the right hemisphere. They also computed a difference score in approach tendency as compared with avoidance tendency. Using these discrepancy scores, the researchers found a positive correlation between frontal lobe asymmetric activity and differences in approach as compared with avoidance. Although the use of discrepancy scores is controversial, these findings suggest that individual differences in approach tendency as compared with avoid tendency are associated with differences in activity at the neural level in the frontal lobes.

ERPs have also been used to examine the relation of individual differences in personality traits to neural processing. In one study, participants completed an auditory oddball task in which they had to identify rare instances of target tones in a series of tones. Participants also completed measures of trait Reward Dependence, Novelty Seeking, and Persistence. As mentioned above, the P300 is an ERP that has been associated with novelty detection and orientation. The magnitude of the response is thought to represent the cognitive resources devoted to information processing. The latency of the response is thought to represent the duration of stimulus evaluation. The researchers found that Reward Dependence was positively associated with P300 magnitude, whereas P300 latency positively correlated with Persistence and negatively correlated with Novelty Seeking. These findings suggest that individual differences in Reward Dependence are associated with differential allocation of neural resources to the processing of a target stimulus and that duration of stimulus evaluation is associated with greater Persistence and less Novelty Seeking at the neural level.

Yet another example of the use of ERPs for understanding personality processes comes from a study examining the moderating effect of Conscientious on task persistence (Pailing & Segalowitz, 2004). In this study, participants completed an association task in which different letters and their fonts were associated with different key and hand responses. The conditions of task completion were manipulated to motivate the participants with monetary reward or no reward. Participants also completed measures of the five major dimensions of personality. The findings show that individual differences in Conscientiousness moderated ERPs associated with error recognition. In particular, individuals low in Neuroticism showed smaller changes in the neural signature of error recognition (i.e., error-related negativity, ERN) across motivation conditions. Individual differences in Neuroticism accounted for differences above and beyond Conscientiousness. These findings were interpreted as support for the association between Emotional Stability and error monitoring.

In contrast to patient approaches, which involve many of the same design principles as other kinds of behavioral research, imaging studies require consideration of a number of additional factors to ensure a strong design. First, although nature has made it easier to examine some brain areas of interest to personality psychologists because of the ridge underlying the orbitofrontal cortex or Urbach-Wiethe, it has made EEG/ERP and fMRI measurements of these areas more difficult than measurements of other brain areas. The orbitofrontal cortex and amygdala lie deep within the brain, making it difficult to get strong EEG signals, and lie next to air cavities, making it difficult to detect the BOLD signal in fMRI measurement. In EEG/ERP recordings, the electrical signals are conducted by the brain, skull, and scalp and are more easily detectable the closer to they are to the scalp. Detecting the BOLD signal in orbitofrontal tissue is difficult for a number of reasons, such as the magnetic field inhomogeneity caused by the proximity of this area to the air cavity of the nasal sinus. However, it is not the case that measurement of every area of interest to personality psychologists will be difficult. For example, the anterior cingulate is easily measured with EEG or fMRI. However, if effects are hypothesized to take place in troublesome regions, it is important to make the necessary parameter adjustments to optimize measurement of these tricky regions. The exact adjustments will vary across equipment and may involve strategies such as exclusively measuring the specific brain area instead of collecting whole-brain measurements, or collecting whole-brain measurements in a manner that optimizes signals from the hypothesized regions. Another strategy is to collect whole-brain data but analyze only regions of interest (ROIs), which is a more powerful way of detecting significant brain activity (see, e.g., Brett, Anton, Valabregue, & Poline, 2002).

Second, comparison conditions in brain imaging studies must be designed so that only the variable of interest differs between the conditions. Although this is true in all experiments, the standards are higher in brain imaging studies. For example, parameters such as word length, picture complexity, difficulty, and stimulus size must be uniform. Differences in brain activity may not reflect differences in the hypothesized personality process, but rather differences in difficulty of the task or some other third variable based on perceptual differences.

Third, whereas many EEG/ERP studies compare waves from scalp electrodes to the objective control of the ear electrode, fMRI does not have an analogous gold standard of control. In fMRI, results are always interpreted in comparison to the control or baseline condition, which is a task designed by the experimenter. There is no way to look at activity from a task condition without using some kind of baseline estimate. Therefore, the baseline condition must be rigorously designed. In fMRI experiments, participants are asked to fixate on a crosshair presented in the middle of the screen and clear their minds. However, there is some debate over whether a fixation point is a reasonable control condition, because participants may self-reflect during such a low-level task and obscure any differences in self-reflective experimental conditions (e.g., making personality judgments about themselves). Another potential problem is that participants' interest may not be held by a crosshair, and therefore they may plan their strategy for the next upcoming trial. The neural activity associated with planning may be similar to that recruited to complete your task and obscure a significant effect.

Another consideration for personality psychologists using brain imaging techniques is how best to include an individual difference measure. Sample sizes tend to be much smaller (15–40 participants) in brain imaging studies than in a typical study of individual differences. Smaller samples may mean less variance in the individual difference of interest. Pilot testing is particularly critical to determine whether normal variance can be found and whether an effect can be detected in such a small sample. In addition, if a trait questionnaire measurement is to be included, it may be best to administer it well before the EEG/ERP or fMRI session instead right after the participant completes the task. If there is an obvious relation between the task and the questionnaire measurement, participants' answers may be confounded by the fresh memory of task performance and not reflect their true disposition. In this case, it would be problematic to interpret correlations between the questionnaire measurement and brain activity as exclusively reflecting individual differences in the trait.

To optimize a brain imaging study, scientists should adopt the imaging method that best suits their purpose. fMRI is much better at resolving the region responsible for the brain activity, whereas EEG/ERPs provide greater temporal information. As with lesion studies, the psychological phenomena studied in brain imaging approaches should be detectable in a small sample size, and this may require considerable pilot testing (see Desmond & Glover, 2002). If variance in an individual difference is needed, then a larger number of participants may have to be prescreened to ensure reasonable variance in the small sample. Both fMRI and ERP measurements have strict timing requirements and require a large number of trials. For example, individual trials tend to last for milliseconds or a few seconds and may be repeated with 40 to 100 trials or more. Therefore, the phenomenon of interest should lend itself to brief trials and continue to yield a psychological effect from a large number of repetitions. In the case of fMRI, researchers must choose between a block design, in which trials are clustered together, and an event-related design, in which brain activity can be associated with a specific stimulus presentation (Aguirre & D'Esposito, 2000; Friston, Zarahn, Josephs, Henson, & Dale, 1999). Block designs give researchers greater power for detecting an effect, but event-related designs give greater precision in tasks in which participants may not always respond the same way within an experimental condition. For example, although a researcher may use a standardized set of emotional stimuli, participants may not respond emotionally to every single picture. Therefore, it is optimal to examine brain activity in relation to only those stimuli that had the desired effect. As mentioned above, the control condition in an fMRI study is particularly important, because any experimental effect is interpreted in relation to the control task. Finally, if interactions between brain areas are relevant for the hypothesis of interest, advanced statistical procedures can be used to test those relations in fMRI studies.

Conclusion

It is certainly not the case that neuroscience methods should replace traditional methods used in personality research. However, neuroscience approaches are other tools that personality psychologists can consider when planning an experiment. These approaches are best used to examine whether personality processes are similar or different from one another (by comparing brain regions recruited for each process) and to examine the relation of individual differences in personality traits to individual differences in cognitive processes (measured at the neural level). The first question a researcher should ask when planning one of these studies is, "What will brain data tell me about the psychological process I'm interested in?" Asking this question as a first step will help prevent the design of studies that do little more than map the human brain. It should be noted that although the patient and imaging methods in this chapter have been described separately, combinations of these approaches are also possible and valuable. Finally, studies showing a relation between individual differences in self-report measurements and individual differences in neural activity will not only help personality psychologists learn about the processes underlying traits, but will make it that much harder for neuroscientists to turn their noses up at self-report measurement.

Recommended Readings

Buxton, R. B. (2002). *Introduction to functional magnetic resonance imaging: Principles and techniques.* New York: Cambridge University Press.

Fabiani, M., Gratton, G., & Coles, M. G. H. (2000). Event-related brain potentials. In J. T. Cacioppo, L. G. Tassinary, & G. G. Berntson (Eds.), *Handbook of psychophysiology* (2nd ed., pp. 53–84). Cambridge, UK: Cambridge University Press.

Gazzaniga, M. S., Ivry, R. B., & Mangun, G. R. (1998). *Cognitive neuroscience: The biology of the mind.* New York: Norton.

Huettal, S. A., Song, A. W., & McCarthy, G. (2004). *Functional magnetic resonance imaging.* Sunderland, MA: Sinauer Associates.

Kolb, B., & Whishaw, I. Q. (2003). *Fundamentals of human neuropsychology.* New York: Worth.

Rorden, C., & Karnath, H. O. (2004). Using human brain lesions to infer function: A relic from a past era in the fMRI age? *Nature Reviews Neuroscience, 5,* 813–819.

References

Aguirre, G. K., & D'Esposito, M. (2000). Experimental design for brain fMRI. In C. T. W. Moonen & P. A. Bandettini (Eds.), *Medical radiology: Functional MRI* (pp. 369–380). New York: Springer.

Beer, J. S., Heerey, E. H., Keltner, D., Scabini, D., & Knight, R. T. (2003). The regulatory function of self-conscious emotion: Insights from patients with orbitofrontal damage. *Journal of Personality and Social Psychology, 85,* 594–604.

Beer, J. S., Knight, R. T., & D'Esposito, M. (2006). Integrating emotion and cognition: The role of the frontal lobes in distinguishing between helpful and hurtful emotion. *Psychological Science, 17,* 448–453.

Beer, J. S., Shimamura, A. P., & Knight, R. T. (2004). Frontal lobe contributions to executive control of cognitive and social behavior. In M. S. Gazzaniga (Ed.), *The newest cognitive neurosciences* (3rd ed., pp. 1091–1104). Cambridge, MA: MIT Press.

Berlin, H. A., Rolls, E. T., & Kischka, U. (2004). Impulsivity, time perception, emotion and reinforcement sensitivity in patients with orbitofrontal cortex lesions. *Brain, 127,* 1108–1126.

Brett, M., Anton, J. L., Valabregue, R., & Poline, J. B. (2002). *Region of interest analysis using an SPM toolbox.* Paper presented at the 8th International Conference on Functional Mapping of the Human Brain, Sendai, Japan.

Bryson S. E., Rogers S. J., & Fombonne E. (2003). Autism spectrum disorders: Early detection and intervention, education, and psychopharmacological management. *Canadian Journal of Psychiatry, 48,* 506–516.

Buxton, R. B. (2002). *Introduction to functional magnetic resonance imaging: Principles and techniques.* New York: Cambridge University Press.

Canli, T., Sivers, H., Whitfield, S. L., Gotlib, I. H., & Gabrieli, J. D. (2002). Amygdala response to happy faces as a function of extraversion. *Science, 296,* 2191.

Canli, T., Zhao, Z., Desmond, J. E., Kang, E., Gross, J., & Gabrieli, J. D. (2001). An fMRI study of personality influences on brain reactivity to emotional stimuli. *Behavioral Neuroscience, 115,* 33–42.

Desmond, J. E., & Glover, G. H. (2002). Estimating sample size in functional MR (fMRI) neuroimaging studies: Statistical power analyses. *Journal of Neuroscience Methods, 118,* 115–128.

Doyle, T. F., Bellugi, U., Korenberg, J. R., & Graham, J. (2004). "Everybody in the world is my friend": Hypersociability in young children with Williams syndrome. *American Journal of Medical Genetics, 124A,* 263–273.

Fabiani, M., Gratton, G., & Coles, M. G. H. (2000). Event-related brain potentials. In J. T. Cacioppo, L. G. Tassinary, & G. G Berntson (Eds.), *Handbook of psychophysiology* (2nd ed., pp. 53–84). Cambridge, UK: Cambridge University Press.

Friston, K. J., Zarahn, E., Josephs, O., Henson, R. N. A., & Dale, A. M. (1999). Stochastic designs in event-related fMRI. *NeuroImage, 10,* 607–619.

Gazzaniga, M. S., Ivry, R. B., & Mangun, G. R. (1998). *Cognitive neuroscience: The biology of the mind.* New York: Norton.

Guillem, F., Rougier, A., & Claverie, B. (1999). Short- and long-delay intracranial ERP repetition effects dissociate memory systems in the human brain. *Journal of Cognitive Neuroscience, 11,* 437–458.

Halgren, E., Baudena, P., Heit, G., Clarke, J. M., Marinkovic, K., Chauvel, P., et al. (1994). Spatio-temporal stages in face and word processing. 2. Depth-recorded potentials in the human frontal and Rolandic cortices. *Journal of Physiology, 88,* 51–80.

Horowitz, A. L. (1995). *MRI physics for radiologists: A visual approach.* New York: Springer-Verlag.

Huettal, S. A., Song, A. W., & McCarthy, G. (2004). *Functional magnetic resonance imaging.* Sunderland, MA: Sinauer Associates.

John, O. P., & Srivastava, S. (1999). The Big Five trait taxonomy: History, measurement, and theoretical perspectives. In L. A. Pervin & O. P. John (Eds.), *Handbook of personality: Theory and research* (2nd ed., pp. 102–138). New York: Guilford Press.

Kolb, B., & Whishaw, I. Q. (2003). *Fundamentals of human neuropsychology.* New York: Worth.

Lannoo, E., de Deyne, C., Colardyn, F., de Soete, G., & Jannes, C. (1997). Personality change following head injury: Assessment with the NEO Five-Factor Inventory. *Journal of Psychosomatic Research, 43,* 505–511.

McCarthy, G., Nobre, A. C., Bentin, S., & Spencer, D. D. (1995). Language-related field potentials in the anterior-medial temporal lobe: I. Intracranial distribution and neural generators. *Journal of Neuroscience, 15,* 1080–1089.

Nobre, A. C., Allison, T., & McCarthy, G. (1994). Word recognition in the human inferior temporal lobe. *Nature, 17,* 260–263.

Ogawa, S., Lee, T., Nayak, A., & Glynn, P. (1990). Oxygenation-sensitive contrast in magnetic resonance image of rodent brain at high magnetic fields. *Magnetic Resonance in Medicine, 14,* 68–78.

Ogawa, S., Tank, D. W., Menon, R., Ellerman, J. M., Kim, S. G., & Merkle, H. (1992). Intrinsic signal changes accompanying sensory stimulation: Functional brain mapping with magnetic resonance imaging. *Proceedings of the National Academy of Sciences USA, 89,* 5951–5955.

Pailing, P. E., & Segalowitz, S. J. (2004). The error-related negativity as a state and trait measure: Motivation, personality, and ERPs in response to errors. *Psychophysiology, 41,* 84–95.

Perry, R. J., Rosen, H. R., Kramer, J. H., Beer, J. S., Levenson, R. L., & Miller, B. L. (2001). Hemispheric dominance for emotions, empathy and social behaviour: Evidence from right and left handers with frontotemporal dementia. *Neurocase, 7,* 145–160.

Polich, J. (2004). Neuropsychology of P3a and P3b: A theoretical overview. In N. C. Moore & K. Arikan (Eds.), *Brainwaves and mind: Recent developments* (pp. 15–29). Wheaton, IL: Kjeilberg.

Rorden, C., & Karnath, H. O. (2004). Using human brain lesions to infer function: A relic from a past era in the fMRI age? *Nature Reviews Neuroscience, 5,* 813–819.

Siebert, M., Markowitsch, H. J., & Bartel, P. (2003). Amygdala, affect and cognition: Evidence from 10 patients with Urbach–Wiethe disease. *Brain, 12,* 2627–2637.

Soltani, M., & Knight, R. T. (2000). Neural origins of the P300. *Critical Reviews in Neurobiology, 14,* 199–224.

Sutton, S. K., & Davidson, R. J. (1997). Prefrontal brain asymmetry: A biological substrate of the behavioral approach and inhibition systems. *Psychological Science, 8,* 204–210.

## CHAPTER 22

Physiological Measures

Lisa M. Diamond
Kimberly D. Otter-Henderson

Historically, psychophysiological measures have made an invaluable contribution to personality psychology. Questions regarding interindividual differences and intraindividual changes in emotion, cognition, motivation, arousal, and attention are core topics within personality psychology, and these questions are particularly amenable to a psychophysiological approach. In particular, psychophysiological measures can help researchers develop more comprehensive, differentiated conceptualizations of temperament and personality dimensions by elucidating biological processes that might serve as precursors, concomitants, markers, or moderators of such differences (see Cacioppo, Tassinary, & Berntson, 2000, for an excellent discussion of the precise distinction between these concepts). Yet integrating psychophysiological measures into personality research involves both logistical and conceptual complexities and may seem daunting to researchers without biology-oriented back-grounds. Our goal in this chapter is to provide an accessible, user-friendly overview of some of the most widely used psychophysiological indices in social-personality psychology and to provide some basic technical and conceptual guidelines as to their use and interpretation. We focus on the hypothalamic–pituitary–adreno-cortical (HPA) axis of the endocrine system (assessed via salivary cortisol), cardiovascular measures of autonomic nervous system (ANS) activity (assessed via heart rate, blood pressure, respiratory sinus arrhythmia, cardiac output, pre-ejection period, and total peripheral resistance), and electrodermal measures of ANS activity (assessed via skin conductance). Space limitations obviously preclude exhaustive treatment of all the relevant biological and technical information, and therefore Table 22.1 provides additional references to which readers can turn for additional information about each measure. This table also includes references for additional psychophysiological parameters

TABLE 22.1. Additional References on Physiological Systems

Basic cardiovascular functioning	Blascovich & Kelsey (1990); Brownley et al. (2000)
Impedance cardiography	Sherwood (1993)
Parasympathetic nervous system functioning (RSA, vagal tone)	Porges (1995); Task Force of the European Society of Cardiology and the North American Society of Pacing and Electrophysiology (1996)
Ambulatory blood pressure measurement	Mussgay & Rüddel (1996)
Electrodermal activity	Blascovich & Kelsey (1990); Dawson et al. (2000); Tranel (2000)
HPA and SAM axis activity	Baum & Grunberg (1995); Blascovich & Tomaka (1996); Lovallo & Thomas (2000)
Other endocrine measures	Baum & Grunberg (1995); Becker, Breedlove, Crews, & McCarthy (2002)
Surface electromyography (EMG)	Tassinary & Cacioppo (2000)
Human startle eyeblink reflex	Dawson, Schell, & Bohmelt (1999)
Electroencephalography (EEG)	Coan & Allen (2003); Davidson, Jackson, & Larson (2000)
Event-related brain potential (ERP)	Fabiani, Gratton, & Coles (2000); Rugg & Coles (1995)
Positron emission tomography (PET)	Dougherty, Rauch, & Fischman (2004); Reiman, Lane, Van Petten, & Bandettini (2000)
Functional magnetic resonance imaging (fMRI)	Davidson (2003); Reiman et al. (2000)
Immune functioning	Maier & Watkins (1998); Segerstrom & Miller (2004); Uchino, Kiecolt-Glaser, & Glaser (2000)
Sexual response	Geer & Janssen (2000); Janssen (2002)

that may be of interest to personality psychologists, but which we do not cover in detail in this chapter, such as muscular activity in the face and other parts of the body via surface electromyography (EMG), measurement of the human startle eyeblink reflex, measures of brain activity, such as electroencephalography (EEG), event-related brain potential (ERP), positron emission tomography (PET), and functional magnetic resonance imaging (fMRI), immune functioning, and genital sexual response. Although these measures are being used with increasing frequency, they typically involve greater technical sophistication and greater expense than the measures covered in this chapter, and are therefore less widely used and less accessible to the average personality psychologist.

Finally, in considering psychophysiological research, it is useful to bear in mind the distinction between "trait-based" and "state-based" investigative approaches. The former focus on stable, trait-like characteristics of individuals (i.e., do neurotic individuals have specific patterns of electrodermal reactivity to stress?), whereas the latter focus on situation-specific changes in affective, cognitive, or physiological state that generalize across individuals (under what conditions does evaluation apprehension reliably trigger HPA reactivity?). The state-based approach is a fundamentally within-person approach (comparing an individual's baseline responses to the same individual's responses under specific conditions, such as stress), whereas the trait-based approach is a fundamentally between-person approach (comparing different individuals' baseline or reactivity responses).

Of course, there is some overlap between the two; most notably, there is between-person variability in the *degree* of within-person reactivity to most laboratory tasks, and thus some trait-based approaches use mixed models that focus on within-person *and* between-person effects. Yet the basic distinction is helpful to bear in mind, as it has important implications for the selection of psychophysiological measures, their integration into research design, and their interpretation. For example, baseline measures of physiology, typically taken during a long quiet resting period, may be of little intrinsic interest to researchers investigating experimentally induced deviations from baseline. Yet for researchers investigating stable interindividual differences, baseline measures may be of considerable interest. Because interindividual differences are the "bread and butter" of personality psychology, we place primary emphasis on the applications of psychophysiology to individual differences.

Finally, researchers who are beginning a program of psychophysiological research may also seek information about where to purchase the necessary equipment. An excellent Web-based resource listing a broad range of U.S. and international companies selling psychophysiological research systems can be found at *www.psychophys.com/company.html*. Companies vary widely in regard to whether they sell integrated, multicomponent systems or whether they sell equipment component by component. Some companies will customize a system based on the researcher's needs. Costs, too, vary widely. Simple systems measuring one or two parameters may be purchased for less than $1,000, whereas more complex, integrated systems may cost 50 times as much. Researchers purchasing equipment for the first time are advised to speak *directly* to customer support personnel at various companies to determine what type of system meets their specific research needs. Another important consideration is technical support: How easy is it to obtain telephone assistance at odd hours (such as evenings and weekends) for unexpected technical problems? If a piece of equipment needs replacement or repair, what is the average turnaround time? Even 3–4 days of "work stoppage" can be a logistical nightmare for laboratories in which subjects are scheduled back-to-back for days or weeks at a time. Finally, many companies will provide, upon request, names of established researchers using their systems and/or lists of published studies conducted with their equipment. Contact a vendor's current clients and find out what type of research they do, why they chose this particular vendor, and whether they would make a different choice now.

General Laboratory Guidelines

Although different psychophysiological measures are appropriate for different types of research questions, certain general guidelines regarding laboratory practice apply to all of these

measures. First, researchers should keep in mind that the entire laboratory environment can play a role in influencing participants' psychophysiological responses from the moment they walk in the door (Christenfeld, Glynn, Kulik, & Gerin, 1998). Does the laboratory resemble a living room, complete with decorative lamps and plants, a comfortable couch, and framed posters on the walls, or does it have a sterile, potentially intimidating feel, with bare walls, rigid chairs, and harsh fluorescent lighting? A good general practice is to tailor the laboratory environment so that it mimics the setting to which one is attempting to generalize the findings. Hence, a clinical setting may be appropriate for assessing individuals' reactivity to work-related or performance-based stressors, whereas a home-like setting may be more appropriate for assessing couples' reactivity during marital squabbles.

If the laboratory visit will involve the administration of a stress task (addressed in more detail below), it is preferable for the person who administers the stress task to be *different* from the person who greets participants, walks them through the informed consent procedure, hooks them up to the equipment, and debriefs them at the end of the assessment. It is ideal to keep constant the sex, general age, and attire of the experimenter, as well as the person who hooks up the participant to the physiological equipment. With child and adolescent participants, it may be advisable to ensure that the research assistant hooking up the physiological equipment is of the *same sex* as the participant.

It is preferable (and critical in the case of cortisol assessments, described in greater detail below) to perform laboratory assessments at approximately the same time of day for all participants. Regardless of time of day, however, participants should be instructed (and reminded) to refrain from smoking, taking over-the-counter medication, eating, and drinking caffeinated beverages for at least 2 hours before coming to the laboratory. Adherence to this request should be confirmed during the informed consent procedure. For lengthy laboratory visits, researchers should consider keeping snacks and beverages on hand to offer to (potentially famished!) participants as soon as they have finished the psychophysiological assessments.

Whether one is interested in basal physiological functioning (i.e., continuous physiological functioning that maintains basic, vital activities of the organism) or task-related reactivity, an accurate baseline assessment is critical. Given that many individuals find the process of coming to a laboratory and getting fitted with physiological equipment to be mildly arousing in and of itself, it is preferable to allow individuals at least 10 minutes to get used to the equipment and their surroundings before officially beginning the baseline assessment, which should last approximately 5–10 minutes. In addition, instead of having participants simply sit quietly during baseline assessment, it is increasingly common to administer what is called a "vanilla" baseline, in which individuals are engaged in a relaxing, nondemanding task that minimally engages their attention, such as rating their liking of a variety of pleasant landscape photographs. Vanilla baselines show greater stability of physiological responding, both within the baseline assessment and across assessments administered to the same person on different occasions (Jennings, Kamarck, Stewart, & Eddy, 1992).

For researchers measuring respiratory sinus arrhythmia (RSA), an index of parasympathetic nervous system (PNS) activity described in greater detail below, an additional baseline assessment during which participants carefully control their respiratory frequency is also ideal. This is because estimates of RSA are sensitive to respiratory rate, and large changes in respiratory parameters can alter the degree of association between RSA and true PNS activity (Berntson et al., 1997). Some researchers therefore statistically control for respiratory rate when analyzing RSA data, yet this is an extremely conservative correction approach, and other researchers maintain that it is not necessary in studies that focus primarily on within-person changes in RSA across different laboratory tasks (Houtveen, Rietveld, & De Geus, 2002). Yet when *between-person* comparisons are the primary focus, as is typically the case with assessments of baseline vagal activity, respiration can be easily standardized by simply having respondents breathe along with a tape recorder or metronome that paces their inhalations and exhalations (respiratory frequencies of 6–8 seconds are suitable for this purpose) for a period of 3–5 minutes.

Two factors that critically affect the interpretation of baseline and reactivity data are *age* and *gender*. Age and gender differences have been documented for all the physiological systems commonly assessed in personality re-

search, and researchers therefore risk misinterpreting their findings unless they take these dimensions into account, either by including them as covariates or selecting their samples for homogeneity. Cross-sectional studies, for example, have found that both parasympathetic and sympathetic nervous system functioning varies markedly from infancy to late adulthood (Korkushko, Shatilo, YuI, & Shatilo, 1991; Uchino, Kiecolt-Glaser, & Cacioppo, 1992), as does HPA activity (Seeman, Singer, Wilkinson, & McEwen, 2001; Walker, Walder, & Reynolds, 2001). In considering the effects of age on HPA activity, it is appropriate to remember that these effects are more a function of *development* than of simple *chronological age*. For example, the developing and changing sleep–wake cycle of the infant is associated with variability in his or her HPA functioning, making it difficult to interpret associations between cortisol, behavior, and emotion (de Weerth, Zijl, & Buitelaar, 2003). Once children reach toddlerhood, their patterns of HPA reactivity are more consistent, allowing for more robust interpretations of individual differences (Gunnar, Sebanc, Tout, Donzella, & van Dulmen, 2003). Nonetheless, patterns of HPA reactivity continue to change from adolescence all the way into late adulthood; for example, the HPA axis is more reactive among younger than older adults (Kudielka, Buske-Kirschbaum, Hellhammer, & Kirschbaum, 2004).

Gender, too, is strongly associated with a variety of differential patterns of both basal and stress-related autonomic (Kiecolt-Glaser & Newton, 2001; Levenson, Carstensen, & Gottman, 1994) and HPA functioning (Otte et al., 2005; Seeman et al., 2001). Hormonal fluctuations over the menstrual cycle also influence cardiovascular and HPA axis activity (Kirschbaum, Kudielka, Gaab, Schommer, & Hellhammer, 1999; Sato, Miyake, Akatsu, & Kumashiro, 1995), and thus a female participant should provide the date of her last menstrual cycle and her average cycle length so that her menstrual phase can be determined and statically controlled.

Choosing Laboratory Stressors

Many psychologists have used psychophysiological measures to assess interindividual differences in physiological reactivity to controlled laboratory manipulations. In some cases, the content of the manipulation is critically important to the research question, as in research on gender differences in responses to imagined scenarios of infidelity (Pietrzak, Laird, Stevens, & Thompson, 2002). In other cases, researchers may simply want to elicit stress and/or anxiety in the most reliable way possible. Although it may seem that "any stressor will do" for such research designs, this is not the case. Rather, operationalizing the construct of stress/anxiety for the purposes of assessing psychophysiological reactivity is a complex task. What type of stress is of interest? Should participants feel challenged and motivated to perform to their highest ability, or should they be led to feel inadequate, evaluated, threatened, or even angry?

Laboratory tasks that elicit different emotional and motivational states are known to have distinctive profiles of reactivity and recovery across different physiological systems (see, e.g., Tomaka, Blascovich, Kelsey, & Leitten, 1993). The most notable effects have been documented for the following characteristics: (1) whether the task requires active effort, watchful attention, or passive participation (Smith, Ruiz, & Uchino, 2000); (2) the incentive or penalty used to elicit task performance (Waldstein, Bachen, & Manuck, 1997); (3) the difficulty, effort requirement, and familiarity of the task (Kelsey et al., 1999); (4) the extent to which individuals can control their own performance and/or the administration of rewards and penalties (Peters et al., 1998); (5) whether participants perceive that they do or do not have the resources to perform the task successfully, denoted as a "challenge" versus a "threat" appraisal (Tomaka, Blascovich, Kibler, & Ernst, 1997).

The distinction between challenging and threatening tasks is particularly tricky, inasmuch as individuals draw upon a variety of explicit and implicit cues—as well as their own stable self-concepts—in making such appraisals. Thus, factors such as self-esteem (Seery, Blascovich, Weisbuch, & Vick, 2004), the presence of an evaluative or nonevaluative audience (Kelsey et al., 2000), person-characteristics of the audience or experimenter (Blascovich, Mendes, Hunter, Lickel, & Kowai-Bell, 2001), the type of feedback given on performance (Earle, Linden, & Weinberg, 1999), and emotional cues (Blascovich & Mendes, 2000) can influence respondents' experiences of challenge versus threat. Thus, researchers should ideally assess participants' appraisals of task difficulty, controllability, and performance both before and after the task in order to validate its intended psychological characteristics.

The tailoring of task characteristics, of course, depends on the aim of the study and the context to which one wants to generalize the research findings. Thus, personality researchers interested in trait-like patterns of reactivity to performance motivation should select a "challenge" task that involves controllable, moderate effort in response to incentive, whereas those interested in trait-like patterns of reactivity to anxiety may want to select a "threat" task that maximizes feelings of apprehension and is perceived as uncontrollable. Perhaps most important, however, whenever variability *across individuals* in trait-like patterns of reactivity is of interest (rather than variability *across tasks or testing situations*), it is generally recommended to administer multiple tasks within the experimental session and average the resultant responses within physiological parameter and within task type (Kamarck, Debski, & Manuck, 2000; Pruessner et al., 1997), thereby yielding (for example) an aggregate measure of heart rate to challenge, heart rate to threat, electrodermal response to challenge, electrodermal response to threat, and so forth. This is important because previous studies have found only mild-to-moderate intertask consistency, test–retest reliability, and longitudinal stability in physiological reactivity (see Kamarck & Lovallo, 2003; Manuck, Kamarck, Kasprowicz, & Waldstein, 1993), raising concerns about the categorization of individuals into "high-reactive" and "low-reactive" groups on the basis of a single task. Some studies have found that correlations between physiological reactivity and various personality dimensions are strengthened when aggregated measures are used (Pruessner et al., 1997).

Another consideration to keep in mind is that some classes of tasks may elicit more consistent within-person response profiles than others (Manuck et al., 1993). Perhaps most notably, tasks that provoke extremely high or low reactivity may fail to elicit the range of variability necessary to identify individual profiles—if a stimulus is threatening enough, everyone will show a robust fight-or-flight response, whereas if it is too mild, nobody will. Thus, researchers interested in idiographic analyses of trait-like response profiles should pilot test and select tasks eliciting moderate reactivity (Kamarck & Lovallo, 2003).

Using Multiple Measures and Analytical Approaches

Individuals who are consistently "high-reactive" in one physiological parameter are not necessarily high-reactive on others, and therefore personality researchers interested in trait-like patterns of reactivity should include not only multiple tasks, but multiple physiological measures to capture different aspects of the overall stress process (such as endocrine vs. cardiovascular reactivity; sympathetic nervous system activation vs. parasympathetic withdrawal; vascular vs. myocardial changes in blood pressure, all of which are addressed in greater detail later below). This will allow the researcher to reliably characterize individuals not only with respect to whether they are consistently high-reactive or low-reactive on one particular physiological parameter, but whether they consistently show certain *combinations* of reactivity patterns, such as high heart rate *in the absence of* correspondingly high HPA reactivity, or parasympathetic withdrawal *plus* myocardial-driven changes in blood pressure. The fact that individuals consistently differ from one another with regard to such response profiles has been termed *individual response stereotypy* (Engel, 1960), and the question of whether certain response patterns are systematically related to psychological traits or health risks is an active topic of current psychophysiological research (Berntson & Cacioppo, 2003).

In addressing such questions, researchers should bear in mind that levels of consistency and reliability vary across different physiological measures. For example, research using different subject populations has consistently found greater test–retest reliability in heart rate than in diastolic blood pressure (Kamarck et al., 1992). Task characteristics also influence reliability: for example, blood pressure readings show greater reliability for nonspeaking than for speaking tasks (Swain & Suls, 1996), and greater reliability when task difficulty is calibrated to each individual subject, typically using computerized task protocols (Kamarck et al., 1992).

Analyses also require careful consideration. Instead of simply comparing individuals' baseline-to-task reactivity, researchers should consider examining other dimensions along which individual differences in reactivity might be manifested: threshold to respond, level of peak response, rise time to peak response, and degree and timing of recovery (Brosschot & Thayer, 1998; Davidson, 1998). Unfortunately, the psychometric characteristics of most of these less widely used parameters are less well established (Davidson, 1998), although there has been increasing research on the appropriate modeling of recovery profiles (Christenfeld, Glynn, & Gerin, 2000). Yet such measures have the potential to significantly refine our capacity to capture meaningful individual and situational differences with potentially important mental and physical health implications (see, e.g., Brosschot & Thayer, 1998).

Finally, in addition to measuring participants' cognitive appraisals of the task, researchers should also include self-report measures of individuals' subjective emotional states, not only immediately before and after the tasks, but also after a fixed recovery period (typically 2–3 minutes). Although it is commonly assumed that psychophysiological measures are, in fact, primarily useful as valid indices of individuals' authentic subjective responses to experimental manipulations, in actuality the relationship between subjective and physiological responses appears to be substantially more complex and inconsistent (Blascovich, Brennan, Tomaka, & Kelsey, 1992). Even setting aside the inevitable ambiguity associated with self-reports of emotion, most individuals are also poor judges of changes in their own physiological states, such as increases in heart rate or body heat (Edelmann & Baker, 2002), as well as sexual arousal (Heiman, 1975). The circumstances under which one does or does not find direct correspondence between self-reports and physiological responses remain to be fully specified and have become an increasing topic of theory and research (see Cacioppo et al., 2000, on the full range of possible relations between psychophysiological measures and psychological constructs). Because discrepancies may be found for some physiological parameters and not others, the measurement of multiple physiological systems can aid researchers in interpreting their meaning; for example, might they stem from dysregulation in one particular physiological system (such as hypocortisolism, reviewed below), or might they reflect a global tendency to misreport or misinterpret subjective experience, in which case self-reports should diverge from *multiple* physiological parameters?

Considering all of these complexities, the ideal research design for identifying individual response profiles would involve the administration of *multiple* tasks eliciting moderate reactivity, classed within different task types (i.e., several active coping tasks *and* several passive coping tasks), repeated across *multiple* testing sessions (different days, different times of day), using a wide range of physiological *and* self-report measures. Of course, this ideal scenario is logistically unfeasible, but it provides a useful template to keep in mind when deciding which design elements are most indispensable for certain hypothesis tests and how such decisions affect the interpretation of these tests. With these general guidelines in mind, we now offer a more detailed discussion of the specific physiological systems likely to be of greatest interest to personality psychologists.

The HPA Axis

The neuroendocrine system balances concentrations of hormones in the body with the psychological and physical demands of the environment. Neuroendocrine responses to environmental demands are observed in two major axes: the sympathetic–adrenal medullary (SAM) axis (involving the release of catecholamines such as norepinephrine and epinephrine), and the HPA axis (involving the release of CRH [corticotropin-releasing hormone], ACTH [adrenocorticotropic hormone], and cortisol, as reviewed in Baum & Grunberg, 1995).

Most personality-oriented research documenting associations between neuroendocrine functioning and psychological traits has focused on the HPA axis, and our review mirrors this emphasis. The disproportionate attention to the HPA axis may be due to the fact that HPA activity in response to environmental demands is associated with appraisals of such demands as threatening (i.e., exceeding the individual's capacity to cope) or affectively negative, whereas SAM activation appears to represent an adaptive response to challenge situations in which the individual feels he or she has sufficient coping resources (for reviews, see Blascovich & Tomaka, 1996; Cacioppo, 1994). Given that investigations into the potential biological correlates of psychological states

and traits tend to cluster around negative phenomena such as anxiety, neuroticism, inhibition, and aggression, the predominant focus on HPA rather than SAM activation is understandable.

Although HPA activation results in the secretion of a variety of hormones, it is most commonly assessed via *cortisol*, which is secreted by the adrenal gland and serves to regulate both homeostatic functioning and stress reactivity. The pathway to cortisol secretion begins in the hypothalamus, where CRH is released into the anterior pituitary in response to environmental demands. CRH secretion triggers the release of ACTH, which causes the synthesis of cortisol in the adrenal gland. The cessation of cortisol production is accomplished through a negative feedback loop. Specifically, once sufficient plasma levels of cortisol have been reached, CRH synthesis is inhibited, thereby down-regulating the chain of events required for additional cortisol production.

Measurement Issues

Cortisol can be measured in blood, urine, or saliva. All three provide reliable indices of cortisol secretion, but measurement in saliva is by far the most commonly used method, largely because it is the most noninvasive (requiring only that participants saturate a sterile swab and store it in a plastic tube) and the most convenient for subjects to self-administer in their natural environments. The latter reason is particularly important because cortisol secretion shows strong diurnal variation (reviewed below), and hence accurate assessment of total cortisol secretion requires collecting multiple samples over the course of the day, ideally for several days. This can be easily accomplished by instructing research subjects to collect and store a series of saliva samples on their own, following a prearranged schedule, but would be logistically problematic for collecting urinary or plasma samples. Common practice in using salivary cortisol samples is to have participants immediately refrigerate or freeze their samples until mailing them back to the researcher. However, as long as they are shipped within 4 days, refrigeration is not necessary. Beyond that point, mold may begin to grow. Some maintain that mold growth compromises the interpretation of the assay, whereas others argue that it does not. The safest course, of course, is to refrigerate or freeze the samples (for long-term storage, it is preferable to freeze the samples at –20° C). If samples are sent off-site to be assayed and shipment delays are anticipated, they can be packed with dry ice. If they can be expected to arrive within 3–4 days, no such precautions are necessary. A number of laboratories in the United States and Europe provide assay services, for fees ranging from $2.50 to $15.00 per sample (two of the most widely used are the Kirschbaum laboratory in Germany, *biopsychologie.tu-dresden.de*, and the Penn State Behavioral Endocrinology laboratory, *bbh.hhdev.psu.edu/labs/behavioral%20endo%20lab/bel.html*). Another option is to conduct assays in-house, using assay kits that are available for purchase. This gives the researcher more control over the process, but requires substantial additional investment in laboratory supplies (such as precision pipettes, centrifuges, etc.), staff training, and quality management. To get a sense of the degree of complexity involved in analyzing one's own samples, and the type of equipment required, see the detailed instructions on the Salimetrics website, at *www.salimetrics.com/ercortisol-kitinsert.htm*. Salimetrics is only one of many companies that sell assay kits. Additional detail on the "nuts and bolts" of collecting and analyzing salivary cortisol can be found on the Kirschbaum and Penn State websites, mentioned above, and in the 2000 report on salivary cortisol measurement produced by the John D. and Catherine T. MacArthur Research Network on Socioeconomic Status and Health, *www.macses.ucsf.edu/Research/Allostatic/notebook/salivarycort.html*.

Unlike measures of autonomic functioning, in which physiological reactivity is immediately measurable after the onset of a psychological stimulus, it takes approximately 20–30 minutes for HPA responses to show up in cortisol concentrations. Thus, in order to assess HPA responses to specific events, researchers should collect cortisol samples 20–30 minutes *after* the event has occurred. This also obviously affects measurement of baseline cortisol levels in laboratory environments. Rather than collecting a baseline sample as soon as the participant has arrived at the laboratory, it is preferable to take his or her baseline sample 20–30 minutes after the participant has had an opportunity to calmly acclimate to the lab environment. For field studies in which participants provide multiple within-day cortisol samples, it is advisable to collect information on the participant's activity level, food consumption, alcohol and tobacco use, and emotional state *20–30 minutes*

before the saliva sample is taken, as these factors are known to influence cortisol levels (Backhaus, Junghanns, & Hohagen, 2004).

Yet by far the most important methodological consideration for cortisol assessment is the time of day. Cortisol secretion shows distinct diurnal variation, typically peaking immediately after waking, significantly dipping before noon, minimally rising again for a period, and then resuming a steady decline into the mid-to-late evening hours (reviewed in Lovallo & Thomas, 2000). The specific shape of this diurnal curve varies from individual to individual (see, e.g., Smyth et al., 1997), and has been of considerable interest for its associations with a variety of psychological states, traits, and conditions (reviewed below). Yet this diurnal profile must also be taken into account for accurately measuring HPA reactivity to both naturally occurring and laboratory stressors. Generally, cortisol reactivity to stress appears greatest when basal cortisol concentrations are low (Dallman et al., 2004), and it is therefore ideal to conduct laboratory stress protocols in the late afternoon or early evening. With respect to naturally occurring stressors, which may occur at any time, researchers should control for the expected cortisol level for the particular time of day before interpreting a certain cortisol level as indicating a low or high stress response.

Basal HPA Functioning

Assessment of individual differences in basal HPA functioning typically focuses on three different outcomes: the overall shape of the diurnal profile, the morning "peak" or "challenge," or the total cortisol concentration over the entire day (sometimes called AUC, or "area under the curve"). Individual differences are observed in each of these domains, and therefore each may be of interest to personality psychologists. As noted earlier, a normal diurnal profile involves a strong morning peak that declines subsequently, with a minimal increase in the early evening. To accurately capture this profile, it is generally recommended that sampling begin with the moment of waking (while the respondent remains in bed), then 30 minutes later, followed by 3 hours after waking, 8 hours after waking, 12 hours after waking, and finally at bedtime (Stewart & Seeman, 2000). This measurement profile provides the most accurate portrait of diurnal fluctuation in cortisol as well as the most accurate assessment of overall cortisol levels throughout the day (AUC). As these dimensions fluctuate to some degree from day-to-day, however, collection of data on at least 2 consecutive days is preferable (Stewart & Seeman, 2000). Increasing the number of within-day measurements as well as the number of days sampled will improve reliability.

Most research on individual differences in cortisol profiles has concerned "flattened" patterns of cortisol release, characterized by a blunted morning peak and/or a minimal decline into the evening and overnight. Because this pattern tends to be produce low measures of total daily cortisol concentration over the day, it has been called "hypocortisolism" (Gunnar & Vazquez, 2001; Heim, Ehlert, & Hellhammer, 2000). Some research suggests that flattened cortisol profiles are associated with adverse early life conditions that produce dysregulation in the HPA axis or dysregulation in cognitive appraisals of stressors (reviewed in Gunnar & Vazquez, 2001). One study, for example, found flattened profiles to be associated with insecure childhood attachment relationships, as assessed retrospectively with the Adult Attachment Interview (Adam & Gunnar, 2001). A blunted morning response has also been associated with lower socioeconomic status (SES) (Brandtstaedter, Baltes-Goetz, Kirschbaum, & Hellhammer, 1991), job burnout (Pruessner, Hellhammer, & Kirschbaum, 1999), and self-reported job stress (Caplan, Cobb, & French, 1979). The previous night's sleep quality is also associated with morning cortisol peaks and should be assessed in investigations of this parameter (Backhaus et al., 2004). Although studies have not found consistent links between personality traits and diurnal profiles (Smyth et al., 1997), this remains an active area for research, specifically with respect to the potential importance of early adverse experiences in permanently altering individuals' psychological and physiological capacities for stress and emotion regulation (Gunnar & Vazquez, 2001; Hart, Gunnar, & Cicchetti, 1996).

Research on flattened diurnal cycles has also proved informative in helping to explain the fact that associations between AUC cortisol concentrations and measures of stress or maladaptation have varied notably across studies and even within samples, such that cortisol levels sometimes appeared elevated in individuals with high stress or negative affectivity (Polk, Cohen, Doyle, Skoner, & Kirschbaum, 2005; Portella, Harmer, Flint, Cowen, & Goodwin, 2005) and sometimes appeared dampened (Anisman, Griffiths, Matheson, Ravindran, & Merali, 2001). Dampened levels have also been associated with aggression and conduct problems in youth (Shoal, Giancola, & Kirillova, 2003). Future research is necessary to pinpoint the specific correlates, antecedents, and implications of atypically high versus atypically low cortisol secretion (Gunnar & Vazquez, 2001; Heim et al., 2000), and this is likely to remain an active topic of interest among personality psychologists. Perhaps the most important consideration for personality researchers is to conduct sufficient descriptive and exploratory analyses to permit identification of different—and sometimes seemingly contradictory—subtypes of HPA response. For example, one study of socially phobic individuals found that a subset of these participants showed significantly *elevated* cortisol stress responses, whereas another subset showed significant *declines* (Furlan, DeMartinis, Schweizer, Rickels, & Lucki, 2001). Computing aggregated correlations between social phobia and cortisol levels would obviously have obscured such a finding.

HPA Reactivity Assessments

There are notable individual differences in HPA stress reactivity that have been the subject of considerable research for their associations with psychological states and traits, as well as with psychiatric conditions such as depression, anxiety, and social phobia (see, e.g., Habra, Linden, Anderson, & Weinberg, 2003; Kirschbaum, Bartussek, & Strasburger, 1992). A comprehensive review of HPA reactivity protocols by Dickerson and Kemeny (2004) found that researchers generally observe the most robust and consistent responses when utilizing stressors that last 15 minutes or longer and which are perceived as uncontrollable and involving social evaluation. A classic example is the Trier Social Stress Test (Kirschbaum, Pirke, & Hellhammer, 1993), a widely used and well-validated task requiring participants to deliver a speech and perform mental arithmetic in front of an evaluative audience. Recovery profiles have also been of interest with respect to HPA stress responses (Roy, Kirschbaum, & Steptoe, 2001), and can be assessed by collecting an additional cortisol sample approximately 41–60 minutes after the initiation of the stressor (Dickerson & Kemeny, 2004). As in the case of laboratory stressors, discussed earlier, it is important to collect data on participants' appraisals of effort, control, anxiety, and emotional state in order to accurately interpret their levels of reactivity (Dickerson & Kemeny, 2004; Polk et al., 2005).

As with diurnal cycles and overall cortisol concentrations, it is important to note that one cannot uniformly interpret high cortisol stress reactivity as indicative of highly negative states or traits. Although studies typically find that heightened cortisol reactivity and attenuated recovery are associated with traits such as negative affectivity and social inhibition (Habra et al., 2003; Kagan, Resnick, & Snidman, 1987) and are typically interpreted as indicative of poor emotion regulation (Scarpa & Raine, 1997), other studies have found that *blunted* patterns of reactivity are also maladaptive (Buske-Kirschbaum et al., 1997) and appear to be linked to early experiences with adversity that might produce dysregulation in the HPA system (Hart, Gunnar, & Cicchetti, 1995). Thus, as with AUC measures, researchers should inspect their data for the possible existence of multiple response profiles rather than averaging together cortisol increases with cortisol decreases.

Overall, studies investigating global associations between HPA reactivity and *personality* dimensions have found inconsistent patterns (Berger et al., 1987; Brandtstaedter et al., 1991; Goodyer, Park, Netherton, & Herbert, 2001), but some have suggested that interpretable associations are more likely to emerge in studies of *habituation* to repeated stressors than in single assessments of stress reactivity (Kirschbaum, Wust, Faig, & Hellhammer, 1992). Repeated exposure to stress generally produces rapid habituation (Kirschbaum et al., 1995), yet some individuals fail to show this effect, instead maintaining sustained levels of high HPA response that can have adverse health consequences (Krantz & Manuck, 1984; Munck, Guyre, & Holbrook, 1984). One study found that individuals whose cortisol responses failed to show habituation to repeated stress were lower in self-esteem and extraversion and higher in neuroticism and physical complaints (Kirschbaum et al., 1995), and another found that such individuals tended to be depressive and harm avoidant (Gerra et al., 2001). Thus, personality researchers interested in cortisol stress reactivity should consider assessing *progressive habituation* to repeated stressors rather than either singular or aggregated stress responses.

ANS Measures

Assessments of ANS functioning are, without question, among the most widely used psychophysiological measures in psychological research. The most common measures are heart rate, blood pressure, electrodermal activity, and respiratory sinus arrhythmia (sometimes referred to as *heart rate variability* or *vagal tone*), but in recent years assessments of pre-ejection period, cardiac output, and peripheral resistance have become more common. In selecting among these measures, researchers should keep two basic distinctions in mind: that between sympathetic nervous system (SNS) and parasympathetic nervous system (PNS) functioning, and that between cardiac and vascular reactivity. Each has relevance to the types of research questions typically asked by personality psychologists.

SNS versus PNS Functioning

The parasympathetic and sympathetic branches of the ANS have antagonistic effects on the physiological processes involved in stress reactivity. The SNS is responsible for redistributing metabolic output in times of external threat, and therefore heightened activation of this system produces the physiological changes most commonly associated with "fight-or-flight" responses: increases in heart rate, blood pressure, sweating, cardiac output, vasoconstriction, and blood flow to the skeletal muscles, myocardium, brain, kidneys, gastrointestinal tract, and skin. In contrast, the parasympathetic system is responsible for maintaining normal growth and restoration of internal organs, processes that are suspended in times of intense stress. Thus, heightened engagement of this system produces the types of physiological changes typically associated with relaxation rather than arousal, such as deceleration in heart rate and blood pressure. These changes function to distribute metabolic energy toward normal maintenance of internal organs and to maintain a state of homeostasis. During periods of stress, however, the PNS typically "withdraws" to shift metabolic and attentional resources to the stressor without requiring overactivation of the SNS (Calkins, 1997). Recovery from stress is typically associated with reinstatement of PNS activity, which functions to reestablish homeostasis.

Thus, all changes in ANS activity are driven by the *coordinated* up-regulation and down-regulation of the PNS and the SNS, rendering meaningless any notion of "generalized autonomic arousal." Stress-related increases in heart rate, for example, may result from heightened SNS activation, PNS withdrawal, or some graded combination of the two. Similarly, poststressor declines in heart rate may result from decreased SNS activity *or* increases in PNS activity. The specific balance of SNS and PNS functioning (sometimes called "autonomic balance") has been shown to vary not only across tasks, but also across individuals (Berntson, Cacioppo, Quigley, & Fabro, 1994), and is thought to be a trait-like individual difference dimension that emerges early in development (Friedman & Thayer, 1998) and that has implications for cardiovascular health risk and psychological functioning.

Specifically, patterns of cardiovascular stress reactivity that are driven by the SNS rather than the PNS are associated with hypertension and other long-term cardiovascular health risks (Kristal-Boneh, Raifel, Froom, & Rivak, 1998), as well as immune deficits (Croiset, Heijnen, Van der Wal, De Boer, & De Wied, 1990; del Rey, Besedovsky, Sorkin, da Prada, & Arrenbrecht, 1981). They have also been associated with a stress-prone, "Type A" personality (Kamada, Miyake, Kumashiro, Monou, & Inoue, 1992). High sympathetic tone has also been found to be associated with inhibition, excitability, emotional liability, a tendency to deny emotions, and susceptibility to psychosomatic complaints (Schweiger, Wittling, Genzel, & Block, 1998).

In contrast, ANS stress responses that involve a greater degree of PNS withdrawal than SNS activation appear to be more rapid, more flexible, and easier to disengage than SNS-dominated responses (Berger, Saul, & Cohen, 1989; Saul, 1990), and thus individuals with more PNS-driven patterns of cardiovascular reactivity are conceptualized as having nervous systems that more flexibly react to and recover from environmental stressors than those with sympathetically mediated patterns (Calkins, 1997; DeGangi, DiPietro, Greenspan, & Porges, 1991; Porges, Doussard-Roosevelt, & Maiti, 1994).

Consistent with this perspective, infants and children with high parasympathetic tone have been characterized as more attentive and reactive to changes in their environment (Healy, 1989; Stifter, Fox, & Porges, 1987), less inhibited (Reznick, Kagan, & Snidman, 1986), and

less prone to misconduct (Kibler, Prosser, & Ma, 2004). High parasympathetic tone has therefore been viewed as a key substrate for the development of effective emotion regulation (Porges, 1991; Porges et al., 1994). Studies on adults provide further support for this perspective, finding associations between high parasympathetic tone and more effective emotional and behavioral responses to stress (Fabes & Eisenberg, 1997). In contrast, low parasympathetic tone has been associated with inhibition, aggression, depression, anger, mental stress, generalized anxiety, and panic anxiety (reviewed in Brosschot & Thayer, 1998; Friedman & Thayer, 1998). Personality psychologists interested in integrating autonomic measures into their research should take care to include independent assessments of PNS and SNS activity so that they can capture such differences.

Measuring PNS Functioning: Respiratory Sinus Arrhythmia

Researchers investigating PNS functioning often speak of measuring *vagal tone* (see Porges, 1991; Porges et al., 1994), which refers to the functioning of the vagus nerve (the 10th cranial nerve, a critical component of the PNS) in maintaining chronotropic control of the heart to regulate metabolic output. Vagal tone is typically indexed by measuring the degree of heart rate variability that occurs in response to respiration, known as *respiratory sinus arrhythmia* (RSA). To explain briefly: Heart rate accelerates slightly with each inhalation and decelerates slightly with each exhalation. This regular oscillation reflects the repeated withdrawal and subsequent reinstatement of vagal influence. The greater the vagal regulation of metabolic activity, the more that heart rate will accelerate and decelerate in response to inhalation and exhalation, producing an RSA waveform with a larger amplitude. It is this amplitude that is used as an index of overall vagal control of heart rate (note, however, that there are considerable variations in terminology—studies assessing PNS functioning may refer to *RSA*, *vagal tone*, *heart rate variability* [HRV], or *high-frequency heart rate variability*).

The different methods of measuring HRV, their technical requirements, and their appropriateness for different research aims are comprehensively reviewed in a task force report on these topics (Task Force of the European Society of Cardiology and the North American Society of Pacing and Electrophysiology, 1996). Presently, most social psychophysiologists use spectral analysis (Porges, 1986) to extract periodicity in the heart period pattern that occurs at the typical respiratory frequency (0.12–40.0 Hz, corresponding to approximately 7.5–24.0 breaths per minute). The variance of the heart period pattern in this bandwidth is calculated as the estimate of RSA. Another technique, called the "peak-to-valley" method (Grossman & Svebak, 1987), uses time series data on heart rate and actual respiratory rate to isolate respiration-induced variability in heart rate on a breath-by-breath basis. There is very high correspondence between measurements obtained using these methods (Grossman, van Beek, & Wientjes, 1990).

Finally, although studies of PNS activity have historically emphasized *basal* parasympathetic tone (measured during a resting baseline), researchers have increasingly investigated stress-related *declines* in PNS activity (often denoted as "suppression") as measures of the capacity to efficiently shift metabolic resources in response to challenge, providing an ancillary index of autonomic and emotional regulation (Cohen et al., 2000; Stifter & Corey, 2001). Supporting this interpretation, individuals with high levels of baseline vagal tone tend to show greater stress-related vagal suppression (DeGangi et al., 1991; El-Sheikh, 2005). Yet these two indices of PNS functioning do not appear to be redundant; studies of children have tended to find that stress-related vagal suppression is a more reliable predictor of adaptive functioning than basal vagal tone (Calkins & Dedmon, 2000).

Furthermore, the degree and direction of task-related change in PNS activity varies according to task characteristics. Whereas stress and negative affect provoke the classic PNS suppression effect, tasks involving nonstressful cognitive attention or social interaction often induce *increases* in PNS activity (Suess & Bornstein, 2000). In addition, some researchers have called attention to poststressor recovery or "rebound" in PNS activity as yet another index of effective regulation (Rottenberg, Wilhelm, Gross, & Gotlib, 2003). Thus, researchers interested in parasympathetic functioning should assess baseline levels as well as stress-induced reactivity and recovery in order to obtain the most complete picture of parasympathetic functioning.

Measuring SNS Functioning: Electrodermal Activity

The most widely used and noninvasive technique for specifically assessing *sympathetic* nervous system activity involves measurement of electrodermal response (EDR), also known as skin conductance (comprehensively reviewed in Dawson, Schell, & Filion, 2000). SNS activation produces greater conductivity in the skin, partly as a result of increased sweat secretion. By passing an electrical current across the skin, one can measure these increases in conductance (also commonly conceptualized as *decreases* in skin resistance). Increases in skin conductance are commonly observed during stress- or anxiety-induced SNS activation, but are also observed as a function of orienting and attention, muscular activity, deep breaths, and thermoregulatory sweating. Hence, in order to reliably interpret skin conductance data, laboratory and stimulus conditions should be carefully controlled.

One of the advantages of assessing skin conductance is that the measure is noninvasive and relatively unobtrusive, and it has shown robust associations with a variety of psychological states and traits in prior research, including repressive coping (Brosschot & Janssen, 1998), anxiety, nervousness, and panic (Carrillo et al., 2001), attachment avoidance (Diamond, Hicks, & Otter-Henderson, 2006; Roisman, Tsai, & Chiang, 2004), harm avoidance (Yoshino, Kimura, Yoshida, Takahashi, & Nomura, 2005), and behavioral inhibition (Fowles, 1988; Raine, Venables, & Williams, 1995). Methodologically, assessment of skin conductance is fairly simple, involving the placement of several electrodes on the individual's nondominant hand, and the primary methodological cautions concern selection of the specific electrode sites, ensuring that respondents wash their hands with a neutral, nonabrasive soap before beginning assessment, and instructing participants to avoid large body movements, which can cause artifacts (for details, see Dawson et al., 2000). The most common electrode sites are the *medial or distal phalanges* of the first and second index fingers. If you turn your hand palm side up and look down at your index finger, the uppermost padded area is the distal phalange. The area just below the crease of the fingertip is the medial phalange. Readings from distal phalanges tend to be higher, and so it is important to report the specific electrode site so that this can be taken into account when comparing the results of different studies.

Assessments of skin conductance yield two parameters: basal skin conductance level (SCL) and phasic skin conductance response (SCR). SCL represents the overall level of conductance during a particular moment in time, or averaged within a specific epoch. SCL typically declines during long assessments as individuals habituate to their surroundings, but this tendency is typically reversed if individuals are exposed to laboratory stressors. SCR, in contrast, represents discrete "spikes" in SCL that can be counted within different epochs and analyzed with respect to their amplitude and latency. SCRs are of particular interest to researchers investigating autonomic responses to specific stimuli, as they are typically observed immediately after stimulus presentation (representing either an orienting or an emotional response— or both—depending on the stimulus). Such responses are called "specific" SCRs. However, SCRs can also be "nonspecific," meaning that they are observed in the absence of any discernible triggering stimulus. Nonspecific SCRs are typically reported as rates (number per minute), and the rate is typically 1–3. Generally, researchers use a 0.05 microsiemen change in skin conductance level as the criterion for detecting an SCR. This value is somewhat arbitrary but has been conventionally adopted, therefore allowing for valid comparisons across different studies. To score SCRs, researchers typically visually inspect the data and verify that each "spike" in SCL meets the selected criterion to be considered a response. Yet in recent years, several computerized scoring programs have been developed that increase the speed and reliability of this process (see Dawson et al., 2000, for details).

Although they are not perfectly correlated, emotional stress tends to be associated with increases in SCL *and* increases in nonspecific SCRs, and thus either parameter may be used as an index of stress reactivity. There are no firm guidelines as to the use of one index versus the other, but assessment of specific SCRs is particularly appropriate for studies assessing responses to time-delimited stimulus presentation (such as images or words). Such research designs should also consider measuring the magnitude of the SCR, the poststimulus latency to respond, and the recovery time. In general, greater response intensity is manifested not only in more frequent SCRs, but in larger responses that reach their peak more quickly (reviewed in Dawson et al., 2000).

Blood Pressure and Impedance Cardiography

Blood pressure is another widely used cardiovascular measure of ANS activity. Systolic and diastolic blood pressure measure the force of blood against arterial walls. Maximum arterial pressure is reached during ventricular contraction, when the heart beats (denoted as systolic blood pressure, or SBP), and minimum arterial pressure is reached during ventricular relaxation, the period between beats (denoted as diastolic blood pressure, or DBP). Numerous studies have detected that stable psychological traits are associated with heightened blood pressure reactivity, sometimes detected in SBP and sometimes in DBP (Carels, Blumenthal, & Sherwood, 2000; Habra et al., 2003).

An important complication in blood pressure assessments is that they can be decomposed into their *vascular* versus *cardiac* (or *myocardial)* components. In short, an increase in blood pressure can result from greater cardiac output (i.e., greater blood being pumped through the heart and therefore pressing against the arterial walls) or increased resistance in the vasculature (i.e., "tightening" of the arteries, such that blood is being pumped through a smaller space, resulting in increased pressure). Blood pressure changes across different situations and different individuals may be of similar magnitude, yet show notably different patterns of cardiac and vascular change (Manuck et al., 1993; Sherwood, Allen, Obrist, & Langer, 1986), often called the "hemodynamic profile." Generally, vascular responses are more closely associated with hypertension than with cardiac responses. Moreover, stress tasks that involve active coping more typically evoke myocardial responses, whereas passive tasks tend to evoke vascular responses (reviewed in Gregg, James, Matyas, & Thorsteinsson, 1999). Researchers are increasingly investigating whether intraindividual variability in *overall* blood pressure reactivity is differentially driven by myocardial versus vascular factors among different individuals (Chen, Matthews, Salomon, & Ewart, 2002; Hawkley, Burleson, Berntson, & Cacioppo, 2003), and this question is likely to be of interest to personality psychologists.

The standard oscillometric methods for assessing blood pressure (involving the familiar inflatable blood pressure cuff) can provide separate assessments of systolic and diastolic pressure, but cannot provide independent assessments of myocardial versus vascular changes. However, *impedance cardiography* is a well-validated technique for doing so that is used with increasing frequency among health psychologists. This technique also allows for the specific measurement of cardiovascular correlates of SNS activity (just as RSA provides for PNS activity).

Impedance cardiography uses external current and voltage electrodes to pass a high-frequency, low-amplitude, alternating current through the thorax and measure changes in electrical resistance. Because blood is a conductor, these changes index the changes in aortic blood volume and flow velocity associated with systole and diastole. The technical specifics of impedance cardiography are beyond the scope of this chapter (for more thorough discussion, see Brownley, Hurwitz, & Schneiderman, 2000; Sherwood, 1993). The key advantage of this technique is that it yields measures of (1) pre-ejection period (PEP), technically defined as the systolic time interval, or the time between the onset of left ventricular depolarization to the moment just before blood is ejected from the left ventricle, (2) stroke volume, which can be multiplied by heart rate to yield a measure of *cardiac output*, the total amount of blood being ejected from the left ventricle, in liters per minute, and (3) total peripheral resistance (TPR), or the resistance to blood flow in the peripheral arteries, calculated as mean arterial blood pressure divided by cardiac output. PEP is of interest because it serves as a measure of sympathetic nervous system activity, as increased sympathetic activation leads to greater contractility of the left ventricle and hence shorter systolic time intervals (i.e., *smaller* PEP readings). Cardiac output and TPR are of interest because each of these dimensions represents, respectively, the myocardial and vascular contributors to blood pressure, as reviewed above. Impedance cardiography is quickly becoming standard practice in behavioral medicine research, but is less commonly used by the average psychologist. Nonetheless, personality psychologists whose research questions require specific isolation of SNS activity or identification of hemodynamic profiles will find it indispensable.

Conclusions

The integration of psychophysiological measures into personality research can make an important contribution to overall multimethod approaches in personality psychology that seek to understand how and why psychological traits are associated with diverse domains of human functioning, from cognition to emotion to behavior to physiology. The increasing availability of noninvasive, well-validated measures of multiple physiological systems makes it relatively easy for personality psychologists interested in psychophysiology—even those with little background in human physiology—to integrate these measures into their research programs, given careful attention to some of the biological and methodological basics we have outlined above. The end result may be a more comprehensive understanding of the complex and diverse patterns of interindividual variability in human functioning across different domains.

Recommended Reading

Cacioppo, J. T., Tassinary, L. G., & Berntson, G. G. (Eds.). (2000). *Handbook of psychophysiology* (2nd ed.). New York: Cambridge University Press. *Note*. Also refer to Table 22.1.

References

Adam, E. K., & Gunnar, M. R. (2001). Relationship functioning and home and work demands predict individual differences in diurnal cortisol patterns in women. *Psychoneuroendocrinology, 26,* 189–208.

Anisman, H., Griffiths, J., Matheson, K., Ravindran, A. V., & Merali, Z. (2001). Posttraumatic stress symptoms and salivary cortisol levels. *American Journal of Psychiatry, 158,* 1509–1511.

Backhaus, J., Junghanns, K., & Hohagen, F. (2004). Sleep disturbances are correlated with decreased morning awakening salivary cortisol. *Psychoneuroendocrinology, 29,* 1184–1191.

Baum, A., & Grunberg, N. (1995). Measurement of stress hormones. In S. Cohen, R. C. Kessler, & L. U. Gordon (Eds.), *Measuring stress: A guide for health and social scientists* (pp. 175–192). New York: Oxford University Press.

Becker, J. B., Breedlove, S. M., Crews, D., & McCarthy, M. M. (2002). *Behavioral endocrinology* (2nd ed.). Cambridge, MA: MIT Press.

Berger, M., Bossert, S., Krieg, J. C., Dirlich, G., Ettmeier, W., Schreiber, W., et al. (1987). Interindividual differences in the susceptibility of the cortisol system: An important factor of the degree of hypercortisolism in stress situations? *Biological Psychiatry, 22,* 1327–1339.

Berger, R. D., Saul, J. P., & Cohen, R. J. (1989). Transfer function analysis of autonomic regulation: I. The canine atrial rate response. *American Journal of Physiology, 256,* H142–H152.

Berntson, G. G., Bigger, J. T. J., Eckberg, D. L., Grossman, P., Kaufmann, P. G., Malik, M., et al. (1997). Heart rate variability: Origins, methods, and interpretive caveats. *Psychophysiology, 34,* 623–648.

Berntson, G. G., & Cacioppo, J. T. (2003). A contemporary perspective on multilevel analyses and social neuroscience. In F. Kessel, P. L. Rosenfield, & N. B. Anderson (Eds.), *Expanding the boundaries of health and social science: Case studies in interdisciplinary innovation* (pp. 18–40). New York: Oxford University Press.

Berntson, G. G., Cacioppo, J. T., Quigley, K. S., & Fabro, V. T. (1994). Autonomic space and psychophysiological response. *Psychophysiology, 31,* 44–61.

Blascovich, J., Brennan, K., Tomaka, J., & Kelsey, R. M. (1992). Affect intensity and cardiac arousal. *Journal of Personality and Social Psychology, 63,* 164–174.

Blascovich, J., & Kelsey, R. M. (1990). Using electrodermal and cardiovascular measures of arousal in social psychological research. In C. Hendrick & M. S. Clark (Eds.), *Research methods in personality and social psychology* (pp. 45–73). Newbury Park, CA: Sage.

Blascovich, J., & Mendes, W. B. (2000). Challenge and threat appraisals: The role of affective cues. In J. P. Forgas (Ed.), *Feeling and thinking: The role of affect in social cognition.* (pp. 59–82). New York: Cambridge University Press.

Blascovich, J., Mendes, W. B., Hunter, S. B., Lickel, B., & Kowai-Bell, N. (2001). Perceiver threat in social interactions with stigmatized others. *Journal of Personality and Social Psychology, 80,* 253–267.

Blascovich, J., & Tomaka, J. (1996). The biopsychosocial model of arousal regulation. In M. Zanna (Ed.), *Advances in experimental social psychology* (Vol. 28, pp. 1–51). New York: Academic Press.

Brandtstaedter, J., Baltes-Goetz, B., Kirschbaum, C., & Hellhammer, D. (1991). Developmental and personality correlates of adrenocortical activity as indexed by salivary cortisol: Observations in the age range of 35 to 65 years. *Journal of Psychosomatic Research, 35,* 173–185.

Brosschot, J. F., & Janssen, E. (1998). Continuous monitoring of affective–autonomic response dissociation in repressors during negative emotional stimulation. *Personality and Individual Differences, 25,* 69–84.

Brosschot, J. F., & Thayer, J. F. (1998). Anger inhibition, cardiovascular recovery, and vagal function: A model of the link between hostility and cardiovascular disease. *Annals of Behavioral Medicine, 20,* 326–332.

Brownley, K. A., Hurwitz, B. E., & Schneiderman, N. (2000). Cardiovascular psychophysiology. In J. T. Cacioppo, L. G. Tassinary, & G. G. Berntson (Eds.), *Handbook of psychophysiology* (2nd ed., pp. 224–264). New York: Cambridge University Press.

Buske-Kirschbaum, A., Jobst, S., Psych, D., Wustmans, A., Kirschbaum, C., Rauh, W., et al. (1997). Attenuated free cortisol response to psychosocial stress in children with atopic dermatitis. *Psychosomatic Medicine, 59,* 419–426.

Cacioppo, J. T. (1994). Social neuroscience: Autonomic, neuroendocrine, and immune responses to stress. *Psychophysiology, 31,* 113–128.

Cacioppo, J. T., Tassinary, L. G., & Berntson, G. G. (2000). Psychophysiological science. In J. T. Cacioppo, L. G. Tassinary, & G. G. Berntson (Eds.), *Handbook of psychophysiology* (2nd ed., pp. 3–23). New York: Cambridge University Press.

Calkins, S. D. (1997). Cardiac vagal tone indices of temperamental reactivity and behavioral regulation in young children. *Developmental Psychobiology, 31,* 125–135.

Calkins, S. D., & Dedmon, S. E. (2000). Physiological and behavioral regulation in two-year-old children with aggressive/destructive behavior problems. *Journal of Abnormal Child Psychology, 28,* 103–118.

Caplan, R. D., Cobb, S., & French, J. R. (1979). White collar work load and cortisol: Disruption of a circadian rhythm by job stress? *Journal of Psychosomatic Research, 23,* 181–192.

Carels, R. A., Blumenthal, J. A., & Sherwood, A. (2000). Emotional responsivity during daily life: Relationship to psychosocial functioning and ambulatory blood pressure. *International Journal of Psychophysiology, 36,* 25–33.

Carrillo, E., Moya-Albiol, L., Gonzalez-Bono, E., Salvador, A., Ricarte, J., & Gomez-Amor, J. S. (2001). Gender differences in cardiovascular and electrodermal responses to public speaking task: The role of anxiety and mood states. *International Journal of Psychophysiology, 42,* 253–264.

Chen, E., Matthews, K. A., Salomon, K., & Ewart, C. K. (2002). Cardiovascular reactivity during social and nonsocial stressors: Do children's personal goals and expressive skills matter? *Health Psychology, 21,* 16–24.

Christenfeld, N., Glynn, L. M., & Gerin, W. (2000). On the reliable assessment of cardiovascular recovery: An application of curve-fitting techniques. *Psychophysiology, 37,* 543–550.

Christenfeld, N., Glynn, L. M., Kulik, J. A., & Gerin, W. (1998). The social construction of cardiovascular reactivity. *Annals of Behavioral Medicine, 20,* 317–325.

Coan, J. A., & Allen, J. J. B. (2003). The state and trait nature of frontal EEG asymmetry in emotion. In K. Hugdahl & R. J. Davidson (Eds.), *Asymmetrical brain* (pp. 565–615). Cambridge, MA: MIT Press.

Cohen, H., Benjamin, J., Geva, A. B., Matar, M. A., Kaplan, Z., & Kotler, M. (2000). Autonomic dysregulation in panic disorder and in post-traumatic stress disorder: Application of power spectrum analysis of heart rate variability at rest and in response to recollection of trauma or panic attacks. *Psychiatry Research, 96,* 1–13.

Croiset, G., Heijnen, C. J., Van der Wal, W. E., De Boer, S. F., & De Wied, D. (1990). A role for the autonomic nervous system in modulating the immune response during mild emotional stimuli. *Life Sciences*, 46, 419–425.

Dallman, M. F., Akana, S. F., Strack, A. M., Scribner, K. S., Pecoraro, N., La Fleur, S. E., et al. (2004). Part III. Neuroendocrine regulation in stress. In K. Pacak, G. Aguilera, E. Sabban, & R. Kvetnansky (Eds.), *Stress: Current neuroendocrine and genetic approaches* (pp. 141–223): New York Academy of Sciences.

Davidson, R. J. (1998). Affective style and affective disorders: Perspectives from affective neuroscience. *Cognition and Emotion*, 12, 307–330.

Davidson, R. J. (2003). Affective neuroscience: A case for interdisciplinary research. In F. Kessel, P. L. Rosenfield, & N. B. Anderson (Eds.), *Expanding the boundaries of health and social science: Case studies in interdisciplinary innovation* (pp. 99–121). New York: Oxford University Press.

Davidson, R. J., Jackson, D. C., & Larson, C. L. (2000). Human electroencephalography. In J. T. Cacioppo, L. G. Tassinary, & G. G. Berntson (Eds.), *Handbook of psychophysiology* (2nd ed., pp. 27–52). New York: Cambridge University Press.

Dawson, M. E., Schell, A. M., & Bohmelt, A. H. (1999). *Startle modification: Implications for neuroscience, cognitive science, and clinical science*. New York: Cambridge University Press.

Dawson, M. E., Schell, A. M., & Filion, D. L. (2000). The electrodermal system. In J. T. Cacioppo, L. G. Tassinary, & G. G. Berntson (Eds.), *Handbook of psychophysiology* (2nd ed., pp. 200–223). New York: Cambridge University Press.

DeGangi, G. A., DiPietro, J. A., Greenspan, S. I., & Porges, S. W. (1991). Psychophysiological characteristics of the regulatory disordered infant. *Infant Behavior and Development*, 14, 37–50.

del Rey, A., Besedovsky, H. O., Sorkin, E., da Prada, M., & Arrenbrecht, S. (1981). Immunoregulation mediated by the sympathetic nervous system, II. *Cellular Immunology*, 63, 329–334.

de Weerth, C., Zijl, R. H., & Buitelaar, J. K. (2003). Development of cortisol circadian rhythm in infancy. *Early Human Development*, 73, 39–52.

Diamond, L. M., Hicks, A. M., & Otter-Henderson, K. A. (2006). Physiological evidence for repressive coping among avoidantly attached adults. *Journal of Social and Personal Relationships*, 23, 205–229.

Dickerson, S. S., & Kemeny, M. E. (2004). Acute stressors and cortisol responses: A theoretical integration and synthesis of laboratory research. *Psychological Bulletin*, 130, 355–391.

Dougherty, D. D., Rauch, S. L., & Fischman, A. J. (2004). Positron emission tomography and single photon emission computed tomography. In D. D. Dougherty, S. L. Rauch, & J. F. Rosenbaum (Eds.), *Essentials of neuroimaging for clinical practice* (pp. 75–91). Washington, DC: American Psychiatric Press.

Earle, T. L., Linden, W., & Weinberg, J. (1999). Differ-

ential effects of harassment on cardiovascular and salivary cortisol stress reactivity and recovery in women and men. *Journal of Psychosomatic Research*, 46, 125–141.

Edelmann, R. J., & Baker, S. R. (2002). Self-reported and actual physiological responses in social phobia. *British Journal of Clinical Psychology*, 41, 1–14.

El-Sheikh, M. (2005). Stability of respiratory sinus arrhythmia in children and young adolescents: A longitudinal examination. *Developmental Psychobiology*, 46, 66–74.

Engel, B. T. (1960). Stimulus–response and individual–response specificity. *Archives of General Psychiatry*, 2, 305–313.

Fabes, R. A., & Eisenberg, N. (1997). Regulatory control in adults' stress-related responses to daily life events. *Journal of Personality and Social Psychology*, 73, 1107–1117.

Fabiani, M., Gratton, G., & Coles, M. G. H. (2000). Event-related brain potentials. In J. T. Cacioppo, L. G. Tassinary, & G. G. Berntson (Eds.), *Handbook of psychophysiology* (2nd ed., pp. 53–84). New York: Cambridge University Press.

Fowles, D. C. (1988). Psychophysiology and psychopathology: A motivational approach. *Psychophysiology*, 25, 373–391.

Friedman, B. H., & Thayer, J. F. (1998). Autonomic balance revisited: Panic anxiety and heart rate variability. *Journal of Psychosomatic Research*, 44, 133–151.

Furlan, P. M., DeMartinis, N., Schweizer, E., Rickels, K., & Lucki, I. (2001). Abnormal salivary cortisol levels in social phobic patients in response to acute psychological but not physical stress. *Biological Psychiatry*, 50, 254–259.

Geer, J. H., & Janssen, E. (2000). The sexual response system. In J. T. Cacioppo, L. G. Tassinary, & G. G. Berntson (Eds.), *Handbook of psychophysiology* (2nd ed., pp. 315–341). New York: Cambridge University Press.

Gerra, G., Zaimovic, A., Mascetti, G. G., Gardini, S., Zambelli, U., Timpano, M., et al. (2001). Neuroendocrine responses to experimentally induced psychological stress in healthy humans. *Psychoneuroendocrinology*, 26, 91–107.

Goodyer, I. M., Park, R. J., Netherton, C. M., & Herbert, J. (2001). Possible role of cortisol and dehydroepiandrosterone in human development and psychopathology. *British Journal of Psychiatry*, 179, 243–249.

Gregg, M. E., James, J. E., Matyas, T. A., & Thorsteinsson, E. B. (1999). Hemodynamic profile of stress induced anticipation and recovery. *International Journal of Psychophysiology*, 34, 147–162.

Grossman, P., & Svebak, S. (1987). Respiratory sinus arrhythmia as an index of parasympathetic cardiac control during active coping. *Psychophysiology*, 24, 228–235.

Grossman, P., van Beek, J., & Wientjes, C. (1990). A comparison of three quantification methods for estimation of respiratory sinus arrhythmia. *Psychophysiology*, 27, 702–714.

Gunnar, M. R., Sebanc, A. M., Tout, K., Donzella, B., & van Dulmen, M. M. H. (2003). Peer rejection, temperament, and cortisol activity in preschoolers. *Developmental Psychobiology, 43,* 346–358.

Gunnar, M. R., & Vazquez, D. M. (2001). Low cortisol and a flattening of expected daytime rhythm: Potential indices of risk in human development. *Development and Psychopathology, 13,* 515–538.

Habra, M. E., Linden, W., Anderson, J. C., & Weinberg, J. (2003). Type D personality is related to cardiovascular and neuroendocrine reactivity to acute stress. *Journal of Psychosomatic Research, 55,* 235–245.

Hart, J., Gunnar, M. R., & Cicchetti, D. (1995). Salivary cortisol in maltreated children: Evidence of relations between neuroendocrine activity and social competence. *Development and Psychopathology, 7,* 11–26.

Hart, J., Gunnar, M. R., & Cicchetti, D. (1996). Altered neuroendocrine activity in maltreated children related to symptoms of depression. *Development and Psychopathology, 8,* 201–214.

Hawkley, L. C., Burleson, M. H., Berntson, G. G., & Cacioppo, J. T. (2003). Loneliness in everyday life: Cardiovascular activity, psychosocial context, and health behaviors. *Journal of Personality and Social Psychology, 85,* 105–120.

Healy, B. T. (1989). Autonomic nervous system correlates of temperament. *Infant Behavior and Development, 12,* 289–304.

Heim, C., Ehlert, U., & Hellhammer, D. H. (2000). The potential role of hypocortisolism in the pathophysiology of stress-related bodily disorders. *Psychoneuroendocrinology, 25,* 1–35.

Heiman, J. R. (1975). The physiology of erotica: Women's sexual arousal. *Psychology Today, 8,* 90–94.

Houtveen, J. H., Rietveld, S., & De Geus, E. J. C. (2002). Contribution of tonic vagal modulation of heart rate, central respiratory drive, respiratory depth and respiratory frequency to respiratory sinus arrhythmia during mental stress and physical exercise. *Psychophysiology, 39,* 427–436.

Janssen, E. (2002). Psychophysiological measurement of sexual arousal. In M. W. Wiederman & B. E. J. Whitley (Eds.), *Handbook for conducting research on human sexuality* (pp. 139–171). Mahwah, NJ: Erlbaum.

Jennings, J. R., Kamarck, T. W., Stewart, C., & Eddy, M. J. (1992). Alternate cardiovascular baseline assessment techniques: Vanilla or resting baseline. *Psychophysiology, 29,* 742–750.

Kagan, J., Resnick, A., & Snidman, N. (1987). The physiology and psychology of behavioral inhibition in children. *Child Development, 58,* 1459–1473.

Kamada, T., Miyake, S., Kumashiro, M., Monou, H., & Inoue, K. (1992). Power spectral analysis of heart rate variability in Type As and Type Bs during mental workload. *Psychosomatic Medicine, 54,* 462–470.

Kamarck, T. W., Debski, T. T., & Manuck, S. B. (2000). Enhancing the laboratory-to-life generalizability of cardiovascular reactivity using multiple occasions of measurement. *Psychophysiology, 37,* 533–542.

Kamarck, T. W., Jennings, J. R., Debski, T. T., Glickman-Weiss, E., Johnson, P. S., Eddy, M. J., et al. (1992). Reliable measures of behaviorally-evoked cardiovascular reactivity from a PC-based test battery: Results from student and community samples. *Psychophysiology, 29,* 17–28.

Kamarck, T. W., & Lovallo, W. R. (2003). Cardiovascular reactivity to psychological challenge: Conceptual and measurement considerations. *Psychosomatic Medicine, 65,* 9–21.

Kelsey, R. M., Blascovich, J., Leitten, C. L., Schneider, T. R., Tomaka, J., & Wiens, S. (2000). Cardiovascular reactivity and adaptation to recurrent psychological stress: The moderating effects of evaluative observation. *Psychophysiology, 37,* 748–756.

Kelsey, R. M., Blascovich, J., Tomaka, J., Leitten, C. L., Schneider, T. R., & Wiens, S. (1999). Cardiovascular reactivity and adaptation to recurrent psychological stress: Effects of prior task exposure. *Psychophysiology, 36,* 818–831.

Kibler, J. L., Prosser, V. L., & Ma, M. (2004). Cardiovascular correlates of misconduct in children and adolescents. *Journal of Psychophysiology, 18,* 184–189.

Kiecolt-Glaser, J. K., & Newton, T. L. (2001). Marriage and health: His and hers. *Psychological Bulletin, 127,* 472–503.

Kirschbaum, C., Bartussek, D., & Strasburger, C. J. (1992). Cortisol responses to psychological stress and correlations with personality traits. *Personality and Individual Differences, 13,* 1353–1357.

Kirschbaum, C., Kudielka, B. M., Gaab, J., Schommer, N. C., & Hellhammer, D. H. (1999). Impact of gender, menstrual cycle phase, and oral contraceptives on the activity of the hypothalamic–pituitary–adrenal axis. *Psychosomatic Medicine, 61,* 154–162.

Kirschbaum, C., Pirke, K. M., & Hellhammer, D. H. (1993). The "Trier Social Stress Test": A tool for investigating psychobiological stress responses in a laboratory setting. *Neuropsychobiology, 28,* 76–81.

Kirschbaum, C., Prussner, J. C., Stone, A. A., Federenko, I., Gaab, J., Lintz, D., et al. (1995). Persistent high cortisol responses to repeated psychological stress in a subpopulation of healthy men. *Psychosomatic Medicine, 57,* 468–474.

Kirschbaum, C., Wust, S., Faig, H. G., & Hellhammer, D. H. (1992). Heritability of cortisol responses to human corticotropin-releasing hormone, ergometry, and psychological stress in humans. *Journal of Clinical Endocrinology and Metabolism, 75,* 1526–1530.

Korkushko, O. V., Shatilo, V. B., YuI, P., & Shatilo, T. V. (1991). Autonomic control of cardiac chronotropic function in man as a function of age: Assessment by power spectral analysis of heart rate variability. *Journal of the Autonomic Nervous System, 32,* 191–198.

Krantz, D. S., & Manuck, S. B. (1984). Acute psychophysiologic reactivity and risk of cardiovascular disease: A review and methodologic critique. *Psychological Bulletin, 96,* 435–464.

Kristal-Boneh, E., Raifel, M., Froom, P., & Rivak, J. (1998). Heart rate variability in health and disease.

Scandinavian Journal of Work and Environmental Health, 21, 85–95.

Kudielka, B. M., Buske-Kirschbaum, A., Hellhammer, D. H., & Kirschbaum, C. (2004). Differential heart rate reactivity and recovery after psychosocial stress (TSST) in healthy children, younger adults, and elderly adults: The impact of age and gender. *International Journal of Behavioral Medicine, 11,* 116–121.

Levenson, R. W., Carstensen, L. L., & Gottman, J. M. (1994). The influence of age and gender on affect, physiology, and their interrelations: A study of long-term marriages. *Journal of Personality and Social Psychology, 67,* 56–68.

Lovallo, W. R., & Thomas, T. L. (2000). Stress hormones in psychophysiological research: Emotional, behavioral, and cognitive implications. In J. T. Cacioppo, L. G. Tassinary, & G. G. Berntson (Eds.), *Handbook of psychophysiology* (2nd ed., pp. 342–367). New York: Cambridge University Press.

Maier, S. F., & Watkins, L. R. (1998). Cytokines for psychologists: Implications of bidirectional immune-to-brain communication for understanding behavior, mood, and cognition. *Psychological Review, 105,* 83–107.

Manuck, S. B., Kamarck, T. W., Kasprowicz, A. S., & Waldstein, S. R. (1993). Stability and patterning of behaviorally evoked cardiovascular reactivity. In J. J. Blascovich & E. S. Katkin (Eds.), *Cardiovascular reactivity to psychological stress and disease* (pp. 111–134). Washington DC: American Psychological Association.

Munck, A., Guyre, P. M., & Holbrook, N. J. (1984). Physiological functions of glucocorticoids in stress and their relation to pharmacological actions. *Endocrine Reviews, 5,* 25–44.

Mussgay, L., & Rüddel, H. (1996). Ambulatory blood pressure monitoring: Promises and limitations in behavioral medicine. In J. Fahrenberg & M. Myrtek (Eds.), *Progress in ambulatory assessment: Computer-assisted psychological and psychophysiological methods in monitoring and field studies.* (pp. 365–374). Seattle, WA: Hogrefe & Huber.

Otte, C., Hart, S., Neylan, T. C., Marmar, C. R., Yaffe, K., & Mohr, D. C. (2005). A meta-analysis of cortisol response to challenge in human aging: Importance of gender. *Psychoneuroendocrinology, 30,* 80–91.

Peters, M. L., Godaert, G. L., Ballieux, R. E., van Vliet, M., Willemsen, J. J., Sweep, F. C., et al. (1998). Cardiovascular and endocrine responses to experimental stress: Effects of mental effort and controllability. *Psychoneuroendocrinology, 23,* 1–17.

Pietrzak, R. H., Laird, J. D., Stevens, D. A., & Thompson, N. S. (2002). Sex differences in human jealousy: A coordinated study of forced-choice, continuous rating-scale, and physiological responses on the same subjects. *Evolution and Human Behavior, 23,* 83–94.

Polk, D. E., Cohen, S., Doyle, W. J., Skoner, D. P., & Kirschbaum, C. (2005). State and trait affect as predictors of salivary cortisol in healthy adults. *Psychoneuroendocrinology, 30,* 261–272.

Porges, S. W. (1986). Respiratory sinus arrhythmia: Physiological basis, quantitative methods, and clinical indications. In P. Grossman, K. H. Janssen, & D. Vaitl (Eds.), *Cardiorespiratory and cardiosomatic psychophysiology* (pp. 101–106). New York: Plenum Press.

Porges, S. W. (1991). Vagal tone: An autonomic mediator of affect. In J. Garber & K. A. Dodge (Eds.), *The development of emotion regulation and dysregulation* (pp. 111–128). New York: Cambridge University Press.

Porges, S. W. (1995). Cardiac vagal tone: A physiological index of stress. *Neuroscience and Biobehavioral Reviews, 19,* 225–233.

Porges, S. W., Doussard-Roosevelt, J. A., & Maiti, A. K. (1994). Vagal tone and the physiological regulation of emotion. In N. Fox (Ed.), The development of emotion regulation: Biological and behavioral considerations. *Monographs of the Society for Research in Child Development, 59*(2–3, Serial No. 240), 167–186.

Portella, M. J., Harmer, C. J., Flint, J., Cowen, P., & Goodwin, G. M. (2005). Enhanced early morning salivary cortisol in neuroticism. *American Journal of Psychiatry, 162,* 807–809.

Pruessner, J. C., Gaab, J., Hellhammer, D. H., Lintz, D., Schommer, N., & Kirschbaum, C. (1997). Increasing correlations between personality traits and cortisol stress responses obtained by data aggregation. *Psychoneuroendocrinology, 22,* 615–625.

Pruessner, J. C., Hellhammer, D. H., & Kirschbaum, C. (1999). Burnout, perceived stress, and cortisol responses to awakening. *Psychosomatic Medicine, 61,* 197–204.

Raine, A., Venables, P. H., & Williams, M. (1995). High autonomic arousal and electrodermal orienting at age 15 years as protective factors against criminal behavior at age 29 years. *American Journal of Psychiatry, 152,* 1595–1600.

Reiman, E. M., Lane, R. D., Van Petten, C., & Bandettini, P. A. (2000). Positron emission tomography and functional magnetic resonance imaging. In J. T. Cacioppo, L. G. Tassinary, & G. G. Berntson (Eds.), *Handbook of psychophysiology* (2nd ed., pp. 85–118). New York: Cambridge University Press.

Reznick, J. S., Kagan, J., & Snidman, N. (1986). Inhibited and uninhibited children: A follow-up study. *Child Development, 57,* 660–680.

Roisman, G. I., Tsai, J. L., & Chiang, K.-H. S. (2004). The emotional integration of childhood experience: Physiological, facial expressive, and self-reported emotional response during the adult attachment interview. *Developmental Psychology, 40,* 776–789.

Rottenberg, J., Wilhelm, F. H., Gross, J. J., & Gotlib, I. H. (2003). Vagal rebound during resolution of tearful crying among depressed and nondepressed individuals. *Psychophysiology, 40,* 1–6.

Roy, M. P., Kirschbaum, C., & Steptoe, A. (2001). Psychological, cardiovascular, and metabolic correlates of individual differences in cortisol stress recovery in young men. *Psychoneuroendocrinology, 26,* 375–391.

Rugg, M. D., & Coles, M. G. H. (1995). *Electrophysiology of mind: Event-related brain potentials and cognition.* New York: Oxford University Press.

Sato, N., Miyake, S., Akatsu, J. I., & Kumashiro, M. (1995). Power spectral analysis of heart rate variability in healthy young women during the normal menstrual cycle. *Psychosomatic Medicine, 57,* 331–335.

Saul, J. P. (1990). Beat-to-beat variations of heart rate reflect modulation of cardiac autonomic outflow. *News in Psychological Science, 5,* 32–37.

Scarpa, A., & Raine, A. (1997). Psychophysiology of anger and violent behavior. *Psychiatric Clinics of North America, 20,* 375–394.

Schweiger, E., Wittling, W., Genzel, S., & Block, A. (1998). Relationship between sympathovagal tone and personality traits. *Personality and Individual Differences, 25,* 327–337.

Seeman, T. E., Singer, B. H., Wilkinson, C. W., & McEwen, B. (2001). Gender differences in age-related changes in HPA axis reactivity. *Psychoneuroendocrinology, 26,* 225–240.

Seery, M. D., Blascovich, J., Weisbuch, M., & Vick, S. B. (2004). The relationship between self-esteem level, self-esteem stability, and cardiovascular reactions to performance feedback. *Journal of Personality and Social Psychology, 87,* 133–145.

Segerstrom, S. C., & Miller, G. E. (2004). Psychological stress and the human immune system: A meta-analytic study of 30 years of inquiry. *Psychological Bulletin, 130,* 601–630.

Sherwood, A. (1993). Use of impedance cardiography in cardiovascular reactivity research. In J. Blascovich & E. S. Katkin (Eds.), *Cardiovascular reactivity to psychological stress and disease* (pp. 157–199). Washington DC: American Psychological Association.

Sherwood, A., Allen, M. T., Obrist, P. A., & Langer, A. W. (1986). Evaluation of beta-adrenergic influences on cardiovascular and metabolic adjustments to physical and psychological stress. *Psychophysiology, 23,* 89–104.

Shoal, G. D., Giancola, P. R., & Kirillova, G. P. (2003). Salivary cortisol, personality, and aggressive behavior in adolescent boys: A 5-year longitudinal study. *Journal of the American Academy of Child and Adolescent Psychiatry, 42,* 1101–1107.

Smith, T. W., Ruiz, J. M., & Uchino, B. N. (2000). Vigilance, active coping, and cardiovascular reactivity during social interaction in young men. *Health Psychology, 19,* 382–392.

Smyth, J. M., Ockenfels, M. C., Gorin, A. A., Catley, D., Porter, L. S., Kirschbaum, C., et al. (1997). Individual differences in the diurnal cycle of cortisol. *Psychoneuroendocrinology, 22,* 89–105.

Stewart, J., & Seeman, T. E. (2000, June). *Salivary cortisol measurement.* Retrieved June 1, 2005, from *www.macses.ucsf.edu/Research/Allostatic/notebook/salivarycort.html*

Stifter, C. A., & Corey, J. M. (2001). Vagal regulation and observed social behavior in infancy. *Social Development, 10,* 189–201.

Stifter, C. A., Fox, N. A., & Porges, S. W. (1987). Facial expressivity and vagal tone in 5- and 10-month-old infants. *Infant Behavior and Development, 12,* 467–474.

Suess, P. E., & Bornstein, M. H. (2000). Task-to-task vagal regulation: Relations with language and play in 20-month-old children. *Infancy, 1,* 303–322.

Swain, A., & Suls, J. (1996). Reproducibility of blood pressure and heart rate reactivity: A meta-analysis. *Psychophysiology, 33,* 162–174.

Task Force of the European Society of Cardiology and the North American Society of Pacing and Electrophysiology. (1996). Heart rate variability: Standards of measurement, physiological interpretation and clinical use. *Circulation, 93,* 1043–1065.

Tassinary, L. G., & Cacioppo, J. T. (2000). The skeletomotor system: Surface electromyography. In J. T. Cacioppo, L. G. Tassinary, & G. G. Berntson (Eds.), *Handbook of psychophysiology* (2nd ed., pp. 163–199). New York: Cambridge University Press.

Tomaka, J., Blascovich, J., Kelsey, R. M., & Leitten, C. L. (1993). Subjective, physiological, and behavioral effects of threat and challenge appraisal. *Journal of Personality and Social Psychology, 65,* 248–260.

Tomaka, J., Blascovich, J., Kibler, J., & Ernst, J. M. (1997). Cognitive and physiological antecedents of threat and challenge appraisal. *Journal of Personality and Social Psychology, 73,* 63–72.

Tranel, D. (2000). Electrodermal activity in cognitive neuroscience: Neuroanatomical and neuropsychological correlates. In R. D. Lane & L. Nadel (Eds.), *Cognitive neuroscience of emotion* (pp. 192–224). New York: Oxford University Press.

Uchino, B. N., Kiecolt-Glaser, J. K., & Cacioppo, J. T. (1992). Age-related changes in cardiovascular response as a function of a chronic stressor and social support. *Journal of Personality and Social Psychology, 63,* 839–846.

Uchino, B. N., Kiecolt-Glaser, J. K., & Glaser, R. (2000). Psychological modulation of cellular immunity. In J. T. Cacioppo, L. G. Tassinary, & G. G. Berntson (Eds.), *Handbook of psychophysiology* (2nd ed., pp. 397–424). New York: Cambridge University Press.

Waldstein, S. R., Bachen, E. A., & Manuck, S. B. (1997). Active coping and cardiovascular reactivity: A multiplicity of influences. *Psychosomatic Medicine, 59,* 620–625.

Walker, E. F., Walder, D. J., & Reynolds, F. (2001). Developmental changes in cortisol secretion in normal and at-risk youth. *Development and Psychopathology, 13,* 721–732.

Yoshino, A., Kimura, Y., Yoshida, T., Takahashi, Y., & Nomura, S. (2005). Relationships between temperament dimensions in personality and unconscious emotional responses. *Biological Psychiatry, 57,* 1–6.

## CHAPTER 23

The Human Genome Project and Personality

What We Can Learn about Our Inner and Outer Selves through Our Genes

Richard P. Ebstein
Rachel Bachner-Melman
Salomon Israel
Lubov Nemanov
Inga Gritsenko

Both genes and environment contribute to the emergence of adult personality. As in research on complex traits such as asthma, hypertension, major mental illness, and others, several basic steps are suggested that provide a useful framework for organizing molecular genetic research around the personality phenotype.

• *Choose a trait.* Personality defines our uniqueness and in its broadest sense encompasses all of the behavioral features that distinguish individual human beings. The myriad facets of personality suggest that, like a set of Legos, this broad phenotype needs to be decomposed into more manageable blocks and narrowed to digestible components for molecular genetic studies.

• *Choose a population.* Because personality is not an aberration and each of us has one, the choice of what population to study is potentially the whole human race. We therefore need to be discriminating and carefully select a subset of people for investigation.

• *Choose an experimental design.* There are several robust genetic designs employed in the study of complex traits, and the choice may be critical to the success of a study.

• *Ascertain samples.* The phenotype needs to be measured or ascertained; the vast majority of personality genetic studies have depended on self-report questionnaires. But which self-report questionnaire to employ?

• *Choose markers.* Having decided on a linkage (linkage studies employ anonymous markers that identify broad chromosomal regions) or an association (candidate genes are examined that a priori are thought to be relevant to personality—e.g., the serotonin transporter to neuroticism), the design imposes the additional burden of deciding what genetic markers to genotype (e.g., microsatellites, single nucleotide polymorphisms, SNPs, repeat regions, candidate genes) and how to choose them.

• *Data analysis.* Finally, having decided all of the above, we need to know what statistical techniques and methods will enable us to evaluate our findings and will ensure robust and reliable conclusions.

Measuring Personality

Most molecular genetic studies rely on a rather narrow definition of personality (Loehlin, 1992). Personality is considered the characteristic manner of an adult individual's behavior distinct from the goals toward which the behavior is directed (motivation) or the machinery of its execution (cognitive and motor skills). In this narrow sense, personality is comparable to temperament, which is defined by Webster's as "the peculiar or distinguishing mental or physical character determined by the relative proportions of the humors according to medieval physiology" (Figure 23.1): choleric (hot tempered), sanguine (related to blood; sturdy and cheerful), phlegmatic (slow and stolid), and melancholy (irascibilie or depressed). Each of the humors was associated with various correspondences and particular physical and mental characteristics and could, moreover, be combined with others for more complex personality types (e.g., choleric-sanguine, etc.). The result was a system that provided a quite elaborate classification of types of personality and, surprisingly, is not very dissimilar from more modern class-

ifications (Eysenck, 1970). For example, Cloninger's Tridimensional Personality Questionnaire (TPQ) (and the newer Temperament Character Index (TCI) (Cloninger, Svrakic, & Prybeck, 1994)) originally distinguished three temperament factors (Novelty Seeking, Harm Avoidance, Reward Dependence; Persistence was later separated from Reward Dependence) (Cloninger, 1987), and the TCI added an additional three so-called character factors: Self-directedness, Cooperativeness, and Self-Transcendance. Eysenck's scheme (Figure 23.1) (Eysenck, 1970) includes stable and unstable types as well as introverted and extroverted axes of personality. The NEO Personality Inventory—Revised (NEO-PI-R; Costa & McCrae, 1992) comprises five factors: Neuroticism, Extraversion, Openness to Experience, Agreeableness, and Conscientiousness.

Non-psychologists, especially neuroscientists and molecular geneticists, are invariably doubtful regarding the reliability of self-report questionnaires and are prone to question whether people reliably and honestly answer questions regarding their personalities and behavior. Despite these caveats, self-report personality tests appear to have good psychometric properties, are reliable across time, and appear to reliably assess the style of our personalities (McCrae et al., 2000).

An important decision to be made in choosing the complex trait to be studied is whether to study discrete, usually dichotomous, traits (in which there are two possible phenotypes, such as having diabetes or not), or continuous, quantitative traits (in which the phenotype can have a range of values, such as blood glucose levels and the so-called QTLs, or quantitative trait loci). Regarding personality traits, they

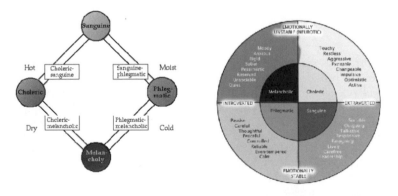

FIGURE 23.1. Eysenck's (1970) view and the Greek view of personality.

are apparently QTLs, and scores on self-report questionnaires readily lend themselves to analysis as straightforward quantitative traits. However, some investigators have used phenotype extremes (e.g., the top percentile of scorers on neuroticism) and convert quantitative scores into categorical traits. Presumably, using subjects with extreme scores reduces genotyping expenses because most of the genetic information is thought to be captured by this strategy (but see Sirota, Greenberg, Murphy, & Hamer, 1999).

Which Questionnaire to Use?

Based on this somewhat restricted view of personality as temperament, a large number of molecular genetic studies have been published in the past 10 years that attempt, with varying degrees of success, to unravel how variants in DNA sequence contribute to individual differences in personality. The phenotype in molecular genetic studies needs to be measured, and some phenotypes are easier, and more reliable, to measure than others. The definition of hypertension appears to be relatively straightforward, based on a simple procedure of measuring blood pressure using a sphygmotonometer cuff. Measuring personality or temperament is no more complex, but substitutes a physiological assessment for a written account. Most genetic studies are based on self-report questionnaires including the NEO-PI-R (Costa & McCrae, 1992), Eysenck's Personality Inventory (Eysenck, 1970), the TPQ/TCI (Cloninger, 1987; Cloninger et al., 1994), and Zuckerman's Sensation Seeking Scale (Zuckerman & Link, 1968). The vast majority of personality genetics studies have used one of these inventories. The two most popular, in terms of numbers of genetic publications, are the TPQ/TCI and the NEO-PI-R.

Another decision to be made before embarking on personality genetics studies is whether to employ more than one questionnaire in a study. Self-report questionnaires purport to measure similar traits, especially Harm Avoidance/Neuroticism and Extraversion/Novelty Seeking; nevertheless, it is notable that gene associations may be test specific. For example, although two recent meta-analysis confirm the association between the serotonin transporter (SLC6A4) promoter region 44 base pair repeat (Lesch et al., 1996) and anxiety-related personality traits, the association appeared to be ro-

bust only for the NEO-PI-R and not for the TPQ (Schinka, Busch, & Robichaux-Keene, 2004; Sen, Burmeister, & Ghosh, 2004).

As noted by Munafo, Clark, and Flint (2005), the findings of the Schinka and Sen meta-analyses (Schinka et al., 2004; Sen et al., 2004) are a challenge to personality genetics inasmuch as the NEO neuroticism demonstrates substantial psychometric form equivalence with TCI/TPQ harm avoidance (De Fruyt, Van De Wiele, & Heeringen, 2000) and, assuming that questionnaire equivalence reflects the measurement of the same underlying biological substrate, each assessment of neuroticism should be associated with the same genetic variants. Failure to provide comparable genetic associations questions the view that different personality measurements measure the same personality trait. In this regard, the reader is referred to a helpful article by Markon, Krueger, and Watson (2005) that delves into the psychometric properties of personality questionnaires and their structural relationships. Munafo and colleagues reexamined the meta-analyses of Schinka and colleagues (2004) and Sen and colleagues (2004). This third analysis concluded that there might be a small association between the serotonin transporter promoter region polymorphism and anxiety-related traits, particularly for TCI/TPQ Harm Avoidance (opposite to the previous two studies!), but found that the effect, if present, is small. It is important to note that in their analysis they excluded subjects collected on psychiatric samples, which they suggest reduced the possibility of confounding an association between the serotonin transporter gene and other psychiatric diseases with anxiety-related traits. Indeed, many studies of personality genetics have inventoried groups with psychiatric comorbidity. Studies of such groups may contaminate the association between genes and temperament; indeed, the observation may be showing association between genes and psychopathology and not genes and personality per se.

Often the reason for studying groups with comorbidity is one of convenience. The investigator has access to groups that have been inventoried for personality in the framework of studies of specific psychopathologies, and such groups are therefore a convenient source of information. For example, the Study on the Genetics of Alcoholism (COGA; Bierut et al., 2002) has generated a series of articles on personality genetics (Cloninger et al., 1998). The question remains whether it is not better to study personality in nonclinical groups, thus avoiding the conundrum of comorbidity. However, some clinical groups represent the extreme of personality phenotypes and may be informative. For example, our studies of fibromyalgia strengthen the association between the serotonin transporter and anxiety-related personality traits (Cohen, Buskila, Neumann, & Ebstein, 2002) and the role of the dopamine d4 receptor in Novelty Seeking or Extraversion (Buskila, Cohen, Neumann, & Ebstein, 2004). Similarly, a German study investigated a high-risk group of adolescents and observed an association between the DRD4 seven repeat and TPQ Novelty Seeking (Becker, Laucht, El-Faddagh, & Schmidt, 2005). This study is of special interest because these adolescents were studied from birth and constitute a group who suffered from a variety of adversities, including psychosocial, economic, and obstetrical complications.

Choosing a Population to Study

The budding investigator of molecular personality genetics, having decided on the personality phenotype and how to measure it, is now faced with the question of what population to study. Age and gender have an impact on human personality. For example, TPQ Novelty Seeking scores modestly decline with age and women score somewhat higher than men on Reward Dependence and Harm Avoidance (Zohar et al., 2001). These considerations suggest that the "cleanest" search for genes contributing to a personality phenotype may best be restricted to subjects within a narrow age range, equally balanced for men and women. An advantage of studying a young population is that parents are available for DNA sampling, allowing the use of a family-based design (discussed below). Of course, if the investigator is interested in the relationships between personality, genes, and health in an aging population, then the focus necessarily shifts to that age group.

Another concern is whether the population should be screened for medical problems, psychopathology, personality disorders, drug and alcohol abuse, major mental illness, and other possibly confounding conditions. How much to screen is a further question. Some studies

employ so-called supernormal controls (Hysi et al., 2005), but that may be an expensive undertaking. In our own studies we do some screening, but the cost of a thorough interview needs to be weighed against the bias introduced into the study by including some individuals who are expected to have undiagnosed personality disorders or medical conditions. Inclusion of such subjects will result in a loss of statistical power. Moreover, in studies of relatively young populations, especially university students, many of the subjects are below the age of onset of some psychopathologies.

Genes, Genes Everywhere

Although the completion of the Human Genome Project was celebrated in April 2003 and sequencing of the human chromosomes is essentially "finished," the exact number of genes encoded by the genome is still unknown. The October 2004 findings from the International Human Genome Sequencing Consortium reduce the estimated number of human protein-coding genes from 35,000 to only 20,000–25,000 (Stein, 2004).

Although this is a surprisingly low number for our species, it is nevertheless a daunting number for personality genetics studies, because as many as half this number are estimated to be expressed in the human brain and a priori any one is a potential candidate for contributing to personality. There is considerable overall uncertainty in selecting what genes to test in personality genetics. When many genes are conjectured to contribute to a complex disorder or trait, but the effect size of any one of these genes likely explains only a small percentage of the individual differences, geneticists have tried to narrow the target by the technique of positional cloning.

Positional cloning is used when the biochemical nature of a disease is unknown or when there are so many reasonable candidates that a genome-wide scan of possibilities is indicated. Marker genes (microsatellites consisting of di- or tetranucleotide repeats and very polymorphic and, nowadays, single nucleotide polymorphisms, or SNPs) not related to the phenotype are used for genome-wide screens that, if successful, can locate the phenotype locus to a chromosome region, which, unfortunately, often includes millions of base pairs and may contain hundreds of genes. Having accomplished this first aim, the next step is to localize the gene and determine its functional and biological role in the disease (disease–map–gene–function). Positional cloning depends on identifying the transfer of chromosomal regions in affecting sibling pairs and require DNA from parents and siblings but measurements of the phenotypes is needed only for affected children (i.e., the proband, Figure 23.2). The method is suitable for both categorical traits (e.g., schizophrenia) and QTLs, such as scores on personality tests. The main stumbling block is the large number of sibling pairs (hundreds if not thousands) required to gain sufficient statistical power (Risch, 2000).

Several studies have employed positional cloning (linkage analysis using anonymous markers that identify often broad chromosomal areas) to search for QTLs contributing to personality traits (Cloninger et al., 1998; Curtis, 2004; Dina et al., 2005; Fullerton et al., 2003; Neale, Sullivan, & Kendler, 2004; Zohar et al., 2003). Three studies (Cloninger et al., 1998; Dina et al., 2005; Fullerton et al., 2003)

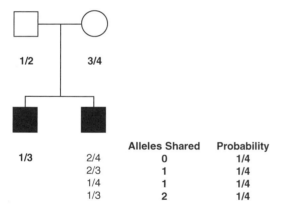

FIGURE 23.2. The affected sib pair method of linkage analysis used in positional cloning (Nyholt, 2000). Nuclear family with an affected sibling pair (ASP) showing inheritd by descent–sharing possibilities for a marker where all four parental alleles, denoted as "1," "2," "3," and "4," can be distinguished. By fixing the first sibling's genotype (1/3) and by listing the other sibling's possible genotypes (2/4, 2/3, 1/4, and 1/3), it can be seen that, under Mendelian inheritance (i.e., L), siblings are expected to share zero, one, and two alleles with a probability of 25%, 50%, and 25%, respectively. The ASP logarithm of the odds score is calculated as $\log_{10}(L_{HA}/L^{H0})$.

have now identified a broad region on chromosome 8p that harbors a locus that contributes to individual differences in a personality trait that is a measure of emotional liability. Two studies, using TPQ, found a linkage to Harm Avoidance (Cloninger et al., 1998; Dina et al., 2005), and Fullerton and colleagues (2003) used Eysenck's EPQ and found a linkage to Neuroticism (Eysenck, 1970). Subjects who score high on Harm Avoidance can be described as worrying and pessimistic, fearful and doubtful, shy and fatigable. High scorers on Eysenck's neuroticism dimension can similarly be described. The Cloninger and colleagues (1998) genome scan used subjects recruited from families with an alcoholic proband as part of the COGA study (Schuckit et al., 2001). The most significant linkage was to a site for Harm Avoidance at 27 cM (centimorgans; a measure of chromosomal distance in crossover units; 1 cM is approximately a million base pairs or DNA "letters," and there may be tens of such genes, or more, in such a region). A British study (Fullerton et al., 2003) genotyped 561 extremely discordant and concordant sibling pairs selected from a large population of 34,580 families. They observed a linkage to Neuroticism at 8 cM. Our own study (Dina et al., 2005; Zohar et al., 2003) observed a main linkage to TPQ Harm Avoidance more centromeric than these two studies, at approximately 60 cM, and therefore the likelihood needs to be considered that it is a distinct locus. The more general question, at what distance do we reject the hypothesis that two location estimates in a genomic region represent the same gene, has been addressed in a computer simulation study by Roberts, MacLean, Neale, Eaves, and Kendler (1999). Their results suggest that, even with relatively large numbers of families, chance variation in the location estimate is substantial. Their findings suggest that variability in position is substantial for complex disorders, with 95% confidence intervals (95% CI) covering long stretches of DNA in samples consisting of relatively large numbers of families. Such theoretical considerations lend credence to the provisional location of a single locus for anxiety-related personality traits in a chromosomal region 8p observed now in three independent studies across ethnic and cultural groups. However, the region highlighted by these three independent groups of investigators is quite large and a great deal of additional work is required before the actual gene is identified.

Choosing Markers

Positional cloning by linkage analysis depended until recently on the availability of microsatellite markers (short tandem repeats, or STR) that are distributed somewhat evenly across the genome and are highly polymorphic. A rule of thumb was to employ 300–400 such markers spaced ~10 cM across the genome in linkage studies. Recently, because of the availability of a dense human SNP map and the ability to assay SNPs by high throughput methods such as microarrays, SNPs appear to be replacing STRs as the marker of choice in both linkage and genome-wide association studies (Lee, Choi, Lee, & Lee, 2005).

In candidate gene and association studies (including genome-wide association studies) markers are chosen on the basis of four criteria: the prior probability of being functional, the correlation with potential causal variants (linkage disequilibrium), missense variants detected by sequencing, and technological considerations including the availability of high-throughput lower-cost preselected SNP sets.

There is a rational method to select SNPs for association studies. SNPs can be chosen to tag other SNPs or multi-SNP haplotypes based on local linkage disequilibrium patterns in reference samples. SNPs can be identified from public databases, such as dbSNP, based on putative function or evolutionary conservation across multiple species (displayed through the University of California, Santa Cruz Genome Browser) (Karolchik et al., 2003). SNPs can be discovered by targeted resequencing (such as exons and splice sites). See, for example, the recent report by the Budapest group on a new SNP in the DRD4 promoter region and a rare 27 bp deletion (Ronai et al., 2004; Szantai, Szmola, Sasvari-Szekely, Guttman, & Ronai, 2005). SNPs may also be preselected as part of large high-throughput (and often lower-cost) genotyping platforms and are obtained through a variety of ascertainment schemes (e.g., Affymetrix GeneChip Human Mapping 100 K Set; *www.affymetrix.com/index.affx*). Below we suggest a step-by-step procedure for SNP and repeat selection.

We first mine SNP and haplotype data from HapMap and Haploview (and SNPbrowser) and wherever possible choose a group of htSNPs for each candidate that define the haplotype block structure and maximize the power of the subsequent tests of association but minimize the actual number of SNPs for genotyping. However, for some of the candidates of interest, there is no haplotype block information currently available in HapMap. This impediment can be circumvented by taking ad-

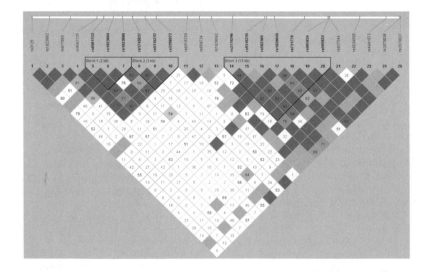

FIGURE 23.3. HTR2a LD PLOT (HaploView) "TAGGER": tagged 25 alleles with mean r^2 of 0.963; 16 SNPs captured 100% of alleles with r^2 > 0.8 using 16 SNPs. Altogether, we would genotype 19 SNPs including the coding regions S and NS.

vantage of the information in the dbSNP database that also includes SNPs with unknown MAF (minor allele frequency). Such SNPs, with undetermined heterozygosity, can be screened using a cost-effective methodology based on a SNaPshot multiplexing. Once the MAF is determined, these SNPs are ready for use in haplotype description and for tests of association. Based on a recent study, it is expected that as many as 50% of screened dbSNPs (Yoshida et al., 2005) will be sufficiently heterozygous to be used in subsequent haplotype analysis.

A Manual of SNP Selection

Log on to the HapMap home page (*www. hapmap.org/cgi-perl/gbrowse/gbrowse/hapmap*) and locate the gene of interest—for example, HTR2A, which spans 66 kilobase pairs. Dump SNP genotype data, which is used in Haplo-View analysis to configure the LD plot and run Tagger. Tagger efficiently identifies htSNPs.

Criteria for SNP Selection

1. Analysis of gene systems with prior evidence for involvement in behavioral disorders (mainly genes involved in regulating neurotransmission of growth factors and arginine vasopressin and serotonergic neurotransmission).
2. All coding SNPs and SNPs that are cited in the literature for association with the phenotype of interest.
3. "Tagging" markers spanning each gene region using Tagger (HaploView) analysis and based in the HAPMAP Caucasian panel.
4. Exclusion of SNPs known to have minor allele frequency (MAF) < .05.
5. Inclusion of validated SNPs whenever possible to fit in with other selection criteria.

Testing a known gene already identified with personality is important because replication of first findings is a critical process in the study of complex diseases. Negative studies especially need to be published toward eventual meta-analyses and the evaluation of the robustness of the original observation. Another worthwhile strategy is to examine new genes that have some functional connection to the gene identified in first findings. For example, having observed an association between DRD4 and

Novelty Seeking, it makes sense to examine other dopamine receptors and other genes involved in dopamine metabolism (Lee et al., 2003; Noble et al., 1998; Thome et al., 1999).

Another important decision is to determine how many markers within the target gene itself are worth genotyping. The complexity of choice is illustrated by the dopamine D4 receptor (DRD4) diagram from the fascinating article by Wang and colleagues (2004) describing the evolutionary history of this gene that we first observed in association with TPQ Novelty Seeking a decade ago (Ebstein et al., 1996) and that marked the onset of the era of molecular genetic personality studies. Although there is increasing interest in the use of SNPs and haplotypes, repeat regions such as the exon3 VNTR and the 120 base pair promoter region repeat in the DRD4 gene continue to be of interest. The exon3 VNTR (Van Craenenbroeck et al., 2005) and the 120 bp promoter tandem duplication (D'Souza et al., 2004) are functional polymorphisms and should be included in any study of this gene. In our enthusiasm for SNPs, STRs should not be overlooked and, as noted by Riley and Krieger (2005), STPs are important targets for evolutionary selection and association with disease. They demonstrate that some untranslated sequence (UTR)-localized STRs exhibit evidence of selection pressure, including STR-coupling preferences, STR conservation, interspecies STR–STR replacements, and STR variants implicated in certain diseases.

Another path toward elucidating the role of a gene in behavior is to examine other phenotypes for association with the gene of interest. For example, the DRD4 is one of the most highly polymorphic human genes and has been associated (in some but not all studies) with many human behavioral phenotypes, including Novelty Seeking (Benjamin, Patterson, Greenberg, Murphy, & Hamer, 1996; Ebstein et al., 1996), Disorganized Attachment (Bakermans-Kranenburg & Van IJzendoorn, 2004; Lakatos et al., 2000), attention-deficit/hyperactivity disorder (ADHD) (Faraone, Doyle, Mick, & Biederman, 2001), Tourette syndrome (Diaz-Anzaldua et al., 2004), fibromyalgia (Buskila et al., 2004), mood disorders (Lopez Leon et al., 2005), substance abuse (Kotler et al., 1997; Luciano et al., 2004; Mel et al., 1998; Muramatsu, Higuchi, Murayama, Matsushita, & Hayashida, 1996), altruism or selflessness (Bachner-Melman et al.,

2005), and eating disorders (Levitan et al., 2004). We suggest that many of these phenotypes are related (perhaps through similar personality profiles), and the emerging picture provides evidence for the robustness of the role of this polymorphic gene in some aspects of human behavior, especially personality.

Population-Based or Family Design Association Studies

A complementary approach to positional cloning by linkage analysis is association or population studies based on candidate genes that make "biological" sense for association with a particular personality trait or traits (see Figure 23.4 for an example of a population-based design). Alternatively, population-based studies may be based on a dense array of SNP markers and haplotypes that are assumed to be in linkage disequilibrium with the true gene that contributes to the trait. Association studies are more powerful statistically than linkage or positional cloning but are thought to generate more false positive results.

An important consideration is whether to use a population design or a family-based approach. A population design facilitates recruitment of subjects but suffers from the conundrum of population stratification (Cardon & Palmer, 2003; Hamer & Sirota, 2000). Population stratification or admixture occurs when there are unknown ethnic groups in the sample that have different allele frequencies as compared with the rest of the subjects. Thus, association between polymorphic genes and personality traits under such circumstances may merely reflect this underlying ethnic diversity rather than true association.

The power and convenience of population-based designs has attracted statistical approaches that detect and/or correct stratification (Bacanu, Devlin, & Roeder, 2000; Pritchard & Rosenberg, 1999). A good example of the application of these statistical designs in personality genetics is the article by Willis-Owen and colleagues (2005). Their article implements Pritchard's method (Pritchard, Stephens, & Donnelly, 2000) for detecting population stratification and used 100 unlinked microsatellite markers derived from the genome-wide scan carried out in this population.

Implementation of these methods needs to be weighed against the cost of additional genotyping and the sample size.

Family-based designs are based on evaluation of the transmission of the associated marker allele from a heterozygous parent to an affected offspring, and testing for deviation from chance transmission under the null hypothesis of no association between the gene and the trait (Spielman, McGinnis, & Ewens, 1993). The transmission disequilibrium test (TDT) design (Figure 23.5) has been extended to genes with multiple alleles such as short tandem repeats (the so-called extended TDT, or ETDT; Sham & Curtis, 1995) as well as quantitative traits (Allison, 1997; Rabinowitz, 1997). The TDT has also been adapted to consider the

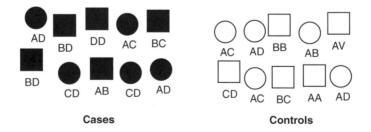

Cases   **Controls**

FIGURE 23.4. Case–control genetic design in population study. The frequency of alleles in the case group is compared with that in the control population. *Allele D is found more frequently among cases than controls.* We can say that a marker allele is associated with a disease if the allele is found more frequently among cases than in the background population, or in a group of unaffected controls. In practical terms, an observed statistical association between an allele and a phenotypic trait will be due to one of three situations: (1) the finding could be due to chance or artifact—for example, confounding or selection bias; (2) the allele is in linkage disequilibrium with an allele at another locus that directly affects the expression of the phenotype; or (3) the allele itself is functional and directly affects the expression of the phenotype.

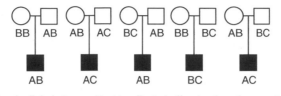

The A allele is transmitted to affected offspring four times out of five.

FIGURE 23.5. Transmission disequilibrium test (TDT). The transmission disequilibrium test was proposed by Spielman et al. (1993) as a robust test for association owing to two loci being tightly linked. To test whether a marker allele exhibits transmission disequilibrium with a disease, parents of affected subjects are observed. If parents who are heterozygous for the allele transmit it to affected subjects on more than 50% of occasions, this is evidence for both linkage and linkage disequilibrium between the marker and disease loci.

effects of more than one genetic loci in contributing to the phenotype, the so-called conditional ETDT (or CETDT) (Koeleman, Dudbridge, Cordell, & Todd, 2000). Many variations of this test are now available, some in relatively user-friendly formats, including the Power-Based Association Test (PBAT; Steen & Lange, 2005), UNPHASED (Dudbridge, 2003), and Quantitative Transmission Disequilibrium Test (QTDT; Abecasis, Cookson, & Cardon, 2000).

Notably in some populations that are claimed to be more ethnically homogenous, such as the Finns (Ekelund, Lichtermann, Jarvelin, & Peltonen, 1999; Ekelund, Suhonen, Jarvelin, Peltonen, & Lichtermann, 2001; Keltikangas-Jarvinen, Raikkonen, Ekelund, & Peltonen, 2004; Lahti et al., 2005; Malhotra et al., 1996), Germans (Becker et al., 2005; Reuter & Hennig, 2005; Soyka, Preuss, Koller, Zill, & Bondy, 2002; Strobel, Gutknecht, et al., 2003; Strobel, Lesch, Jatzke, Paetzold, & Brocke, 2003; Strobel, Spinath, Angleitner, Reiman, & Lesch, 2003), and Japanese (Kato et al., 2005; Matsuzawa, Hashimoto, Shimizu, Fujisaki, & Iyo, 2005; Okuyama et al., 2000; Ronai et al., 2001), many molecular genetic studies are population based, whereas studies in North America with ethnically diverse populations are best based on a family design or, alternatively, a genomic control design should be used.

Haplotype Analysis

Analyses of haplotypes (set of particular alleles at separate loci on the same transmitted chromosome) are predicted to capture more genetic information than single locus analyses, and testing of association between haplotypes and behavioral traits is becoming a mainstay of genetic analysis.

An example of haplotype analysis is a study of the role of catechol-o-methyltransferase (COMT) in neuroticism (Stein, Fallin, Schork, & Gelertner, 2005). Although evidence suggests that rs4680 val108met activity is the predominant factor determining COMT activity in the prefrontal cortex (J. Chen, Lieska, et al., 2004), other variants in the COMT gene may also contribute to the transcriptional efficiency of this gene. In particular, the rs165599 SNP (located near the 3'-UTR of the gene) has been strongly associated with schizophrenia, especially in women, in a large case—control study (Shifman et al., 2002). Those investigators found that a haplotype consisting of rs165599 (3' UTR)—rs4680 (val108met)—rs737865 (near exon #1) was very strongly associated with schizophrenia. In Irish families, a different haplotype, composed of the same three markers but having only the "val" allele in common, was recently reported to be preferentially transmitted to schizophrenic probands (Chen, Wang, O'Neill, Walsh, & Kendler, 2004). These observations are of particular interest because this haplotype is associated with reduced COMT expression in the human brain (Bray et al., 2003).

Stein and colleagues (2005) extended their investigation of the COMT gene and its relationship to neuroticism to include the three SNPs that comprise the haplotype associated with schizophrenia. They also examined a second personality trait, extraversion. Two of the SNPs (rs4680 ("val/met") and rs737865) were significantly associated with (low) extraversion and, less consistently, with (high) neuroticism, with effects confined to women. A significant association between COMT haplotype and (low) extraversion and (high) neuroticism was also observed. Formal testing showed that population stratification did not explain the findings. These data suggest that involvement of the COMT locus in susceptibility to anxiety-related traits (i.e., low extraversion and high neuroticism) is unlikely to be wholly accounted for by the well-studied rs4680 (val108met) polymorphism. Other functional variants may exist that contribute to this relationship. Possible sex-specific effects remain to be further studied and explained.

Gene × Gene Interactions

Single genes account for only a small percentage of the variance in complex traits, and many genes of relatively high prevalence in the population, each of small effect size, are thought to contribute to these phenotypes (Risch, 2000). The importance of gene × gene interaction in complex traits suggests that it is worthwhile to genotype more than one gene rather than relying on the information provided by a single locus.

In our continuing studies of TPQ Novelty Seeking, we examined three common polymorphisms, the DRD4, COMT, and HTTLPR serotonin transporter promoter region deletion/ insertion (Benjamin et al., 2000) in group of 455 nonclinical subjects. Significant interactions (Figure 23.6) were observed by multivariate analysis (COMT × HTTLPR: Hotelling's Trace = 2.3, P = 0.02) and by subsequent univariate three-way analysis of variance (ANOVA) when Novelty Seeking (NS) was the dependent variable: HTTLPR × D4DR (F = 6.18, P = 0.03) and COMT × HTTLPR (F = 4.42, P = 0.03). In the absence of the short HTTLPR allele and in the presence of the high enzyme activity COMT val/ val genotype, NS scores were higher in the presence of the DRD4 seven-repeat allele. The effect of these three polymorphisms on NS was confirmed using a within-families design. Strobel, Lesch, and colleagues (2003) confirmed these findings in a German population. They found that in the group defined by HTTLPR long/long genotype and the COMT val/val genotype, individuals with the DRD4 exon III 7-repeat allele would have higher Novelty Seeking scores than those without the 7-repeat allele.

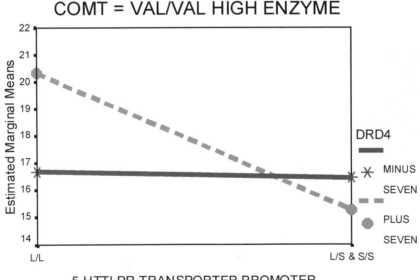

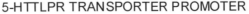

FIGURE 23.6. TPQ Novelty Seeking scores grouped by three polymorphisms: DRD4 exon3 (presence or absence of 7 repeat), the serotonin transporter promoter region short/long 44 bp insertion/deletion, and the COMT val108met SNP. The figure shows how the effect of three genes contribute to the personality trait of Novelty Seeking. Only in the presence of the *COMT* val/val *and SLC6A4* short/short promoter region genotype is the effect of the DRD4 exon III seven repeat observed on TPQ Novelty Seeking.

Power Analysis

Power analyses in behavioral genetics studies are used both prospectively to decide the sample size required to achieve sufficient power and post hoc to interpret the findings, especially important when negative associations are reported. A good example of the value of post hoc analysis is the failure to replicate the role of BDNF in neuroticism personality traits, as discussed in the following paragraph.

Brain-derived neurotrophic factor (BDNF) is important in synaptic plasticity and is involved in stress regulation and physiological response to antidepressant treatment. BDNF is therefore a likely candidate gene for several mood-related phenotypes as well as the personality trait neuroticism (Sen et al., 2003). Willis-Owen and colleagues (2005) failed to replicate the findings of Sen and colleagues (2003) regarding the role of BDNF and anxiety-related personality traits and used a post hoc power analysis to show that their negative study had sufficient power to observe an effect. Simulations of statistical power demonstrated that their sample held sufficient power to enable the detection of extremely small genotypic effects; this population retained 100% power to detect a 0.75% effect size for the main effect and a 4% effect for the gene × environment interaction.

The reader is referred to another good example of the use of post hoc power analysis as part of a critical evaluation of a published study of the serotonin transporter promoter region polymorphism and depression in a presumably ethnically homogeneous German sample (Hoefgen et al., 2005).

Useful Internet sites/programs for genetic power analyses include the Genetic Power Calculator at *webvpn.huji.ac.il/http/0/statgen.iop.kcl.ac.uk/gpc/#qtdt_ins* (Purcell, Cherny, & Sham, 2003), Quanto at *hydra.usc.edu/gxe* (Gauderman, 2003), and PBAT (Steen & Lange, 2005).

Using Environmental Information to Enrich Genetic Association Studies of Personality

Caspi and his colleagues elegantly demonstrated experimentally the long-held notion that the inclusion of environmental information in the genetic model could be critical in showing an association between genes and behavioral traits (Caspi et al., 2002, 2003).

Following Caspi and colleagues, the budding personality geneticist needs to decide whether early environmental information can be assessed in his or her sample. Longitudinal studies are ideal, but have the drawback of entailing high cost and long-term support from granting agencies. A drawback of cross-sectional studies is that they rely on recalled events and environmental factors that may be inaccurately reported by subjects and their parents. Only a few of us are fortunate enough to be able to exploit ongoing longitudinal studies toward unraveling the role of environmental challenges in shaping the gene × environment interactions in personality determination. Others will have to depend on retrospective accounts of early environment or ignore environmental information.

A Finnish study (Keltikangas-Jarvinen et al., 2004) was the first, to our knowledge, to use environmental information toward strengthening the genetic model in the analysis of the role of the dopamine D4 receptor (DRD4) exon3 repeat region and Novelty Seeking (NS). A sample of children drawn from a representative population sample of healthy young Finns ($N = 2149$) was studied from childhood to adulthood over 14 years to determine whether the childhood environment moderated the effect of the DRD4 polymorphism on NS. A significant interaction between the DRD4 alleles and environmental variables was observed. When the childrearing environment was more hostile (emotional distance, low tolerance of the child's normal activity, and strict discipline), the participants carrying any two- or five-repeat alleles of the DRD4 gene had a significantly greater risk of exhibiting NS scores that were above the 10th percentile on a population distribution of 2,149 adult Finnish women and men. The genotype had no effects on NS when the childhood environment was more favorable. Although the results are preliminary, pending replication, they nevertheless provide important information on the long-term effects of nurture and nature on NS temperament. Notably, the exon3 alleles identified in the Finnish study with NS are not the same alleles that we originally observed (Ebstein et al., 1996). This is not an unusual occurrence, and the reader is referred to an insightful article by Neale and Sham (2004), who discuss the somewhat novel concept of gene-based analysis and replication.

The investigation by Willis-Owen and colleagues (2005), discussed above, is also notable for their use of environmental information to enrich the genetic analysis. ANOVA was used to test for gene–environment interaction through the inclusion of a 1 *df* cross-product interaction term. This assumed an additive genetic mode of action and included childhood circumstances (classified as 0, 1, and 2 or more) and adult life events/long-term difficulties (classified as 0, 1, 2, 3, and 4 or more) as continuous variables. Interestingly, although both childhood and adult life events were found to be strongly predictive of adult neuroticism scores, no interaction could be detected between BDNF val66met genotype and either childhood adversity or life events and difficulties of the past 5 years.

Future Directions

The molecular genetic study of personality, similar to the study of other complex traits, stands today at the threshold of a second revolution determined by the high throughput technologies that allow the efficient exploitation of the increasingly dense SNP and haplotype maps now becoming available on public-access Internet sites. We may expect that investigations of personality genetics will employ large populations, using either family-based designs or association studies using checks for population stratification. Extensive genotyping based on an efficient SNP, and repeat selection procedures using the latest bioinformatic methods and coupled with ever more sophisticated statistical techniques for testing association and linkage, should lead to major advances in personality genetics. Although gene × environmental interactions have captured the imagination of behavioral geneticists following the publications by Caspi and his colleagues (Caspi et al., 2002, 2003; Moffitt, Caspi, & Rutter, 2005), we predict that gene × gene interactions also hold great promise for unraveling the genetic contribution to complex behavioral phenotypes.

Acknowledgments

This research was partially supported by the Israel Science Foundation, established by the Israel Academy of Sciences and Humanities, and a Distinguished Investigator grant from the National Alliance for Research on Schizophrenia and Depression (both to Richard P. Ebstein).

Recommended Readings

Benjamin, J., Ebstein, R. P., & Belmaker, R. H. (2002). Genes for human personality traits: Endophenotypes of psychiatric disorders. In J. Benjamin, R. P. Ebstein, & R. H. Belmaker (Eds.), *Molecular genetics and the human personality* (pp. 333–344). Washington, DC: American Psychiatric Publications.

Borecki, I. B., & Suarez, B. K. (2001). Linkage and association: Basic concepts. *Advances in Genetics, 42,* 45–66.

Glazier, A. M., Nadeau, J. H., & Aitman, T. J. (2002). Finding genes that underlie complex traits. *Science, 298,* 2345–2349.

Hariri, A. R., & Weinberger, D. R. (2003). Imaging genomics. *British Medical Bulletin, 65,* 259–270.

Kendler, K. S. (2005). "A gene for": The nature of gene action in psychiatric disorders. *American Journal of Psychiatry, 162*(7), 1243–1252.

Savitz, J. B., & Ramesar, R. S. (2004). Genetic variants implicated in personality: A review of the more promising candidates. *American Journal of Medical Genetics B: Neuropsychiatric Genetics, 131*(1), 20–32.

References

Abecasis, G. R., Cookson, W. O., & Cardon, L. R. (2000). Pedigree tests of transmission disequilibrium. *European Journal of Human Genetics, 8*(7), 545–551.

Allison, D. B. (1997). Transmission-disequilibrium tests for quantitative traits *American Journal of Human Genetics, 60*(3), 676–690.

Bacanu, S. A., Devlin, B., & Roeder, K. (2000). The power of genomic control. *American Journal of Human Genetics, 66*(6), 1933–1944.

Bachner-Melman, R., Gritsenko, I., Nemanov, L., Zohar, A. H., Dina, C., & Ebstein, R. P. (2005). Dopaminergic polymorphisms associated with self-report measures of human altruism: A fresh phenotype for the dopamine D4 receptor. *Molecular Psychiatry, 10*(4), 333–335.

Bakermans-Kranenburg, M. J., & Van IJzendoorn, M. H. (2004). No association of the dopamine D4 receptor (DRD4) and -521 C/T promoter polymorphisms with infant attachment disorganization. *Attachment and Human Development, 6*(3), 211–218; discussion 219–222.

Becker, K., Laucht, M., El-Faddagh, M., & Schmidt, M. H. (2005). The dopamine D4 receptor gene EXON III polymorphism is associated with novelty seeking in 15-year-old males from a high-risk community sample. *Journal of Neural Transmission, 112*(6), 847–858.

Benjamin, J., Li, L., Patterson, C., Greenberg, B. D., Murphy, D. L., & Hamer, D. H. (1996). Population and familial association between the D4 dopamine receptor gene and measures of novelty seeking. *Nature Genetics, 12*(1), 81–84.

Benjamin, J., Osher, Y., Kotler, M., Gritsenko, I., Nemanov, L., Belmaker, R. H., et al. (2000). Association between Tridimensional Personality Questionnaire (TPQ) traits and three functional polymorphisms: Dopamine receptor D4 (DRD4), serotonin transporter promoter region (5-HTTLPR) and catechol o-methyltransferase (COMT). *Molecular Psychiatry, 5*(1), 96–100.

Bierut, L. J., Saccone, N. L., Rice, J. P., Goate, A., Foroud, T., Edenberg, H., et al. (2002). Defining alcohol-related phenotypes in humans: The collaborative study on the genetics of alcoholism. *Alcohol Research and Health, 26*(3), 208–213.

Bray, N. J., Buckland, P. R., Williams, N. M., Williams, H. J., Norton, N., Owen, M. J., et al. (2003). A haplotype implicated in schizophrenia susceptibility is associated with reduced comt expression in human brain. *American Journal of Human Genetics, 73*(1), 152–161.

Buskila, D., Cohen, H., Neumann, L., & Ebstein, R. P. (2004). An association between fibromyalgia and the dopamine D4 receptor EXON III repeat polymorphism and relationship to novelty seeking personality traits. *Molecular Psychiatry, 9*(8), 730–731.

Cardon, L. R., & Palmer, L. J. (2003). Population stratification and spurious allelic association. *Lancet, 361*(9357), 598–604.

Caspi, A., McClay, J., Moffitt, T. E., Mill, J., Martin, J., Craig, I. W., et al. (2002). Role of genotype in the cycle of violence in maltreated children. *Science, 297,* 851–854.

Caspi, A., Sugden, K., Moffitt, T. E., Taylor, A., Craig, I. W., Harrington, H., et al. (2003). Influence of life stress on depression: Moderation by a polymorphism in the 5-HTT gene. *Science, 301,* 386–389.

Chen, J., Lipska, B. K., Halim, N., Ma, Q. D., Matsumoto, M., Melhem, S., et al. (2004). Functional analysis of genetic variation in catechol-o-methyltransferase (COMT): Effects on MRNA, protein, and enzyme activity in postmortem human brain. *American Journal of Human Genetics, 75*(5), 807–821.

Chen, X., Wang, X., O'Neill, A. F., Walsh, D., & Kendler, K. S. (2004). Variants in the catechol-o-methyltransferase (COMT) gene are associated with schizophrenia in Irish high-density families. *Molecular Psychiatry, 9*(10), 962–967.

Cloninger, C. R. (1987). A systematic method for clinical description and classification of personality variants: A proposal. *Archives of General Psychiatry, 44*(6), 573–588.

Cloninger, C. R., Svrakic, D. M., & Prybeck, T. R. (1994). *The Temperament and Character Inventory* (TCI): A guide to its development and use. St. Louis, MO: Center for Psychobiology of Personality.

Cloninger, C. R., Van Eerdewegh, P., Goate, A., Edenberg, H. J., Blangero, J., Hesselbrock, V., et al. (1998). Anxiety proneness linked to epistatic loci in genome scan of human personality traits. *American Journal of Medical Genetics, 81*(4), 313–317.

Cohen, H., Buskila, D., Neumann, L., & Ebstein, R. P. (2002). Confirmation of an association between fibromyalgia and serotonin transporter promoter region (5-HTTLPR) polymorphism, and relationship to anxiety-related personality traits. *Arthritis and Rheumatism, 46*(3), 845–847.

Costa, P. T., & McCrae, R. R. (1992). *Revised NEO Personality Inventory and the NEO Five Factor model.* Odessa, FL: Psychological Assessment Resources.

Curtis, D. (2004). Re-analysis of collaborative study on the genetics of alcoholism pedigrees suggests the presence of loci influencing novelty-seeking near d12s391 and d17s1299. *Psychiatric Genetics, 14*(3), 151–155.

De Fruyt, F., Van De Wiele, L., & Van Heeringen, C. (2000). Cloninger's psychobiological model of temperament and character and the five-factor model of personality. *Personality and Individual Differences, 29,* 441–452.

Diaz-Anzaldua, A., Joober, R., Riviere, J. B., Dion, Y., Lesperance, P., Richer, F., et al. (2004). Tourette syndrome and dopaminergic genes: A family-based association study in the French Canadian founder population. *Molecular Psychiatry, 9*(3), 272–277.

Dina, C., Nemanov, L., Gritsenko, I., Rosolio, N., Osher, Y., Heresco-Levy, U., et al. (2005). Fine mapping of a region on chromosome 8p gives evidence for a QTL contributing to individual differences in an anxiety-related personality trait: TPQ harm avoidance. *American Journal of Medical Genetics B: Neuropsychiatric Genetics, 132*(1), 104–108.

D'Souza, U. M., Russ, C., Tahir, E., Mill, J., McGuffin, P., Asherson, P. J., et al. (2004). Functional effects of a tandem duplication polymorphism in the 5'flanking region of the DRD4 gene. *Biological Psychiatry, 56*(9), 691–697.

Dudbridge, F. (2003). Pedigree disequilibrium tests for multilocus haplotypes. *Genetic Epidemiology, 25*(2), 115–121.

Ebstein, R. P., Novick, O., Umansky, R., Priel, B., Osher, Y., Blaine, D., et al. (1996). Dopamine d4 receptor (D4DR) EXON III polymorphism associated with the human personality trait of novelty seeking. *Nature Genetics, 12*(1), 78–80.

Ekelund, J., Lichtermann, D., Jarvelin, M. R., & Peltonen, L. (1999). Association between novelty seeking and the type 4 dopamine receptor gene in a large Finnish cohort sample. *American Journal of Psychiatry, 156*(9), 1453–1455.

Ekelund, J., Suhonen, J., Jarvelin, M. R., Peltonen, L., & Lichtermann, D. (2001). No association of the -521 C/T polymorphism in the promoter of DRD4 with novelty seeking. *Molecular Psychiatry*, 6(6), 618–619.

Eysenck, H. J. (1970). *The structure of human personality* (3rd ed.). London: Methuen.

Faraone, S. V., Doyle, A. E., Mick, E., & Biederman, J. (2001). Meta-analysis of the association between the 7-repeat allele of the dopamine D(4) receptor gene and attention deficit hyperactivity disorder. *American Journal of Psychiatry*, 158(7), 1052–1057.

Fullerton, J., Cubin, M., Tiwari, H., Wang, C., Bomhra, A., Davidson, S., et al. (2003). Linkage analysis of extremely discordant and concordant sibling pairs identifies quantitative-trait loci that influence variation in the human personality trait neuroticism. *American Journal of Human Genetics*, 72(4), 879–890.

Gauderman, W. J. (2003). Candidate gene association analysis for a quantitative trait, using parent–offspring trios. *Genetic Epidemiology*, 25(4), 327–338.

Hamer, D., & Sirota, L. (2000). Beware the chopsticks gene. *Molecular Psychiatry*, 5(1), 11–13.

Hoefgen, B., Schulze, T. G., Ohlraun, S., von Widdern, O., Hofels, S., Gross, M., et al. (2005). The power of sample size and homogenous sampling: Association between the 5-HTTLPR serotonin transporter polymorphism and major depressive disorder. *Biological Psychiatry*, 57(3), 247–251.

Hysi, P., Kabesch, M., Moffatt, M. F., Schedel, M., Carr, D., Zhang, Y., et al. (2005). Nod1 variation, immunoglobulin e and asthma. *Human Molecular Genetics*, 14(7), 935–941.

Karolchik, D., Baertsch, R., Diekhans, M., Furey, T. S., Hinrichs, A., Lu, Y. T., et al. (2003). The UCSC genome browser database. *Nucleic Acids Research*, 31(1), 51–54.

Kato, C., Kakiuchi, C., Umekage, T., Tochigi, M., Kato, N., Kato, T., et al. (2005). Xbp1 gene polymorphism (-116c/g) and personality. *American Journal of Medical Genetics B: Neuropsychiatric Genetics*, 136(1), 103–105.

Keltikangas-Jarvinen, L., Raikkonen, K., Ekelund, J., & Peltonen, L. (2004). Nature and nurture in novelty seeking. *Molecular Psychiatry*, 9(3), 308–311.

Koeleman, B. P., Dudbridge, F., Cordell, H. J., & Todd, J. A. (2000). Adaptation of the extended transmission/disequilibrium test to distinguish disease associations of multiple loci: The conditional extended transmission/disequilibrium test. *Annals of Human Genetics*, 64(Pt. 3), 207–213.

Kotler, M., Cohen, H., Segman, R., Gritsenko, I., Nemanov, L., Lerer, B., et al. (1997). Excess dopamine D4 receptor (D4DR) EXON III seven repeat allele in opioid-dependent subjects. *Molecular Psychiatry*, 2(3), 251–254.

Lahti, J., Raikkonen, K., Ekelund, J., Peltonen, L., Raitakari, O. T., & Keltikangas-Jarvinen, L. (2005). Novelty seeking: Interaction between parental alcohol use and dopamine D4 receptor gene EXON III

polymorphism over 17 years. *Psychiatric Genetics*, 15(2), 133–139.

Lakatos, K., Toth, I., Nemoda, Z., Ney, K., Sasvari-Szekely, M., & Gervai, J. (2000). Dopamine D4 receptor (DRD4) gene polymorphism is associated with attachment disorganization in infants. *Molecular Psychiatry*, 5(6), 633–637.

Lee, H. J., Lee, H. S., Kim, Y. K., Kim, L., Lee, M. S., Jung, I. K., et al. (2003). D2 and D4 dopamine receptor gene polymorphisms and personality traits in a young Korean population. *American Journal of Medical Genetics B: Neuropsychiatric Genetics*, 121(1), 44–49.

Lee, J. E., Choi, J. H., Lee, J. H., & Lee, M. G. (2005). Gene snps and mutations in clinical genetic testing: Haplotype-based testing and analysis. *Mutation Research*, 573(1–2), 195–204.

Lesch, K. P., Bengel, D., Heils, A., Sabol, S. Z., Greenberg, B. D., Petri, S., et al. (1996). Association of anxiety-related traits with a polymorphism in the serotonin transporter gene regulatory region. *Science*, 274, 1527–1531.

Levitan, R. D., Masellis, M., Lam, R. W., Muglia, P., Basile, V. S., Jain, U., et al. (2004). Childhood inattention and dysphoria and adult obesity associated with the dopamine D4 receptor gene in overeating women with seasonal affective disorder. *Neuropsychopharmacology*, 29(1), 179–186.

Loehlin, J. C. (1992). *Genes and environment in personality development*. Newbury Park, CA: Sage.

Lopez Leon, S., Croes, E. A., Sayed-Tabatabaei, F. A., Claes, S., Van Broeckhoven, C., & van Duijn, C. M. (2005). The dopamine D4 receptor gene 48-base-pair-repeat polymorphism and mood disorders: A meta-analysis. *Biological Psychiatry*, 57(9), 999–1003.

Luciano, M., Zhu, G., Kirk, K. M., Whitfield, J. B., Butler, R., Heath, A. C., et al. (2004). Effects of dopamine receptor D4 variation on alcohol and tobacco use and on novelty seeking: Multivariate linkage and association analysis. *American Journal of Medical Genetics*, 124B(1), 113–123.

Malhotra, A. K., Virkkunen, M., Rooney, W., Eggert, M., Linnoila, M., & Goldman, D. (1996). The association between the dopamine D4 receptor (D4DR) 16 amino acid repeat polymorphism and novelty seeking. *Molecular Psychiatry*, 1(5), 388–391.

Markon, K. E., Krueger, R. F., & Watson, D. (2005). Delineating the structure of normal and abnormal personality: An integrative hierarchical approach. *Journal of Personality and Social Psychology*, 88(1), 139–157.

Matsuzawa, D., Hashimoto, K., Shimizu, E., Fujisaki, M., & Iyo, M. (2005). Functional polymorphism of the glutathione peroxidase 1 gene is associated with personality traits in healthy subjects. *Neuropsychobiology*, 52(2), 68–70.

McCrae, R. R., Costa, P. T., Jr., Ostendorf, F., Angleitner, A., Hrebickova, M., Avia, M. D., et al. (2000). Nature over nurture: Temperament, personality, and life span development. *Journal of Personality and Social Psychology, 78*(1), 173–186.

Mel, H., Horowitz, R., Ohel, N., Kramer, I., Kotler, M., Cohen, H., et al. (1998). Additional evidence for an association between the dopamine D4 receptor (D4DR) EXON III seven-repeat allele and substance abuse in opioid dependent subjects: Relationship of treatment retention to genotype and personality. *Addiction Biology, 3*, 473–481.

Moffitt, T. E., Caspi, A., & Rutter, M. (2005). Strategy for investigating interactions between measured genes and measured environments. *Archives of General Psychiatry, 62*(5), 473–481.

Munafo, M. R., Clark, T., & Flint, J. (2005). Does measurement instrument moderate the association between the serotonin transporter gene and anxiety-related personality traits?: A meta-analysis. *Molecular Psychiatry, 10*(4), 415–419.

Muramatsu, T., Higuchi, S., Murayama, M., Matsushita, S., & Hayashida, M. (1996). Association between alcoholism and the dopamine D4 receptor gene. *Journal of Medical Genetics, 33*(2), 113–115.

Neale, B. M., & Sham, P. C. (2004). The future of association studies: Gene-based analysis and replication. *American Journal of Human Genetics, 75*(3), 353–362.

Neale, B. M., Sullivan, P. F., & Kendler, K. S. (2004). A genome scan of neuroticism in nicotine dependent smokers. *American Journal of Medical Genetics, 132*, 65–69.

Noble, E. P., Ozkaragoz, T. Z., Ritchie, T. L., Zhang, X., Belin, T. R., & Sparkes, R. S. (1998). D2 and D4 dopamine receptor polymorphisms and personality. *American Journal of Medical Genetics, 81*(3), 257–267.

Nyholt, D. R. (2000). All lods are not created equal. *American Journal of Human Genetics, 67*(2), 282–288.

Okuyama, Y., Ishiguro, H., Nankai, M., Shibuya, H., Watanabe, A., & Arinami, T. (2000). Identification of a polymorphism in the promoter region of DRD4 associated with the human novelty seeking personality trait. *Molecular Psychiatry, 5*(1), 64–69.

Pritchard, J. K., & Rosenberg, N. A. (1999). Use of unlinked genetic markers to detect population stratification in association studies. *American Journal of Human Genetics, 65*(1), 220–228.

Pritchard, J. K., Stephens, M., & Donnelly, P. (2000). Inference of population structure using multilocus genotype data. *Genetics, 155*(2), 945–959.

Purcell, S., Cherny, S. S., & Sham, P. C. (2003). Genetic power calculator: Design of linkage and association genetic mapping studies of complex traits. *Bioinformatics, 19*(1), 149–150.

Rabinowitz, D. (1997). A transmission disequilibrium test for quantitative trait loci. *Human Heredity, 47*(6), 342–350.

Reuter, M., & Hennig, J. (2005). Association of the functional catechol-o-methyltransferase val158met polymorphism with the personality trait of extraversion. *NeuroReport, 16*(10), 1135–1138.

Riley, D. E., & Krieger, J. N. (2005). Short tandem repeat (STR) replacements in UTRS and introns suggest an important role for certain STRS in gene expression and disease. *Gene, 344*, 203–211.

Risch, N. J. (2000). Searching for genetic determinants in the new millennium. *Nature, 405*, 847–856.

Roberts, S. B., MacLean, C. J., Neale, M. C., Eaves, L. J., & Kendler, K. S. (1999). Replication of linkage studies of complex traits: An examination of variation in location estimates. *American Journal of Human Genetics, 65*(3), 876–884.

Ronai, Z., Szantai, E., Szmola, R., Nemoda, Z., Szekely, A., Gervai, J., et al. (2004). A novel a/g SNP in the -615th position of the dopamine D4 receptor promoter region as a source of misgenotyping of the -616 c/g snp. *American Journal of Medical Genetics B: Neuropsychiatric Genetics, 126*(1), 74–78.

Ronai, Z., Szekely, A., Nemoda, Z., Lakatos, K., Gervai, J., Staub, M., et al. (2001). Association between novelty seeking and the -521 c/t polymorphism in the promoter region of the DRD4 gene. *Molecular Psychiatry, 6*(1), 35–38.

Schinka, J. A., Busch, R. M., & Robichaux-Keene, N. (2004). A meta-analysis of the association between the serotonin transporter gene polymorphism (5-HTTLPR) and trait anxiety. *Molecular Psychiatry, 9*(2), 197–202.

Schuckit, M. A., Edenberg, H. J., Kalmijn, J., Flury, L., Smith, T. L., Reich, T., et al. (2001). A genome-wide search for genes that relate to a low level of response to alcohol. *Alcoholism Clinical and Experimental Research, 25*(3), 323–329.

Sen, S., Burmeister, M., & Ghosh, D. (2004). Meta-analysis of the association between a serotonin transporter promoter polymorphism (5-HTTLPR) and anxiety-related personality traits. *American Journal of Medical Genetics, 127B*(1), 85–89.

Sen, S., Nesse, R. M., Stoltenberg, S. F., Li, S., Gleiberman, L., Chakravarti, A., et al. (2003). A bdnf coding variant is associated with the NEO personality inventory domain neuroticism, a risk factor for depression. *Neuropsychopharmacology, 28*(2), 397–401.

Sham, P. C., & Curtis, D. (1995). An extended Transmission/Disequilibrium Test (TDT) for multi-allele marker loci. *Annals of Human Genetics, 59*(Pt. 3), 323–336.

Shifman, S., Bronstein, M., Sternfeld, M., Pisante-Shalom, A., Lev-Lehman, E., Weizman, A., et al. (2002). A highly significant association between a comt haplotype and schizophrenia. *American Journal of Human Genetics, 71*(6), 6.

Sirota, L. A., Greenberg, B. D., Murphy, D. L., & Hamer, D. H. (1999). Non-linear association between the serotonin transporter promoter polymorphism and neuroticism: A caution against using extreme samples to identify quantitative trait loci. *Psychiatric Genetics, 9*(1), 35–38.

Soyka, M., Preuss, U. W., Koller, G., Zill, P., & Bondy, B. (2002). Dopamine D4 receptor gene polymorphism and extraversion revisited: Results from the Munich Gene Bank Project for Alcoholism. *Journal of Psychiatric Research, 36*(6), 429–435.

Spielman, R. S., McGinnis, R. E., & Ewens, W. J. (1993). Transmission test for linkage disequilibrium: The insulin gene region and insulin-dependent diabetes mellitus (IDDM). *American Journal of Human Genetics, 52*(3), 506–516.

Steen, K. V., & Lange, C. (2005). Pbat: A comprehensive software package for genome-wide association analysis of complex family-based studies. *Human Genomics, 2*(1), 67–69.

Stein, L. D. (2004). Human genome: End of the beginning. *Nature, 431,* 915–916.

Stein, M. B., Fallin, M. D., Schork, N. J., & Gelernter, J. (2005). COMT polymorphisms and anxiety-related personality traits. *Neuropsychopharmacology, 30,* 2092–2102.

Strobel, A., Gutknecht, L., Rothe, C., Reif, A., Mossner, R., Zeng, Y., et al. (2003). Allelic variation in 5-HT(1A) receptor expression is associated with anxiety- and depression-related personality traits. *Journal of Neural Transmission, 110*(12), 1445–1453.

Strobel, A., Lesch, K. P., Jatzke, S., Paetzold, F., & Brocke, B. (2003). Further evidence for a modulation of novelty seeking by DRD4 EXON III, 5-HTTLPR, and COMT VAL/MET variants. *Molecular Psychiatry, 8*(4), 371–372.

Strobel, A., Spinath, F. M., Angleitner, A., Riemann, R., & Lesch, K. P. (2003). Lack of association between polymorphisms of the dopamine D4 receptor gene and personality. *Neuropsychobiology, 47*(1), 52–56.

Szantai, E., Szmola, R., Sasvari-Szekely, M., Guttman, A., & Ronai, Z. (2005). The polymorphic nature of the human dopamine D4 receptor gene: A comparative analysis of known variants and a novel 27 BP deletion in the promoter region. *BioMed Genetics, 6*(1), 39.

Thome, J., Weijers, H. G., Wiesbeck, G. A., Sian, J., Nara, K., Boning, J., et al. (1999). Dopamine D3 receptor gene polymorphism and alcohol dependence: Relation to personality rating. *Psychiatric Genetics, 9*(1), 17–21.

Van Craenenbroeck, K., Clark, S. D., Cox, M. J., Oak, J. N., Liu, F., & Van Tol, H. H. (2005). Folding efficiency is rate-limiting in dopamine D4 receptor biogenesis. *Journal of Biological Chemistry, 280*(19), 19350–19357.

Wang, E., Ding, Y. C., Flodman, P., Kidd, J. R., Kidd, K. K., Grady, D. L., et al. (2004). The genetic architecture of selection at the human dopamine receptor D4 (DRD4) gene locus. *American Journal of Human Genetics, 74*(5), 931–944.

Willis-Owen, S. A., Fullerton, J., Surtees, P. G., Wainwright, N. W., Miller, S., & Flint, J. (2005). The Val66Met coding variant of the brain-derived neurotrophic factor (BDNF) gene does not contribute toward variation in the personality trait neuroticism. *Biological Psychiatry, 58*(9), 738–742.

Yoshida, R., Fukami, M., Sasagawa, I., Hasegawa, T., Kamatani, N., & Ogata, T. (2005). Association of cryptorchidism with a specific haplotype of the estrogen receptor {alpha} gene: Implication for the susceptibility to estrogenic environmental endocrine disruptors. *Journal of Clinical Endocrinology and Metabolism, 90*(8), 4716–4721.

Zohar, A. H., Dina, C., Rosolio, N., Osher, Y., Gritsenko, I., Bachner-Melman, R., et al. (2003). Tridimensional personality questionnaire trait of harm avoidance (anxiety proneness) is linked to a locus on chromosome 8p21. *American Journal of Medical Genetics, 117B*(1), 66–69.

Zohar, A. H., Lev-Ari, L., Benjamin, J., Ebstein, R., Lichtenberg, P., & Osher, Y. (2001). The psychometric properties of the Hebrew version of Cloninger's Tridimensional Personality Questionnaire. *Personality and Individual Differences, 30*(8), 1297–1309.

Zuckerman, M., & Link, K. (1968). Construct validity for the sensation-seeking scale. *Journal of Consulting and Clinical Psychology, 32*(4), 420–426.

PART III

Analyzing and Interpreting Personality Data

## CHAPTER 24

Toward Modern Psychometrics

Application of Item Response Theory Models in Personality Research

Julien Morizot
Andrew T. Ainsworth
Steven P. Reise

Measurement is central to the work of personality and psychopathology researchers. Traditionally, psychometric analyses have rested on *classical test theory* (CTT) methods. However, an alternative psychometric framework, emerging from cognitive abilities and aptitude assessment domains, also exists: *item response theory* (IRT; Embretson & Reise, 2000; Hambleton, Swaminathan, & Rogers, 1991). IRT is a set of mathematical models designed to conduct psychometric analyses. As such, IRT provides an alternative approach to CTT in terms of evaluating item and scale psychometric properties, scoring individuals, and creating and administering personality scales. Moreover, as we hope to demonstrate, IRT methods can also be used to address substantive issues in personality theory and to indirectly improve the quality of personality research through improving the quality of measurement operations. IRT methods are often referred to as *modern psychometrics* because in large-scale

educational assessment, licensure testing programs, and professional testing firms, they have essentially replaced CTT methods. In contrast, IRT methods have been infrequently applied in personality research.

IRT, like many quantitative methods (e.g., factor analysis), is conceptually simple but technically highly complex. In this overview chapter, we ignore the technical details and nuances of IRT in favor of introducing the basic concepts and applications of IRT methods to personality data. However, it is only fair to warn readers that the judicious use of IRT methods depends highly on familiarity with its more technical aspects (e.g., parameter estimation, prior distributions). Moreover, we focus our discussion on a few simple IRT models applicable to dichotomously scored items. Because the basic ideas do not change when using more complicated IRT models, we do not discuss more complex models applicable to dichotomously scored items, or the half dozen or so potential models for polytomously scored items. Interested readers are directed to the recommended readings provided at the end of this chapter.

Basics of IRT

We begin by outlining three fundamental features that distinguish IRT from CTT, namely, (1) the item response function, (2) the item and scale information functions, and (3) the property of item and person invariance. Throughout the following discussion, we make reference to the concept of a "latent trait" assumed to underlie and, in a sense, cause item responses. One of the key differences between IRT and CTT is that in the latter, individual differences are represented by raw scores, whereas in the former, individual differences are represented by relative standing on a latent variable. It is generally assumed that the latent trait variable representing the construct of interest has a mean of 0 with a standard deviation of 1, and thus individual latent trait estimates typically range from –3 to 3, just like the well-known z-scores. In IRT jargon, the latent trait level is typically denoted by the Greek letter theta (θ).

Item Response Function

The first step in applying an IRT model is to estimate an *item response function* (IRF) for each item of a scale. An IRF is simply a curve that describes how the probability of responding to an item changes as a function of an individual's level on a latent variable. To illustrate, Figure 24.1 displays an IRF for a dichotomously scored item. The horizontal axis represents individual differences in trait level, and the vertical axis represents the probability of responding to the item in the keyed direction. The IRF can be thought of as the fundamental unit in IRT, and establishing an IRF for each item on a scale is the basic goal of an IRT application. In turn, IRFs serve as building blocks to derive other important psychometric properties.

All the various IRT models are simply different equations for modeling the shape and location of an IRF. The simplest of these models is the one-parameter logistic model (1PLM), also called the Rasch model.[1] In a 1PLM model, IRFs are allowed to vary in their *difficulty* or

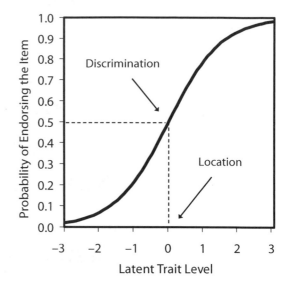

FIGURE 24.1. Item response function (IRF) for an illustrative dichotomous item.

location. An item's location is defined as how much of the latent trait is needed to have a .50 probability of endorsing the item. In practice, item location parameters typically range in value from –2.5 (item endorsed by nearly everyone) to 2.5 (item endorsed only by those very high in the trait). In the IRT literature, the Greek letter beta (β), or simply b, is often used to represent this parameter. Items with high positive locations require higher levels of the trait in order to have a high probability of endorsement. In contrast, items with negative locations elicit high endorsement rates even for individuals with low levels of the latent trait. Figure 24.2 shows two illustrative items from a 1PLM.

More complex IRT models, such as the 2-parameter logistic model (2PLM), allow IRFs to vary in both their location and their steepness. In CTT, the extent to which items vary in the strength of their relation with the construct is usually indexed by an item–test correlation or by the relative size of a factor loading. In IRT, items can vary in their *discrimination*, which is defined as the steepness of the IRF at the item's location. The Greek letter alpha (α), or simply a, is often used to represent this parameter. Items with high discrimination, represented by a steep IRF, are better at differentiating individuals in the latent trait range around the point of inflection. A low discrimination,

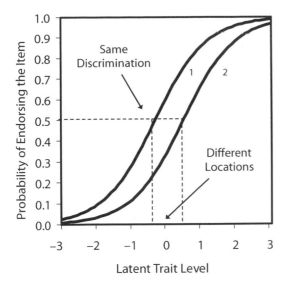

FIGURE 24.2. Two illustrative item response functions (IRFs) from a 1PLM.

represented by a flat IRF, means that the endorsement rates do not change much as a function of individual differences on the latent trait. Item discrimination typically ranges between .50 and 2.0 in personality scales. Figure 24.3 displays two illustrative items from a 2PLM. Notice that these items vary both in their location and in their discrimination.

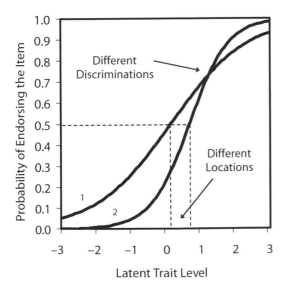

FIGURE 24.3. Two illustrative item response functions (IRFs) from a 2PLM.

Item and Scale Information Functions

In traditional CTT practice, the precision of test scores is often indexed by a sample specific measure of reliability, that is, an estimate of the degree to which observed score variation can be attributed to true score variation. In IRT, the concept of reliability is replaced by that of item and scale information. Once the parameters (i.e., location and discrimination) for an IRF have been estimated, each IRF can then be transformed into an *item information function* (IIF). The IIF indexes the degree to which an item is able to differentiate between individuals at different trait levels. Different items, with different sets of item parameters, provide different amounts of information across the trait continuum. The amount of information an item provides is determined by the discrimination parameter, and where that information is concentrated along the latent trait is determined by the location parameter.

Figure 24.4 displays example IIFs for four dichotomous items. Item 1 has a location parameter of about 0.0 and a discrimination of about 1.0 (a typical value for a personality item). This item best differentiates between individuals with average standing on the latent trait. Item 2 has a similar location as item 1, but a much lower item discrimination value (i.e., 0.25), and thus it provides less information. Item 3 has a very high discrimination value (2.0) and thus provides the most precision, but only in a limited range of the latent trait. Because item 3 has a location parameter above zero, the information is peaked in the

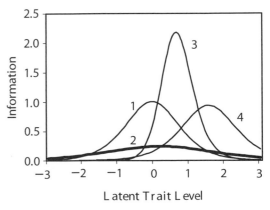

FIGURE 24.4. Item information function (IIF) of four illustrative items.

average-high end of the latent trait. Finally, item 4 has a discrimination of about 1.0 and thus provides an average level of information. However, item 4 has the most positive location parameter, and thus it provides information at the high end of the latent trait. Item 4 would be an excellent candidate for differentiating between high trait individuals, but it would be worthless for differentiating between low trait individuals.

The concept of item information is a critical one in IRT because it plays an important role in two applications. First, the concept of information is useful in scale construction and modification (for further information on the utility of IRT in scale construction, see Simms & Watson, Chapter 14, this volume). For example, a researcher wishing to build a scale to best differentiate between individuals high in the trait would select items with information in the high trait range. Alternatively, if a researcher desired a scale that would provide roughly equal precision across the trait range, a judicious selection of items with different information functions could potentially be used to achieve this goal. A second application of item information is in the domain of computerized adaptive testing (CAT). In a CAT, individuals are administered an item, and then they are "scored" after each response. By scored, we mean that their location on the latent trait continuum is estimated after every item response. Our goal here is not to review the technical details of implementing IRT-based CAT, but merely to note that item information is used to select which items to administer next in a CAT. Specifically, items are administered to individuals that maximize the information at their current trait level estimate.

IIFs are additive, such that the sum of all IIFs forms a *scale information function* (SIF). The SIF shows the precision of a scale across all levels of the latent trait. In IRT, standard errors can vary for individuals at different trait ranges. More precisely, the standard error of measurement is 1 divided by the square root of the scale information at a given trait level. Thus, if scale information varies at different trait levels, standard errors will also differ at different trait levels. Figure 24.5 shows an illustrative SIF and its corresponding standard errors (dotted line). Clearly, this scale better differentiates individuals who are just above average on the latent trait continuum and is less differentiating at either extreme. Figure 24.5 also shows that there are relatively larger

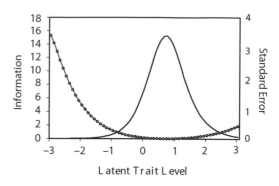

FIGURE 24.5. Scale information function (SIF) and its corresponding standard errors for an illustrative scale.

measurement errors for individuals with very low scores on the latent trait.

Information is arguably the most important feature of IRT for the comparison, construction, and modification of scales. For development or improvement of scales, researchers should inspect the SIF in order to determine where potential measurement gaps exist on the latent trait. The SIF can suggest what kind of new or replacement items would be needed to assess individual differences with more precision across the entire latent trait continuum. Information can also be fruitfully used to shorten scales. By overlaying simultaneously the IIFs from an item pool, a researcher can eliminate items with low information or items that duplicate each other in terms of the information provided. Items can then be retained based on the magnitude and the desired location of the information provided.

Invariance Property

One of the most important advantages of IRT methods rests with the property of item and person parameter invariance. This property underlies many applications of IRT introduced later in this chapter. For instance, the efficient linking of different scales of the same construct, the implementation of CAT, and conducting differential item functioning analysis are directly reliant on the fact that the property of invariance holds.

Invariance in IRT essentially means two things. First, an individual's latent trait level can be estimated on the basis of his or her responses to any set of items with known IRFs.

This person parameter invariance is a tricky concept to understand without delving into the more technical details of IRT. Nevertheless, we find it useful to consider the following. In CTT, there is no person parameter invariance because a person's "true" score depends solely on what items are administered to him or her. This is because the true score scaling is defined by a given set of items. If the items change, the true score scaling would change and people could not be compared with one another if they responded to different sets of items. In IRT, in contrast, the scaling of the latent trait does not depend on any particular set of items. In turn, an individual's "true" standing on the latent trait does not depend on a particular set of items. More critically, and technically, in IRT the parameters of an IRF (i.e., location, discrimination) are defined with respect to the latent trait scaling. Consequently, a response to any set of items can be used to estimate an individual's location on the latent trait.

The second aspect of invariance is item parameter invariance, namely, the idea that the location and discrimination of an item do not depend on the characteristics of the sample. Note that this property never holds in CTT, in which item means, item–test correlations, and test score reliability estimates are all critically influenced by properties of the sample such as the mean level and variability on the construct. In IRT, item parameter estimates are also influenced by the mean level and variability of the sample used to estimate those item parameters. Even in IRT, if a measure of IQ were administered to a group of very low ability, the estimated item location parameters would all be high, whereas if the same measure were given to a high-ability group, the estimated item location parameters would be relatively low. In this sense, IRT item parameter estimates are just as sample bound and noninvariant as CTT indices, such as an item mean and item–test correlation.

However, in IRT, item parameter estimates are assumed invariant, but that invariance is defined *only within a linear transformation*. Consider again an IQ measure. With traditional psychometrics, there would be no way to compare the item statistics across low- and high-ability samples. It would also not be possible to compare item and scale statistics calculated across different samples of individuals (gender, ethnic groups, clinical groups) if those groups are different in level and variability on

the construct. However, in IRT item parameters can be estimated in different samples of individuals, and if the IRT model holds, those item parameter estimates can be transformed, via a linear transformation, to be on a common metric even when the groups differ in mean level and variability on the construct. The IRT item parameter invariance property is of paramount importance in the assessment of differential item functioning, and in scale linking, as discussed further subsequently.

A Step-by-Step Guide for the Application of IRT Models

There is no set script to follow for conducting an IRT analysis. Generally, the process proceeds from data collection, to evaluating assumptions, selecting and fitting a model, and determining the fit, and then finishes with applications. Typically, a researcher works back and forth among these basic stages. In the following sections, we briefly discuss several of the major steps necessary to conduct an IRT analysis. Throughout, some IRT computer programs are cited.

Sample Size Requirements

Although the question, "How many respondents do I need for an IRT analysis?" is frequently asked, there is no gold standard or magic number that can be proposed. The critical issue in an IRT analysis is how well (i.e., precisely) the item parameters (location, discrimination) are estimated. Another way of stating this is to ask, "How well do the estimated item parameters reflect their true population values?" The sample size needed to achieve accurate item parameter estimation depends on a number of factors, including (1) model complexity (e.g., dichotomous items versus polytomous items), (2) the structure of the data (e.g., whether the items are highly discriminating and reflect a single construct), (3) the heterogeneity of the sample, and (4) the particular estimation (e.g., maximum likelihood, Bayesian method used) and imposed constraints (e.g., strength of imposed priors in Bayesian estimation). Given these considerations, some general guidelines can be provided.

First, IRT models with fewer estimated parameters (e.g., 1PLM, Rasch) require smaller samples. For items that are dichotomously scored, some authors suggest that as few as 100 individuals are needed for the 1PLM or Rasch model. More complex models require larger samples. Some authors have suggested as few as 200 respondents for the 2PLM, but a study by Tsutakawa and Johnson (1990) suggests that at least 500 respondents are required. Second, because increasing the number of response categories increases the number of location parameters that need to be estimated, IRT models for polytomous items generally require much larger sample sizes. However, Reise and Yu (1990) reported acceptable item parameter estimates with sample sizes of 500 and more for items with 5-point response formats.

Related to sample size is an additional concern that is especially important in IRT modeling. Recall from the previous discussion that the latent trait scale in IRT is often arbitrarily specified to have a mean value of 0 and a standard deviation of 1 within a specific population (note: a similar identification is generally specified on latent factors in confirmatory factor analysis). Recall also that the IRF (i.e., discrimination and location) is defined with respect to this latent trait scaling. Consequently, defining a priori who the population is, and obtaining a representative sample from that population, is critically important in IRT. It is important because interpreting the item parameter values depends on fully understanding what population was used to identify the latent trait scaling and to estimate the values of the item parameters. The item parameter invariance property discussed previously does not mean that the sample used to estimate the item parameters in IRT is irrelevant. In fact, sample composition in IRT has the same importance as it does in the establishment of *t*-score norms in traditional norming studies for a standardized test.

Computing Basic Descriptive CTT Statistics

The first task is to compute all the basic descriptive CTT statistics. The item means (i.e., proportion endorsed for each response category), interitem and item–total correlations, and internal consistency should be computed. It is important to make sure that there are responses in every category for all items. The total score (i.e., raw summed score) should also be computed, along with its mean, standard deviation, and distributional statistics (i.e., skew-

ness and kurtosis). It is important to conduct these basic analyses because if some items show poor psychometric properties with CTT statistics, they will almost certainly not be good for IRT modeling either. At this stage, if there are only a few items with poor properties, they may be discarded.

Evaluating IRT Model Assumptions

All commonly applied "unidimensional" (one latent trait) IRT models rest on a series of fundamental assumptions. There are two key assumptions that must be evaluated before applying an IRT model, namely, monotonicity of responses and unidimensionality.

Assessing Monotonicity

IRT models such as the 1PLM or 2PLM stipulate that the item responses and the latent trait are related by a monotonic logistic function. That is, as latent trait level increases, the probability of endorsing an item also increases (see Figures 24.1 through 24.3 for examples). Because IRFs are monotonically increasing functions, the data need to be consistent with the model, or else the application of the model makes little sense. To evaluate whether a set of item responses is monotonic, so-called nonparametric IRT models are particularly useful. *Nonparametric* simply means that the estimation of an IRF is dictated by the data only, without the forcing of a specific "parametric" function such as a 1PLM or 2PLM onto the data.

Nonparametric methods assess monotonicity of item response through the analysis of an "empirical" IRF. These methods constitute tests of monotonicity at the raw score level, which provides evidence of monotonicity at the latent trait level (Thissen & Orlando, 2001). For example, programs such as MSP5 (Molenaar & Sijtsma, 2000) or TEST-GRAF (Ramsey, 2000) can be used to evaluate monotonicity. Specifically, MSP5 computes a rest-score (total raw scale score minus the item score = the total of the "rest" of the items) for each item. Then, the proportion of respondents in each rest-score group endorsing the item is tabulated. In other words, the conditional item mean is computed for each rest-score value. MSP5 then computes a statistical test to determine whether these conditional means are monotonically increasing. Apart from sampling fluctuation, the item endorsement rate should increase as the rest-score increases. If this predicted order is violated, that is, if the probability of endorsing the item decreases at some point on the empirical IRF, there is a violation of monotonicity. Such items need to be discarded prior to applying an IRT model. Alternatively, nonparametric (Meijer & Baneke, 2004) or unfolding (Stark, Chernyshenko, Drasgow, & Williams, 2006) IRT models may need to be considered, but these are beyond the scope of this discussion.

Assessing Unidimensionality

It is perhaps tautological to say that a key requirement in the application of a unidimensional (i.e., people differ on only one latent trait) IRT model is to meet the assumption of unidimensionality. A scale is unidimensional when a single latent trait accounts for all the common variance among item responses; that is, one and only one common factor (or latent variable) accounts for the covariance among the items. More technically, unidimensionality is defined through the property of local independence (McDonald, 1999). *Local independence* means that once the latent trait level is controlled for, there are no significant correlations left among the items.

The unidimensionality/local independence constraint is often not a realistic model in practice for complex personality constructs. Acknowledging this, the key question is not whether an item set is strictly "unidimensional or not," but rather whether it is "unidimensional enough." That is, is there enough common variance among the items, such that item parameter estimates are unbiased and accurate? Moreover, can the estimated IRT model be used for scaling individuals on a common trait without that scaling being biased by multidimensionality? We advise readers to not get unduly absorbed with the statistical evaluation of whether an item set is unidimensional or not—no statistic is satisfactory, and the premise that an item response can have one and only one common cause is unrealistic. In our view, one should expect some multidimensionality and focus on the evaluation of how this may bias item parameter estimates, the scaling of individual differences, or the interpretation of applications of IRT.

That being said, there are dozens of methods to assess unidimensionality (Hattie, 1985). As a

general rule, because no single statistical method ever provides a definitive answer about unidimensionality, we recommend the use of several approaches. First, exploratory factor analyses should be conducted (for a review of factor analysis, see Reise, Waller, & Comrey, 2000; Lee & Ashton, Chapter 25, this volume). Alternatively, a scree plot of eigenvalues can be plotted. If a clear knee point emerges after the first factor, this is a sign of unidimensionality. Another commonly used strategy is to compute the ratio of the first to the second eigenvalues. There is no gold standard on what ratio is indicative of unidimensionality, but usually a ratio of 3 or more is considered adequate. Moreover, after extracting a single factor in a confirmatory factor model, residual correlations should be inspected for signs of multidimensionality. Residual correlations above .20 should certainly receive special attention and consideration.

We believe that a fruitful approach for evaluating dimensionality is to use a bifactor modeling approach (Reise & Haviland, 2005; Reise, Morizot, & Hays, in press). In a bifactor model, all items are free to load on a general factor. In addition, each item may load on one secondary or "group" factor. The group factors are specified to be uncorrelated with each other and with the general factor. The bifactor model can be fit with TESTFACT (Wood et al., 2003), which is an IRT-based factor analysis program. Alternatively, more general programs such MPLUS (Muthén & Muthén, 2006) also allows fitting a bifactor model.

We have found in our own research that many existing personality and psychopathology scales are consistent with a bifactor representation. That is, items have strong loading on a general factor, but also have significant loadings on secondary group factors. Frequently, the existence of group factors arises because a scale contains clusters of items with very similar content (Steinberg & Thissen, 1996). For example, a scale of a complex trait like Extraversion may include a set of items dealing with Sociability, a set dealing with Energy, another set dealing with Sensation Seeking, and so on. These item content clusters can induce multidimensionality. The question then becomes, to what degree is that multidimensionality important? There are several ways in which conducting a bifactor analysis can assist in addressing this question.

First, a researcher can compare the factor loadings from a unidimensional factor analysis with those taken from the general factor of the bifactor analysis. If the item loadings are nearly the same across the two models, this suggests that multidimensionality is not biasing the parameters. It can then be considered safe to go ahead and fit a unidimensional IRT model to these data. On the other hand, if the factor loadings are different across the two models, then this suggests that the latent trait (i.e., factor) in the unidimensional model is contaminated by the multidimensionality. In this case, a researcher must consider more complex models such as multidimensional IRT models (Wang, Chen, & Cheng, 2004). Again, however, a discussion of these models is beyond the scope of this chapter.

Second, a bifactor analysis can be used to judge the degree to which the general trait (the one the researcher is trying to measure) accounts for the common variance among the items. Specifically, for a dataset to be appropriate for IRT modeling, the general factor should explain most of the common variance and the group factors should explain relatively little of it. In other words, reliable item response variation should be mostly influenced by the common general construct. For example, Reise and Haviland (2005) applied a unidimensional IRT model to a cognitive problems scale despite the fact that traditional exploratory and confirmatory factor models demonstrated that the scale was highly multidimensional. Their justification was that a bifactor analysis showed the general factor to dominate responses. Specifically, 75% of the common variance was due to the general cognitive problem factor, 3.4% to a memory factor, 1.7% to a concentration factor, 2.6% to a confusion factor, 1.9% to a slow mental functioning factor, 4.2% to an indecision factor, and 0.5% to an unspecified problems group factor.

Local dependence (i.e., multidimensionality) is a very important problem in IRT that must be dealt with (Steinberg & Thissen, 1996). When local dependencies occur, by definition item responses do not depend only on the latent trait of interest, but are also explained by other factors. When local dependencies occur in a scale, it can be problematic for several reasons. First, it can distort item parameter estimates, for example, by resulting in item discrimination parameters that are larger than they should be. In turn, the inflated item discrimination parameters will artificially boost item and scale information, which leads to a scale appearing more precise than it really is. Finally, and most important, the clusters of items that are locally dependent (i.e., highly correlated even after controlling for the common trait) can distort the latent trait, which is obviously a big problem in terms of construct validity. For example, let us say a scale contains an item pair that have almost exactly the same content. In turn, the correlation between these two items is .90, whereas the average correlation between the remaining items is .40. When applying an IRT model (or a factor model), the item pair with the disproportional intercorrelation will define and thus distort the latent trait. That is, these items will have huge item discrimination parameters (or factor loadings in a factor analysis) and appear, falsely, to be the best indicators of the common dimension.

Model Selection and Estimation of Item Parameters

If item response data are deemed appropriate for IRT modeling, the next question is then, which IRT model should be applied? To a large extent the choice of IRT model is driven by the item response format. For dichotomous items, a researcher may select between the 1PLM or 2PLM previously described. There are also more complicated IRT models for dichotomous items that allow the lower asymptote of the IRF to be a non-zero value (i.e., the probability of endorsement for low-trait individuals asymptotes at some non-zero value), or for the upper asymptote of the IRF to be a non-one value (i.e., the probability of endorsement for high-trait individuals asymptotes at some none-one value). Interested readers should see Reise and Waller (2003) for further discussion and substantive interpretation of these more complex three- and four-parameter logistic IRT models.

For items with polytomous formats, a researcher has more options in terms of models to select from. However, the main choice is between models that are extensions of the 1PLM and 2PLM for dichotomous items. The bottom line is that regardless of item format, the researcher has to make a decision between the more parsimonious (but possibly worse-fitting) model, where items vary in their location only, and more complex (but possibly better-fitting) models, where items vary in their location and in their discrimination. Selecting among various IRT models requires an evaluation of the fit of the estimated model to the data. The topic of evaluating fit is covered in the next section.

After selecting a model to estimate, the next step is to use a software program to estimate the item parameters. Item parameter estimation is a very technically complex topic that we cannot do justice to here. Again, interested readers should see the recommendations at the end of this chapter for further reading. Nonetheless, we want to note that programs such as BILOG-MG (Zimowski, Muraki, Mislevy, & Bock, 2003), MULTILOG (Thissen, Chen, & Bock, 2003) and PARSCALE (Muraki & Bock, 2003) are commonly used to estimate IRT model parameters for a wide variety of IRT models. IRT models from the Rasch (1PLM) family can be estimated with programs such as WINSTEPS (Linacre, 2005), CON-QUEST (Wu, Adams, & Wilson, 1998), and RUMM2010 (Andrich, Sheridan, & Luo, 2004). Finally, note also that generalized latent variable modeling programs such as MPLUS (Muthén & Muthén, 2006) and GLLAMM (Skrondal & Rabe-Hesketh, 2004) can also calibrate various kinds of IRT models.

Evaluating Model–Data Fit

Although IRT models have important advantages over CTT, a researcher can use an IRT model with confidence only if it is shown that the estimated model fits the data. All applications of IRT (see the section on applications below), such as evaluating differential functioning of items and scales across different groups (e.g., ethnic groups), linking scores from different scales to be comparable, and computerized adaptive testing, assume that the IRT model fits the data.

In evaluating model–data fit, the basic question is, how well do the estimated item parameters recover the original data? This question is much more tractable in structural equations modeling (SEM) than in IRT modeling (for further information about SEM, see Hoyle, Chapter 26, this volume). In SEM, a researcher wants to know how well a "reproduced" (from the estimated model parameters) covariance matrix agrees with the observed sample covariance matrix. In SEM, a wide variety of fit indices are available to guide the researcher in evaluating how well an estimated model fits the

data. In contrast, in IRT the basic issue is, on an item-by-item basis, how well do the estimated item parameters recover the observed item responses?

As Embretson and Reise (2000) noted, there are no gold standard indices or methods for assessing model–data fit in IRT. Generally, assessment of model–data fit must be thought of as similar to "relative fit" assessment in SEM, because researchers must use various descriptive and inferential statistical tests, theoretical arguments, and their best judgment (see Hambleton et al., 1991). The fit of an IRT model is generally assessed at two different levels, namely, at the item and person levels.

Item Fit

Typically, two methods are used to assess item fit. The first are chi-square tests comparing expected (based on the model) and observed response proportions. Unfortunately, because of their oversensitivity to sample size, the results of these fit tests are generally not considered as strong evidence of model fit. Indeed, with large samples, even minimal differences between expected and observed frequencies may be flagged as significant. Some authors proposed that a better method is to compute chi-square tests for pairs and triplets of items (Chernyshenko, Stark, Chan, Drasgow, & Williams, 2001). Because pairs and triplets are more sensitive to different kinds of misfit, these tests provide a stronger test of item fit. Chernyshenko and colleagues (2001) demonstrated that although several items can show adequate fit based on single-item tests, many item pairs and triples can still show significant misfit. The MODFIT (Stark, 2001) program computes chi-square tests for singles, pairs, and triplets of items.

Graphical methods are also routinely used to inform the study of item fit. In order to build a fit plot, one uses the estimated latent trait levels and separates the individuals into, say, 10 or more strata. Then, the empirical IRF for each item is calculated as follows. For each stratum, the number of individuals who endorsed the item is divided by the total number of individuals. Thus, the data points in the empirical IRF are the proportion of individuals who endorsed the item at different points along the latent trait continuum. Then, the estimated IRF is superimposed with this empirical IRF, and large discrepancies between the two curves are indicative of item misfit. The MODFIT (Stark, 2001) program also builds fit plots for dichotomous and polytomous items.

Person Fit

Another way of examining model–data fit in IRT is at the person level. In person–fit analysis, the focus is on evaluating the degree of consistency between the individual's item response pattern and the estimated item parameters. For example, if an individual with low trait level endorses several items with high location, while he or she does not endorse any item with low location, this response pattern would be considered very unlikely. Several person–fit statistics have been developed for detecting aberrant or highly unlikely item response patterns (Meijer, 2003). These indices quantify the degree to which a response pattern is statistically unlikely, given the estimated IRT model parameters. Some of these indices are available in the WPERFIT program (Ferrando & Lorenzo, 2000).

Evaluating Differential Functioning of Items and Scales

Ultimately, estimated item parameters (location, discrimination) are used for scaling individual differences on a latent trait. Therefore, it is critical that the estimated item parameters be valid for all members of the population under consideration. In other words, a hidden assumption of IRT models is that the IRFs are a valid representation of the relation between trait level and item endorsement rates for all members of the population. If item parameters (i.e., IRFs) are not valid for different groups of individuals (e.g., gender groups), this is termed *differential item functioning* (DIF). Note that DIF does not simply mean a difference in the proportion of endorsement of an item. An item shows DIF if individuals from different groups with the same latent trait level do not have the same probability of endorsing the item.

An important step in evaluating IRT model fit is to determine whether the same set of item parameters can be used to scale all individuals in the population. In other words, conducting an analysis of DIF across different groups of individuals (e.g., gender, ethnic, clinical) is an important part of establishing model fit and, ultimately, its applicability. If some items display

DIF, it may well be impossible to use a common set of item parameters to scale individual differences and to compare scores between individuals from different groups.

It is beyond the scope of this chapter to present detailed guidelines for IRT-based DIF assessment. Interested readers may consult Camilli and Shepard (1994) and Holland and Wainer (1993). In this section we simply outline one common approach to investigating differential item functioning. Specifically, after estimating item parameters separately within two or more groups, using the item parameter invariance property described previously, a linear transformation that places the item parameters estimated separately in each group onto a common metric is found (see Kolen & Brennan, 2004). If there is no DIF, then the item parameters estimated within each group, after transformation, should be exactly the same within sampling error. Many tests for DIF, as well as effect size statistics, are implemented in the DIFpack (William Stout Institute, 1999) and DFIT (Raju, van der Linden, & Fleer, 1995) programs.

If DIF is identified, researchers have three options: (1) Allow the IRFs to vary across groups when scoring individuals, (2) form separate scales for different groups, or (3) delete DIF items from the scale. However, before any of these options are considered, it is imperative to systematically evaluate the impact of DIF items at the overall scale level. Raju and colleagues (1995) developed a method for calculating the impact of DIF items on a scale, that is, to identify *differential scale functioning* (DSF). Indeed, DIF effects can cumulate and have a significant impact at the overall scale level (and thus distorting group comparisons on a common trait), or DIF effects can cancel each other out and ultimately have no impact at the scale level. DSF indices can be estimated with the DFIT program (Raju et al., 1995).

Examples of IRT Applications in Personality Research

As mentioned in the introduction to this chapter, IRT is fundamentally an alternative psychometric framework for the analyses of psychological scales. Nevertheless, IRT methods can also be used as an alternative to CTT for various important applications. In addition, we argue that IRT methods, when applied to certain contexts, can be useful in terms of gaining better traction for studying substantive problems in personality research. For example, as argued below, IRT can potentially provide a superior metric for studying continuity and change.

In the following section, we review some examples of IRT applications in personality research. The goal is not to provide a detailed review of all published work, but rather to point the reader to a few key examples. Six basic applications of IRT are illustrated: (1) evaluation of psychometric properties, (2) scale construction and modification, (3) evaluation of differential functioning of items and scales, (4) linkage of different scales of a common construct, (5) computerized adaptive testing, and (6) improving substantive research using IRT-based scores.

Evaluation of Psychometric Properties

Psychometric tools for analyzing the properties of a scale in a given sample have existed for more than a century. In the last 15 years several researchers have taken a fresh look at personality and psychopathology scales using an IRT perspective. For example, in one of the first studies to apply IRT in a personality research context, Reise and Waller (1990) examined the applicability of IRT models to traits measured by the Multidimensional Personality Questionnaire. More recently, these same authors (Reise & Waller, 2003) examined homogeneous clusters of MMPI-2 items and comparatively evaluated the fit of several IRT models.

Yet those studies are not optimal examples of the value of looking at a scale from an IRT psychometric perspective. In our judgment, a study that exemplifies the value of IRT is the Gray-Little, Williams, and Hancock (1997) examination of the psychometric properties of the Rosenberg Self-Esteem Scale. Among their many interesting findings was that the information function of the Rosenberg Scale is highly skewed and that thus the scale is much better at discriminating individuals with low trait levels than those with high trait levels. Note that this finding implies that summarizing the precision of measurement on this scale via an index such as coefficient alpha would be potentially misleading. Perhaps most interesting was their examination of the IRFs for the Rosenberg items. Inspection of these curves clearly shows that even individuals below average in self-esteem have high probability of responding in the high categories (e.g., responding 4 on a 5-point scale). We believe such findings have substantive consequence in terms of interpreting what scores mean on that scale.

Scale Construction and Modification

There is a paucity of research using IRT to develop new personality scales. Most of what can be found in the literature revolves around two lines of work, namely, developing a new scale using items from existing scales, and shortening existing scales. Typically, scale development and modification using IRT centers on the inspection of item and scale information functions. For example, in community-based research with representative samples, a researcher may desire a relatively flat SIF in order to differentiate individuals with low, average, and high levels of a trait with the same degree of precision. In a clinical context, however, a researcher may desire peaked scale information at the high end of the continuum in order to best differentiate between individuals with very high levels of the trait.

In an instructive study, Fraley, Waller, and Brennan (2000) used IRT to demonstrate how traditional scaling of individuals on adult attachment scales can lead to erroneous conclusions about individual differences. The authors fit an IRT model to different well-known attachment scales and showed that most provide low levels of information. Moreover, most scales provide information at only one end of the latent trait continuum (i.e., the secure [versus insecure] end). Using a pool of 323 items, the authors selected items with information evenly distributed across the entire latent trait continuum in order to develop a new scale of adult attachment with more precision than all the existing scales they studied.

In a recent study, Krueger and colleagues (2004) used symptoms from different existing alcohol problems inventories to develop a new alcohol problems scale. There were a total of 110 symptom items dichotomously scored. The authors fit the 2PLM to identify the location (which they called severity) and discrimination parameters for all symptom items. The SIF revealed that the majority of symptoms provided the most information at the high end of the alcohol problems continuum. The authors also examined the SIF for the different alcohol problems scales separately. They showed that all the alcohol problems scales they studied provided peaked information at the high end of the continuum. Thus, using their large pool of symptoms, the authors constructed a new alcohol problems scale by selecting 12 symptoms that provided optimal information across the entire trait continuum. As argued by the authors, this scale would be best suited for use in large community-sample screening because it provides more precision at all ranges of the alcohol problems continuum.

Differential Functioning of Items and Scales

Testing group differences is a central endeavor in personality psychology. For example, numerous publications specifically address the question of whether there are mean differences in personality between gender, ethnic, or clinical groups. However, in order to draw conclusions regarding substantive differences between groups, researchers must be certain that their scale is not biased (i.e., scores mean the same thing in two or more groups). Using IRT and its inherent item parameter invariance assumption, differential item functioning is rather easy to define. Specifically, an item displays DIF when the IRFs are different for two or more groups. In order to compare people on the same continuum, or to compare groups on the same scale, items must function the same way across the groups. If some items have different IRFs for different groups (i.e., display DIF), this could greatly compromise the evaluation of group mean differences. For this reason, perhaps the most commonly observed application of IRT methods is for the identification of differential item and scale functioning.

For example, Orlando and Marshall (2002) studied DIF with a Spanish translation of the Posttraumatic Stress Disorder Checklist (PTSDC) in a sample of Spanish and English speakers. In order to detect DIF, for each studied item, the authors fit an IRT model constraining item parameters to be equal across the two language groups and then a second model allowing the item parameters to be freely estimated within each group. Six out of 10 items showed DIF for the location parameters, but no item showed DIF in discrimination. This finding indicates that for many items, the response categories do not have the same meaning (i.e., reflect the same severity) across the two language versions. Interestingly, the authors then evaluated the practical impact of

DIF at the scale level. Their analysis revealed that Spanish speakers tend to score slightly lower on the 6 DIF items at the low end of the latent trait, and English speakers tend to score slightly lower at the high end of the trait. However, these differences do not seem to be practically important because they tend to cancel each other out at the scale level.

Waller, Thompson, and Wenk (2000) examined DIF and DSF in the Minnesota Multiphasic Personality Inventory—2nd edition (MMPI-2) scales across Black and White ethnic groups. The authors used two different IRT-based methods to identify DIF. They first calibrated all scales separately for Blacks and Whites using the 2PLM, and then the scores of both groups were linked onto a common metric. Chi-square tests revealed that, on average, up to 38% of the items showed DIF between Blacks and Whites. Nonetheless, the authors showed that this relatively large number of DIF items does not seem to have a significant impact at the scale level. Indeed, although some MMPI-2 traits showed slight differential scale functioning, the authors concluded that these differences should not be considered clinically significant because they did not systematically favor one group over another.

Linking Scores from Different Scales

For important constructs like depression, extraversion, or self-esteem there are many competing scales. Although some may consider this an embarrassment of riches, too many scales all purporting to measure the same construct can cause problems in communication, and maybe even in scientific progress. Similar types of transportability problems occur when ostensibly "gold-standard" scales receive substantial revisions. For example, a longitudinal study may begin, but then 10 years down the line an important scale is revised with new items added and old items deleted. Should the researcher use the new and improved scale and lose comparability with the old one, or should the researcher use the old scale again—the one that needed to be revised? More important, we believe that a major problem in the field is that it is often challenging to intelligently compare results across different studies that use different scales of the same construct. This problem is especially pertinent now because researchers are asking more challenging (and costly) questions about the relation between personality and psychopathology or brain functioning, for example. Hypothetically, will this research make important progress if results change whenever a different scale is used?

IRT cannot solve all measurement problems. However, it does allow researchers to gain traction in resolving certain types of problems. A major potential advantage of IRT is that it can be used to "link" different scales of the same construct onto the same metric. As a consequence, individuals who participate in different studies that use different scales, or in longitudinal studies that use different scales at different ages, can be compared. Note that the ability to link items onto a common metric is the basis of computerized adaptive testing (CAT) used by large-scale testing companies that change the item content of their test banks on a nearly constant basis. Note also that the use of IRT to link scales onto a common metric also makes use of the person parameter invariance property described earlier.

Again, the details of linking two or more scales are complex, and this is not the proper context for providing detailed discussion (for an excellent overview, see Kolen & Brennan, 2004). Here we simply provide an example taken from Orlando, Sherbourne, and Thissen (2000). These authors used an IRT method to link two versions of the Center for Epidemiologic Studies Depression Scale (CES-D). Both versions of the scale were first calibrated (i.e., IRT item parameters were estimated). Then the scales were placed on a common metric using an IRT-based linking procedure. The authors then built a transformation table presenting IRT-based latent trait estimates derived from raw scores. Finally, raw scores that were comparable in both versions of the CES-D were determined. The authors were also able to determine a clinical cutoff score for the new version that was comparable to the original one.

Computerized Adaptive Testing

Another advantage of IRT over CTT is the possibility of conducting CAT (Wainer, 2000). In order to conduct CAT, the researcher needs to have an item pool in which each item has known item parameters (e.g., known IRFs). When a scale is administered through CAT, a standard procedure is to first administer a few items of average location. After obtaining the responses, the computer then estimates the in-

dividual's position on that latent trait. The new estimate is used to select the next item to be presented that provides the most psychometric information, given the individual's current trait level estimate. For this reason, CAT is also frequently called *tailored testing*.

Several researchers have used IRT to develop item pools for CAT in domains such as large-scale educational assessment and health outcome assessment. In these domains, IRT-based CAT has been shown to be at least twice as efficient as paper-and-pencil testing, with little loss of information (Weiss, 2004). Only a handful of researchers examined the applicability of CAT with personality scales. For example, Reise and Henson (2000) examined the performance of a CAT version of the NEO Personality Inventory—Revised (NEO-PI-R). The 30 primary traits of the NEO-PI-R were first calibrated with a polytomous IRT model. The authors showed that with CAT, it is possible to identify the latent trait level of each primary trait by using only four items, rather than the eight items of the paper-and-pencil version, with little loss in measurement precision.

Simms and Clark (2005) studied the applicability of CAT with the Schedule for Adaptive and Non-Adaptive Personality (SNAP). The authors randomly assigned individuals to one of four experimental groups: two consecutive paper-and-pencil administrations, two consecutive CAT administrations, one paper-and-pencil administration followed by a CAT administration, and one CAT administration followed by a paper-and-pencil administration. They showed that with the number of items held constant, both forms of administration provided similar estimates for descriptive statistics, rank ordering of individuals, reliability, and concurrent validity. However, almost 90% of the individuals exposed to both forms of administration preferred the CAT version. Moreover, CAT required approximately 35% fewer items and 60% less testing time. The authors concluded that these are important advantages of CAT, given the fact that the SNAP may be too long (375 items) for most applied or research contexts.

Substantive Research Using IRT-Based Scores

Another application involves the use of IRT-based latent trait levels to explore substantive research questions. Recall that CTT raw summed scores do not provide an interval metric, that is, the distances between adjacent raw scores often vary. IRT-based scoring, on the contrary, transforms the scores into a logit scaling, which is, arguably, closer to an interval scaling. This is important because most statistical methods commonly used in personality and developmental research assume an interval scale (e.g., latent curve modeling). In the following discussion, we cite research that illustrates how the improved scale properties of IRT can result in different substantive conclusions, as compared with the traditional raw summed score.

The study of continuity and change has always been controversial in psychology. This is perhaps the domain where the availability of a "true" interval metric is most important (Khoo, West, Wu, &, Kwok, 2006). In a study cited above, Fraley and colleagues (2000) provided a clear example of the potential advantages of IRT scaling in terms of continuity and change research. First, Fraley and colleagues demonstrated that the measurement precision of commonly used adult attachment scales is concentrated on one side of the latent trait continuum. They then argued that this can lead to biased estimates of rank-order continuity if raw scale scores were used. More critically, using simulation studies, they demonstrated that analyses of change at the raw score level may even lead to opposite conclusions, as compared with analyses using the latent trait scores.

In another study that examined the relation between raw score and IRT latent trait estimates, Reise and Haviland (2005) demonstrated that equal changes on the IRT latent trait continuum do not correspond to equal changes in raw scores on a cognitive problems scale. Specifically, equal changes in raw scores do not imply equal changes on that latent trait. In some trait ranges, a large change in raw scores could translate into a large change in the latent trait, but in other trait ranges, a large change in raw scores implies very little change in the latent trait. Again, these types of findings result from having highly peaked information functions such that some levels of the latent trait are measured with great precision but other levels are measured poorly. Regardless, the critical point is that both the Fraley and colleagues (2000) and Reise and Haviland studies call into question the blind trust researchers often place in raw summed scores as indicators of change.

A second domain where the IRT-based scaling has shown its superiority is in the detection of moderation and mediation effects. The identification of moderators and mediators is a critical task in personality research (for further information, see Chaplin, Chapter 34, this volume). Some recent studies showed that using a latent trait metric is probably superior to using the raw scores. Specifically, simulation research by Embretson (1996) and by Kang and Waller (2005) demonstrates that using the raw score metric can lead to the identification of spurious interactions, whereas using the IRT metric does not. In both studies, the authors noted that this phenomenon is most likely to occur if there is a mismatch between item locations and individual trait levels (e.g., a negative emotionality scale is administered to normal undergraduates).

Conclusion

IRT is an intriguing alternative to traditional CCT methods of analyzing scales and scoring individuals. After presenting the fundamental concepts in IRT and reviewing methods of conducting an IRT analysis, we offered examples of research that illustrate some of the relative strengths of IRT. In summary, IRT potentially can provide (1) a technically superior scaling for measuring individual differences, (2) the ability to compare people who have been administered different scales of the same construct, (3) the ability to create an item pool in order to implement CAT, (4) a clear view of whether measurement precision is or is not equivalent for individuals who are at different levels on a trait, (5) relatedly, tools for intelligently modifying a scale to have certain measurement properties, and (6) a solid method for investigating whether items and scales are functioning the same across different populations.

That is the promise of IRT, but like many advanced and technically sophisticated techniques, there are many devils in the details. Introductory chapters, like this one, cannot possibly review all the potential stumbling blocks. However, as we mentioned in the introduction, it is only fair to warn readers that applying IRT can often present some major challenges, and familiarity with technical topics (e.g., prior distributions, dimensionality assessment) is almost mandatory in order to carry out a competent analysis. More critically, the positive features of IRT, such as DIF assessment, linking scales, and CAT, require that (1) the data meet the assumptions (e.g., unidimensionality, monotonicity) of IRT modeling, (2) the model fits the data (in all groups if studying DIF), and (3) attention be given to a host of other technical requirements that depend on the context. For example, in all linking and CAT, it is important for an item set to have a good spread in the item location parameters.

Beyond these technical concerns, there are also substantive issues that create challenges when applying IRT to personality and psychopathology scales. Recall that IRT originated and is mostly used in large-scale aptitude testing. Consider a typical aptitude construct like spelling or algebra skill. It is easy to think of an almost infinite number of items that could be written to assess individual differences on a spelling or algebra trait. This greatly facilitates the creation of an item pool for CAT. Moreover, substantive knowledge of the cognitive skills involved in, say, algebra, would make the creation of items of low, average, or high difficulty rather straightforward. In turn, being able to create items with a good spread of location parameters would greatly facilitate the creation of a scale that has good information across the entire trait continuum. Finally, with algebra (or spelling, etc.) types of questions, about the only way to obtain a correct response to a difficult item (beyond guessing) is to actually be high on the trait—that is, to know how to solve the problem. It is hard to imagine a scale of a construct like algebra being anything but highly unidimensional.

Now consider a personality construct like extraversion, for example. Once a few questions about participation in social groups, interests in social and exciting activities, and positive affects have been asked, there is not much more to ask. There are only so many ways to ask whether a person generally prefers to spend his or her free time by him- or herself versus being with others. In short, we argue that personality and psychopathology constructs have a limited number of nonredundant indicators, at least as compared with cognitive ability constructs. Thus, it is also much more challenging to create items with location parameters that span the entire trait continuum. For example, what would be a good item to differentiate between individuals very low in depression, or to

differentiate between individuals very high in extraversion? It is also sometimes not quite clear what a high (or low) score on a personality scale might really mean in terms of underlying psychological processes. For example, if a person scores high on a self-esteem scale, it could reflect valid positive self-appraisals, or alternatively, it could result from a defensive reaction. Finally, substantively important personality constructs can be complex and conceptually broad, which may, in turn, tend to produce scales that are multidimensional. Our point is not to bash personality constructs relative to cognitive ability constructs. Rather, we simply want to point out that certain features of constructs more naturally lend themselves to an IRT perspective to psychometrics, whereas certain aspects of personality constructs may create challenges for the application of IRT models.

In summary, the preceding paragraphs were not meant to scare people away from IRT, but to merely give warning—it is not as easy at is sounds. In fact, we strongly encourage the application of IRT models in personality and psychopathology research. As mentioned previously, this is a critical time for measurement. In modern times, personality and clinical researchers are asking interesting, important, and challenging questions about social and biological systems and genetics and how they relate to personality characteristics. Moreover, powerful statistical models are being developed to study important topics such as continuity and change. These new research domains and statistical methods require the best possible measurement tools. We strongly encourage researchers to use IRT to contribute to this exciting future.

Note

1. The 1PLM and Rasch model are mathematically equivalent. In the 1PLM, the person mean is set to 0, and in the Rasch model, the item location mean is set to 0. Some authors (e.g., Wright, 1999) would argue that the Rasch model has nothing to do with other logistic IRT models, but is rather a derivation from measurement axioms. Although arguments contrasting the Rasch model with other logistic IRT models have some merits, we do not discuss this complex issue further and assume that the two models are equivalent.

Recommended Readings

Introductory/Didactical

Embretson, S. E., & Reise, S. P. (2000). *Item response theory for psychologists.* Mahwah, NJ: Erlbaum.

Hambleton, R. K., Swaminathan, H., & Rogers, H. J. (1991). *Fundamentals of item response theory.* Newbury Park, CA: Sage.

Thissen, D., & Wainer, H. (Eds.). (2001). *Test scoring.* Mahwah, NJ: Erlbaum.

Wainer, H. (2000). *Computerized adaptive testing: A primer* (2nd ed.). Mahwah, NJ: Erlbaum.

Advanced/Technical

Baker, F. B., & Kim, S.-H. (2004). *Item response theory: Parameter estimation techniques* (2nd ed.). New York: Marcel Dekker.

van der Linden, W. J., & Hambleton, R. K. (Eds.). (1997). *Handbook of modern item response theory.* New York: Springer-Verlag.

References

Andrich, D., Sheridan, B. E., & Luo, G. (2004). *RUMM2010: Rasch unidimensional measurement models: A Windows-based computer program* [Computer software]. Perth, Australia: Murdoch University.

Camilli, G., & Shepard, L. A. (1994). *Methods for identifying biased test items.* Thousand Oaks, CA: Sage.

Chernyshenko, O. S., & Stark, S., Chan, K. Y., Drasgow, F., & Williams, B. (2001). Fitting item response theory models to two personality inventories: Issues and insights. *Multivariate Behavioral Research, 36,* 523–562.

Embretson, S. E. (1996). Item response theory models and spurious interaction effects in factorial ANOVA design. *Applied Psychological Measurement, 20,* 201–212.

Embretson, S. E., & Reise, S. P. (2000). *Item response theory for psychologists.* Mahwah, NJ: Erlbaum.

Ferrando, P. J., & Lorenzo, U. (2000). WPERFIT: A program for computing parametric person–fit statistics and plotting person response curves. *Educational and Psychological Measurement, 60,* 479–487.

Fraley, R. C., Waller, N. G., & Brennan, K. A. (2000). An item response theory analysis of self-report measures of adult attachment. *Journal of Personality and Social Psychology, 78,* 350–365.

Gray-Little, B., Williams, V. S. L., & Hancock, T. D. (1997). An item response theory analysis of the Rosenberg Self-Esteem Scale. *Personality and Social Psychology Bulletin, 23,* 443–451.

Hambleton, R. K., Swaminathan, H., & Rogers, H. J. (1991). *Fundamentals of item response theory.* Newbury Park, CA: Sage.

Hattie, J. A. (1985). Methodology review: Assessing unidimensionality of tests and items. *Applied Psychological Measurement, 9,* 139–164.

Holland, P. W., & Wainer, H. (Eds.). (1993). *Differential item functioning.* Hillsdale, NJ: Erlbaum.

Kang, S.-M., & Waller, N. G. (2005). Moderated multiple regression, spurious interaction effects, and IRT. *Applied Psychological Measurement, 29,* 87–105.

Khoo, S. T., West, S. G., Wu, W., & Kwok, O. I. (2006). Longitudinal methods. In M. Eid & E. Deiner (Eds.), *Handbook of psychological measurement: A multimethod perspective* (pp. 301–317). Washington, DC: American Psychological Association.

Kolen, M. J., & Brennan, R. L. (2004). *Test equating, scaling, and linking: Methods and practices* (2nd ed.). New York: Springer.

Krueger, R. F., Nichol, P. E., Hicks, B. M., Markon, K. E., Patrick, C. J., Iacono, W. G., et al. (2004). Using latent trait modeling to conceptualize an alcohol problems continuum. *Psychological Assessment, 16,* 107–119.

Linacre, J. M. (2005). *A user's guide to WINSTEPS / MINISTEPS: Rasch-model computer program* (Version 3.60) [Computer software]. Chicago: MESA Press.

McDonald, R. P. (1999). *Test theory: A unified approach.* Mahwah, NJ: Erlbaum.

Meijer, R. R. (2003). Diagnosing item score patterns on a test using item response theory-based person–fit statistics. *Psychological Methods, 8,* 72–87.

Meijer, R. R., & Baneke, J. J. (2004). Analyzing psychopathology items: A case for nonparametric item response theory modeling. *Psychological Methods, 9,* 354–368.

Molenaar, I. W., & Sijtsma, K. (2000). *MSP5 for Windows: A program for Mokken scale analysis for polytomous Items* (Version 5) [Computer software]. Groningen, Netherlands: ProGAMMA.

Muraki, E., & Bock, R. D. (2003). *PARSCALE: IRT-based test scoring and item analysis for graded items and rating scales* (Version 4) [Computer software]. Lincolnwood, IL: Scientific Software International.

Muthén, L. K., & Muthén, B. O. (2006). *Mplus user's guide* (Version 4) [Computer software]. Los Angeles: Muthén & Muthén.

Orlando, M., & Marshall, G. N. (2002). Differential item functioning in a Spanish translation of the PTSD checklist: Detection and evaluation of impact. *Psychological Assessment, 14,* 50–59.

Orlando, M., Sherbourne, C. D., & Thissen, D. (2000). Summed-score linking using item response theory: Application to depression measurement. *Psychological Assessment, 12,* 354–359.

Raju, N. S., van der Linden, W. J., & Fleer, P. F. (1995). IRT-based internal measures of differential measures of items and tests. *Applied Psychological Measurement, 19,* 353–368.

Ramsey, J. O. (2000). *TESTGRAF: A program for the graphical analysis of multiple-choice test and questionnaire data* [Computer software]. Montreal: Department of Psychology, McGill University.

Reise, S. P., & Haviland, M. (2005). Item response theory and the measurement of clinical change. *Journal of Personality Assessment, 84,* 228–238.

Reise, S. P., & Henson, J. M. (2000). Computerization and adaptive administration of the NEO-PI-R. *Assessment, 7,* 347–364.

Reise, S. P., Morizot, J., & Hays, R. D. (in press). The role of the bifactor model in resolving dimensionality issues in health outcomes measures. *Quality of Life Research.*

Reise, S. P., & Waller, N. G. (1990). Fitting the two-parameter model to personality data. *Applied Psychological Measurement, 14,* 45–58.

Reise, S. P., & Waller, N. G. (2003). How many IRT parameters does it take to model psychopathology items? *Psychological Methods, 8,* 164–184.

Reise, S. P., Waller, N. G., & Comrey, A. L. (2000). Factor analysis and scale revision. *Psychological Assessment, 12,* 287–297.

Reise, S. P., & Yu, J. Y. (1990). Parameters recovery in the graded-response model using MULTILOG. *Journal of Educational Measurement, 27,* 133–144.

Simms, L. J., & Clark, L. A. (2005). Validation of a computerized adaptive version of the Schedule for Nonadaptive and Adaptive Personality (SNAP). *Psychological Assessment, 17,* 28–43.

Skrondal, A., & Rabe-Hesketh, S. (2004). *Generalized latent variable modeling: Multilevel, longitudinal, and structural equation models.* Boca Raton, FL: Chapman-Hall/CRC.

Stark, S. (2001). *MODFIT: A computer program for model-data fit.* Urbana-Champaign: Department of Psychology, University of Illinois.

Stark, S., Chernyshenko, O. S., Drasgow, F., & Williams, B. A. (2006). Examining assumptions about item responding in personality assessment: Should ideal point methods be considered for scale development and scoring? *Journal of Applied Psychology, 91,* 25–39.

Steinberg, L., & Thissen, D. (1996). Uses of item response theory and the testlet concept in the measurement of psychopathology. *Psychological Methods, 1,* 81–97.

Thissen, D., Chen, W-H., & Bock, R. D. (2003). *MULTILOG: Multiple-category item analysis and test scoring using item response theory* (Version 7) [Computer software]. Lincolnwood, IL: Scientific Software International.

Thissen, D., & Orlando, M. (2001). Item response theory for items scored in two categories. In D. Thissen & H. Wainer (Eds.), *Test scoring* (pp. 73–140). Mahwah, NJ: Erlbaum.

Tsutakawa, R. K., & Johnson, J. (1990). The effect of uncertainty of item parameter estimation on ability estimates. *Psychometrika, 55,* 371–390.

Wainer, H. (2000). *Computerized adaptive testing: A primer* (2nd ed.). Mahwah, NJ: Erlbaum.

Waller, N. G., Thompson, J. S., & Wenk, E. (2000). Using IRT to separate measurement bias from true group differences on homogeneous and heterogeneous scales: An illustration with the MMPI. *Psychological Methods, 5,* 125–146.

Wang, W., Chen, P., & Cheng, Y. (2004). Improving measurement precision of test batteries using multidimensional item response models. *Psychological Methods, 9,* 116–136.

Weiss, D. J. (2004). Computerized adaptive testing for effective and efficient measurement in counseling and education. *Measurement and Evaluation in Counseling and Development, 37,* 70–84.

William Stout Institute for Measurement. (1999). *DIFPACK—Dimensionality-based DIF/DBF package: SIBTEST, POLY-SIBTEST, CROSSING SIBTEST, DIFSIM, DIFCOMP* [Computer software]. Urbana-Champaign, IL: Author.

Wood, R., Wilson, D. T., Gibbons, R., Schilling, S., Muraki, E., & Bock, R. D. (2003). *TESTFACT: Test scoring, item statistics, and item factor analysis* (Version 4) [Computer software]. Lincolnwood, IL: Scientific Software International.

Wright, B. D. (1999) Fundamental measurement for psychology. In S. E. Embretson & S. L. Hershberger (Eds.), *The new rules of measurement: What every educator and psychologist should know* (pp. 65–104). Hillsdale, NJ: Erlbaum.

Wu, M., Adams, R. J., & Wilson, M. (1998). *ACER ConQuest: Generalized item response modeling software* [Computer software]. Hawthorn, Australia: Australian Council for Educational Research.

Zimowski, M. F., Muraki, E., Mislevy, R. J., & Bock, R. D. (2003). *BILOG-MG: Multiple-group IRT analysis and test maintenance for binary items* (Version 3) [Computer software]. Lincolnwood, IL: Scientific Software International.

## CHAPTER 25

Factor Analysis in Personality Research

Kibeom Lee
Michael C. Ashton

The personality researcher frequently works with a large set of variables that correlate with each other to varying extents. The complexity of such a variable set can create difficulties for data analysis and for conceptual understanding, and one way to reduce this complexity is to use *factor analysis*. Briefly, factor analysis summarizes the relations between many variables by expressing each variable as some unique combination of a few basic dimensions, known as factors. In this way, a group of correlated variables can often be treated as examples of a single, broad factor that is distinct from other factors that summarize other groups of correlated variables. By reducing many variables to a few factors, factor analysis provides a convenient method of simplifying one's variable set for the purpose of examining relations with outside criteria. In addition, factor analysis may stimulate insights into the nature of the variables themselves, by allowing the researcher to identify some common element among variables belonging to the same factor.

In this chapter, we describe the use of factor analysis in personality research and related contexts. First, we begin with a very brief and nontechnical explanation of the mathematical basis of factor analysis. Then we proceed to a discussion of the many decisions to be made by the researcher when using this technique, with special attention to some of the more complex issues that frequently arise. Next, we show an example of factor analysis using real data from a published personality study; readers may prefer to examine this example before reading the more abstract description given immediately below. Finally, we add some closing remarks about the use of this technique.

An Overview of Factor Analysis

Factor analysis attempts to reduce many correlated variables to a few broader dimensions (i.e., factors) that summarize the correlations between those variables.[1] The process of factor analysis generally begins with the calculation of a matrix of correlations among the variables that have been assessed in one's participant sample. This correlation matrix allows one to find the linear combination of variables that will produce the first and largest factor. (See Table 25.1 for an example correlation matrix, derived from a dataset introduced toward the end of this chapter.) Specifically, participants' scores on the first factor can be derived by finding the linear combination of standardized scores (i.e., z-scores) on the variables that has the maximum possible variance. The variance of the factor obtained in this way is known as the *eigenvalue*, and this value thus represents the size of the factor. Because the variance of any linear combination is a function of the correlations among the variables involved, the more strongly correlated the variables are, the larger the first eigenvalue will be. Consequently, those variables that correlate substantially with many other variables in the dataset are likely to be the variables that will be weighted heavily in producing the first factor. (Note that negatively correlated variables will have opposite-signed weights in the equation that produces the first factor.)

The second factor is derived in precisely the same way, except that the variance of the first factor has first been completely removed from all variables in the dataset, so that the correlation matrix being factor analyzed is actually a matrix of residual correlations after the removal of that variance. As a consequence, the second factor is uncorrelated with the first. This process of extracting additional uncorrelated factors can continue until all of the variance of every variable in the analysis is completely exhausted.

In the initial factoring stage, therefore, the variances of k variables are completely redistributed to produce as many as k orthogonal factors, each of which represents the largest possible factor after the preceding ones, and each of which is successively smaller. These characteristics are very useful in making a decision as to how many dimensions are needed to best represent the data (i.e., how many factors to extract), because the first m factors always provide the best summary of the variable set that could be achieved by any possible set of m dimensions. As we discuss later in this chapter, the task of determining the number of factors is one of the most important and difficult in factor analysis, and most decision rules involve in

some way the use of eigenvalues obtained in the initial factor extraction stage.

If we extract a certain number of factors (m), these factors can be described in terms of their correlations with the observed variables. The correlations between variables and factors are called *factor loadings*, and a matrix showing these values is called a *factor loading matrix* (see Table 25.2 in the example at the end of this chapter).[2] A useful way to imagine the factors is to draw them as vectors of unit length drawn at right angles to all other vectors; in this way, a variable's loading on a factor is its projection on a vector, and any given variable can be located by a set of coordinates (i.e., its factor loadings) in the space that is spanned by those factors or dimensions. (See a hypothetical example in Figure 25.1, which shows the locations of six variables within the space of two dimensions, the unrotated factors I and II.)

Note that the variance of each factor (i.e., each *eigenvalue*) can be obtained from a factor loading matrix by finding the column-wise sums of squared factor loadings. For example, in the dataset introduced later in this chapter (see Table 25.2), the eigenvalue of the first unrotated factor (i.e., 4.48) can be obtained by finding $(-.83)^2 + .72^2 + .63^2 + \ldots + (-.26)^2 + .09^2 + .50^2$. On the other hand, the row-wise sums of squared factor loadings are called *communalities*, each of which corresponds to the proportion of variance in a variable that is accounted for by the retained factors. For example, in Table 25.2, the communality of Fun Seeking (.58) can be obtained by finding $.72^2 + .20^2 + .16^2$. If the communality of a given variable is particularly small, this suggests that the variable is poorly accommodated within the space spanned by the retained factors (i.e., dimensions).

Another important feature of the factor loading matrix is that a correlation between any two variables can be estimated by finding the sum of cross-products of factor loadings of the two variables on the same factors. For example, in Table 25.2, the correlation between Neuroticism and Psychoticism can be estimated by calculating the expression $(-.53)(.50) + (.59)(-.01) + (.44)(.55)$. All of the other correlations among variables can be estimated in an analogous way, and the resulting correlation matrix (i.e., often called a *reproduced correlation matrix*) is sometimes compared against the *observed correlation matrix*. Specifically, the reproduced correlation matrix can be sub-

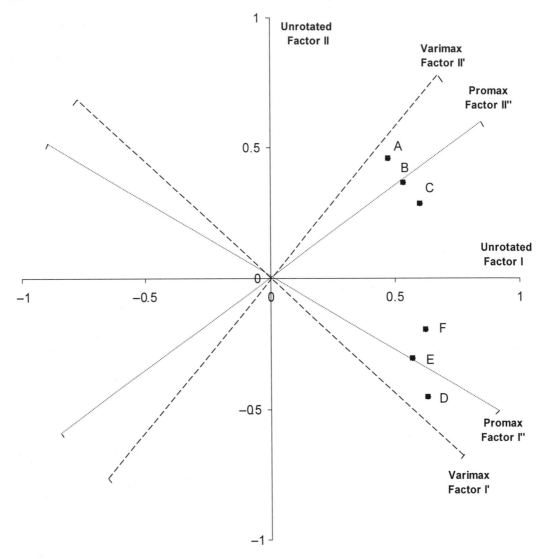

Hypothetical Factor Pattern Matrices

Variables	Unrotated		Varimax Rotated		Promax Rotated ($r_{I''II''} = .43$)	
	I	II	I′	II′	I″	II″
A	.47	.46	.05	.66	−.11	.70
B	.53	.36	.16	.63	.02	.64
C	.60	.28	.26	.61	.13	.60
D	.63	−.45	.77	.08	.81	−.10
E	.57	−.31	.63	.15	.64	.01
F	.62	−.20	.60	.26	.58	.14

FIGURE 25.1. A graphical illustration of factor rotation.

tracted from the observed correlation matrix to produce a *residual correlation matrix*. If all of the elements in the residual matrix are fairly small, one can conclude that the obtained factor structure provides a reasonably good approximation to the data.

The factor loading matrix obtained in the initial factoring process usually produces factors that each show substantial loadings for many variables, rather than very strong loadings for only a few variables each. As a result, inspection of this matrix usually does not allow simple interpretations of the nature of the factors. However, this result is not unexpected, given that the factors obtained in this stage are linear combinations derived exclusively by a criterion of variance maximization, with no attempt made to simplify their meaning.[3] To improve the interpretability of components, the axes of factors can be *rotated* in such a way that each factor will have high loadings for a few variables, and low loadings for the (many) others. (See again the hypothetical results shown in Figure 25.1, where the original factor axes, I and II, have been rotated to new positions, I′ and II′ and also I″ and II″.) Many methods of factor rotation are available, some of which are introduced later in this chapter. As a result of rotation, a new factor loading table is created, and on the basis of this table (see Table 25.3, as derived from the personality dataset described later in the chapter), the rotated factors are interpreted and labeled in such a way as to summarize the common elements of the variables that define each factor. As with eigenvalues, the variances of the *rotated* factors can also be obtained by summing the squared loadings within each factor. These figures are usually labeled *sums of squared loadings (SSLs)* to distinguish them from eigenvalues.

It is important to note that *orthogonally* rotated solutions are mathematically equivalent to each other. This means that the reproduced correlation matrix among variables estimated from such solutions is invariant, that the communality of a variable is invariant, and that the total of the SSLs within a given space is invariant, regardless of the rotational positions of the orthogonal axes. Rotation involves, however, the redistribution of variances in the retained factors, and hence the SSL for each of the factors taken individually will change, depending on the locations of factor axes.

Finally, after the rotated factors are interpreted (and labeled), scores on the factors can be computed for each participant for use in subsequent analyses. A widely used method of obtaining such scores is to compute a mean score across the variables that load strongly on each factor. Other, more sophisticated methods generate a set of factor scoring coefficients that are applied to individuals' scores on the original variables to produce factor scores. The most widely used such method is called the regression approach. In principal components analysis, factor scores obtained from the regression approach have a mean of 0 and a standard deviation of 1; when the factors are orthogonal, these regression-based factor scores will also be orthogonal.

Decision Steps and Complexities

Variable Set

Factor analysis is sometimes conducted simply for the purpose of data reduction, in the sense of summarizing scores on many variables in terms of scores on only a few factors. For example, if a factor defined by several highly intercorrelated personality variables were found to be correlated with some outside criterion, it would be simpler to report this single finding than to report individually the relations of each of those personality variables in turn with the criterion.[4]

Beyond serving the purpose of data reduction, factor analysis can also play a crucial role in identifying a set of basic dimensions that underlie the domain of personality itself. In other words, factor analysis may be used in the search for a few broad dimensions of personality that in combination will summarize the relations among the full array of personality characteristics. But when factor analysis is used for this purpose, the composition of the variable set is of crucial importance: If some aspects of the personality domain are under- or overrepresented, then one's factor solution is likely to omit some important factors or to include extra factors defined by trivially redundant variables. Because personality inventories assess relatively small numbers of variables selected according to the preferences of the test developer, it is highly doubtful that the variables of any inventory (or even any combination of inventories) will provide a representative sampling of the personality domain. For this reason, even the repeated recovery of a given factor solution from a personality inventory does not constitute evidence regarding the structure of personality variation more generally (cf. McCrae & Costa, 1997). It may sometimes be of interest to examine the factors underlying the scales of a given inventory (e.g., Ashton, Jackson, Helmes, & Paunonen, 1998), but again, the obtained factors are chiefly of local interest.

To find the set of major dimensions that summarize the domain of personality variation, it is necessary to analyze a set of variables that comprehensively represents the full personality domain. The only strategy that has thus far been proposed for this purpose is based on the Lexical Hypothesis (e.g., Goldberg, 1981), which is the idea that personality characteristics having importance in person description tend to become encoded in languages as single words (typically as adjectives, or as their corresponding attribute nouns). Following the logic of the Lexical Hypothesis, a complete list of the common personality-descriptive adjectives of a language would approximate a representative sampling of the domain of personality characteristics. Therefore, a factor analysis of ratings on those adjectives should produce a structure corresponding closely to the structure of personality variation itself. Interestingly, there has been some consistency in the factor structures obtained thus far from lexical studies of personality structure conducted in several diverse languages (see, e.g., Ashton, Lee, & Goldberg, 2004; Ashton, Lee, Perugini, et al., 2004; Ashton & Lee, in press).[5]

Between the extremes of simple data reduction and of identifying the structure of the personality domain, the use of factor analysis can also be applied to the exploration of some specified region of the personality domain. For example, a researcher may want to identify and to interpret a few factors that will provide a useful conceptual summary, say, of traits associated with social interactions, or with gender differences, or with cognitive styles. One such case is described later in this chapter, where an examination by Zelenski and Larsen (1999) of affect- and impulse-related traits is reviewed.

Participant Sample

When conducting psychological research, one ought to select a participant sample for which the obtained results will generalize to the population of interest. Ideally, one should have a participant sample that is not only very large but also very similar to the target population in terms of demographic variables that may conceivably influence the factor structure of the variable set in question. But it is also important to keep in mind that the factor structure of a given domain may differ, depending on how broadly one defines the population of interest. For example, large sex differences on some variables may cause those variables to correlate more strongly within a mixed-sex sample than within a sample of men only or of women only. As a result, these sex-correlated variables may define a factor of their own within the mixed-sex sample (or may attract a factor axis upon simple-structure rotation), even though those variables may instead define several different factors within a single-sex sample. Similarly, when participants are drawn from more than one language, cultural, or racial group, or when there are wide variations in the ages or in the socioeconomic statuses of participants, factor structures may also differ from those derived from samples that are homogeneous with regard to those variables.

It is also possible, of course, that the effects of demographic variables in the context of a given variable set will be trivially small. Nevertheless, the researcher should be aware of the potential for sample heterogeneity to influence factor structures. In addition, the researcher should also consider which result is of greater theoretical interest: the solutions derived from samples that are homogeneous on the demographic variable in question, or the solutions derived from heterogeneous samples. The answer to this question will likely depend on how the researcher views the demographic variable in terms of its influence on the variable set to be factor analyzed. If that demographic variable is viewed as a source of variation that is qualitatively different from (and perhaps quantitatively much stronger than) the sources of variation within demographic groups, then the results based on homogeneous samples will likely be of greater interest. But if the demographic variable is instead viewed simply as a contributor of some additional variation on certain personality variables—variation of the same kind as that occurring within demographic groups—then the results based on heterogeneous samples will likely be of greater interest.

Scaling and Distributions of Variables

When the variables to be factor analyzed are individual items rather than multi-item scales, the nature of the item response format influences the distribution of responses to the items and, as a result, may influence the magnitude of the observed relations between those items. For example, when the item response format is dichotomous (e.g., true/false), the maximum possible correlation between items having different response distributions is sharply limited (e.g., an upper bound of $r = .25$ between items having 80% true versus 20% true responses). This problem is reduced somewhat when items use a multipoint response format, such as a 5-, 7-, or 9-point scale. For this reason, we recommend the use of multipoint, rather than dichotomous, item response formats, even though the latter can still be used for factor-analytic purposes. The precise number of response options is not especially important, but participants may prefer an odd number, which allows for exactly neutral responses to some items. An item format having more response options (e.g., 9 points as opposed to 5) will allow for slightly greater precision in responses, but is also slightly more difficult for participants to use.

Depending on the nature of the variable set to be analyzed, researchers may consider the use of *ipsatized* scores (i.e., scores that have been standardized *within subjects*) instead of raw scores when calculating the correlation matrix. The purpose of using ipsatized scores is to prevent the potential distortion of factor analytic results that may result from individual differences in the overall elevation or extremity of responses to items. For example, because participants differ in their average level of endorsement of items, *independently of the content of the items*, variables will tend to correlate positively with each other. As a result, variables that are inherently opposite in nature may be roughly uncorrelated, thus producing two unipolar factors (e.g., *A* and *not A*) rather than one bipolar factor (*A versus not A*). The use of ipsatized scores eliminates this problem, but an important caution should be noted: If one's variable set tends to represent only one pole of each potential factor—for example, if one has many more items for *A* than for *not A*, and for *B* than for *not B*—then ipsatization will tend to remove variance associated with the content areas themselves, in addition to (or instead of) variance due to elevation and extremity of responses.

The decisions discussed above regarding item response options and the ipsatization of variables tend to be somewhat less important when the variables to be analyzed are multi-item scales rather than individual items.[6] First, concerns about the distributions of items are usually less serious, because the averaging or summing of responses across several items tends to produce distributions that approach normality. Second, if the multi-item *scales* each consist of several items, with each scale roughly balanced in terms of positive- and negative-keyed items, then ipsatization of those scales is unnecessary and is likely even to distort the results, unless the scales themselves are scored in such a way as to represent high and low levels of broad underlying factors about evenly.

Inspection of Data

Before conducting a factor analysis, it is important to ensure that one's data have been properly entered and coded; for example, one should check that all participants' responses to an item fall within the possible range of values. Data should also be inspected with a view to identifying the extent to which there are missing data for each participant and each item. In general, when a participant fails to respond to a substantial fraction of the items, this suggests that the data for this participant may be less than meaningful (perhaps due to inattention or to noncompliance) and ought therefore to be removed. Similarly, if a large fraction of participants fail to respond to a given item, this suggests that the data for this item may be less than meaningful (perhaps due to ambiguity or to obscurity) and ought therefore to be removed. When a participant misses only a small fraction of items, or when an item has missing data for only a small fraction of participants, methods such as mean substitution, listwise deletion, or pairwise deletion are usually adequate ways of handling the problem of missing data.

We should briefly note the problem of statistical outliers: When a participant's responses are vastly different from those of other participants—say, being 4 standard deviations (*SDs*) from the mean—*this may suggest that the participant's response is not due to the same sources of variation as those that underlie the distribution of the variable in general. As a re-*

sult, *the researcher may decide to discard the outlier participant's data. Outliers may also be removed on the basis of bivariate relations, as, for example, when a participant has very high levels of two variables that are otherwise strongly negatively correlated. However, we recommend a very* conservative approach to the removal of outlier participants, especially bivariate outliers; if a too liberal threshold is used, the researcher may distort the relations between variables by discarding participants who truly do have relatively unusual combinations of levels of the variables in question.

Stability of Results: Sample Size, Variable Intercorrelations, and Variables per Factor

Factor analyses are usually computed from a matrix of correlations between variables, and the extent to which obtained correlations will fluctuate across samples varies with the square root of sample size. Therefore, larger sample sizes will produce more stable factor analytic results, in terms of the loadings of variables on factors extracted from a correlation matrix.

In addition to sample size, there are other influences on the stability of factor analytic results. Because the sampling fluctuation of a correlation coefficient is smaller when the population value of the correlation coefficient is very large, factor loadings are more stable when the variables defining each factor tend to be strongly intercorrelated (and hence highly loaded on their respective factors). Moreover, because a variable will show less sampling fluctuation in its average correlation with many other variables than in its average correlation with few other variables, factor analytic results are more stable when each factor is defined by many variables. The above features have been demonstrated empirically by Guadagnoli and Velicer (1988), who showed in a series of simulation studies that the stability of factor analytic results depended on (1) the absolute sample size, (2) the loadings of variables on factors in the population, and to a lesser extent, (3) the number of variables per factor.

Many sources suggest that a certain minimum ratio of sample size to number of variables (e.g., 5 to 1, 10 to 1, etc.) is needed to ensure the stability of factor analytic results. These suggestions are entirely misguided. Having a larger number of variables in a factor analysis does *not* undermine the stability of factor analytic results, and neither does the ratio of sample size to number of variables influence the stability of results. Because the sampling error of a correlation coefficient depends on the sample size rather than on the number of other correlation coefficients being calculated, the factor analysis of a large variable set does not require an especially large sample size (see Guadagnoli & Velicer, 1988, for an empirical demonstration).

Component Model versus Factor Model

One decision to be made in conducting a factor analysis is whether to use a *component* model (Hotelling, 1933) or a *factor* model (Pearson, 1901; Spearman, 1904) of factor extraction. For practical purposes, the chief difference between these models is that the component model uses values of 1 in the diagonal elements of the correlation matrix that is factor analyzed, whereas the factor model uses smaller values, typically representing the variance shared between each variable and the rest of the variable set (as indexed, for example, by the squared multiple correlation of each variable with the remaining variables).

When there are many variables to be factor analyzed, the differences between the results yielded by these two methods tend to be small. This is especially so when there is a large ratio of variables to factors, and when the correlations between the variables tend to be large. In such a situation, it does not matter which model is used as a basis for extracting factors.

In the opposing situation, in which there are few variables (and, especially, few variables per factor) and relatively weak correlations between them, then the results obtained from the two methods do tend to diverge, insofar as the component model tends to produce larger loadings for the variables. On one hand, this may be viewed as a disadvantage of the component model, insofar as the loadings obtained in the component model are inflated by variance that is unique to each variable (including error variance), whereas the loadings obtained in the factor model represent more accurately the amount of variance common to the variables. On the other hand, one may view the "inflated" loadings of the component model as advantageous in the sense that they draw one's attention to potential factors that may be underrepresented in a given variable set, and particularly to the variables that are most isolated in the sense of having few strong correlates within that variable set. That is, the factor model provides a faithful representation of the variance shared among the variables, whereas the component model provides a faithful representation of the total variance of the variable set.

How Many Factors to Extract?

The question of how many factors to extract involves a tradeoff between parsimony and completeness in summarizing the relations between the variables. Ideally, one would hope to account for the relations between the variables with only one factor, but then one would need to consider whether the extraction of a second factor would provide a substantially more accurate summary of the relations between the variables. If so, then the same question would be asked regarding the extraction of a third factor, and so on until the extraction of an additional factor would provide such a small increment in accuracy of one's summary that it would not justify the loss of parsimony.

This logic is embodied in the use of several rules for deciding the number of factors to extract. One such rule is simply to extract only those factors whose eigenvalues exceed a certain minimum size. Kaiser (1960) suggested that only factors with eigenvalues of at least 1 should be extracted, because further factors would account for less variance than that of any one variable, and therefore would not help in reducing the variable set to a smaller number of dimensions. However, a fundamental flaw of the eigenvalue-1 criterion is that the number of factors extracted will depend heavily on the number of variables in the analysis, even though the number of variables representing a domain does not change the dimensionality of that domain. More generally, any criterion based solely on eigenvalue size is also highly problematic insofar as one will often extract some factors whose eigenvalues exceed only very slightly those of other factors that are not extracted.

A more defensible strategy for deciding on the number of factors to extract is to consider the *differences* between eigenvalue sizes for successive factors. To use this method, known as the "scree test" (Cattell, 1966), one begins by inspecting the sizes of the eigenvalues of all *k* possible factors in an analysis of *k* variables,

or by inspecting a graph of those eigenvalues (i.e., a scree plot). One then looks, moving from the *k*th factor to the *k* 1th, to the *k* 2th, and so forth, at the increases in the sizes of the eigenvalues. In most datasets, these increases are very small until one is within the ten (or fewer) largest factors. But when there appears the first noteworthy increase or "jump" in the sizes between the eigenvalues of two successive factors, say, the fourth and the third (see the example in Figure 25.2), this suggests that (in this case) three factors should be extracted. According to the logic of the scree test, one would be justified in ceasing the extraction of factors at three, because the extraction of the third factor provides a notably greater increase in accuracy than does the extraction of the fourth factor. In contrast, if one were to extract a fourth factor, there would be little reason not to extract a fifth factor also, or a sixth, and so on.

Although we agree with the reasoning behind the scree test, we should point out that it is sometimes difficult to judge exactly where the first real "jump" in eigenvalues does occur. (For example, even in the example in Figure 25.2, a case may be made for the extraction of four factors, based on the small jump between the fifth and fourth factors.) Sometimes the scree test suggests two or more alternative numbers of factors to extract; for example, a fairly small jump between the eighth and seventh eigenvalues and a much larger jump between the fifth and fourth would suggest the extraction of either four or seven factors. But rather than being a shortcoming of the scree test, this is likely to be a reflection of reality, as a given variable set may be meaningfully summarized, for example, by a set of four larger factors or by a set of seven smaller factors.

Alternative methods for deciding on the number of factors to extract include the parallel test (Horn, 1965), the minimum average partial method (Velicer, 1976), and the chi-square test (Bartlett, 1950, 1951). The parallel test involves the comparison of eigenvalues obtained from the observed correlation matrix with the average eigenvalues obtained from correlation matrices generated at random from a population in which all correlations equal zero and in which the numbers of variables and participants are the same as those of the observed data. One then retains only those factors that have eigenvalues exceeding those of their corresponding random eigenvalues. The minimum average partial method (Velicer, 1976) is

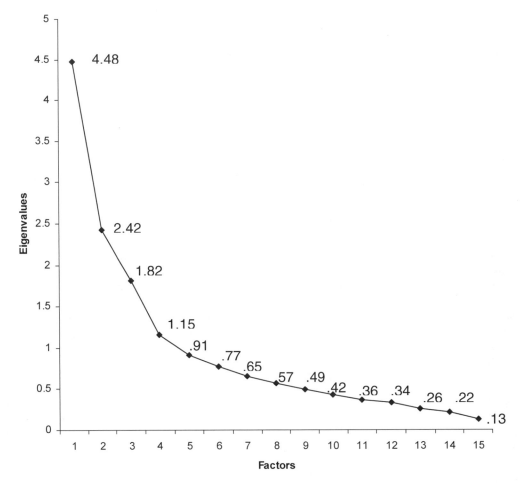

FIGURE 25.2. Scree plots of eigenvalues of factors from the Zelenski and Larsen (1999) dataset.

based on the changes in partial correlations between variables after successive factors are extracted. In this method, components are successively partialled out from the original correlation matrix, and for each resulting matrix of partial correlations, the average of the squared partial correlations is calculated. The optimal number of factors is reached at the point when this average value reaches a minimum.[7]

Finally, a chi-square significance test can be used to determine the number of factors if one adopts the maximum likelihood (or generalized least squares) factor extraction method (cf. the Bartlett test for principal components analysis). In this method, a goodness-of-fit test (i.e., a chi-square test) for a given number of factors is provided by comparing the reproduced correlations between the variables (as derived from the obtained factors) with the observed correla-

tions. Beginning with a one-factor solution, the researcher continues to extract factors until a statistical test first produces a nonsignificant result, because this indicates that the reproduced and observed correlations are not statistically significant. This method, however, has been known to have two crucial problems. First, it requires the assumption of multivariate normality. Second, it is sensitive to sample size, because of its reliance on statistical significance testing. For example, when the sample size is very large, the first solution to produce a nonsignificant result may include a large number of factors, and such a solution would be unparsimonious and unlikely to be replicated in other participant samples or other variable sets.

Once the number of factors to be extracted is determined, it is informative to report the per-

Factor Analysis **433**

centage of the total variance that is accounted for by the retained factors. However, we do not suggest any wholesale guideline regarding the minimum proportion of total variance that should be accounted for by a factor solution, because this proportion depends on the reliabilities of the variables being analyzed and on whether the variables have been selected as "markers" that strongly define a given set of factors. For example, the largest replicated factor solutions found in lexical studies of personality structure, based on relatively unreliable ratings on single adjectives representing the entire personality domain, typically account for 20–30% of total variance. In contrast, the largest replicated factor solutions in investigations of omnibus personality inventories, based on relatively reliable scores on multi-item scales developed specifically as factor markers, typically account for 50–75% of total variance.

Factor Replicability and the Number of Factors to Extract

The aforementioned methods of deciding on the number of factors to extract are all based on attempts to identify a point at which further extraction of factors would provide little improvement in the summary of the relations between the variables. An alternative approach is to identify the largest number of factors that can be replicated across subsamples of participants (see Everett, 1983, for a widely used test of factor replicability). We recommend against the use of such methods as applied to *random split-halves* of a given sample, for the simple reason that the replicability of any factor structure derived from a given variable set is a function of sample size: With a small enough sample, any structure will sometimes fail to be recovered from random split-halves of that sample; conversely, with a large enough sample, any structure will be consistently recovered from random split-halves of that sample.

However, we do recommend the use of tests of factor replicability for the comparison of factor structures obtained from participant samples that differ in some substantive way, such as in their demographic composition or the source of the data. For example, if one wishes to compare factor structures from men and from women, or from Australians and from Americans, or from self-ratings and from peer ratings, then methods such as Everett's test will allow one to determine whether or not a given structure replicates across different types of samples. When a given factor structure is found to replicate across demographic groups or across rating sources, this provides much more impressive evidence of replicability than does any result based on random split-halves of a given sample. (Moreover, if a given solution replicates across demographic groups or across rating sources, then that solution is obviously a meaningful one, regardless of any failure to replicate that solution across the much smaller subsamples created by random split-half divisions of a given sample.) Note that the use of tests to find the number of replicable factors requires the use of very large samples; otherwise, a factor structure may fail to replicate across demographic groups or across rating sources simply because of sampling error.

As noted above, tests of factor replicability can be useful for deciding on the number of factors to extract from a given variable set, at least when replicability is evaluated across very large samples consisting of *different types of participants*. But if one has the more ambitious aim of discovering the dimensionality of a given domain—not simply the dimensionality of a particular variable set taken from that domain—then there is a much more important issue than that of the replicability of a solution across different samples. The important issue, instead, is whether a solution is replicable *across different variable sets* that are each selected to be roughly representative of the domain of interest. If, for example, a given factor structure of personality characteristics is found to be very similar across various sets of indigenous personality-descriptive adjectives taken from different languages, then this provides very impressive evidence of the replicability of the solution, regardless of any results derived from comparisons of samples on the basis of a single variable set. When investigating the dimensionality of a given domain, it is important to remember that one is sampling not only from a population of participants, but also from a population of variables.

A few additional remarks are warranted regarding the decision of the number of factors to extract. First, although it is obviously of much interest to find the "ideal" factor solution underlying one's variable set, it is also useful to examine the nature of the dimensions obtained in solutions involving different numbers of factors (Goldberg, 2006). The researcher can proceed systematically by first examining the first unrotated factor, then the rotated two-factor solution, three-factor solution, and so on, until a solution is reached in which some of the factors become too small and too weakly defined to be interpretable. This exercise is likely to provide the researcher with a deeper understanding of the relations among his or her variables and of the plausibility of various solutions; furthermore, by reporting these results at least briefly, the investigator allows future researchers to compare obtained solutions involving a given number of factors with corresponding solutions derived from other variable sets. And finally, if a given factor solution is of particular interest because of its relevance to the researcher's theoretical expectations, then he or she may well decide to examine that solution in detail, regardless of the results of more algorithmic procedures described earlier in this section.

Rotation of Factors and Simple Structure

After extracting a given number of factors, the researcher will want to interpret those factors. However, when more than one factor is extracted, the patterns of factor loadings of the variables are often quite complex, with many factors being defined modestly by many variables, and with many variables showing moderate loadings on many factors. To better understand the factor space that summarizes the relations among a set of variables, it is convenient to reorient the factor loading matrix to a mathematically equivalent position in which each factor is defined strongly by a few variables and not at all by most variables, and in which each variable defines one factor strongly and the other factors not at all. That is, the researcher rotates the obtained factor axes (or vectors) so that the new positions of those vectors will produce a "simple structure" that allows easier interpretation of the factors, by categorizing variables more neatly within the various factors.

The first decision that must be made when rotating factors is whether to use an orthogonal rotation, in which all vectors will remain at right angles to each other after rotation, or an oblique rotation, in which the angles between the vectors will be allowed to deviate from orthogonality. That is, the factors remain mutually uncorrelated in the case of orthogonal rotations, but are permitted to correlate with each other in the case of oblique rotations. The choice of an orthogonal or an oblique rotation depends mainly on the expected pattern of relations among the variables. If one expects that the domain of variables being analyzed contains at least two roughly independent dimensions (e.g., when analyzing a wide array of personality variables), then an orthogonal rotation is preferred, in order to obtain a simple representation of the location of each variable within the space of those dimensions. If one expects instead that the domain of variables being analyzed is dominated by a single large general factor (e.g., when analyzing cognitive ability variables, or personality variables thought to be facets of one personality dimension), then an oblique rotation is preferred, in order to identify clusters of variables that are particularly closely linked and to indicate the extent to which those clusters are intercorrelated.[8]

When an orthogonal rotation is used, the researcher obtains a single set of factor loadings for each variable on each of the uncorrelated factors. When an oblique rotation is used, there are two matrices representing the relations between the factors and the variables (see Table 25.4, based on data introduced later in this chapter). One matrix, known as the pattern matrix, shows regression coefficients associated with the factors on each variable; therefore, these values represent the unique contributions of the factors to the variance in each variable. The other matrix, known as the structure matrix, shows the correlations between the variables and the factors. (Note that when all factors are uncorrelated, regression coefficients and correlations are identical, which is why orthogonal rotation methods generate only one factor-loading matrix.) It is the pattern matrix that most clearly expresses the simple structure achieved by an oblique rotation; therefore, this matrix should be reported whenever oblique rotations are performed. However, the structure matrix is also informative, by showing how strongly each variable is correlated with each factor; sometimes, a variable having low regression coefficients on a factor will nevertheless be strongly correlated with that factor, if factors are correlated substantially and if the variable has high regression weights on the other factors. In addition to the pattern and structure matrices, a matrix showing correlations between the factors is also generated when one performs an oblique rotation. When space is limited, a researcher may report only the pattern matrix and the factor correlation matrix, because the structure matrix is obtained by finding the product of the pattern matrix and the factor correlation matrix.

For both orthogonal and oblique rotations, there are several alternative algorithms that can be used, depending on one's strategy for achieving simple structure. For orthogonal rotations, the most widely used algorithm is varimax (Kaiser, 1958), which rotates the factors so that the variances of the squared factor loadings on *each factor* are maximized. In other words, varimax simplifies *each factor* by forcing the variables to show either strong loadings or near-zero loadings on a given factor. Another orthogonal rotation algorithm is quartimax (see, e.g., Neuhaus & Wrigley, 1954), which rotates the factors so that the variances of the squared factor loadings of *each variable* are maximized. In other words, quartimax simplifies *each variable* by forcing it to show a strong loading on one factor and near-zero loadings on the other factor(s). A third orthogonal rotation algorithm is equamax (Saunders, 1962), which represents a compromise between the varimax and quartimax algorithms. For most variable sets, the solutions yielded by these algorithms are very similar. However, varimax is usually preferred over quartimax (or the equamax hybrid), because the researcher is usually more interested in simplifying the interpretation of the factors than in simplifying the location of the variables. Moreover, varimax rotations produce rotated factors that are more nearly equal in size (as indexed by the sums of squared loadings) than are those produced by quartimax rotations. Figure 25.1 shows the varimax rotation (see axes I′ and II′) as applied to a hypothetical two-factor space.

For oblique rotations, two of the more widely used algorithms are promax (Hendrickson & White, 1964) and direct oblimin (Jennrich & Sampson, 1966). Promax proceeds by taking a varimax factor-loading matrix and then creating a new matrix by raising the factor loadings to some exponent (but without changing the sign of the loadings). The exponent, called *kappa*, is typically assigned a value of 4; when loadings are transformed in this way, they all become much smaller, but the *ratios* between the (originally) higher and lower loadings become much greater, with the latter becoming vanishingly small and thus simplifying the structure. The factors are then rescaled to return them to their original length, and the

original (varimax) factor axes are rerotated in such a way as to be as close as possible to the factor axes of the new matrix. Note that when variables originally showed substantial secondary loadings, and hence were located in the interstitial factor space rather than along any one factor axis, the newly rotated factor axes will be "pulled" from the original orthogonal positions toward those interstitial regions in which variables are clustered, thereby reducing secondary loadings. As a result, those axes become oblique, as seen in the hypothetical example of axes I″ and II″ in Figure 25.1.

Direct oblimin proceeds by finding a rotation of the initial extracted factors that will minimize the cross products of the factor loadings; this generates a simple-structured solution because those cross products are small when many of the loadings are close to zero. The extent of the correlation among factors in a direct oblimin solution is influenced by a parameter, usually called *delta*, which is typically assigned a value of 0 but can range from large negative values (producing near-orthogonal solutions) to positive values (producing more oblique solutions) that hypothetically range as high as 4/3, but cannot exceed 0.8 in some computer statistical packages. In our experience, the differences between promax and direct oblimin solutions tend to be fairly small, but we tend to prefer promax because of its (relative) conceptual and computational simplicity.

As explained above, the purpose of factor rotation is usually to produce a "simple structure" solution in which each factor is defined by only a few variables, and each variable defines only one factor. For many variable sets, rotational algorithms can approach the ideal of simple structure quite closely, so that there are few variables that divide their loadings across two or more factors. But for many other variable sets, it is inevitable that many variables will divide their loadings across factors, despite the best efforts of rotation algorithms. This reflects the fact that many individual difference variables tend to be distributed throughout the space defined by two or more dimensions, not grouped neatly along a single set of axes within that space. For example, personality characteristics involving interpersonal behaviors and emotional reactions tend to be spread almost evenly throughout a *space* of at least three dimensions (e.g., Saucier, 1992), rather than being isolated along orthogonal axes. As a result, rotational algorithms may yield quite different results depending on the particular set of variables being analyzed, or even depending on the sample on which the variables are measured. It is not entirely clear whether the space mentioned above would be summarized more elegantly by a set of three orthogonal axes representing bossiness, friendliness, and anxiety, or by another set of three orthogonal axes representing shyness, irritability, and sentimentality. In such cases, one may ultimately decide on the preferred factor axis locations by finding the solution that seems to recur most frequently across variable sets and subject samples, or by finding the solution that one finds simplest to interpret theoretically.

In addition to the strategies mentioned above, there is another strategy for factor rotation to be noted, which does not involve a search for simple structure within a given dataset, but rather an attempt to match a previously obtained (or theoretically expected) factor structure as closely as possible. This approach involves the use of a targeted rotation (also called a Procrustes rotation), in which the researcher specifies a "target" matrix of loadings expected on the basis of prior data or theory, and then rotates the obtained factors in such a way as to maximize similarity to the specified target matrix. When applied to oblique factors, this method is highly problematic, because the obtained matrix can be rotated to almost any target solution, no matter how implausible, if the correlations between the factors are allowed to be extreme. When applied to orthogonal factors, however, a close approximation to the target matrix can be achieved only when the obtained matrix is indeed nearly a rotational variant of the target matrix. Formulas for calculating the similarity, or congruence, between the target matrix and the matrix calculated by targeted (Procrustes) rotation of the obtained matrix are provided by Paunonen (1997). The use of orthogonal Procrustes rotation is especially useful when a variable set is not especially simple-structured, and tends to produce rotated factor axes whose locations vary from one sample to another.

Factor Scores or Scale Scores?

After conducting a factor analysis, the researcher often wants to calculate scores for each participant on the obtained factors. When one performs a principal components analysis followed by an orthogonal rotation, perfectly uncorrelated *factor scores* can be calculated (and can be provided by statistical computing packages). When one performs a common factor analysis followed by an orthogonal rotation, the factor scores can only be estimated, usually by multiple regression, so the obtained scores will usually not be precisely uncorrelated. An alternative to calculating (or estimating) factor scores is to calculate *scale scores* corresponding to the obtained factors, by finding the unit-weighted sums of the variables that define each factor most strongly. Even when applied to orthogonal factors, however, this method will usually produce somewhat correlated factors. This is because some of the variables that define a given factor will have nontrivial secondary loadings on another factor, and rarely will these secondary loadings be perfectly balanced between positive and negative values. The fact that one can obtain orthogonal scores by calculating factor scores, but not by calculating scale scores, may be seen as an advantage of the former approach over the latter. However, a disadvantage of calculating factor scores is that the values of the factor scoring matrix are sample dependent and in small samples may fluctuate widely; this problem obviously does not afflict the calculation of scale scores via unit-weighted combinations of items.

Confirmatory Factor Analysis?

Researchers interested in testing hypotheses regarding the factor structure of a given variable set frequently employ confirmatory factor analysis (CFA). In CFA, one specifies a priori one's hypotheses regarding the number of factors, the loadings of variables on factors, and the correlations (if non-zero) between the factors. Using the covariance matrix calculated on the basis of the data obtained from one's subject sample, the CFA algorithm evaluates the extent to which the hypothesized structure matches the observed relations between the variables, reporting one or more "goodness-of-fit" statistics. Since the 1980s, CFA has been widely used in psychological research, including personality research. Despite the widespread popularity of CFA, however, we believe that researchers should be cautious in their use of this method in personality research, for the reasons that we explain here.

First, if the researcher has a large variable set—for example, the several hundred adjectives typically investigated in lexical studies of personality structure—it is implausible that the researcher would be able to specify accurately, on theoretical grounds, the behavior of so many variables. Instead, it is likely that for many of the variables the researcher would either have no real hypothesis or would misspecify their locations.

Alternatively, if the researcher has a smaller variable set—for example, the 10 to 50 scales of a typical omnibus personality inventory—the specification of the theoretically expected loadings of variables is much more feasible. Unfortunately, CFA frequently fails in these cases, by rejecting even those factor structure models that clearly replicate across different types of participant samples and clearly include all of the large factors underlying the variable set. In the case of CFA models that assume perfectly simple-structured, perfectly orthogonal factors, the obtained levels of fit are usually very poor, because most personality variables are not associated univocally with only one factor; however, even when substantial secondary loadings and/or factor intercorrelations are incorporated, the obtained levels of fit still tend to be somewhat poor (see, e.g., McCrae, Zonderman, Costa, Bond, & Paunonen, 1996). One can obtain models having somewhat better levels of fit by incorporating *all* nontrivial secondary loadings, but this undermines the purpose of testing a theoretically driven structure.

As an example of these problems, consider the NEO Personality Inventory—Revised (NEO-PI-R), whose 30 facet-level scales consistently produce the same five large factors in exploratory factor analyses, albeit with some variation in the varimax-rotated locations of two of the factor axes. When CFA is applied to even large-sample data for the NEO-PI-R scales, the result is a rejection of the five-factor model that is hypothesized on a priori grounds, even when the factors are allowed to correlate and even when substantial secondary loadings are specified (McCrae et al., 1996). In contrast, the use of targeted orthogonal Procrustes rotation (described above; see Paunonen, 1997) does support the structural model underlying the NEO-PI-R (McCrae et al., 1996).

Case Example: Zelenski and Larsen (1999)

As an example of the use of factor analysis, consider the dataset of Zelenski and Larsen (1999), who extracted and rotated three factors from a variable set consisting of 15 self-report questionnaire scales, based on responses of 86 persons. Those variables were selected to represent the constructs of the personality theories of Eysenck, Gray, and Cloninger, and together span a variety of traits related to positive and negative emotions and to impulse expression versus control. Note that, because this variable set was selected with the express aim of defining a specified (three-dimensional) factor space, the results of this analysis would not be expected to reveal the structure of the personality domain more generally. However, the analysis would be very useful for the purposes of locating each variable within this theoretically specified subspace of the personality domain, and of providing factor scores that would allow these variables' common relations with external criteria to be summarized concisely.

The correlations between the variables are shown in Table 25.1. Although Zelenski and Larsen reported results based on common factor analysis (specifically, principal-axis factoring), we show here the results based on principal components analysis. As can be seen in the list of eigenvalues and the scree plot in Figure 25.2, the differences in size between adjacent eigenvalues increase noticeably between the fourth and third factors, thus suggesting a three-factor solution. (Actually, as noted earlier, a weaker case may also be made for a four-factor solution, but here we report the three-factor solution, which allows comparison with the theoretically guided analysis by Zelenski and Larsen (1999).)

Table 25.2 shows the loadings and communalities of the variables in the unrotated factor solution. Notice that it is difficult to find a simple interpretation of these factors, as each factor shows moderately high loadings for many diverse variables. For example, the first unrotated factor is defined by variables related to positive affect, to impulse expression, and to (low) negative affect. The second unrotated factor is defined in part by variables related to negative affect, but also by other variables, such as Reward Responsiveness, Reward De-

TABLE 25.1. Correlations between the Personality Variables of Zelenski and Larsen (1999)

	1	2	3	4	5	6	7	8	9	10	11	12	13	14	15
1. Drive	1.00														
2. Behavior Inhibition	-.09	1.00													
3. Reward Responsiveness	.46	.27	1.00												
4. Fun Seeking	.35	-.28	.40	1.00											
5. Extraversion	.30	-.13	.25	.39	1.00										
6. Neuroticism	-.06	.61	.21	-.23	-.24	1.00									
7. Psychoticism	.28	-.27	.12	-.33	.10	-.01	1.00								
8. Punishment Expectancy	.03	.23	.02	-.02	-.08	.50	.00	1.00							
9. Reward Expectancy	.46	-.23	.30	.30	.46	-.40	.10	-.20	1.00						
10. Impulsiveness	.33	-.19	.28	.50	.29	-.07	.57	-.06	.17	1.00					
11. Venturesomeness	.23	-.33	.12	.46	.32	-.33	.32	-.09	.35	.35	1.00				
12. Novelty Seeking	.18	-.28	.21	.43	.35	-.19	.37	-.14	.18	.59	.25	1.00			
13. Harm Avoidance	-.32	.53	-.17	-.52	-.54	.60	-.32	.22	-.54	-.32	-.40	-.52	1.00		
14. Persistence	.30	.22	.29	.07	.17	.07	-.14	.10	.33	-.13	.16	-.33	-.14	1.00	
15. Reward Dependence	.00	.45	.30	.13	.19	.24	-.05	.12	.16	-.06	-.01	.03	.08	.12	1.00

TABLE 25.2. Loadings and Communalities of the Variables in the Unrotated Factor Solution

Variables	Factors 1	2	3	h^2
Harm Avoidance	−.83	.15	.20	.75
Fun Seeking	.72	.20	.16	.58
Novelty Seeking	.63	−.08	.47	.63
Impulsiveness	.63	.09	.56	.72
Reward Expectancy	.63	.20	−.49	.68
Venturesomeness	.63	−.01	−.06	.40
Extraversion	.62	.23	−.20	.47
Drive	.53	.41	−.08	.46
Reward Responsiveness	.35	.70	.04	.62
Behavior Inhibition	−.53	.67	.05	.73
Reward Dependence	−.02	.61	−.03	.37
Neuroticism	−.53	.59	.44	.82
Punishment Expectancy	−.26	.40	.28	.31
Persistence	.09	.52	−.59	.62
Psychoticism	.50	−.01	.55	.55
Eigenvalues	4.48	2.42	1.82	

pendence, and Persistence. The third unrotated factor is defined by variables related to impulse expression, and also by (low) Persistence and (low) Reward Expectancy.

When these three factors are rotated to a varimax solution (see Table 25.3), the interpretation of factors becomes much clearer. The factors of the rotated solution are defined by variables assessing (1) positive affect and sensitivity to rewards, (2) impulsivity and thrill-seeking, and (3) negative affect and sensitivity to punishments, respectively. Comparison of the varimax-rotated principal components of Table 25.2 with the varimax-rotated common (principal axis) factors reported by Zelenski and Larsen (1999, Table 2) reveals a very similar pattern of results, apart from an (unimportant) change in the order of the first and second *rotated* factors. Factor loadings are somewhat higher in the principal components analysis than in the common factor analysis (see the earlier section on the factor and component models), but even in the current example the differences are rather minor, in spite of the small number of variables per factor and the somewhat low proportions of common variance for some of those variables. Note that although we have not reported the communalities of the variables in Table 25.3, these values are identical to those of Table 25.2, because the process of rotating factors does not change the communalities of variables.

Alternatively, an oblique rotation of the factors may be performed. Table 25.4 shows the results of a promax rotation of the three extracted factors. For this oblique rotation, we have reported three matrices: first, the pattern matrix shows the regression weights of each factor on each variable; second, the structure matrix shows the correlations of each factor with each variable; third, the factor correlation matrix shows the correlations between the three factors. Note that the correlations between the three factors are rather small, with the highest correlations having absolute values of approximately .30; the pattern and structure matrices are thus relatively similar to each other and to the rotated matrix from the varimax solution of Table 25.4. In this case, the use of an orthogonal rotation (rather than oblique) seems justified: Given that there is little indication of a general higher-order factor, and given that most variables show a reasonably simple structure with respect to the varimax factor axes, there is little need to abandon the conceptual simplicity of the solution defined by mutually orthogonal factors.

The factor analysis reported by Zelenski and Larsen (1999) illustrates both the conceptual and the practical usefulness of the technique. From a conceptual standpoint, the three factors represent the major constructs that are shared among several theories of the causal basis of individual differences in emotion- and impulse-

TABLE 25.3. Loadings of the Variables in the Varimax-Rotated Factor Solution

Variables	Factors 1	2	3
Reward Expectancy	.76	.03	−.30
Persistence	.66	−.40	.16
Extraversion	.62	.24	−.16
Drive	.61	.27	.07
Reward Responsiveness	.61	.25	.44
Venturesomeness	.42	.36	−.30
Impulsiveness	.16	.84	.01
Novelty Seeking	.11	.77	−.16
Psychoticism	.03	.74	−.02
Fun Seeking	.48	.59	−.09
Neuroticism	−.22	−.02	.88
Behavior Inhibition	.03	−.32	.79
Harm Avoidance	−.54	−.39	.56
Punishment Expectancy	−.08	.04	.55
Reward Dependence	.35	−.04	.49
Sum of squared loadings (SSL)	3.07	2.93	2.72

TABLE 25.4. Pattern and Structure Coefficients of the Variables in the Promax-Rotated Factor Solution, and Correlations between the Factors

Variables	Pattern coefficients 1	2	3	Structure coefficients (factor loadings) 1	2	3
Reward Expectancy	.78	−.15	−.28	.77	.18	−.36
Persistence	.76	−.52	.14	.57	−.32	.17
Reward Responsiveness	.62	.23	.51	.61	.27	.35
Extraversion	.61	.13	−.11	.66	.35	−.24
Drive	.60	.20	.13	.65	.35	−.02
Venturesomeness	.37	.26	−.25	.49	.45	−.39
Impulsiveness	.04	.87	.13	.30	.84	−.13
Psychoticism	−.08	.79	.08	.15	.74	−.14
Novelty Seeking	−.01	.78	−.06	.24	.79	−.29
Fun Seeking	.41	.53	.00	.58	.66	−.22
Neuroticism	−.18	.16	.90	−.27	−.17	.88
Behavior Inhibition	.12	−.21	.78	−.07	−.41	.83
Punishment Expectancy	−.06	.14	.58	−.10	−.05	.54
Reward Dependence	.40	−.03	.52	.31	−.06	.47
Harm Avoidance	−.48	−.23	.51	−.63	−.53	.65
Sum of squared loadings (SSL)				3.48	3.45	3.05

	Factor correlations 1	2	3
Factor 1	1.00		
Factor 2	.32	1.00	
Factor 3	−.15	−.30	1.00

related personality traits. From a practical standpoint, the calculation of factor scores for the three rotated factors allowed Zelenski and Larsen an efficient means of examining the relations between this variable set and various dependent variables, including participants' emotional responses to a laboratory mood induction.

Summary

Factor analysis is a useful tool in the study of personality and of individual differences more generally. The purpose of this technique is to reduce a large set of correlated variables to a much smaller set of dimensions. Each of those dimensions, or factors, can be calculated as a linear combination of the variables, and each variable can be located within the space that is defined by those dimensions. This method is useful for the purposes of simplifying one's variable set and of understanding the common nature of the variables that jointly define a given factor.

When conducting a factor analysis, it is best to use a large participant sample that is representative of the population being examined, as well as a variable set that is representative of the domain being studied. The process of factor analysis begins with the computation of a matrix of correlations between those variables. One then extracts factors, each of which accounts in turn for the maximum amount of variance between the variables, and all of which are mutually uncorrelated. Several criteria exist for deciding how many factors to extract; these methods generally aim to find the optimal tradeoff between parsimony and completeness in explaining the covariances between the variables (in the case of the common-factor model) or the variance of the entire variable set (in the case of the component model). After extracting the desired number of factors, one may then rotate those factors in such a way as to produce a "simple structure," in which each factor is to be defined strongly by a few variables only, thus facilitating the interpretation of factors. In rotating factors, one may choose an orthogonal solution (in which all factors remain uncorrelated) or an oblique solution (in which factors will be correlated). Finally, one may choose among various methods of computing or estimating participants' scores on the factors.

Acknowledgments

This research was supported by Social Sciences and Humanities Research Council of Canada Grant Nos. 410-2003-0946 and 410-2003-1835. We thank John Zelenski for providing the data from the Zelenski and Larsen (1999) study. We also thank Richard Robins and John Zelenski for helpful comments on an earlier version of this chapter.

Notes

1. At this point, we do not yet draw any distinction between common factor analysis and principal components analysis. The fundamental processes involved in these two forms of analysis are similar except insofar as their treatment of the unique aspects of the variables' variances are concerned, as we discuss below. For the sake of simplicity, we use the term *factor* to apply both to common factors and to principal components.

2. Note that these factor loadings are not the same as the weights that are applied to the variables in calculating scores on these factors. Instead, the factor loadings can be understood as weights that are applied to factor scores to predict standardized scores on each variable.

3. However, the first unrotated factor obtained in the initial factoring process—the largest factor— usually carries important and meaningful information. For example, in factor analyses of cognitive ability tests, the first unrotated factor is usually a vector representing general intelligence (Spearman, 1904); moreover, in factor analyses of personality variables, the first unrotated factor is usually a vector contrasting socially desirable and socially undesirable characteristics.

4. However, there will be cases in which a researcher would predict, on rational grounds, that one or more personality variables defining a factor should be *especially* strongly correlated with a given criterion. In these cases, the use of factor analysis as a data reduction tool should not preclude the examination of the individual variable(s) having special a priori interest.

5. For related domains of individual differences, the problem of obtaining a representative sampling of variables within the domain also applies. Attempts to produce a complete structure of cognitive abilities (e.g., Carroll, 1993) have paid far too little attention to the problem of delineating the domain and sampling it in a representative fashion, but admittedly this problem may be difficult to solve. Researchers attempting to recover the structure of other domains may have an easier task. For example, it is conceivable that a nearly complete list of the occupations (or hobbies) practiced in a given time and place could be obtained and sampled, thus allowing a systematic

exploration of the structure of vocational (or recreational) interests. Similarly, a nearly complete list of the salient political issues in a given time and place may also be identifiable, thus allowing meaningful study of the structure of political attitudes.

6. As described here, a multi-item scale includes not only a predefined personality scale but also an ad hoc item parcel. See Bandalos and Finney (2001) and Kishton and Widaman (1994) for issues related to item parceling procedures commonly used in structural equation modeling.

7. One difficulty in the implementation of both of the above methods is that commonly used statistical computing packages do not provide algorithms for their use.

8. An example of the choice between orthogonal and oblique rotations involves analyses of the structure of hierarchically organized personality inventories, in which several broad factor scales each consist of several narrower trait (or facet) scales, each of which in turn consists of several items. If one wishes to examine the structure of the variables within any one of the presumed factor-level scales within the inventory, then one should apply an oblique rotation to factors derived from an analysis of all *items* within all facet scales belonging to that factor scale. If one wishes to examine the structure of the entire inventory, then one should apply an orthogonal rotation to factors derived from an analysis of all *facet scales* of the inventory. Note also that a factor analysis of all items within a well-constructed inventory would likely produce a few broad factors similar to those defined by the facet-level scales. However, a factor analysis of the same set of items would be extremely unlikely to generate a very large number of narrow factors that would correspond cleanly to the entire array of facet scales included in the inventory, no matter how well constructed that inventory might be. This fact argues against the suggestion (Carroll, 2002) that hierarchical factor analysis be applied to item-level personality variables.

Recommended Readings

Goldberg and Digman (1994) and Goldberg and Velicer (2006) give a very clear and thorough introduction to the use of exploratory factor analysis.

Nunnally (1978) also provides a reader-friendly introduction to factor analysis, including a pedagogically useful example of how to perform factor analysis by using the centroid method, a technique similar to principal components analysis. Nunnally and Bernstein (1994) give an expanded discussion of several aspects of factor analysis.

McCrae and colleagues (1996) demonstrate the difficulties associated with the application of confirmatory factor analysis to personality research, and also give a nice example of targeted orthogonal Procrustes rotation, the use of which is explained by Paunonen (1997).

For readers interested in the mathematical basis of factor analysis, textbooks on this topic include Harman (1976), Gorsuch (1983), and Cureton and D'Agostino (1983).

References

Ashton, M. C., Jackson, D. N., Helmes, E., & Paunonen, S. V. (1998). Joint factor analysis of the Personality Research Form and the Jackson Personality Inventory: Comparisons with the Big Five. *Journal of Research in Personality, 32,* 243–250.

Ashton, M. C., & Lee, K. (in press). Empirical, theoretical, and practical advantages of the HEXACO model of personality structure. *Personality and Social Psychology Review.*

Ashton, M. C., Lee, K., & Goldberg, L. R. (2004). A hierarchical analysis of 1,710 English personality-descriptive adjectives. *Journal of Personality and Social Psychology, 87,* 707–721.

Ashton, M. C., Lee, K., Perugini, M., Szarota, P., De Vries, R. E., Di Blas, L., et al. (2004). A six-factor structure of personality-descriptive adjectives: Solutions from psycholexical studies in seven languages. *Journal of Personality and Social Psychology, 86,* 356–366.

Bandalos, D. L., & Finney, S. J. (2001). Item parceling issues in structural equation modeling. In G. A. Marcoulides & R. E. Schumaker (Eds.), *Advanced structural equation modeling: New developments and techniques* (pp. 269–296). Mahwah, NJ: Erlbaum.

Bartlett, M. S. (1950). Tests of significance in factor analysis. *British Journal of Psychology, 3,* 77–85.

Bartlett, M. S. (1951). A further note on tests of significance in factor analysis. *British Journal of Psychology, 4,* 1–2.

Carroll, J. B. (1993). *Human cognitive abilities: A survey of factor-analytic studies.* New York: Cambridge University Press.

Carroll, J. B. (2002). The five-factor personality model: How complete and satisfactory is it? In H. I. Braun, D. N. Jackson, & D. E. Wiley (Eds.), *The role of constructs in psychological and educational measurement* (pp. 97–126). Mahwah, NJ: Erlbaum.

Cattell, R. B. (1966). The scree test for the number of factors. *Multivariate Behavioral Research, 1,* 245–276.

Cureton, E. E., & D'Agostino, R. B. (1983). *Factor analysis: An applied approach.* Hillsdale, NJ: Erlbaum.

Everett, J. E. (1983). Factor comparability as a means of determining the number of factors and their rotation. *Multivariate Behavioral Research, 18,* 197–218.

Goldberg, L. R. (1981). Language and individual differences: The search for universals in personality lexicons. In L. Wheeler (Ed.), *Review of personality and social psychology* (Vol. 2, pp. 141–165). Beverly Hills, CA: Sage.

Goldberg, L. R. (2006). Doing it all bass-ackwards: The development of hierarchical factor structures from the top down. *Journal of Research in Personality, 40,* 347–358.

Goldberg, L. R., & Digman, J. M. (1994). Revealing structure in the data: Principles of exploratory factor analysis. In S. Strack & M. Lorr (Eds.), *Differentiating normal and abnormal personality* (pp. 216–242). New York: Springer.

Goldberg, L. R., & Velicer, W. F. (2006). Principles of exploratory factor analysis. In S. Strack (Ed.), *Differentiating normal and abnormal personality* (2nd ed., pp. 209–237). New York: Springer.

Gorsuch, R. L. (1983). *Factor analysis.* Hillsdale, NJ: Erlbaum.

Guadagnoli, E., & Velicer, W. F. (1988). Relation of sample size to the stability of component patterns. *Psychological Bulletin, 103,* 265–275.

Harman, H. H. (1976). *Modern factor analysis* (3rd ed., rev.). Chicago: University of Chicago Press.

Hendrickson, A. E., & White, P. O. (1964). Promax: A quick method of rotation to oblique simple structure. *British Journal of Statistical Psychology, 17,* 65–70.

Horn, J. L. (1965). A rationale and test for the number of factors in factor analysis. *Psychometrika, 30,* 179–185.

Hotelling, H. (1933). Analysis of a complex of statistical variables into principal components. *Journal of Educational Psychology, 24,* 417–441, 498–520.

Jennrich, R. I., & Sampson, P. J. (1966). Rotation for simple loadings. *Psychometrika, 31,* 313–323.

Kaiser, H. F. (1958). The varimax criterion for analytic rotation in factor analysis. *Psychometrika, 23,* 187–200.

Kaiser, H. F. (1960). The application of electronic computers to factor analysis. *Educational and Psychological Measurement, 20,* 141–151.

Kishton, J. M., & Widaman, K. F. (1994). Unidimensional versus domain representative parceling of questionnaire items: An empirical example. *Educational and Psychological Measurement, 54,* 757–765.

McCrae, R. R., & Costa, P. T., Jr. (1997). Personality trait structure as a human universal. *American Psychologist, 52,* 509–516.

McCrae, R. R., Zonderman, A. B., Costa, P. T., Jr., Bond, M. H., & Paunonen, S. V. (1996). Evaluating replicability of factors on the revised NEO Personality Inventory: Confirmatory factor analysis versus Procrustes rotation. *Journal of Personality and Social Psychology, 70,* 552–566.

Neuhaus, J. O., & Wrigley, C. (1954). The quartimax method: An analytical approach to orthogonal simple structure. *British Journal of Statistical Psychology, 7,* 81–91.

Nunnally, J. C. (1978). *Psychometric theory* (2nd ed.). New York: McGraw-Hill.

Nunnally, J. C., & Bernstein, I. H. (1994). *Psychometric theory* (3rd ed.). New York: McGraw-Hill.

Paunonen, S. V. (1997). On chance and factor congruence following orthogonal Procrustes rotation. *Educational and Psychological Measurement, 57,* 33–59.

Pearson, K. (1901). On lines and planes of closest fit to systems of points in space. *Philosophical Magazine, Series 6, 2,* 559–572.

Saucier, G. (1992). Benchmarks: Integrating affective and interpersonal circles with the Big-Five personality factors. *Journal of Personality and Social Psychology, 62,* 1025–1035.

Saunders, D. R. (1962). Trans-varimax. *American Psychologist, 17,* 395.

Spearman, C. (1904). General intelligence, objectively determined and measured. *American Journal of Psychology, 15,* 201–293.

Velicer, W. F. (1976). Determining the number of components from the matrix of partial correlations. *Psychometrika, 41,* 321–327.

Zelenski, J. M., & Larsen, R. J. (1999). Susceptibility to affect: A comparison of three personality taxonomies. *Journal of Personality, 67,* 761–791.

## CHAPTER 26

Applications of Structural Equation Modeling in Personality Research

Rick H. Hoyle

Structural equation modeling is a general statistical technique for testing multivariate hypotheses about the relations between variables. Two capabilities set structural equation modeling apart from more commonly used statistical techniques in personality research. First, it is not only possible to test hypotheses involving multiple independent and multiple dependent variables; it is possible to test hypotheses about relations *between* independent and *between* dependent variables. Second, it is possible to evaluate these relations at the construct rather than variable level; that is, variables (e.g., questionnaire items, observer ratings) can be treated as fallible representations of constructs (e.g., extraversion, neuroticism), allowing for hypothesis tests that are not contaminated by many forms of measurement error. In addition to these distinctive capabilities, structural equation modeling can be used to test any hypothesis that could be tested using *t*-test, analysis of variance, multivariate analysis of variance, correlation analysis, multiple regression analysis, or factor analysis. The flexibility and generality of structural equation modeling coupled with a capacity for simultaneously testing many, interrelated hypotheses makes it an attractive statistical alternative for personality researchers.

Overview

The goal of most applications of structural equation modeling is to model the relations between a set of variables. *Model*, in this context, can take on different meanings (Jöreskog, 1993). In a *strictly confirmatory* application of structural equation modeling, the goal is to evaluate the degree to which a single, a priori model accounts for a set of observed relations. For example, a researcher may evaluate the degree to which self-ratings on a set of adjectives selected to represent five personality domains conform to a model in which each adjective loads on only one of five correlated factors. Alternatively, instead of focusing on a single model, structural equation modeling may be used to compare two or more competing models in an *alternative models* application. To continue the example, in addition to a model with five correlated factors, the researcher may consider a model with five uncorrelated factors, a model with a single factor, and/or a second-order model in which three of the factors load on one superordinate factor and the other two factors load on a second, correlated one. Finally, the application of structural equation modeling may involve *model generating*. If, for example, the researcher's proposed five-factor model does not adequately explain self-ratings on the adjectives, and there are no obvious alternative models, rather than abandoning the data, the researcher may use it to generate an explanatory model. Of course, using the data to generate a model of the data is inferentially risky (MacCallum, Roznowski, & Necowitz, 1992); however, careful modification of an a priori model with the goal of finding a model that accounts for the data can lead to discoveries that, if replicated, advance our understanding of personality assessment, structure, or process.

It is useful to distinguish two general components of a model that may appear individually or together in a given application of structural equation modeling (Anderson & Gerbing, 1988). One concerns those aspects of the model that reflect the relations between variables and the constructs they represent. (Models in which all constructs are measured or otherwise operationally defined using one variable do not include this component because, in such models, variables and constructs are isomorphic.) Collectively, these relations are referred to as the *measurement model*. Measurement models include two kinds of variables and three kinds of parameters. In terms of variables, there are indicators and latent variables. *Indicators* are measured but fallible representations of constructs. Ideally, the dataset includes at least three indicators of each construct. Indicators can take the form of individual items, arbitrarily grouped subsets of items (i.e., parcels), subscales, or complete scales. If fallibility attributable to method variance is to be modeled, then indicators should be operationally defined using different methods (e.g., self-report, physiological activity, implicit measure). *Latent variables*, traditionally referred to as factors, are unmeasured variables that are related to the indicators. Although latent variables can be caused by their indicators, in virtually all operational definitions in personality research, latent variables cause their indicators (Bollen & Lennox, 1991). Although a person's standing on an indicator is assumed to be caused by a latent variable of interest, it is caused by other, unintended factors as well. Collectively, these factors are referred to as uniquenesses. *Uniquenesses* reflect both random variance and systematic variance not shared with the remaining indicators of the latent variable (i.e., specificity)—that is, all the variance in the indicator not attributable to the latent variable.

Beyond indicators, latent variables, and uniquenesses, measurement models include three kinds of parameters, or coefficients. *Loadings* are coefficients that result from the regression of each indicator on its latent variable. In standardized form, these are the equivalent of factor loadings in exploratory factor analysis. In addition, each latent variable has a variance and each uniqueness has a variance. In the standard measurement model, variance in each indicator is apportioned into a component attributable to the latent variable it represents and its uniqueness. Traditionally, the uniqueness component has received relatively little attention from personality researchers because the exploratory factor model requires that uniquenesses be independent. This requirement can be relaxed in measurement models analyzed using structural equation modeling, allowing for the examination of covariances between uniquenesses as well as relations between uniquenesses and other variables in a model (e.g., Newcomb, 1994). Measurement model parameters are listed and defined in the top half of Table 26.1.

A second component of models concerns the relations between constructs, defined as either latent or measured variables. Collectively, these relations are referred to as the *structural model*. Structural models comprise three kinds of variables and four kinds of parameters. In structural models, variables are either measured or latent. *Measured variables* are those for which there are actual scores in the data matrix and can include scores on individual items, sets of items, or complete scales. They also can include scores produced by any method of measurement or scores that indicate

TABLE 26.1. Parameters in Structural Equation Models

Parameter	Definition
Measurement model	
Loading	Coefficient resulting from the regression of an indicator on a latent variable; typically reported in standardized form
Variance, latent variable	Variance of a latent variable as specified in a model
Variance, uniqueness	Variance of the uniqueness component associated with an indicator of a latent variable; variance in the indicator not attributable to the latent variables on which it loads
Structural model	
Variance, independent variables	Variance of a measured or latent variable that is not predicted by other variables in the model
Variance, disturbance	Variance of a measured or latent variable that is predicted by other variables in the model but is not attributable to those predictors
Nondirectional path	Indicates the degree of covariance (or, in standardized form, correlation) between two variables
Directional path	Indicates the amount of change in an outcome attributable to a predictor controlling for other relations in the model

standing on experimentally manipulated variables. That structural models can include latent variables is a key strength of structural equation modeling. Because indicator-level uniqueness has been removed from latent variables, the estimates of relations between latent variables more closely approximate population values than estimates of relations between their measured counterparts. In addition to measured and latent variables, structural models include *disturbances*, which are components of variance in dependent variables not explained by the model. In multiple regression parlance, these are error terms.

Structural models can include four kinds of parameters. Associated with each independent variable and each disturbance is a variance. In addition, coefficients are associated with two kinds of *paths*, which reflect the assumed nature of the relation between variables (including disturbances). *Nondirectional paths* reflect noncausal relations between variables, the equivalent of correlations. *Directional paths* reflect assumed causal relations, differentiating between the putative cause and effect. Coefficients associated with nondirectional paths are covariances or, in standardized form, correlation coefficients. Coefficients associated with directional paths are regression coefficients, which can be presented and interpreted in either unstandardized or standardized form. Structural model parameters are listed and defined in the bottom half of Table 26.1.

Applications of structural equation modeling that focus strictly on the measurement model are referred to as *confirmatory factor analyses*. Applications that focus strictly on the structural model—that is, they include no latent variables—are referred to as *path analyses*. Structural equation modeling is used to fullest advantage in models that include both measurement and structural components, providing estimates of the relations between constructs from which measurement error has been removed. Specific applications of confirmatory factor analysis, path analysis, and full structural equation modeling are described later in the chapter.

Steps in an Application of Structural Equation Modeling

All applications of structural equation modeling involve five steps; most involve an additional step followed by one or more cycles through earlier steps. These steps are shown in Figure 26.1 and detailed in the remainder of this section of the chapter.

Specification

The application of structural equation modeling begins with the specification of a model. A *model* is a formal, statistical hypothesis regarding the mechanisms that produced the observed

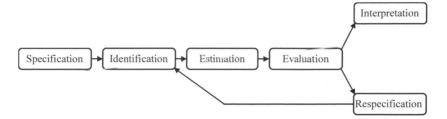

FIGURE 26.1. Steps in the application of structural equation modeling in personality research.

associations between a set of variables. Those mechanisms can include the theoretical processes that motivated the research as well as features of the sample and design. *Specification* involves designating the variables, relations between variables, and status of the parameters in a model. In terms of designating variables, the decisions are which variables in a data matrix to include as measured variables and which latent variables, if any, to model. In terms of designating the relations between variables, the researcher must decide which variables are related and, for those that are related, whether the relation is nondirectional or directional. Finally, the status of parameters in a model must be specified. In general, a parameter can be either fixed or free. *Fixed parameters* are those whose values are set by the researcher, whereas *free parameters* are those whose values are estimated from the data given the model. For instance, when variables are specified as unrelated in a model, a parameter (either covariance or directional path) fixed at zero is implied.

The activity of specification typically involves expressing a model either as a diagram or as a set of equations. *Path diagrams* make use of a relatively small number of graphical components and minimal notation to capture all aspects of model specification. The specification of a simple measurement model using a path diagram is illustrated in Figure 26.2. In the diagram, squares represent indicators, ellipses represent latent variables (including uniquenesses), straight arrows represent directional effects, and double-headed arrows that originate and terminate with the same variable represent variances. A final component, not shown in Figure 26.2, is the double-headed arrow that originates with one variable and terminates with another, representing a nondirectional relation, or covariance. In the way of notation, asterisks represent free parameters

and numeric values next to a path indicate the value of a fixed parameter. The measurement model in Figure 26.2 indicates a specification in which six indicators, *v1* to *v6*, are influenced by a single latent variable, extraversion. Each indicator is influenced by one of six uniqueness components, *u1* to *u6*. The variances of the latent variable and the indicators are shown. The asterisks indicate that all the variances and five of the six loadings are free parameters. The value of one loading is fixed at 1.0. The uniquenesses do not covary; the covariances between them are, in effect, fixed at zero.

An alternative approach to specifying a model is through a set of equations. For example, here are the *measurement equations* that correspond to the path diagram in Figure 26.2:

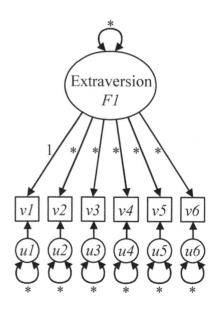

FIGURE 26.2. Latent variable model of extraversion showing indicators (*v1* to *v6*), uniquenesses (*u1* to *u6*), and free parameters (**'s).

$$v1 = 1F1 + u1$$
$$v2 = {}^*F1 + u2$$
$$v3 = {}^*F1 + u3$$
$$v4 = {}^*F1 + u4$$
$$v5 = {}^*F1 + u5$$
$$v6 = {}^*F1 + u6$$

In order for the specification to be complete, we must include the variances of F1 and the uniquenesses, which, using double-label notation, are indicated as follows:

$$F1,F1 = {}^*$$
$$u1,u1 = {}^*$$
$$u2,u2 = {}^*$$
$$u3,u3 = {}^*$$
$$u4,u4 = {}^*$$
$$u5,u5 = {}^*$$
$$u6,u6 = {}^*$$

Like the path diagram, the equation representation makes evident all variables in the model, which variables are related to which others, and the location of free and fixed parameters.[1]

There are variations on both the path diagram and equation approaches to model specification, but the goal is always the same: to make explicit the full set of statistical hypotheses encompassed by a model.

Identification

It is possible to specify a model for which suitable values of the free parameters cannot be estimated. Such a model would be described as *unidentified*. Thus, in addition to accurately reflecting the theoretical processes that motivated a study and known features of the sample and design, a model must be specified in such a way that it is identified. An *identified model* is one in which a unique value can be obtained for each free parameter through a manipulation of the observed data given the model specification. Determining the identification status of a specified model can be a challenge, sometimes requiring the determination of whether the specification meets one or more technical criteria. Those criteria are detailed in comprehensive treatments of structural equation modeling (e.g., Bollen, 1989). In some instances, those criteria manifest as relatively straightforward rules of thumb. For instance, in order for the variance of a latent variable to be defined, it

must be fixed either to a specific value (e.g., 1.0) or to the value of the common portion of one of the indicators, which is accomplished by fixing the loading for that indicator to a value of 1.0 (Steiger, 2002). Another rule of thumb concerns the number of indicators per latent variable. If a latent variable is modeled as uncorrelated with other variables in a model (e.g., a one-factor model or a model with orthogonal factors), it must have at least three indicators in order to be identified. This is because of the general identification rule that a model cannot have more free parameters than the number of nonredundant elements in the observed covariance matrix.[2] For present purposes, it is important only to understand that, although structural equation modeling is very flexible in terms of the kinds of relations between variables that can be specified, that flexibility is limited somewhat by technical considerations having to do with how parameters are estimated.

Estimation

If a specified model is identified, then values of its free parameters can be estimated. The means by which estimates are derived depend on which of a number of possible estimators are used. For most applications, the maximum likelihood estimator is the best choice. The goal of *maximum likelihood estimation* is to find a set of estimates for the free parameters that, when the fixed parameters are taken into account, maximize the likelihood of the data, given the specified model (Myung, 2003). Maximum likelihood estimation is an iterative procedure that begins with a somewhat arbitrary set of *start values* for the free parameters and updates these values until the difference between the observed data and the data implied by the model is minimized. At this point, the estimation procedure is said to have *converged*, and the adequacy of the resultant model is evaluated.

The use of estimators other than maximum likelihood usually is motivated by one or more characteristics of the data that do not meet the assumptions of maximum likelihood estimation. Principal among these is multivariate normality and sufficiently large samples (a minimum of 200–400, depending on model complexity and other factors). Alternative estimators include unweighted least squares, generalized least squares, weighted least squares, and asymptotically distribution-free estimators. Because the validity of model evaluation rests most fundamentally on the integrity of estimates, a critical concern for researchers is whether maximum likelihood estimation is appropriate and, if it is not, which alternative estimator overcomes the limitations of maximum likelihood without introducing additional concerns about the integrity of estimates (see Chou & Bentler, 1995, and Ullman, 1996, for relevant discussions).

Evaluation

When estimates have been obtained for a properly specified model, the adequacy of the model as an explanation for the data can be evaluated. The degree to which a model explains a set of data is termed the *fit* of the model to the data. How close a fit is necessary in order for a model to be accepted is a point of lively debate (see, e.g., MacCallum, 2003; Meehl & Waller, 2002). In order to appreciate the concern, a bit of background regarding the nature of statistical tests of fit in the structural equation modeling context is useful.

The "raw data" in structural equation modeling is not the set of individual scores on the measured variables, but rather the covariance matrix of the measured variables.[3] Thus, the evaluation of fit in structural equation modeling is an evaluation of how well a model accounts for the observed covariances. This can be determined most directly by comparing the observed covariance matrix with the covariance matrix implied by the model. This *implied covariance matrix* is obtained through manipulations of the fixed parameter values and estimated values of the free parameters. The subtraction of each value in the implied covariance matrix from its corresponding value in the observed covariance matrix yields the *residual matrix*. If a model perfectly accounts for the observed data, all values in the residual matrix will be zero. If the values in the residual matrix significantly depart from zero, there is evidence of *misspecification* in the model; that is, one or more relations are over- or underestimated by the model.

Although examination of the residual matrix is important and, for the experienced user, a means of determining where misspecification might be located in a model with unacceptable fit, it does not provide a statistical test of the sort to which personality researchers are accus-

tomed. A statistic that, under specific conditions, is distributed as a χ^2 can be generated, but it has for two reasons fallen into disfavor as a means of evaluating model fit. First, it assumes characteristics of the data and model that rarely are met in practice. Second, it tests a hypothesis of limited interest—that the model perfectly fits the data. Thus, although this statistic is routinely included in reports of structural equation modeling results, it rarely is interpreted.[4]

Because of the limited value of the test based on the χ^2 statistic, alternative means of evaluating model fit are required. A common strategy involves comparing the fit of a specified model against the fit of a model that specifies no relations between the variables (Bentler & Bonett, 1980). This *comparative fit* strategy typically yields a value between 0 and 1.0 that is interpreted as a proportion. These values are indices, not statistics, and therefore are descriptive rather than inferential. The most widely used is the comparative fit index (Bentler, 1990). An alternative strategy is to index the *absolute fit* of a model by summarizing the residuals. The root mean square error of approximation (RMSEA) is a commonly used index of this sort (Steiger & Lind, 1980). The RMSEA has the additional benefits of including a correction for model complexity and an interpretation that allows for tests of close, rather than exact, fit.

Consultation of these indexes of fit is sufficient for evaluating the fit of models when the strictly confirmatory or model-generating approaches are taken; however, when the alternative models approach is taken, model comparisons are required. In the ideal case, two or more models representing incompatible theoretical models are statistically compared. A statistical comparison is possible if the two models are *nested*—that is, the free parameters in one model are a subset of the free parameters in the other. For instance, suppose that two theoretical models of a particular personality domain disagree as to whether the domain comprises one or two dimensions. A one-dimensional model can be produced from a two-dimensional model by fixing the free covariance between factors representing the two dimensions to a value that would standardize to 1.0 (i.e., a perfect correlation). The one-dimensional model is nested in the two-dimensional model, having one fewer free parameter; thus, a statistical test can be used to choose one over the other. There is no definitive strategy for statistically comparing models that are not nested.

An often neglected aspect of evaluating the fit of a model is consideration of the parameter estimates. The standard hypothesis regarding parameter estimates is that they differ from zero. This hypothesis is tested by the *critical ratio*, which, as in other statistical contexts, is the ratio of the unstandardized estimate to its standard error. The observed value of the critical ratio is evaluated against critical values from the z-distribution.

Respecification

As indicated in Figure 26.1, there are two potential directions the application of structural equation modeling can take following evaluation of fit. If the fit of the model is adequate and/or the application is strictly confirmatory, then the results are interpreted as described in the next section of this chapter. If, however, the fit of the model is inadequate and the researcher is not committed to the strictly confirmatory approach, then the next step is to respecify the model with the goal of improving fit.

Decisions regarding how to respecify a model are based on *specification searches*, which involve looking for sources of misspecification among the fixed and free parameters in the initially specified model. For instance, a parameter fixed at zero may result in significant underestimation of the observed covariance between two variables, leading to a significant difference between the observed and implied values of the relevant covariance. Freeing a parameter to allow this covariance to be accounted for would result in a closer match between the observed and implied covariance matrices and therefore a reduction in misspecification. Specification searches can be manual, which involves an informal examination of the residual matrix, or statistical, which involves the use of a statistical algorithm that evaluates the incremental improvement in fit if each fixed parameter is freed or each free parameter is fixed.

Because decisions about respecification are made with reference to the data, the likelihood of Type I error is unacceptably high, and therefore fit statistics and indices cannot be taken at face value (MacCallum et al., 1992). Thus, although investigators may be tempted to confidently interpret the results from estimation of

respecified models that produce acceptable values of fit indices, they should instead proceed with caution, because the likelihood that the model fits the data in hand, but would not fit another set of data from the same population, is unacceptably high (i.e., > .05). In order to draw an inference about the population from which the sample was drawn, the investigator would need to demonstrate satisfactory fit of the respecified model to data from an independent sample from the same population.

Interpretation

When statistical support for a model has been obtained, then the results of estimation can be interpreted. If the researcher is committed to a strictly confirmatory application of structural equation modeling, the focus of interpretation is the parameter estimates. The magnitude and sign of estimates that are significantly different from zero can be interpreted in light of predicted values. Whether the unstandardized or standardized estimates will be presented and interpreted is a matter of whether the measurement scales have inherent meaning (e.g., dollars, pounds) and what is typical in the literature. In the personality literature, measurement scales rarely have inherent meaning, and the presentation and interpretation of standardized values is typical.

A key consideration in interpretation is whether a statistically defensible model provides a *uniquely* satisfactory account of the data. When the alternative models approach to structural equation modeling is used, competing models of theoretical interest are specified before the data are analyzed and compared to the focal model. In addition to models of theoretical interest, however, certain models are of inferential interest because they are equivalent to the focal model. *Equivalent models* are those with the same number of fixed and free parameters but with one or more paths changed either in type (e.g., directional to nondirectional) or direction (MacCallum, Wegener, Uchino, & Fabrigar, 1993). Equivalent models produce identical fit statistics and therefore provide equally defensible statistical accounts of the data. For example, in a simple study involving two variables, x and y, the model that specifies x as a cause of y cannot be distinguished in terms of fit from a model that specifies y as a cause of x or x and y as simply correlated. Sometimes this inferential conundrum can be resolved through design (e.g., x is manipulated) or a consideration of what the variables represent (e.g., x is a biological characteristic). Otherwise, the researcher can infer only that the results provide necessary, but not sufficient, support for the focal model.

As suggested by the discussion of equivalent models, although researchers may be tempted to use causal language when describing relations in structural equation models, such language must be used with caution. Because of its capacity for isolating putative causal variables and modeling data from longitudinal designs, structural equation modeling offers a stronger basis for inferring causality than commonly used statistical techniques. In the end, however, statistics yield to design when it comes to causal inferences, and therefore data generated by experimental or carefully designed quasi-experimental designs with a longitudinal component are required.

Specific Applications

Although a full implementation of structural equation modeling involves at least five of the six steps shown in Figure 26.1, the focus in this section is limited to the specification step. It is at the specification step—where hypotheses about personality structure and process are translated into statistical form—that the rich potential of structural equation modeling for personality research is realized.

Rather than provide a cursory account of the many possible specifications relevant to personality research, I focus in some detail on a single comprehensive example that allows for an integrated presentation of applications most likely to be used in personality research. The example is drawn from research by Graziano and colleagues, who take a hierarchical level-of-analysis approach (McAdams, 1995), linking personality to adjustment and behavior through specific strategies and motives (e.g., Graziano, Hair, & Finch, 1997; Graziano, Jensen-Campbell, & Finch, 1997). In one study, Graziano, Jensen-Campbell, and Finch (1997) examined the influence of personality as conceptualized in the five-factor model on adolescents' adjustment in the school setting. They were interested in the extent to which observed relations between personality and adjustment could be attributed to self-evaluation in the domain relevant to the adjustment domain. Al-

though their analysis involved multiple personality, self-evaluative, and adjustment domains, for present purposes only one of each is needed.

Specifically, I focus on a portion of one of their models predicting an effect of extraversion on peer relations transmitted through social self-evaluation. Extraversion was assessed using 10 items, but the number of indicators was reduced to 3 through parceling; that is, 3 composites were created by summing sets of 3, 3, and 4 items. Social self-esteem was assessed using 6 self-report items, each serving as an indicator. The quality of peer relations was assessed using teachers' ratings of same-sex and other-sex relations with peers at the beginning and at the end of the school year. The beginning-of-year and end-of-year ratings were combined, yielding 2 indicators of peer relations. Thus, the dataset comprises 11 indicators presumed to reflect 3 latent variables. The model linking the indicators to latent variables and the latent variables to each other is displayed in Figure 26.3.[5]

Measurement Model Applications

An advantage of structural equation modeling is its explicit focus on the relations between indicators and latent variables. This focus allows for a set of interesting applications that logically precede applications that focus on the relations between latent variables. The most fundamental of these applications concerns whether the data are consistent with a model in which each indicator is influenced by a specific latent variable and is not influenced by the remaining latent variables. Referring to Figure 26.3, imagine that the directional paths between latent variables were replaced by nondirectional paths, leaving directional paths only between latent variables and indicators. This model would have no structural component, thereby shifting the focus strictly to measurement concerns. The most basic concern is whether the measurement model is correct. This concern has two primary components: (1) whether three is the correct number of latent variables and (2) whether, given three latent variables, the pattern of loadings is correct. A secondary concern is whether the implicit assumption that the uniquenesses are uncorrelated is tenable, given the data. Each of the considerations can be approached empirically.

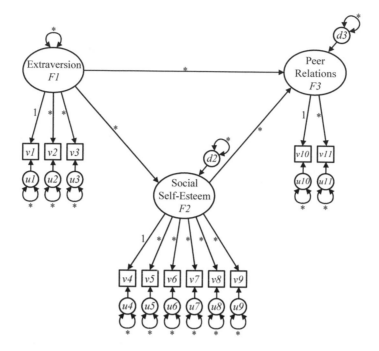

FIGURE 26.3. A portion of the model tested by Graziano, Jensen-Campbell, and Finch (1997), which is used to illustrate an array of applications of structural equation modeling.

If there is reason to believe that three is not the correct number of latent variables, a series of unrestricted factor models can be estimated that differ only in how many sources of commonality they propose. A virtue of this model is that by allowing all indicators to load on all factors, it eliminates pattern of loadings as a potential contributor to lack of fit (Hoyle & Duvall, 2004). Stated differently, unrestricted factor models deconfound number of factors and pattern of loadings as potential sources of misspecification. Once the number of factors has been established, either on conceptual (as in our example) or empirical grounds, the focus can shift to the pattern of loadings.

A property of the model depicted in Figure 26.3 is that it manifests a *simple structure* pattern of loadings; that is, each indicator is free to load on one factor but, implicitly, its loadings on the remaining factors are fixed to zero. Thus, for instance, *v3* is an indicator of extraversion but not of social self-esteem or peer relations. If we feel confident that we have the number of latent variables correct but a model does not evince adequate fit to a set of data, we might consider whether the simple structure pattern of loadings is not tenable. For example, an examination of the residual matrix may re-

veal nontrivial residual association between *v9*, *v10*, and *v11*, suggesting that *v9* should be allowed to load on *F3* as well as *F2*.

What if an examination of the residual matrix indicates unexplained correlation between *v9* and *v10* but not *v9* and *v11*? This misspecification would not be appropriately addressed by allowing *v9* to load on *F3*, because this specification would lead to an overestimation of the *v9–v11* relation. An alternative means of addressing this nonzero residual would be to allow *u9* and *u10* to covary.

That example concerns two indicators that covary but are not presumed to reflect the same latent variable. More commonly, inspection of the residual matrix reveals unexplained association between two variables presumed to reflect the same latent variable. At first blush, this pattern may seem impossible, given that association between the two variables is modeled through their common loadings on a single latent variable. It is important to recognize, however, that the latent variable accounts only for the commonality between the two variables that is shared with the other variables that reflect the latent variables. For instance, it is possible that a portion of the correlation between *v4* and *v5* is not explained by *F2* because it is not shared with *v6–v9*. This residual covariation could be modeled as a freed covariance between *u4* and *u5*.

This discussion suggests that free parameters can be added to measurement models at will. In reality, the freeing of parameters such as cross-loadings and correlated uniquenesses clearly moves the analysis from strictly confirmatory to model generating. Although applications of the latter sort are valuable, they make use of the data to model the data and therefore risk capitalization on chance. Thus, unless a clear logical or theoretical rationale can be offered for such modifications, these aspects of a measurement model should be considered tentative until replicated and explained.

In addition to concerns about the basic associations between latent variables and their indicators are concerns related to the degree to which those associations hold between groups, across situations, and over time. For instance, in the Graziano, Jensen-Campbell, and Finch (1997) study from which our example is drawn, data were provided by 189 girls and 128 boys. If one of our research questions concerns gender differences in the structural portion of the model, our confidence in analyses relevant to that question would be higher if we first established that our model of the constructs is equally valid for girls and boys. If our study were longitudinal, with each construct measured at each of three time points separated by a year, we may also be concerned that the indicators are interpreted in different ways during different developmental periods (e.g., before vs. after puberty), leading to a different measurement model at different time points. As a class, these issues concern *measurement invariance* (Widaman & Reise, 1997).

Measurement invariance falls along a continuum; thus, we do not describe a measurement model as invariant or not. Rather, we determine the degree of invariance in a measurement model by focusing on the equivalence of sets of parameters between groups, across situations, or over time (Byrne, Shavelson, & Muthén, 1989). For illustration purposes, let us return to the measurement model involving extraversion, social self-esteem, and peer relations and the question of whether the same model holds for girls and boys in the sample. The most basic concern is that the same number of latent variables is reflected by the indicators. Beyond that, we are interested in whether the items load on the latent variables according

to the same pattern; that is, do *v1* to *v3* reflect *F1*; *v4* to *v9*, *F2*; and *v10* and *v11*, *F3* for girls and boys? If we find support for these elements of invariance, our next concern is the magnitude of the parameter estimates. For instance, is *v5* an equivalently strong indicator of *F2* for boys and girls? We can ask this of each set of parameter estimates—the loadings, the uniquenesses, the variances of the latent variables, and the covariances between the latent variables. Invariance in the number of latent variables and pattern of loadings, and at least partial invariance in the magnitude of loadings, is necessary for meaningful between-group comparisons of structural parameters involving the latent variables (Byrne et al., 1989). The presence of at least partial invariance also affords the possibility of comparing *structured means*—that is, means of the indicators and latent variables in the context of the model.

Structural Model Applications

Once support has been obtained for the measurement component of a model, attention turns to the structural component. In our example, this involves the direct effect of extraversion on peer relations and the indirect effect of extraversion on peer relations through social self-esteem. Referring again to Figure 26.3, note that *F2* and *F3* are influenced by both other latent variables in the model and a disturbance term. Thus, for instance, the observed variance in social self-esteem is partitioned into a portion attributable to extraversion—captured by the path from *F1* to *F2*—and a portion that is not explained by the model—captured by the variance associated with *d2*. When this structural component is added to the measurement model, five new parameters are introduced. Three directional paths replace the nondirectional paths between latent variables, and the variances of *F2* and *F3* are replaced by *d2* and *d3*, respectively.

The structural component of this model is not unlike a multiple regression model, with the *s on the directional paths corresponding to partial regression coefficients and the *d*s corresponding to residuals. Despite these similarities, applications focused on the structural portion of models estimated using structural equation modeling differ from applications of multiple regression analysis in three important ways. First, as noted earlier in the chapter, parameter estimates in structural equation modeling typically are obtained using maximum likelihood, not ordinary least squares, estimation. Second, both predictors and outcomes are modeled as latent, not observed, variables. Third, the multiple equations comprised by most structural models are estimated simultaneously.

The most basic concern in regard to applications focused on the structural model are the estimates of parameters corresponding to directional paths between variables. When, as in our example, the variables are modeled as latent variables, these estimates are corrected for measurement error. Thus, our estimate of the effect of extraversion on social self-esteem is not influenced by random error or systematic error unique to a subset of the indicators of these latent variables.

As was true of the measurement model, we may be interested in whether the structural paths are equivalent for girls and boys. In order to pursue this interest, we could separate the data for boys and girls and run a multigroup analysis. In *multigroup analyses*, as in analyses of between-group measurement invariance, a model is simultaneously fit to two or more covariance matrices. This analytic strategy allows for direct comparisons of specific parameters and sets of parameters. For example, if our interest is whether the effect of social self-esteem on peer relations is the same for girls and boys, we could test this by statistically comparing two multigroup models, one in which the parameter corresponding to that path is equal for girls and boys and another in which that parameter is free to vary between groups. This comparison corresponds to the standard test of an interaction effect, but is more powerful because the effects are not attenuated by measurement error. A benefit of this strategy is that it rules out the possibility that the parameter estimates differ for girls and boys but only because the reliability of the variables varies for the two groups.

Additional Applications

Beyond these basic applications of structural equation modeling are a growing number of more sophisticated applications of particular relevance to personality researchers. In many instances, these applications represent the only statistical means of addressing a specific hypothesis. In some instances, they suggest interesting hypotheses that otherwise may not have been evident to personality researchers. The applications are too numerous to present in full. Instead, I describe four that are particularly useful for personality researchers.

Structural equation modeling is well suited for modeling sources of commonality in multitrait–multimethod matrices (Campbell & Fiske, 1959). In the prototypic multitrait–multimethod matrix, three traits are measured using three methods, yielding nine observed variables. Returning to our running example, early in the research program represented by the model in Figure 26.3, we may have had concerns about the validity of our measure of social self-esteem. Specifically, we may have questioned whether social self-esteem is distinct from two related constructs, social desirability and social anxiety, and whether some portion of the variability in scores on our measure can be attributed to the self-report mode of measurement. To address these concerns, we could conduct a validation study in which social self-esteem, social desirability, and social anxiety are measured using self-reports, peer reports, and observer ratings. We could then specify a model in which each score is influenced by two latent variables, one corresponding to the relevant trait and one corresponding to the relevant method (see Marsh & Grayson, 1995). In this application, each measure of social self-esteem—including the self-report measure on which our research is based—is partitioned into a portion attributable to the construct regardless of how it is measured (monotrait–heteromethod), a portion attributable to how it was measured without reference to the constructs (heterotrait–monomethod), and a portion attributable to neither the trait nor the method (error). This application also yields estimates of the correlations between the three constructs, eliminating correlation attributable to shared method variance. This sophisticated application of the measurement model is a formal, flexible means of mining multitrait–multimethod and similar matrices (e.g., Panter, Tanaka, & Hoyle, 1994).

An alternative partitioning of variance in scores on a measure distinguishes variance in a construct that is stable across contexts and time from reliable variance that is subject to change across context or time. The partitioning is accomplished in trait–state–error measurement models (e.g., Kenny & Zautra, 1995). The value of this partitioning can be seen by reconsidering the structural model with latent variables shown in Figure 26.3. In this model, peer relations are assumed to covary with extraversion; that is, as extraversion increases, the quality of peer relations increases. If, however, peer relations are trait-like, they are, by definition, not causally influenced by other variables. Thus, it is to our advantage to determine whether peer relations, as we have measured them, include a state component. Applying the trait–state–error model, we can model the variance in peer relations in terms of components that correspond to a trait, a state, and error. It is the state component that would be subject to influence by extraversion. Like measurement models for multitrait–multimethod matrices, the trait–state–error model uses structural equation modeling to disentangle variance components in a measure of a construct, allowing for cleaner, more focused tests of hypotheses involving the construct.

In addition to distinguishing trait and state components of peer relations, we may be interested in the pattern of change in the quality of students' peer relations over time. In pursuing this interest, our focus shifts from variances to means and a class of applications referred to as *latent growth curve modeling* (Willett & Sayer, 1994). Like trend analysis in repeated measures analysis of variance, latent growth curve models focus on modeling patterns of means over time. For instance, if we acquired data on students' peer relations at the beginning of their last 2 years in middle school and their first 2 years of high school, we could examine the trajectory, or growth curve, of mean peer relations during these transitional years. As in repeated measures analysis of variance, we can evaluate the first $k - 1$ order curves, with k indicating the number of repeated assessments.

A virtue of latent growth-curve modeling in the structural equation modeling context is the ability to focus on individual growth (Willett & Sayer, 1994). For instance, in our example, let us assume that, in general, the peer relations trajectory during the period we are studying is linear. This outcome would be determined by observing acceptable fit of relevant portions of a model in which the means are fit to a straight line. If estimation yields support for this model, then the focus turns to variability in growth parameters—the slope and intercept of the linear trajectory. These growth parameters are modeled as variances of latent variables; hence, the label, *latent* growth-curve modeling. If, for instance, there is, in effect, no variability in the

slope parameter, we may infer that the trajectory is normative. If there is variability in this parameter or the intercept parameter, then we can move to an interesting set of questions that concern the explanation or consequences of this variability. At this point, the model is referred to as a *conditional growth model*, because we are acknowledging that the growth parameters vary across individuals as a function of some characteristic of those individuals or the circumstances in which they live. This general strategy—determining the shape of the trajectory of change in a construct over time, then attempting to explain individual variability in trajectories—is particularly useful for testing process-oriented hypotheses about personality-influenced development or change.

Shifting the focus to the structural model, I now consider an application that sheds light on the direction of influence between two variables that are associated—the cross-lagged panel model. In the simplest cross-lagged panel model, two constructs are measured at two points in time. For instance, to continue the illustrative example, assume that social self-esteem and peer relations are measured on two occasions 2 months apart and the question is whether there is a causal relation between the two and, if so, which construct is the cause. The name derives from the fact that, in addition to estimating autoregressive effects—the effect of the construct on itself at a later time (i.e., stability)—we are estimating the effect of each construct on the other construct at a later time. These latter effects, which are the focal part of the model, are the cross-lagged paths.

Structural equation modeling is particularly well suited for the analysis of data generated by such designs. The ability to model both constructs on both occasions as latent variables is important because it ensures that no path coefficients are attenuated due to measurement error. This is a particular advantage in this context because the cross-lagged path coefficients are to be compared, and it is important that any observed differences in coefficients be attributable to differences in the actual strength of the relations between constructs as opposed to differential attenuation of path coefficients due to measurement error. Another concern is that the cross-lagged path coefficients are estimated controlling for stability, which ensures that the cross-lagged paths do not reflect the covariation between stable components of the two constructs.

Returning to our example, in which social self-esteem and peer relations are modeled as latent variables on two occasions separated by 2 months, the focus is on four structural parameters—two stability and two cross-lagged coefficients. The magnitude of the stability coefficients reveals how much of the variance in time-2 measures is subject to influence by the time-1 measures. The cross-lagged coefficients indicate the directional influence of each variable on the other. If we can demonstrate, by statistical test, that one of these coefficients is larger in magnitude than the other, then we have evidence for a specific direction of influence. For instance, given the specification displayed in Figure 26.3, we would expect the cross-lagged path running from time-1 social self-esteem to time-2 peer relations to be significant and stronger than the path running from time-1 peer relations to time-2 social self-esteem. It is important to note that these paths are not influenced by measurement error or covariation between stable components of the two constructs.

Issues and Concerns

Although structural equation modeling is uniquely well suited for addressing many personality research questions, it is not without important limitations. In general, these limitations are of two types: those that concern technical aspects of the procedure, and those that concern interpretation of results produced using the procedure.

Sample size is a fundamental concern in applications of structural equation modeling. The theoretical properties of the maximum likelihood estimator typically used in applied structural equation modeling assume arbitrarily large samples. The practical question for personality research is, What minimum number of observations is necessary for valid estimation? Although there are qualifying factors, and the number is somewhat variable as a function of the particular outcome in question (e.g., parameter estimates, fit indices), simulation studies point to about 400 as the number of observations at which the outcomes of maximum likelihood estimation correspond to expectation (e.g., Bentler, 1990). The stability of parameter estimates is questionable in all but the simplest models (i.e., fewer than 10 variables)

with fewer than 200 observations (Loehlin, 1992). This number increases as the distributions of the variables depart from normality and as models become more complex. The minimum number is substantially larger for estimators that do not assume normality and/or continuous measurement.

Another fundamental assumption of the maximum likelihood estimator is continuous measurement of variables (Jöreskog, 1994). Strictly speaking, this assumption is not met by most measures in personality research. Typically, research participants are provided a relatively small number of response options arrayed along a continuum defined by two extreme options. Such response formats produce variables that, at best, evince interval scale properties. Although violation of this assumption seems almost certain in the typical application of structural equation modeling, the consequences of violating the assumption in the manner typical of personality research (i.e., 5- or 7-point Likert scales) do not appear to be severe (e.g., Tepper & Hoyle, 1996). Nonetheless, the more coarsely categorized a measurement scale, the greater the cause for concern, and estimation from data gathered on response scales with fewer than five options is best carried out using an estimator for ordered categorical variables (e.g., Muthén, 2001).

A second set of limitations associated with applications of structural equation modeling in personality research concerns interpretation. The most fundamental of these are inferences about the suitability of a given model as an explanation for a set of data. Assuming that the technical assumptions associated with fit statistics and indices have been met, the validity of such inferences is a function of the basis for the specification in question. If the model was specified and estimated without consulting the data, then inferences based on fit statistics and indices are valid. If, as is more often the case, the model was respecified following an unfavorable result from estimation of a hypothesized model, then inferences based on fit statistics and indices are not valid (MacCallum et al., 1992).

As noted earlier in this chapter, interpretation of results from estimation of a model must also take into account the possibility that other models provide an equally tenable account of the data (MacCallum et al., 1993). For instance, imagine a measurement model for a

nine-item measure of self-esteem in three domains. We might posit a second-order factor
model in which a general self-esteem factor
accounts for the correlation between three
first-order domain-specific factors. Although
suitable absolute fit of this model would be
consistent with our hypothesis, the fit of this
model would be identical to the fit of a model
in which the three factors were simply allowed
to correlate (i.e., no second-order factor). This
issue is of greater concern in structural models,
for which equivalent models can often be generated that posit directional paths running in
opposite directions. In many instances, statistically equivalent models can be ruled out
through research design strategies such as manipulation of variables and longitudinal measurement.

A specific instance of equivalent models is
worth further consideration. I use our running
example to illustrate this concern. In the model
depicted in Figure 26.3, we posit that social
self-esteem causes peer relations. Yet, if the
data from which this model is estimated were
gathered at one point in time and neither variable was manipulated, other plausible specifications are possible. For instance, it could be
posited that social self-esteem is a result of the
quality of peer relations. Or we might assume
that both social self-esteem and peer relations
are a product of family support, for which we
do not have data. As with equivalent models,
the solution to this conundrum is research design. For instance, if we had data on social self-
esteem and peer relations at two points in time,
we might specify and estimate a cross-lagged
panel model. Or we might randomly assign students to levels of a manipulated variable, leaving only one plausible direction of influence
(Spencer, Zanna, & Fong, 2005). From this example, it is evident that structural equation
modeling alone cannot be used to determine
the direction of association between two constructs. The advantages structural equation
modeling offers over other statistical approaches in this regard are the capacity to
model relations between latent variables and,
in quasi- or nonexperimental studies, to isolate
putative causes and effects from extraneous
variables.

These technical and interpretational limitations are often not acknowledged and addressed in applications of structural equation
modeling, leading to criticism of the strategy
and questioning of certain findings produced
by it (see, e.g., Breckler, 1990; MacCallum et
al., 1993). As illustrated in this chapter, structural equation modeling is a valuable approach
to research on personality; however, it is not
without limitations. The credibility of findings
from applications of structural equation modeling in personality research hinges on careful
attention to statistical assumptions and the limits of what can be inferred, given the design of
the study that generated the data.

Conclusions

The flexibility and generality of structural
equation modeling makes it an attractive alternative to traditional statistical strategies such
as analysis of variance, multiple regression
analysis, and exploratory factor analysis for
personality researchers. As is true for all statistical procedures, there are technical limitations
associated with structural equation modeling.
Some of these, such as the requirement that a
model must be specified so that all parameters
are identified before it can be estimated, cannot
be overcome. Other technical limitations are
gradually being eliminated by advances in the
generality and robustness of estimators. For instance, widely available software now includes
estimators for categorical variables and variables that are not normally distributed (e.g.,
Bentler, 1995; Muthén & Muthén, 2004).
Moreover, simulation research indicates that
under certain conditions, estimators such as
maximum likelihood can produce valid results
with relatively small samples typical of some
personality research (Hoyle, 1999). Finally,
novel applications of potential relevance for
personality research questions appear regularly
in the methodology literature (e.g., Bollen &
Curran, 2004; Cole, Martin, & Steiger, 2005;
Marsh, Wen, & Hau, 2004). These recent developments, coupled with increasingly user-
friendly software, stamps structural equation
modeling as a core statistical strategy for addressing personality research questions.

Acknowledgment

During the writing of this chapter, I was supported
by Grant No. P20-DA017589 from the National Institute on Drug Abuse.

Notes

1. An alternative, more technical, approach to representing the model is using matrix notation. For this simple model, the matrix notation is

$$
\begin{bmatrix} x_1 \\ x_2 \\ x_3 \\ x_4 \\ x_5 \\ x_6 \end{bmatrix} = \begin{bmatrix} 1 \\ \lambda_{21} \\ \lambda_{31} \\ \lambda_{41} \\ \lambda_{51} \\ \lambda_{61} \end{bmatrix} \xi_1 + \begin{bmatrix} \delta_1 \\ \delta_2 \\ \delta_3 \\ \delta_4 \\ \delta_5 \\ \delta_6 \end{bmatrix}
$$

or, more compactly,

$$
\mathbf{x} = \lambda_x \xi + \delta
$$

In addition, we need a representation for the variance of the latent variable, which would be ϕ_{11}, the lone element in the Φ matrix, and one for covariances among the uniquenesses, which would be the θ_δ matrix,

$$
\begin{bmatrix} \theta_{\delta_{11}} \\ 0 & \theta_{\delta_{22}} \\ 0 & 0 & \theta_{\delta_{33}} \\ 0 & 0 & 0 & \theta_{\delta_{44}} \\ 0 & 0 & 0 & 0 & \theta_{\delta_{55}} \\ 0 & 0 & 0 & 0 & 0 & \theta_{\delta_{66}} \end{bmatrix}
$$

The diagonal elements in this matrix correspond to the δs in the expanded matrix equation.

Comparing the expanded matrix equation and accompanying matrices to the notation in Figure 26.2, the xs are the same as the vs, the λs are the same as the *s on the paths from the latent variable to the indicators, ξ_1 is the same as *F1*, the δs are the same as the us, and ϕ_{11} is the same as the * indicating the variance of *F1*. One advantage of the expanded matrix notation is that it reveals all possible parameters. For instance, we can see that in addition to the variances of the uniqueness, there are parameters that capture the covariances among them. As is evident in the notation, these covariances are fixed to zero.

2. A single latent variable that is not correlated with other variables in a model is just identified with three indicators. This is because the observed covariance matrix includes six nonredundant elements (three variances and three covariances) and the model includes six free parameters—the variance of the latent variable, two loadings (one is fixed at 1.0), and three uniquenesses. An isolated latent variable with two indicators is unidentified because it has four free parameters—the variance

of the latent variable, one loading, and two uniquenesses—but the observed covariance matrix has only three nonredundant elements (two variances and one covariance). In the two-indicator case, the model will be identified if the latent variable is specified as either directionally or nondirectionally related to at least one other variable in a model and the estimate of the parameter for that relation is significantly different from zero.

3. The term *raw data* as I use it here refers to the data that are used in estimation, as opposed to the data that are read by the software program used to do the analysis—the "input file." On the latter count, individual scores on the observed variables or a correlation matrix accompanied by standard deviations can be provided as input. In either case, a covariance matrix is computed before estimation begins. If means are to be modeled, the observed means will need to be included with either the covariance matrix or the correlation matrix with standard deviations. An advantage to providing individual scores on the observed variables is that the parameters that describe the distributions of variables can be derived for use in estimators that make use of that information.

4. Why report a statistic that is not interpreted? Although the χ^2 statistic is not valid for judging the absolute fit of a model, it is useful for comparing certain alternative models and for the construction of certain indices of fit that might not have been included in the report.

5. For this model, the matrix notation requires two equations because the model includes both measurement and structural components. For the measurement model, the equation is

$$
\begin{bmatrix} x_1 \\ x_2 \\ x_3 \\ x_4 \\ x_5 \\ x_6 \\ x_7 \\ x_8 \\ x_9 \\ x_{10} \\ x_{11} \end{bmatrix} = \begin{bmatrix} 1 & 0 & 0 \\ \lambda_{21} & 0 & 0 \\ \lambda_{31} & 0 & 0 \\ 0 & 1 & 0 \\ 0 & \lambda_{52} & 0 \\ 0 & \lambda_{62} & 0 \\ 0 & \lambda_{72} & 0 \\ 0 & \lambda_{82} & 0 \\ 0 & \lambda_{92} & 0 \\ 0 & 0 & 1 \\ 0 & 0 & \lambda_{11,3} \end{bmatrix} \begin{bmatrix} \xi_1 \\ \xi_2 \\ \xi_3 \end{bmatrix} + \begin{bmatrix} \delta_1 \\ \delta_2 \\ \delta_3 \\ \delta_4 \\ \delta_5 \\ \delta_6 \\ \delta_7 \\ \delta_8 \\ \delta_9 \\ \delta_{10} \\ \delta_{11} \end{bmatrix}
$$

or, as before, more compactly,

$$
\mathbf{x} = \lambda_x \xi + \delta
$$

Because there are multiple latent variables that, in an evaluation of the measurement model, would be allowed to covary, we need an additional matrix that includes those covariances, Φ:

$$\begin{bmatrix} \phi_{11} & & \\ \phi_{21} & \phi_{22} & \\ \phi_{31} & \phi_{32} & \phi_{33} \end{bmatrix}$$

In this matrix, the parameters on the diagonal of the matrix are the variances of the latent variables, and the parameters below the diagonal are the covariances between the latent variables. As in the earlier example, the 11×11 θ_δ matrix would include the variances of the uniquenesses on the diagonal (corresponding to the δs in the expanded equation) and, given that we are specifying that none of the uniquenesses covary, zeroes below the diagonal.

In order to specify the structural model using matrix notation, I must distinguish between latent variables that are independent variables (*F1*) and those that are dependent variables (*F2* and *F3*). The former retain their label from the measurement model, ξ, but the latter take on a new label, η. The directional relations between these latent variables are expressed in matrix notation as

$$\begin{bmatrix} \eta_1 \\ \eta_2 \end{bmatrix} = \begin{bmatrix} 0 & 0 \\ \beta_{21} & 0 \end{bmatrix} \begin{bmatrix} \eta_1 \\ \eta_2 \end{bmatrix} + \begin{bmatrix} \gamma_{11} \\ \gamma_{21} \end{bmatrix} \begin{bmatrix} \xi_1 \end{bmatrix} + \begin{bmatrix} \zeta_1 \\ \zeta_2 \end{bmatrix}$$

or, more compactly,

$$\eta = B\eta + \Gamma\xi + \zeta$$

Comparing the expanded matrix equation to relevant aspects of the notation in Figure 26.3, ξ_1 corresponds to *F1* and η_1 and η_2 correspond to *F2* and *F3*, respectively. β_{21} corresponds to the * on the path from *F1* to *F2*, and γ_{11} and γ_{21} correspond to *s on paths from *F1* to *F2* and *F2* to *F3*, respectively. ζ_1 and ζ_2 correspond to the *s indicating the variances of *F2* and *F3*, respectively.

Recommended Readings

Bollen, K. A., & Lennox, R. D. (1991). Conventional wisdom on measurement: A structural equation perspective. *Psychological Bulletin, 110*, 305–314.

Breckler, S. J. (1990). Applications of covariance structure modeling in psychology: Cause for concern? *Psychological Bulletin, 107*, 260–273.

Hoyle, R. H. (2000). Confirmatory factor analysis. In H. E. A. Tinsely & S. D. Brown (Eds.), *Handbook of applied multivariate statistics and mathematical modeling* (pp. 465–497). New York: Academic Press.

Hoyle, R. H., & Smith, G. T. (1994). Formulating clinical research hypotheses as structural equation mod-

els: A conceptual overview. *Journal of Consulting and Clinical Psychology, 62*, 429–440.

Kline, R. B. (2005). *Principles and practice of structural equation modeling* (2nd ed.). New York: Guilford Press.

McDonald, R., & Ho, M.-H. R. (2002). Principles and practice in reporting structural equation analyses. *Psychological Methods, 7*, 64–82.

References

Anderson, J. C., & Gerbing, D. W. (1988). Structural equation modeling in practice: A review and recommended two-step approach. *Psychological Bulletin, 103*, 411–423.

Bentler, P. M. (1990). Comparative fit indices in structural models. *Psychological Bulletin, 107*, 238–246.

Bentler, P. M. (1995). *EQS structural equations program manual*. Encino, CA: Multivariate Software.

Bentler, P. M., & Bonett, D. G. (1980). Significance tests and goodness-of-fit in the analysis of covariance structures. *Psychological Bulletin, 88*, 588–606.

Bollen, K. A. (1989). *Structural equations with latent variables*. New York: Wiley.

Bollen, K. A., & Curran, P. J. (2004). Autoregressive latent trajectory (ALT) models: A synthesis of two traditions. *Sociological Methods and Research, 32*, 336–383.

Bollen, K. A., & Lennox, R. D. (1991). Conventional wisdom on measurement: A structural equation perspective. *Psychological Bulletin, 110*, 305–314.

Breckler, S. J. (1990). Applications of covariance structure modeling in psychology: Cause for concern? *Psychological Bulletin, 107*, 260–273.

Byrne, B. M., Shavelson, R. J., & Muthén, B. (1989). Testing for the equivalence of factor covariance and mean structures: The issue of partial measurement invariance. *Psychological Bulletin, 105*, 456–466.

Campbell, D. T., & Fiske, D. W. (1959). Convergent and discriminant validation by the multitrait–multimethod matrix. *Psychological Bulletin, 56*, 81–105.

Chou, C. P., & Bentler, P. M. (1995). Estimates and tests in structural equation modeling. In R. H. Hoyle (Ed.), *Structural equation modeling: Concepts, issues, and applications* (pp. 37–55). Thousand Oaks, CA: Sage.

Cole, D. A., Martin, N. C., & Steiger, J. H. (2005). Empirical and conceptual problems with longitudinal trait–state models: Introducing a trait–state–occasion model. *Psychological Methods, 10*, 3–20.

Graziano, W. G., Hair, E. C., & Finch, J. F. (1997). Competitiveness mediates the link between personality and group performance. *Journal of Personality and Social Psychology, 73*, 1394–1408.

Graziano, W. G., Jensen-Campbell, L. A., & Finch, J. F. (1997). The self as a mediator between personality and adjustment. *Journal of Personality and Social Psychology, 73,* 392–404.

Hoyle, R. H. (Ed.). (1999). *Statistical strategies for small sample research.* Thousand Oaks, CA: Sage.

Hoyle, R. H., & Duvall, J. L. (2004). Determining the number of factors in exploratory and confirmatory factor analysis. In D. Kaplan (Ed.), *Handbook of quantitative methodology for the social sciences* (pp. 301–315). Thousand Oaks, CA: Sage.

Jöreskog, K. G. (1993). Testing structural equation models. In K. A. Bollen & J. S. Long (Eds.), *Testing structural equation models* (pp. 294–316). Thousand Oaks, CA: Sage.

Jöreskog, K. G. (1994). On the estimation of polychoric correlations and their asymptotic covariance matrix. *Psychometrika, 59,* 381–389.

Kenny, D. A., & Zautra, A. (1995). The trait–state–error model for multiwave data. *Journal of Consulting and Clinical Psychology, 63,* 52–59.

Loehlin, J. C. (1992). *Genes and environment in personality development.* Thousand Oaks, CA: Sage.

MacCallum, R. C. (2003). Working with imperfect models. *Multivariate Behavioral Research, 38,* 113–139.

MacCallum, R. C., Roznowski, M., & Necowitz, L. B. (1992). Model modifications in covariance structure analysis: The problem of capitalization on chance. *Psychological Bulletin, 111,* 490–504.

MacCallum, R. C., Wegener, D. T., Uchino, B. N., & Fabrigar, L. R. (1993). The problem of equivalent models in applications of covariance structure analysis. *Psychological Bulletin, 114,* 185–199.

Marsh, H. W. & Grayson, D. (1995). Latent variable models of multitrait-multimethod data. In R. H. Hoyle (Ed.), *Structural equation modeling: Concepts, issues, and applications* (pp. 177–198). Thousand Oaks, CA: Sage.

Marsh, H. W., Wen, Z., & Hau, K.-T. (2004). Structural equation models of latent interactions: Evaluation of alternative estimation strategies and indicator construction. *Psychological Methods, 9,* 275–300.

McAdams, D. P. (1995). What do we know when we know a person? *Journal of Personality, 63,* 365–396.

Meehl, P. E., & Waller, N. G. (2002). The path analysis controversy: A new statistical approach to strong appraisal of verisimilitude. *Psychological Methods, 7,* 283–300.

Muthén, B. O. (2001). Second-generation structural equation modeling with a combination of categorical and continuous latent variables: New opportunities for latent class/latent growth modeling. In L. M. Col-lins & A. Sayer (Eds.), *New methods for the analysis of change* (pp. 291–322). Washington, DC: American Psychological Association.

Muthén, L. K., & Muthén, B. O. (2004). *Mplus user's guide* (3rd ed.). Los Angeles: Muthén & Muthén.

Myung, J. (2003). Tutorial on maximum likelihood estimation. *Journal of Mathematical Psychology, 47,* 90–100.

Newcomb, M. D. (1994). Drug use and intimate relationships among women and men: Separating specific from general effects in prospective data using structural equation models. *Journal of Consulting and Clinical Psychology, 62,* 463–476.

Panter, A. T., Tanaka, J. S., & Hoyle, R. H. (1994). Structural models for multimode designs in personality and temperament research. In C. F. Halverson, G. A. Kohnstamm, & R. P. Martin (Eds.), *The developing structure of temperament and personality from infancy to adulthood* (pp. 111–138). Hillsdale, NJ: Erlbaum.

Spencer, S. J., Zanna, M. P., & Fong, G. T. (2005). Establishing a causal chain: Why experiments are often more effective than mediational analyses in examining psychological processes. *Journal of Personality and Social Psychology, 89,* 845–851.

Steiger, J. H. (2002). When constraints interact: A caution about reference variables, identification constraints, and scale dependencies in structural equation modeling. *Psychological Methods, 7,* 210–227.

Steiger, J. H., & Lind, J. C. (1980, May). *Statistically based tests for the number of common factors.* Paper presented at the annual meeting of the Psychometric Society, Iowa City, IA.

Tepper, K., & Hoyle, R. H. (1996). Latent variable models of need for uniqueness. *Multivariate Behavioral Research, 31,* 467–494.

Ullman, J. B. (1996). Structural equation modeling. In B. G. Tabachnick & L. S. Fidell (Eds.), *Using multivariate statistics* (3rd ed., pp. 709–819). New York: HarperCollins.

Widaman, K. F., & Reise, S. P. (1997). Exploring the measurement invariance of psychological instruments: Applications in the substance use domain. In K. J. Bryant, M. Windle, & S. G. West (Eds.), *The science of prevention: Methodological advances from alcohol and substance abuse research* (pp. 281–323). Washington, DC: American Psychological Association.

Willett, J. B., & Sayer, A. G. (1994). Using covariance structure analysis to detect correlates and predictors of individual change over time. *Psychological Bulletin, 116,* 363–381.

## CHAPTER 27

The Importance of Being Valid

Reliability and the Process of Construct Validation

Oliver P. John
Christopher J. Soto

The truth is rarely pure and never simple. Modern life would be very
tedious if it were either.
—OSCAR WILDE, *The Importance of Being Earnest*

The empirical sciences all design measurement procedures to obtain accurate information about objects, individuals, or groups. When astronomers measure the behavior of planets and stars, when molecular biologists assay the expression of hormones in cells, when medical doctors assess how much amniotic fluid is left late in a pregnancy, they all worry whether their measurement procedures provide the kind of information they are looking for—that is, is the information generally applicable and does it capture the phenomenon they are interested in? Across all these disciplines, reliability and validity are fundamental concepts that help researchers evaluate how well their measures work.

Consider the amniotic fluid test doctors use to determine whether a fetus may be at risk late in a pregnancy. Exact measurement, as in some of the physical sciences, is not possible here; the doctor can hardly pump out all the amniotic fluid that is left in the mother's amniotic sack to measure its volume exactly (which would indeed put the fetus at risk). Instead, medical researchers have developed an ingenious multistep procedure, using two-dimensional ultrasound images to estimate the three-dimensional volume of fluid present in the uterus. The test is administered by a technician, who produces a single number, which doctors then rely on to make critical treatment decisions. However, as doctors well know (but most patients do not), these numbers are hardly perfect. Two different technicians assessing the same woman do not always come up with the same number; the same technician assessing the same group of women on 2 subsequent days may come up with different results, and in some cases a low amniotic fluid score is obtained even though other measures confirm that the fetus is not at risk. In measurement terms, doctors worry about the degree to which their tests show interjudge agreement, retest reliability, and predictive validity, respectively,

461

and expectant parents (and patients more generally) should be equally worried about these issues. As this example shows, having a keen understanding of issues related to reliability and validity may be important to your own health or that of your loved ones, and this chapter is intended to provide both historical and contemporary ideas about these key measurement issues. In addition, this chapter also provides answers to questions commonly asked by students of personality psychology, such as whether an alpha reliability of .50 is high enough, why we should care whether a scale is unidimensional, and what one should do to show that a measure is valid.

Some Basic Considerations in Evaluating Measurement Procedures

These questions all illustrate the fundamental concern of empirical science with *generalizability*, that is, the degree to which we can make inferences from our measurements or observations in regard to other samples, items, measures, methods, outcomes, and so on (Cronbach, Gleser, Nanda, & Rajaratnam, 1972; see also Brennan, 2001). If we cannot make such generalizations, our measurements are obviously much less useful than if we can provide explicit evidence for generalizability.

Good measurement implies not only that we can reproduce or replicate a certain score, but that we can trust that the measurement has a particular *meaning*—we want to be able to make inferences about other variables that interest us. In the amniotic fluid test example, the volumetric measurements would be useless if they failed to help doctors predict which babies are at risk and should be delivered soon. Another basic idea is that all measures—self-reports, observer ratings, even physiological measures—are prone to errors and that we cannot simply assume that a single measurement will generalize. Any one measurement may be distorted by numerous sources of error (e.g., the medical technician may have made a human error, or the position of the fetus and the umbilical cord may have been unusual, etc.), and the resulting observation (or score) is therefore related only imperfectly to what we want to measure, namely, the risk to the baby. To counteract this limitation of single measurements, psychologists aim to obtain multiple measurements (e.g., across different stimuli, experimenters, or observers) and then aggregate them into a more generalizable composite score.

Personality Measurement: Formulating and Evaluating Models in the Psychometric Tradition

What is measurement and how may it be defined? Early on, Stevens (1951) suggested that measurement is the assignment of numbers to objects or events according to rules. More recently, Dawes and Smith (1985) and others have argued that measurement is best understood as the process of building models that represent phenomena of interest, typically in quantitative form. The raw data in personality research initially exist only in the form of minute events that constitute the ongoing behavior and experience of individuals. Judd and McClelland (1998, pp. 3–4) suggest that

> measurement is the process by which these infinitely varied observations are reduced to compact descriptions or *models* that are presumed to represent meaningful regularities in the entities that are observed ... Accordingly, measurement consists of rules that assign scale or variable values to entities to represent the constructs that are thought to be theoretically meaningful. (emphasis added)

Like most models, measurement models (e.g., tests or scales) have to be reductions or simplifications to be useful. Although they should represent the best possible approximation of the phenomena of interest, we must expect them, like all "working models," to be eventually proven wrong and to be superseded by better models. For this reason, measurement models must be specified explicitly so that they can be evaluated, disconfirmed, and improved. Moreover, we should not ask whether a particular model is true or correct; instead, we should build several plausible alternative models and ask, Given everything we know, which models can we rule out and which model is currently the best at representing our data? Or, even more clearly, which model is the *least wrong*? This kind of comparative model testing (e.g., Judd, McClelland, & Culhane, 1995) is the best strategy for evaluating and improving our measurement procedures.

Organization of This Chapter

This chapter is organized into three major parts. We begin with historically early conceptions of reliability, then move on to increasingly complex views that emphasize the construct validation process, and finally consider model testing as an integrative approach. Specifically, we first consider issues traditionally discussed under the heading of *reliability*, review still-persistent "types" of reliability coefficients, then suggest generalizability theory as a broader perspective, and finally discuss in some detail the problems and misuses of coefficient alpha, the most commonly used psychometric index in personality psychology. Second, we discuss five kinds of evidence that are commonly sought in the process of *construct validation*, which we view as the most crucial issue in psychological measurement. In the third part, we consider *model testing in the context of construct validation*; following a brief introduction to measurement models in structural equation modeling (SEM), we discuss an empirical example that presents the issue of dimensionality as an aspect of structural validity.

From a Focus on "Reliability Coefficients" to Generalizability Theory

As our introductory examples illustrate, most measurement procedures in psychology and other empirical disciplines are subject to "error." In personality psychology, the observations, ratings, or judgments that constitute the measurement procedure are typically made by humans who are subject to a wide range of frailties. Research participants may become careless or inattentive, bored or fatigued, and may not always be motivated to do their best. The particular conditions and point in time when ratings are made or recorded may also contribute error. Further errors may be introduced by the rating or recording forms given to the raters; the instructions, definitions, and questions on these forms may be difficult to understand or require complex discriminations, again entering error into the measurement.

These various characteristics of the participant, the testing situation, the test or instrument, and the experimenter can all introduce measurement error and thus affect what has traditionally been called *reliability*. Reliability refers to the consistency of a measurement procedure, and indices of reliability all describe the extent to which the scores produced by the measurement procedure are reproducible.

Reliability in Classical Test Theory

Issues of reliability have traditionally been treated within the framework of classical test theory (Gulliksen, 1950; Lord & Novick, 1968). If a given measurement X is subject to error e, then the measurement without the error, $X - e$, would represent the accurate or "true" measurement T. This seemingly simply formulation, that each observed measurement X can be partitioned into a true score T and measurement error e, is the fundamental assumption of classical test theory. Conceptually, each true score represents the mean of a very large number of measurements of a specific individual, whereas measurement error represents all of the momentary variations in the circumstances of measurement that are unrelated to the measurement procedure itself. Such errors are assumed to be random (a rather strong assumption, to which we return later), and it is this assumption that permits the definition of error in statistical terms.

Conceptions of reliability all involve the notion of repeated measurements, such as over time or across multiple items, observers, or raters. Classical test theory has relied heavily on the notion of *parallel tests*—that is, two tests that have the same mean, variance, and distributional characteristics and correlate equally with external variables (Lord & Novick, 1968). Under these assumptions, true score and measurement error can be treated as independent. It follows that the variance of the observed scores equals the sum of the variance of the true scores and the variance of the measurement error:

$$\sigma_X^2 = \sigma_{T+e}^2 = \sigma_T^2 + \sigma_e^2$$

Reliability can then be defined as the ratio of the true-score variance to the observed-score variance, which is equivalent to 1 minus the ratio of error variance to observed-score variance:

$$r_{xx} = \frac{\sigma_T^2}{\sigma_X^2} = 1 - \frac{\sigma_e^2}{\sigma_X^2}$$

If there is no error, then the ratio of true-score

variance to total variance (and hence reliability) would be 1; if there is only error and no true-score variance, then this ratio (and hence reliability) would be 0.

Costs of Low Reliability, and Correcting Observed Correlations for Attenuation Due to Low Reliability

Classical test theory (Lord & Novick, 1968) suggests that researchers ought to work hard to attain high reliabilities because the reliability of a measure constrains how strongly that measure may correlate with another variable (e.g., an external criterion). If error is truly random, as classical test theory assumes, the upper limit of the correlation for a measure is not 1.0 but the square root of its reliability (i.e., the correlation of the measure with itself). Thus, the true correlation between the measure and another variable may be underestimated (i.e., attenuated) when reliability is inadequate. In other words, low reliability comes at a cost.

Students sometimes ask questions like "My scale has a reliability of .70—isn't that good enough?" and are frustrated when the answer is, "That depends." Although it would be quite convenient to have a simple cookbook for measurement decisions, there is no minimum or optimum reliability that is necessary, adequate, or even desirable in all contexts. Over the years a convention seems to have evolved, often credited to Nunnally (1978), that regards "reliabilities of .7 or higher" (p. 245) as sufficient. However, a reliability of .70 is *not* a benchmark every measure must pass. In the words of Pedhazur and Schmelkin (1991),

> Does a .5 reliability coefficient stink? To answer this question, no authoritative source will do. Rather, *it is for the user to determine what amount of error variance he or she is willing to tolerate, given the specific circumstances of the study.* (p. 110, emphasis in original)

We wondered, then, is there something useful in the widely shared view of .70 as the "sweet spot" of reliability? To find out, we examined the relative costliness of various levels of reliability, as presented in Table 27.1. We derived the numbers in Table 27.1 by rewriting the formula traditionally used to correct observed correlations for attenuation due to unreliability (Cohen, Cohen, West, & Aiken, 2003; Lord & Novick, 1968) and solving it for the observed

correlations. This equation estimates the expected observed correlation (r_{XY}), given the true correlation between the constructs measured by X and Y (ρ_{XY}) and the geometric average of the two measures' reliabilities (r_{XX} and r_{YY}):

$$r_{XY} = \rho_{XY} \sqrt{r_{XX} r_{YY}}$$

As shown in Table 27.1, if X and Y both have a high reliability of .90 (or an average reliability of .90), then the losses are modest. For example, a true correlation of .70 (an unusually large effect size) would result in an observed correlation of .63 and a true correlation of .30 (a common effect size) would still result in an observed correlation of .27. In short, the loss due to unreliability would be quite small, with observed correlations being 90% of the true correlations—that is, only 10% lower. At an average reliability of .70 (a common situation in personality research), the losses would be more pronounced: A true correlation of .70 would be reduced to .49, and a true correlation of .30 to .21, with observed correlations being only 70% of the true correlations—a loss of 30%. At an average reliability of .50, the losses would be drastic: A true correlation of .70 would become a mere .35, and a true correlation of .30 would be reduced to .15—a 50% loss.

It is easy to see that with small sample sizes and true effect sizes typically in the .15–.40 range, discovering real effects with unreliable measurements becomes increasingly difficult,

TABLE 27.1. The Cost of Low, Medium, and High Reliability: Observed Correlations as a Function of True Correlations and Three Levels of Reliability

True correlation	Mean reliability of X and Y		
	.50	.70	.90
.70	.35	.49	.63
.60	.30	.42	.54
.50	.25	.35	.45
.40	.20	.28	.36
.30	.15	.21	.27
.20	.10	.14	.18
.10	.05	.07	.09

Note. Table entries are observed correlations estimated via equation for the correction of attenuation due to unreliability (see text).

making the costs of reliabilities in the .50 range prohibitive. For example, with a sample of 100 participants and true correlations in the .30 range, an average reliability of .70 is barely large enough to observe statistically significant correlations. If we assume that this scenario is quite common in the field, then the benchmark reliability of ".70 or above" makes some sense; certainly one would not want to accept reliabilities lower than .70 if that means being unable to detect expected correlations in the .30 range.

However, the costs of reliabilities lower than .70 can be at least partially offset. As Table 27.1 shows, if true-correlation sizes are large (or sample sizes are large), lower reliabilities are more easily tolerated because expected effects would still be detected at conventional significance levels. Nonetheless, it must be emphasized that even under these favorable conditions, the true effect sizes will be severely underestimated—a grave disadvantage, given that obtaining replicable estimates of the size of a correlation is now deemed much more important than its statistical significance in any one sample (see Fraley & Marks, Chapter 9, this volume).

Researchers sometimes use reliability indices to *correct* observed correlations between two measures for attenuation due to unreliability. The correction formula (Cohen et al., 2003; Lord & Novick, 1968) involves dividing the observed correlation by the square root of the product of the two reliabilities:

$$\rho'_{XY} = \frac{r_{XY}}{\sqrt{r_{XX}r_{YY}}}$$

This correction expresses the size of the association relative to the maximum correlation attainable, given the imperfect reliabilities of the two measures. This kind of correction is sometimes used to estimate the true correlation between the latent constructs underlying the measures (see also the section on SEM below), thus indicating what the observed correlation would be if both constructs were assessed with perfect reliability. Correction for attenuation can also be useful when researchers want to compare effect sizes across variables or studies that use measures of varying reliabilities, as in meta-analyses (see Roberts, Kuncel, Viechtbauer, & Bogg, Chapter 36, this volume). Another application is in contexts where researchers want to distinguish the long-term stability of personality and attitudes from the reliability of measurement.

However, the ease with which this correction is made should not be seen as a license for sloppy measurement. In many situations, low reliability will create problems for estimating effect sizes, testing hypotheses, and estimating the parameters in structural models—problems that cannot be overcome by simply correcting for attenuation due to unreliability. This is especially true in multivariate applications, such as multitrait–multimethod matrices (discussed below), where unequal reliabilities might bias conclusions about convergent and discriminant validity (West & Finch, 1997). In general, then, researchers are well-advised to invest the time and effort needed to construct reliable measures and consult Table 27.1 to gauge the amount of measurement error that they are willing to tolerate, given the goals of their research.

Evidence for Reliability: Traditional Types of "Reliability Coefficients"

The three most common procedures to assess reliability are shown in Table 27.2: internal consistency (or split-half), retest (or stability), and interrater agreement designs. The American Psychological Association (APA) committee on psychological tests articulated these types of designs to clarify that "reliability is a generic term referring to many types of evidence" (American Psychological Association, 1954, p. 28). Clearly, the different study designs in Table 27.2 assess rather different sources of error. *Internal consistency* procedures offer an estimate of error associated with the particular selection of items; error is high (and internal consistency is low) when items are heterogeneous in content and lack content saturation and when respondents change how they respond to items designed to measure the same characteristic (e.g., owing to fatigue). *Retest* (or stability) designs estimate how much responses vary within individuals across time and situation, thus reflecting error due to differences in the situation and conditions of test administration or observation.[1] *Interrater* or *interjudge agreement* designs estimate how much scores vary across judges or observers (see von Eye & Mun, 2005), thus reflecting error due to disagreements between raters and to individual differences among raters in response styles, such as the way they scale their responses. It is important to note that, as Table 27.2 shows, there are several different reliabil-

TABLE 27.2. Traditional Reliability Coefficients: Study Design, Statistics, Sources of Error, and Facets of Generalizability

Traditional reliability coefficient	Study design	Reliability statistic	Major sources of error	Facet of generalizability
Internal consistency	Measure participants at a single time across multiple items	Cronbach's coefficient alpha (split-half correlations rarely used today)	Heterogeneous item content; participant fatigue	Items
Retest	Measure the same participants across two or more occasions or times using the same set of items	Correlation between participants' scores at the two times	Change in participants' responses; change in measurement situation	Occasions
Interrater (interjudge)	Obtain ratings of a set of stimuli (individuals, video recordings, transcribed interviews) from multiple raters (e.g., observers, coders) at one time	1. Mean pairwise interrater agreement correlation (for reliability of a typical single rater) 2. Cronbach's coefficient alpha (for reliability of the mean rating) 3. Cohen's kappa (for agreement of categorical ratings)	Disagreement among raters; variation in raters' response styles	Raters

ity indices, and not all of them are based on correlations; therefore, different criteria for evaluating the reliability of a measure will be needed. Values approaching 1.0 are not expected for all reliability indices—for example, Cohen's kappa, which measures agreement among categorical judgments (see, e.g., von Eye & Mun, 2005).

Moving beyond the Classical Conception of Reliability: Generalizability Theory

The distinctions among "types of reliability coefficients" had a number of unfortunate consequences. First, what had been intended as heuristic distinctions became reified as *the* stability coefficient or *the* alpha coefficient even though the notion of reliability was intended as a general concept. Second, the classification itself was too simple, equating particular kinds of reliability evidence with only one source of error and resulting in a restrictive terminology that cannot fully capture the broad range and combination of multiple error sources that are of interest in most research and measurement applications (e.g., Shavelson, Webb, & Rowley, 1989). For example, as we show in Table 27.2, retest reliability involves potential changes over

time in both the research participants and the testing conditions (e.g., prior to vs. just after September 11, 2001).

Third, the types-of-reliability approach masked a major shortcoming of classical test theory: If all these measures were indeed parallel and all errors truly random, then all these approaches to reliability should yield the same answer. Unfortunately, they do not, because reliability depends on the particular *facet* of generalization being examined (Cronbach, Rajaratnam, & Gleser, 1963). For example, to address the need for superbrief scales of the Big Five trait domains for use in surveys and experimental contexts, researchers have recently constructed scales consisting of only two or four items each (Gosling, Rentfrow, & Swann, 2003; Rammstedt & John, 2006, 2007). These items were not chosen to be redundant in meaning but instead to represent the broad Big Five domains, as well as to balance scoring by including both true-scored and false-scored items. Not surprisingly, the resulting scales had very low internal consistency (alpha) reliabilities. Does this mean that these scales are generally unreliable? Not at all. They do show impressive reliability when other facets of generalizability are considered. For example, with less than one-quarter of the items of the full-length 44-item Big Five Inventory (BFI; see John & Srivastava, 1999), the BFI-10 scales can still represent the content of the full scales with an average part–whole correlation of .83; 6-week retest correlations average .75. In short, different types of reliability have conceptually distinct meanings that do not necessarily cohere.

Therefore, the American Psychological Association (e.g., 1985) recommended in subsequent editions of the *Standards for Educational and Psychological Testing* that these distinctions and terminology be abolished and replaced by the broader view advocated by generalizability theory (Cronbach et al., 1963). Regrettably, however, practice has not changed much over the years, and generalizability theory has not fully replaced these more simplistic notions. Note that the last column in Table 27.2 spells out the *facet of generalizability* that is being varied and studied in each of these generalizability designs.

Generalizability theory holds that we are interested in the "reliability" of an observation or measurement because we wish to *generalize* from this observation to some other class of observations. For example, Table 27.2 shows that a concern with interjudge reliability may actually be a concern with the question of how accurately we can generalize from one judge to another (pairwise agreement) or from a given set of judges to another set (generalizability of aggregated or total scores). Or we may want to know how well scores on an attitude scale constructed according to one set of procedures generalize to another scale constructed according to different procedures. Or we may want to test how generalizable is a scale originally developed in English to a Chinese language and cultural context.

All these facets of generalizability represent legitimate research concerns (see the later section on construct validation), and they can be studied systematically in generalizability designs, both individually and together. These designs allow the researcher to deliberately vary the facets that potentially influence observed scores and estimate the variance attributable to each facet (Cronbach et al., 1972). In other words, whereas classical test theory tries to estimate the portion of variance that is attributable to "error," generalizability theory aims to estimate the extent to which specific sources of variance contribute to test scores under carefully defined conditions. Thus, instead of the

traditional reliability coefficients listed in Table 27.2, we should use more general estimates, such as intraclass correlation coefficients (Shrout & Fleiss, 1979), to probe particular aspects of the dependability of measures. For example, intraclass coefficients can be used to index the generalizability of one set of judges to a universe of similar judges (von Eye & Mun, 2005).

Generalizability theory *should* hold considerable appeal for psychologists because the extent to which we can generalize across items, instruments, contexts, groups, languages, and cultures is crucial to the claims we can make about our findings. Despite excellent and readable introductions (e.g., Brennan, 2001; Shavelson et al., 1989), generalizability theory is still not used as widely as it should be. A recent exception is the flourishing research on the determinants of consensus among personality raters (e.g., Kenny, 1994; see also John & Robins, 1993; Kashy & Kenny, 2000; Kwan, John, Kenny, Bond, & Robins, 2004).

Generalizability theory is especially useful when data are collected in nested designs and multiple facets may influence reliability, as illustrated by King and Figueredo's (1997) research on chimpanzee personality differences. The investigators collected ratings of chimpanzees, differing in age and sex (subject variables) on 40 traits (stimulus variables) at several different zoos (setting variables), from animal keepers familiar with the animals to varying degrees (observer variables). They then used a generalizability design to show how these facets affected agreement among the judges. It is unfortunate that generalizability theory, as well as Kenny's (1994) social relations model, have been perceived as "technical." With clear and accessible introductions available, it is high time that these important approaches to variance decomposition achieve greater popularity with a broader group of researchers.

Coefficient Alpha: Personality Psychology's Misunderstood Giant

Cronbach's (1951) coefficient alpha is an index of internal consistency that has become the default reliability index in personality research. Any recent issue of a personality journal will show that alpha is the index of choice when researchers want to claim that their measure is reliable. Often it is the only reliability evidence considered, contrary to the recommendations in the *Standards* (American Psychological Association, 1985).

We suspect that alpha has become so ubiquitous because it is easy to obtain and compute. Alpha does not require collecting data at two different times from the same subjects, as retest reliability does, or the construction of two alternate forms of a measure, as parallel-form reliability (now rarely used) would require. Alpha is a "least effort" reliability index—it can be used as long as the same subjects responded to multiple items thought to indicate the same construct. And, computationally, SPSS and other statistical packages now allow the user to view the alpha of many alternative scales formed from any motley collection of items with just a few mouse clicks. Unfortunately, whereas alpha has many important uses, it also has important limitations—long known to methodologists, these limitations are less well appreciated by researchers and thus worth reviewing in some detail.

Alpha Is Determined by Both Item Homogeneity (Content Saturation) and Scale Length

The alpha coefficient originated as a generalization of split-half reliability, representing the corrected mean of the reliabilities computed from all possible split-halves of a test. As such, alpha is a function of two parameters: (1) the homogeneity or interrelatedness of the items in a test or scale (as indexed by the mean intercorrelation of all the items on the test, $\bar{r}_{ij}$) and (2) the length of the test (as indexed by the number of items on the test, k). The formula is

$$\alpha = \frac{k\bar{r}_{ij}}{k\bar{r}_{ij} + (1 - \bar{r}_{ij})}$$

Conceptually, note that the term on the top of the fraction allows alpha to increase as the number of items on the scale goes up and as the mean intercorrelation between the items on the scale increases. However, to constrain alpha to a range from 0 to 1, the same term repeats at the bottom of the fraction *plus* a norming term $(1 - \text{mean } r_{ij})$ that increases the divisor as the mean interitem correlation decreases. If that interitem correlation were indeed 1, the norming term would reduce to 0 and alpha would be at its maximum of 1.0 regardless how many items were on the scale. Conversely, if the interitem correlation were 0, the numerator would become 0 and so would alpha, again re-

gardless of the number of items on the scale. Finally, alpha is defined meaningfully only for $K \geq 2$ because at least 2 items are needed to compute the mean interitem correlation required for the formula. Consider a questionnaire scale with 9 items and mean $r_{ij} = .42$: alpha would be $(9 \times .42)/(9 \times .42 + [1 - .42]) = 3.78/(3.78 + .58) = .87$.

What exactly does alpha mean, then? An alpha of .87 means, in plain English, that the *total score derived from aggregating these 9 items would correlate .87 with the total score derived from aggregating another (imaginary) set of 9 equivalent items; that is, alpha captures the generalizability of the total score from one item set to another item set.* The term *internal consistency* is therefore a misleading label for alpha: The homogeneity or interrelatedness of the items on the scale and the length of the scale have been aggregated and thus integrated into the total score, and the generalizability of this total score (i.e., alpha) can therefore no longer tell us anything concrete about the internal structure or consistency of the scale. The hypothetical data presented in Table 27.3 were designed to make these points as concrete and vivid as possible.

Table 27.3 shows the interitem correlation matrices for three hypothetical questionnaire scales. Following Schmitt (1996), we constructed our examples in correlational (rather than covariance) terms for ease of interpretation. Scale A is the one we just considered, with 9 items, a mean interitem correlation of .42, and an alpha of .87. Scale B has 6 items, and it has the same alpha of .87 as Scale A. But note that Scale B attained that alpha in a rather different way. Scale B has 3 fewer items, but that deficiency is offset by the greater homogeneity or content saturation of its items: They are more highly intercorrelated (mean $r_{ij} = .52$) than are the 9 items of Scale A (mean $r_{ij} = .42$).

This example illustrates the idea that test length can compensate for lower levels of interitem correlation, an idea that is formalized in the Spearman–Brown prophecy formula, which specifies the relation between test length and reliability (see, e.g., Lord & Novick, 1968). For any mean interitem correlation, the formula computes how many items are needed to achieve a certain level of alpha. Figure 27.1 shows this relation for mean interitem correlations of .20, .40, .60, and .80. Three points are worth noting. First, the alpha reliability of the total scale always increases as the number of

TABLE 27.3. Interitem Correlation Matrix for Three Hypothetical Scales with Equal Coefficient Alpha Reliability

Scale A: 9 items, mean interitem correlation = .42, α = .87

	1	2	3	4	5	6	7	8	9
1	—								
2	.42	—							
3	.42	.42	—						
4	.42	.42	.42	—					
5	.42	.42	.42	.42	—				
6	.42	.42	.42	.42	.42	—			
7	.42	.42	.42	.42	.42	.42	—		
8	.42	.42	.42	.42	.42	.42	.42	—	
9	.42	.42	.42	.42	.42	.42	.42	.42	—

Scale B: 6 items, mean interitem correlation = .52, α = .87

	1	2	3	4	5	6
1	—					
2	.52	—				
3	.52	.52	—			
4	.52	.52	.52	—		
5	.52	.52	.52	.52	—	
6	.52	.52	.52	.52	.52	—

Scale C: 6 items, mean interitem correlation = .52, α = .87

	1	2	3	4	5	6
1	—					
2	.70	—				
3	.70	.70	—			
4	.40	.40	.40	—		
5	.40	.40	.40	.70	—	
6	.40	.40	.40	.70	.70	—

Note CFA analyses showed that for Scale A, all items load .648 on a single factor; fit is perfect. For Scale B, all items load .721 on a single factor; fit is perfect. In contrast, Scale C is not unidimensional; for the one-factor model, all items load .721 and standardized root mean residual (RMR) is only .124. For two-factor models for Scale C, all items load .837 on their factor; the interfactor correlation is .571 and fit is perfect.

items increases (as long as adding items does not lower the mean interitem correlation). Second, the utility of adding ever more items diminishes quickly, so that adding the 15th item leads to a much smaller increase in alpha than adding the 5th item, just as consuming the 15th beer or chocolate bar adds less enjoyment than consuming the earlier ones. Third, less is to be gained from adding more items if those items are highly intercorrelated (e.g., mean r_{ij} = .60) than when they show little content saturation (e.g., mean r_{ij} = .20). The lesson here is that we need to be careful in interpreting alpha; we must recognize that a given magnitude of alpha may be achieved via many possible combinations of content saturation and scale length.

These considerations make clear that alpha is a statistic that applies only to the total score (mean or sum) derived by aggregating across multiple items, observations, or even observers. Often researchers are more concerned about the homogeneity of the items, and the only way to estimate that is a direct index of item content saturation, the simplest being the mean interitem correlation (r_{ij}). We strongly recommend that researchers routinely compute both alpha and the mean interitem correlation (available in the SPSS Reliability program under statistics). The two indexes provide different information: The mean interitem correlation tells us about the items—how closely are they related? how unique versus redundant is the variance

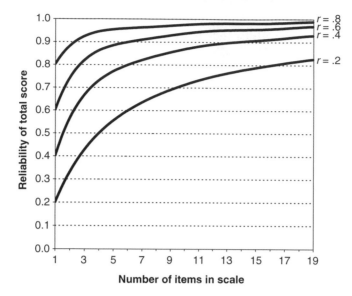

FIGURE 27.1. Cronbach's coefficient alpha reliability as a function of the number of items on a scale (k) and the mean of the correlations among all the items (mean r_{ij}); see the text for the formula used to generate this graph.

they are capturing?—whereas alpha tells us about the total or aggregated scale score.

Alpha Does Not Index Unidimensionality

The third scale in Table 27.3 highlights a second issue with alpha. Contrary to popular belief, alpha does *not* indicate the degree to which the interitem intercorrelations are homogeneously distributed, nor does a high alpha indicate that a scale is unidimensional. In fact, although Scale C in Table 27.3 has the same alpha and mean interitem correlation as Scale B, it differs radically in the dispersion (or variance) of the correlations between its items. For Scale B, the correlations are completely homogeneous (all are .52, with a standard deviation, *SD*, of 0 in this hypothetical example), whereas for Scale C they vary considerably (from .40 to .70, with an *SD* of .15). Because computation of alpha does not consider this variability, Cortina (1993) derived an index that reflects the spread of the interitem correlations and argued that this index should be reported along with alpha. A large spread in interitem correlations is a bad sign because it suggests that either the test is multidimensional or the interitem correlations are distorted by substantial sampling error. In our example, the pattern of item intercorrelations for Scale C suggests that the problem is multidimensionality.

Clearly, the responses to these 6 items are a function of not one, but two, factors: Items 1, 2, and 3 correlate much more substantially with each other (mean r = .7) than they correlate (mean r = .4) with items 4, 5, and 6, which in turn correlate more highly among themselves (mean r = .7). Alpha completely disguises this rather important difference between Scales C and B.

Because alpha cannot address it, unidimensionality needs to be established in other ways, as we describe in later sections of this chapter on structural validity and on model testing; there we also discuss factor analyses of the example data in Table 27.3. Here, it is important to emphasize that the issue of error (or unreliability) present in an item is separate from the issue of multidimensionality. In other words, unidimensionality does not imply lower levels of measurement error (i.e., unreliability), and multidimensionality does not imply higher levels of error. Once we know that a test is not unidimensional, can we go ahead and still use alpha as a reliability index? Unfortunately, the answer is no. The reliability of a multidimensional scale can be estimated only through parallel forms, which must have the same factor structure (Cronbach, 1947, 1951). In fact, if the test is not unidimensional, then alpha *underestimates* reliability (see Schmitt, 1996, for an example). Thus, if a test is found to be multidimensional, one should score two unidimensional subscales and then use alpha to index their reliabilities separately.[2]

Evaluating the Size of Alpha

According to Classical Test Theory, increasing alpha can have only beneficial effects. As discussed previously, higher reliability means that a greater proportion of the individual differences in measurement scores reflect variance in the construct being assessed (as opposed to error variance), thus increasing the power to detect significant relations between variables. In reality, however, instead of assuming that a bigger alpha coefficient is always better, alpha must be interpreted in terms of its two main parameters—interitem correlation and scale length—and in the context of how these two parameters fit the definition of the particular construct to be measured. In any one context, a particular level of alpha may be too high, too low, or just right.

Alpha and Item Redundancy

Consider a researcher who wants to measure the broad construct of neuroticism—which includes anxiety, depression, and hostility as more specific facets (see Figure 27.2). The researcher has developed a scale with the following items: "I am afraid of spiders," "I get anxious around creepy-crawly things," "I am not bothered by insects" (reverse scored), and "Spiders tend to make me nervous." Note that these items are essentially paraphrases of each other and represent the same item content (arachnophobia or being afraid of insects) stated in slightly different ways. Cattell (1972) considered scales of this kind to be "bloated specifics"—they have high alphas simply because the item content is extremely redundant and the resulting interitem correlations are very high. Thus, alphas in the high .80's or even .90's, especially for short scales, may not indicate an impressively reliable scale but instead signal redundancy or narrowness in item content. Such measures are susceptible to the so-called *attenuation paradox*: Increasing the internal consistency of a test beyond a certain point will not enhance validity and may even come at the expense of validity when the added items emphasize one narrow part of the construct over other important parts.

An example of a measure with high item redundancy is the 10-item Rosenberg (1979) self-esteem scale, which has alphas approaching .90 and some interitem correlations approaching .70 (Gray-Little, Williams, & Hancock, 1997; Robins, Hendin, & Trzesniewski, 2001). Not surprisingly, some of these items turn out to be almost synonymous, such as "I certainly feel useless at times" and "At times I think I am no good at all." Although such redundant items increase alpha, they do not add unique (and thus incremental) information and can often be omitted in the interest of efficiency, suggesting that the scale can be abbreviated without much loss of information (see, e.g., Robins et al., 2001). More recently, considerable item redundancy was noted by the authors of the original and revised Experiences in Close Relationships questionnaires (ECR and ECR-R; Brennan, Clark, & Shaver, 1998; Fraley, Waller, & Brennan, 2000). One example of a redundant item pair, from the ECR anxiety scale, is "I worry about being abandoned" and "I worry a fair amount about losing my partner." A second example, from the ECR avoidance scale, is "Just when my partner starts to get close to me, I find myself pulling away" and "I want to get close to my partner, but I keep pulling back." We have observed interitem correlations in excess of .70 for each of these pairs (Soto, Gorchoff, & John, 2006).

The fear-of-insects items on the hypothetical neuroticism scale illustrate how easy it is to boost alpha by writing redundant items. However, unless one is specifically interested in insect phobias, this strategy is not very useful. The narrow content representation (i.e., high content homogeneity) would make this scale less useful as a measure of the broader construct of neuroticism. Although the scale may predict the intensity of emotional reactions to spiders with great precision (or fidelity), it is less likely to relate to anything else of interest because of its very narrow bandwidth. Conversely, broadband measures (e.g., a neuroticism scale) can predict a wider range of outcomes or behaviors but generally do so with lower fidelity. This phenomenon is known as the bandwidth–fidelity tradeoff (Cronbach & Gleser, 1957) and has proven to be of considerable importance in many literatures, including personality traits (Epstein, 1980; John, Hampson, & Goldberg, 1991) and attitudes (Eagly & Chaiken, 1993; Fishbein & Ajzen, 1974). In general, predictive accuracy is maximized when the trait or attitude serving as the predictor is measured at a similar level of abstraction as the criterion to be predicted.

The close connection between the hierarchical level of the construct to be measured and the content homogeneity of the items is illustrated in Figure 27.2. Anxiety, depression, and hostility are three trait constructs that tend to be positively intercorrelated and together define the broader construct of neuroticism (e.g., Costa & McCrae, 1992). (Our initial example of the insect phobia scale might be represented as an even lower-level construct, one of many more specific components of anxiety.) Consider now the anxiety scale on the left side of Figure 27.2. Because its six items represent a narrow range of content (e.g., being fearful, nervous, and worrying), item content should be relatively homogeneous, leading to a reasonably high mean interitem correlation and, with 6 items, a reasonable alpha reliability. Similar expectations should hold for the six-item depression and hostility scales.

Researchers rarely publish or even discuss interitem correlations, and so far we have focused on hypothetical data to illustrate general issues. How high are typical interitem correlations on personality questionnaire scales? Are

they closer to .70, indicating a high level of redundancy, or to .30, suggesting more modest overlap? Table 27.4 provides real data from a sample of University of California–Berkeley undergraduates ($N = 649$); for this illustration, we used their responses to a subset of 12 neuroticism items selected from Costa and McCrae's (1992) NEO Personality Inventory—Revised (NEO-PI-R) anxiety (A) and depression (D) facet scales. In the NEO-PI-R, each of the Big Five personality domains is defined by 6 "facet" scales that each have 8 items; the resulting 48-item Big Five scales are very long and thus all have alphas exceeding .90.

We examine the reliability of the anxiety and depression facet scales first. Consider the relevant within-facet interitem correlations that are set in **bold** in Table 27.4. All these correlations were positive and significant; their mean was .38 for the 6 anxiety items and .39 for the 6 depression items, as shown in Figure 27.2. That is, even for these lower-level facet scales, the items on the scale correlated only moderately with each other. With these moderate interitem correlations, the 6-item facet scales attained alphas of .78 for anxiety and .79 for depression (Figure 27.2).

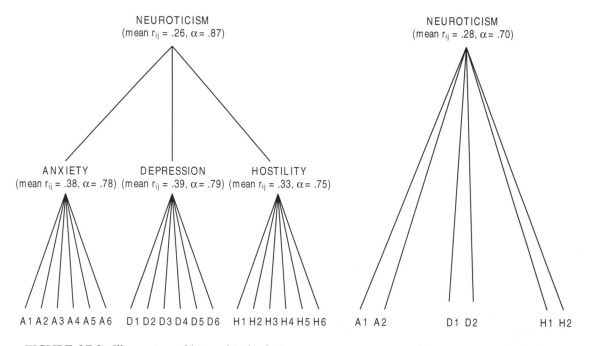

FIGURE 27.2. Illustration of hierarchical relations among constructs and homogeneity of item content: A general neuroticism factor and more specific 6-item facets of anxiety (A), depression (D), and hostility (H); the results of internal consistency (alpha) analyses for each scale are shown in parentheses ($N = 649$).

TABLE 27.4. How High Are Interitem Correlations on Personality Questionnaire Scales?: Correlations among 12 Neuroticism Items Selected from the NEO-PI-R Anxiety (A) and Depression (D) Facet Scales

	A1	A2	A3	A4	A5	A6	D1	D2	D3	D4	D5	D6
A1	—											
A2	.39	—										
A3	.44	.43	—									
A4	.33	.31	.51	—								
A5	.32	.22	.40	.27	—							
A6	.43	.36	.47	.44	.34	—						
D1	.26	.19	.37	.35	.33	.31	—					
D2	.21	.27	.33	.42	.20	.34	.45	—				
D3	.25	.20	.40	.39	.27	.32	.59	.48	—			
D4	.21	.23	.24	.30	.14	.30	.29	.39	.25	—		
D5	.28	.23	.29	.32	.14	.40	.24	.43	.29	.29	—	
D6	.22	.34	.29	.37	.21	.30	.38	.61	.43	.30	.44	—

Note. N = 649. For all correlations, $p < .01$. Items A1–A6 are the first six items of the eight-item NEO-PI-R (Costa & McCrae, 1992) anxiety facet scale; D1–D6 are the first six items of the eight-item depression scale. False-keyed items have been reverse-scored here. Within-facet interitem correlations (mean $r = .38$) are set in **bold**, whereas between-facet interitem correlations (mean $r = .28$) are set in regular type. The interitem correlations for item A4 that are shown in *italics* illustrate discriminant-validity problems; specifically, three within-facet correlations (with anxiety items 1, 2, and 4) were lower than four of its cross-facet correlations (with depression items 1, 2, 3, and 6). The broader theoretical structure model for these data, and the mean interitem correlations and alpha reliabilities for the resulting scales, are shown in Figure 27.2, and the results of exploratory factor analysis (EFA) and CFA analyses in Figures 27.3 and 27.4, respectively.

Now consider the between-facet interitem correlations, set in regular type; their mean was .28, lower on average than the (**bold**) within-facet correlations. This is as expected: Although all 12 of these neuroticism items should intercorrelate, the cross-facet (or discriminant) correlations of anxiety items with depression items should be lower than the within-facet (or convergent) correlations. This convergent–discriminant pattern generally held for the individual items, but there was at least one problematic item, A4 ("I often feel tense and jittery"). Consider the *italicized* interitem correlations for A4. Three of its within-facet correlations (with A1, A2, and A5) were lower than four of its cross-facet correlations (with D1, D2, D3, and D6), indicating that this item did not clearly differentiate anxiety from depression.

The hierarchical-structure model in Figure 27.2 implies that the facet scales should cohere as components of the broader neuroticism domain but also differentiate anxious from depressed mood. How high, then, should facet intercorrelations be? In our student sample, the anxiety scale and depression scale correlated .58; even when corrected for attenuation due to unreliability, the estimated true correlation of .74 remained clearly below 1.0. More generally, using the full-length 8-item NEO-PI-R

facet scales, the mean correlation between facets within the same superordinate Big Five domain was .40, indicating that same-domain facet scales share some common variance but also retain some uniqueness. This moderate correlation also reminds us that superordinate dimensions can be measured reliably with relatively heterogeneous "building blocks" as long as there are enough such blocks—six facets per Big Five domain in the case of the NEO-PI-R.

Finally, scales for broadband constructs like neuroticism must address issues of item heterogeneity. Consider a 6-item neuroticism scale (shown on the right side of Figure 27.2), consisting of two anxiety items, A1 and A2; two depression items, D1 and D2; and two hostility items, H1 and H2. As compared with the lower-level facet scales, the item content on this superordinate scale is much more heterogeneous, which should lead to a lower mean interitem correlation and thus a lower alpha, given that scale length is constant at 6 items. Indeed, the analyses in our student sample bear out this prediction; the mean interitem correlation was only .28 and alpha .70.

One implication of Figure 27.2 is that if one wants to measure broader constructs such as neuroticism, one should probably include a larger number of items to compensate for the greater content heterogeneity. For example, one might use all 18 items, from A1 to H6, to measure the superordinate neuroticism construct defined on the left side of Figure 27.2. As one would expect, the mean interitem correlation for the 18-item scale was .26, just as low as that for the 6-item neuroticism scale, but this longer scale had an impressive alpha of .87. As we discuss next, however, the strategy of increasing alpha by increasing scale length can be taken too far.

Alpha and Scale Length

Whereas scales with unduly redundant item content have conceptual limitations, scales that bolster alpha by including a great many items have practical disadvantages. Overlong scales or assessment batteries can produce respondent fatigue and therefore less reliable responses (e.g., Burisch, 1984). Lengthy scales also consume an inordinate amount of participants' time, making it likely that researchers will use them only if their interests lie solely with the construct being measured. Recognition of these disadvantages has led to a growing number of very brief measures.

Indeed, for very brief scales, alpha may not be a sensible facet of generalizability at all. For example, in our discussion of generalizability theory, we noted that very brief Big Five scales did not have high interitem correlations, because the items were chosen to represent very broad constructs as comprehensively as possible (e.g., Rammstedt & John, 2006, in press). Not surprisingly, these scales had paltry alphas; more important, they showed substantial retest reliability and predicted the longer scales that they were designed to represent quite well, findings that also hold for other innovative short measures, such as the single-item self-esteem scale (Robins et al., 2001).

Resisting the Temptation of Too-High Alphas

What can be done to prevent the construction of scales whose internal consistencies are too high? Some rules of thumb can serve as a start. We suggest that scale developers review all pairs of items that intercorrelate .60 or higher to decide whether one item in the pair may be eliminated. Ultimately, however, there is no foolproof empirical solution; as scale developers, only good judgment can save us from the siren song of inappropriately maximized alphas. Specifically, we must keep in mind that,

beyond a certain point, the length of a scale will be inversely related to its usefulness for many researchers—researchers are operating under constraints on the recruitment and assessment of participants. We must also control our desire to maximize interitem correlations by way of item redundancy. We can achieve this by making sure that, throughout the scale development process, the breadth of the construct we intend to measure is reflected in the breadth of the scale items we intend to measure it with.

Item Response Theory

Classical test theory has also been criticized by advocates of item response theory (IRT; e.g., Embretson, 1996; Embretson & Reise, 2000; Mellenbergh, 1996). In classical theory, the characteristics of the individual test taker and those of the test cannot be separated (Hambleton, Swaminathan, & Rogers, 1991). That is, the person's standing on the underlying construct is defined only in terms of responses on the particular test; thus, the same person may appear quite liberal on a test that includes many items measuring extremely conservative beliefs but quite conservative on a test that includes many items measuring radical liberal beliefs. The psychometric characteristics of the test also depend on the particular sample of respondents; for example, whether a belief item from a conservatism scale reliably discriminates high and low scorers depends on the level of conservatism of the sample, so that the same test may work well in a very liberal student sample but fail to make reliable distinctions among the relatively more conservative respondents in an older sample. In short, classical test theory does not apply if we want to compare individuals who have taken different tests measuring the same construct or if we want to compare items answered by different groups of individuals.

Another limitation of classical test theory is the assumption that the degree of measurement error is the same for all individuals in the sample—an implausible assumption, given that tests and items differ in their ability to discriminate among respondents at different levels of the underlying construct (Lord, 1984). Moreover, classical theory is test-oriented rather than item-oriented and thus does not make predictions about how an individual or group will perform on a particular item.

These limitations can be addressed in IRT (see Morizot, Ainsworth, & Reise, Chapter 24, this volume). Briefly put, IRT provides quantitative procedures to describe the relation of a particular item to the latent construct being measured in terms of difficulty and discrimination parameters. This information can be useful for item analysis and scale construction, permitting researchers to select items that best measure a particular level of a construct and to detect items biased for particular respondent groups. IRT is increasingly being applied to personality measures, such as self-esteem (Gray-Little et al., 1997) and romantic attachment (Fraley et al., 2000).

To summarize, in this section we focused on classical test theory approaches to reliability, the costs associated with low reliability and the practice of correcting for attenuation, specific types of reliability indices, and issues with coefficient alpha (test length, unidimensionality, and construct definitions). In our discussion, we mentioned such concepts as latent (or underlying) constructs, construct definitions, dimensionality, criterion variables, and discriminant relations, but did not discuss them systematically. These concepts are complex and go beyond the classical view of reliability, emphasizing that the meaning and interpretation of measurements is crucial to evaluating the quality of our measurements. Traditionally, issues of score meaning and interpretation are discussed under the heading of validity, to which we now turn.

Construct Validation

Measurements of psychological constructs, such as neuroticism, rejection sensitivity, or smiling, are fundamentally different from basic physical measurements (e.g., mass), which can often be based on concrete standards—such as the 1-kilogram chunk of platinum and iridium that standardizes the measurement of mass. Unfortunately, the behaviorist movement sparked a preoccupation with "gold standards" (or platinum-and-iridium standards) for psychological measures (e.g., Cureton, 1951) that lasted into the 1970s (see Kane, 2004). Eventually researchers came to recognize that for most psychological concepts there exists no single, objective, definitional criterion standard against which all other such measures can be compared.

In the absence of such criterion standards, personality psychologists have long been concerned with ways to conceptualize the validity of their measurement procedures. Although the first American Psychological Association committee on psychological tests distinguished initially among several "types" of validity, Cronbach and Meehl (1955) had already recognized that all validation of psychological measures is fundamentally concerned with what they called construct validity—evidence that scores on a particular measure can be interpreted as reflecting variation in a particular construct (i.e., an inferred characteristic) that has particular implications for human behavior, emotion, and cognition.

Process and Evidence

The idea of construct validity has been elaborated upon over time by such investigators as Loevinger (1957), Cronbach (1988), and Messick (1995), and it is now generally recognized as *the central concern* in psychological measurement (see also Braun, Jackson, & Wiley, 2002; Kane, 2004). The 1999 edition of the *Standards for Educational and Psychological Testing* (American Educational Research Association, American Psychological Association, & National Council on Measurement in Education, 1999) emphasizes that "validation can be viewed as developing a scientifically sound validity argument to support the intended interpretation of test scores and their relevance to the proposed use" (p. 9). Yet construct validity continues to strike many of us, from graduate students to senior professors, as a rather nebulous or "amorphous" concept (Briggs, 2004), perhaps because there is no such thing as "the construct validity coefficient," no single statistic that researchers can point to as proof that their measure is valid. Because of this, it may be easier to think of construct validity as a process (i.e., the steps that one would follow to test whether a particular interpretation of a particular measure is valid) than as a property (i.e., the specific thing that a measurement interpretation must have in order to be valid).

Keeping with this emphasis on construct validity as a process rather than a property, Smith (2005b) articulated four key steps in the validation process. First, a definition of the theoretical construct to be measured is proposed. Second, a theory, of which the construct in question is a part, is translated into hypotheses about how a valid measure of the construct would be expected to act. Third, research designs appropriate for testing these hypotheses are formulated. Fourth, data are collected using these designs and observations based on these data are compared to predictions. (For a similar, process-oriented approach based on definition and evidence, see Kane, 2004.)

A fifth step, revision of the theory, construct, or measure (and repetition of steps one through four), highlights the idea that the construct validation process is a basic form of theory testing: "To validate a measure of a construct is to validate a theory" (Smith, 2005a, p. 413). As with any other theory or model, the validity of the particular score interpretation can never be fully established but is always evolving to form an ever-growing "nomological network" of validity-supporting relations (Wiggins, 1973).

Given that multiple pieces of evidence are needed to cumulatively support the hypothesized construct, it is often difficult to quickly summarize the available validity evidence. For example, Snyder (1987) wrote an entire book to summarize the validity argument (Cronbach, 1988) for his self-monitoring construct, drawing on everything that had been learned about this construct in more than 15 years of empirical research and construct development. More recently, meta-analytic techniques have proven useful to make such data summaries more manageable and objective (Schmidt, Hunter, Pearlman, & Hirsch, 1985). Westen and Rosenthal (2003) proposed two heuristic indices to operationalize construct validity in terms of the relative fit of observations to hypotheses, thus addressing the fourth step in Smith's (2005b) process model. Nonetheless, attempts to quantify construct validity remain controversial (cf. Smith, 2005a, 2005b; Westen & Rosenthal, 2005).

Another way to elaborate the notion of construct validity in personality psychology is to consider the kinds of evidence that personality psychologists typically seek as part of the construct validation process (cf. Messick, 1989, 1995). Here we focus on five major forms of

TABLE 27.5. Five Commonly Sought Forms of Evidence for Construct Validity and Some Examples

Forms of evidence for construct validity	Examples of study designs
1. *Generalizability:* Evidence that score properties and interpretations generalize across population groups, settings, and tasks	*Reliability and replication:* Test whether score properties are consistent across occasions (i.e., retest reliability), samples, and measurement methods (e.g., self-report and peer report)
2. *Content validity:* Evidence of content relevance, representativeness, and technical quality of items	*Expert judgments and review:* Test whether experts agree that items are relevant and represent the construct domain; use ratings to assess item characteristics, such as comprehensibility and clarity
3. *Structural validity:* Evidence that the internal structure of the measure reflects the internal structure of the construct domain	*Exploratory or confirmatory factor analysis:* Test whether the factor structure of the measure matches the hypothesized structure of the construct
4. *External validity:* Evidence that the measure relates to other measures and to nontest criteria in theoretically expected ways	*Criterion correlation:* Test whether measurement scores correlate with relevant criteria (e.g., membership in a criterion group)
	Multitrait–multimethod matrix: Test whether different measures of the same construct correlate more strongly than do measures of different constructs that use the same and different methods (e.g., instruments, data sources)
5. *Substantive validity:* Evidence that measurement scores meaningfully relate to theoretically postulated domain processes	*Mediation analysis:* Test whether measurement scores mediate the relationship between an experimental manipulation and a behavioral outcome in an expected way

evidence; they are listed and defined briefly in Table 27.5.[3] We emphasize at the outset that this list is not meant to constrain the kinds of evidence that should be considered in the validation process, that particular kinds of evidence may be more or less important for supporting the validity of a particular measurement interpretation, and that these five kinds of evidence are not intended as mutually exclusive categories.

Evidence for Generalizability

Generalizability evidence is needed in a test validation program to demonstrate that score interpretations apply across tasks or contexts, times or occasions, and observers or raters (see Table 27.2). The inclusion of generalizability evidence here makes explicit that construct validation includes consideration of "error associated with the sampling of tasks, occasions, and scorers [that] underlie traditional reliability concerns" (Messick, 1995, p. 746). That is, the notion of generalizability encompasses traditional conceptions of both reliability and criterion validation; they may be considered on a continuum, differing only in how far generalizability claims can be extended (Thorndike, 1997). Traditional reliability studies provide relatively weak tests of generalizability, whereas studies of criterion validity provide stronger tests of generalizability.

For example, generalizing from a test score to another test developed with parallel procedures (e.g., a Form A and Form B of the same test) does increase our confidence in the test but does so only modestly (i.e., providing evidence of parallel-form equivalence). If we find we can also generalize to other times or occasions, our confidence is further strengthened, but not by quite as much as when we can show generalizability to other methods or even to nontest criteria related to the construct the test was intended to measure. Thus, generalizability can be thought of as similar to an onion— not because it smells bad, but because it involves layers. The inner layers represent relatively modest levels of generalization, and the outer layers represent farther-reaching generalizations to contexts that are more and more removed from the central core (i.e., dissimilar from the initial measurement operation).

The kind of validity evidence Messick (1989) considered under the generalizability rubric is crucial for establishing the limits or boundaries beyond which the interpretation of the measure cannot be extended. An issue of particular importance for personality researchers is the degree to which findings generalize from "convenience" samples, such as American college students, to groups that are less educated, older, or come from different ethnic or cultural backgrounds.

Evidence for Content Validity

A second form of validational evidence involves content validity; such evidence is provided most easily if the construct has been explicated theoretically in terms of specific aspects that exhaust the content domain to be covered by the construct. Common problems involve underrepresenting an important aspect of the construct definition in the item pool and overrepresenting another one. An obvious example is the multiple-choice exams we often construct to measure student performance in our classes; if the exam questions do not sample fairly from the relevant textbook and lecture material, we cannot claim that the exam validly represented what students were supposed to learn (i.e., the course *content*).

Arguments about content validity arise not only between professors and students, but also in research. The Self-Monitoring Scale (see Snyder, 1974) is a good example because it began with a set of 25 rationally derived items; when evidence later accumulated regarding the structure and external correlates of these items, Snyder (e.g., 1987) made revisions to both the construct and the scale, excluding a number of items measuring other-directed self-presentation. As a result, behavioral variability and attitude–behavior inconsistency were represented to a lesser extent in the revised scale. Because all items measuring public performing skills were retained, the construct definition in the new scale shifted toward a conceptually unrelated construct, extraversion (John, Cheek, & Klohnen, 1996). This example shows that discriminant aspects are also important in content validation: To the extent that the items measure aspects not included in the construct definition, the measure would be contaminated by construct-irrelevant variance. For example, when validating scales to measure coping or emotion regulation, the item content on such scales should not assess variance that must be attributed to distinct constructs, such as psychological adjustment or social outcomes that are theoretically postulated to be direct consequences of the regulatory processes the scales are intended to assess (see, e.g., John & Gross, 2004, 2007).

To address questions about content validity, researchers may use a number of validation procedures (see also Smith & McCarthy, 1995). Researchers might ask expert judges to review the match between item representation and construct domain specification, and these conceptual–theoretical judgments can then be used to add or delete items. For example, Jay and John (2004) adopted the *Diagnostic and Statistical Manual of Mental Disorders* (4th ed.) (DSM-IV) symptom list for major depression as an explicit construct definition for their California Psychological Inventory (CPI)–based Depressive Symptom (DS) scale. Advanced graduate students in clinical psychology then provided expert judgments classifying all the proposed DS items as well as the items of several other depression self-report scales according to the DSM symptoms. Moreover, in an effort to address discriminant validity early in the scale construction process, the judges were also given the choice to classify items as *more* relevant to anxiety than to depression, reasoning that depression needs to be conceptually differentiated from anxiety and therefore anxiety items should not appear on a depressive symptom scale. In this way, Jay and John (2004) were able to (1) focus their scale on item content uniquely related to depression rather than anxiety symptoms, (2) examine how comprehensively their DS item set represented the intended construct (e.g., they found that only one DSM symptom cluster, suicidal ideation, was not represented), and (3) compare the construct representation of the DS items with those of other, commonly used depression scales. This theoretically based approach, when applied to questionnaire construction, has become known as the rational–intuitive approach; it has been widely used by personality and social psychologists focused on measuring theoretically postulated constructs (e.g., Burisch, 1986). Probably the most explicitly rational approach to construct definition in personality psychology is Buss and Craik's (1983) act frequency approach: Selection of act items was based not on an abstract theoretical definition of each trait construct but on folk wisdom, captured in terms of college students' aggregated judgments of the prototypicality

(or relevance) of a large number of acts for a particular trait (Buss & Craik, 1983).

Content validity can also be considered in the context of the quality and adequacy of formal or technical aspects of items. In the domain of self-reports and questionnaires, it is important to recognize that the researcher is trying to communicate accurately and efficiently with the research participants, and thus formal item characteristics, such as the clarity of wording, easy comprehensibility, low ambiguity, and so on, are crucial linguistic and pragmatic concerns in the design of items (e.g., Angleitner, John, & Lohr, 1986).

Evidence for Structural Validity

Structural validity requires evidence that the correlational (or factor) structure of the items on the measure is consistent with the hypothesized internal structure of the construct domain. We noted the issue of multidimensionality in the section on reliability, pointing out that coefficient alpha does not allow inferences about the dimensionality of a measure. The structure underlying a measure or scale is not an aspect of reliability; rather, it is central to the interpretation of the resulting scores and thus needs to be addressed as part of the construct validation program. Researchers have used both exploratory and confirmatory factor analysis for this purpose; we return to this important issue below in the context of evaluating measurement with structural equations models.

Evidence for External Validity: Convergent and Discriminant Aspects

External validity has been at the core of what most personality psychologists think validity is all about: How well does a test predict conceptually relevant behaviors, outcomes, or criteria? Wiggins (1973, p. 406) argued that prediction "is the sine qua non of personality assessment," and Dawes and Smith (1985, p. 512) suggested that "the basis of all measurement is empirical prediction." Obviously, it makes sense that a test or scale should predict construct-relevant criteria. It is less apparent that we also need to show that the test does *not* predict conceptually unrelated criteria. In other words, a full demonstration of external aspects of construct validation requires a demonstration of both what the test measures and what it does *not* measure.

*Predicting Criterion Group Membership
and Nontest (External) Criterion Variables*

One long-popular method for demonstrating
the external validity of a measure was to test
whether the measure can successfully distinguish between criterion groups—groups that
are presumed to differ substantially in their
mean levels of the construct to be measured.
Historically, the Minnesota Multiphasic Personality Inventory (MMPI; Hathaway & Mc-
Kinley, 1943) and CPI (Gough, 1957) were the
first personality inventories developed according to the criterion (or contrast) group approach. For example, items were selected for
the MMPI depression scale if they could discriminate patients hospitalized with a diagnosis
of major depression from nonpsychiatric control subjects. Gough (1957) selected items for
his subsequent achievement via conformance
scale if they predicted grade point average
(GPA) in high school (assumed to reflect conventional achievement requiring rule following) and for his achievement via independence
scale if they predicted GPA in college (assumed
to reflect more autonomous pursuit of achievement goals and interests). More recently,
Cacioppo and Petty (1982) developed the need
for cognition scale to measure individual differences in the preference and enjoyment of
effortful thinking. As part of their construct
validation program, they conducted a study
contrasting college professors (assumed to need
cognition) and assembly line workers (assumed
not to need cognition). Consistent with the interpretation of their measure as reflecting individual differences in need for cognition, the
mean score of the professors was much higher
than the mean score of the assembly line workers. Gosling, Kwan, and John (2003) validated
owners' judgments of their dogs' Big Five personality traits by showing that these judgments
predicted relevant behavior in a dog park, as
rated by strangers who interacted with the dogs
for an hour.

A critical issue with the use of such external
criteria is the "gold standard" problem mentioned earlier—that the convergent and discriminant construct validity of the criterion itself is typically not well established. For
example, patients with a diagnosis of major depression may be comorbid with other disorders
(e.g., anxiety) or may have been hospitalized
for construct-irrelevant reasons (e.g., depressed
individuals lacking social or financial support
are more likely to be hospitalized), just as col-

lege professors likely differ from assembly
workers in more ways than just their personal
need for cognition. In recognition of this problem, Gosling, Kwan, and John (2003) tried to
rule out potential confounds, such as that the
observers' behavior ratings of the dogs in the
park were not based simply on appearance and
breed stereotypes that may be shared by both
owners and strangers.

Multitrait–Multimethod Matrix

Campbell and Fiske (1959) introduced the
terms *convergent* and *discriminant* to distinguish demonstrations of what a test measures
from demonstrations of what it does not measure. The convergent validity of a self-report
scale of need for cognition could be assessed by
correlating the scale with independently obtained peer ratings of the subject's need for cognition and with frequency of effortful thinking
measured by "beeping" the subject several
times during the day. Discriminant validity
could be assessed by correlating the self-report
scale with peer ratings of extraversion and a
beeper-based measure of social and sports activities. Campbell and Fiske were the first to
formalize these ideas of convergent and discriminant validity into a single systematic design that crosses multiple traits or constructs
(e.g., need for cognition and extraversion) with
multiple methods (e.g., self-report, peer ratings, and beeper methodology). They called
this design a multitrait–multimethod (MTMM)
matrix, and the logic of the MTMM is both intuitive and compelling.

What would we expect for our need for cognition example? Certainly, we would expect
sizable convergent validity correlations between the need for cognition measures across
the three methods (self-report, peer report,
beeper); because these correlations involve the
same trait but different methods, Campbell and
Fiske (1959) called them monotrait–heteromethod coefficients. Moreover, given that need
for cognition is theoretically unrelated to extraversion, we would expect small discriminant
correlations between the need for cognition
measures and the extraversion measures. This
condition should hold even if both traits are
measured with the same method, leading to so-
called heterotrait–monomethod correlations.
Certainly, we want each of the convergent correlations to be substantially higher than the discriminant correlations involving the same trait.
And finally, the same patterns of intercorre-

lations between the constructs should emerge, regardless of the method used; in other words, the relations between the constructs should generalize across methods.

Method Variance

An important recognition inherent in the MTMM is that we can never measure a trait or construct by itself; rather, we measure the trait intertwined with the method used: "Each measure is a trait–method unit in which the observed variance is a combined function of variance due to the construct being measured and the method used to measure that construct" (Rezmovic & Rezmovic, 1981, p. 61). The design of the MTMM is so useful because it allows us to estimate variance in our scores that is due to *method* effects—that is, errors systematically related to our measurement methods and thus conceptually quite different from the notion of random error in classical test theory. These errors are systematic because they reflect the influence of unintended constructs on scores, that is, unwanted variance—something we did not wish to measure but that is confounding our measurement (Ozer, 1989).

Method variance is indicated when two constructs measured with the same method (e.g., self-reported attitudes and self-reported behavior) correlate more highly than when the same constructs are measured with different methods (e.g., self-reported attitudes and behavior coded from videotape). Response styles, such as acquiescence, may contribute to method variance when the same respondent completes more than one measure (Soto, John, Gosling, & Potter, 2006). Another example involves positivity bias in self-perceptions, which some researchers view as psychologically healthy (Taylor & Brown, 1988). However, if positivity bias is measured with self-reports and the measure of psychological health is a self-report measure of self-esteem, then a positive intercorrelation between these measures may not represent a valid hypothesis about two constructs (positivity bias and psychological health), but shared self-report method variance associated with narcissism (John & Robins, 1994); that is, individuals who see themselves too positively may be narcissistic and also rate their self-esteem too highly. Discriminant validity evidence is needed to rule out this alternative hypothesis, and the construct validity of the positivity bias measure would be strength-ened considerably if psychological health were measured with a method other than self-report, such as ratings by clinically trained observers (Jay & John, 2004).

LOTS: Multiple Sources of Data

Beginning with Cattell (1957, 1972), psychologists have tried to classify the many sources researchers can use to collect data into a few broad categories. Because each data source has unique strengths and limitations, the construct validation approach emphasizes that we should collect data from *lots* of different sources, and so the acronym LOTS has particular appeal (Block & Block, 1980; see also Craik, 1986).

L data refer to life event data that can be obtained fairly objectively from an individual's life history or life record, such as graduating from college, getting married or divorced, moving, socioeconomic status, memberships in clubs and organizations, and so on. Examples of particularly ingenious measures derived from *L* data are counts of bottles and cans in garbage containers to measure alcohol consumption (Webb, Campbell, Schwartz, Sechrest, & Grove, 1981), police records of arrests and convictions to measure antisocial behavior (Caspi et al., 2005), and the use of occupational, marital, and family data to score the number of social roles occupied by an individual (Helson & Soto, 2005).

O data refer to observational data, ranging from observations of very specific aspects of behavior to more global ratings (see Bakeman, 2000; Kerr, Aronoff, & Messé, 2000). Examples are careful and systematic observations recorded by human judges, such as in a particular laboratory setting or carefully defined situation; behavior coded or rated from photos or videos; and, broader still, reports from knowledgeable informants, such as peers, roommates, spouses, teachers, and interviewers that may aggregate information across a broad range of relevant situations in the individual's daily life. *O* data obtained through unobtrusive observations or coded later from videotape can be particularly useful to make inferences about the individual's attitudes, prejudices, preferences, emotions, and other attributes of interest to social scientists. Harker and Keltner (2001) used ratings of emotional expressions in women's college yearbook photos to predict marital and well-being outcomes 30 years later. Gross and Levenson (1993) used frequency of blinking while watching a disgust-eliciting film as an index of distress. Fraley and Shaver (1998) observed and coded how different romantic couples behaved as they were saying good-bye to one another at an airport and found that separation behavior was related to adult attachment style. Another nice illustration is a study that recorded seating position relative to an outgroup member to measure ethnocentrism (Macrae, Bodenhausen, Milne, & Jetten, 1994).

T data refer to information from test situations that provide standardized measures of performance, motivation, or achievement, and from experimental procedures that have clear and objective rules for scoring performance. A timed intelligence test is the most obvious example; other examples include assessments of the length of time an individual persists on a puzzle or delays gratification in a standardized situation (Ayduk et al., 2000). Reaction times are frequently used in studies of social cognition, providing another kind of objective measure of an aspect of performance. Recently, the Implicit Association Test (IAT; Greenwald, McGhee, & Schwartz, 1998), which uses reaction-time comparisons to infer cognitive associations, has become a popular method of assessing implicit aspects of the self-concept; Greenwald and Farnham (2000) provided evidence for the external and discriminant validity of IAT measures of self-esteem and masculinity–femininity.

Finally, *S* data refer to self-reports. *S* data may take various forms. Global self-ratings of general characteristics and *true–false* responses to questionnaire items have been used most frequently. However, self-reports are also studied in detailed interviews (see Bartholomew, Henderson, & Marcia, 2000), in narratives and life stories (see Smith, 2000), and in survey research (Visser, Krosnick, & Lavrakas, 2000). Daily experience sampling procedures (see Reis & Gable, 2000) can provide very specific and detailed self-reports of moment-to-moment functioning in particular situations.

The logic underlying *S* data is that individuals are in a good position to report about their psychological processes and characteristics—unlike an outside observer, they have access to their private thoughts and experiences and they can observe themselves over time and across situations. However, the validity of self-reports depends on the ability and willingness of individuals to provide valid reports, and self-

reports may be influenced by various constructs other than the intended one. Systematic errors include, most obviously, individual differences in response or rating scale use, such as acquiescence (see McCrae, Herbst, & Costa, 2001; Soto, John, Gosling, & Potter, 2006; Visser et al., 2000) and response extremeness (Hamilton, 1968). Another potential source of error is reconstruction bias, in which individuals' global or retrospective ratings of emotions and behaviors differ substantially from their real-time or "online" ratings (Scollon, Diener, Oishi, & Biswas-Diener, 2004).

Moreover, some theorists have argued that self-reports are of limited usefulness because they may be biased by social desirability response tendencies. Two kinds of desirability biases have been studied extensively (for a review, see Paulhus, 2002; also Paulhus & Vazire, Chapter 13, this volume). *Impression management* refers to deliberate attempts to misrepresent one's characteristics (e.g., "faking good") whereas *self-deceptive enhancement* reflects honestly held but unrealistic self-views. Impression management appears to have little effect in research contexts where individuals participate anonymously and are not motivated to present themselves in a positive light; self-deception is not simply a response style but related to substantive personality characteristics, such as narcissism (Paulhus & John, 1998).

Fortunately, although personality psychologists still use self-report questionnaires and inventories most frequently, other methods are available and used (Craik, 1986; Craik, Chapter 12, this volume; Robins, Tracy, & Sherman, Chapter 37, this volume). Thus, measures based on *L*, *O*, and *T* data can help evaluate and provide evidence for the validity of more easily and commonly obtained self-report measures tapping the same construct. Unfortunately, research using multiple methods to measure the same construct has not been very frequent. Overall, multimethod designs have been underused in construct validation efforts. Researchers seem more likely to talk about the MTMM approach than to go to the trouble of actually using it.

There is an extensive and useful methodological literature on the MTMM, which began in the mid-1970s when SEM became available and provided powerful analytical tools to estimate separate trait and method factors (e.g., Kenny, 1976; Schwarzer, 1986; Wegener

& Fabrigar, 2000). A number of excellent reviews and overviews are also available. For example, Judd and McClelland (1998) describe a series of examples that illustrate Campbell and Fiske's (1959) original principles of convergent and discriminant validation as well as the application of SEM techniques to estimate separate trait and method effects. For specific issues in fitting SEM models, see Kenny and Kashy (1992) and Marsh and Grayson (1995). Hypothetical data may be found in West and Finch (1997), who illustrate three scenarios: (1) convergent and discriminant validity with minimal method effects, (2) strong method effects, and (3) effects of unreliability and lack of discriminant validity. John and Srivastava (1999) modeled trait and instrument effects with data for three commonly used Big Five instruments.

Evidence for Substantive Validity

The final form of validational evidence in Table 27.5 involves substantive validity. Substantive validation studies make use of substantive theories and process models to further support the interpretation of the test scores. The strongest evidence for substantive validity comes from studies that use experimental manipulations that directly vary the processes in question. For example, Petty and Cacioppo (1986) showed that the process of attitude change was mediated by need for cognition. Individuals scoring high on the scale were influenced by careful examination of the arguments presented in a message, whereas those scoring low were more influenced by extraneous aspects of the context or message (e.g., the attractiveness of the source of the message). Another example is Paulhus, Bruce, and Trapnell's (1995) use of experimental data to examine an aspect of the substantive validity of two social desirability scales. When subjects were asked to intentionally present themselves in a favorable way (e.g., as they might during a job interview), the self-presentation scale showed the predicted increase over the standard "honest self-description" instruction, but the self-deception scale did not, just as one would expect for a scale designed to measure unrealistically positive self-views that the individual believes are true of him or her.

Substantive validity, then, is really about testing theoretically derived propositions about how the construct in question should function in particular kinds of contexts and how it should influence the individual's behavior, thoughts, or feelings. In that sense, studies of substantive validity are at the boundary between validational concerns and broader concerns with theory building and testing. The concept of substantive validity thus serves to illustrate the back and forth (dialectic) of theory and research. That is, when a study fails to show the effect predicted for a particular construct, it is unclear whether the problem involves a validity issue (i.e., the measure is not valid), or faulty theorizing (i.e., the theory is wrong), or both.

The consideration of substantive aspects of validity illustrates that ultimately measurement cannot be separated from theory, and a good theory is one that includes an account of the relevant measurement properties of its constructs. For example, a theory of emotion might distinguish among multiple emotion components, such as subjective experience, emotion-expressive behavior, and physiological response patterns (see, e.g., Gross, 1999), and specify how these components are most validly measured, such as emotion experience with particular kinds of self-report measures, emotion expressions with observer codings from video recordings of the individual, and physiological responding with objective tests. How exactly these three emotion components ought to be related to each other is foremost a theoretical issue but also involves substantive validity issues; for example, if a study were to show zero correlations between measures of sadness experience and measures of sadness expression, the theoretical notion of emotion as a unitary and coherent construct may have to be modified because method variance and systematic factors (e.g., display rules; individual differences in expressivity) might influence the coherence of emotion experience and expression for particular emotions and particular individuals (see, e.g., Gross, John, & Richards, 2000). Substantive validity, then, is the broadest of all five forms of validational evidence and, ultimately, indistinguishable from using theory-testing to build the nomological network for a construct.

Construct Validation: Summary and Conclusions

To summarize, in this section we reviewed five forms of evidence central to a program of construct validation (see Table 27.5). We considered one of them, external validation, in some detail, highlighting the need to consider both convergent and discriminant aspects and illustrating the multitrait–multimethod approach, the nature of method variance, and multiple sources of data. Clearly, these five forms of validational evidence are not perfectly delineated and they overlap somewhat. Consider, for example, a study finding a high 2-year retest correlation. For a measure of a trait like extraversion, that finding could be considered as evidence both for generalizability (because scores were consistent across time and testing situations) and for substantive validity (because extraversion is conceptualized as a trait construct predicted to show substantial levels of temporal stability). In contrast, finding the same high retest correlation for a measure of an emotional state would not be reassuring but would undermine its substantive validity because specific emotional states are assumed to fluctuate across time and situations (e.g., Watson & McKee Walker, 1996).

Nonetheless, despite their imperfections, these five forms of validational evidence include most of the validity concerns that are important to personality research; thus, Table 27.5 provides a reasonably comprehensive and heuristically useful list for personality researchers to consider as they plan a program of validational research. More specifically, we want to reiterate two important points that are clear to methodologists but have not yet been widely adopted in our empirical journals: (1) Evidence concerning traditional issues of reliability ought to be part of the construct validation program, under the heading of generalizability, and (2) evidence about dimensionality must also be included in validation research, under the heading of structural validity. In the following section, we reconsider these issues, now from the perspective of the measurement model in SEM.

Model Testing in Construct Validation and Scale Construction

The measurement model in structural equation modeling (SEM; Jöereskog & Sörbom, 1981; see also Bentler, 1980) is based on confirmatory factor analysis (CFA). Kline (2004), Loehlin (2004), McArdle (1996), and Bollen and Long (1993) have provided readable introductions. CFA is particularly promising be-

cause it provides a general analytic approach to assessing construct validity. As will become clear, convergent validity, discriminant validity, and random error can all be addressed within the same general framework. To illustrate these points, we return to our earlier numerical examples (Tables 27.3 and 27.4) and show how these data can be analyzed and understood using CFA-based measurement models.

Measurement Models in SEM: Convergent Validity, Discriminant Validity, and Random Error

Like all factor analytic procedures (Floyd & Widaman, 1995; Tinsley & Tinsley, 1987; see also Lee & Ashton, Chapter 25, this volume), CFA assumes that a large number of observations or items are a direct result (or expression) of a smaller number of *latent* sources (i.e., unobserved, hypothetical, or inferred constructs). However, CFA eliminates some of the arbitrary features often criticized in exploratory factor analysis (Gould, 1981; Sternberg, 1985). First, CFA techniques require the researcher to specify an explicit model (or several competing models) of how the observed (or measured) variables are related to the hypothesized latent factors. Second, CFA offers advanced statistical techniques that allow the researcher to test how well the a priori model fits the particular data; even more important, CFA permits comparative model testing to establish whether the a priori model fits the data better (or worse) than plausible alternative or competing models.

CFA models can also be displayed graphically, allowing us to effectively communicate the various assumptions of each model. Two examples are shown in Figure 27.3. Figure 27.3a shows a common-factor model in which a single underlying construct (neuroticism, shown as an ellipse at the top) is assumed to give rise to the correlations between all 12 items, or responses A1 to D6 (the observed variables, shown in squares). Following convention (Bentler, 1980), ellipses are used to represent latent variables, whereas squares represent measured (or manifest) variables; arrows with one head represent directed or regression parameters, whereas two-headed arrows (which are often omitted) represent covariance of undirected parameters. Note that each measured variable has two arrows leading to it. The arrow from the latent construct is a factor

A

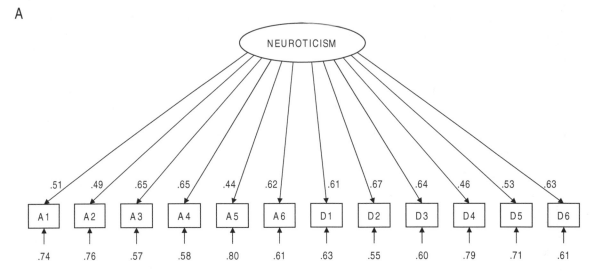

B

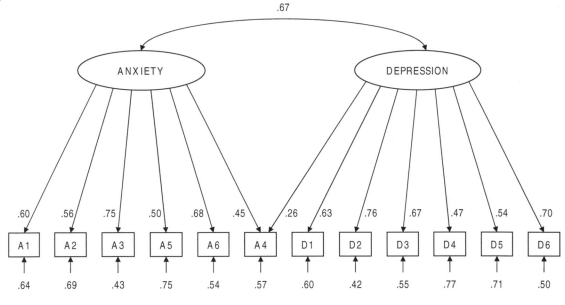

FIGURE 27.3. Two confirmatory factor analysis models of 12 NEO-PI-R neuroticism items (6 from the anxiety (A) and 6 from the depression (D) facet scale (see Table 27.4 and Figures 27.2 and 27.4). N = 649. In each panel, the top row of values represents estimates of standardized regression coefficients (i.e., factor loadings in correlational metric). The bottom row of values provides estimates of error variances (i.e., uniquenesses expressed in variance terms). Panel (a) shows parameter estimates for the general neuroticism factor model (Model 1 in Table 27.6); panel (b) shows parameter estimates for the best-fitting two-correlated-factors model with item A4 ("I often feel tense and jittery") allowed to load on both the anxiety and depression factors (Model 4 in Table 27.6).

loading L_m that represents the strength of the effect that the latent construct has on each observed variable. The other arrow involves another latent variable for each observed variable—these are unique factor scores (e_m) that represent the unique or residual variance (U^2) remaining in each observed variable.

Conceptually, this model captures a rather strong structural hypothesis, namely, that the 12 observed variables covary only because they all measure the same underlying construct, neuroticism. In other words, we hypothesize that the only thing the items have in common is this one latent construct, and all remaining or residual item variance is idiosyncratic to each item and thus unshared. This structural model provides a new perspective on how to define two important terms we have used in this chapter: the convergent validity of the item and random error. In particular, the loading of an item on the construct of interest represents the convergent validity of the item, whereas its unique variance represents random error. However, in this simple measurement model, we cannot address discriminant validity.

Compare the measurement model in Figure 27.3a to the one in Figure 27.3b, which postulates two factors (anxiety and depression) influencing responses to the same 12 items. Here we are hypothesizing two distinct constructs, rather than one. This model incorporates another condition, known as *simple structure*. The convergent validity loadings (represented by arrows from the latent constructs to the observed items) indicate that the first 5 items are influenced by the first construct but not the second construct, whereas the last 6 items are influenced only by the second construct and not the first. In other words, 11 of these items (all except item A4) can be uniquely assigned to only one construct, thus greatly simplifying the measurement model.

With two constructs in the measurement model, we can also address issues of discriminant validity. Whereas an item's loading on the construct of interest represents convergent validity and its unique variance random error, its loading on a construct *other* than the intended one speaks to its discriminant validity. For item A4, our earlier correlational analyses had suggested discriminant validity problems (see Table 27.4), and we therefore examined one model (Model 4, which is shown in Figure 27.3b) that allowed item A4 to have both a

convergent loading (on its intended anxiety factor) and a discriminant loading (on the depression factor).

Note that this model includes an arrow between the two constructs, indicating a correlation (or covariance); the two constructs are not independent (orthogonal) but related (oblique). This correlation tells us about discriminant validity at the level of the constructs. If the correlation is very high (e.g., .90), we would worry that the two constructs are not sufficiently distinct and that we really have only one construct. If the correlation is quite low (e.g., .10), we would be reassured that the two concepts show good discriminant validity with respect to each other. There is another possibility here, namely, that the two constructs are substantially correlated (e.g., .70) because they are both facets, or components, of a broader, superordinate construct that includes them both, which, of course, is the hierarchical model of the NEO-PI-R from which this example was taken. Note that here we are addressing issues that involve questions about the dimensionality and internal structure of the constructs being measured. We discussed these issues earlier in the section on reliability, especially coefficient alpha, but, as we argued in the section on validity, dimensionality issues should be considered part of the construct validation program (see Table 27.5) because they concern the structural validity of the interpretation of our measures.

Structural Validity Examined with SEM

Structural validity issues resurface with great regularity in the personality literature. Some of the most popular constructs have endured protracted debates focused on their structural validity: self-monitoring, attributional style, hardiness, Type A coronary-prone behavior pattern, and, most recently, need for closure (e.g., Hull, Lehn, & Tedlie, 1991; Neuberg, Judice, & West, 1997). Part of the problem is that many of these constructs, and the scales designed to measure them, were initially assumed to be unidimensional, but later evidence challenged those initial assumptions. It is therefore instructive to consider how SEM approaches can help address the underlying issues and to provide some numerical examples to illustrate the issues.

Testing the Unidimensionality of Scales: What Coefficient Alpha Reliability Cannot Do

As we noted earlier, coefficient alpha does not address whether a scale is unidimensional. For this purpose, factor analyses are needed; CFA provides the most rigorous approach because it can test how well the interitem correlation matrix for a particular scale fits a single-factor, rather than multifactor, model. In other words, how well can the loadings on a single factor reproduce the correlation matrix actually observed?

Consider again the three scales for which we presented interitem correlation data in Table 27.3; all had alphas of .87. What do CFAs of these correlation matrices tell us about their dimensionality? One-factor models perfectly fit the data pattern for both Scales A and B, just as expected for these unidimensional scales. CFA also estimates factor loadings for the items, providing an index of content saturation. For Scale A (which had nine items all intercorrelating .42), the items all had the same factor loading of .648 (i.e., the square root of .42, which was the size of the interitem correlations in this example). For Scale B (six items all intercorrelating .52), the factor loadings were all .721; this slightly higher value reflects that the interitem correlations (and thus content saturation) were slightly higher for Scale B than for Scale A.

In contrast, for Scale C (which had heterogeneous interitem correlations of .40 and .70, averaging .52) the fit of the one-factor model was unacceptable (for N = 200, CFI = .726, and root mean square error of approximation [RMSEA] = .263). Note, however, that the item loadings were all .721 (i.e., the square root of .52, which was the mean of the interitem correlations), the same as for the truly unidimensional Scale B. As expected, the two-factor model fit Scale C better than did the one-factor model, and perfect fit was obtained when we allowed the factors to correlate. Reflecting their .70 correlations with each other, Scale C items 1, 2, and 3 loaded .837 on factor 1 and 0 on factor 2, whereas items 4, 5, and 6 loaded 0 on factor 1 and .837 on factor 2. The interitem correlation of .40 across the two subsets of items was reflected in an estimated correlation of .571 between the two latent factors.

These results highlight that the error (or unreliability) present in an item is separate from the issue of multidimensionality. In these CFA measurement models, the item loadings represent how much of the item variance is shared across items (and is thus generalizable). Error is captured by the residual item variance (i.e., 1 minus the squared loading) indicating how much variance is unique to that item; the proportion of shared to total item variance is often referred to as *content saturation*. Dimensionality, however, is captured by the relative fit of the one-factor model versus multiple-factor models. Comparing Scales A and C in Table 27.3, the longer Scale A is clearly more unidimensional than C, yet its items do not show greater content saturation (i.e., higher factor loadings and lower error terms). In other words, unidimensionality does not imply lower levels of measurement error (i.e., unreliability), and vice versa.

Comparative Tests of Measurement Models: Testing Alternative Models for the Neuroticism Example

The general model is shown in Figure 27.2, along with the mean interitem correlations and alpha reliability coefficients we obtained when we applied the traditional canon of internal consistency analysis to these scales: a 12-item superordinate neuroticism scale with 6-item anxiety and depression facets.

The traditional method in the analysis of structural validity is exploratory factor analysis. When applied to this example (see the interitem correlation matrix given in Table 27.4), we expected evidence for both a general neuroticism factor (the first unrotated principal component) and two rotated factors representing the anxiety and depression items, respectively. Indeed, principal components analyses resulted in eigenvalues that made it difficult to decide between the one- and two-factor solutions: The first unrotated component accounted for 39% of the total variance, almost four times the size of the second component, which accounted for only 10.8%. After varimax rotation, however, the two factors were almost identical in size, accounting for 26% and 23% of the variance.

The loadings for the two rotated factors are shown in Figure 27.4, with the x-axis representing the anxiety factor and the y-axis the depression factor. Overall, there was some evidence of simple structure, in that the items tended to cluster close to their anticipated fac-

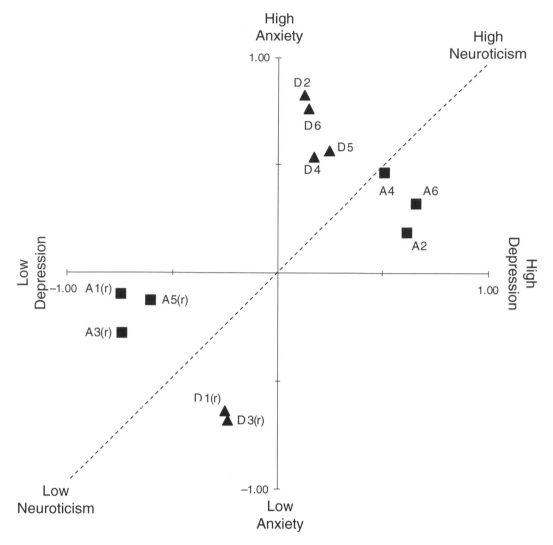

FIGURE 27.4. Loading plot for exploratory factor (principal components) analysis of 12 NEO-PI-R neuroticism items, with 6 items each from the anxiety (A) and depression (D) facet scales (see Table 27.4 and Figure 27.2). N = 649 college students. An "(r)" following the item number indicates items to be re-verse-keyed (i.e., items measuring low anxiety or low depression). The dashed line indicates the first unrotated component representing the general neuroticism factor. Note how the loadings for item A4 ("I often feel tense and jittery") place it about halfway between the anxiety and depression factor axes and close to the general neuroticism factor, suggesting that this item is a better indicator of general distress (Watson et al., 1995) shared by both anxiety and depression than a unique (or primary) indicator of anxiety.

tor locations (e.g., all 3 low-anxiety items fall together just below the low-anxiety pole). But the simple structure is not perfect; as expected, the items formed a positive manifold (all items are either in the high-high or low-low quadrant), with the two a priori facet scales forming reasonably separable anxiety and depression clusters, especially in the lower-left quadrant that includes the low-anxiety and low-depression (reverse-keyed) items.

The dashed line represents the location of the first unrotated component, that is, the general neuroticism factor that accounted for almost 40% of the item variance; all 7 true-keyed items had substantial positive loadings on it, and all 5 false-keyed items had substantial negative loadings. This factor clearly captures the positive correlation ($r = .58$) between the two item sets. Note how the loadings for item A4 ("I often feel tense and jittery") place it about halfway between the orthogonal anxiety and depression factor axes and rather close to the general neuroticism factor; this item may be a better indicator of general distress (Watson et al., 1995) shared by both anxiety and depression than a unique indicator of anxiety.

These exploratory factor analyses leave us with some alternative hypotheses that we can test formally using CFA. The CFA results are summarized briefly in Table 27.6. We begin with the one-factor model because it is the simplest or "compact model" (Judd et al., 1995). Because the models are all nested, we can statistically compare them with each other, testing the relative merits of more complex (i.e., full or augmented) models later. Without going into detail, the model-comparison results show that we can clearly reject Model 1 (one general neuroticism factor only) and Model 2 (two uncorrelated anxiety and depression factors), as both had substantially and significantly higher χ^2 values than Model 3, which defines anxiety and depression as two distinct but correlated factors. Model 4, shown in Figure 27.3b, also takes into account the discriminant validity problems of item A4 by allowing it to load on the depression factor; this model fits significantly better than the simpler Model 3, though the change in χ^2 was not large in size. These conclusions were also consistent with a wide variety of absolute and relative fit indices, like the Goodness-of-Fit Index (GFI) and the Comparative Fit Index (CFI). Table 27.6 also presents the estimated correlation between the two latent factors, which was .71 in Model 3. This value was, as expected, higher than the

simple observed correlation of .58 between the unit-weighted scales and just a tad below the estimate of .74 for the correlation corrected for attenuation due to unreliability.[4]

More Complex Models Including External Validity

In a fully developed construct validation program, of course, we would not stop here. Next, one might begin studies of external validity, modeling the relations of these two correlated CFA-based constructs with other measures of anxiety and depression, preferably drawn from other data sources, such as interview-based judgments by clinical psychologists (Jay & John, 2004). Using an MTMM design to address external validity, we would gather evidence about both convergent validity (e.g., self-reported anxiety with measures of anxiety drawn from another data source) and discriminant validity (e.g., self-reported anxiety with measures of depression drawn from another data source). Again, we would use SEM procedures for these additional validation steps, because one can model the measurement structure we have discussed so far, along with a predictive (or convergent) validity relation. Note that this model addresses the criterion problem that seemed so intractable in the early treatments of validity. The criterion itself is not treated as a "gold standard" but is modeled as a construct that must also be measured with fallible observed indicator variables. We should note that the models used to represent trait and method effects in MTMM matrices are considerably more complex than the simple models considered here. For example, McArdle (1996, Fig. 2) provides an elegant model for a more complete representation of the construct validation program.

TABLE 27.6. Using CFA to Examine Structural Validity: Comparative Model Fit for a General Neuroticism Factor as Well as Anxiety and Depression Facets

Model	χ^2	df	$\Delta\chi^2$	GFI	CFI	Interfactor correlation	Mean loading
1. One general factor: neuroticism	504.5	54	212.1*	.87	.81	N/A	.57
2. Two uncorrelated factors: anxiety and depression	547.5	54	255.1*	.89	.79	.00	.62
3. Two correlated factors: anxiety and depression	292.4	53	N/A	.92	.90	.71	.62
4. Two correlated factors, plus one cross-loading item	271.9	52	20.5*	.93	.91	.67	.58

Note. $\Delta\chi^2$: compared with Model 3; GFI, Goodness-of-Fit Index (Jöereskog & Sörbom, 1981); CFI, Comparative Fit Index (Bentler, 1980); mean loading, mean of the standardized loading of each item on its factor(s).
* $p < .05$.

Implications of Construct Validation for Scale Construction

So far, we have discussed construct validation as if the measure to be validated already existed. However, construct validation issues are central not only during the evaluation of existing measures but also during each stage of their development (see Simms & Watson, Chapter 14, this volume). Most modern scale construction efforts have adopted, implicitly or explicitly, many of the features of the construct validation program discussed in this chapter. In fact, much of our presentation here has spelled out the kinds of issues that researchers constructing a new measure must consider. There is no simple formula, but the integrated conception of construct validity and the various validation procedures summarized in Table 27.5 provide a blueprint for the kinds of evidence to be gathered and procedures to be followed.

Questionnaire construction, like measurement more generally, involves theory building and thus requires an iterative process. It begins with (1) generating hypotheses, (2) building a model and plausible alternatives, (3) generating items, using construct definitions, generalizability facets, and content validation procedures as guides (for information about item and response formats, see Visser et al., 2000), (4) gathering and analyzing data, (5) confirming and disconfirming the initial models, (6) generating alternative hypotheses leading to (7) improved models, (8) additional and more content-valid items, (9) more data gathering, and so on. The cycle continues, until a working model has been established that is "good enough"—one that the investigator can live with, for now, given the constraints and limits of real-life research. In other words, scale construction and construct validation go hand in hand, one cannot be separated from the other, and both fundamentally involve theory-building and theory-testing efforts.

Some Final Thoughts

In this chapter we have tried to strike a balance between description and prescription, between "what is" and "what should be" the practice of measurement and construct validation in personality research. We reviewed the traditional reliability coefficients but urged the reader to think instead about facets of generalizability such as time, items, and observers. We railed against some of our pet peeves, such as overreliance on coefficient alpha, articulating its limitations and arguing for a more nuanced understanding of this ubiquitous index. We advocated for a more process-oriented conception of construct validity, suggesting that the validation process deserves the same thoughtful consideration as any other form of theory testing. We illustrated, briefly, the power of no-longer new SEM techniques to help model measurement error, as well as convergent and discriminant validity.

This chapter has noted some shortcomings of current measurement conventions, practices that ought to be changed. Nonetheless, we are upbeat about the future. Specifically, over the past years we have become persuaded by the logic of comparative model testing; we now see it as *the* best strategy for evaluating and improving our measurement procedures. We are confident that as a new generation of personality researchers "grows up" using model comparison strategies, and as more of the old dogs among us learn this new trick, comparative model testing will continue to spread and help improve the validity of our measures. And because valid measures are a necessary precondition for good research, *everything* that we do as scientists comes back, in the end, to the importance of being valid.

Acknowledgments

The preparation of this chapter was supported, in part, by a grant from the Retirement Research Foundation and by a Faculty Research Award from the University of California–Berkeley. We are indebted to Monique Thompson, Josh Eng, and Richard W. Robins for their helpful comments on earlier versions.

Notes

1. Table 27.2 shows that both Pearson and intraclass correlations can be used to index retest stability. Pearson correlations reflect changes only in the relative standing of participants from one time to the other, which is typically the prime concern in research on individual differences. When changes in mean levels or variances are of interest too, then the intraclass correlation is the appropriate index.
2. In one context, this internal consistency concep-

tion does not apply. In most psychological measurement, the indicators of a construct are seen as effects caused by the construct; for example, individuals endorse items about liking noisy parties because of underlying individual differences in extraversion. However, as Bollen (1984) noted, constructs such as socioeconomic status (SES) are different. SES indicators, such as education and income, cause changes in SES, rather than SES causing changes in education or income. In these cases of "cause indicators," the indicators are not necessarily correlated and the internal consistency conception does not apply.

3. As an additional, distinct form of validity evidence, Messick (1989) included what he called *consequential validity*, which addresses the personal and societal consequences of interpreting and using a particular measure in a particular way (e.g., using an ability test to decide on school admissions). It requires the test user to confront issues of test bias and fairness and is of central importance when psychological measures are used to make important decisions about individuals. This type of validity evidence is generally more relevant in applied research and in educational and employment settings than in basic personality research, in which scale scores have little, if any, consequence for the research participant.

4. The mean loadings in Table 27.6 indicate that loadings were substantial in all models, with the general-factor model falling just below the two-factor models. Figure 27.3b shows the final parameter estimates for Model 4; consistent with the discriminant-validity problems apparent in Table 27.4 and Figure 27.4, item A4 had significant loadings on both the anxiety and depression latent factor.

Recommended Readings

Campbell, D. T., & Fiske, D. W. (1959). Convergent and discriminant validation by the multitrait-multimethod matrix. *Psychological Bulletin, 56,* 81–105.

Cronbach, L. J. (1988). Five perspectives on the validity argument. In H. Wainer & H. I. Braun (Eds.), *Test validity* (pp. 3–17). Hillsdale, NJ: Erlbaum.

Cronbach, L. J., & Meehl, P. E. (1955). Construct validity in psychological tests. *Psychological Bulletin, 52,* 281–302.

Gosling, S. D., Kwan, V. S. Y., & John, O. P. (2003). A dog's got personality: A cross-species comparative approach to personality judgments in dogs and humans. *Journal of Personality and Social Psychology, 85,* 1161–1169.

Judd, C. M., & McClelland, G. H. (1998). Measurement. In D. T. Gilbert, S. T. Fiske, & G. Lindzey (Eds.), *Handbook of social psychology* (Vol. 2, pp. 180–232). Boston: McGraw-Hill.

Loevinger, J. (1957). Objective tests as instruments of psychological theory. *Psychological Reports, 3,* 635–694.

McArdle, J. J. (1996). Current directions in structural factor analysis. *Current Directions in Psychological Science, 5,* 11–18.

Messick, S. (1995). Validity of psychological assessment. *American Psychologist 50,* 741–749.

Wiggins, J. S. (1973). *Personality and prediction: Principles of personality assessment.* Menlo Park, CA: Addison-Wesley.

References

American Educational Research Association, American Psychological Association, and National Council on Measurement in Education. (1999). *Standards for educational and psychological testing.* Washington, DC: American Educational Research Association.

American Psychological Association. (1954). Technical recommendations for psychological tests and diagnosis techniques. *Psychological Bulletin, 51,* 201–238.

American Psychological Association. (1985). *Standards for educational and psychological testing.* Washington, DC: Author.

Angleitner, A., John, O. P., & Lohr, F. J. (1986). It's what you ask and how you ask it: An itemmetric analysis of personality questionnaires. In A. Angleitner & J. S. Wiggins (Eds.), *Personality assessment in questionnaires* (pp. 61–108). Berlin: Springer-Verlag.

Ayduk, O., Mendoza-Denton, R., Mischel, W., Downey, G., Peake, P. K., & Rodriguez, M. (2000). Regulating the interpersonal self: Strategic self-regulation for coping with rejection sensitivity. *Journal of Personality and Social Psychology, 79,* 776–792.

Bakeman, R. (2000). Behavioral observation and coding. In H. T. Reis & C. M. Judd (Eds.), *Handbook of research methods in social and personality psychology* (pp. 138–159). New York: Cambridge University Press.

Bartholomew, K., Henderson, A. J. Z., & Marcia, J. E. (2000). Coded semistructured interviews in social psychological research. In H. T. Reis & C. M. Judd (Eds.), *Handbook of research methods in social and personality psychology* (pp. 286–312). New York: Cambridge University Press.

Bentler, P. M. (1980). Multivariate analysis with latent variables: Causal modeling. *Annual Review of Psychology, 31,* 419–456.

Bentler, P. M. (1990). Comparative fit indices in structural models. *Psychological Bulletin, 107,* 238–246.

Block, J. H., & Block, J. (1980) The role of ego-control and ego-resiliency in the organization of behavior. In W. A. Collins (Ed.), *Development of cognition, affect, and social relations: The Minnesota Symposia on Child Psychology* (Vol. 13, pp. 40–101). Hillsdale, NJ: Erlbaum.

Bollen, K. A. (1984). Multiple indicators: Internal consistency or no necessary relationship? *Quality and Quantity, 18,* 377–385.

Bollen, K. A., & Long, J. S. (Eds.). (1993). *Testing structural equation models.* Newbury Park, CA: Sage.

Braun, H. I., Jackson, D. N., & Wiley, D. E. (2002). *The role of constructs in psychological and educational measurement.* Mahwah, NJ: Erlbaum.

Brennan, K. A., Clark, C. L., & Shaver, P. R. (1998). Self-report measurement of adult attachment: An integrative overview. In J. A. Simpson & W. S. Rholes (Eds.), *Attachment theory and close relationships* (pp. 46–76). New York: Guilford Press.

Brennan, R. (2001). An essay on the history and future of reliability from the perspective of replications. *Journal of Educational Measurement, 38,* 295–317.

Briggs, D. C. (2004). Comment: Making an argument for design validity before interpretive validity. *Measurement: Interdisciplinary Research and Perspectives, 2,* 171–191.

Burisch, M. (1984). You don't always get what you pay for: Measuring depression with short and simple versus long and sophisticated scales. *Journal of Research in Personality, 18,* 81–98.

Burisch, M. (1986). Methods of personality inventory development: A comparative analysis. In A. Angleitner & J. S. Wiggins (Eds.), *Personality assessment via questionnaire* (pp. 109–120). Berlin: Springer-Verlag.

Buss, D. M., & Craik, K. H. (1983). The act frequency approach to personality. *Psychological Review, 90,* 105–126.

Cacioppo, J. T., & Petty, R. E. (1982). The need for cognition. *Journal of Personality and Social Psychology, 42,* 116–131.

Campbell, D. T., & Fiske, D. W. (1959). Convergent and discriminant validation by the multitrait-multimethod matrix. *Psychological Bulletin, 56,* 81–105.

Caspi, A., McClay, J., Moffitt, T., Mill, J., Martin, J., Craig, I. W., et al. (2005). Role of genotype in the cycle of violence in maltreated children. *Science, 297,* 851–854.

Cattell, R. B. (1957). *Personality and motivation structure and measurement.* New York: World Book.

Cattell, R. B. (1972). *Personality and mood by questionnaire.* San Francisco: Jossey-Bass.

Cohen, J., Cohen, P., West, S. G., & Aiken, L. S. (2003). *Applied multiple regression/correlation analysis for the behavioral sciences* (3rd ed.). Mahwah, NJ: Erlbaum.

Cortina, J. M. (1993). What is coefficient alpha? An examination of theory and applications. *Journal of Applied Psychology, 78,* 98–104.

Costa, P. T., & McCrae, R. R. (1992). *NEO-PI-R. The Revised NEO Personality Inventory.* Odessa, FL: Psychological Assessment Resources.

Craik, K. H. (1986). Personality research methods: An historical perspective. *Journal of Personality, 54,* 18–51.

Cronbach, L. J. (1947). Test "reliability": Its meaning and determination. *Psychometrika, 12,* 1–16.

Cronbach, L. J. (1951). Coefficient alpha and the internal structure of tests. *Psychometrika, 16,* 297–334.

Cronbach, L. J. (1988). Five perspectives on the validity argument. In H. Wainer & H. I. Braun (Eds.), *Test validity* (pp. 3–17). Hillsdale, NJ: Erlbaum.

Cronbach, L. J., & Gleser, G. C. (1957). *Psychological tests and personnel decisions.* Urbana: University of Illinois.

Cronbach, L. J., Gleser, G. C., Nanda, H., & Rajaratnam, N. (1972). *The dependability of behavioral measurements: Theory of generalizability for scores and profiles.* New York: Wiley.

Cronbach, L. J., & Meehl, P. E. (1955). Construct validity in psychological tests. *Psychological Bulletin, 52,* 281–302.

Cronbach, L. N., Rajaratnam, N., & Gleser, G. C. (1963). Alpha coefficients for stratified-parallel tests. *Educational and Psychological Measurement, 25,* 291–312.

Cureton, E. E. (1951). Validity. In E. F. Lindquist (Ed.), *Educational measurement* (pp. 621–694). Washington, DC: American Council on Education.

Dawes, R. M., & Smith, T. L. (1985). Attitude and opinion measurement. In G. Lindzey & E. Aronson (Eds.), *Handbook of social psychology* (Vol. 1, pp. 509–566). New York: Random House.

Eagly, A. H., & Chaiken, S. (1993). *The psychology of attitudes.* Fort Worth, TX: Harcourt Brace Jovanovich.

Embretson, S. E. (1996). The new rules of measurement. *Psychological Assessment, 8,* 341–349.

Embretson, S. E., & Reise, S. P. (2000). *Item response theory for psychologists.* Mahwah, NJ: Erlbaum.

Epstein, S. (1980). The stability of behavior: II. Implications for psychological research. *American Psychologist, 35,* 790–806.

Fishbein, M., & Ajzen, I. (1974). Attitudes toward objects as predictors of single and multiple behavioral criteria. *Psychological Review, 81,* 59–74.

Floyd, F. J., & Widaman, K. F. (1995). Factor analysis in the development and refinement of clinical assessment instruments. *Psychological Assessment, 7,* 286–299.

Fraley, R. C., & Shaver, P. R. (1998). Airport separations: A naturalistic study of adult attachment dynamics in separating couples. *Journal of Personality and Social Psychology, 75,* 1198–1212.

Fraley, R. C., Waller, N. G., & Brennan, K. A. (2000). An item response theory analysis of self-report measures of adult attachment. *Journal of Personality and Social Psychology, 78,* 350–365.

Gosling, S. D., Kwan, V. S. Y., & John, O. P. (2003). A dog's got personality: A cross-species comparative approach to personality judgments in dogs and humans. *Journal of Personality and Social Psychology, 85,* 1161–1169.

Gosling, S. D., Rentfrow, P. J., & Swann, W. B. (2003). A very brief measure of the Big Five personality domains. *Journal of Research in Personality, 37,* 504–528.

Gough, H.G. (1957). *The California Psychological Inventory administrator's guide.* Palo Alto, CA: Consulting Psychologists Press.

Gould, S. J. (1981). *The mismeasure of man.* New York: Norton.

Gray-Little, B., Williams, S. L., & Hancock, T. D. (1997). An item response theory analysis of the Rosenberg Self-Esteem Scale. *Personality and Social Psychology Bulletin, 23,* 443–451.

Greenwald, A. G., & Farnham, S. D. (2000). Using the Implicit Association Test to measure self-esteem and self-concept. *Journal of Personality and Social Psychology, 79,* 1022–1038.

Greenwald, A. G., McGhee, D. E., & Schwartz, J. L. K. (1998). Measuring individual differences in implicit cognition: The Implicit Association Test. *Journal of Personality and Social Psychology, 74,* 1464–1480.

Gross, J. J. (1999). Emotion and emotion regulation. In L. A. Pervin & O. P. John (Eds.), *Handbook of personality: Theory and research* (2nd ed., pp. 525–552). New York: Guilford Press.

Gross, J. J., John, O. P., & Richards, J. M. (2000). The dissociation of emotion expression from emotion experience: A personality perspective. *Personality and Social Psychology Bulletin, 26,* 712–726.

Gross, J. J., & Levenson, R. W. (1993). Emotional suppression: Physiology, self-report, and expressive behavior. *Journal of Personality and Social Psychology, 64,* 970–986.

Gulliksen, H. (1950). *Theory of mental tests.* New York: Wiley.

Hambleton, R. K., Swaminathan, H., & Rogers, H. J. (1991). *Fundamentals of item response theory.* Newbury Park: Sage.

Hamilton, D. L. (1968). Personality attributes associated with extreme response style. *Psychological Bulletin, 69,* 192–203.

Harker, L., & Keltner, D. (2001). Expressions of positive emotions in women's college yearbook pictures and their relationship to personality and life outcomes across adulthood. *Journal of Personality and Social Psychology, 80,* 112–124.

Hathaway, S. R., & McKinley, J. C. (1943). *The Minnesota Multiphasic Personality Inventory* (rev. ed.). Minneapolis: University of Minnesota Press.

Helson, R., & Soto, C. J. (2005). Up and down in middle age: Monotonic and nonmonotonic changes in roles, status, and personality. *Journal of Personality and Social Psychology, 89,* 194–204.

Hull, J. G., Lehn, D. A., & Tedlie, J. C. (1991). A general approach to testing multi-faceted personality constructs. *Journal of Personality and Social Psychology, 61,* 932–945.

Jay, M., & John, O. P. (2004). A depressive symptom scale for the California Psychological Inventory: Construct validation of the CPI-D. *Psychological Assessment, 16,* 299–309.

Jöereskog, K. G., & Sörbom, D. (1981). *LISREL V: User's guide.* Chicago: National Educational Resources.

John, O. P., Cheek, J. M., & Klohnen, E. C. (1996). On the nature of self-monitoring: Construct explication via Q-sort ratings. *Journal of Personality and Social Psychology, 71,* 763–776.

John, O. P., & Gross, J. J. (2004). Healthy and unhealthy emotion regulation: Personality processes, individual differences, and life span development. *Journal of Personality, 72,* 1301–1333.

John, O. P., & Gross, J. J. (2007). Individual differences in emotion regulation. In J. J. Gross (Ed.), *Handbook of emotion regulation* (pp. 351–372). New York: Guilford Press.

John, O. P., Hampson, S. E., & Goldberg, L. R. (1991). The basic level in personality-trait hierarchies: Studies of trait use and accessibility in different contexts. *Journal of Personality and Social Psychology, 60,* 348–361.

John, O. P., & Robins, R. W. (1993). Determinants of interjudge agreement on personality traits: The Big Five domains, observability, evaluativeness, and the unique perspective of the self. *Journal of Personality, 61,* 521–551.

John, O. P., & Robins, R. W. (1994). Accuracy and bias in self-perception: Individual differences in self-enhancement and the role of narcissism. *Journal of Personality and Social Psychology, 66,* 206–219.

John, O. P., & Srivastava, S. (1999). The Big Five trait taxonomy: History, measurement, and theoretical perspectives. In L. A. Pervin & Oliver P. John (Eds.), *Handbook of personality: Theory and research* (2nd ed., pp. 102–139). New York: Guilford Press.

Judd, C. M., & McClelland, G. H. (1998). Measurement. In D. T. Gilbert, S. T. Fiske, & G. Lindzey (Eds.), *Handbook of social psychology* (Vol. 2, pp. 180–232). Boston: McGraw-Hill.

Judd, C. M., McClelland, G. H., & Culhane, S. E. (1995). Data analysis: Continuing issues in the everyday analysis of psychological data. *Annual Review of Psychology, 46,* 433–465.

Kane, M. (2004). Certification testing as an illustration of argument-based validation. *Measurement: Interdisciplinary Research and Perspectives, 2,* 135–170.

Kashy, D. A., & Kenny, D. A. (2000). The analysis of data from dyads and groups. In H. T. Reis & C. M. Judd (Eds.), *Handbook of research methods in social and personality psychology* (pp. 451–477). New York: Cambridge University Press.

Kenny, D. A. (1976). An empirical application of confirmatory factor analysis to the multitrait–multimethod matrix. *Journal of Experimental Social Psychology, 12,* 247–252.

Kenny, D. A. (1994). *Interpersonal perception: A social relations analysis.* New York: Guilford Press.

Kenny, D. A., & Kashy, D. A. (1992). Analysis of the multitrait–multimethod matrix by confirmatory factor analysis. *Psychological Bulletin, 112,* 165–172.

Kerr, N. L., Aronoff, J., & Messé, L. A. (2000). Methods of small group research. In H. T. Reis & C. M. Judd (Eds.), *Handbook of research methods in social and personality psychology* (pp. 160–189). New York: Cambridge University Press.

King, J. E., & Figueredo, A. J. (1997). The five-factor model plus dominance in chimpanzee personality. *Journal of Research in Personality, 31,* 257–271.

Kline, R. B. (2004). *Principles and practices of structural equation modeling* (2nd ed.). New York: Guilford Press.

Kwan, V. S. Y., John, O. P., Kenny, D. A., Bond, M. H., & Robins, R. W. (2004). Reconceptualizing individual differences in self-enhancement bias: An interpersonal approach. *Psychological Review, 111,* 94–110.

Loehlin, J. C. (2004). *Latent variable models: An introduction to factor, path, and structural analysis* (4th ed.). Mahwah, NJ: Erlbaum.

Loevinger, J. (1957). Objective tests as instruments of psychological theory. *Psychological Reports, 3,* 635–694.

Lord, F. (1984). Standard errors of measurement at different ability levels. *Journal of Educational Measurement, 21,* 239–243.

Lord, F., & Novick, M. R. (1968). *Statistical theories of mental tests.* New York: Addison-Wesley.

Macrae, C. N., Bodenhausen, G. V., Milne, A. B., & Jetten, J. (1994). Out of mind but back in sight: Stereotypes on the rebound. *Journal of Personality and Social Psychology, 67,* 808–817.

Marsh, H. W., & Grayson, D. (1995). Latent variable models of multitrait–multimethod data. In R. H. Hoyle (Ed.), *Structural equation modeling: Concepts, issues, and applications* (pp. 177–198). Thousand Oaks, CA: Sage.

McArdle, J. J. (1996). Current directions in structural factor analysis. *Current Directions in Psychological Science, 5,* 11–18.

McCrae, R. R., Herbst, J. H., & Costa, P. T., Jr. (2001). Effects of acquiescence on personality factor structures. In R. Riemann, F. M. Spinath, & F. Ostendorf (Eds.), *Personality and temperament: Genetics, evolution, and structure* (pp. 217–231). Berlin: Pabst Science.

Mellenbergh, G. J. (1996). Measurement precision in test score and item response models. *Psychological Methods, 1,* 293–299.

Messick, S. (1989). Validity. In R. L. Linn (Ed.), *Educational measurement* (3rd ed., pp. 13–103). New York: Macmillan.

Messick, S. (1995). Validity of psychological assessment. *American Psychologist, 50,* 741–749.

Neuberg, S. L., Judice, T. N., & West, S. G. (1997). What the need for closure scale measures and what it does not: Toward differentiating among related epistemic motives. *Journal of Personality and Social Psychology, 72,* 1396–1412.

Nunnally, J. C. (1978). *Psychometric theory* (2nd ed.). New York: McGraw-Hill.

Ozer, D. J. (1989). Construct validity in personality assessment. In D. M. Buss & N. Cantor (Eds.), *Personality psychology: Recent trends and emerging directions* (pp. 224–234). New York: Springer-Verlag.

Paulhus, D. L. (2002). Socially desirable responding: The evolution of a construct. In H. I. Braun, D. N. Jackson, & D. E. Wiley (Eds.), *The role of constructs in psychological and educational measurement* (pp. 49–69). Mahwah, NJ: Erlbaum.

Paulhus, D. L., Bruce, M. N., & Trapnell, P. D. (1995). Effects of self-presentation strategies on personality profiles and their structure. *Personality and Social Psychology Bulletin, 21,* 100–108.

Paulhus, D. L., & John, O. P. (1998). Egoistic and moralistic biases in self-perception: The interplay of self-deceptive styles with basic traits and motives. *Journal of Personality, 66,* 1025–1060.

Pedhazur, E. J., & Schmelkin, L. P. (1991). *Measurement, design, and analysis: An integrated approach.* Hillsdale, NJ: Erlbaum.

Petty, R. E., & Cacioppo, J. T. (1986). *Communication and persuasion: Central and peripheral routes to attitude change.* New York: Springer-Verlag.

Rammstedt, B., & John, O. P. (2006). Short version of the Big Five Inventory: Development and validation of an economic inventory for assessment of the five factors of personality. *Diagnostica, 51,* 195–206.

Rammstedt, B., & John, O. P. (2007). Measuring personality in one minute or less: A 10-item short version of the Big Five Inventory in English and German. *Journal of Research in Personality, 41,* 203–212.

Reis, H. T., & Gable, S. L. (2000). Event-sampling and other methods for studying everyday experience. In H. T. Reis & C. M. Judd (Eds.), *Handbook of research methods in social and personality psychology* (pp. 190–222). New York: Cambridge University Press.

Rezmovic, E. L., & Rezmovic, V. (1981). A confirmatory factor analysis approach to construct validation. *Educational and Psychological Measurement, 41,* 61–72.

Robins, R. W., Hendin, H. M., & Trzesniewski, K. H. (2001). Measuring global self-esteem: Construct validation of a single-item measure and the Rosenberg self-esteem scale. *Personality and Social Psychology Bulletin, 27,* 151–161.

Rosenberg, M. (1979). *Conceiving the self.* New York: Basic Books.

Schmidt, F. L., Hunter, J. E., Pearlman, K, & Hirsch, H. R. (1985). Forty questions about validity generalization and meta-analysis. *Personnel Psychology, 38,* 697–798.

Schmitt, N. (1996). Uses and abuses of coefficient alpha. *Psychological Assessment, 8,* 350–353.

Schwarzer, R. (1986). Evaluation of convergent and discriminant validity by use of structural equations. In A. Angleitner & J. S. Wiggins (Eds.), *Personality assessment via questionnaire* (pp. 192–213). Berlin: Springer-Verlag.

Scollon, C. N., Diener, E., Oishi, S., & Biswas-Diener, R. (2004). Emotions across cultures and methods. *Journal of Cross-Cultural Psychology, 35*, 304–326.

Shavelson, R. J., Webb, N. M., & Rowley, G. L. (1989). Generalizability theory. *American Psychologist, 44*, 922–932.

Shrout, P. E., & Fleiss, J. L. (1979). Intraclass correlations: Uses in assessing rater reliability. *Psychological Bulletin, 86*, 420–428.

Smith, C. P. (2000). Content analysis and narrative analysis. In H. T. Reis & C. M. Judd (Eds.), *Handbook of research methods in social and personality psychology* (pp. 313–335). New York: Cambridge University Press.

Smith, G. T. (2005a). On the complexity of quantifying construct validity: Reply. *Psychological Assessment, 17*, 413–414.

Smith, G. T. (2005b). On construct validity: Issues of method and measurement. *Psychological Assessment, 17*, 296–408.

Smith, G. T., & McCarthy, D. M. (1995). Methodological considerations in the refinement of clinical assessment instruments. *Psychological Assessment, 7*, 300–308.

Snyder, M. (1974). Self-monitoring of expressive behavior. *Journal of Personality and Social Psychology, 30*, 526–537.

Snyder, M. (1987). *Public appearances, private realities: The psychology of self-monitoring.* New York: Freeman.

Soto, C. J., Gorchoff, S., & John, O. P. (2006). *Adult attachment styles and the Big Five: Different constructs or different contexts?* Manuscript in preparation.

Soto, C. J., John, O. P., Gosling, S. D., & Potter, J. (2006). *Developmental psychometrics: The structural validity of Big-Five personality self-reports in late childhood and adolescence.* Unpublished manuscript.

Sternberg, R. J. (1985). Human intelligence: The model is the message. *Science, 230*, 1111–1118.

Stevens, S. S. (1951). Mathematics, measurement, and psychophysics. In S. S. Stevens (Ed.), *Handbook of experimental psychology* (pp. 1–49). New York: Wiley.

Taylor, S. E., & Brown, J. (1988). Illusion and well-being: A social psychological perspective on mental health. *Psychological Bulletin, 103*, 193–210.

Thorndike, R. M. (1997). *Measurement and evaluation in psychology and education* (6th ed.). Upper Saddle River, NJ: Prentice-Hall.

Tinsley, H. E., & Tinsley, D. J. (1987). Uses of factor analysis in counseling psychology research. *Journal of Counseling Psychology, 34*, 414–424.

Visser, P. S., Krosnick, J. A., & Lavrakas, P. J. (2000). Survey research. In H. T. Reis & C. M. Judd (Eds.), *Handbook of research methods in social and personality psychology* (pp. 223–252). New York: Cambridge University Press.

von Eye, A., & Mun, E. Y. (2005). *Analyzing rater agreement: Manifest variable methods.* Mahwah, NJ: Erlbaum.

Watson, D., Clark, L. A., Weber, K., Assenheimer, J. S., Strauss, M. E., & McCormick, R. A. (1995). Testing a tripartite model: II. Exploring the symptom structure of anxiety and depression in student, adult, and patient samples. *Journal of Abnormal Psychology, 104*, 15–25.

Watson, D., & McKee Walker, L. (1996). The long-term stability and predictive validity of trait measures of affect. *Journal of Personality and Social Psychology, 70*, 567–577.

Webb, E. J., Campbell, D. T., Schwartz, R. D., Sechrest, L., & Grove, J. B. (1981). *Nonreactive measures in the social sciences* (2nd ed.). Boston: Houghton-Mifflin.

Wegener, D. R., & Fabrigar, L. R. (2000). Analysis and design for nonexperimental data: Addressing causal and noncausal hypotheses. In H. T. Reis & C. M. Judd (Eds.), *Handbook of research methods in social and personality psychology* (pp. 412–450). New York: Cambridge University Press.

West, S. G., & Finch, J. F. (1997). Measurement and analysis issues in the investigation of personality structure. In R. Hogan, J. Johnson, & S. Briggs (Eds.), *Handbook of personality psychology* (pp. 143–164). Dallas, TX: Academic Press.

Westen, D., & Rosenthal, R. (2003). Quantifying construct validity: Two simple measures. *Journal of Personality and Social Psychology, 84*, 608–618.

Westen, D., & Rosenthal, R. (2005). Improving construct validity: Cronbach, Meehl, and Neurath's ship. *Psychological Assessment, 17*, 409–412.

Wiggins, J. S. (1973). *Personality and prediction: Principles of personality assessment.* Menlo Park, CA: Addison-Wesley.

## CHAPTER 28

Evaluating Effect Size in Personality Research

Daniel J. Ozer

To provide an understanding of the origins and consequences of individual differences in personality, research commonly includes two or more variables and addresses the question: Are these variables related? Do persons high in agreeableness have more satisfying romantic relationships? Do those high in conscientiousness perform better at work? If such relations are thought to exist, one might ask the effect size question: What is the magnitude of the relationship between two variables (or groups of variables)? Questions of this kind are fundamental in personality research. Indeed, with the exception of univariate descriptive statistics and the statistical methods associated with hypothesis testing, most other quantitative methods used in personality research can be understood in the context of effect size estimation. Differences between means, correlation coefficients, regression coefficients, and the parameters of structural equation models are all example of effect size estimates. This chapter

provides an account of effect size statistics as they are used in personality research. The primary focus is on the interpretation of these statistics, with estimation discussed only (and especially) insofar as interpretation depends on understanding how the effect size statistic has been generated.

What Do We Mean by "Effect Size"?

The term *effect size* has it origins in the statistical methods used to analyze experiments—"magnitude of experimental effect" (Friedman, 1968) is an equivalent label. Here, "effect" is used to refer to the impact of the causal, independent variable that is observed on the dependent variables. In the less than full rank analysis of variance model (Kirk, 1995, pp. 240), where Y_{ij} is the score of the ith person in the jth group, μ is the population mean (estimated by the grand mean of Y), α_j is the *effect* of treatment j (estimated as the difference between the mean of the jth group and the grand mean), and ε_{ij} is a residual, error value (estimated by the difference between the individual i's score and the group's mean): $y_{ij} = \mu + \alpha_j + \varepsilon_{ij}$. Thus, one basic notion of effect size is $\alpha_j = \bar{y}_j - \bar{y}$—the difference between a group mean and a grand mean.

In the two group case, particularly where one is a treatment group and the other is a control, defining effect size as the difference between means, $\bar{y}_{Treatment} - \bar{y}_{Control}$, is an attractive alternative. In either case, the concept of effect size arises in the context of a bivariate relation between independent and dependent variables. Although adaptations to multivariate circumstances are possible, the straightforward simplicity of the bivariate case is considerably diminished as additional variables are included.

In personality research, it is frequently the case that quasi-experimental or correlational research designs are used, and in such designs the use of the term *effect* may be more analogical than literal. So, for example, if one examines the relationship between conscientiousness and job performance, one might refer to the magnitude of the obtained relation as the "effect size" despite the absence of a manipulated, independent variable. There is an implicit causal model that is untested in the research that provides a context for the assumption, and the estimate of effect size is contingent on the model. This broader, liberal use of causal language absent evidence in support of causality is adopted here, but it is important to remember that in this usage, as in personality research more generally, *effect size* may be a reference only to covariation between variables of interest.

Types of Effect Size Measures

This section describes two broad and widely applied types of effect size measures (raw and standardized) and briefly notes a third class of measures that are here labeled "criterion referenced" to parallel the meaning of that term in the context of testing.

Raw Measures of Effect Size

The most straightforward measure of effect size is simply the difference between two means. The interpretation of this measure depends on the units of measure and whether they are intrinsically meaningful. Most measures used in personality research are not directly and simply interpretable, and so raw measures of effect size have certain immediate disadvantages. Despite this drawback, raw effect size measures do have important uses because they are unaffected by sample standard deviations. When variables do have meaningful units, raw measures of effect size may be preferable.

When effect size is understood as degree of association, one occasionally useful effect size measure is the covariance. The sample covariance, computed as $s_{xy} = \sum (x - \bar{x})(y - \bar{y})/n$, is difficult to interpret because the meaning of the units in which it is expressed is entirely opaque. It is worth mentioning here only because the covariance is an important ingredient of the correlation coefficient that is the most widely used measure of effect in personality research. Unlike the correlation, the covariance has no upper or lower bound, and so the confidence interval surrounding sample estimates of population values are symmetric. For some purposes (e.g., in structural equation modeling), this property is sufficiently important to lead analysts to prefer the covariance rather than the correlation when inferential rather than descriptive goals are pursued.

Among the more common and useful raw measures of effect size is the unstandardized, or raw, regression coefficient: $b_{yx} = s_{xy}/s_x^2$, the ratio of the covariance to the variance of the predictor variable. This raw coefficient is the estimated change in y per unit change in x. In the special case where x is a dichotomy, with values of "0" and "1" a unit change in x is the difference between the two levels of the dichotomy, so the value b_{yx} is the mean difference in y between x units coded "1" and x units coded "0." For example, if a trait self-rating is obtained on a single 1–9 Likert scale and is regressed on participant gender (males arbitrarily assigned "1" and females arbitrarily assigned "0"), then the regression intercept is the mean of females on the self-rating, and the raw regression coefficient b_{yx} is the difference between females and males on the self-rating variable. So in this limited case, where x is a dichotomy and dummy coding is employed, the raw regression coefficient b_{yx} is simply the difference between two means.

When the predictor variable x is continuous, b_{yx} is the change in y associated with a unit change in x. It should be clear that the value of b_{yx}, which is expressed in the units of y, depends on the scaling of x. The change in weight associated with a unit change in height will depend on whether height is measured in inches, feet, or yards.

Standardized Measures of Effect Size

In the two group case, a raw effect size measure of some interest is the difference between group means: $\bar{y}_1 - \bar{y}_2$. As is generally the case, if the variable y is measured in interpretable units, then this raw effect size measure has much to recommend it. But when the units are not interpretable, this difference between means may be rescaled to reflect a standardized difference between means: $(\bar{y}_1 - \bar{y}_2)/s$. Depending on how the standard deviation, s, is calculated, this formula provides one of three different statistics. One approach developed for meta-analytic purposes comparing treatment and control groups (Glass, 1977; Glass, McGaw, & Smith, 1981) utilizes the estimate of the population standard deviation of the control group for s (i.e., sum of squared deviations from the control group mean divided by $n_{control} - 1$). Hedges g statistic (Hedges & Olkin, 1985) uses the estimate of the population standard deviation of both groups to obtain a pooled standard deviation estimate. The most frequently used effect size measure based on the standardized difference between means is Cohen's d, where s is the pooled sample standard deviations calculated with n rather than $n - 1$ in the formula for s (Cohen, 1977). To the extent that the variances of the two groups are the same, and as sample size gets large, these three measures of effect size converge; for most purposes, they may be given the same interpretation: The difference between sample means expressed in standard deviation units (i.e., the mean of either groups expressed as a z-score in the distribution of the other group).

Perhaps the most important and frequently used statistic in personality research is the Pearson coefficient of correlation, an effect size measure that expresses degree of association. Two formulas serve a definitional function for the correlation

$$r = \frac{\sum Z_x Z_y}{n} = \frac{s_{xy}}{s_x s_y}$$

The first expression shows that the correlation is the average cross-product of z-scores, or the covariance of a set of z scores. In the second expression, the correlation is seen as the ratio of the covariance to the product of standard deviations. It is helpful to know that the maximum possible value of the covariance is the product of standard deviations, so the correlation is the percent of maximum possible covariance that is obtained in the data.

A frequent interpretation of r is based on its equivalence to β, the standardized regression coefficient, when there is but a single predictor variable in the regression equation. Thus, the correlation is the slope of the regression line relating scores on z_y to z_x.

Criterion-Referenced Measures of Effect Size

By a "criterion-referenced" measure of effect size, I mean a measure of effect that is tied to some meaningful standard outside the original units. It is a deliberate (but, I hope, useful) misnomer to refer to these as criterion-referenced measures of effect, because the measures of effect to be discussed here are in fact precisely those discussed above as raw measures of effect size. It is the units of measurement that are criterion referenced. This parallels the relation between standardized and raw effect-size measures—the scores are standardized and then effect size is determined.

A widely applicable kind of criterion-referenced effect size measure is based on "Percent of Maximum Possible" (Cohen, Cohen, Aiken & West, 1999), or POMP. Such scores are defined as $100 \times$ (Observed score – Minimum score)/(Maximum score – Minimum score). This linear transformation of raw scores preserves several of the benefits of using raw scores while also providing several of the benefits associated with standardized scores. Consider a hypothetical case where the raw-regression coefficient based on POMP scores is .25. In this case, the difference or change on y associated with the difference or change on the entire possible range (maximum–minimum values) on x is the .25 value. That is, the maximum possible range of x is associated with one-quarter the maximum possible range on y. As in a standardized measure, this value is not dependent on the particular original units of the variables, but as in a raw measure, the results are not sample dependent, so that selection of samples with broader or narrower ranges of observed scores should not alter the estimated effect size.

One concern that POMP scores suggest is the difficulty in knowing a small, medium, or large change or difference on a predictor variable x. A result like .25, above, is clear in relative terms: A difference of 1 unit on x is associated with a .25 unit difference on y; but it is quite possible that .25 on y is larger or more meaningful than a full unit on x. It is this phenomenon that makes Rosenthal's (1990) critique of standards used to assess effect size so powerful. There are instances where small or apparently minor treatments have dramatic effects (e.g., aspirin consumption on heart attacks). POMP measures are no more successful than other procedures in accommodating to certain kinds of interpretive weaknesses in our measures.

At least some kinds of interpretive difficulties can be resolved by importing a different kind of meaning into scores—meaning defined by the human observer. The just noticeable difference (jnd) of classical psychophysics provides a basis for interpreting the units of some scores, and methods for estimating scores in jnd units requires reference samples where the only information needed is the judge agreement, expressed as an average interjudge correlation and the validity of the judgment against the scale of interest (Ozer, 1993).

Other Methods of Characterizing Effect Size Measures

Broadly categorizing types of effect size measures in terms of the units used (raw, standardized, criterion referenced) is surely not the only approach, and there is benefit to considering alternatives. Vacha-Haase and Thompson (2004) suggest a different tripartite scheme—standardized mean differences, variance-accounted-for statistics, and corrected measures of effect size—to better estimate population values. All three of these types fall into my standardized or "norm-referenced" category, and it is certainly the case that if one wants to roughly divide the actual usage of effect size measures into roughly equal categories, the Vacha-Haase and Thompson approach does a better job than that employed above. Raw and criterion-referenced effect size measures are rarely used. Neither approach promotes consideration of partialled versus unpartialled estimates as a primary con-

sideration, though this is certainly a matter of interpretative importance. Yet making distinctions between mean and correlation-based measures, or between sample values and estimates of population effects, or partialled and unpartialled effects, seems to place statistical matters first. Effect size estimation is at least in part a measurement problem, and if effect size values are to be understood, the first order of business is to understand the units used to express the effect. Following Cohen and colleagues (1999), I contend that reliance on standardized, norm-referenced units limits the potential accomplishments (e.g., any quantitative expression designed to describe or predict behavior or experience, using such units, will necessarily lack generality). Meaningful units of measure provide an opportunity for meaningful measures of effect.

The Interpretation of Effect Size Measures

Cohen (1962, 1977) originally proposed standards of "small" ($r = .1$, $d = .2$), "medium" ($r = .3$, $d = .5$), and "large" ($r = .5$, $d = .8$) to provide a rough interpretation of the magnitude of effects. In much of personality research, r^2 rather than r is used and interpreted as "percent of variance accounted for." Indeed, in its list of effect size measures, the APA (American Psychological Association, 2001) publication manual lists r^2 but not r (pp. 25–36) as an effect size measure. Rosenthal and Rubin (1982), Ozer (1985), Ahadi and Deiner (1989), and Abelson (1985), among others, have suggested that Cohen's standards may sell effects short and that squaring r exacerbates this tendency. It would seem that institutional guidelines and informal, traditional practice are each likely to lead to an underestimation of treatment effects and association among variables.

Abelson (1985) describes how intuitions about the meaning of "variance accounted for" can and frequently do create misconceptions about effect size. In an informal, but illustrative case, he shows how skill in batting accounts for substantially less than 1% of the variance in the outcome of a major league baseball at-bat. When Abelson polled colleagues to guess the percent of variance explained in an at-bat by batting skill, they overestimated the effect by a factor of 75! Either Abelson's colleagues are lacking knowledge about baseball (but then so too are baseball fans, players, managers, and team owners who greatly value, each in their own currency, each increment in batting skill) or the variance-accounted-for metric seriously distorts judgments about effect size. Curiously, Abelson never fully resolves the question as to whether the variance-accounted-for measure or our lay intuition about this effect size is flawed. He does, however, suggest that when the natural causal structure of the world creates outcomes based on aggregated performance, the percent-variance-explained metric applied to a single unaggregated outcome will distort our understanding of effect size. Batting skill explains much more of the variance in a season's performance than in single at-bats. Likewise, extraversion may explain little variance in a measure of "new friends made today," but if there is any effect at all, the impact of extraversion on number of friends made in a year will be substantially larger.

Ahadi and Diener (1989) report two simulations showing that even when traits are the sole determinant of an outcome, if there are multiple causal traits, the correlation between any one trait and the outcome had an upper bound in the .45–.50 range. Interpreting the correlation between a trait and behavior of .21, the average effect size reported in the social and personality literature (Richard, Bond, & Stokes-Zoota, 2003) must be understood in this context. Given the myriad determinants of single behaviors under controlled circumstances, not to mention consequential outcomes reflecting years of effort and performance (e.g., measures of career success), a correlation of .25 suggests that the most potent, influential determinant of the outcome of interest has been successfully identified.

The correlation coefficient, r, and the coefficient of determination, r^2, are each a transparent nonlinear transformation of the other, and so at first glance it may seem that there could be little basis for preferring one or the other as a measure of effect size. Both r^2 and the absolute value of r range from 0.00 to 1.00, and so each statistic may appear to invite a percentage or proportion interpretation. Nearly all statistics textbooks and nearly all psychological researchers would endorse this practice insofar as it pertains to r^2 (as per the "coefficient of determination" name for this quantity and its interpretation as the percent of variance accounted for). But these same textbooks and researchers would deny that r has any meaningful or useful

percentage interpretation. In this view, $r_{xy} = .2$ means that 4% of the variance in y is explained by x; and no meaningful interpretation of the relation between x and y invokes the quantity 20%. Some may go so far as to claim that half of a perfect correlation is not .5, but rather .707, because $r = .707$ yields a value of .50 for r^2. Why is the interpretation of r denied the privilege of a percentage interpretation that is granted to r^2?

The measure of variation with the property of additivity is the variance. This derives from the variance sum law, which states that the variance of a sum is the sum of all variances plus twice all covariances. Thus, r^2 is the percent of variance accounted for; $1 - r^2$ is percent of variance not accounted for (the variance of the residual values). One cannot form a parallel relation on the scale of correlation. That is, r can be thought of as the proportion of standard deviation accounted for, but the standard deviation of the residuals is $\sqrt{(1 - r^2)}$, not $1 - r$. This additivity on the scale of r^2 is especially important in multiple regression contexts. If predictor variables x and z are uncorrelated, then $R_{y.xz}^2 = r_{yx}^2 + r_{yz}^2$. This result enables the researcher to partition the total effect of a set of independent or predictor variables into parts attributable to each of the variables in the predictor set so that the sum of the effects of the parts are equal to the total effect. There is no such simple partitioning of effects on the scale of r, and it is this property of the scale of r^2 that accounts for the preference of textbooks and researchers for this metric.

Yet the validity of interpreting the partitioning of the squared multiple correlation, R^2, in terms of the r^2 (or squared, hierarchical semipartial correlations when predictors are correlated) values of the predictor variables is only rarely evaluated. Darlington (1990) develops an example that deeply undermines the use of the squared correlation metric for examining the relative importance of each variable. In this example, a nickel and a dime are (independently) tossed, and an outcome of a head results in winning the coin; if the outcome is a tail, nothing is won. In a single trial, there are four possible outcomes, each with a probability of .25: gains of nothing, 5¢, 10¢, and 15¢. Over multiple trials, it should be apparent that all the variance in winnings can be explained from the outcomes of the coin tosses, and the results for the dime coin are twice as important as the nickel coin results. Imagine the regression of winnings (possible values on any trial are 0, 5, 10, and 15) on the predictor variable "nickel result" (head coded 1, tail coded 0) and the predictor variable "dime result" (dummy coded in a parallel fashion). The expected results (nickel and dime outcomes independent and each of the four outcomes equally represented) are that the r^2 values for predicting winnings from the nickel and dime outcomes are .20 and .80, respectively. On the scale of r^2, it seems that dimes are four times more important than nickels in determining winnings, when it was clear, from the outset, that dimes should be only twice as important as nickels. Are regression statistics meaningless? Not when the appropriate statistic is used: The square roots of .2 and .8 are, respectively, .4472 and .8944. On the scale of r, dimes are exactly twice as important as nickels in determining winnings.

There is also a less widely known type of additivity associated with effect size on the scale of r. Consider the following thought experiment. Suppose that one wanted to generate a sample of observation pairs where the correlation between the pairs was exactly half of perfect. One might imagine creating one sample where the relation is perfectly present ($r = r^2 = 1.00$) and another sample, of the same size, where the relation is perfectly absent ($r = r^2 = 0.00$). What is the correlation in the combined, concatenated sample? The correlation, r, is .50, or half of perfect. This demonstration is depicted in Table 28.1. Under the specified conditions, additivity across variables accrues on the scale of r^2, but additivity over sampling units accrues on the scale of r. Although an explanation of additivity on the scale of r^2 is widely understood, additivity on the scale of r, as depicted in Table 28.1, has been a well-kept secret.

Final Comments

Measures of effect size figure prominently in the analysis of data collected in personality research. The reliability and validity of personality measures are most often evaluated with correlational measures of effect size, and personality structure is examined by factor analytic methods that rely on correlations among variables and provide correlations between variables and factors in the guise of factor loadings. But if any task is central to the enduring research program of personality psychology, it is the prediction of important life outcomes (Ozer & Benet-Martínez, 2006; Wiggins, 1973). Evaluating the success of this enterprise, in general, or the success of any particular prediction from a personality measure requires that measures of effect size be appropriately interpreted. Where it was once common practice to square a correlation coefficient and to interpret this diminished quantity uncritically on a simple percentage scale, it is now recognized that r as well as r^2 is needed to properly evaluate research progress (Rosenthal, 1990).

TABLE 28.1. The Additivity of Correlations over Sample Mixtures

	X	Y	
Sample A	1	1	
	1	3	
	2	2	$r_{xy} = .00$ in Sample A
	2	2	
	3	3	
	3	1	
			$r_{xy} = .50$ in combined sample
Sample B	1	1	
	1	1	
	2	2	$r_{xy} = 1.00$ in Sample B
	2	2	
	3	3	
	3	3	

Note. This demonstration of additivity of r over sample mixtures depends on the equality of means and standard deviations of each of the two variables across the samples.

Recommended Readings

Cohen, J., Cohen, P., West, S. G., & Aiken, L. S. (2003). *Applied multiple regression/correlation analysis for the behavioral sciences* (3rd ed.). Mahwah, NJ: Erlbaum.

Grissom, R. J., & Kim, J. J. (2005). *Effect sizes for research: A broad practical approach.* Mahwah NJ: Erlbaum.

Meyer, G. J., Finn, S. E., Eyde, L. D., Kay, G. G., Moreland, K. L., Dies, R. R., et al. (2001).Psychological testing and psychological assessment: A review of evidence and issues. *American Psychologist, 56,* 128–165.

Rosenthal, R., Rosnow, R. L., & Rubin, D. B. (2000) *Contrasts and effect sizes in behavioral research: A correlational approach.* Cambridge, UK: Cambridge University Press.

References

Abelson, R. P. (1985). A variance explanation paradox: When a little is a lot. *Psychological Bulletin, 97,* 129–133.

Ahadi, S., & Diener, E. (1989). Multiple determinants and effect size. *Journal of Personality and Social Psychology, 56,* 398–406.

American Psychological Association. (2001). *Publication manual of the American Psychological Association* (5th ed.). Washington DC: Author.

Cohen, J. (1962). The statistical power of abnormal-social psychological research: A review. *Journal of Abnormal and Social Psychology, 65,* 145–153.

Cohen, J. (1977). *Statistical power analysis for the behavioral sciences* (rev. ed.). New York: Academic Press.

Cohen, P., Cohen, J., Aiken, L. S., & West, S. G. (1999). The problem of units and the circumstances for POMP. *Multivariate Behavioral Research, 34,* 315–346.

Darlington, R. B. (1990). *Regression and linear models.* New York: McGraw-Hill.

Friedman, H. (1968). Magnitude of experimental effect and a table for its rapid estimation. *Psychological Bulletin, 70,* 245–251.

Glass, G. V. (1977). Integrating findings: The meta-analysis of research. *Review of Research in Education, 5,* 351–379.

Glass, G. V., McGaw, B., & Smith, M. L. (1981). *Meta-analysis in social research.* Beverly Hills, CA: Sage.

Hedges, L. V., & Olkin, I. (1985). *Statistical methods for meta-analysis.* San Diego, CA: Academic Press.

Kirk, R. (1995). *Experimental design: Procedures for the behavioral sciences.* Pacific Grove, CA: Brooks/Cole.

Ozer, D. J. (1985). Correlation and the coefficient of determination. *Psychological Bulletin, 97,* 307–315.

Ozer, D. J. (1993). Classical psychophysics and the assessment of agreement and accuracy in judgments of personality. *Journal of Personality, 61,* 739–767.

Ozer, D. J., & Benet-Martínez, V. (2006). Personality and the prediction of consequential outcomes. *Annual Review of Psychology, 57,* 401–421.

Richard, F. D., Bond, C. F., & Stokes-Zoota, J. J. (2003). One hundred years of social psychology quantitatively described. *Review of General Psychology, 7,* 331–363.

Rosenthal, R. (1990). How are we doing in soft psychology? *American Psychologist, 45,* 775–777.

Rosenthal, R., & Rubin, D. B. (1982). A simple general purpose display of magnitude of experimental effect. *Journal of Educational Psychology, 74,* 166–169.

Vacha-Haase, T., & Thompson, B. (2004). How to estimate and interpret various effect sizes. *Journal of Counseling Psychology, 51,* 473–481.

Wiggins, J. S. (1973). *Personality and prediction: Principles of personality assessment.* Reading MA: Addison-Wesley.

CHAPTER 29

Multilevel Modeling
in Personality Research

John B. Nezlek

Increasingly, personality researchers are creating hypotheses and collecting data that require multilevel analyses, or more formally, multilevel modeling. For example, hypotheses may concern how trait level characteristics moderate within-person relationships. Do people who are more neurotic react more strongly to stressful situations than those who are less neurotic? Answering such questions requires data at both the trait level (e.g., a single measure of neuroticism) and multiple data points at the within-person level (e.g., repeated assessments of stress and some measure of reactions to stress). Such data should be analyzed using multilevel modeling, because multilevel modeling can simultaneously take into account influences at both levels of analysis. For example, how stressed a person feels in a particular situation can reflect some type of stable individual characteristic (e.g., neuroticism) and it can reflect situational characteristics (e.g., if performance is being evaluated or not).

In this chapter, I provide a rationale for a type of multilevel analysis known as multilevel random coefficient modeling (MRCM); I describe how to do such analyses and interpret the results using an example dataset. I also discuss various aspects of MRCM that need to be considered when designing studies, analyzing data, and reporting results. The examples and discussion rely on analyses using the program HLM 6 (Raudenbush, Bryk, Cheong, & Congdon, 2004), although other programs can be used to do the same analyses. These topics are also covered in Nezlek (2001, 2003, 2005), and general introductions to MRCM can be found in Kreft and de Leeuw (1998), Raudenbush and Bryk (2002), and Snijders and Bosker (1999).

Multilevel Data Structures and Analyses

The defining characteristic of a multilevel data structure is that observations at one level of analysis are nested within observations at another level. Across different disciplines what is nested within what can vary considerably. In educational settings, students might be nested within classes; in industrial/organizational (I/O) settings, workers might be nested within work groups. For personality psychologists, the most common nesting will probably be observations nested within persons, observations that might be generated by some sort of experience-sampling technique (see Conner, Feldman Barrett, Tugade, & Tennen, Chapter 5, this volume).

Such nesting means that the variability of a set of observations, for example, measures of how extraverted people feel on different occasions, can be understood in terms of within-person and between-person differences. When explaining differences among a set of observations, explanatory variables at both levels of analysis can be used. Differences in measures of state extraversion can be understood in terms of state level (within-person) variables such as situational factors, and they can also be understood in terms of trait level (between-persons) variables such as trait extraversion. And as discussed below, explanations can involve combinations of factors at both levels.

There is an emerging consensus that such multilevel data structures need to be analyzed with techniques specifically designed for multilevel data, techniques known collectively as MRCM. One way to think of these analyses is as a series of hierarchically nested regression equations in which the coefficients from one level of analysis become the dependent measures at the next level of analysis. For example, assume a study in which data are collected every day for a sample of individuals. Hypotheses of interest might concern relationships between traits and means of these daily measures, or they might concern relationships between daily measures (within-person relationships such as between stress and mood), or they might concern individual differences in such within-person relationships. Structurally similar data would be persons nested within cultures, in which hypotheses of interest might concern within-culture coefficients (means and relationships between person-level variables) and how such means and relationships vary as a function of cultural level differences.

Within a multilevel framework, mean states (daily measures) can be represented by the intercept of one equation, and relationships between this intercept and trait level measures can be examined. Or, a within-person (state level) relationship between two daily measures can be represented by a coefficient (referred to as a slope), and relationships between this slope and trait level measures can be examined. Technically, MRCM analyses rely on one equation including terms from all levels of analysis; nevertheless, following the treatment of Raudenbush and Bryk (2002), for explanatory purposes the analyses are conceptualized in terms of a series of nested equations. I focus primarily on two-level models, that is, observations nested within persons, although more levels can be used.

Such analyses beg questions about why one should use MRCM when (conceptually) it may appear to be just as appropriate to conduct standard ordinary least squares (OLS) regression analyses for each person and use these coefficients as dependent measures in another analysis. There are numerous reasons for this, the most important of which has to do with the way in which OLS analyses model error. Assume a study in which a set of observations is collected for each person. In most studies of this type, little importance is placed on the specific occasions when the measures are collected. Measures may be collected so that certain situations are represented (e.g., home vs. work), but typically it does not matter much which specific occasions are measured. The assumption is that occasions are randomly sampled from the universe (or universes) of possible occasions.

Within such a study, coefficients for an individual estimated from one set of observations should be similar to coefficients based on another set of measures, although it is not likely that the two sets of coefficients will be identical. That is, there is some error associated with the sampling of occasions, and therefore there is random error associated with the estimates of state level coefficients. It is the random error associated with the sampling of observations that creates problems for multilevel OLS analyses. For example, if OLS regression analyses are used to estimate within-person coefficients (intercepts or slopes), and such coefficients are used as dependent measures in a between-persons analysis, the random error associated with these estimated coefficients is not taken into account. Moreover, this is not simply a matter of reliability, it is a matter of how error is modeled in an analysis. OLS analyses cannot estimate two related error terms simultaneously, and because of this, they provide less accurate parameter estimates than comparable MRCM analyses. The advantages of MRCM over OLS for analyzing multilevel data structures commonly collected by personality psychologists, including advantages not discussed here, are discussed in Nezlek (2001).

One of the important advantages of MRCM over comparable OLS analyses is the separation of true and random (error) variance. Classical measurement theory posits that the variance of a set of observations has two components: true variance and random (or error) variance. Observations may vary because, in fact, the underlying construct varies (true variance), or they may vary randomly because of factors such as measurement error. Typically, both types of variance contribute to observed variance. In MRCM, the variance of a coefficient can be separated into fixed (true) and random (error) variance. Note the *can* in this sentence. As discussed below, there are times when the data will not provide a basis for distinguishing these two types of variance.

In this chapter, MRCM models and analyses are described using the nomenclature that is fairly standard for multilevel analysis. This includes specific terms (e.g., level 1, not lower level) and specific letters (e.g., β, not b or B). Although potentially cumbersome at first, the use of these conventions facilitates communication. Multilevel analyses are inherently more complex than most single-level analyses, and the use of different terms and symbols by different authors to refer to the same entities is likely to increase readers' confusion.

The analytic techniques described in this chapter are all available in the program HLM (Version 6; Raudenbush et al., 2004), and the analyses described here were conducted using this program. These analyses could have been conducted using other multilevel programs such as MLwiN (Rabash et al., 2000), a multilevel module in LISREL 8, SAS PROC MIXED (Singer, 1998), and others. Some of the terms and symbols may vary from program to program, but for the most part the terms used here should provide readers a good introduction. Finally, many of the analytic conventions (e.g., precision weighting—discussed later) used by HLM are also used by other programs. That is, when the same models are specified, different programs can give identical results. This chapter describes results from HLM analyses because HLM is a popular multilevel program.

Conducting MRCM Analyses

Various aspects of conducting MRCM analyses are illustrated through the analyses of a hypothetical dataset, presented in Appendix 29.1. Conceptualized as a study of personality, there are nine people (level-2 observations) and between 8 and 13 measurement occasions for each person (level-1 observations). For each person, a trait level variable (Anxiety) was measured, and for each occasion, three different measures were taken, extraversion and agreeableness, measured on 10-point scales, and whether the person talked or not, a dichotomous measure. The level-1 dataset in the appendix also contains additional variables that are discussed in different sections.

It is important to note that in MRCM analyses, it is possible to have varying (even widely varying) numbers of observations for each person (i.e., different numbers of level-1 observations for each level-2 unit). Moreover, when creating raw data files, one does not need to have the same number of observations for each person—that is, one does not need blank records or records with all missing data. This is one of the advantages of MRCM over some OLS techniques such as repeated measures ANOVA (analysis of variance), which requires the same number of observations per person and is relatively intolerant of missing data.

The first step in any MRCM analysis should be running what is called a null or unconditional model. Such a model is presented below.

Level 1: $y_{ij} = \beta_{0j} + r_{ij}$

Level 2: $\beta_{0j} = \gamma_{00} + \mu_{0j}$

In the level-1 (within-person) model, there are i observations for j individuals of a variable y that are modeled as a function of the intercept for each person (β_{0j}, the mean of y) and error (r_{ij}), and the variance of r_{ij} is the level-1 random variance. In the level-2 (between-persons) model, the mean of y for each of j persons (β_{0j}) is modeled as a function of only the grand mean (μ_{00}) and error (μ_{0j}), and the variance of μ_{0j} is the level-2 variance. Such models are referred to as unconditional because y is not modeled as a function of another variable at level 1 or level 2.

Although unconditional models typically do not test hypotheses, they can provide useful information. For example, they describe how much of the total variance of y is at each level of analysis. In a two-level model, the total variance is the sum of the variances of r_{ij} and of μ_{0j}, and the distribution of the total variance of y suggests the levels at which further analyses might be productive. For example, if all the variance is at level 1, it may be difficult to model variance at level 2. The variance estimates provided by unconditional models also provide baselines that can be used to estimate effect sizes, which is discussed below. Note: HLM provides robust and nonrobust estimates of fixed effects (Raudenbush & Bryk, 2002, pp. 276–279). Owing to the small number of level-2 observations in the test dataset, nonrobust estimates are reported in this chapter.

Particularly for those unfamiliar with reading the results of multilevel analyses, the following may be helpful. In an HLM output, the variance estimates are presented after the tests of the fixed effects in a section with the heading "Final estimation of variance components." For the test data, the between-persons (level-2) variance is labeled "INTRCPT1, U0," and the within-person (level-1) variance is labeled "level-1, R." "U0" and "R" are the English alphabet equivalents of the Greek mu (μ_{0j}) and rho (r_{ij}) from the equations above.

Significance tests of fixed effects are presented in two sections labeled "Final estimation of fixed effects" (the first being nonrobust, the second section robust). The test of a specific coefficient is on a line corresponding to the name and notation for an effect. For example, the test of the hypothesis that the intercept is different from 0 is on a line labeled " INTRCPT2, G00." The "2" in INTRCPT2 indicates that this is a mean of a level-1 coefficient (i.e., a level-2 intercept), and the G00 is the English alphabet equivalent of γ_{00}, the Greek gamma. The level-1 coefficient is on the line above this, for example, "INTRCPT1, B0" (the level 1 intercept, Greek beta, β_{0j}).

An unconditional model of extraversion from the sample data produced the following estimates (all rounded to two decimals): Mean, 5.10; level-1 variance, 3.11; level-2 variance, 0.73. The significance test of the mean (γ_{00}) tests if the mean is significantly different from 0, an unimportant result in the present case, given that the scale has no 0 point. The significance test of the random error term indicates if the random and fixed variability of the intercept can be reliably separated. Interpreting error terms is discussed below.

Most modelers argue that level-1 models should be finalized before examining how the coefficients from level 1 vary as a function of level-2 variables. In the sample dataset, this will consist of predicting extraversion from agreeableness. The equations are below:

Level 1: $y_{ij} = \beta_{0j} + \beta_{1j} \, (\text{Agre}) + r_{ij}$

Level 2: $\beta_{0j} = \gamma_{00} + \mu_{0j}$
          $\beta_{1j} = \gamma_{10} + \mu_{1j}$

In the level-1 (within-person) model, β_{1j} is a coefficient, called a slope to distinguish it from an intercept, representing the relationship between extraversion and agreeableness. Interpreting this slope and the intercept depends on how agreeableness is centered, a topic discussed below. For the analyses discussed here, agreeableness was group-mean centered. Group mean centering, which for data structures such as this means centering predictors around person level means because people are the groups in such analyses, is the type of centering that I think makes the most sense for continuous variables for the types of hypotheses studied by most personality researchers. Centering is discussed in a subsequent section.

This model produced the following estimates: intercept of the intercept, $\gamma_{00} = 5.08$; intercept of the slope (lines labeled "AGRE slope, B1," "INTRCPT2, G10" in the fixed effects section), $\gamma_{10} = 0.86$; level-1 variance, 0.27; level-2 variance of the intercept, 1.05; level-2 variance of the slope, 0.34 (line labeled "AGRE slope, U1" in the estimation of variance component section). Note that the level-1 variance is considerably lower than it was in the unconditional model, and perhaps surprisingly, the variance of the intercept is greater. The significance test of the mean slope (γ_{10}) tests if the mean slope is significantly different from 0, which it was, $p < .001$. The significance test of the random error term for the slope indicates if the random and fixed variability of the slope can be reliably separated. If the random error term associated with a slope is not significant, the random error term should be eliminated. This is called fixing the slope, and is discussed below.

As will be seen from the examples below, the key to interpreting the results of MRCM analyses—that is, understanding what the coefficients mean—is to generate expected or predicted values. Interpreting the slope is fairly straightforward, keeping in mind that MRCM analyses estimate only *unstandardized* coefficients. A slope of 0.86 means that, on average, for every 1 unit increase in agreeableness, extraversion increased 0.86. The critical issue here is "on average." For some people the slope might be larger than this, and for some it might be smaller. Some believe that you can understand how much a slope varies by examining the significance of the random error term associated with the slope. A nonsignificant error term is presumed to indicate that the slopes do not vary. Although this is true in a very narrow sense, this sense does not include the hypotheses in which most personality researchers are probably interested. A nonsignificant random error term indicates that a coefficient does not vary randomly; however, slopes *can vary without an associated random error term*, something that is called nonrandom variation. That is, one can analyze individual differences in within-person relationships (slopes) when the random error term for a slope is not significant. To claim that a slope does not vary at all would require examining relationships between that slope and all possible level-2 (trait level individual difference measures) and finding that there were no relationships. This issue is discussed below.

The strength of the relationships between two variables can be evaluated in two ways. The first, and least controversial, is simply to interpret the size of the coefficient. In the present case, extraversion and agreeableness change almost point for point. Analysts interested in estimating changes in terms of standard deviations (*SD*'s) will have to estimate the within-person *SD* for the predictor, much as one would do in single-level regression. This is *not* done, however, using simple single-level descriptive statistics that ignore grouping. The estimated within-person *SD* can, and should, be derived from an unconditional analysis of the predictor. It is the level-1 *SD*, or the square root of the level-1 variance if the *SD* is not provided directly. For the sample dataset, this is 2.19. By the way, simply taking the *SD* of all the level-1 observations produces an estimate of 2.59. Estimated extraversion when agreeableness is +1 *SD* would be 5.08 + (.86*2.19) = 6.96. Estimated extraversion when agreeableness is −1 *SD* would be 5.08 − (.86*2.19) = 3.20.

Another way of evaluating the slope is to estimate the percent of variance in the dependent measure accounted for by the predictor. To do this, one compares the level-1 variance from the totally unconditional model (3.11) to the level-1 variance with the predictor included (0.27). In this analysis, the two variables share just over 90% of the variance, which translates into an average within-subject correlation of about .95. Moreover, reversing the equation (predicting agreeableness from extraversion) produces approximately the same numbers.

Using residual variances to estimate the strength of relationships is a somewhat controversial topic among multilevel modelers. For example, although Kreft and de Leeuw (1998) discuss R^2, they advise caution when interpreting such estimates of effect sizes: "In general, we suggest not setting too much store by the calculation of R_B^2 [level-2 variance] or R_W^2 [level-1 variance]." Part of this is due to the fact that adding significant level-1 predictors does not necessarily lead to a reduction in residual variances. Unlike the case in OLS analyses, in which significance tests are based on reductions in error variance, in MRCM analyses, significance tests concern the fixed effect (or component) of a coefficient, whereas error variances concern the random effect, and these two effects are estimated separately. In some cases, residual variances may increase with the addition of predictors, a mathematical impossibility in OLS. There are also questions about how centering affects such estimates, a topic discussed below. My advice in this regard is to follow Kreft and deLeeuw and be cautious. For the moment, it will suffice to note that it appears that models with single predictors at level 1 with no level-2 variables provide a reasonably stable estimate of the variance shared by two level-1 variables.

Once the level-1 model is finalized, variables can be included at level 2. Finalizing the level-1 model also entails specifying the error structure (the random error terms), which for the present model was straightforward. Specifying error structure may not always be straightforward, however, and specifying random error terms is discussed below. The simplest two-level model involves examining the relationship between a level-1 intercept (e.g., the mean for a person) and a trait variable at level 2. The equations for such a model are presented below.

Level 1: $y_{ij} = \beta_{0j} + r_{ij}$
Level 2: $\beta_{0j} = \gamma_{00} + \gamma_{01}$ (Anxiety) $+ \mu_{0j}$

The results of this analysis found that Anxiety was not significantly related to the intercept, $\gamma_{01} = .07$, $p = .55$ (line labeled "ANXIETY, G01," underneath "INTRCPT1, B0," in the fixed effects section). Assuming that it was significant, the relationship could be explained in terms of the size of the coefficient using predicted values +/− 1 *SD*. Recall that the *SD* for Anxiety was 2.50. Therefore, for someone +1 *SD* on Anxiety, the estimated intercept (mean extraversion score) would be 5.09 + (0.07*2.50) = 5.26, and for someone −1 *SD*, it would be 4.91.

These results could also be understood in terms of a reduction in error variance. For this, one would normally compare the level-2 variance (variance of the intercept) from the unconditional model with the level-2 variance from the analysis and estimate the shared variance. Using the sample dataset, however, such a comparison is not particularly sensible because the variance from the second model is greater than the variance from the unconditional model (0.84 vs. 0.73). If the level-2 predictor is significant, the variance from a conditional model is usually less than the variance from an unconditional model. Nevertheless, the fact that the variance from a conditional model was greater than the variance from the unconditional model, even though the predictor was not significant, highlights the caution offered by Kreft and deLeeuw about using variance estimates from MRCM analyses.

Level-1 slopes can also be analyzed at level 2 using the same type of model. Individual differences in the slope between extraversion and agreeableness would be analyzed as follows, with agreeableness entered group-mean centered and Anxiety entered grand-mean centered:

Level 1: $y_{ij} = \beta_{0j} + \beta_{1j}$ (Agre) $+ r_{ij}$
Level 2: $\beta_{0j} = \gamma_{00} + \gamma_{11}$ (Anxiety) $+ \mu_{0j}$
           $\beta_{1j} = \gamma_{10} + \gamma_{21}$ (Anxiety) $+ \mu_{1j}$

Note that the level-2 variable, Anxiety, is in both equations. There is broad agreement among multilevel modelers that the same predictors should be included, at least initially, in all level-2 equations. The primary reason for this is that MRCM analyses rely on covariance

matrices. If a variable is not included in an equation, the tacit assumption is that it is not significant and that there is not any meaningful covariation between the coefficients across the equations. Analysts will need to make their own decisions about the coefficients in final models.

The results of this analysis for the intercept were very similar to those of the model that did not have agreeableness at level 1: γ_{00} (mean of the intercept) = 5.08, γ_{11} (relationship of Anxiety to intercept) = 0.07, variance of the intercept = 1.15. This will be the case when continuous level-1 predictors are entered group-mean centered and continuous level-2 predictors are grand-mean centered. The intercept for the slope (γ_{10}) was 0.87, identical (within rounding) to the estimate from the analysis with no level-2 predictors. This will be the case when continuous level-2 predictors are grand-mean centered.

For many researchers, the γ_{21} coefficient, representing the relationship between the slope and the trait level variable, Anxiety, will be the most interesting coefficient. Such relationships can be called *cross-level interactions* or *moderated relationships*. For the sample dataset, Anxiety moderated the relationship between extraversion and agreeableness, $\gamma_{21} = -.18$, $p = .018$ (line labeled "ANXIETY, G11," underneath "AGRE slope, B1," in the fixed effects section). Similar to interpreting other coefficients, interpreting this relationship involves generating predicted values, perhaps for people +/− 1 *SD* on Anxiety. Recall that the *SD* for Anxiety was 2.50. The intercept for the slope (γ_{10}) was 0.87; for a person +1 *SD* the estimated slope would be 0.42 [0.87 + (−0.18*2.50)]. For a person −1 *SD*, the estimated slope would be 1.32 [0.87 − (−0.18*2.50)].

The moderating relationship can also be evaluated using a reduction in the error variance of the slope. From the analysis in which Anxiety was not included at level 2 (referred to as unconditional at level 2), the error variance for the slope was 0.34. When Anxiety was included, it was 0.16, corresponding to a shared variance of 53%. Despite the apparent common sense of this estimate, I urge analysts to exercise caution when using such estimates. Moreover, as explained below, such estimates are not possible when coefficients are fixed, that is, when no random error term is estimated.

For the sake of simplicity, these examples have included only one continuous predictor at each level of analysis. Nonetheless, as in OLS multiple regression, any combination of continuous and categorical variables can be used at either or both levels of analysis. In fact, as discussed and illustrated below, with the proper selection of options, a very broad range of relationships can be examined and hypotheses tested, much broader than that offered by single-level OLS analyses. Regardless, given this broad range of options and the complexity inherent in multilevel analyses, analysts are strongly encouraged to anticipate estimating predicted values as they plan their models and analyses.

Fixed and Random Effects

Understanding random and fixed effects in MRCM can be confusing, given the ways in which they have been described. First, it is important to note that for most purposes, researchers will be interested in the fixed effects of the predictor variables included in their models. For example, the significance test of the extraversion-agreeableness slope (was it different from 0?) in the previous example was a test of the fixed effect. The significance test of the random effect associated with a predictor indicates if true and random variance can be reliably separated. As explained below, it does not formally test if level-2 units vary in some way—for example, do all people have the same slope?

The absence or presence of a random error term needs to be understood within the context of random and nonrandom variation. Coefficients that have a random error term are described as "randomly varying" or as random coefficients. Coefficients that do not have a random error term can be what is described as "nonrandomly varying." In the previous example, the extraversion-agreeableness slope was modeled as randomly varying. If the random error term is deleted, the slope is "fixed" (and is called a fixed coefficient), although one can still model variability in the slope at level 2— that is, nonrandomly varying.

Repeating the analyses of the extraversion-agreeableness slope with the slope fixed leads to the following results. The intercept of the slope when Anxiety was not included was 0.68,

somewhat different from the slope when the random error term was included (0.86). It is not unusual for the fixed part of a coefficient to change when a random term is eliminated. When Anxiety was included, the γ_{11} coefficient representing the moderating relationship was -0.09, $p = .06$. That is, fixing the slope did not prevent modeling variability in the slope. Note: The ability to model the variability in this slope without modeling it as a random coefficient was not a function of the fact that there was a significant random error term when the slope was modeled as random. When slopes that do not have a significant random effect are fixed, the variability in these slopes can be modeled.

The meaning of fixing a coefficient can also be understood by looking at estimated values for coefficients. In the HLM program, these are in residual files, and for the sample dataset, the level-2 residual file contains the person level estimates of the intercepts and slopes (and other statistics that are not relevant at this point). For the analysis in which the agreeableness slope was fixed and Anxiety was not included as a predictor, the "fitted value" for the slope was .68 for all the level-2 units (i.e., people). This may appear to suggest that all people had the same slope; however, this is not exactly true. When Anxiety was included in the model, the fitted values for the agreeableness slope varied across persons. They varied as a function of Anxiety; they were varying nonrandomly. When the slope was fixed and Anxiety was not included, the variability among the slopes was not being modeled. This is not the same as saying that the slopes did not vary.

It is inappropriate to conclude on the basis of a nonsignificant random error term that a level-1 coefficient (usually a slope) does not vary at all. Such a conclusion would require modeling the coefficient with an infinite number of level-2 predictors. Short of this, a nonsignificant random error term means that an analyst can conclude only that the coefficient does not vary randomly, and if level-2 predictors are included, that it does not vary as a function of these level-2 variables. A significant random error term means that a coefficient varies randomly, which formally means that there is enough information to separate true and random variability for that coefficient. For researchers interested in variability per se, the presence of a significant random error term means that level-2 units (usually people) vary;

however, the absence of a significant random error term does not mean that they do not vary.

Although random error terms typically do not test hypotheses per se (at least for personality researchers), they must be properly specified before examining significance tests of fixed effects, which are usually the focus of most researchers. The "error structure" (as the covariance matrix of random terms is called) must be specified properly because an improper error structure creates a "misspecified" model, which, in turn, can lead to inaccurate significance tests of the fixed effects. Moreover, the direction of this inaccuracy cannot be predicted. That is, fixing an effect that should be modeled as random (deleting a random term that should be included) can make the fixed part of a coefficient significant when it should not be, or vice versa, just as when a random effect is included that should not be included.

Theoretically and conceptually, most coefficients in personality studies should probably be modeled as random. Nevertheless, it may not be possible to estimate reliably all the random error terms in a model. Keep in mind that most MRCM analyses also estimate the covariances among all the error terms. Most multilevel modelers argue that nonreliable error terms should be eliminated, although a minority argue that some estimate of the random error should be made, based on information from other sources, such as previous studies. At this point, most researchers will be on solid ground if they eliminate unreliable random error terms from their models, keeping in mind, of course, that fixed coefficients can vary nonrandomly.

Guidelines for making decisions about random error terms are provided in Nezlek (2001). Three bases are suggested for making decisions about whether to model coefficients as fixed or random: theoretical, statistical, and practical. Theoretically (or conceptually), it is possible (although not typical) that some coefficients should be fixed because they have a narrow "breadth of inference" or "inference space"— that is, they are meant to describe a very specific population. As already discussed, coefficients can be fixed if the random error term is not statistically significant. Finally, coefficients may be fixed if estimating them (and their covariances with other error terms) prevents a model from converging—a practical issue. In this regard, informally, many multilevel modelers look for models to converge in less than 500 iterations.

Centering

Centering refers to the reference value from which deviations are taken, and it is critical that analysts choose the appropriate method to center predictors. Centering changes the meaning of coefficients and can change estimates and significance tests of both fixed and random effects. For analysts whose primary experience is OLS regression, it may take some time to understand and appreciate the importance of centering. OLS regression analyses are almost invariably mean centered. In other words, the mean of a variable is subtracted from every individual's score. As such, the intercept represents the expected score for an observation at the mean of a predictor or set of predictors. Other options exist in MRCM.

At level 1 in a two-level model (and levels 1 and 2 in a three-level model), there are three options: uncentered (sometimes called zero-mean centering), group-mean centering, and grand-mean centering. When a predictor is *uncentered*, relationships between the dependent measure and deviations of the predictor from 0 are modeled. Modeling predictors as uncentered makes little sense when 0 is not a valid value for a predictor—for example, when a predictor is a continuous variable measured on a 1–7 scale. In contrast, modeling predictors as uncentered makes much more sense when predictors are coded variables for which 0 is a valid value or for continuous variables for which 0 is a valid value. Moreover, by subtracting a constant, 0 can become a valid value for a continuous variable. For example, an analyst interested in using age as a predictor can subtract a certain number of years from a measure of age so that a certain age is represented by 0.

For continuous variables for which 0 is not a valid value, and in some cases for coded variables, predictors may be either group- or grand-mean centered. When predictors are *group-mean centered*, the reference value from which deviations are taken is the mean of a predictor for each group. "Group" in this instance refers to a level-2 unit of analysis, which for many personality psychologists will be the person. This option is the closest (functionally) to conducting individual multiple regression analyses for each group (i.e., each person) and using these resulting coefficients as dependent measures in another analysis (i.e., at level 2). When predictors are group-mean centered, the estimated value of the intercept will not vary (aside from rounding) from the value from a totally unconditional model, nor will the variance estimates associated with intercept. In addition, analysts who are interested in using changes in level error variances should use group-mean centered predictors because group-mean centered predictors do not "bring down to level 1" variability from level-2 differences in predictors. That is, when predictors are group-mean centered, level-2 differences in level-1 predictors are not part of the model and do not contribute to parameter estimates, a topic discussed below.

Grand-mean centering is the third centering option at level 1. When predictors are *grand-mean centered*, the reference value from which deviations are taken is the grand mean of a predictor across all groups (e.g., all people in a study in which observations are nested within persons). When predictors are grand-mean centered, the estimated value of the intercept and variance estimates associated with the intercept will vary from the values from a totally unconditional model as a function of level-2 differences in group means of level-1 predictors. The larger the level-2 differences in means of level-1 predictors, the greater the differences, because these level-2 differences will contribute to estimates of level-1 parameters.

Such differences are illustrated by comparing group- and grand-mean centered analyses of the test dataset. Recall that the group-mean centered analyses described above produced the following estimates: intercept of the intercept, $\gamma_{00} = 5.08$; intercept of the slope, $\gamma_{10} = 0.86$; level-1 variance, 0.27; level-2 variance of the intercept, 1.05; level-2 variance of the slope, 0.34. When agreeableness was grand-mean centered, the following estimates were produced: intercept of the intercept, $\gamma_{00} = 5.46$; intercept of the slope, $\gamma_{10} = 0.86$; level-1 variance, 0.27; level-2 variance of the intercept, 4.40; level-2 variance of the slope, 0.33. Note that the mean slopes estimated by the two analyses were very similar, whereas the intercepts and their variances differed.

The fact that group-mean centering controls for level-2 differences in level-1 predictors can be illustrated more dramatically by making level-2 differences in level-1 predictors larger. For these analyses, a new variable, agre2 was created. For subjects *a*, *b*, *c*, and *d*, agre2 was the same as the variable from the original analyses. For subjects *e*, *f*, *g*, *h*, and *i*, 100 was

added to the original variable to create agre2. When agre2 was group-mean centered, the results were *identical* to those from the original analyses. The level-2 differences in agre2 were controlled. In contrast, when agre2 was grand-mean centered, the following estimates were produced: intercept of the intercept, $\gamma_{00} = -8.04$; intercept of the slope, $\gamma_{10} = 0.35$; level-1 variance, 1.61; level-2 variance of the intercept, 323.6; level-2 variance of the slope, 0.14. Moreover, both random error terms were not significant. Clearly, allowing the level-2 differences in agre2 to contribute to the parameter estimates destabilized the model and led to inappropriate parameter estimates. Rarely are level-2 differences as pronounced as the differences in this example; however, this example makes the point that such differences contribute to parameter estimates.

Nevertheless, some analysts argue that group-mean centering predictors leads to misspecified models because level-2 differences in level-1 predictors are not part of the model; that is, they are artificially eliminated. Some suggest that one way to reintroduce such differences is to group-mean center predictors but include group means (i.e., person-level means) as predictors at level 2. Unfortunately, such a procedure may not be a panacea. If the previous analysis with agre2 as a grand-mean centered level-1 predictor is repeated with the mean of agre2 as a level-2 predictor (grand-mean centered as described below), the following estimates are produced: intercept of the intercept, $\gamma_{00} = 7.53$; intercept of the slope, $\gamma_{10} = 0.70$; level-1 variance, 0.60; level-2 variance of the intercept, 137.5; level-2 variance of the slope, 0.07. It should be noted the intercept was not significantly different from 0.

Although these estimates are improvements over the estimates from the analysis without the mean of agre2 as a level-2 predictor, they are quite different from the estimates of the group-mean centered analysis and they are probably not good estimates. Admittedly, this is a harsh example. There are few level-2 observations, and the level-2 differences in agre2 are much greater than one would expect in a real dataset. Moreover, no level-2 unit was actually at (or near) the mean for agre2, diminishing the representativeness of estimating a coefficient for someone at the grand mean. MRCM analyses rely on covariance matrices to estimate parameters, and when variances vary dramatically across observations, estimation algorithms can break down.

In my own work, I group-mean center continuous level-1 predictors because I want the analyses to be as close as possible (conceptually) to individual regression equations for each person. Moreover, I have compared the results of group- and grand-mean centered analyses, and for my data, typically, they are quite similar. This is due in part to the fact that there are not pronounced level-2 differences in the means of the level-1 predictors in my models. As these examples illustrate, making decisions about centering can be complex. Analysts may want to conduct group- and grand-mean centered analyses (and perhaps uncentered if appropriate) and compare the results, trying to understand whatever differences exist between or among them. As Bryk and Raudenbush (1992, p. 27) noted, "No single rule covers all cases," and analysts will need to make decisions about centering based on their specific situations.

Fortunately, centering at level 2 is much less complicated. At level 2 (or level 3 in a three-level model) there are two options: uncentered (sometimes called zero-mean centering) and grand-mean centering. Grand-mean centering is functionally equivalent to the type of centering used in most OLS regression analyses. The intercept represents the expected score for an observation (i.e., a person) at the mean of a predictor (or set of predictors). Zero centering at level 2 has the same meaning as zero centering at level 1. The intercept represents the expected score for an observation with 0 on the predictor. In addition to being less complicated, centering at level 2 tends to have less dramatic effects on the model as a whole than centering at level 1.

Coding and Categorical Variables as Predictors

The previous discussion has concerned continuous variables, and although much personality research concerns continuous measures, categorical measures are also of interest. This section concerns the use of categorical variables as predictors. Using categorical variables as dependent measures is discussed below. The logic underlying the use of categorical predictors in MRCM is conceptually similar to the logic underlying the use of categorical predictors in OLS regression, although there are some important differences between the two in terms of how categories are represented and compared.

One of the important differences I have found between the two is the use in MRCM of zero intercept (or no intercept) models, accompanied by follow-up tests of fixed effects (described below). Although it is technically possible, rarely is the intercept dropped from an OLS analysis. In contrast, there may be compelling reasons to do so in MRCM. In this section I describe the use of contrast and dummy coded measures and the use of no intercept models with dummy codes as predictors to estimate means for groups or types of situations. These topics are also discussed in Nezlek (2001, 2003).

The sample dataset contains a level-1 variable named Talk, which for the present purposes represents if the subject talked or not, coded 1 = talked, 0 = no talk. Many analysts would enter this variable as a level-1 predictor, and if the coefficient was significant, conclude that there was a difference in the dependent measure as a function of whether the person talked or not. Running this analysis on the sample dataset, with Talk entered uncentered at level 1, produces a model that converges in more than 1,300 iterations, with nonsignificant error terms for both the intercept and the slope. Repeating the analysis with the slope fixed creates a more stable model that converges in 4 iterations with the following estimates: intercept of the intercept, $\gamma_{00} = 4.61$; intercept of the slope, $\gamma_{10} = 0.90$; level-1 variance, 2.92; level-2 variance of the intercept, 0.82; and because the slope was fixed, there is no level-2 variance of the slope. The slope was significant ($p < .001$), leading to the conclusion that when people were talking they felt more extraverted. In terms of predicted values, the intercept represents the expected score when talk = 0, and the estimated score for talking situations is 5.51 = 4.61 + 1*.90, that is, when talk = 1.

There is nothing wrong with such a procedure; however, it is important to keep in mind exactly what the coefficients represent. The intercept represents the mean for not talking, and the slope represents the difference between talking and not talking. The mean for talking per se is not specifically estimated in the model. Therefore, relationships between extraversion when talking and level-2 individual differences cannot be examined. This can be done by predicting extraversion with the variable ntalk, coded 1 = not talk and 0 = talk. When extr is predicted by ntalk, the intercept now represents the estimated mean for situations involving talking. Now, however, the mean for not talking is not directly represented in the model.

Means for talking and not talking can be directly estimated in the same model using what I call a dual dummy code with no intercept. In terms of the sample dataset, the model looks like this:

Level 1: $y_{ij} = \beta_{1j} (\text{Talk}) + \beta_{2j} (\text{Ntalk}) + r_{ij}$

Level 2: $\beta_{1j} = \gamma_{10} + \mu_{1j}$

$\quad\quad\quad \beta_{2j} = \gamma_{20} + \mu_{2j}$

The intercept must be deleted from the model to avoid linear dependence among the predictors. The level-1 predictors must be entered uncentered. Notice the changes in the subscripts to indicate that there is no intercept. Allowing both slopes to vary randomly indicated that the slope for talk could be fixed ($p > 0.20$), and repeating the analysis with talk fixed created a more stable model that converged in 7 iterations. The slope for talk, which represents the estimated mean for talk, was 5.49, and the slope for ntalk was 4.55. In such a model, relationships between a level-2 variable, such as Anxiety, and extraversion during talking and not talking situations can be examined simultaneously and, as described below in the section on tests of fixed effects, can be compared.

Level 2: $\beta_{1j} = \gamma_{10} + \gamma_{11} (\text{Anxiety}) + \mu_{1j}$

$\quad\quad\quad \beta_{2j} = \gamma_{20} + \gamma_{21} (\text{Anxiety}) + \mu_{2j}$

Such an analysis found that Anxiety was not significantly related to either extraversion during talk or not talk ($\gamma_{11} = 0.01$, $\gamma_{21} = 0.28$; p's = 0.90, 0.23, respectively).

Within such a framework, it is also possible to compare the two means (γ_{10} and γ_{20}) using the tests of fixed effects described below. It is important to note that although the results of such comparisons will typically be similar to the results of the significance test of a level-1 coefficient representing the difference between two categories, the results may not be exactly the same. This is because when differences are modeled at level 1 with a contrast variable or a single dummy code, the model is estimating a difference score for each person and then estimating the mean difference score. When dummy codes are used with a no intercept

model, means for each category are estimated and then the difference of these means is tested.

This type of analysis is possible only when observations can be classified using a mutually exclusive system—that is, an observation falls into one and only one category. The number of categories is not limited, but they must all be mutually exclusive. There is also one important caveat regarding the validity of relationships between level-1 slopes (which in this instance represent means) and level-2 variables. The estimates of means for each category are stable even when some level-2 units do not have observations in all categories. Assume a four-category system, and that 50% of participants do not have observations in the fourth of these categories. The means (level-1 slopes) for category 4 estimated from an analysis of all participants, and from an analysis restricted to only those who have some observations in category 4, are identical; however, estimates of relationships between level-2 variables and means for this category are not the same. When a substantial number of participants (perhaps 10% or more) are missing observations in a category, analysts should conduct separate analyses on subsets of participants who have observations in all categories, and those who do not, to determine if the subsamples differ meaningfully in other ways.

Analysts may also be interested in using non-exclusive, overlapping categories as level-1 predictors (e.g., talking and arguing). One way to deal with such categories is to combine them into mutually exclusive categories (e.g., talking and arguing, talking but no arguing, etc.), and then use dummy codes for each category and proceed as above. This may not always be practical or desirable, and categorical predictors can be represented with contrast (or effect) codes. In the sample dataset, there is variable ctalk, which is a contrast variable coded as 1 = talk, −1 = not talk.

If extr is modeled as a function of ctalk (uncentered), the random error term for ctalk is not significant ($p > 0.5$). Fixing ctalk leads to an estimate of the intercept of 5.06 and a slope (difference score) of 0.46 ($p < .01$). Using these coefficients to estimate predicted values for talking and not talking provides estimates identical to those from the original analysis in which extr was modeled as a function of the talk dummy-coded variable. The difference between the two analyses is what the intercept represents. In the original, it was either talk or not talk (depending on the predictor). In this analysis, the intercept is the mean for each person, adjusted for the relative distribution of the talk and no talk; that is, the expected score when the contrast variable is zero.

An important advantage of contrast coding is that it allows individual differences in difference scores to be modeled. Moreover, multiple contrasts can be included simultaneously, including contrasts when there are more than two categories. When using multiple contrast codes, analysts need to be mindful of the fact that the coefficients are adjusted for each other, meaning that the estimate of a specific contrast may vary as a function of the other contrasts in a model. A disadvantage of contrast coding is that it does not allow differences in relationships between category means and level-2 variables to be examined.

I recommend that analysts prepare both dummy and contrast codes for categorical variables, and model dependent measures in different ways. If contrast and dummy-coded analyses provide dramatically different conclusions about mean differences, this should be investigated, because they should not. The two types of coding provide different advantages, and analysts will need to understand when to use these two approaches. This topic is discussed in somewhat more detail in Nezlek (2001, 2003).

Interactions

In MRCM, interactions can be either within or between levels or can blend the two. Between-level interactions, often referred to as cross-level interactions, represent a type of moderated relationship. Put simply, a cross-level interaction occurs when a level-1 relationship varies as a function of a level-2 variable. The example from the test dataset of how the extraversion–agreeableness relationship varied as a function of Anxiety represents a cross-level interaction.

Within-level interactions are a bit more complex, particularly at level 1. At level 2, setting up and interpreting within-level interactions is very similar to setting up and conducting interactions in OLS regression. See Aiken and West (1991) for a thorough description of how to do this. Moreover, just as a single level-2 variable can moderate a level-1 relationship, level-1 relationships can vary as a joint function of two (or more) level-2 variables.

At level 1, setting up within-level interactions follows the same guidelines as setting up OLS interactions, but with a few caveats. Most important, continuous variables need to be centered within each group (i.e., within each person). For example, in the sample dataset, to create an interaction involving agre, the mean of each person's score on agre would be subtracted from the raw agre score, and this centered score would be used as part of the interaction. For subject *a*, this would 2.75, for subject *b*, it would be 3.67, and so forth. The interaction terms are then entered *uncentered* into the model because they have been centered. Other terms would be entered group-mean centered. This makes generating predicted values easier.

Generating predicted scores representing level-1 interactions can be particularly challenging. If the standard +/– 1 *SD* is used, keep in mind that within-person *SD*'s must be used, and these must be generated using variance estimates from unconditional models. Moreover, level-1 interactions may also vary as a function of level-2 variables. In such cases, different sets of level-1 coefficients need to be generated, representing participants at level 2. This could entail different groups at level 2 or individuals who are +/– 1 *SD* on a level-2 variable. Analyses of within-person interactions and modeling of individual differences in within-person interactions can be found in Nezlek and Plesko (2003).

Comparing Coefficients: Tests of Fixed Effects and Standardization of Measures

In addition to testing the significance of individual coefficients, MRCM allows sophisticated and powerful tests that can compare coefficients. Such comparisons can involve slopes or intercepts. The logic of these tests (called tests of fixed effects in HLM) relies on examining the impact of constraints on a model. In HLM6, such constraints are tested by clicking on "Other Settings" then "Hypothesis Testing." Each box that appears allows for a constraint, which may include multiple coefficients and multiple comparisons.

For example, as shown below, assume a dependent measure *y* and two continuous level-1 independent measures X1 and X2.

Level 1: $y_{ij} = \beta_{0j} + \beta_{1j} (X1) + \beta_{2j} (X2) + r_{ij}$
Level 2: $\beta_{0j} = \gamma_{00} + \mu_{0j}$
$\beta_{1j} = \gamma_{10} + \mu_{1j}$
$\beta_{2j} = \gamma_{20} + \mu_{2j}$

The relative strength of the relationships between y and X1 and X2 can be examined by comparing the γ_{10} and γ_{20} coefficients, representing the mean slopes for X1 and X2, respectively. This is done by imposing a constraint on the model, in this instance, constraining γ_{10} and γ_{20} to be equal. If the constraint leads to a significant decrease in the fit of the model, then one can conclude that the coefficients (the mean slopes) are not the same. The significance test is a chi-square with 1 *df*. Note that such a procedure can be used to compare the means for talking and not talking in the examples using dummy-coded predictors.

These procedures are infinitely flexible and can be used to compare all sorts of relationships. For example, assume that the unconditional level-2 model in the previous example is conditional. There is a level-2 predictor, L2, that is being used to model individual differences in the X1 and X2 slopes.

Level 2: $\beta_{0j} = \gamma_{00} + \gamma_{10} (L2) + \mu_{0j}$
$\beta_{1j} = \gamma_{10} + \gamma_{11} (L2) + \mu_{1j}$
$\beta_{2j} = \gamma_{20} + \gamma_{21} (L2) + \mu_{2j}$

The strength of the moderating relationships of L2 on X1 and X2 can be compared by comparing the γ_{10} and γ_{20} coefficients, representing the moderating relationships for X1 and X2, respectively. This is the functional equivalent of comparing within-person correlations, a particularly vexing procedure in most OLS analyses.

These examples have focused on comparisons of only two coefficients, but constraints can involve more than two coefficients. Assume that there are three level-1 predictors in the preceding example. This would generate four fixed effects at level 2, one for the intercept (γ_{00}) and one for each of the three slopes (γ_{10}, γ_{20}, and γ_{30}). A constraint could compare the average of the first two with the third (γ_{10}, γ_{20}, vs. γ_{30}), which could be coded -1, -1, 2. Similarly, the moderating relationships of L2 on each of these could be compared.

Constraints can also have more than 1 *df*. Assume the broad hypothesis is that the X1, X2, and X3 slopes are different, much like the

null hypothesis of an ANOVA with more than two groups. This hypothesis could be tested with a 2 *df* constraint, perhaps coded as 1, -1, 0, and 1, 0, -1 for γ_{10}, γ_{20}, and γ_{30}, respectively. Keep in mind that just like the *F*-test from an ANOVA, such a constraint would not indicate precisely what the differences were between the three slopes.

These examples represent only the tip of the iceberg. I believe that these tests of fixed effects are severely underutilized in research using MRCM. Through the creative combination of coding schemes and constraints, analysts can use MRCM to conduct ANOVA-like analyses for categorical variables, they can compare the strength of relationships without having to rely on variance estimates of questionable meaning, and so forth. One reason I have emphasized the careful understanding of exactly what each coefficient in a model represents is to encourage analysts to create models in anticipation of using these tests.

There is one important caveat to keep in mind when using these tests. MRCM estimates only unstandardized coefficients. Therefore, the variances of measures contribute to the results of such comparisons. For example, assume a model in which there are two level-2 predictors of a level-1 intercept. Changing the variance of these predictors will change the results of the comparison of the level-2 coefficients. Tests of the individual effects will not change, but chi-squared tests of constraints will. Similarly, the variances of level-1 predictors contribute to tests of constraints of their means at level 2.

At level 2, the solution is fairly simple, particularly for personality researchers: Standardize level-2 (trait or person level) variables before analyses. This does two things. First, it eliminates the contribution to significance tests of differences in the variances of variables. Second, it makes generating predicted values easier. When they are standardized, coefficients involving these variables will represent 1 *SD*.

At level 1, the situation is not so straightforward. First, it is best to avoid such problems by designing studies so that measures have similar variances—for example, use the same scale for different measures. This is not always possible, however (e.g., the data may have been collected), and so measures can be transformed to reduce or eliminate differences in variances. Analysts should avoid (or consider very carefully) standardizing *within* persons (i.e., calculating an *SD* for each person) and representing observations in terms of *SD*'s from each person's own mean. Such standardization eliminates mean differences in intercepts, artificially setting the mean for all persons to 0 and eliminating any variance in the intercept.

Estimating Reliability of Scales

It is not uncommon for researchers to administer scales (or a series of items intended to measure the same construct) or a series of such scales on a repeated basis. For example, each day for a few weeks, participants in a study might complete four items measuring their self-esteem. In such a study, a researcher might be interested in the reliability of this scale. How consistently do the four items measure same construct? It is instructive to discuss how this should *not* be done before discussing the proper technique, because there appears to be considerable misunderstanding about this.

First, it is incorrect to estimate the reliability of this scale by creating an aggregate score (e.g., the mean of the four items), conducting an unconditional analysis, and examining the reliability of the intercept produced by this analysis. Such a reliability is an indication of how reliably the true and random variance of the intercept can be separated; it is not a measure of the consistency of responses to the four items. Second, it is incorrect to calculate within-person means (across the days of the study) for each of the items and then estimate Cronbach's alpha using these means as person-level item scores. This is equivalent to using correlations between within-person means to examine within-person relationships between two constructs, and it ignores within-person variability, which in a study such as I am discussing, is a critical component. Third, it is incorrect to treat each day of a study as a "mini-study," calculate a Cronbach's alpha for each day, and then combine these alphas. Assuming that day 1 for person 1 should be matched with day 1 for person 2 ignores the random error associated with the sampling of days. Moreover, such a procedure does not take into account between-day variance because each day is treated separately.

The reliability of our hypothetical four items should be estimated by conducting a three-level

model in which items are nested within days and days are nested within people. The level-1 model would consist of responses to each item (four per day). In HLM, the reliability of the level-1 coefficient is the reliability of the scale. See Nezlek and Gable (2001) for an example of this procedure.

Multivariate Analyses

There are times when researchers want to analyze several dependent measures simultaneously. Unlike a multivariate analysis of variance (MANOVA) or cannonical correlation, multivariate analyses in MRCM require multiple (at least two) observed measures for each construct of interest. If there are not two items, true and random variance cannot be distinguished. Similar to the analyses of reliability described above, such data require a level of nesting in which items are nested within occasions. Observations at the first level of analysis consist of responses to individual items, and for each construct, dummy-coded variables representing the particular construct an item measures.

Assume a study in which negative affect is measured every day with eight items, four for negative active affect (NA, e.g., nervous) and four for negative deactive affect (ND, e.g., sad). In addition, stress is measured each day. These data can be analyzed using a three-level model in which items are nested within days and days are nested within people. For these data, there are eight responses for each day, four for NA and four for ND, and each of these eight responses is modeled as a function of two dummy-coded variables, one representing NA and the other representing ND. One dummy-coded variable is set to 1 for each measure of NA and 0 for each measure of ND, whereas the other is set to 1 for each measure of ND and 0 for each measure of NA.

The level-1 model is a no intercept model, and y_{ijk} represents the i-th response on day j for person k and the level-1 coefficients, π_{1jk} and π_{2jk}, represent daily mean scores of NA and ND, respectively.

$$y_{ijk} = \pi_{1jk} (NA) + \pi_{2jk} (ND) + e_{ijk}$$

Such a model estimates the reliability of both NA and ND and allows for comparing the strength of relationships between NA and daily stress and between ND and daily stress at level 2. The level-2 model that provides the basis for this is

$$\text{NA: } \pi_{1jk} = \beta_{11k} \text{ (Stress)} + r_{1jk}$$
$$\text{ND: } \pi_{2jk} = \beta_{21k} \text{ (Stress)} + r_{2jk}$$

The within-person relationship between NA and Stress is represented by the β_{11k} coefficient, and the within-person relationship between ND and Stress is represented by the β_{21k} coefficient. The strength of these relationships is compared by placing a constraint on the model, that the two coefficients are equal, and examining the impact of this constraint on the overall fit of the model. See Nezlek and Gable (2001) for an example of testing the strength of coefficients using this technique.

Moderation and Mediation

Within MRCM, moderation is relatively straightforward, at least conceptually. As described previously, between levels, moderation can be examined through significance tests of level-2 predictors of level-1 slopes. Within a level, terms can be created representing interactions of predictors, very much like what is done in OLS regression. Moreover, within level 2, interpreting such the results of such analyses is very much like interpreting the results of OLS analyses: Significant interaction terms indicate moderation.

Evaluating moderation within level 1 is a little trickier because there is the possibility that coefficients representing moderation will vary. That is, significance tests evaluate the mean moderation effect. It is possible that moderation may be stronger or weaker for different people. Moreover, such a possibility cannot necessarily be deduced from the significance test of the random error term. For example, Nezlek and Plesko (2003) found that a level-2 variable moderated a level-1 moderating effect for some measures even when the coefficient representing the level-1 moderating effect had no significant random error term.

Evaluating mediation in multilevel models is particularly challenging. Within level 2, various decision rules about mediation in OLS regression can probably be applied fairly straightforwardly. Within level 1, the situation is particu-larly complex, despite recent attempts to provide guidelines (e.g., Kenny, Korchmaros, & Bolger, 2003). First, similar to evaluating moderation within level 1, coefficients representing mediation within level 1 may vary across level-2 units (people). Kenny et al. rely on significance tests of the random error terms associated with slopes to determine if such coefficients vary; however, they do not consider the possibility that slopes representing mediational effects may vary nonrandomly. Second, as noted earlier, there is some confusion regarding the meaning of changes in level-1 residual variances as a means of evaluating effect sizes. To the extent that explanations of mediation rely on changes in variances, such explanations need to be evaluated cautiously.

At present, it is difficult to provide clear guidelines regarding lower-level mediation in multilevel models. The traditional OLS rule (see, e.g., Baron & Kenny, 1986), that mediation occurs when including a second predictor in a model (that is itself related to the outcome and the first predictor) renders the original predictor nonsignificant, seems like a good place to start because such a procedure relies on significance tests rather than variance estimates. Nevertheless, analysts need to be aware of the possibility that all of the relationships needed to establish mediation may vary across level-2 units.

Interpreting Results

For analysts whose experience is primarily with single-level OLS analyses that produce standardized coefficients, developing a sense of how to interpret the results of MRCM analyses will take some time. Listed below are some important considerations.

1. MRCM analyses produce two (or more) sets of coefficients, and in the case of cross-level interactions (described below), coefficients at lower levels of analysis may need to be interpreted in light of coefficients at higher levels of analysis. More levels create a more thorough understanding, but they also create more complexity.

2. Most coefficients in most analyses will be unstandardized. (See the section below on standardization.) Although analysts can still rely on significance tests to determine if relationships are significantly different from 0 or different

from each other, the fact that coefficients are unstandardized must be kept in mind.

3. Significance tests of the fixed effect of a coefficient can vary as a function of the inclusion or exclusion of a random error term for that coefficient. Before evaluating the results of significance tests of fixed effects (the tests that are most relevant for most personality researchers), the error terms must be specified properly. For most analyses, this will mean that error terms that are significant should be retained, whereas those that are not should be eliminated (i.e., the effect should be "fixed").

4. The meaning of coefficients depends directly on how variables are centered, and different centering options will produce different (sometimes dramatically different) results, including the results of significance tests. Unlike the specification of error structures, which often has a post hoc component (i.e., eliminating error terms that cannot be estimated reliably), centering is something that should be done completely in advance. Analysts should know in advance what they want each coefficient to represent and should select the centering options that represent these quantities.

With these considerations in mind, the key to understanding the results of MRCM analyses is to generate predicted/expected values as I have done with the analyses of the sample dataset. In the case of categorical measures this would mean expected values for each category, whereas for continuous measures, one might chose to estimate values for observations +/1 SD on predictors. Given the potential complexity of the results, the importance of generating predicted values cannot be overstated. Such an emphasis contrasts sharply with the emphasis in many single-level OLS analyses on significance tests of standardized coefficients.

Reporting Results

It is probably best for authors to follow the adage "less is more" when describing MRCM results. All too often, articles contain too many statistics and results that are not central to the primary hypotheses, hypotheses that invariably concern fixed effects. For example, authors who describe random error terms in detail and make claims about the lack of variability in a coefficient often misunderstand what random error terms mean. It may be useful to describe

briefly what effects were modeled as random and what effects were fixed, and why they were fixed, but for most purposes, random error terms are of peripheral interest.

Some authors also present elaborate comparisons of models, very similar to what is done when presenting standard equation modeling (SEM) analyses. Although MRCM models can be compared, and there can be good reasons to do so, for most purposes it should suffice simply to report the results of significance tests of individual fixed coefficients (e.g., slopes). Comparisons of two models, one with and one without a predictor, includes not only the fixed coefficient for the predictor (is the predictor different from 0?). It also includes the random error term for the predictor and the covariances between this random error term and the other random error terms in the model. Model comparison procedures can be useful when evaluating the retention or deletion of a group of random error terms; however, it is probably overkill for evaluating the significance of a single predictor. Moreover, with some exceptions, descriptions of MRCM analyses tend to focus on individual parameters more than the overall fit of a model, whereas in SEM, the overall fit of a model is typically the focus of the analyses.

When reporting the results of tests of individual coefficients, it will usually suffice to describe the fixed coefficient (usually a γ of some kind), the significance level associated with the test of the hypothesis that the coefficient is 0, and perhaps the t-value. There is no need to report both the t-value and the standard error, as the t-value is simply the coefficient divided by the standard error. Analysts may want to report degrees of freedom, although the p-values associated with reported t-values do not vary as a function of degrees of freedom as they would in an OLS analyses, because the t-values in MRCM are approximations. Some other tests, such as multiparameter tests, produce chi-squares indicating differences in model fits. For such tests, reporting the chi-squared and its associated degrees of freedom and p-value is appropriate.

Regardless, authors are encouraged to illustrate their results with descriptions of predicted values, particularly for complex findings such as cross-level interactions. Such descriptions may not be particularly important for readers who are familiar with MRCM, but they may be invaluable for readers who are not.

Nonlinear Outcomes

Thus far, the discussion has assumed that dependent measures are continuous and more or less normally distributed; however, personality research may concern measures that are not continuous or not normally distributed. Analyses of percents and other measures that are by definition not normally distributed (e.g., binomial data, categorical measures, highly skewed count data) rely on the same logic as analyses of normally distributed measures but use different algorithms. Different algorithms are necessary because the means and variances of such measures are not independent, which violates a critical assumption. For example, the variance of a binomial is npq, where n = number of observations, p = the probability of the more common outcome, and $q = 1 - p$. As the mean (expected value, p) changes, the variance changes.

Analyses of nonlinear outcomes are structurally similar to the analyses of linear outcomes, albeit with certain transformations that will vary as a function of the type of outcome. For example, in the sample dataset, there is a variable Talk, which indicates if the person talked, and the percent of occasions during which a person talked can be examined using a Bernoulli model with $n = 1$. The model is below.

$$\text{Prob}(y = 1 | \beta_{0j}) = \phi$$

The coefficient from this analysis, the log-odds of talking, is .16 (unit-specific, nonrobust estimate), corresponding to a percent of 0.54, which in this case was not significantly different from 0. Keep in mind that in an analysis of percents, the null hypothesis that the coefficient is 0 corresponds to a null of 50%. Although the null hypothesis is always that a coefficient is different from 0, different nonlinear outcomes will have different substantive null hypotheses depending on what 0 represents.

Predictors can be added at levels 1 and 2 in the same way they can be added to analyses of linear outcomes, and the results of the analyses are interpreted similarly. For example, if Anxiety is included in the level-2 model (grand-mean centered), the resulting coefficient is –0.13, which is not significant ($p = 0.30$). Assuming that it was significant, one way to interpret the relationship would be to generate predicted values for people +/– 1 SD. The SD of Anxiety is 2.50, so a person +1 SD would have a predicted log-odds of –0.15 = 0.18 + (2.50*–0.13), corresponding to 46%. A person –1 SD would have a predicted log-odds of 0.51 = 0.18 – (2.50*–0.13), corresponding to 63%. Note that although Anxiety was grand-mean centered, the intercept in this analysis is slightly different from the intercept in the unconditional model.

When analyzing nonlinear outcomes, analysts should be aware of the following:

1. Be particularly cautious when conducting and interpreting nonlinear analyses. Although transformations may be clearly described in the manuals that accompany software, producing predicted values, which are needed to understand the coefficients, can be quite vexing for those who are not familiar with working with log-odds. I use a spreadsheet with a series of steps corresponding to each term of the equation that is needed to generate point estimates from log-odds.

2. Analyses of nonlinear outcomes do not produce estimates of level-1 variances. This is due to the nature of the algorithms used in these analyses.

3. For analyses of nonlinear outcomes, HLM produces two sets of coefficients, unit-specific and population-average, and such coefficients can be meaningfully different. For nonlinear outcomes, estimating coefficients requires a "link function," and different options for this function are available. Detailed discussion of link functions is well beyond the scope of this chapter. It may suffice to note that unit-specific coefficients are intended to describe relationships such a as slope (e.g., the change due to a one-unit change in a predictor) at the discrete unit (e.g., person), whereas population-average coefficients are intended to describe relationships as they exist in the population. Although blanket recommendations are not possible, it seems likely that many personality researchers will be interested in unit-specific coefficients more than population-average coefficients. Interested readers are encouraged to consult Raudenbush and Bryk (2002).

Model Building

Seemingly, there are two traditions in OLS regression: one characterized by careful hypothesis testing in which some predetermined set of predictors are all included, regardless of their statistical significance, and another approach, more exploratory in nature, in which all predictors are included and those that are significant are retained. Certainly, other possibilities exist and are used. Nevertheless, neither of these approaches may be appropriate for MRCM, particularly when the number of predictors is large.

This difference between OLS regression and MRCM reflects one of the critical differences between the two techniques. In OLS regression, for each predictor only a fixed effect is estimated, and only one error term is estimated for the whole model. In contrast, in MRCM, for each level-1 predictor, a fixed effect and a random effect are estimated, and the covariances among the random error terms are also estimated. In MRCM, this means that the number of parameters being estimated increases nonlinearly as predictors are added. With a level-1 model with no predictors, two parameters are estimated: fixed and random effects for the intercept. With one predictor, five parameters are estimated: fixed and random effects for the intercept and the slope, and the covariances between the two errors. With three predictors, nine parameters are estimated: fixed and random effects for the intercept and the two slopes, and the covariances between the three errors—and so on.

When thinking of the complexity of a model, statisticians colloquially refer to the "carrying capacity" of the data. How many parameters can a dataset estimate? In this regard, it is useful to think of a data structure as an information bank and to think of parameters in terms of the amount of information that is available to estimate them. Assuming the same data structure, the more parameters one estimates, the less information there is available for each parameter. At some point, the data are stretched too thin and there is not enough information to estimate all the parameters.

In light of this aspect, multilevel modelers tend to recommend forward-stepping algorithms—that is, adding predictors one at a time and deleting those that are not significant, or testing smaller models first and adding to them as needed. In contrast are the backward-stepping algorithms, in which many predictors are included and those that are not significant are deleted. The forward-stepping approach tends to build smaller models with fewer, but more stable, parameter estimates than backward-stepping algorithms. Of course, individual analysts will have to be guided by the specific situations they face. Nevertheless, analysts who are accustomed to including numerous predictors in a model will have to come to terms with the possibility that they cannot include as many (perhaps not nearly as many) predictors in their level-1 models as they may want to include.

Using Estimated Coefficients in Other Analyses

The coefficients estimated in a MRCM analysis can be saved and used in other analyses; however, analysts are urged to be cautious when using such estimates in this way. First, as is the case with any technique involving multiple predictors, the estimates from any specific analysis will reflect the covariances among the variables that are included in the analysis. Moreover, with MRCM, such estimates will also reflect whatever error structure was in the model and the level-2 variables that were included. Analysts need to keep in mind that although it may be useful to think of MRCM models as series of nested equations, in fact, MRCM analyses rely on a single equation that simultaneously includes predictors at all levels. Second, if shrunken estimates are used (based on a Bayesian analysis, something commonly used in MRCM programs), they are typically highly correlated with OLS estimates. They differ from OLS estimates in terms of their variances, and so for pure correlational analyses, there may not be much difference in results using the two. Third, unless the coefficients are used in an analysis in which random error can be modeled, the analysis will not reflect this aspect of the multilevel analysis, undermining the value of using MRCM to estimate the coefficients.

In light of this caution, analysts are encouraged to think creatively about how to examine their hypotheses of interest within the multilevel framework. For example, questions of changes across time can frequently be addressed by including some kind of time variable at level 1. All sorts of group comparisons can be made by creating variables at level 2. Analysts should exhaust all reasonable possibilities before using MRCM to estimate coefficients that are then used in some single-level analysis.

Software Options

The increasing popularity of MRCM is reflected in the increasing number of programs that can perform such analyses, too many to discuss here. For analysts who are familiar with random coefficient models and the subtleties of MRCM, the selection of software can be guided by familiarity and accessibility. If an analyst knows what he or she is doing, virtually all programs will provide the same estimates, *provided the same models are specified*. For analysts who are not familiar with MRCM or random coefficient models in general, the situation is somewhat different. For such analysts, I recommend programs that are specifically designed to conduct MRCM such as HLM and MlwiN, with HLM probably being the easiest to use. This recommendation is based on my experience in giving workshops, the ease with which models can be specified (error terms, centering, etc.), and the ease with which the output can be interpreted, as compared with that of all-purpose programs such as SAS or SPSS. For analysts who are not familiar with random coefficient models and/or multilevel models, the array of options in many all-purpose programs can be confusing and may lead analysts to specify (unwittingly) inappropriate or incorrect models.

The availability of these different software options highlights the importance of referring to the analyses discussed in this chapter as *multilevel random coefficient models* instead of *hierarchical linear models* (HLM). In the multilevel world, HLM is a specific program that conducts MRCM, and authors should be careful to distinguish the statistical technique they used (MRCM) from the program that was used to implement this technique (e.g., HLM, SAS).

Some Concluding Thoughts

The growth in the use of MRCM in personality research is likely to continue over the next few years, and perhaps longer. The technique provides a comprehensive analytic framework for investigating topics that have not been investigated in the past—because researchers did not know how or have used a hodge-podge of techniques that had no firm basis in statistical theory. My goal in writing this chapter was to describe some of the applications of the basic techniques of multilevel modeling to the study of personality. Certainly, there are other applications (e.g., time series analysis) that could have been described. Nevertheless, this review should provide enough information to allow researchers who are unfamiliar with the technique to consider using MRCM, or at the least, provide them with enough information to understand the results of studies using MRCM.

Recommended Readings

Resources for Understanding and Applying Multilevel Models

Kreft, I. G. G., & de Leeuw, J. (1998). *Introducing multilevel modeling*. Newbury Park, CA: Sage.—A very informative guide organized in terms of frequently asked questions.

Nezlek, J. B. (2001). Multilevel random coefficient analyses of event and interval contingent data in social and personality psychology research. *Personality and Social Psychology Bulletin, 27*, 771–785.—A basic introduction to multilevel modeling written specifically for personality and social psychologists.

Nezlek, J. B. (2003). Using multilevel random coefficient modeling to analyze social interaction diary data. *Journal of Social and Personal Relationships, 20*, 437–469.—An introduction to multilevel modeling written specifically for research involving social interaction diaries. The techniques can be readily applied to other types of diaries.

Raudensbush, S. W., & Bryk, A. S. (2002). *Hierarchical linear models* (2nd ed.). Newbury Park, CA: Sage.—A meaningful revision of the first edition. A classic reference that goes hand-in-hand with the program HLM.

Raudenbush, S. W., Bryk, A., Cheong, Y. F., & Congdon, R. (2004). *HLM 6: Hierarchical linear and nonlinear modeling*. Lincolnwood, IL: Scientific Software International.—The help screens in this program almost consist of a tutorial in how to conduct multilevel modeling. Very thorough. Very helpful.

Snijders, T., & Bosker, R. (1999). *Multilevel analysis*. London: Sage.—A solid introduction to multilevel modeling.

Examples of Good Practice

Barnett, R. C., Brennan, R. T., Raudenbush, S. W., & Marshall, N. L. (1993). Gender and the relationship between marital role-quality and psychological distress: A study of dual-earner couples. *Journal of Personality and Social Psychology, 64*, 794–806.—A useful example of how to analyze couple data using multilevel modeling.

Nezlek, J. B., & Leary, M. R. (2002). Individual differences in self-presentational motives and daily social interaction. *Personality and Social Psychology Bulle-*

tin, 28, 211–223.—This article contains multilevel analyses of relationships between trait level variables and social interaction.

Nezlek, J. B., & Plesko, R. M. (2003). Affect- and self-based models of relationships between daily events and daily well-being. *Personality and Social Psychology Bulletin, 29*, 584–596.—This article contains multilevel analyses of within-person interactions and trait level moderation of within-person relationships.

Vansteelandt, K., Van Mechelen, I., & Nezlek, J. B. (2005). The co-occurrence of emotions in daily life: A multilevel approach. *Journal of Research in Personality, 39*, 325–335.—This article contains analyses illustrating the application of the dummy-coded technique for multilevel, multivariate analyses discussed in this chapter.

References

Aiken, L. S., & West, S. G. (1991). *Multiple regression: Testing and interpreting interactions*. Newbury Park, CA: Sage.

Baron, R. M., & Kenny. D. A. (1986). The moderator–mediator distinction in social psychological research: Conceptual, strategic, and statistical considerations. *Journal of Personality and Social Psychology, 51*, 1173–1182.

Bryk, A. S., & Raudenbush, S. W. (1992). *Hierarchical linear models*. Newbury Park, CA: Sage.

Kenny, D. A., Korchmaros, J. D., & Bolger, N. (2003). Lower level mediation in multilevel models. *Psychological Methods, 8*, 115–128.

Kreft, I. G. G., & de Leeuw, J. (1998). *Introducing multilevel modeling*. Newbury Park, CA: Sage.

Nezlek, J. B. (2001). Multilevel random coefficient analyses of event and interval contingent data in social and personality psychology research. *Personality and Social Psychology Bulletin, 27*, 771–785.

Nezlek, J. B. (2003). Using multilevel random coefficient modeling to analyze social interaction diary data. *Journal of Social and Personal Relationships, 20*, 437–469.

Nezlek, J. B. (2005). *A multilevel framework for understanding relationships among traits, states, situations, and behaviors*. Unpublished manuscript, College of William and Mary.

Nezlek, J. B., & Gable, S. L. (2001). Depression as a moderator of relationships between positive daily events and day-to-day psychological adjustment. *Personality and Social Psychology Bulletin, 27*, 1692–1704.

Nezlek, J. B., & Plesko, R. M. (2003). Affect- and self-based models of relationships between daily events and daily well-being. *Personality and Social Psychology Bulletin, 29*, 584–596.

Rabash, J., Browne, W., Goldstein, H., Yang, M., Plewis, I., Healy, M., et al. (2000). *MLn: Command reference guide*. London: Institute of Education.

Raudensbush, S. W., & Bryk, A. S. (2002). *Hierarchical linear models* (2nd ed.). Newbury Park, CA: Sage.

Raudenbush, S. W., Bryk, A., Cheong, Y. F., & Congdon, R. (2004). *HLM 6: Hierarchical linear and nonlinear modeling*. Lincolnwood, IL: Scientific Software International.

Singer, J. D. (1998). Using SAS PROC MIXED to fit multilevel models, hierarchical models, and individual growth models. *Journal of Educational and Behavioral Statistics, 23*, 323–355.

Snijders, T., & Bosker, R. (1999). *Multilevel analysis*. London: Sage.

APPENDIX 29.1. SAMPLE DATASETS

LEVEL-1 DATA

subj$	extr	agre	agre2	talk	ntalk	ctalk
a	1	1	1	0	1	−1
a	2	2	2	1	0	1
a	3	2	2	1	0	1
a	4	3	3	1	0	1
a	5	3	3	0	1	−1
a	6	3	3	1	0	1
a	7	4	4	1	0	1
a	8	4	4	1	0	1
b	2	2	2	0	1	−1
b	2	2	2	0	1	−1
b	3	2	2	0	1	−1
b	3	4	4	0	1	−1
b	4	4	4	1	0	1
b	4	4	4	1	0	1
b	5	5	5	1	0	1
b	6	5	5	0	1	−1
b	6	5	5	0	1	−1
e	1	4	104	0	1	−1
e	2	5	105	1	0	1
e	3	6	106	0	1	−1
e	4	6	106	0	1	−1
e	5	6	106	1	0	1
e	6	7	107	0	1	−1
e	7	8	108	1	0	1
e	8	9	109	1	0	1
e	9	10	110	0	1	−1
e	9	10	110	0	1	−1
f	1	1	101	0	1	−1
f	1	2	102	0	1	−1
f	4	5	105	0	1	−1
f	4	6	106	1	0	1
f	5	7	107	1	0	1
f	5	8	108	1	0	1
f	5	9	109	0	1	−1
f	6	10	110	0	1	−1
i	6	4	104	0	1	−1
i	6	4	104	0	1	−1
i	6	5	105	0	1	−1
i	6	6	106	0	1	−1
i	7	7	107	1	0	1
i	7	7	107	1	0	1
i	7	8	108	1	0	1
i	7	9	109	1	0	1
i	8	10	110	0	1	−1
i	8	10	110	0	1	−1

subj$	extr	agre	agre2	talk	ntalk	ctalk
c	3	3	3	0	1	−1
c	3	3	3	1	0	1
c	3	3	3	0	1	−1
c	4	6	6	1	0	1
c	4	6	6	1	0	1
c	4	6	6	1	0	1
c	5	8	8	1	0	1
c	5	8	8	0	1	−1
c	5	9	9	1	0	1
c	6	9	9	1	0	1
d	2	1	1	0	1	−1
d	3	2	2	1	0	1
d	4	3	3	1	0	1
d	4	4	4	0	1	−1
d	5	5	5	1	0	1
d	6	6	6	1	0	1
d	6	7	7	1	0	1
d	7	8	8	1	0	1
d	8	9	9	1	0	1
d	9	10	10	1	0	1
g	5	2	102	0	1	−1
g	5	2	102	0	1	−1
g	5	2	102	0	1	−1
g	6	3	103	0	1	−1
g	6	3	103	1	0	1
g	6	3	103	1	0	1
g	7	4	104	1	0	1
g	7	4	104	1	0	1
g	7	5	105	0	1	−1
g	8	6	106	0	1	−1
h	4	1	101	0	1	−1
h	4	1	101	0	1	−1
h	4	2	102	1	0	1
h	5	2	102	1	0	1
h	5	3	103	1	0	1
h	5	4	104	0	1	−1
h	6	5	105	1	0	1
h	6	5	105	1	0	1
h	6	6	106	1	0	1
h	6	7	107	0	1	−1
h	7	5	105	1	0	1
h	7	5	105	1	0	1

LEVEL-2 DATA

subj$	Anxiety	agre2
a	8	2.75
b	12	3.6667
c	14	6.1
d	9	5.5
e	12	107.1
f	14	106
g	12	103.4
h	15	103.83
i	15	107

## CHAPTER 30

Studying Personality Processes

Explaining Change in between-Persons Longitudinal and within-Person Multilevel Models

William Fleeson

The purpose of this chapter is to guide the use of analytic models for studying the processes underlying personality variables. It is important that personality psychologists have available powerful and widely understood methods for studying processes, for at least three reasons (Cervone & Mischel, 2002; Fleeson, 2004; Funder, 2001; Pervin, 1994). First, interest in process has always been strong among personality psychologists (Allport, 1937; Cattell, 1966; Larsen, 1989), but has grown recently as personality psychologists become increasingly interested not only in what personality is but also in how it works (Funder, 2001; McCrae & Costa, 1999; Mischel, 2004). Second, such advancement in understanding process is the hallmark of a mature science and reflects the field's growing self-confidence. Finally, advancement in describing processes will reveal the potential for personality change as well as promising opportunities to effect such change. Meeting this growing interest in studying processes have been assessment, com-

puting, and conceptual advances that make studying processes more practical. This chapter provides initial guidance in implementing these advances.

Process refers to a combination of actions, changes, or events that bring about an outcome. The outcome can be the creation of something new or a change in the existing level of a variable. Personality psychologists typically investigate the latter, with research directed at explaining change in existing variables such as traits, well-being, behavior, or life events. Processes can be simple, such as when one change brings about another change, or they can be complex, such as when multiple events cascade in a temporal sequence to bring about an ultimate outcome. Processes can also be ongoing, in cases when the outcome fluctuates and its value at any given time is determined by other concurrent events in a mathematically describable manner. By identifying the steps or changes that bring about an outcome, processes describe how things work (the mechanism) and identify points at which interventions can efficiently produce changes in the outcome.

Structure is the complement to process; a structure consists of the variables or parts of personality and their typical or fixed relationship to each other. Processes operate on and within these structures. Although the term *structure* is often used as a shorthand for *covariance structure*, referring to the correlations between individual differences in traits such as the Big Five, it is also used more generally to refer to any set of variables and their relationships. A complete description of personality requires knowledge of both the structures being operated on and the processes operating on them. Personality psychology primarily has focused on identifying variables and their covariance structures, but it is also necessary to enhance research on processes (Cervone, 2004; Fleeson, in press).

Most psychological processes happen within a person, but processes can be studied by a between-persons or by a within-person approach (Epstein, 1983; Lamiell, 1997).[1] The traditional between-persons approach usually investigates simpler processes, attempting to explain change in one variable by changes in or actions of only one or a few other variables. Between-persons approaches do so by testing whether differences between people in an outcome variable are related to corresponding differences between people in an explanatory variable. For example, researchers may investigate whether extraversion leads to happiness by testing whether happier people are that way because they are more extraverted than other people (Costa & McCrae, 1980). Once such a relationship is identified between persons, it is inferred that a process occurred within each individual to lead to their respective levels on the outcome variable. However, the correspondence between between-persons relationships and within-person processes is complex. Sometimes the directly analogous process is inferred to operate within persons. For example, because individuals who use problem-focused coping methods have less stress, it is inferred that when each individual uses a problem-focused coping method, his or her stress will be reduced. At other times the between-persons relationship indicates where to look for a within-person process. For example, extraverts' higher level of happiness has directed some researchers to investigate what it is that extraverts do that leads to happiness (e.g., Rusting & Larsen, 1998). At still other times, the process can be studied only between persons, because the explanatory variable changes so rarely or so slowly that within-person approaches are impractical. For example, extraverts may be happier because of enhanced functioning of the dopamine system, as determined early in development (Depue & Collins, 1999).

Within-person approaches investigate processes by assessing each individual on multiple occasions and comparing those occasions to each other, one individual at a time. The degree to which the outcome and explanatory variable covary across occasions is calculated for each individual, and the average of these covariances describes the within-person relationship (averaging is necessary because individuals show slightly different relationships owing to chance alone). Within-person approaches may reveal different answers than between-persons approaches reveal, because variables may vary across persons for different reasons than they vary within people across occasions (Robinson, 1950). For example, across persons the relationship between extraversion and positive affect is strong and positive, but this may not mean that the relationship within persons between extraversion and positive affect is positive. In fact, changing the amount anyone acts extraverted may have no impact on that person's happiness, because extraversion and positive affect may vary within people for different reasons than they vary between people (Fleeson, Malanos, & Achille, 2002). Often the within-person processes are the processes of primary interest to psychologists, because psychologists are interested in how the mind works. However, personality psychologists tend to use the more practical between-persons approaches and then make inferences about the processes happening within a person.

This chapter describes both between-persons approaches and within-person approaches, with the goal of promoting the study of process. Although process is studied with many types of psychological variables, this chapter is directed at researchers interested in personality concepts, such as traits, goals, attachment styles, well-being, personality disorders, self-concepts, and coping. I hope to provide enough detail to guide the actual use of these methods. However, rather than focus on technical details, I focus on how statistical techniques can be used to answer interesting questions about how personality works.

Between-Persons Approaches to Studying Change

All research investigating process shares the goals of identifying the causes and consequences of personality variables and of discovering how personality variables work. When studied between persons, the effort is usually known as studying "change." This is mainly because the common longitudinal method is to measure the outcome twice and test whether an explanatory variable predicts changes in the outcome variable from the first occasion to the second. It is a between-persons approach because it tests whether differences between individuals in the explanatory variable are aligned with differences between individuals in change. For example, Carver and Scheier (1994) investigated whether individual differences in coping are correlated with individual differences in stress change from a semester beginning to a semester end. An important advantage of studying change is that, when done correctly, it enhances the ability to make conclusions about causality. Thus, researchers can not only identify the variables that are involved in the process of change, but can also have confidence that the direction of causality flows from the explanatory variables to the outcome, rather than the reverse.

This section of the chapter describes methods that allow conclusions about causality and change and diverts the reader away from some tempting but ultimately less effective methods. Although researchers often use regression to study change, explications of the appropriate methodological and analytic procedure are not widely published and researchers are hard-pressed to find guidance on these issues (Darlington & Smulders, 2001). Because change is so critical to personality theory and because suboptimal analytic techniques are occasionally used, it is important for the appropriate analyses to be available to personality researchers.

Step-by-Step Guide

Longitudinal designs are the designs of choice for at least two reasons: (1) They provide a more rigorous test of causal hypotheses than is possible using concurrent designs, and (2) they allow time to pass so that the processes in question have an opportunity to produce change. Longitudinal designs entail at least two times of measurement of the same participants. For example, a researcher may measure coping and stress at both the beginning of a semester (time 1) and the end of the semester (time 2), or measure extraversion and happiness each at the beginning of the study (time 1) and then again 10 years later (time 2). The hypothesis tested in such designs is that the explanatory variable is responsible for change in the outcome—more precisely, that differences in the explanatory variable will produce changes in the outcome.

At least four variables are needed to test this hypothesis: a participant identification variable, the explanatory variable (EV; also known as the independent variable) measured at time 1, and the outcome (also known as the dependent variable) measured both at time 1 and at time 2. Figure 30.1 shows this design and three possible regressions for investigating the effect of the explanatory variable on the outcome. It is well known that the first regression, a standard cross-sectional regression in which the time 1 outcome is predicted from the time 1 explanatory variable, is not sufficient for determining causal direction, because any relationship between the two variables could be due to the explanatory variable causing the outcome, the outcome causing the explanatory variable, or a third variable causing both.

A second possibility, improved but still not sufficient, is to predict the outcome at time 2 rather than at time 1. This analysis, part of the cross-lagged approach, is an improvement because the future cannot affect the past—the outcome at time 2 cannot have caused the explanatory variable at time 1, so any revealed relationship between them cannot be due to the outcome from time 2 causing the explanatory variable. However, the explanatory variable in such an analysis is not independent of influence from the outcome, because it is not independent of the outcome at time 1. If the outcome is stable at all from time 1 and to time 2, the joint influence of the time-1 outcome on the explanatory variable and the stability of the outcome is more than enough to produce a spurious relationship between the explanatory variable and the time-2 outcome, even if the explanatory variable does not cause the outcome. Thus, the causal direction between the explanatory variable and the outcome remains ambig-

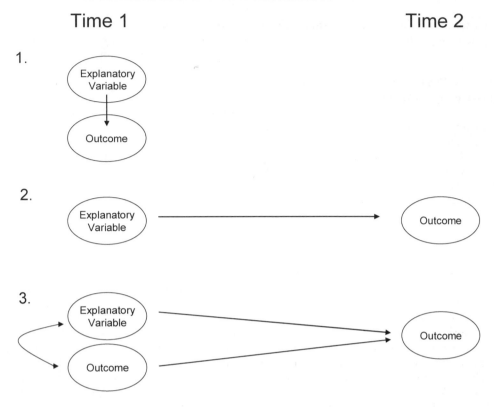

FIGURE 30.1. Three possible regressions for investigating the effect of the explanatory variable on the outcome. The bottom represents the recommended analysis.

uous in such an analysis. To fix this problem, the explanatory variable must be made independent of the outcome from time 1.

The final and recommended analysis is a multiple regression, predicting the time-2 outcome simultaneously from two variables: the time-1 explanatory variable and the time-1 outcome. Whenever multiple independent variables (IVs) are included in a simultaneous multiple regression, the relationships are calculated for only part of each IV, namely, the part of each IV that is independent of the other IVs. In the recommended analysis, this means that the relationship for the explanatory variable is calculated for the part of the explanatory variable that is independent of the time-1 outcome (allowing for imperfection in measurement of the time-1 outcome). If this relationship exists, it cannot be due to the time-1 outcome causing the explanatory variable (because the regression made the explanatory variable independent of the time-1 outcome) and it cannot be due to the time-2 outcome causing the explanatory variable (because the future cannot affect the past), so it must go in the other causal direction (or be due to a third variable).

The magnitude and direction of the relationship are described by the unstandardized beta for the explanatory variable (the slope). In particular, an unstandardized beta communicates the number of points the time-2 outcome, changes for every point the part of the explanatory variable that is independent of the time-1 outcome changes (these points are the points on the scales of the explanatory variable and the outcome). In this case, the multiple regression makes the explanatory variable independent of the time-1 outcome and then predicts the time-2 outcome from that independent part. Because the explanatory variable is independent of the time-1 outcome, any relationship between the explanatory variable and the time-2 outcome must have arisen between times 1 and 2, and thus cannot be caused by the outcome.

This analysis supports conclusions both about change and about causal direction. Because the analysis "equates" the participants statistically on the outcome at time 1, it is in fact predicting change in the outcome. That is, the analysis reveals what happens to the time 2 outcome among individuals who at time 1 have the same level on the outcome but different levels on the explanatory variable. If the outcome changes from time 1 to time 2, and these changes are caused by the explanatory variable, then people who started with the same standing on the outcome will change to a standing on the outcome as a consequence of their time-1 explanatory variable standing. By conducting a multiple regression in this fashion, the researcher has directly tested whether the process creating change in the outcome involves this particular explanatory variable.

Case Examples

Extraversion and Positive Affect

An important personality finding of the last 20 years is that positive affect is associated more strongly to extraversion than to any other variable, including objective circumstances (Costa & McCrae, 1980; Lucas & Baird, 2004; Staudinger, Fleeson, & Baltes, 1999). This finding was first discovered by Costa and McCrae in 1980, when they proposed that internal personality factors might be one component in the process that results in happiness. Even though the process was presumed to work within the one individual, Costa and McCrae used a between-persons method. They used a longitudinal design, measuring extraversion at time 1 and positive affect 10 years later at time 2. Unfortunately, they did not have positive affect measures available at time 1, so they could use only the second of the analysis techniques illustrated in Figure 30.1. They found that extraversion predicted positive affect even 10 years later ($r = 0.23$). That is, individuals who differed from each other in extraversion at time 1 had corresponding differences in positive affect 10 years later. Because they could not control for time-1 positive affect, it is possible that this correlation was due to positive affect causing extraversion rather than extraversion causing positive affect. Even though Costa and McCrae were unable to determine unambiguously the direction of causality, the suggestion that extraversion might be involved in the process determining happiness was so important that it inspired decades of research to further investigate the process. Only recently has an experimental

approach been used to conclude that extraversion in fact causes positive affect (McNiel & Fleeson, 2006).

Coping and Mental Health Symptomology

Stressors impact mental health, but do so differently for different people. The way an individual copes with stressors has been proposed as an important part of the process affecting change in mental health symptomology (Lazarus, 2000). In particular, trying to avoid the problem has been proposed to be generally less effective at reducing symptomology than is acknowledging or trying to solve the problem that led to the stressor. Aldwin and Revenson (1987) tested whether coping affected change in symptomology with a between-persons longitudinal approach. They measured symptoms (on a 0–44 scale) two times about a year apart, along with several ways of coping (on 1–4 scales) at the first time point.

They predicted time-2 symptoms (the outcome) in a multiple regression with the several time-1 ways of coping (the explanatory variables) and time-1 symptoms as the independent variables. Three of the coping styles had significant relationships to time-2 symptoms. Because time-1 symptoms were controlled in the analysis and time-2 symptoms cannot affect the past, these significant relationships cannot be due to symptoms causing ways of coping, but rather must be due to ways of coping (or a third variable) causing symptoms. In particular, escapism (0.45) and social support mobilization (0.20) predicted increased symptoms at time 2, whereas instrumental action (–0.18) predicted reduced symptoms. These betas describe the changes in symptoms for each point change in the respective ways of coping, independent of all other ways of coping and of time-1 symptoms (it was unspecified in the article whether these betas were unstandardized betas). Thus, the results show that coping is likely to be an important variable in the process affecting changes in mental health symptomology.

Complexities

The basic analyses as described above are fairly straightforward, but there are several complications that may arise in the course of any particular study. Here I discuss two important and frequent complications that arise from researchers attempting other less optimal ways to measure change and two important caveats to the conclusions based on these methods. For additional complexities and possibilities, see Darlington (1990).

Difference Scores as Outcomes

An intuitively appealing but less effective technique for predicting change is to compute the difference in the outcome variable between time 1 and time 2 and then use the difference score as the dependent variable. Such a method appears to measure change, because time-1 scores on the outcome are subtracted from time-2 scores on the outcome so that positive numbers indicate increases in the outcome and negative numbers indicate declines in the outcome.

What undermines this technique is that difference scores are usually correlated with time-1 scores on the outcome. Participants who scored higher on the outcome at time 1 are more likely to have a low or negative difference score (more likely to decline), and those who scored higher on the outcome at time 1 are more likely to have a high or positive difference score (more likely to increase on the outcome).

This correlation between time-1 scores and difference scores creates two problems. The first problem is an ambiguity about what the outcome is. When the difference scores are correlated with time-1 scores, the difference scores reflect two variables (i.e., change over time and the time-1 score). Thus, it will not be clear which of these two concepts is responsible for any observed association to the explanatory variable. In particular, the time-1 outcome may be associated with the explanatory variable and so produce a spurious association of the explanatory variable to the difference score when it actually has no relationship to change on the outcome. The way to disambiguate this is to partial the time-1 outcome out of the explanatory variable, as explained above. The second problem is that the causal direction of the effect cannot be specified. Because the difference score contains variance of the time-1 outcome, any relationship between the difference score and the explanatory variable may be due to the time-1 outcome rather than to the explanatory variable. What is desired by the researcher is to predict change that is independent of the time-1 outcome—the analysis for doing so is the recommended analysis described above (replacing the time-2 outcome by

difference scores in the recommended analysis will not change the unstandardized beta for the explanatory variable).

In contrast to this position, Rogosa (1995) makes a spirited defense of the raw difference score as the best measure of change, partly because it straightforwardly assesses whether each individual changed on the outcome. However, correlations between an explanatory variable and the difference score are almost always ambiguous as to whether they are due to the value of the time-1 outcome or to change. Specifically, if the explanatory variable is related to the outcome at time 1, and the outcome at time 1 in turn is negatively related to change, this will introduce a spurious negative component to the association between the explanatory variable and change. The spurious negative component may mask an underlying positive effect of the explanatory variable on the time-2 scores. The way to check for this is to compare those individuals with the same value of the outcome at time 1 but different values of the explanatory variable, and to observe whether they end up with different resulting scores of the time-2 outcome (i.e., to conduct the recommended analysis). However, I do agree with Rogosa that analyzing change at the individual level has many advantages, as is explicated in the subsequent section "Within-Person Multilevel Models for Studying Process."

Residualized Change Scores as Outcomes

Recognition of the problems with difference scores has led to occasional use of residualized change scores. Also derived from longitudinal designs, residualized change scores are created before the main analysis by conducting a preliminary multiple regression in which the time-2 outcome is predicted from the time-1 outcome. The residuals are saved from this analysis and are similar to difference scores in that they describe the direction and magnitude of change from time 1 to time 2. However, residuals are improved over difference scores in that they are independent of the time-1 outcome (the residualizing removes the dependency). Thus, participants are no more likely to have a positive direction of change only because of starting low and no more likely to have a negative direction of change only because of starting high.

However, residualized change scores still are not recommended for studying change for at least two reasons. First, removing the time-1 outcome from the time-2 outcome (by residualizing) but not removing it from the explanatory variable will leave irrelevant and obscuring variance in the explanatory variable (namely, variance related to the outcome at time 1). This irrelevant variance may seriously reduce the explanatory variable's apparent effect (Darlington & Smulders, 2001; Furr, 2005) and underestimate its role in producing change in almost all cases. Because the recommended analysis does not have this problem, and already reveals the explanatory variable's effect specifically on change in the outcome, it is almost always superior. (Removing the time-1 outcome from both the explanatory variable and the time-2 outcome produces the same unstandardized beta as does the recommended analysis above.)

Second, no modification to the outcome is necessary for testing hypotheses about change in the outcome. This is because it is very difficult for an explanatory variable to have a causal impact on a time-2 outcome score without changing that score. Thus, the recommended analysis already predicts change in the outcome, even without directly calculating a change score.

It is possible, however, as some researchers propose, that the variables that cause change in an outcome are different from those that cause the creation or level of the outcome. Such researchers are proposing a moderator variable, because they are proposing that the effect of the explanatory variable on the outcome depends on some other factor, such as time. Testing a moderator hypothesis requires identifying that moderator variable, assessing it, and using an interactive term to test the theory (see Chaplin, Chapter 34, this volume), not partialling the outcome on an earlier time. For example, a researcher may propose that the outcome is created at a young age by one set of variables and then changed at older ages by another set of variables (e.g., Sroufe, Egeland, Carlson, & Collins, 2005); here age is proposed as a moderator of the effect of those variables on the outcome. Linear changes to the outcome do not represent moderation and do not adequately test such theories (Cronbach & Furby, 1970; Darlington, 1990).

In sum, residualized change scores may result in inaccurate results and gain little conceptually in regard to predicting change rather than level (Cronbach & Furby, 1970; Darling-

ton, 1990). The only potential gain is a reduction in total variance in the time-2 outcome, which may increase percentages of explained variance under some conditions.

Measurement Error in the Outcome

The final two complexities present limitations to the conclusions that can be drawn from these analyses. First, inevitable measurement error in the outcome prevents absolute certainty about causal direction. The ability to conclude causality depends on removing the time-1 outcome from the explanatory variable, so that any remaining relationship to the later outcome is entirely independent of the earlier standing on the outcome. However, this is accomplished only imperfectly. Researchers must use a measurement of the time-1 outcome rather than the true standing. All measurements have error, so this procedure does not entirely remove the true standing on the earlier outcome from the explanatory variable—it removes most but not all of it. Thus, the explanatory variable may remain slightly contaminated by the time-1 outcome. This slight contamination is unlikely to account for observed relationships between the explanatory variable and the time-2 outcome and is not usually a serious problem, but it is important to be aware of this problem, particularly in the case of outcomes that have poor reliability.

The Ecological Fallacy

The second caution concerns making conclusions about processes within individuals on the basis of differences between individuals (what Robinson, 1950, called the ecological fallacy). Between-persons research investigates psychological processes by relating differences (variances) across individuals and determining whether individuals who differ on the explanatory variable also differ systematically on an outcome variable. Part of the value in identifying between-persons relationships comes from the inference that the same relationship holds up within people. For example, the finding that individuals who use instrumental action to cope with problems accrue fewer symptoms down the road obtains value partly from the inference that individuals will reduce their symptoms when they use instrumental action. However, this inference changes *what* the differences are across, and this change may weaken the inference. Rather than relating differences across individuals, within-person relationships relate differences across occasions, within each person taken one at a time. Differences across occasions may occur for different reasons than those producing differences across people; thus, the relationships among those differences are not likely to be the same as the relationships among differences across people.

The recommended between-subjects analysis goes a long way in rectifying this problem; this is one reason the recommended analysis is promoted in this chapter. However, direct inferences to a within-person process are still vulnerable to the ecological fallacy. Part of the reason for this is that between-persons and within-person designs typically differ in time frame, and different processes may operate at different speeds. Additionally, between-persons designs are sensitive to both long- and short-term processes, even when the occasions differ only by a short time. Another reason is that between-persons designs are vulnerable to between-person third variables such as response styles (within-person designs are also vulnerable to some third variables).

For example, within individuals, amount of exercise is likely positively associated with fatigue, because an individual will be more fatigued on occasions he or she exercises than on occasions he or she does not. However, between individuals, amount of exercise may be negatively associated with fatigue, because individuals who exercise more than others will likely reduce their overall fatigue (Puetz, O'Connor, & Disham, 2006). Thus a between-persons design may lead to the conclusion that exercise reduces or does not affect fatigue whereas a within-person design may lead to the conclusion that exercise increases fatigue. This may be true even if the recommended between-persons design is employed and even if the occasions in the between-persons design are the same as the occasions in the within-person design.

Another example is the between-persons relationship between extraversion and positive affect: Individuals who are higher than others on extraversion tend to be higher than others on positive affect. This relationship partly obtains value from the inference that individuals may have a route to enhanced life quality, in that variation within each person across occasions in his or her extraversion may predict variation in positive affect. However, extraversion variation within individuals across hours may not be associated with variation within individuals in positive affect, because extraversion variation within a person across hours may occur for different reasons than does extraversion variation between individuals. If extraverts' greater happiness than introverts' is due to a greater number of dopamine neurons (Depue & Collins, 1999), within-person variations in how extraverted a person is acting at the moment would not have an impact on positive affect. In this case, a between-person design would lead to the conclusion that extraversion predicts increases in happiness, whereas the within-person design would lead to the conclusion that extraversion has no effect on happiness.

Finally, Marco, Neale, Schwartz, Shiffman, and Stone (1999) tested whether the times the average individual used problem-focused coping showed reduced stress as compared with the times the same individual did not use problem-focused coping. Every hour for 2 days, participants described whether a stressor occurred in the previous hour, how they coped with it, and their current mood. A within-person analysis revealed no significant predictions of later mood from the coping strategies used. Thus, the between-persons approach led to the conclusion that problem-focused coping lowers negative affect, whereas the within-person approach led to the conclusion that problem-focused coping does not lower negative affect. It is unknown whether this was due to the time frame used (the positive effects of problem-focused coping may take a while to manifest), to the ineffectiveness of coping in reducing negative affect, or to some other cause.

In many cases, the inference from a between-persons relationship to the within-person relationship will be accurate at least in direction. Correspondence increases in likelihood if the occasions in the two designs are more similar. However, the inference is rarely likely to be accurate in the precise magnitude and occasionally will be inaccurate even in direction (Robinson, 1950). For these reasons, researchers need to be cautious when making this inference.

Within-Person Multilevel Models for Studying Process

The goal of within-person approaches to studying process is to identify the causes and consequences of personality variables and to discover how personality works. By studying within-person processes directly, observing changes within one individual unfolding over time, within-person approaches avoid the ecological fallacy.[2] The basic plan is to observe a (usually small) number of individuals each over a period of time, measuring a few variables repeatedly. Then the variations and covariations of those variables are analyzed to characterize each individual in terms of his or her particular patterns of variability and his or her own particular functional processes (Allport, 1937; Epstein, 1983; Lamiell, 1997; Nesselroade, 1991; Tennen, Affleck, Armeli, & Carney, 2000). Patterns and processes can also be compared across individuals to identify common processes that operate within all individuals. This section describes multilevel modeling of experience-sampling data as an ideal method for studying process within persons. However, processes can be studied with other within-person approaches as well, such as dynamic *p*-factor analysis, spectral analysis, and triple-typology analysis (see Singer & Willett, 2002; Larsen, 1989; Nesselroade, 1991; Vansteelandt & VanMechelen, 2004).

Within-person approaches to process can address the same kinds of questions as are addressed by between-persons approaches. A few examples are whether extraversion predicts positive affect (Fleeson et al., 2002), whether stressors increase stress and whether coping reduces stress (Marco et al., 1999; Mroczek & Almeida, 2004), and whether situations influence trait-manifesting behavior (Fleeson, in press). There are several important ways in which within-person approaches differ from between-persons approaches. First, the outcome variable both increases and decreases over time within the same individual. The intention accordingly shifts from trying to predict whether and in which direction the outcome changes, to trying to predict what level the outcome will have at any moment, given the concurrent values of the explanatory variables. Second, within-person approaches are most effective at studying rapid processes and rapidly varying outcomes. The research goal often is to predict changes that occur over the course of days, hours, or even seconds rather than over years. Third, it is more difficult to assess direction of causality because the explanatory variables and outcomes are measured simultaneously, and the lags of causal effect are often shorter than the intervals between measurements. Fourth, the within-person approach

starts with the individual: It characterizes one individual at a time by his or her own particular processes and functions. Then, it also allows generalization across individuals and quantification of differences between individuals in their processes. Fifth, as a result of these characteristics, within-person approaches focus on assessing the ongoing psychological functioning of individuals as they live their lives in naturalistic settings. They aim to obtain mathematical functions to describe and predict what state an individual will be in at each and every given moment.

Multilevel modeling facilitates addressing at least two types of theoretical question. The first type of question concerns what the within-person process is. The within-person process is the relationship between variables across occasions, taking each individual one at a time and then averaging across them. Averaging across individuals is necessary because chance and other factors will lead to each individual revealing a slightly different relationship between the variables in any particular study. Averaging cancels out these chance variations. Multilevel modeling produces one answer to this question, which describes the within-person relationship between the variables for the average or typical individual. This one answer may be different from the answer provided by a between-persons approach because different psychological principles may determine variance and covariance across occasions than the principles that determine variance and covariance across persons.

The second type of question starts with taking the differences between individuals in the within-person relationship seriously and investigates whether those differences are due to more than just chance. Such differences in the covariance relationship may in fact represent differences between people in how they function psychologically. This question marks a radical distinction from between-persons approaches. Between-persons approaches assume that the same psychological process operates within all individuals; it may not be evident in a given individual in a given study, but that is due to chance or to other processes masking the operation of the one principle. In contrast, multilevel modeling addresses the possibility that the psychological process operates differently for different people and that these differences describe enduring characteristics of the individuals' personalities. Multilevel modeling tests this possibility by testing whether differences between individuals in the relationship between the variables are more than would be expected from chance.

Step-by-Step Guide

Multilevel modeling (MLM) is actually quite simple, just like the ordinary least squares (OLS) regression that is routine for most personality psychologists. However, MLM was developed for a wide diversity of purposes, and the computer programs were written to accommodate the many possible purposes. This diversity of options and capabilities in applying MLM to a specific case can be overwhelming. The purpose of this section is to provide a guide specifically focused on applying MLM to the particular case of studying personality processes. There are other excellent guides to MLM (e.g., Bolger, Davis, & Rafaeli, 2003; Kreft & de Leeuw, 1998; Nezlek, Chapter 29, this volume) that are more general and written for the multiple diverse applications that MLM is capable of.

The data for this technique typically consist of a few explanatory variables and a few outcomes measured for only a few participants (20–50 participants are usually enough) on a large number of occasions for each participant (e.g., 25–200 per participant). For example, 50 participants may report how extraverted they acted and how much positive affect they experienced every 3 hours for 2 weeks. The power of these studies comes from the large number of occasions per participant rather than from the large number of participants.

I provide specific instructions for conducting MLM in SPSS, because this is a widely used program and because it embeds MLM into a wide array of data manipulation and analytic capabilities. Some familiarity with SPSS is assumed; I am basing instructions on SPSS 14, so details may vary in other versions (commands appear to be identical in SPSS 15.0). However, there are other excellent programs available, such as HLM 6 (Raudenbush, Bryk, & Congdon, 2004) and SAS. MLM requires some preparatory work. The first step is to make sure the data are in the correct form. Each row must correspond to one occasion, with occasions sorted by participant. Thus, each participant will have many rows. There should be one column for each variable, plus one additional column indicating the participant who generated the occasion (e.g., the participant's ID

number). If, alternatively, the data are organized such that each participant has only one row, with different variables for each occasion, the "restructure" dialogue box in the SPSS data menu can restructure the data into the correct order.

Centering is an important consideration, and how it should be done depends on the particular interest of the researcher (Kreft & de Leeuw, 1998). However, when trying to discover within-person processes, it is almost always best to center the explanatory variables within each person, to be sure that between-persons variance does not contaminate the result and that it is a pure description of within-person processes. To center variables within people, use the aggregate command in the "data" menu (after putting the data in the correct form). Put the participant ID into the "break variable" box and the explanatory variable into the "summaries of variables" box, and make sure "add aggregated variables to active dataset" is checked. If this has successfully created a new variable, with each participant's mean on the explanatory variable indicated for each of his or her occasions, then subtract this new variable from the original explanatory variable to make the centered explanatory variable that will be used in subsequent analyses. Open the compute dialogue under the transform menu, type the name of the explanatory variable (followed by "_centered") in the "target variable" box, and put the explanatory variable, a minus sign, and the newly aggregated mean variable in the "numeric expression" box.

The analysis program in SPSS is called Mixed Models–Linear and was designed very broadly to be able to accomplish a wide variety of purposes. Getting it to conduct a within-person MLM is a bit awkward. After opening Mixed Models—Linear in the Analyze drop-down menu, put the participant ID in the "subjects" box and click "continue"; put the outcome in the "dependent variable" box and the centered explanatory variable in the "covariate" box (factors are used when the explanatory variable is a categorical variable). In the "fixed . . . " dialogue, add the explanatory variable to the "model" box, and make sure that "include intercept" is checked. In the "random . . . " box, choose unstructured for the covariance type, add the explanatory variable to the "model" box, and check "include intercept." Also move the participant ID to the combinations box (this step is easy to overlook because a similar step was completed earlier). In the "statistics . . . " dialog check "parameter estimates" and "tests for covariance parameters."

"Fixed" and "random" are used in multiple ways in statistics and in MLM. In this case, a *fixed effect* refers to an effect that is the same for all participants and a *random effect* refers to an effect that is allowed to vary randomly across participants. In most cases, in investigating personality processes, the effect of the explanatory variable will be assumed to have both a fixed and a random part. The fixed part refers to the average or universal effect of the predictor on the outcome for people; the random effect refers to the fact that the effect of the predictor may differ across individuals for reasons particular to each individual. In terms of the intercept, the fixed part refers to the overall average level of the outcome for people in general; the random part refers to individual aspects of each participant that give him or her a different average level of the outcome across occasions.

The "covariance type" refers to the constraints put on the matrix describing the variances and covariances among the coefficients (the intercept and one for each beta) across participants. This matrix indicates how much participants differed in their intercepts or effects of the explanatory variable, and how much the effects of the explanatory variable were related to each other and to the intercept. Choosing "unstructured" for the covariance type means that there are no constraints and that the matrix will be determined by the variances and covariances in the data.

Before interpreting the results, it is important to look for warnings or errors. If there are warnings, it is best to try to resolve them because, otherwise, they may mean that the output is incorrect. For example, if the analysis fails to converge, try increasing the number of iterations in the estimation dialog box. Other reasons for nonconvergence include too many parameter estimates or setting up the analysis incorrectly. Compare your syntax to that in Table 30.1 to identify possible errors.

MLM provides a coefficient to address the first type of question, whether the explanatory variable predicts changes in the outcome variable for the average or typical person. The coefficient is just like an unstandardized coefficient from regression, with magnitude and direction to indicate whether and how strongly the explanatory variable predicts changes in the outcome. This coefficient is the first entry in the row labeled by the explanatory variable, in the "estimates of fixed effects" table. Because the coefficient is unstandardized, it describes the number of points the outcome changes for the average person when the explanatory variable changes one point (these points are the points on the scales of the predic-

---

TABLE 30.1. Example Syntax Generated by Pasting from a Successful Multilevel Model Run in SPSS

```
sort cases by ID.

AGGREGATE
 /OUTFILE=*
 MODE=ADDVARIABLES
 /BREAK=ID
 /extra_mean = MEAN(extra).

COMPUTE extra_centered = extra - extra_mean .
EXECUTE .

MIXED
 positiveaffect WITH extra_centered
 /CRITERIA = CIN(95) MXITER(100) MXSTEP(5) SCORING(1)
 SINGULAR(0.000000000001) HCONVERGE(0, ABSOLUTE) LCONVERGE(0, ABSOLUTE)
 PCONVERGE(0.000001, ABSOLUTE)
 /FIXED = extra_centered | SSTYPE(3)
 /METHOD = REML
 /PRINT = SOLUTION TESTCOV
 /RANDOM INTERCEPT extra_centered | SUBJECT(ID) COVTYPE(UN) .
```

tor and outcome). The rest of the row for the explanatory variable provides a significance test on this coefficient. A significant coefficient means that an ongoing process has been identified that describes and predicts the variation in the outcome.

The intercept row describes the average person's score on the outcome on those occasions when the explanatory variable has a score of 0. If the explanatory variable was centered as recommended, this describes the average person's score on the outcome on the average occasion.

MLM provides a variance to address the second type of question, the extent to which the explanatory variable predicts changes in the outcome variable differently for different people. This variance is just like any other variance that describes how much a quantity varies across people. The quantity in this case is the coefficient that describes the relationship between the explanatory variable and the outcome. The novel, exciting, and sometimes daunting concept is that a finding (a relationship or a coefficient) can vary across people, just like any other quantity can. Normally, personality psychologists conceive of personality as consisting of differences in levels on variables; this quantity describes personality as consisting of differences in relationships between variables. That is, the psychological process relating the outcome to the explanatory variable can be different for different people. This variance is the statistic that describes whether the general principle relating two variables does not apply to some people, does apply to most people but in different strengths, or is even completely reversed for some people.

This variance is listed in the "UN (2,2)" row of the "estimates of covariance parameters" table (if there are more predictors, each subsequent predictor's variance is found in a row that has a number higher than 2 repeated in the parentheses, for example, "UN (3,3)"). The estimate is the variance—it is usually best to take the square root of this number (which will make it much larger if the variance is less than 1) and turn it into the more interpretable standard deviation (SD). The larger the SD, the more individuals differ in the process (i.e., in the direction, presence, or magnitude of the process). These numbers often appear to be very small even when they represent large differences between individuals in the strength or direction of the process. The way to evaluate their magnitude is to compare them to the

value of the beta they modify. Most such betas are also less than 1, so SD's on them will be smaller than that. If the distribution is relatively normal, approximately two-thirds of the participants will have a process coefficient within plus or minus 1 SD of the typical individual's process coefficient. Thus, an SD of even 0.20 or so on a typical beta of 0.30 describes substantial variation in the strength of the process across individuals.

The rest of the row provides a significance test on the variance; if the variance is significant, it means that individuals differ from each more than would be expected by chance sampling of occasions. This implies at least three overlapping interpretations. First, the process differs in its weight in the psychological functioning of individuals, and perhaps does not constitute the psychological functioning of some individuals at all. Second, the strength and relevance of this particular explanatory variable in this process differs across individuals. Third, differences between individuals in processes are reliable individual difference variables that describe part of the individual's personality (Fleeson, 2007; Mischel & Shoda, 1995). Note that a nonsignificant variance does not mean that individuals do not differ from each other—it means only that this particular study did not provide evidence to allow concluding that they differ reliably. Note also that the accuracy of this significance test is still being improved (Raudenbush & Bryk, 2002).

I suggest the following guidelines for reporting the results of MLM. Because MLM is a relatively new technique, researchers have often included equations in their articles. However, as the technique becomes more common, this practice should fade and become no more common than writing out equations for regressions is now. Second, tables are recommended for presenting the key results, but it is usually best to include only the important information; including only the important information enhances communication and interpretation of the results. Again because MLM is new, there is a temptation to overreport information, cluttering the tables and reducing the reader's comprehension. Rather, report the process coefficient and its significance for the average individual, and the SD across individuals in the process coefficient and the SD's significance, for each explanatory variable. If the intercept is reported, it should follow the same format, with its value for the average individual and the standard deviation (*SD*) across individuals (the standard deviation is the square root of the variance estimate in the "UN(1,1)" row). Finally, when reporting results, use similar terms to those used in this chapter rather than the Greek letters or technical names for the coefficients. For example, report the "typical individual's relationship," rather than γ_{10}.

Case Example: Extraversion and Positive Affect

Most work on the relationship between extraversion and positive affect has been between persons, leaving it unclear whether this work translated into a within-persons process, such that individuals can become happier by acting more extraverted. In fact, there is reason to believe it may not translate; for example, introverted individuals may not derive happiness from the same activities as do extraverts, and even extraverts' happiness may not come from how they are acting. Fleeson and colleagues (2002) conducted a within-person process study to address this question directly. In an experience-sampling study, participants reported how extraverted they were acting (the explanatory variable) and how much positive affect they were experiencing (the outcome) every few hours.

This section provides a walk-through of the steps in MLM for these data. In order to facilitate the reader's following along, artificial data based on a real dataset (10 participants and 8–20 occasions per participant) are provided in Appendix 30.1 (the data can also be e-mailed upon request to Fleesonw@wfu.edu). Note that each row corresponds to one occasion and shows the extraversion and positive affect reported on that occasion, as well as an arbitrary identification number of the participant to which the occasion belongs. Each participant has multiple rows, one per occasion (the data are shown in multiple columns to save space, but in SPSS each row should have three entries). Note that a typical study would have more occasions and more participants.

Because state extraversion varied both between and within participants, and because the interest is in the correlates of within-person variation in state extraversion, the first step is to center extraversion on each person's mean. This allows the results to be interpreted as describing within-person processes only. Open the "aggregate . . . " dialog in the data menu,

move ID to the "break variable" box, extra to the "summaries of variables" box, and make sure the "add aggregated variables to active dataset" box is checked. After clicking "ok," check that extra_mean is included in the data file and that all occasions for a given participant have the same value. Finally, subtract extra_mean from extra to create extra_centered.

In the MLM analysis, the effects of extraversion were assumed to be both fixed (part of the effect was common to all participants) and random (part of the effect of acting extraverted was allowed to differ across individuals). The same was assumed for the intercept (it was assumed that there was a common average level of positive affect for all participants and that each participant had unique factors that adjusted his or her own particular average level of positive affect). To run the MLM analysis, open the mixed models-linear dialog in the analyze menu. Move ID to the "subjects" box and click "continue"; move positiveaffect to the "dependent variable" box and extra_centered to the "covariate" box. In the "fixed . . . " dialog, add extra_centered to the "model" box and make sure that "include intercept" is checked. This step instructs the analysis to generate both the average level of positive affect (PA) for the typical participant (by clicking "include intercept") and the association between extraversion and positive affect for the typical participant (by adding extra_centered to the model). In the "random . . . " dialog, choose unstructured for the covariance type, add extra_centered to the "model" box, and check "include intercept"; this step allows both the average level of positive affect and the association between extraversion and positive affect to differ by participant. In addition, move ID to the combinations box to instruct the analysis to group the cases by participant. In the "statistics . . . " dialog, check "parameter estimates" and "tests for covariance parameters." Table 30.1 shows the syntax generated by clicking "paste" for a correctly entered model, including centering. If problems are encountered, generate syntax by clicking the "paste" button and compare it in detail with this example.

Running the MLM analysis revealed the output shown in Table 30.2 and the results shown in Table 30.3. The fixed effects table in the output shows the results for the average participant. The intercept row describes the average person's positive affect on those occasions when extra_centered had a score of 0. Because

TABLE 30.2. Selected Output Generated by Running the Syntax in Table 30.1 on the Sample Data

Estimates of Fixed Effects(a)

Parameter	Estimate	Std. Error	df	t	Sig.	95% Confidence Interval	
						Lower Bound	Upper Bound
Intercept	4.037936	.328432	8.961	12.295	.000	3.294480	4.781391
extra_centered	.603568	.096111	7.192	6.280	.000	.377527	.829609

a Dependent Variable: positiveaffect.

Estimates of Covariance Parameters(a)

Parameter		Estimate	Std. Error	Wald Z	Sig.	95% Confidence Interval	
						Lower Bound	Upper Bound
Residual		.614374	.079300	7.747	.000	.477050	.791227
Intercept + extra_centered [subject = ID]	UN (1,1)	1.030863	.509549	2.023	.043	.391253	2.716091
	UN (2,1)	−.101249	.123736	−.818	.413	−.343767	.141269
	UN (2,2)	.038032	.044154	.861	.389	.003908	.370137

a Dependent Variable: positiveaffect.

extraversion was centered, this means that the average person's score on positive affect on an average day was 4.04. The row for extra_centered addresses the first type of question, the degree to which extraversion predicts changes in positive affect for the average or typical person. The coefficient, 0.60, is just like an unstandardized coefficient from a regression, with magnitude and direction to indicate whether and how strongly extraversion predicted changes in positive affect. Because the coefficient is unstandardized, it means that, for

TABLE 30.3. The Within-Person Process Relating Extraversion to Positive Affect: Results from a Multilevel Model on a Small Subset of Data

Process	Typical individual	Standard deviation across individuals
Association of extraversion to PA	.60**	.19
Average PA	4.04**	1.02*

Note. The outcome is positive affect (PA), and the association of extraversion to PA for the typical individual means that every point the typical individual changes in extraversion across occasions is associated with a .60 increase in positive affect. In the full sample, the *SD* across individuals in this association was significant, *p* < .01, meaning that individuals differed reliability in the association of extraversion to PA.

* *p* < .05; ** *p* < .001.

the typical or average individual, each point he or she increased his or her momentary level of extraversion was associated with a little more than a half point increase in his or her level of positive affect (both extraversion and positive affect were on 1–7 scales). This result was significant, meaning that the within-person association between extraversion and positive affect is greater than expected by chance and that an ongoing process describing variation in positive affect has been identified.

Thus, this is a case in which the between-persons approach and the within-person approach produced answers in the same direction but different magnitude. Specifically, extraversion and positive affect are positively related both across people and across occasions within each person. However, the relationship is stronger within people than it is across people. This result is surprising, because this is a case in which the inference from the between-persons relationship to the within-persons relationship is not as plausible, and it is easily imaginable that the relationship would not hold up within people (it is easy to imagine that acting extraverted would not have the same impact on happiness that actually being an extravert would have). However, not only does this relationship describe within-person variation, it does so even more strongly than it does between people. Thus, this result demonstrates the need to examine within-person processes directly, because it shows that the result may be different than expected on the basis of the between-subjects research.

The next set of output, in the "covariance parameters" table, concerns how applicable these average effects are to each of the individuals and how much individuals differed from each other in these effects. The "estimate" column provides variances (and covariances) across participants in each of the fixed effects described above. The variance across individuals in average positive affect is printed in the row for UN(1,1)—the intercept is parameter number 1, and 1,1 means that the estimate is its covariance with itself, that is, its variance. The variance of 1.03 means that individuals differ quite a bit in how much positive affect they experience on an average day. Taking the square root of the variance to create a standard deviation and assuming a relatively normal distribution leads to the conclusion that about two-thirds of the participants have an average positive affect between 3.02 and 5.06 and about one-third have an average positive affect outside that range. This variance is significant, meaning that these participants differ from each other more than would be expected from chance.

The variance listed in the UN(2,2) row indicates how much individuals differed from each other in the coefficient relating positive affect to extraversion. This variance is exciting because it indicates whether and to what extent different individuals are described by different psychological processes. In this case, the question is whether the psychological process that relates positive affect to extraversion is different for different people. Because this estimate is a variance, it is usually best to take its square root and turn it into the more interpretable *SD*, 0.19 in this case. Assuming a relatively normal distribution, approximately two-thirds of the participants have an association between extraversion and positive affect between 0.41 and 0.79. The significance test on this variance shows that this difference was not greater than expected by chance, and so this reduced dataset did not produce evidence that individuals differ in this process more than would be expected by chance (e.g., due to more than the particular occasions sampled). However, in the actual data (Fleeson et al., 2002) the *SD* was 0.14 and significant, *p* < 0.01, meaning that individuals differed from each other in the process relating positive affect to extraversion. Some individuals experience a very strong positive affect

boost at those times when they act extraverted, and some individuals experience only a moderate boost. These differences are not large, but because they are significant they reflect reliable aspects of these individuals' personalities. That is, it is possible to generalize from the particular occasions sampled for each individual to enduring differences between these individuals in their psychological processes regarding extraversion and positive affect.

Table 30.3 shows a way to report these results intended to maximize clarity, communication, and interpretation without cost to accuracy. The column for the typical individual shows the fixed effects that describe the process on average and whether the fixed effects differ significantly from zero. The column for the SD shows the random effects that describe how much individuals differed from each other and whether those differences are greater than expected from chance.

Complexities

In the interest of clarity, the preceding discussion described a relatively straightforward use of MLM. This section briefly extends MLM in ways that are more complex.

Using OLS Rather than MLM

It is possible to address almost the same hypotheses with the ordinary least squares (OLS) regression that most personality researchers use regularly and routinely. This would be accomplished by conducting a regression separately for each participant, predicting the outcome from the explanatory variable. Then, each participant's beta would be entered into a new data file. The average of these betas provides the average or typical individual's process coefficient (which can be tested against zero with a one-sample *t*-test). The *SD* across these coefficients indicates how much individuals differ from each other in the process. Using OLS in this method is familiar to researchers and provides an intuitive grasp of what MLM does. However, MLM has at least three advantages over OLS. First, MLM is more convenient, because the OLS procedure requires entering the betas from the regressions in a new data file. Second, MLM weights participants by the reliability of their coefficients, so more reliable data contribute more to the conclusion. OLS weights participants equally. Third and most important, MLM provides a significance test on the variability across participants' process coefficients. This is the key issue for personality psychologists, because it tests whether individual differences in the processes are greater than expected from chance and, rather, due to different psychological processes operating for different individuals (Fleeson, in press; Magnusson, 1999; Mischel & Shoda, 1995).

Predicting Individual Differences in the Process

A very exciting possibility of MLM is the opportunity to explain and predict individual differences in processes. Recall that MLM provides a coefficient describing the typical individual's process and a variance describing how much individuals differ from each other in that coefficient (in that process). A significant variance in the coefficient, establishing that individuals differ reliably in the process, is a very important first step because it suggests that the nature of personality includes individual differences in how processes operate. The next step is to explain why there are differences in those processes. One way to do this is to invoke other personality variables. For example, extraversion might predict the strength of the within-person process relating acting extraverted to happiness.

To test this kind of hypothesis, in which a personality variable is proposed to be related to individual differences in the process, the researcher adds the personality variable as a column in the dataset, with each participant's value on the personality variable repeated in each row for that participant. The personality variable should be centered across participants (this can be accomplished by subtracting the mean of the personality variable from the personality variable). This variable is called a person-level or level-2 variable because it does not vary within a person, only across persons. In the mixed models command, first add the personality variable as another covariate. Then, in the "fixed . . . " dialog, highlight both predictors, make sure "factorial" is selected, click "add," and run the analysis.

A significant interaction term in the "estimates of fixed effects" table means that the personality variable predicted individual differences in the process coefficient: A positive interaction means that individuals higher on the personality variable had a more positive re-

lationship between the explanatory variable and the outcome, whereas a negative interaction means that the individuals lower on the personality variable had a more positive relationship between the explanatory variable and the outcome. The estimate for the explanatory variable in the fixed effects table has a new interpretation in this type of analysis—it is now the effect of the explanatory variable for participants with a personality variable score of 0 (the mean if it was centered). Finally, the estimate for the personality variable is its effect on individuals' average levels of the outcome. The significance for the variance in the process coefficient indicates whether there is evidence for remaining individual differences in the process beyond the variance explained by the personality variable.

In following this procedure, Fleeson and colleagues (2002) found in fact that trait extraversion significantly predicted the coefficient relating acting extraverted to positive affect, but that the prediction was negative. That is, introverts experienced a larger positive affect boost when acting extraverted than did extraverts.

Additional Explanatory Variables

More than one explanatory variable can be tested simultaneously. This works similarly to adding additional explanatory variables in multiple regression. Add the additional variables to the covariates box, to the fixed effects box, and to the random effects box. To recreate a typical multiple regression, do not add them as factorials but only as main effects. The resulting coefficients can be interpreted as in a multiple regression, revealing the effect of each explanatory variable while controlling for the other explanatory variables. However, because MLM estimates variances and covariances among all coefficients and intercepts, these models become unstable with only a few variables. Caution is urged.

Causal Direction

Finally, it is possible to address causal direction between the explanatory variable and the outcome. This invokes a similar procedure to that used in between-persons analyses: The explanatory variable and the outcome at time 1 are used to predict the outcome at time 2. However, times 1 and 2 are usually successive occasions only hours apart. If there is a significant relationship between the explanatory variable and the time-2 outcome, this cannot be due to the outcome causing the explanatory variable, because the future cannot affect the past and because the explanatory variable was made independent of the earlier time-1 outcome in the model. However, two difficulties arise in using this method. First, because of the rapid variations in the explanatory variable and in the outcome, having the correct time lag between time 1 and time 2 is crucial and may be very difficult. For example, if the effect of the explanatory variable on the outcome is immediate and short-lived, a lag of a few hours between occasions may not pick up that effect. Second, studies of this sort typically have missing occasions. Missing occasions break the chain of lags between occasions, and so reduce power. Not only does this create missing data, the analysis will erroneously skip ahead to the next occasion to fill in the lag unless the researcher prepares the data ahead of time.

Future Directions

There are at least five future directions for this method. First, software improvements are continually improving the convenience of this analytic tool. What is needed most is software simultaneously integrated with other software so that data transformations are easy to do within the same program, and targeted at studying within-person processes (such as HLM) rather than written broadly to include all possible uses of mixed models (such as SPSS). Also needed are labels and instructions that are intuitively compelling to researchers familiar with regression and other common statistical techniques.

Second, it is critical to be able to include multiple predictors and their interactions in these models. Personality psychologists typically need to control many possible third variables and desire to test complex process models. Current packages become unstable quickly under such conditions. Future software and statistical advances should be directed at solving these problems.

Third, a high priority is to improve the reliability of or replace the significance test on the variances across individuals (i.e., determining whether individuals differ reliably in the direction, presence, or magnitude of the process). The standard errors as currently calculated may be inaccurate with low N's (although most experience sampling methods (ESM) studies may have sufficient N's). More work is needed to establish a universally accepted and accurate test of the significance of individual differences in the process (Raudenbush & Bryk, 2002).

Fourth, factor analyses may benefit from a similar treatment. Currently, factor analyses primarily are applied to all individuals equally. What would be valuable would be the ability to conduct factor analyses for each individual uniquely at the same time that the analyses are compared across individuals. This concept, called p-technique factor analysis by Cattell (1952), is currently possible but is also less convenient than it could be. P-technique is very promising for discovering factor structures that differ from individual to individual, and may possibly be integrated into the MLM framework. Personality psychology may make significant advances with p-technique if it could be more convenient to use.

A final future direction is for process to become normal personality research. The *Journal of Personality and Social Psychology* covers two personality topics: personality processes and individual differences. In the past, attention to individual differences has been predominant, but recently attention to process has grown. Understanding process is critical to explaining how personality works and to identifying the mechanisms underlying personality. In addition, detailing the steps in a process often locates opportunities, in the form of modifiable actions or events, for altering or improving processes to result in improved mental health. Both between-persons and within-person approaches are critical in the study of process. Recent developments in software and equipment make within-person approaches more accessible, adding them to the set of personality psychologists' techniques and thereby reducing the need for inferences from between-person designs to within-person processes. These recent developments in software and equipment, combined with texts to guide their use and interpretation, may make for a process revolution in personality psychology.

Acknowledgments

Preparation of this chapter was supported by National Institute of Mental Health Grant No. R01 MH70571. I would like to thank Mike Furr and Eric Stone for discussions about change, Sarah Ross and

Martin Lynch for comments on earlier drafts, and Faye Reece for assistance in preparing the manuscript.

Notes

1. Many important processes happen between individuals; those processes should be studied between individuals. The point being made here is that the processes that are theorized to occur within individuals are often studied by comparing between individuals rather than by comparing within individuals over time.
2. However, within-person approaches are vulnerable to a kind of reverse ecological fallacy, namely the inference that a process demonstrated to operate in the short term operates similarly in the long term. This inference is not always valid.

Recommended Readings

Aldwin, C. M., & Revenson, T. A. (1987). Does coping help? A reexamination of the relation between coping and mental health. *Journal of Personality and Social Psychology, 53,* 337–348.

Cronbach, L. J., & Furby, L. (1970). How should we measure change—Or "should" we? *Psychological Bulletin, 74,* 68–80.

Darlington, R. B. (1990). *Regression and linear models.* New York: McGraw-Hill.

Fleeson, W., Malanos, A., & Achille, N. (2002). An intra-individual process approach to the relationship between extraversion and positive affect: Is acting extraverted as "good" as being extraverted? *Journal of Personality and Social Psychology, 83,* 1409–1422.

Kreft, I., & de Leeuw, J. (1998). *Introducing multilevel modeling.* Thousand Oaks, CA: Sage.

Lamiell, J. T. (1997). Individuals and the differences between them. In R. Hogan, J. A. Johnson, & S. R. Briggs (Eds.), *Handbook of personality psychology* (pp. 117–141). San Diego, CA: Academic Press.

Singer, J. D., & Willett, J. B. (2002). *Applied longitudinal data analysis.* New York: Oxford University Press.

References

Aldwin, C. M., & Revenson, T. A. (1987). Does coping help? A reexamination of the relation between coping and mental health. *Journal of Personality and Social Psychology, 53,* 337–348.

Allport, G. W. (1937). *Personality: A psychological interpretation.* Oxford, UK: Holt.

Bolger, N., Davis, A., & Rafaeli, E. (2003). Diary methods: Capturing life as it is lived. *Annual Review of Psychology, 54,* 579–616.

Carver, C. S., & Scheier, M. F. (1994). Situational coping and coping dispositions in a stressful transaction. *Journal of Personality and Social Psychology, 66,* 184–195.

Cattell, R. B. (1952). The three basic factor-analytic research designs—their interrelations and derivatives. *Psychological Bulletin, 49,* 499–520.

Cattell, R. B. (1966). *Handbook of multivariate experimental psychology.* Chicago: Rand McNally.

Cervone, D. (2004). The architecture of personality. *Psychological Review, 111,* 183–204.

Cervone, D., & Mischel, W. (2002). Personality science. In D. Cervone & W. Mischel (Eds.), *Advances in personality science* (pp. 1–26). New York: Guilford Press.

Costa, P. T., Jr., & McCrae, R. R. (1980). Influence of extraversion and neuroticism on subjective well-being: Happy and unhappy people. *Journal of Personality and Social Psychology, 38,* 668–678.

Cronbach, L. J., & Furby, L. (1970). How should we measure change—Or "should" we? *Psychological Bulletin, 74,* 68–80.

Darlington, R. B. (1990). *Regression and linear models.* New York: McGraw-Hill.

Darlington, R. B., & Smulders, T. V. (2001). Problems with residual analysis. *Animal Behaviour, 62,* 599–602.

Depue, R. A., & Collins, P. F. (1999). Neurobiology of the structure of personality: Dopamine, facilitation of incentive motivation, and extraversion. *Behavioral and Brain Sciences, 22,* 491–569.

Epstein, S. (1983). A research paradigm for the study of personality and emotions. In R. Dienstbier (Series Ed.) & M. M. Page (Vol. Ed.), *Nebraska Symposium on Motivation: Vol. 30. Personality: Current theory and research* (pp. 91–154). Lincoln: University of Nebraska Press.

Fleeson, W. (2004). Moving personality beyond the person–situation debate: The challenge and the opportunity of within-person variability. *Current Directions, 13,* 83–87.

Fleeson, W. (2007). Using experience sampling and multilevel linear modeling to study person–situation interactionist approaches to positive psychology. In A. D. Ong & M. van Dulmen (Eds.), *Oxford handbook of methods in positive psychology* (pp. 501–514). New York: Oxford University Press.

Fleeson, W. (in press). Situation-based contingencies underlying trait-content manifestation in behavior. *Journal of Personality.*

Fleeson, W., Malanos, A., & Achille, N. (2002). An intra-individual process approach to the relationship between extraversion and positive affect: Is acting extraverted as "good" as being extraverted? *Journal of Personality and Social Psychology, 83,* 1409–1422.

Funder, D. C. (2001). Personality. *Annual Review of Psychology, 52,* 197–221.

Furr, R. M. (2005). *The analysis of change across two time points: A comparison of difference scores, residualized change scores, and multiple regression.* Winston-Salem, NC: Wake Forest University.

Kreft, I., & de Leeuw, J. (1998). *Introducing multilevel modeling.* Thousand Oaks, CA: Sage.

Lamiell, J. T. (1997). Individuals and the differences between them. In R. Hogan, J. A. Johnson, & S. R. Briggs (Eds.), *Handbook of personality psychology* (pp. 117–141). San Diego, CA: Academic Press.

Larsen, R. J. (1989). A process approach to personality psychology: Utilizing time as a facet of data. In D. M. Buss & N. Cantor (Eds.), *Personality psychology: Recent trends and emerging directions* (pp. 177–193). New York: Springer-Verlag.

Lazarus, R. S. (2000). Toward better research on stress and coping. *American Psychologiset, 55,* 665–673.

Lucas, R. E., & Baird, B. M. (2004). Extraversion and emotional reactivity. *Journal of Personality and Social Psychology, 86,* 473–485.

Magnusson, D. (1999). Holistic interactionism: A perspective for research on personality development. In L. A. Pervin & O. P. John (Eds.), *Handbook of personality: Theory and research* (2nd ed., pp. 219–248). New York: Guilford Press.

Marco, C. A., Neale, J. M., Schwartz, J. E., Shiffman, S., & Stone, A. A. (1999). Coping with daily events and short-term mood changes: An unexpected failure to observe effects of coping. *Journal of Consulting and Clinical Psychology, 67,* 755–764.

McCrae, R. R., & Costa, P. T., Jr. (1999). A five-factor theory of personality. In O. P. John & L. A. Pervin (Eds.), *Handbook of personality: Theory and research.* (2nd ed., pp. 139–153). New York: Guilford Press.

McNiel, J. M., & Fleeson, W. (2006). The causal effects of extraversion on positive affect and neuroticism on negative affect: Manipulating state extraversion and state neuroticism in an experimental approach. *Journal of Research in Personality, 40,* 529–550.

Mischel, W. (2004). Toward an integrative science of the person. *Annual Review of Psychology, 55,* 1–22.

Mischel, W., & Shoda, Y. (1995). A cognitive-affective system theory of personality: Reconceptualizing situations, dispositions, dynamics, and invariance in personality structure. *Psychological Review, 102,* 246–268.

Mroczek, D. K., & Almeida, D. M. (2004). The effects of daily stress, personality, and age on daily negative affect. *Journal of Personality, 72,* 355–378.

Nesselroade, J. R. (1991). Interindividual differences in intraindividual change. In L. M. Collins & J. L. Horn (Eds.), *Best methods for the analysis of change* (pp. 92–105). Washington, DC: American Psychological Association.

Pervin, L. A. (1994). A critical analysis of current trait theory. *Psychological Inquiry, 4,* 122–130.

Puetz, T. W., O'Connor, P. J., & Dishman, R. K. (2006). Effects of chronic exercise on feelings of energy and fatigue: A quantitative synthesis. *Psychological Bulletin, 132,* 866–876.

Raudenbush, S. W., & Bryk, A. S. (2002). *Hierarchical linear models: Applications and data analysis methods* (2nd ed., Vol. 1). Thousand Oaks, CA: Sage.

Raudenbush, S. W., Bryk, A. S., & Congdon, R. (2004). Hierarchical linear and non-linear modeling (Version 6.0) [Computer software]. Lincolnwood, IL: Scientific Software International.

Robinson, W. S. (1950). Ecological correlations and the behavior of individuals. *American Sociological Review, 15,* 351–357.

Rogosa, D. (1995). Myths and methods: "Myths about longitudinal research" plus supplemental questions. In J. M. Gottman (Ed.), *The analysis of change* (pp. 3–66). Mahwah, NJ: LEA.

Rusting, C. L., & Larsen, R. J. (1998). Personality and cognitive processing of affective information. *Personality and Social Psychology Bulletin, 24,* 200–213.

Singer, J. D., & Willett, J. B. (2002). *Applied longitudinal data analysis.* New York: Oxford University Press.

Sroufe, L. A., Egeland, B., Carlson, E. A., & Collins, W. A. (2005). *The development of the person: The Minnesota Study of Risk and Adaptation from Birth to Adulthood.* New York: Guilford Press.

Staudinger, U. M., Fleeson, W., & Baltes, P. B. (1999). Predictors of subjective physical health and global well-being: Similarities and differences between the United States and Germany. *Journal of Personality and Social Psychology, 76,* 305–319.

Tennan, H., Affleck, G., Armeli, S., & Carney, M. A. (2000). A daily process approach to coping: Linking theory, research, and practice. *American Psychologist, 55,* 626–636.

Vansteelandt, K., & Van Mechelen, I. V. (2004). The personality triad in balance: Multidimensional individual differences in situation–behavior profiles. *Journal of Research in Personality, 38,* 367–393.

APPENDIX 30.1. SAMPLE DATA

ID	Extra	Positive Affect	ID	Extra	Positive Affect	ID	Extra	Positive Affect
1.00	2.00	3.25	18.00	3.25	5.50	31.00	5.00	5.50
1.00	3.50	3.25	18.00	3.25	4.50	31.00	4.75	4.75
1.00	2.00	2.25	18.00	2.75	4.75	33.00	4.50	4.50
1.00	3.25	3.00	18.00	4.00	5.75	33.00	3.00	2.75
1.00	2.50	2.50	18.00	3.25	5.50	33.00	5.50	5.25
1.00	2.00	2.25	18.00	3.50	4.75	33.00	2.50	2.00
1.00	3.50	3.25	18.00	2.75	5.00	33.00	4.00	1.25
1.00	3.50	3.25	22.00	5.25	6.75	33.00	5.00	6.50
2.00	4.50	5.25	22.00	4.75	6.50	33.00	5.00	3.00
2.00	2.00	2.50	22.00	5.50	6.50	33.00	3.25	2.50
2.00	3.50	4.50	22.00	5.50	7.00	33.00	4.25	3.00
2.00	3.75	4.00	22.00	5.00	5.75	33.00	5.50	4.50
2.00	2.50	2.75	22.00	4.50	6.00	35.00	4.75	4.25
2.00	2.00	1.75	22.00	4.75	6.75	35.00	4.75	4.25
2.00	4.25	3.25	22.00	4.75	6.50	35.00	4.00	4.25
2.00	4.75	4.50	22.00	6.00	6.50	35.00	5.25	4.25
2.00	4.50	4.50	22.00	4.50	5.00	35.00	5.00	4.25
2.00	5.75	5.00	22.00	3.75	5.75	35.00	7.00	6.25
2.00	2.75	3.50	22.00	6.25	6.50	35.00	6.75	5.75
2.00	3.00	2.00	26.00	3.00	2.25	35.00	7.00	5.50
2.00	2.00	2.50	26.00	3.00	3.50	35.00	6.00	3.25
2.00	5.75	5.75	26.00	2.25	3.25	35.00	5.50	5.00
2.00	4.25	2.75	26.00	4.75	3.50	35.00	6.00	5.00
2.00	2.25	2.25	26.00	5.00	3.50	35.00	6.00	4.25
2.00	4.50	5.50	26.00	4.00	2.50	35.00	5.50	5.25
9.00	2.75	3.75	26.00	1.25	1.25	35.00	5.00	5.50
9.00	5.75	3.00	26.00	2.75	2.75	35.00	5.25	5.33
9.00	5.00	5.75	26.00	1.50	1.25	35.00	6.00	5.25
9.00	4.50	4.75	26.00	2.00	1.75	35.00	5.25	3.00
9.00	4.00	4.50	26.00	3.00	1.75	35.00	5.50	2.75
9.00	3.25	3.00	26.00	2.50	3.00	37.00	3.00	3.25
9.00	4.25	2.50	26.00	2.75	3.00	37.00	3.75	4.00
9.00	3.50	3.25	26.00	4.50	4.50	37.00	3.25	3.50
9.00	3.00	3.50	26.00	3.00	2.50	37.00	2.75	3.00
9.00	1.75	4.50	26.00	2.00	4.50	37.00	2.33	2.50
9.00	3.00	2.50	26.00	2.50	4.25	37.00	3.00	3.50
9.00	3.50	3.75	26.00	4.00	5.00	37.00	4.00	4.00
18.00	3.25	4.50	26.00	3.25	2.75	37.00	2.50	2.50
18.00	2.75	4.75	26.00	1.25	1.00	37.00	3.00	2.75
18.00	3.75	5.50	31.00	6.00	4.00	37.00	3.50	3.00
18.00	2.75	3.75	31.00	3.00	3.25	37.00	2.75	3.50
18.00	3.00	4.00	31.00	5.00	4.75	37.00	3.50	2.75
18.00	6.00	5.50	31.00	1.00	1.75	37.00	3.25	3.50
18.00	4.50	4.50	31.00	5.50	4.75	37.00	3.75	4.00
18.00	3.00	4.50	31.00	5.75	5.00	37.00	4.00	4.75
			31.00	5.75	5.75	37.00	4.00	4.00
			31.00	4.75	5.00	37.00	4.00	4.50

## CHAPTER 31

The Analysis of Longitudinal Data in Personality Research

Daniel K. Mroczek

Longitudinal studies are fundamental to research on personality. Whether a particular aspect of personality is hypothesized to change over time or remain stable, it is longitudinal data that verify the answer. There is no substitute for longitudinal information in answering these questions; it is the gold standard when it comes to understanding consistency and change. However, researchers who use longitudinal data often meet with difficulty with respect to analyzing these sometimes complicated data. Longitudinal data analysis can be tricky. This chapter gives a broad overview of the most common types of data analysis that are used in longitudinal research on personality. It starts with some basic and more traditional ways of analyzing longitudinal data and then moves to more complex techniques. The analytic tools presented here are by no means exhaustive of the available techniques, but the reader is assured that these are the ones he or she will most likely encounter when reading the literature (see Table 31.1).

Traditional Data-Analytic Techniques for Longitudinal Data

After obtaining longitudinal data, the first step should be to apply some of the older and more traditional analytic techniques. First among these should be the repeated-measures analysis of variance (ANOVA) and the stability coefficient. These will establish whether there is any change in the overall sample means or in the relative positioning of individuals in the distribution over time, respectively. Much of the important early work on personality stability and change used one or both of these statistical techniques (Conley, 1984, 1985; Costa & Mc-

TABLE 31.1. Common Techniques Used to Describe and Analyze Longitudinal Personality Data

Technique	What it yields	When to use
Repeated-measures ANOVA	Can discern mean differences between measurement occasions.	When the research question focuses on sample (or group-level) change or stability in absolute level of variable.
Stability coefficients	Tells the extent to which two measurements of the same variable are correlated; is the Pearson r among any two measurement occasions.	When the research question focuses on relative or rank-order stability among people in a sample.
Trajectory or growth-curve models: MLM-based	Trajectories of stability/change, both overall (sample-level) and individual differences in trajectories; uses all occasions of measurement in a single model.	When the focus is on both sample-level stability/change and individual differences in stability/change. Also, when there are considerable individual differences in the spacing of measurement occasions.
Trajectory or growth-curve models: SEM-based	Same as above; can also model error via a measurement model.	Same as above, but has greater difficulty in estimation when there are considerable individual differences in the spacing of measurement occasions.

Crae, 1988; Finn, 1986), and much of it has now been synthesized via meta-analysis (Roberts & DelVecchio, 2000).

Repeated-Measures ANOVA

The repeated-measures ANOVA is useful for determining whether there are any significant changes between means for as many measurement occasions that have been obtained. For example, if you have obtained four measurement occasions, you can use the repeated-measures ANOVA to test whether the overall trend deviates significantly from a flat line (indicating stability), and if so, which of the four means differ from one another. Covariates can be added to the model (analysis of covariance, or ANCOVA) to determine whether the overall trend or any pairwise mean difference is influenced by the presence of the covariate. Suppose the following example: A researcher found an overall increase in impulse control over five measurement occasions in a sample of early adolescents. However, when controlling for gender, the effect went away. Breaking out the trend lines for girls and boys revealed that girls accounted for the entire effect, as the boys (on average) did not show an increase in impulse control whereas girls (again, on average) showed a large increase.

This fictional example illustrates the kind of useful analyses that repeated-measures ANOVA makes possible. However, there are some major drawbacks to this venerable old technique. The repeated-measures ANOVA has some very restrictive assumptions. First, it requires that the elapsed time periods between measurements are of equal length (e.g., 6 months between each measurement occasion and the next). Second, it requires that the N is the same at all occasions, meaning that if anyone misses an occasion, all of his or her data must be thrown out of the analysis. Finally, it assumes homogeneity of variance across all occasions. Rarely are these three assumptions met in longitudinal research. The reality of conducting longitudinal studies dictates that the researcher will not be able to measure everyone at every occasion and that often the measurements cannot be equally spaced. The schedules of participants and investigators, along with the uncertainties of research funding, make equal spacing between occasions difficult to obtain in practice unless the investigation is a very short-term longitudinal study (e.g., weeks or months). However, most questions regarding personality stability and change cannot be answered by studies as short as weeks or months. In the long-term, multiyear studies employed by many personality researchers, the assumptions of the repeated-measures ANOVA are likely to be violated. This is a serious downside to the technique.

Stability Coefficients

A stability coefficient is nothing more than the Pearson product–moment correlation between two measurements of the same variable (at two different points in time) on the same people. The magnitude of the coefficient reveals the extent of stability in rank ordering of the people in the distribution. If everyone retains the same ranking within the distribution, even if everyone has increased or decreased by the same amount (e.g., mean change), then the stability coefficient would be 1.00. Stability coefficients in excess of .60 have traditionally been interpreted as indicating a high degree of continuity (Costa & McCrae, 1988). Many personality variables have shown stabilities of more than .70 or .80 over periods of 1–5 years (Costa & McCrae, 1994). Over longer periods of time (6–10 years), the coefficients tend to be somewhat smaller, but typically still in excess of .50. This indicates a substantial degree of stability in personality.

However, stability coefficients have a number of drawbacks as well. The calculation of stabilities requires deletion of cases that lack measurements on any pair of measurement occasions. Indeed, most software packages will automatically do such pairwise deletions when running the coefficients. Thus, a researcher possessing five measurement occasions on some personality variable will have a total of 10 unique stability coefficients (between times 1 and 2, times 1 and 3, times 1 and 4, etc.). However, if there are some missing observations at each measurement occasion, the N's will jump around as the software applies pairwise deletion to the calculation of each coefficient. Occasionally, one sees researchers engaging in listwise deletion to even the N for each correlation, but that can often lead to an unnecessarily low N and biased coefficients.

However, the most serious drawback of stability coefficients is the inability to combine multiple measurements. A researcher can consider only two pairs of measurements at a time. This is quite limiting if one has four or five measurement occasions and is interested in using all of that information to determine the amount of stability or change over time with respect to rank ordering of individuals. That

stability coefficients can yield a single, aggregate number that sums up how stable a variable is over time is a very positive aspect of this statistic. Yet, it is a double-edged sword, because that simplicity and parsimony comes at the cost of not being able to use all information. In fact, the aggregate nature of stability coefficients and repeated-measures means is a key limitation, which is discussed next.

Limitations of Traditional Techniques

Means and correlations are useful because they aggregate information. The mean describes the arithmetic center of a distribution. The stability coefficient describes the degree of relatedness between two distributions of measurements. As useful as this information is, it hides the variability in the distributions. It is this variability among people within a distribution that is one of the main foci of personality psychology. Aggregate statistics such as means and correlations obscure the individual differences inherent in any distribution. In contrast, means and correlations tell us whether a personality variable increases or decreases over time, or whether people maintain the same rank order over time, *in a sample or population.* Repeated-measures means and correlations, valuable as they are, conceal the individual differences in personality stability (Aldwin, Spiro, Levenson, & Bossé, 1989; Lamiell, 1981). Some individuals may be stable, and others changing, but this is hidden by the aggregate nature of means and correlations.

There is actually great irony with respect to this issue. The techniques typically employed to estimate rank-order and mean-level stability in personality variables conceal important information on individual differences. Yet personality psychology is the science of individual differences in psychological characteristics. The phenomenon of individual differences in the rate of change of personality variables has until recently been largely overlooked. However, developmentalists interested in personality discussed this issue almost 30 years ago. Lifespan developmentalists have long advocated the idea of *individual differences in intraindividual change* (Baltes, Reese, & Nesselroade, 1977). Depending on the variable, some people can potentially go up, while others go down or remain stable. Indeed, some variables may be expected to show the same pattern of change (or no change) for all or almost all people. However, for many variables, one should observe variability in rates of change. For example, not everyone gains impulse control at the same rate as childhood gives way to adolescence and young adulthood. Owing to variability in genes, socializing environments, and their interactions, different people should show different rates of change in the development of impulse control, as well as host of other personality characteristics. These kinds of changes are important for understanding personality and its development, yet traditional repeated-measures ANOVAs and stability coefficients are too crude to provide sufficient answers.

The concept of individual differences in intraindividual change remained a largely theoretical notion for much of the late 1970s and 1980s because the statistical models that would permit adequate testing of the concept did not reach maturity until the early 1990s (Bryk & Raudenbush, 1992; Rogosa, Brandt, & Zimowski, 1982). Once these techniques became widely available, more complex and accurate ways of conceptualizing stability and change in personality were within the grasp of researchers. In the next section, these models are described and their potential for advancing the science of personality is discussed.

Analyzing Multiple-Occasion Studies

Why are multiple measurement occasions (more than two) required for the adequate estimation of change in a personality variable, or any other variable for that matter? A bit of history helps in understanding this complex issue. For many years prior to the 1970s, most studies of change used a two-occasion design in which the differences were calculated between two measurements of the same variable over time. These differences were called *change scores*, sometimes called *gain scores*, and were usually treated as outcome variables in statistical analyses. However, in 1970, Cronbach and Furby published an influential article in the *Psychological Bulletin* that severely criticized the use of change scores (Cronbach & Furby, 1970). This article, along with other commentary since then, made clear that two measurement occasions are suboptimal for estimating change—in particular, prohibiting the accurate

estimation of rate of change, or slope (Cronbach & Furby, 1970; Raudenbush & Bryk, 2002; Rogosa et al., 1982; Singer & Willett, 2003). In later articles, Rogosa and others (e.g., McArdle, 1991) showed that three measurements is really the minimum for any accurate estimate of change. Three measurement occasions permit the calculation of residuals between a person's actual observations and the line or curve that best fits his or her set of measurements (hence, the term *growth curve*). If only two occasions are present, the trajectory is simply the line that connects the two points. No residual can be calculated.

This lack of information is one of the main reasons why two occasions is considered inadequate for estimating change (Rogosa et al., 1982). In fact, the more measurement occasions obtained, the more accurate the estimate of the trajectory over time. This concept is not unlike that of traditional reliability in psychometrics. A one-item measure of some concept, say, IQ or extraversion, is typically considered inadequate. A researcher cannot even calculate coefficient alpha on a single item. Two items is marginally better; three, better yet. Four, five, or ten is even better. However, there does come a point of diminishing returns. The same is true of growth curves (Singer & Willett, 2003). The more measurement occasions obtained, the better and more accurate the estimate of change in whatever variable a researcher is tracking. Yet, monthly measurements for 10 years is probably overkill. The bottom line is that at least three measurement occasions is the starting point for any estimate of growth curves, although for estimation of curvilinear models (e.g., quadratic, cubic) more waves are required. So, before applying a growth model, the researcher must first obtain longitudinal data with at least three measurement occasions.

Two Approaches to Growth-Curve Modeling: Multilevel and Structural Equation Modeling

Most of the techniques for modeling change over time can be divided into those that are grounded in a structural equation modeling (SEM) framework (McArdle, 1991; Meredith & Tisak, 1990; Muthén, 2002) or a multilevel modeling (MLM) approach (Raudenbush & Bryk, 2002; Rogosa et al., 1982; Singer &

Willett, 2003; von Eye & Nesselroade, 1992). The former is often called *latent growth-curve* modeling, whereas the latter unfortunately has many names, promoting confusion in the literature. Other names for MLM include random coefficient modeling, random effect modeling, generalized estimating equations, mixed modeling, and hierarchical linear modeling (Raudenbush & Bryk, 2002; Singer & Willett, 2003).

Several recent efforts have built bridges between the SEM and MLM approaches for estimating change (Curran, 2003; Mehta & Neale, 2005; Muthén, 2002; Raudenbush & Sampson, 1999; Rovine & Molenaar, 2000). These newer efforts build on some notable attempts from the moderately distant past (Goldstein & McDonald, 1987; McDonald, 1993; Muthén & Satorra, 1995). No study of personality change has used these techniques yet, mainly because they have yet to move fully out of the technical literature. However, many longitudinal personality studies have employed either one or the other of the SEM and MLM approaches. Some good examples of studies that have examined personality stability and change via SEM techniques are Small, Hertzog, Hultsch, and Dixon (2003) and Jones and Meredith (1996). However, most of the studies that have estimated growth curves of personality have employed MLM techniques. These include Helson, Jones, and Kwan (2002), Jones, Livson, and Peskin (2003), Mroczek and Spiro (2003a), Mroczek and Spiro (2005), Roberts and Chapman (2000), and Srivastava, John, Gosling, and Potter (2003). Therefore, the description of MLM approaches is more extensive in this chapter than the description of SEM approaches. I first compare the MLM and SEM techniques for estimating change using multiple measurement occasions.

MLM modeling techniques for estimating change are often called individual growth models. This is because the parameters that define trajectories (intercepts, slopes, curvatures, etc.) are estimated at the level of the individual, in contrast to specifying and modeling latent constructs for these parameters. In SEM, these latent constructs for intercept, slope, and other data are usually estimated from sample-based variances and covariances, but not always (see Mehta & Neale, 2005). As noted above, SEM estimations of change are usually called latent growth curve (LGC) models. The greatest advantage of SEM over MLM approaches is that the former permits measurement models, allowing better estimation of error structures. Another advantage of SEM-based approaches is that mediation can be examined more directly via path models. Looking at the other side of the coin, the advantage of MLM over SEM is flexibility in handling missing data and unequal spacing between measurement occasions. In many longitudinal studies, the intervals between measurements are often unequal across participants, either by circumstance or by design, creating spaces between measurement occasions that are of varying lengths. MLM approaches have no problem with such data structures (Singer & Willett, 2003). However, several researchers have been working to solve the interval spacing issue in the SEM framework, with increasing success (Curran, 2003; McDonald, 1993; Mehta & Neale, 2005; Muthén, 2002; Rovine & Molenaar, 2000).

Yet many investigators still find the MLM approach to growth curves more intuitively appealing than the SEM approach. It is easier for many researchers to imagine a trajectory or growth curve for each individual in their samples (and an overall trajectory that is a weighted average of the N individual trajectories) than to conceive of change as defined by a latent intercept and a slope that resides at the sample level. Because stability and change in a variable occurs at the level of the individual, it is simply more conceptually appealing for many to think of change within an MLM framework as opposed to an SEM framework.

A researcher should weigh the relative importance of flexibility in handling missing data versus superior estimation of measurement error in making a decision about whether to use MLM- or SEM-based approaches to growth curves. However, the constraints of the available data may force this decision on the researcher.

Growth Curves in an SEM Framework

As noted earlier, most of the examinations of personality change using growth-curve approaches have used the MLM framework; this approach is discussed in detail below. However, it is worth spending at least some time on the SEM approach to growth curves. As in any structural equation model, the latent growth model begins with the specification of a structural model (in contrast to the measurement model). In particular, a latent intercept and a latent slope are specified. That is, the latent trajectory of the observed scores over time is described by the level of the variable (intercept) and the rate of change (slope). The latent intercept and slope, along with the errors on each measurement occasion, are specified to account for the data. If the slope is anything other than zero, this indicates latent change in the variable over time. Curvilinearity can be modeled in the same way, by specifying a latent curvature variable. The model should also be assessed for fit, using some of the standard fit indices for SEM such as the Goodness of Fit Index (GFI, Adjusted Goodness of Fit Index [AGFI]; Bentler & Bonett, 1980) or Akaike's information criterion (AIC; Akaike, 1974). Fit indices give a sense of how well data fit the specified model, relative to some null model or a simpler model. In addition, in the latent growth model, the standard deviations around the latent intercept and slope variables can be estimated, giving the researcher an idea of the extent of the individual differences surrounding the overall latent trajectory, or growth curve. This is the SEM counterpart to the random effects in MLM (see below).

As addressed above, the major advantage of using SEM to model change is its superior ability to model error via the measurement model. However, many investigators do not like the indirectness of specifying latent variables to estimate change. It is a top-down approach, in a sense in which overarching, higher-order latent constructs account for individual-level trajectories. Many find this approach counterintuitive and prefer a more bottom-up approach in which trajectories are estimated for each person. In such a model, the many individual trajectories are used to estimate the overall trajectory. The end result is largely the same (an estimate of an overall growth curve as well as the variability around it), but the approach starts with the individual as opposed to the group or sample. This idea forms the basis of the other major technique for estimating growth curves, the MLM approach.

Growth Curves in an MLM Framework

One of the key differences between the MLM and SEM approaches to growth curves is the way data are set up prior to analysis. When using the MLM approach, the longitudinal measurements for each person must be arranged

in "person-time" (alternatively, a "person-period" file; Singer & Willett, 2003; see also Mroczek, Spiro, Almeida & Pafford, 2006). This requires nesting measurements within persons. Each measurement occasion for a person must be placed on a separate row in the data matrix, with the participant ID serving to identify the multiple observations for a single individual during the analysis. This is sometimes called a "stacked" data structure. It means that each person in a study has his or her own data matrix that, in turn, is nested within the larger data matrix. In this type of data arrangement, participants can vary not only with respect to length of measurement interval, but also with regard to number of measurements. Some people may have three measurements, others four, others five or more, and some individuals may have only one or two. Incidentally, this is not a problem if data are missing at random (for more information on missingness, see Little & Rubin, 1987). This reflects the reality of longitudinal studies, in which participants are often not available at the desired times of measurement or drop out during the follow-up period. This kind of variability in spacing of measurements, common in long-term studies, present no data-analytic problem for growth curves estimated in a MLM modeling framework. However, it violates key assumptions in the repeated-measures ANOVA model; it also poses some difficulties for latent growth models estimated via SEM.

Fixed Effects

Any estimation of growth curves or trajectories using the MLM approach yields fixed and random effects. *Fixed effects* refers to the coefficients that characterize the overall trajectory of the variable of interest over time. In contrast, *random effects* refers to parameters that describe the variability around the fixed effects (i.e., interindividual differences). These random effects are discussed below (see also Mroczek et al., 2006). In a simple linear growth-curve model, where there is no quadratic term to describe curvature, there are two fixed effects, an intercept and a slope. In a quadratic model that includes an estimate of curvature, there obviously would be three fixed effect coefficients: an intercept, a slope, and a curvature term.

The intercept is the average amount of outcome (e.g., extraversion, conscientiousness) where the temporal metameter (time, age, etc.) equals zero. If the temporal metameter is years passed since an event (e.g., birth, baseline assessment, intervention), then the intercept defines the leftmost point of the trajectory. It is where the growth curve or trajectory passes through the y-axis. However, if age is the temporal metameter, then the intercept is the amount of that personality dimension when age equals zero, and it obviously makes little sense to think of a newborn having developed a psychological construct such as extraversion or conscientiousness.

Therefore, it is often desirable to recenter the temporal variable in order to place the zero point at a more conceptually meaningful spot (Biesanz, Debb-Sossa, Papadukis, Bollen, & Curran, 2004; Mroczek et al., 2006). This could be the mean entry age of people in a longitudinal study, the mean overall age across all time points, or even the mean age at study exit. The temporal metameter could also be person-centered, in which each participant's personality measurements over time are centered at a value specific to each person, for example, his or her mean age across all occasions. In such a model, change in personality is interpreted as change from the person's own average. It represents the amount that the person varies from him- or herself over time. In contrast, re-centering age around the grand mean for all people in the study has the effect of placing the intercept in the middle of the entire age distribution. As a result, the intercept is the predicted amount of the personality dimension at a fixed age. Grand-mean and person-mean centering are the most common recentering techniques in growth modeling, and each has its advantages and disadvantages. Regardless of the choice a researcher makes, recentering should have the effect of improving interpretation of the intercept or average level (Biesanz et al., 2004).

The fixed effect for slope represents the amount of change in the personality dimension of interest per unit of time. For example, if time is clocked in years, then the slope represents amount of personality change per year. The fixed effect for slope quantifies rate of change. In a linear model, the intercept and slope together define the overall trajectory (in the quadratic model, there would also be a curvature term). The fixed effects for intercept and slope tell the investigator whether a personality variable increases, decreases, or remains stable over the study time period. The slope also tells the researcher the rate of change. It indicates how quickly or slowly a variable increases or decreases. The fixed effects for intercept and slope, however, define only the overall, sample-level trajectory. Yet MLM models yield more than this. They also estimate the individual differences around the intercept and slope. These are the random effects, which is why some statisticians label these techniques "random coefficient models."

Random Effects

Random effects estimate individual variability around a growth parameter (such as the intercept or slope). The random effect for the intercept is the estimate of variance around the intercept parameter. It simply captures individual differences in the level of the personality variable that is examined. This is usually not very interesting because, at least in the case of personality dimensions, we typically know that they differ significantly across people. Most of the time, the researcher finds the random effect for slope much more interesting and informative. This is because it tells us whether the rate of change varies by person.

As an example, imagine change in neuroticism over a 20-year period. Some people may have trajectories that rise or fall steeply; these individuals demonstrate large slopes. Others display less steep slopes. Still others may show no change and show flat (zero) slopes over time. A slope of zero implies stability (Mroczek & Griffin, 2007; Mroczek & Spiro, 2003a, 2003b). What this illustrates is a range of slopes—some large, some small, some zero, some positive, and some negative.

Such individual differences in rate of change are not only empirically important in many areas of personality research, they are also theoretically important. For example, the existence of considerable individual differences in change, whether it be in cognitive, social, or personality variables, gives support to the theoretical lifespan principle of interindividual differences in intraindividual change (Baltes et al., 1977). In other areas, if individual differences in rate of change are found when none were expected, this can alter theory in such areas. It would imply that many people do not change in the way the theory predicts. The theory would need to take into account these individual differences. The reverse can happen as well.

If individual differences in rate of change in a variable are expected but not found, then this would tell researchers and theorists that there is more uniformity in change than was previously thought.

Estimating Growth-Curve Models in Personality: Level-1 Models

The first step in estimating a growth trajectory for a personality variable is to establish a baseline. Thus, the initial model that should be estimated in any analysis of change is an *unconditional means model* (Singer & Willett, 2003). This baseline model goes by a couple of other names, such as the *intercept-only model* (Raudenbush & Bryk, 2002) or the *empty model*. This model fits only an overall mean, as well as a variance around that mean across all persons and measurement occasions. The temporal metameter, or time variable, is not included in the equation at this step (Singer & Willett, 2003). Interpreting the fixed and random effects in the unconditional means model is fairly straightforward. Only one fixed effect is yielded from this model, and it represents simply the grand mean across all measurements. One random effect is estimated as well. This is the variance around the grand mean. This captures the between-persons differences in intercept, or the individual differences in level of the personality variable of interest, irrespective of measurement occasion. The remaining variability is the within-person variance, plus error (this is sometimes labeled the residual). These estimates of between-persons and within-person variances are useful in that the former tells how much of the variability is due to between-persons differences, and the latter represents how much people vary from themselves. Most important, the unconditional means model also provides a benchmark that the researcher can use to evaluate successive models—for example, by comparing a measure of model fit such as the log likelihood or the Akaike information criterion (Raudenbush & Bryk, 2002).

Next, the researcher adds the time variable (the temporal metameter). In the *linear growth model* where the temporal metameter is age, a formal definition of the model using the personality trait neuroticism can be expressed as

$$\text{Neuroticism}_{ij} = \pi_{0i} + \pi_{1i}(\text{age}_{ij}) + \epsilon_{ij} \quad (1)$$

The amount of neuroticism for individual *i* at measurement occasion *j* is a function of the person's age at that measurement occasion (age_{ij}). The intercept, π_{0i}, is the predicted amount of neuroticism where age = 0 (or, if recentered, at some non-zero age). The linear coefficient, π_{1i}, is the rate of change (slope); it is the predicted annual amount of change in neuroticism for person *i*. ϵ_{ij} represents the errors on each person *i* at occasion *j*. In a sample, each participant's trajectory is described by this equation. Together, these intercepts and slopes define the overall, sample-level intercept and slope. In other words, these are the fixed effects. The variability in intercepts and slopes across *i* persons are the random effects.

A linear growth model may prove adequate for characterizing change in some personality variables, but it is possible that a more complex model is needed for others. By adding a squared function of our temporal variable to the linear growth model, we create the *quadratic growth model*, which is capable of estimating curvilinearity. More formally, and using the personality characteristic self-efficacy, the quadratic model can be expressed as

$$\text{Self-efficacy}_{ij} = \pi_{0i} + \pi_{1i}(\text{age}_{ij}) + \pi_{2i}(\text{age}^2_{ij}) + \epsilon_{ij}(2)$$

The addition of the quadratic coefficient, $?_{2i}$, estimates amount of curvature for person *i*. Note that three parameters are estimated in the quadratic model: intercept, slope, and curvature. Because an extra term is estimated in the quadratic growth model, it is generally recommended that four or more measurement occasions be used (Mroczek et al., 2006; Raudenbush & Bryk, 2002; Singer & Willett, 2003). This is larger than the usual minimum of three. Now, a researcher can fit an MLM model with at least two or three observations on some subjects, as long as a large portion of the subjects have four or more occasions to permit estimation of the level-1 model. Similarly, if cubic functions of time are estimated, to test for a second bend in the curve, at least five measurement occasions on most participants are required. In any case, the usual progression in growth-curve modeling is to test simpler models first and then gradually move toward more complex models, if higher-order models are conceptually justified (Mroczek et al., 2006; Singer & Willett, 2003). An unconditional means model should be estimated first, then a linear growth model, then a quadratic growth model, and if theoretically or conceptually justified, only then cubic or higher models. As argued elsewhere (Mroczek & Griffin, 2007) in the behavioral sciences, complex phenomena such as cubic growth are rare, and it is rarer still to find theories that predict such phenomena.

Explaining Individual Differences in Growth Curves: Level-2 Models

The growth-curve models (both linear and quadratic) described above are level-1 models in the parlance of multilevel modeling (Raudenbush & Bryk, 2002). In the framework of MLM they reside at the first level. They describe the within-person temporal pattern of a personality characteristic or some other type of variable, along with certain between-persons parameters. Typically, if the slope or curvature variance (random effects) is significant at level 1, the investigator has license to proceed to estimation of level-2 models. At level 2, the investigator introduces predictors or other explanatory variables that may account for the observed individual differences in personality change. In doing so, the investigator can potentially answer important conceptual questions in personality development or personality psychology in general. Significance predictors can hint at or even establish why some people change on a given personality dimension while others remain stable.

The use of level-2 models is illustrated in a recent study that applied individual growth models to personality trait data (Mroczek & Spiro, 2003a). Death of spouse was used to predict change in neuroticism over a 12-year period in older adults. The level-1 model determined that there was statistically significant variability among persons in neuroticism slopes over 12 years. At level 2, death of spouse was introduced into the model as a between-persons variable. In a sample of older men, some had experienced the death of a spouse within the 2 years prior to the 12-year longitudinal period, and others had not. This dichotomous variable significantly predicted both intercept and slope of neuroticism. People whose spouses had died started out higher on neuroticism than those who had not endured this tragic life experience, but then displayed slopes that went down at a faster rate over the next 12

years. In other words, neuroticism was temporarily elevated immediately after the death of a person's spouse, but then reverted in the years following. The between-persons variable "death of spouse" accounted for some, but not all, of the individual variability in neuroticism slopes over a 12-year period. This finding indicates that rates of change in traits can be modified, depending on life circumstances. It also speaks to the possibility that certain traits, like neuroticism, may have components that are sensitive to context, in addition to the genetic sources of variance that are stable over time. In this sense, level-2 growth-curve models allow us to more fully understand the ways in which personality dimensions develop over time.

Shorter-Term Change in Personality: Process Approaches and Experience Sampling Designs

With respect to personality traits, growth-curve models are most fruitfully used when long-term data (over years) are available. Traits do change for some people, but such change is usually observable only over long periods of time. Traits do not change quickly, so studies need to stretch many years to permit observable changes.

However, other nontrait types of personality variables may change over shorter periods. Many of the nontrait areas of personality hypothesize changes that occur over weeks, days, or even within a single day. The "process" approach to personality focuses on these shorter durations (Fleeson, 2001, 2004). Although process approaches hypothesize change, it is not change in the sense of trajectories declining over periods of years. The type of change assessed in the process approach is dynamic action. This is, in part, a remnant of the process approach's lineage in classic behaviorism, with its emphasis the unfolding of behavior over short periods of time (e.g., studies of learning curves and reinforcement schedules). Daily diary and experience sampling studies, hallmarks of the process approach, similarly seek to determine the characteristic ways in which people respond to different situational stimuli. The trait approach, with its emphasis on structure, is less concerned with reactions to situations, and in some ways, the structure (trait) and process approaches to personality reflect the distinction immortalized in Cronbach's (1957) "two disciplines of scientific psychology (Mroczek & Spiro, 2003b).

Mroczek and colleagues (2006) have likened these two approaches to personality, structure, and process, to the structural and dynamic components of an automobile. The analogy is worth repeating here. Cars have structural components that do not contain any moving parts, such as the chassis, frame, headlights, windshield, and windows. These make up the basic structure of a vehicle and are analogous to basic structural features of personality, such as the Big Five traits (Goldberg, 1993). Cars also have dynamic components that either contain moving parts or involve a chemical or physical process. Examples of dynamic components include the transmission, the steering and braking systems, and the internal combustion engine. These parts have structural elements, of course, but they differ from purely structural elements in that they involve processes that unfold over time. To brake a car takes time and invokes a dynamic process as calipers are engaged, friction is applied, and wheels are slowed down gradually. Braking is a process (governed by physical principles) in this sense. Other dynamic components involve chemical processes. Inside an internal combustion engine, gasoline is fed into cylinders, where the dynamic action of pistons explodes the fuel, creating heat and energy that powers and propels the vehicle. Although this process involves structures, such as the engine block itself, it is in essence a chemical reaction. The burning of fuel to create energy and motion is not structural, but a process that occurs over a period of time—in this case, over a period of seconds. In essence, there is a stimulus (fuel), action (explosion of fuel), and a response (energy). This also implies a time element; a stimulus occurs first, some action happens, and there is a response—this takes some time, even if it is just seconds.

Personality also involves stimulus–response processes such as those that occur inside a car. Coping styles are processes that are invoked by stressors and unfold over time (Lazarus & Folkman, 1984). The stimulus (stressor) leads to action (the feeling of stress or threat) and a response (negative affect, problem-solving behavior). This is not a structure, but structural elements of personality, such as trait neuroticism, certainly influence this reaction to stimuli

that encompass coping, as well as reactivity to stress (Almeida, 2005; Bolger & Schilling 1991; Mroczek & Almeida, 2004; Tennen, Affleck, Armeli, & Carney, 2000). Defense mechanisms also involve stimuli that invoke a response (Cramer, 2003). The response is the defense itself, and the process of stimulus invoking response unfolds over time, although usually a short period of time. Goal attainment and goal-focused behaviors, a popular set of variables among social-cognitive personality researchers, involve processes that occur over longer periods of time, usually days or weeks, making daily diary and experience sampling methods common in this area (Christensen, Feldman-Barrett, Bliss-Moreau, Lebo, & Kaschub, 2003; Fleeson, 2001). In all these examples, the process is dynamic, involving a sequence of events. Just as the physical and chemical processes that power a car are not discrete events but rather a sequence of events, personality processes involve particular sequences of events over some period of time.

Cattell recognized this distinction between structure and process and incorporated these ideas in his concept of the data box (Cattell, 1966). In the three-dimensional data box, persons make up one dimension, occasions (or situations) a second, and variables a third. Pairs of data-box dimensions can be combined to represent a distinct type of data and a unique way of conceptualizing personality. For example, R-technique focuses on variability across persons on a set of variables, holding occasion constant. R-technique is the essence of the structure approach to personality. It concentrates on variability across persons, or between-persons variance. Or the researcher may choose to focus on within-person variability across occasions (or situations), on a single variable; Cattell called this S-technique. S-technique is the essence of the process approach to personality. It concentrates on variability within persons. The data box, although 40 years old, is an invaluable tool for understanding how structure and process approaches to personality relate to one another (Mroczek & Almeida, 2004; Mroczek & Spiro, 2003b; Mroczek, Spiro, & Almeida, 2003; Nesselroade, 1988). Despite this value, few have used the Cattellian data box to understand personality development, although Ozer (1986) has made the most thorough and notable attempt thus far.

Analyzing Personality Processes with Daily Diary or Experience Sampling Data

To investigate personality processes, many investigators have turned to daily diary or experience sampling designs. These provide the type of short-term but intensive measurements that can capture the dynamic action that interest process-oriented personality psychologists. The typical researcher who samples people's thoughts, feelings, or behaviors once or more a day for some duration finds him- or herself in a similar situation as the researcher who has multiple measurement occasions over many years in a long-term longitudinal study. In both cases, data are nested within persons. However, the investigator interested in personality processes is not usually interested in modeling change in a single variable over time, as in the case of trait change. More common is an interest in whether two or more variables influence one another over the course of a day, or a week, or a month. For example, do daily stressors impact the rise and fall of negative affect over the course of a day or series of days? Or does social interaction impact people's feelings of well-being over the course of a day or week? These are process questions (Fleeson, 2004).

Process studies that utilize daily diary or experience sampling designs yield data that are in "person-time." Within a given person, the researcher has some number of daily, or multiple daily, observations. Usually there are observations of many different variables at each measurement occasion. There is actually very little difference between the data arrangement in longitudinal designs and the data arrangement in diary or experience-sampling designs. The main difference is the length of time between measurement occasions. In most growth-curve studies of personality, the spacing is at least several months and is usually years. Another difference is the use or nonuse of a time variable. In a growth-curve model, the association being modeled is between some measure of time (the aforementioned "temporal meta-meter") and multiple measurements of some variable (e.g., extraversion). In a diary or experience-sampling design, it is typical for the investigator to model the association between two substantive variables over the measurement occasions. In other words, time is usually not part of the model.

For example, many daily experience studies have focused on the association between stressors and emotion (Bolger & Schilling 1991; Mroczek & Almeida, 2004; Suls, 1995; Tennen, Affleck, Armeli, & Carney, 2000). These data are commonly arranged in "person-days," nesting stressor and emotion measurements within persons across some number of days, often over a week or two. Therefore, stressor occurrence and emotion could vary over days within persons. The relationship between the occurrence of a stressor and the emotion can be analyzed in an MLM framework. Specifically, this relationship would comprise a level-1 model. Once the level-1 (within-person) associations are modeled, the researcher could move to a level-2 model that introduces between-persons variables, such as neuroticism. More formally, such level-1 and level-2 models can be expressed as:

Level 1: Negative emotion$_{ij}$ = π_{0i} + π_{1ij}(stress$_{ij}$) + $\in_{ij}$

Level 2: π_{0j} = $\tilde{a}_{00}$ + $\tilde{a}_{01}$(neuroticism) + μ_{0j}
π_{1j} = $\tilde{a}_{10}$ + μ_{1j}

At level 1, the outcome, negative emotion$_{ij}$ is the amount of negative emotion on day i for person j. It is a function of π_{0j}, the person's own intercept, and π_{1j}, the person's own slope, which characterizes the association between stress and negative emotion for that individual. Stress$_{ij}$ is amount of stress on day i for person j, and $\in_{ij}$ is a within-person error or residual term. At Level 2, μ_{0j} is shown as a function of the between-persons intercept ($\tilde{a}_{00}$), the effect of the between-persons variable neuroticism ($\tilde{a}_{01}$), and a between-persons error term (μ_{0j}). The within-person slopes, π_{1j}, are a function of the between-persons slopes ($\tilde{a}_{10}$) and between-persons error term (μ_{1j}) that captures individual differences in the stress–negative emotion slopes.

In simpler terms, within each person in the study there is a relationship between stressor occurrence and negative emotion. This relationship can vary across people. So for some people, there is a tight relationship between experiencing a stressor and feeling negative affect. These are the people who may be labeled stress-reactive. However, for other people experiencing a stressor is not necessarily linked to experiencing negative emotion. These are the "cool cucumbers." These are people who do not become panicked when life gets stressful.

In the MLM framework, the relationship between stressor occurrence and negative emotion can vary just as any regression coefficient can vary. Some people will have a high-magnitude coefficient, others low-magnitude or zero. This variability then becomes the substantive variance for level-2 models, as expressed in a more formal way in the equations above. Much of the process research in personality asks questions regarding variability across individuals in some kind of level-1 (within-person) relationship. The MLM framework is ideal for analyzing data for answering these types of research questions.

This chapter is focused on longitudinal analysis of personality data, and although daily diary or experience-sampling designs are not longitudinal in the traditional sense, the data yielded from such studies have much in common with longer-term longitudinal data. In this sense, there is a clear relationship between analyses of both types of data.

Conclusion

Longitudinal studies of personality are, fortunately, increasing in number. As more and more longitudinal personality databases accumulate, and as statistical techniques for analyzing these data diffuse more widely, the area will see many more sophisticated studies in the future. This chapter was not exhaustive in its treatment of the myriad techniques available to researchers for analyzing longitudinal data. For example, proportional hazards modeling is becoming widely used in certain areas of personality research, particularly in the growing area of personality and mortality (Mroczek & Spiro, in press). Yet it did examine in depth a small number of major techniques that have enjoyed wide use and will likely continue to be heavily used in the future. It is hoped that the expositions of the data-analytic tools contained in this chapter will prove useful to personality researchers.

Acknowledgment

This work was supported by grants from the National Institute on Aging (Nos. R01-AG18436 and P01-AG020166).

Recommended Readings

Biesanz, J. C., Debb-Sossa, N., Papadukis, A. A., Bollen, K. A., & Curran, P. J. (2004). The role of coding time in estimating and interpreting growth curve models. *Psychological Methods, 9,* 30–52.

Cattell, R. B. (1966). The data box: Its ordering of total resources in terms of possible relational systems. In R. B. Cattell (Ed.), *Handbook of multivariate experimental psychology.* Chicago: Rand-McNally.

Mroczek, D. K., & Spiro, A, III. (2003). Modeling intraindividual change in personality traits: Findings from the Normative Aging Study. *Journals of Gerontology: Psychological Sciences, 58B,* 153–165.

Raudenbush, S. W., & Bryk, A. S. (2002). *Hierarchical linear models: Applications and data analysis methods* (2nd ed.). Thousand Oaks, CA: Sage.

Roberts, B. W., & DelVecchio, W. F. (2000). The rank order consistency of personality traits from childhood to old age: A quantitative review of longitudinal studies. *Psychological Bulletin, 126,* 3–25.

Singer, J. D., & Willett, J. B. (2003). *Applied longitudinal analysis: Modeling change and event occurrence.* New York: Oxford University Press.

References

Akaike, H. (1974). A new look at the statistical model identification. *IEEE Transactions on Automatic Control, AC-19,* 716–723.

Aldwin, C. M., Spiro, A., III, Levenson, M. R., & Bossé, R. (1989). Longitudinal findings from the Normative Aging Study: 1. Does mental health change with age? *Psychology and Aging, 4,* 295–306.

Almeida, D. M. (2005). Resilience and vulnerability to daily stressors assessed via diary methods. *Current Directions in Psychological Science, 14,* 64–68.

Baltes, P. B., Reese, H. W., & Nesselroade, J. R. (1977). *Lifespan developmental psychology: Introduction to research methods.* Monterey, CA: Brooks/Cole.

Bentler, P. M., & Bonett, D. G. (1980). Significance tests and goodness of fit in the analysis of covariance structures. *Psychological Bulletin, 88,* 588–600.

Biesanz, J. C., Debb-Sossa, N., Papadukis, A. A., Bollen, K. A., & Curran, P. J. (2004). The role of coding time in estimating and interpreting growth curve models. *Psychological Methods, 9,* 30–52.

Bolger, N., & Schilling, E. A. (1991). Personality and problems of everyday life: The role of neuroticism in exposure and reactivity to daily stressors. *Journal of Personality, 59,* 356–386.

Bryk, A. S., & Raudenbush, S. W. (1992). *Hierarchical linear models in social and behavioral research: Applications and data analysis methods.* Newbury Park, CA: Sage.

Cattell, R. B. (1966). The data box: Its ordering of total resources in terms of possible relational systems. In R. B. Cattell (Ed.), *Handbook of multivariate experi-*

mental psychology (pp. 355–402). Chicago: Rand-McNally.

Christensen, T. C., Feldman Barrett, L., Bliss-Moreau, E., Lebo, K., & Kaschub, C. (2003). A practical guide to experience-sampling procedures. *Journal of Happiness Studies, 4,* 53–78.

Conley, J. J. (1984). The hierarchy of consistency: A review and model of longitudinal findings on adult individual differences in intelligence, personality, and self-opinion. *Personality and Individual Differences, 5,* 11–26.

Conley, J. J. (1985). Longitudinal stability of personality traits: A multitrait–multimethod–multioccasion analysis. *Journal of Personality and Social Psychology, 49,* 1266–1282.

Costa, P. T., & McCrae, R. R. (1988). Personality in adulthood: A six-year longitudinal study of self-reports and spouse ratings on the NEO Personality Inventory. *Journal of Personality and Social Psychology, 54,* 853–863.

Costa, P. T., & McCrae, R. R. (1994). Set like plaster? Evidence for the stability of adult personality. In T. F. Heatherton & J. L. Weinberger (Eds.), *Can personality change?* (pp. 21–40). Washington, DC: American Psychological Association.

Cramer, P. (2003). Personality change in adulthood is predicted by defense mechanism use in early adulthood. *Journal of Research in Personality, 37,* 76–104.

Cronbach, L. J. (1957). The two disciplines of scientific psychology. *American Psychologist, 12,* 671–684.

Cronbach, L. J., & Furby, L. (1970). How we should measure "change"—Or should we? *Psychological Bulletin, 74,* 68–80.

Curran, P. (2003). Have multilevel models been structural equation models all along? *Multivariate Behavioral Research, 38,* 529–569.

Finn, S. E. (1986). Stability of personality self-ratings over 30 years: Evidence for an age/cohort interaction. *Journal of Personality and Social Psychology, 50,* 813–818.

Fleeson, W. (2001). Toward a structure- and process-integrated view of personality: Traits as density distributions of states. *Journal of Personality and Social Psychology, 80,* 1011–1027.

Fleeson, W. (2004). Moving personality beyond the person–situation debate: The challenge and opportunity of within-person variability. *Current Directions in Psychological Science, 13,* 83–87.

Goldberg, L. R. (1993). The structure of phenotypic personality traits. *American Psychologist, 48,* 26–34.

Goldstein, H., & McDonald, R. P. (1987). A general model for the analysis of multilevel data. *Psychometrika, 53,* 455–467.

Helson, R., Jones, C. J., & Kwan, S. Y. (2002). Personality change over 40 years of adulthood: Hierarchical linear modeling analyses of two longitudinal samples. *Journal of Personality and Social Psychology, 83,* 752–766.

Jones, C. J., Livson, N., & Peskin, H. (2003). Longitudinal hierarchical linear modeling analyses of California

Psychological Inventory data from age 33 to 75: An examination of stability and change in adult personality. *Journal of Personality Assessment, 80,* 294–308.

Jones, C. J., & Meredith, W. (1996). Patterns of personality change across the life-span. *Psychology and Aging, 11,* 57–65.

Lamiell, J. T. (1981). Toward an idiothethic psychology of personality. *American Psychologist, 36,* 276–289.

Lazarus, R. S., & Folkman, S. (1984). *Stress, appraisal and coping.* New York: Springer.

Little, R. A. J., & Rubin, D. (1987). *Statistical analysis with missing data.* New York: Wiley.

McArdle, J. J. (1991). Structural models of development theory in psychology. *Annals of Theoretical Psychology, 7,* 139–159.

McDonald, R. P. (1993). A general model for two level data with responses missing at random. *Psychometrika, 58,* 575–585.

Mehta, P. D., & Neale, M. C. (2005). People are variables, too: Multilevel structural equations modeling. *Psychological Methods, 10,* 259–284.

Meredith, W., & Tisak, J. (1990). Latent curve analysis. *Psychometrika, 55,* 107–122.

Mroczek, D. K., & Almeida, D. M. (2004). The effects of daily stress, personality, and age on daily negative affect. *Journal of Personality, 72,* 355–378.

Mroczek, D. K., & Griffin, P. (2007). Growth-curve modeling in positive psychology. In A. Ong & M. H. M. Van Dulmen (Eds.), *Handbook of methods in positive psychology* (pp. 467–476). New York: Oxford University Press.

Mroczek, D. K., & Spiro, A., III. (2003a). Modeling intraindividual change in personality traits: Findings from the Normative Aging Study. *Journals of Gerontology: Psychological Sciences, 58B,* 153–165.

Mroczek, D. K., & Spiro, A., III. (2003b). Personality structure and process, variance between and within: Integration by means of developmental framework. *Journals of Gerontology: Psychological Sciences, 58B,* 305–306.

Mroczek, D. K., & Spiro, A., III. (2005). Change in life satisfaction over 20 years during adulthood. *Journal of Personality and Social Psychology, 88,* 189–202.

Mroczek, D. K., & Spiro, A., III. (in press). Personality change influences mortality in older men. *Psychological Science.*

Mroczek, D. K., Spiro, A., & Almeida, D. M. (2003). Between- and within-person variation in affect and personality over days and years: How basic and applied approaches can inform one another. *Ageing International, 28,* 260–278.

Mroczek, D. K., Spiro, A., Almeida, D. M., & Pafford, C. (2006). Intraindividual change in personality. In D. K. Mroczek & T. D. Little (Eds.), *Handbook of personality development* (pp. 163–180). Mahwah, NJ: Erlbaum.

Muthén, B. O. (2002). Beyond SEM: General latent variable modeling. *Behaviormetrika, 29,* 81–117

Muthén, B. O., & Satorra, A. (1995). Complex sample data in structural equation modeling. In P. Marsden

(Ed.), *Sociological methodology* (pp. 216–316). Boston: Blackwell.

Nesselroade, J. R. (1988). Sampling and generalizability: Adult development and aging issues examined within the general methodological framework of selection. In K. W. Schaie, R. T. Campbell, W. M. Meredith, & S. C. Rawlings (Eds.), *Methodological issues in aging research*. New York: Springer.

Ozer, D. J. (1986). *Consistency in personality: A methodological framework*. Berlin: Springer.

Raudenbush, S. W., & Bryk, A. S. (2002). *Hierarchical linear models: Applications and data analysis methods* (2nd ed.). Thousand Oaks, CA: Sage.

Raudenbush, S. W., & Sampson, R. (1999). Assessing direct and indirect effects in multilevel designs with latent variables. *Sociological Methods and Research, 28*, 123–153.

Roberts, B. W., & Chapman, C. N. (2000). Change in dispositional well-being and its relations to role quality: A 30-year longitudinal study. *Journal of Research in Personality, 34*, 26–41.

Roberts, B. W., & DelVecchio, W. F. (2000). The rank order consistency of personality traits from childhood to old age: A quantitative review of longitudinal studies. *Psychological Bulletin, 126*, 3–25.

Rogosa, D. R., Brandt, D., & Zimowski, M. (1982). A growth curve approach to the measurement of change. *Psychological Bulletin, 92*, 726–748.

Rovine, M. J., & Molenaar, P. C. (2000). A structural modeling approach to a multilevel random coefficients model. *Multivariate Behavioral Research, 35*, 51–88.

Singer, J. D., & Willett, J. B. (2003). *Applied longitudinal analysis: Modeling change and event occurrence*. New York: Oxford University Press.

Small, B. J., Hertzog, C., Hultsch, D. F., & Dixon, R. A. (2003). Stability and change in adult personality over 6 years: Findings from the Victoria Longitudinal Study. *Journals of Gerontology: Psychological Sciences and Social Sciences, 58B*, 166–176.

Srivastava, S., John, O. P., Gosling, S. D., & Potter, J. (2003). Development of personality in early and middle adulthood: Set like plaster or persistent change? *Journal of Personality and Social Psychology, 84*, 1041–1053.

Suls, J. (2001). Affect, stress and personality. In J. P. Forgas (Ed.), *Handbook of affect and social cognition* (pp. 392–409). Mahwah, NJ: Erlbaum.

Tennen, H., Affleck, G., Armeli, S., & Carney, M. A. (2000). A daily process approach to coping: Linking theory, research and practice. *American Psychologist, 55*, 626–636.

von Eye, A., & Nesselroade, J. R. (1992). Types of change: Application of configural frequency analysis in repeated measurement designs. *Experimental Aging Research, 18*, 169–183.

## CHAPTER 32

Person-Centered Structural Analyses

James W. Grice

Allport's early vision of personality psychology was distinctly person centered, as he defined personality as "the dynamic organization within the individual of those psychophysical systems that determine his unique adjustments to his environment" (p. 48, 1937). The locus of investigation in Allport's seminal definition is clearly the psychological life of the individual. Yet in contrast to this person-centered (or within-person) emphasis, a majority of contemporary theories and methodologies found in personality psychology are between-persons in character. Modern trait theories, for example, have emerged from the systematic analysis of aggregate statistics (e.g., means and correlations) computed from numerous samples of individuals. The properties of traits, such as their organization and stability across cultures, are therefore of a between-persons rather than within-person nature.

In this chapter the logical and empirical distinctions between the between-persons and within-person approaches to personality are reviewed and briefly compared to the idiographic–nomothetic controversy. A number of historically important methods for empirically assessing within-person personality structure are also reviewed. The rest, and greater part of this chapter, is then devoted to a little-known method of confirmatory component analysis, multiple-group confirmatory components analysis (MGCCA). MGCCA is introduced, explained, and demonstrated using genuine data obtained from a single person. It will be shown that MGCCA is an effective tool for examining the within-person structure of how individuals view themselves and others along common traits and unique personal constructs. Finally, specific challenges to the future of MGCCA and person-centered analyses are discussed.

Between- and within-Person Distinction

In her classic article "Where Is the Person in Personality Research?" Rae Carlson argued that personality psychology had, by 1971, become a discipline that was ironically disinterested in the study of the individual person. Indeed, in her review of 226 articles, "not a single published study attempted even minimal inquiry into the organization of personality variables within the individual" (p. 209 [original emphasis]; see also Carlson, 1984). One could certainly argue that Carlson's question is still relevant today, as modern personality psychologists rely heavily on aggregate analysis strategies in which data collected from a given person are relevant only to the extent that they contribute to some computational process that averages across individuals (for example, computing means, standard deviations, correlations, etc.). Perhaps nowhere is this aggregating process more clearly seen than in modern trait models of personality. As is well known, for instance, Cattell's 16 PF and the five-factor model were born from factor analyses of individuals' ratings of themselves on adjective terms culled from an English language dictionary (see McCrae & John, 1992). The factor analyses themselves were conducted on measures of bivariate, linear association (typically correlations) that were computed across individual responses. Countless such analyses were conducted over the years to refine and replicate the trait models. In examining this literature one finds tables of structure coefficients, pattern coefficients, factor correlations, indices of model fit, and so forth, but nary any data that can be connected to a single person in a given study. Unlike the literature of the late 1800s and early 1900s, when individual participants were routinely referred to in journal articles (Danziger, 1990, pp. 69–70), modern trait literature is instead saturated with statistics that are derived across—rather than within—individuals to convey relationships between variables. Cervone (2005) thus rightly argues that modern aggregate statistical models are primarily concerned with between-persons personality structure, which is quite distinct from models that seek to capture within-person personality structure. Echoing the thoughts of Carlson, Cervone also suggests the modern drive to develop interindividual taxonomic systems at the expense of searching for intraindividual personality structures and dynamic processes has caused us to forget "the topic that historically was the defining concern of personality psychology: the psychological life of the individual" (p. 425).

The between- versus within-person distinction articulated by Cervone is reminiscent of the idiographic–nomothetic terminology introduced to personality psychologists by Allport in 1937. Properly understood, the term *nomothetic* refers to general laws created by scientists to cover distinct classes of phenomena (Lamiell, 1997, 1998). As general laws they are intended to cover all of the instances of the class, given a number of framing conditions; for instance, when Kelly (1955) postulated that human reasoning is fundamentally dialectical, he was reasoning nomothetically. Kelly considered dialectical reasoning to be common to the psychological domains of all persons with normally developed and functional brains, and he employed this nomothetic concept causally in his explanations of various psychological states such as anxiety and hostility. As a general principle, the dialectical foundation of human reasoning transcends both time and context, and it is explicitly intended by Kelly to aid in the elucidation of the lives of individual persons. Of course, such general laws will never allow for the full description or explication of the life of a given person, because each person has a unique life trajectory that flows through a given interval of time and particular historical and social contexts. What qualifies a construct as nomothetic therefore is not its capacity to fully explicate the life of a person, but rather its generality or commonality to all persons, given a set of specified framing conditions. Conversely, the term *idiographic* refers to explicit, systematic knowledge of a group of people or a single individual that is historical in nature and thus bound by time, context, and culture (Lamiell, 1998, p. 28). Again considering Kelly's personal construct psychology, an idiographic analysis of a person would entail developing a case history as well as cataloging the important constructs the individual uses to make sense of his or her world. Even these latter efforts have a fundamentally historical quality. How did the individual develop his or her personal constructs over time? What constructs does the person use to make sense of his or her own unique circumstances? How are this person's constructs organized into a system? The answers to such questions for any single person will obviously not generally be true for all persons.

Unfortunately, confusion has arisen over the years regarding the meanings of the idiographic and nomothetic terms, particularly the latter. Danziger (1990) refers to "the triumph of the aggregate" that occurred in the early 1900s as the study of individual persons gave way to statistical analysis of group data. During this time "nomothetic" came to be incorrectly equated with the results from aggregate statistical analyses—what was true *on average* was considered to be true *in general* (see Lamiell, 1997, 1998). Where, then, is the person in personality research (Carlson, 1971)? It would seem that the person has not been hidden from view by abstract nomothetic constructs and theories, but has instead been at least partially buried by aggregate research methodology and its accompanying conceptual framework.

The person-centered approach to personality can be viewed as an effort to reverse the historical triumph of the aggregate by placing the psychological life of the individual back on center stage. It is necessarily a nomothetic and idiographic approach that recognizes the pursuit of covering laws as an essential feature of scientific investigation. Such covering laws must, however, aid our understanding of individual persons—not aggregates—if they are to be considered valid or even pragmatically useful. Moreover, the person-centered approach is faithful to Allport's (1937) original within-person definition of personality psychology cited above. This congruence can be seen particularly in person-centered methods for exploring "the dynamic organization within the individual of those psychophysical systems that determine his unique adjustments to his environment processes." Some of these methods can be used to model the dynamic, time-dependent changes that occur within persons (e.g., Molenaar, 2004, 2005), whereas other methods focus on the intra-individual *structural* features of personality in order to explain how people interpret and shape their life experiences (e.g., Cervone, 1997; Shoda, Mischel, & Wright, 1994). It is these latter methods that are explored in the following discussion.

Notable Person-Centered Structural Analyses

Arguably in a state of frustration over the turmoil created by the nomothetic–idiographic distinction he introduced to personality psychology, Allport (1961, 1962) attempted to de-

fuse the debate surrounding this dichotomy with the concept of morphogenesis. While acknowledging the existence of common traits that occur in all individuals, Allport argued that studying the patterning or organization of traits at the individual level resulted in a more complete picture of the person. This intra-individual patterning was referred to as *morphogenesis*, and Allport hoped it would replace the term *idiographic* (1962, p. 100). It never really caught on, however, partly because of Allport's implicit and unfortunate equating of nomothetic and aggregate (see Lamiell, 1998), but morphogenesis did draw attention to the multivariate and *structural* nature of the person-centered view of personality.

Personality structure refers "not to adjectives that co-vary, but to interacting cognitive, affective, and motivational processes that guide an individual's responses in various situations" (Westen, 1996, p. 401). Several aspects of this definition are worth highlighting. First, an important distinction is drawn between variables that co-vary at the aggregate level, and variables that combine at the level of the individual. Second, a structural approach to understanding the "architecture of personality" (Cervone, 2004) is distinctly multivariate in nature, involving data collection for numerous variables such as an individual's personal constructs or the cognitive, affective, and motivational variables referred to in the definition. Finally, a person can be studied without reference to any context, or a person can be studied within specific contexts. With the latter orientation, the different cognitive and affective resources that a person brings to bear on a given experience may differ from context to context, and this variation constitutes an important aspect of the person's personality. In either case, the notion of personality structure is to be understood intrapersonally, and the focus of both theory and research is thus the person and not the aggregate.

Stephenson's Q-sort (1953) is one early embodiment of this notion. In the typical Q-sort a person is given 100 cards, each containing a separate statement (e.g., "I am intelligent," "I despise myself"), and is asked to sort the cards into nine piles that reflect the extent to which the statements are "least like me" to "most like me." The person is also asked to sort the cards in such a way as to approximate a normal distribution. The person can also sort the cards according to "least like my ideal self" versus "most like my ideal self," and the researcher or therapist can set about examining the intra-individual distributions of the cards. In a famous case study by Rogers (1954), for example, the correlation between a female client's self-sort and ideal self-sort was shown to increase over the course of therapy. From Rogers's point of view, the increased similarity between the woman's actual and ideal selves indicated that she had resolved incongruities in the *structure* of her phenomenal field, or self-concept. This conclusion was reached without recourse to between-persons analyses or reference to any sample of individuals. Block (1961) later tied *Q*-sort methodology explicitly to the study of human personality, and the Shelder–Westen Assessment Procedure—200 (Westen, 1996) is a more recent derivative of Stephenson's original technique that explores individual sorts as potential indicators of clinical syndromes.

In 1957, Osgood, Succi, and Tannenbaum published their influential book *The Measurement of Meaning*, in which they reviewed the methodology and research of their semantical differential scaling technique. Their original methodology was comprised of 50 bipolar adjective terms (e.g., "happy–sad," "hard–soft," "slow–fast") that anchored 7-point rating scales. The items were grouped into three categories or dimensions that Osgood et al. considered relevant to understanding an individual's phenomenological realm of meaning: *evaluative, potency*, and *activity*. An individual completing the semantic differential items could rate him- or herself, other known people, objects, various self-images (e.g., the ideal self or one's body image), or concepts (e.g., democracy, government, religion), producing a matrix of ratings that could then be analyzed with a variety of statistical methods. Osgood and colleagues reported a number of interesting results from studies of personality, psycholinguistics, and communication. Equally important, Osgood and colleagues reviewed a number of empirical issues regarding within-person structural analyses. For instance, they discussed different measures of pattern similarity such as intra-individual correlation coefficients and Euclidean distances. They also discussed graphing techniques for presenting results and the use of factor analysis to explore the structure of individual rating matrices. In one particularly interesting application, they examined the factor structures of three different personalities generated by a person diagnosed with multiple-personality disorder (pp. 258–271).

The application of factor analysis to a single person's responses is often credited to Cattell (1943, 1946), who defined the *P*-technique as a type of factor analysis performed on the correlations of a person's scores across different occasions. George Kelly cites Cattell and Osgood when discussing his repertory grid technique (1955; see Chap. 6), which he developed explicitly to assess how individuals construe themselves, others, and their worlds. To complete the original form of Kelly's grid technique, a person first provides the names of individuals who fit specified roles (e.g., "your father, or someone who has been like a father to you," "a person with whom you worked and did not get along with"). The person then elicits a determined number of bipolar personal constructs (e.g., "friendly–unfriendly," "generous–stingy," "cruel–sympathetic") by comparing and contrasting sets of three individuals. For instance, the person may be asked to consider self, mom, and dad and to identify how two of the people are similar to each other but different from the third. The person may respond, "Mom and I both like pets, whereas Dad does not like pets," thus producing the bipolar construct "likes pets/does not like pets." Unlike the semantic differential approach, which incorporates a common list of adjectives, the repertory grid thus requires each person to elicit his or her own unique set of bipolar adjectives. The person finally indicates which pole of each personal construct best describes the named individuals, yielding a matrix of dichotomous ratings. Kelly developed a relatively crude form of nonparametric factor analysis to explore the interrelationships between the binary personal construct ratings and to make a person's construct system public. By so doing he hoped to provide a tool for clinical psychologists to better understand their clients' constructs. For instance, the meaning of "like pets/does not like pets" can be better understood by examining its relationships with other constructs as well as how it is used to discriminate between different people.

In the 1970s, Patrick Slater (1977) pioneered the application of eigenvalue-eigenvector decomposition to repertory grid data, which was an important accomplishment because the traditional parametric methods of principal components analysis and common factor analysis are both based on eigenvalue-eigenvector decompositions. Slater also introduced a variety of other analysis techniques for repertory grid data, as well as methods for simultaneously graphing personal constructs and the rated people or things in two- or three-dimensional plots. These techniques, which are shown below, prove to be particularly useful for elucidating the within-person structure of personality.

Multiple-Group Confirmatory Components Analysis

Description of Analysis Procedures

MGCCA is a simple modeling strategy in which the researcher defines a component or set of components on an a priori basis. Once the components are defined, standard factor analytic output (e.g., structure, pattern, and component correlation matrices; see Lee & Ashton, Chapter 25, this volume) can be examined to determine if the model fits the data well. The analysis itself relies on a simple least squares algorithm to generate values for the different parameters in the component model. The equations can be found in Guttman (1952) and Gorsuch (1983, pp. 80–93).

The question for the investigator using MGCCA is, "What combination or grouping of variables permits me to effectively rank order the rated targets (e.g., the rated people in a repertory grid) on the hypothesized component?" Note that "group" in MGCCA refers to groups of variables, *not* groups of rated targets or people. As with traditional confirmatory factor analysis, the investigator must start with a conception of the components, but he or she works from the variables to the components in MGCCA rather than from the components to the variables. Once the components are defined, the pattern and structure coefficients can be generated from the analysis and reported along with other common statistics, which are discussed below. Pattern coefficients are regression weights for predicting the original ratings from the components, and structure coefficients are the bivariate correlations between the rated items and the components. Of course, it is well known that the pattern and structure coefficients will be identical when the components are orthogonal.

MGCCA, like traditional exploratory principal components analysis, is based on two-dimensional matrices of numerical values. The values are typically obtained from rating scales, such as semantic differential, Likert-type, or binary scales. For aggregate types of analyses, the ratings can be collected from numerous people

and combined in some fashion (e.g., averaging), but for the current purpose the ratings can be collected from a single person. As an example, consider the ratings obtained from a male participant in a recent study by Grice, Jackson, and McDaniel (2006). The participant, "Mark," rated himself, his ideal self, and 22 other individuals on 20 marker items (see Table 32.1) for the Big Five personality traits (Extraversion, Agreeableness, Conscientiousness, Neuroticism, Openness) using a 5-point Likert-type scale.

From a confirmatory analysis perspective, one might wish to assess how well the Big Five trait model fits Mark's ratings. Between-persons analyses conducted by Goldberg (1992, 1999) have established the utilized items as strong and unambiguous indicators of their respective components in aggregated data. The question here is, how well does the five-factor model fit this particular person's ratings of the 24 people (self, ideal self, and 22 others) on the 20 marker items? The MGCCA thus begins with deciding on the number of components to create and assigning the items to their respective components. In this example five components are created to represent the Big Five traits, and each component is comprised of the appropriate four marker items. With other types of grid data the investigator must draw on experience, theory, or prior research to build the component model.

The second step concerns the determination of weights for the marker items of each component. In other words, *the second step involves fixing the component score coefficients to some specified value.* Component score coefficients are regression weights for predicting the components from the original ratings (see Grice, 2001). Typically, the items are weighted with 1, –1, or 0, as shown for the four extraversion items:

$$\text{Extraversion component} = (1)\,(E_1) + (-1)\,(E_2)$$
$$+ (-1)\,(E_3) + (1)\,(E_4)$$
$$+ (0)\,(N_1) + \ldots + (0)\,(I_6)$$

Note that the reverse-keyed extraversion items (i.e., E_2 = "is a very private person," E_3 = "does not talk a lot") are given weights (i.e., score coefficients) of –1, whereas all of the nonextraversion items are given weights of 0, essentially excluding them from the definition of the extraversion component. Given this weighting scheme, then, high scores on this component indicate extaversion whereas low scores indicate introversion. A more complex weighting or scoring coefficient scheme could be used. For example, if the "feels at ease with people" item is considered central to defining the extraversion component, then this item could be given a weight of 2 rather than 1 in the equation above. Although such complex weighting schemes can be used, there is considerable debate regarding potential increases in precision and validity over simple weighting schemes based on 1's, –1's, and 0's. This latter, simple weighting scheme also has a long history in the factor analytic and general multivariate literature (see Grice, 2001; Rozeboom, 1979; Wainer, 1978). Consequently, the simple weighting scheme employed in the equation above was used to combine the four marker items for each of the Big Five components for Mark's grid.

The third decision in an MGCCA regards basing the analysis on standardized scores or centered scores, which is equivalent to choosing between analyzing the correlation or covariance matrices, respectively. This decision is similar to the decision confronting the confirmatory factor analyst to opt for the standardized or unstandardized factor solution (see Loehlin, 1998). The standardized solution based on the correlations is typically easier to interpret, as the structure coefficients will be reported as bivariate correlations, and the pattern coefficients will typically—but not necessarily—range between –1 and 1. A benefit of using the covariance matrix, however, is that ratings for marker items that show no variability (e.g., the 24 people are all rated "2" on the item) will not be excluded from the analysis, whereas the correlations for such items are undefined and must subsequently be deleted from the MGCCA. Given that the standardized solution is more easily interpreted and Mark's ratings were variable for each of the Big Five marker items, the correlation matrix was analyzed herein.

Once the components are defined by fixing the score coefficients and the correlation or covariance matrix is chosen, the investigator must decide to constrain the components to orthogonality or to allow the components to intercorrelate. Again, this decision is faced by the confirmatory factor analyst, and as in the general literature, the investigator must base the decision on theory or on the goals of the investigation. An important issue in MGCCA to consider when making this decision is that when the components are constrained to orthogonality, the order in which the components are defined will impact the results. For example, if the five components in the current example are constrained to orthogonality and defined in order as *extraversion*, *agreeableness*, *conscientiousness*, *neuroticism*, and *openness*, the component variances and structure coefficients derived from the MGCCA will differ from the same values computed from the components defined in any other order. The reason for these differences is that the analysis works sequentially on residual correlation or covariance matrices. The variance of the first defined component is removed from the matrix, the variance of the second component is then removed from the resulting residual matrix, and the subsequent components are likewise removed in order from residual matrices. For orthogonal components, the investigator must therefore decide which component will get the first crack at the item correlations or covariances, which will come second, and so on. When the components are defined obliquely, however, the order in which they are defined will not impact the results in any manner whatsoever, because they can share, rather than compete for, item variance. For Mark's grid the components were defined obliquely in order to assess the orthogonality assumption of the Big Five traits for his ratings. As recently discussed by Saucier (2002), the Big Five traits have historically been assumed to be orthogonal even though many studies of aggregate data have shown different pairs of traits to be moderately correlated. At the level of the person, the traits may be correlated as well.

Example Analysis Results

Idiogrid (Grice, 2002) was used to conduct an MGCCA of Mark's Big Five ratings. Arguably, the most relevant output from the analysis is the matrix of pattern coefficients. As stated above, pattern coefficients are regression weights for predicting the items from the components, and they play an important role in any confirmatory factor or components analysis. The pattern coefficients (λ's) are routinely referred to as loadings, and when the correlation matrix is analyzed, as in this example, they will typically range between –1 and +1 in value. Values near zero indicate particularly weak predictive relationships. As shown in Table

TABLE 32.1. Pattern Coefficients, Squared Multiple Correlations, and Component Variances and Correlations for Example Grid

	Components					
	E	A	C	N	O	SMC
Big Five items						
Takes charge	**.85**	−.39	.79	−.25	−.18	.65
Is a very private person	**−.58**	−.29	.54	−.11	.13	.86
Does not talk a lot	**−.94**	.04	.01	−.06	−.09	.78
Feels at ease with people	**.87**	.14	−.23	.08	.22	.79
Thinks of others first	−.20	**.72**	.15	−.08	.16	.93
Is hard to get to know	−.62	**−.61**	.51	−.33	.05	.79
Takes time out for others	−.28	**.96**	.12	−.06	−.11	.95
Feels little concern for others	.14	**−.76**	−.24	.19	.01	.91
Makes a mess of things	.06	.11	**−1.03**	−.04	.12	.83
Makes plans and sticks to them	−.01	.04	**.94**	−.02	−.03	.91
Does things in a halfway manner	.01	−.15	**−.91**	.00	.11	.88
Pays attention to details	.08	−.08	**.82**	−.02	.26	.88
Gets overwhelmed by emotions	−.08	.64	−.75	**.72**	.08	.51
Gets irritated easily	−.24	.12	−.43	**.86**	.06	.82
Rarely gets irritated	−.17	.73	−.20	**−.53**	−.05	.68
Is relaxed most of the time	−.15	.02	−.98	**−.20**	.19	.71
Has a rich vocabulary	.05	−.03	−.02	.10	**1.01**	.95
Avoids difficult reading material	.12	.18	−.29	.22	**−.70**	.76
Catches on to things quickly	−.01	−.24	−.15	.07	**1.12**	.83
Does not have a good imagination	−.09	−.45	.12	−.05	**−.70**	.89
Component variances and correlations						
(E)xtraversion	4.73					
(A)greeableness	.12	6.14				
(C)onscientiousness	−.40	.64	8.43			
(N)euroticism	−.45	−.11	.24	2.35		
(O)penness	−.36	.62	.76	.10	7.50	

Note. Target loadings are printed in **boldface** type.

32.1, the pattern coefficients for Mark's grid reveal consistent and distinct ratings for the 24 people on the Big Five marker items. Specifically, using a salience criterion of .40, the four extraversion items tend to load more highly (in absolute value) on the first component than the other three components, the agreeableness items tend to load highly only on the second component, and so on for the remaining items and components. In the parlance of factor analysis, the high absolute target loadings and relatively infrequent cross-loadings in Table 32.1 indicate reasonably good *simple structure*. A number of exceptions are noteworthy, however: The items "takes charge" and "is a very private person" load highly on conscientiousness (λ = .79 and .54, respectively), as well as their hypothesized extraversion component (λ = .85 and −.58, respectively), and "is hard to get to know" and "gets overwhelmed by emotions" load on three components. It is also important to note that

"rarely gets irritated" loads more highly on agreeableness (λ = .73) than neuroticism (λ = −.53), and "is relaxed most of the time" loads more highly on conscientiousness (λ = −.98) than neuroticism (λ = −.20). Although overall the pattern coefficients support the fit of the five-factor model, these departures from simple structure and expectation reveal person-specific ways in which Mark understands the items as they apply to the people in the grid. In a more technical sense, the between-persons components that have been shown to successfully model aggregated responses to these Big Five marker items do not perfectly model the within-person ratings provided by Mark. The structure coefficients, which represent the correlations between the components and items, can also be examined to evaluate the fit of the component model (see Thompsen, 1997). The values computed from Mark's grid, although not shown, are generally consistent with the pattern coefficients in terms of relative magnitude and yield the same overall interpretation regarding the fit of the five-factor model.

The squared multiple correlations (SMCs) are reported in Table 32.1, and they indicate the extent to which the defined components explain the variance of each Big Five item. In Mark's case, many of the SMCs are above .80 and most are above .70. The only item whose variance appears to be somewhat unique is "gets overwhelmed by emotions," which yielded an SMC equal to .51. Still, as expected, the pattern coefficient for this item is salient on the neuroticism component ($\lambda = .72$). It also yields salient loadings on the agreeableness ($\lambda = .64$) and conscientiousness ($\lambda = -.75$) components.

Table 32.1 also reports the component variances as well as the correlations between pairs of components. The former values indicate that the components differ somewhat in strength. Whereas neuroticism is the weakest component (2.35), conscientiousness (8.43) and openness (7.50) are the strongest components and explain the largest proportions of variance among the Big Five item ratings. In other words, Mark discriminated most among the 24 people with respect to the conscientiousness and openness components, and least with respect to neuroticism. In regard to the component correlations, Mark's ratings indicate that conscientiousness and openness are highly correlated ($r = .76$), as are agreeableness and openness ($r = .62$) and agreeableness and conscientiousness ($r = .64$). Most of the components are correlated above .20 in absolute magnitude, and the median absolute correlation is .38, indicating that the components are clearly not orthogonal in Mark's individual grid.

Finally, an index of overall fit, the *root mean squared residual*, can be computed for an MGCCA. A result near zero indicates that the five components explain most of the variances and correlations for the Big Five marker items. For Mark's ratings, the root mean squared residual is equal to .11, which is a small value as compared to zero and represents an 85% reduction in the root mean squared value (.71) for the original, unreduced correlation matrix.

Two-dimensional plots that show the relationships among the items and the rated individuals are attractive features of MGCCA. Using techniques outlined by Slater (1977), the items and individuals can be plotted in two-dimensional spaces created from the compo-

nents. The top image in Figure 32.1 shows an example plot constructed from the extraversion and openness components for Mark's ratings. As can be seen, Mark views himself as primarily introverted and slightly high, relative to others, on openness, which is negatively correlated with extraversion (i.e., introverts are typically higher on the openness component). Mom is viewed as highest on the openness component, although being slightly extraverted, whereas Scott, Sam, Mira, and Jess are clearly the extraverted/low-openness individuals. Mark (self) is most similar to Bob, and Mark views his ideal self as less introverted and slightly higher on the openness component than his actual self. As noted, extraversion is negatively correlated with openness in Mark's grid, and the cosine of the angle formed by the two components is equal to their correlation ($r = -.36$). The bottom image in Figure 32.1 shows the agreeableness and conscientiousness components from Mark's ratings. Sam, Mira, and Jess are again seen as highly similar and distinct from self. They are joined by Troy, who is most extremely disagreeable and nonconscientious, although he and the others are "relaxed most of the time"! Paul and Dad, in comparison, are viewed as most agreeable and conscientious, and the two components are obviously highly correlated ($r = .64$). At least in the context of these 24 rated individuals, agreeableness and conscientiousness tend to go hand-in-hand.

All other combinations of the Big Five components could be examined via this graphical method. Three-dimensional graphs shaped as spheres could also be created and viewed (see Slater, 1977, pp. 106–107, 117–119). In this way, the individuals and items could be considered in three-dimensional spaces formed from different combinations of Big Five components. Even with only two dimensions, however, these graphs serve as powerful summaries of the grid data as they offer a window into the way Mark views himself, his ideal self, and the 22 other individuals. Perhaps more than the numerical values reviewed above and presented in the tables herein, these graphs demonstrate the notion of exploring within-person personality structure with MGCCA.

Extension Analysis

Because MGCCA is a confirmatory type of analysis, it is extremely easy to "extend" a

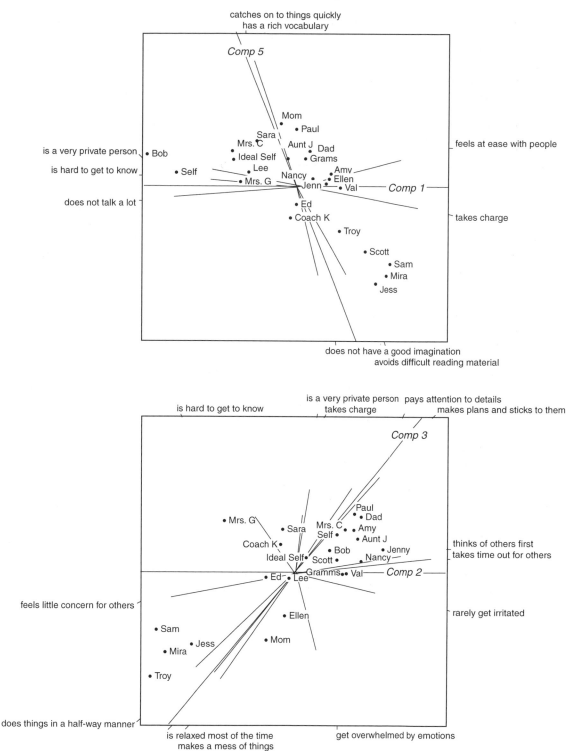

FIGURE 32.1. Two-dimensional plots of example Big Five trait ratings. Axes range from −1.15 to +1.15. "Comp 1" represents Extraversion and "Comp 5" represents Openness in the top image; "Comp 2" represents Agreeableness and "Comp 3" represents Conscientiousness in the bottom image. Only salient Big Five items are shown in both images.

model defined for a set of items to include ratings separately collected for additional items. As part of Grice and colleagues' (2006) study, Mark was in fact asked to elicit 12 of his own bipolar personal constructs in a separate repertory grid task. He was then asked to rate the same 24 individuals (self, ideal self, and 22 others), using the same 5-point scale on each of the constructs. The Big Five components defined in the MGCCA can be extended to include Mark's personal constructs within their multivariate space. Technically, this procedure is referred to as an extension analysis (see Dwyer, 1937, and Gorsuch, 1997), which can be quite complex in the context of common factor analysis. In the context of a priori components, however, extension analysis is straightforward and can be conducted through simple concatenation of the two separate sets of ratings. In the current example, Mark's personal construct ratings are simply concatenated to his Big Five ratings. Because the 24 individuals are common across the two sets of ratings, they are concatenated vertically (i.e., the Big Five grid is stacked on top of the personal construct grid) to form a large 32 by 24, item by individual, grid. The five components are then defined via the score coefficients exactly as described above, and the MGCCA is conducted on the concatenated grid.

The resulting pattern and structure coefficients for the Big Five items are identical to the values for the original ratings reported above. The component correlations are also equivalent to those reported in Table 32.1. What is uniquely reported are component variances and the pattern and structure coefficients for the extended personal constructs. For the sake of brevity, only the pattern coefficients are reported in Table 32.2 in addition to the SMCs for the constructs. As can be seen, most of the SMCs are above .70, indicating that at least 70% of the variability in those particular personal construct ratings is explained by the Big Five components. In comparison, one construct, "not bothered by others/too sensitive," does not fit very well into the five-component space (SMC = .46), and approximately 40% of the variance in the "outgoing/reserved," "reserved/outspoken," and "funny/boring" personal constructs is unexplained by the five components (SMCs = .62, .62, and .58, respectively). Examination of the pattern coefficients reveals the specific details regarding the location of the personal constructs in the component space. For example, "considerate" and "loving" load primarily on the agreeableness component, and "calm" loads almost exclusively on conscientiousness. Because the constructs are bipolar, "selfish" and "hateful" are disagreeable poles and "crazy" is a nonconscientious pole. Other personal constructs were functions of more than one component. For instance, "outgoing/reserved" was best predicted by a function of extraversion, openness, and low conscientiousness, and "has good morals/has bad morals" was a function of agreeableness and conscientiousness. Most of Mark's constructs load at least .50 on one or more of the extraversion, agreeableness, and conscientiousness components, and the location of the constructs in the component space

TABLE 32.2. Extension Analysis Pattern Coefficients and Squared Multiple Correlations for Personal Constructs from Example Grid

| Personal constructs | Components | | | | | SMC |
	E	A	C	N	O	
Considerate : selfish	−.11	.68	.18	−.19	.18	.93
Outgoing : reserved	.64	.14	−.52	.00	.45	.62
Reserved : outspoken	−.64	.00	.26	.06	−.04	.62
Funny : boring	.05	.83	−.68	−.08	.29	.58
Loving : hateful	−.20	.85	.01	−.05	.11	.89
Carefree : worries too much	.36	.42	−.86	−.12	.25	.77
Free-spirited : uptight	.52	.24	−.84	.16	.29	.73
Calm : crazy	−.20	−.23	.97	−.02	−.07	.82
Thinks of others : self-centered	−.12	.67	.16	−.03	.20	.88
Caring about others: cares only for self	−.21	.47	.29	−.12	.24	.88
Has good morals : has bad morals	−.23	.56	.57	−.30	−.23	.83
Not bothered by others : too sensitive	.37	−.29	.44	−.23	−.54	.46

Note. E, Extraversion; A, Agreeableness; C, Conscientiousness; N, Neuroticism; O, Openness.

can be examined visually. As shown in the top image of Figure 32.2, the personal constructs, "outgoing/reserved," "free-spirited/uptight," "not bothered by others/too sensitive," and "reserved/outspoken" load in the extraversion/openness component space. As can be seen in the bottom image of Figure 32.2, nine of Mark's twelve personal constructs load in the agreeableness/conscientiousness component space.

Summary of MGCCA

The relative mathematical simplicity of MGCCA, as compared to, for example, structural equation modeling, makes it an intriguing tool for modeling multivariate data obtained from a single person. In the analysis above, MGCCA was used to test the fit of a personality trait model to ratings of self and others obtained from Mark, a participant in a recent study by Grice and colleagues (2006). The model under consideration, the five-factor model, is arguably the most popular of all contemporary trait models. It was developed through numerous factor analyses, both exploratory and confirmatory, of aggregated self-report ratings on adjectives culled from an English language dictionary (McCrae & John, 1992). The example MGCCA of Mark's grid, discussed above, stands in contrast to these aggregate studies. Instead of fitting a model to a correlation matrix derived from hundreds or thousands of individuals, a component model was fit to correlations computed from ratings obtained from a single person. Although the results showed some support for the fit of the aggregate factor model to Mark's ratings, a number of incongruities were noted that represented nuances of Mark's construal of himself and others. In previous between-persons analyses, for instance, "is relaxed most of the time" has been shown to be a reliable and unambiguous indicator of low neuroticism. For Mark, however, this item was predicted by low scores on the conscientiousness component, as was the neuroticism item "gets overwhelmed by emotions." The extension analysis furthermore revealed that people low in conscientiousness (such as Sam, Jess, Mira, and Troy in the bottom image of Figure 32.2) were "free-spirited," "carefree," and "outgoing." It seems that Mark's particular meaning for low conscientiousness is akin to a "carefree spirit." Such people are relaxed, free, and gre-

garious, but they tend to be sloppy and fail to demonstrate a true concern for the welfare of others (note the positive correlation between conscientiousness and agreeableness). On the other end of the spectrum, conscientious people (such as Paul, Mrs. C, and Bob in the bottom image of Figure 32.2) tend to be "calm," to have "good morals," and to be agreeable. Examining the construct poles associated with conscientiousness, Mark also saw these people as "uptight," "worries too much," and "reserved." It is interesting to note that Mark's conscientiousness component accounted for the greatest amount of variability in his ratings (see Table 32.1). It was also highly correlated with openness, which revealed the second highest component variance. In Mark's view, then, people in the grid who were conscientious also tended to be high in openness, and these two dimensions played important roles in discriminating among the 24 people.

An important lesson to learn from the analysis of Mark's two sets of ratings is that a model developed on the basis of aggregated responses from a sample of individuals will not necessarily fit at the level of the person. Mark's ratings were examined through the lense of a trait model that was itself created through repeated analyses of between-persons data. The picture produced by this lense was found to be incomplete, as the specific meanings that he attached to the marker items for the Big Five traits were clearly evident in the pattern coefficients and in the relationships between Mark's own personal constructs and the marker items. The picture was furthermore incomplete on the basis of the uniqueness found in his personal constructs, which failed to map clearly into the Big Five component space. Two of Mark's unique dimensions for discriminating among the 24 people were "not bothered by others/too sensitive" and "funny/boring." Grice (2004) and Grice and colleagues (2006) discussed other examples of constructs that were outside the purview of the Big Five and also pointed out that the fit of the five-factor model varied greatly from person to person in their studies. For some participants, not all of the five components clearly emerge, and for others, many of the marker items did not load as expected or the components were highly correlated (e.g., $r > .80$). In contrast, clear support for the fit of the Big Five trait model to the aggregated ratings matrices was reported. In other words, what was found true for the aggregate was not

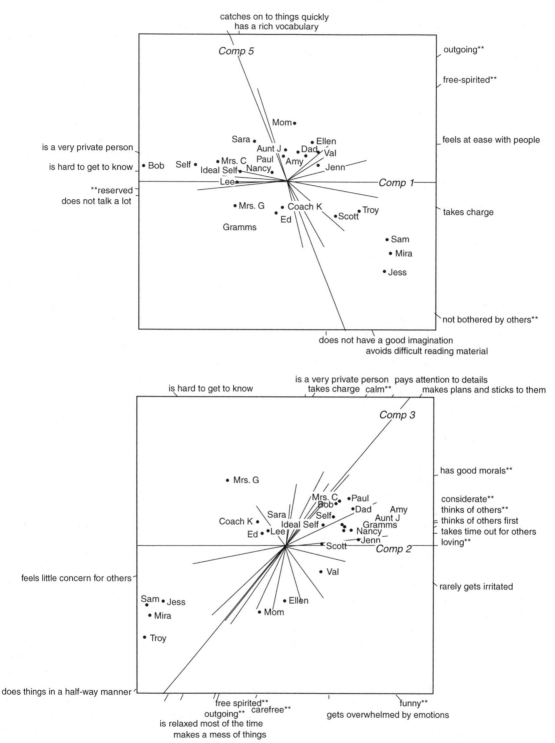

FIGURE 32.2. Two-dimensional plots of example Big Five trait ratings. Axes range from −1.50 to +1.50. "Comp 1" represents Extraversion and "Comp 5" represents Openness in the top image; "Comp 2" represents Agreeableness and "Comp 3" represents Conscientiousness in the bottom image. Only salient Big Five items are shown in both images. Only salient Big Five items and personal constructs (denoted by asterisks) are shown in both images.

necessarily found true for the individuals in the study. The between-persons and within-person distinction is therefore not an esoteric abstraction with little scientific merit, but an empirically demonstrable idea. Sidman (1952; see also Bakan, 1967, Chap. 2) in fact demonstrated long ago the difference between individual and averaged functions describing learning curves. More recently, Molenaar (2004) has shown analytically that crossing the bridge from the aggregate to the individual may in fact be impossible except under restricted conditions.

The Future of Person-Centered and Multiple-Group Analyses

Utility and Context

In the broader personality literature the potential increase in explanatory power associated with person-centered methods has generated a great deal of controversy, as can be seen in the so-called idiographic–nomothetic debate in personality psychology (e.g., see Jaccard & Dittus, 1990; Kenrick & Stringfield, 1980; Rushton, Jackson, & Paunonen, 1981). Controversy regarding the type and trait approaches to personality is also related to the within-person and between-persons distinction (e.g., see Asendorpf, 2003; Robins, John, & Caspi, 1998). Typologies are, by their nature, configural or multivariate conceptualizations of personality, and it is this feature that, some suggest, makes them superior to trait models.

The most recent discussion to arise from the person-centered approach, however, has been centered on social-cognitive models of personality (see, e.g., Cervone, 2004; Mischel, 2004). Like all person-centered approaches, these models are multivariate in nature. With their cognitive–affective processing system model, for instance, Mischel and Shoda (1995, p. 11) consider human personality as "the person's construal and representation of self, people, and situations, enduring goals, expectations-beliefs, and feeling states, as well as memories of people and past events." Furthermore, when assessing such constructions, the context in which the person finds him- or herself is important and must also be assessed. In other words, a hallmark of the social-cognitive approach is an emphasis on context. Mark was asked in his Big Five and personal construct rating tasks to consider himself and the other people generally,

free of any context. From the social-cognitive perspective, the data obtained from Mark are thus only superficially useful because they cannot convey the situational variability that is bound to occur in Mark's constructions. A particular recommendation in the social-cognitive approach would therefore be to ask Mark to conduct his ratings with respect to a particular context or contexts. Grice, Burkley, Burkley, Wright, and Slaby (2004) recently demonstrated that person-centered methods can be easily modified to assess differences in an individual's constructions of him- or herself and others in different contexts, thus providing a more dynamic assessment of the person. As a confirmatory procedure, MGCCA could prove useful for assessing changes in structure across situations. A client, for instance, could rate a constant set of people or targets on a constant set of items over the course of therapy. The component structure of the first set of ratings could be determined with exploratory components analysis and then examined for stability over time with MGCCA. Specific structural changes in the person's view of him- or herself and others could then be empirically assessed. Whether studies such as this, or the social-cognitive approach in general, will finally demonstrate the utility of the person-centered approach, however, is debatable. The accepted—and entrenched—viewpoint in personality psychology is decidedly between-persons in theory and method, and Funder (2001) argues that perhaps only by integration with trait theory will social-cognitive approaches gain widespread appeal (however, see Cervone & Shoda, 1999).

Technical Issues for MGCCA

Even without considering the importance of context or the dynamic aspect of personality, MGCCA itself faces a number of challenges. In this chapter and in the studies by Grice and his colleagues (Grice, 2004; Grice et al., 2006), a component model was used rather than a common factor model. Some authors have argued, however, that the common factor model may be more appropriate for person-centered factor analyses (Pruzek, 1988). As in the general literature, the choice between the component and common factor models hinges on item error and factor score indeterminacy. Common factor analysis provides the means for incorporating measurement error into the factor model, but this advantage comes with a high price, namely, factor score indeterminacy (Grice, 2001). Regardless of these differences, the issue of sample size plays an important role in the current context. In Mark's grid, for instance, 24 people were rated on 20 marker items. The sample size for the MGCCA was therefore 24. In other person-centered studies the number of rated people or targets may even be fewer than the dimensions on which they are rated. Small sample sizes generally lead to difficulties when computing communalities for a multiple-group confirmatory factor analysis. A communality represents the proportion of variance in a given item that is explained by the common factors. With small sample sizes these values will often exceed 1, which is a conceptual impossibility (often referred to as a Heywood case). Moreover, when the number of rated persons exceeds the number of dimensions, initial communality estimates, computed as squared multiple correlations, cannot be derived. A suboptimal method for computing communalities, such as selecting the highest bivariate correlation for each item, must therefore be chosen. With the component model, communality estimation is not an issue and these difficulties are consequently avoided.

Another challenge facing MGCCA regards model fit. In mainstream uses of confirmatory factor analysis, researchers have developed various rules of thumb for assessing the root mean squared residual (RMSR) and other indicators of overall model fit (see Marsh, Hau, & Wen, 2004). These rules of thumb are not without controversy, but the studies on which they are based nonetheless provide a frame of reference for researchers to judge the fit of their factor models. No such social conventions exist at this point for MGCCA or its common factor counterpart. The RMSR for Mark's grid above, for instance, was .11. Does this value constitute good fit? How does it compare to other studies or simulated data under similar conditions? As another index of model fit, Grice (2004) computed congruence coefficients between the pattern coefficients and score coefficients but similarly noted that rules of thumb for interpreting such coefficients in the context of MGCCA do not exist. Future studies are therefore needed on the topic of model fit in component and common factor multiple-group models. These studies could emulate the work conducted in the mainstream confirmatory factor analytic

literature, but a thorny issue would need to be addressed if probability values are sought. Specifically, what constitutes the population with the person-centered approach? Mark's Big Five matrix, for instance, was based on a sample of items and a sample of people. Does the population consist of all people known to Mark, past, present, and future, as well as all possible Big Five marker items? Even so, under what conditions would a researcher or practitioner be interested in generalizing beyond the content of the ratings matrix? Any attempts to develop p-values in the person-centered approach must address questions such as these.

Finally, a related question regarding the person-centered approach and MGCCA concerns the stability of results. On one hand, one would expect the results of an MGCCA conducted on ratings tasks like those completed by Mark to be stable over short periods of time (e.g., < 24 hours). Mark was asked to think of himself and others generally when considering the Big Five marker items and his own personal constructs. In other words, he was prompted to think in terms of dispositions rather than states. The stability of MGCCA results derived from such judgments, however, has not been specifically tested. On the other hand, the person-centered approach recognizes that persons change over time and across contexts. As discussed above, it is therefore expected that the MGCCA results may differ over time and across contexts. With regard to the latter, for instance, one might expect the structure of ratings to change in the context of a party, a rock-climbing expedition, a funeral, a sporting event, or other circumstances. In either case, this issue needs to be addressed. Such work with MGCCA in the future could prove fruitful for advancing a truly person-centered approach toward human personality.

Recommended Readings

Grice, J. W. (2004). Bridging the idiographic-nomothetic divide in ratings of self and others on the Big Five. *Journal of Personality, 72,* 203–242.

Grice, J. W., Jackson, B., & McDaniel, B. (2006). Bridging the idiographic–nomothetic divide: A follow-up study. *Journal of Personality, 74,* 1191–1218.

Guttman, L. (1952). Multiple methods for common-factor analysis: Their basis, computation, and interpretation. *Psychometrika, 17,* 209–222.

References

Allport, G. W. (1937). *Personality: A psychological interpretation*. New York: Holt.

Allport, G. W. (1961). *Pattern and growth in personality*. New York: Holt.

Allport, G. W. (1962). The general and the unique in psychological science. In G. W. Allport, *The person in psychology* (pp. 81–102). Boston: Beacon Press.

Asendorpf, J. B. (2003). Head-to-head comparison of the predictive validity of personality types and dimensions. *European Journal of Personality, 17*, 327–346.

Bakan, D. (1967). *On method*. San Francisco: Jossey-Bass.

Block, J. (1961). *The Q-sort method in personality assessment and psychiatric research*. Springfield, IL: Charles C. Thomas.

Carlson, R. (1971). Where is the person in personality research? *Psychological Bulletin, 75*, 203–219.

Carlson, R. (1984). What's social about social psychology? Where's the person in personality research? *Journal of Personality and Social Psychology, 47*, 1304–1309.

Cattell, R. B. (1943). The description of personality: I. Foundations of trait measurement. *Psychological Review, 50*, 559–592.

Cattell, R. B. (1946). *Description and measurement of personality*. New York: World Book.

Cervone, D. (1997). Social-cognitive mechanisms and personality coherence: Self-knowledge, situational beliefs, and cross-situational coherence in perceived self-efficacy. *Psychological Science, 8*, 43–50.

Cervone, D. (2004). The architecture of personality. *Psychological Review, 111*, 183–204.

Cervone, D. (2005). Personality architecture: Within-person structures and process. *Annual Review of Psychology, 56*, 423–452.

Cervone, D., & Shoda, Y. (Eds.). (1999). *The coherence of personality: Social-cognitive bases of consistency, variability, and organization*. New York: Guilford Press.

Danziger, K. (1990). *Constructing the subject: Historical origins of psychological research*. Cambridge, UK: Cambridge University Press.

Dwyer, P. S. (1937). The determination of the factor loadings of a given test from the known factor loadings of other tests. *Psychometrika, 2*, 173–178.

Funder, D. C. (2001). Personality. *Annual Review of Psychology, 52*, 197–221.

Goldberg, L. R. (1992). The development of markers for the Big-Five factor structure. *Psychological Assessment, 4*, 26–42.

Goldberg, L. R. (1999). A broad-bandwidth, public-domain, personality inventory measuring the lower-level facets of several five-factor models. In I. Mervielde, I. Deary, F. De Fruyt, & F. Ostendorf (Eds.), *Personality psychology in Europe* (Vol. 7, pp. 7–28). Tilburg, The Netherlands: Tilburg University Press.

Gorsuch, R. L. (1983). *Factor analysis* (2nd ed.). Hillsdale, NJ: Erlbaum.

Gorsuch, R. L. (1997). New procedures for extension analysis in exploratory factor analysis. *Educational and Psychological Measurement, 57*, 725–740.

Grice, J. W. (2001). Computing and evaluating factor scores. *Psychological Methods, 6*, 430–450.

Grice, J. W. (2002). Idiogrid: Software for the management and analysis of repertory grids. *Behavior Research Methods, Instruments, and Computers, 34*, 338–341.

Grice, J. W. (2004). Bridging the idiographic–nomothetic divide in ratings of self and others on the Big Five. *Journal of Personality, 72*, 203–242.

Grice, J., Burkley, E., Burkley, M., Wright, S., & Slaby, J. (2004). A sentence completion task for eliciting personal constructs in specific domains. *Personal Construct Theory and Practice, 1*, 60–75.

Grice, J. W., Jackson, B., & McDaniel, B. (2006). Bridging the idiographic–nomothetic divide: A follow-up study. *Journal of Personality, 74*, 1191–1218.

Guttman, L. (1952). Multiple group methods for common-factor analysis: Their basis, computation, and interpretation. *Psychometrika, 17*, 209–222.

Jaccard, J., & Dittus, P. (1990). Idiographic and nomothetic perspectives on research methods and data analysis. In C. Hendrick & M. Hendrick (Eds.), *Research methods in personality and social psychology* (pp. 312–351). Newbury Park, CA: Sage.

Kelly, G. A. (1955). *The psychology of personal constructs*. New York: Norton.

Kenrick, D. T., & Stringfield, D. O. (1980). Personality traits and the eye of the beholder: Crossing some traditional philosophical boundaries in the search for consistency in all of the people. *Psychological Review, 87*, 88–104.

Lamiell, J. T. (1997). Individuals and the differences between them. In R. Hogan, J. Johnson, & S. Briggs (Eds.), *Handbook of personality psychology* (pp. 118–141). San Diego, CA: Academic Press.

Lamiell, J. T. (1998). "Nomothetic" and "idiographic": Contrasting Windelband's understanding with contemporary usage. *Theory and Psychology, 8*, 23–38.

Loehlin, J. C. (1998). *Latent variable models: An introduction to factor, path, and structural analysis* (3rd ed.). Hillsdale, NJ: Erlbaum.

Marsh, H. W., Hau, K. T., & Wen, Z. (2004). In search of golden rules: Comment on hypothesis testing approaches to setting cutoff values for fit indexes and dangers in overgeneralising Hu & Bentler's (1999) findings. *Structural Equation Modelling, 11*, 320–341.

McCrae, R. R., & John, O. P. (1992). An introduction to the five-factor model and its applications. *Journal of Personality, 60*, 175–215.

Mischel, W. (2004). Toward an integrative science of the person. *Annual Review of Psychology, 55*, 1–22.

Mischel, W., & Shoda, Y. (1995). A cognitive-affective

system theory of personality: Re-conceptualizing situations, dispositions, dynamics, and invariance in personality structure. *Psychological Review, 102,* 246–268.

Molenaar, P. C. M. (2004). A manifesto on psychology as idiographic science: Bringing the person back into scientific psychology, this time forever. *Measurement, 2,* 201–218.

Molenaar, P. C. M. (2005). How generalization works through the single case: A simple idiographic process analysis of an individual psychotherapy. *International Journal of Idiographic Science, 1,* 1–20.

Osgood, C., Suci, G., & Tannenbaum, P. (1957). *The measurement of meaning.* Urbana: University of Illinois Press.

Pruzek, R. M. (1988). Latent variable methods for analyzing grid structures. In J. C. Mancuso & M. L. Shaw (Eds.), *Cognition and personal structure* (pp. 279–302). New York: Praeger.

Robins, R. W., John, O. P., & Caspi, A. (1998). The typological approach to studying personality. In R. B. Cairns, J. Kagan, & L. Bergman (Eds.), *The individual in developmental research: Essays in honor of Marian Radke-Yarrow* (pp. 135–160). Beverly Hills, CA: Sage.

Rogers, C. R. (1954). The case of Mrs. Oak: A research analysis. In C. Rogers & R. Dymond (Eds.), *Psychotherapy and personality change* (pp. 259–348). Chicago: University of Chicago Press.

Rozeboom, W. W. (1979). Sensitivity of a linear composite of predictor items to differential item weighting. *Psychometrika, 44,* 289–296.

Rushton, J., Jackson, D., & Paunonen, S. (1981). Personality: Nomothetic or idiographic? A response to Kenrick and Stringfield. *Psychological Review, 88,* 582–589.

Saucier, G. (2002). Orthogonal markers for orthogonal factors: The case of the Big Five. *Journal of Research in Personality, 36,* 1–31.

Shoda, Y., Mischel, W., & Wright, J. (1994). Intraindividual stability in the organization and patterning of behavior: Incorporating psychological situations into the ideographic analysis of personality. *Journal of Personality and Social Psychology, 67,* 674–687.

Sidman, M. (1952). A note on functional relations obtained from group data. *Psychological Bulletin, 49,* 263–269.

Slater, P. (1977). *The measurement of intrapersonal space by grid technique: Vol. 2. Dimensions of intrapersonal space.* London: Wiley.

Stephenson, W. (1953). *The study of behavior.* Chicago: University of Chicago Press.

Thompson, B. (1997). The importance of structure coefficients in structural equation modeling confirmatory factor analysis. *Educational and Psychological Measurement, 57,* 5–19.

Wainer, H. (1978). Estimating coefficients in linear models: It don't make no nevermind. *Psychological Bulletin, 83,* 213–217.

Westen, D. (1996). A model and a method for uncovering the nomothetic from the idiographic: An alternative to the five-factor model? *Journal of Research in Personality, 30,* 400–413.

## CHAPTER 33

Multiple Regression

Applications of the Basics and Beyond in Personality Research

Stephen G. West
Leona S. Aiken
Wei Wu
Aaron B. Taylor

Multiple regression (MR) is a very flexible data analytic technique that addresses questions about the relationship between one or more independent variables (IVs) and a single dependent variable (DV). The IVs can include qualitative (categorical) variables (e.g., gender, experimental treatment conditions, personality types), quantitative variables (e.g., personality traits, mood states, abilities), or both. MR is typically applied in personality research only when the DV is a quantitative measure; however, extensions of the model to other types of DVs can be considered (e.g., categorical variables). Consideration of multiple DVs is possible through the use of contrasts or composite variables. The specification of the form of the relationship between the IVs and the DV may range from a simple linear relationship, to a complex curvilinear relationship, to an interaction involving the combined effects of two or more IVs.

In this chapter we take a broad perspective following that of Cohen, Cohen, West, and Aiken (2003); this perspective encompasses all of what statisticians term the *general linear model* and more. In this framework, analysis of variance (ANOVA) and correlational analysis are treated as special cases within the framework of MR. This breadth and flexibility makes MR a useful statistical technique that can provide answers to many of the central questions faced by researchers. Indeed, the use of MR is now so ubiquitous in many areas of psychology that it has been called "psychology's data analytic workhorse" and "everyday data analysis." For example, of 36 total articles published in 2004 (Volumes 86 and 87) in the *Journal of Personality and Social Psychology: Personality Processes and Individual Differences* (*JPSP:PPID*), 32 (89%) reported at least one MR, correlation, or ANOVA. In addition, many of the newer analyses such as multilevel modeling or growth curve modeling (reported in 33% of the articles) and mediational analyses (reported in about 15% of the articles) can be seen as extensions of the basic MR model (Cohen et al., 2003).

Our goal in this chapter is to consider the use of MR in personality psychology and to provide some insights into this data-analytic workhorse. We present only a brief review of the basics of MR, assuming that readers have had previous exposure elsewhere, most commonly in their first-year graduate course in psychological statistics. Readers without such prior exposure may wish to first read a comprehensive introductory chapter (e.g., Aiken, West, & Pitts, 2003) or another source.[1] Here, we consider basic issues in MR that continue to present challenges for personality researchers. How should interactions and curvilinear effects be modeled? How should categorical IVs be represented and interpreted? How can we diagnose and address problems that result when the model is not correctly specified or when there are problems in the data (e.g., outliers, missing data)? We consider the issues of statistical power and needed sample size, issues that continue to be all too often neglected in personality research. We then consider new developments that broaden the application of the multiple regression framework: How should repeated measures and other forms of data in which observations are not independent be treated? At the end of each section we include comments that address issues that arise in that section.

Multiple Regression: The Basics

In personality psychology, MR is nearly always used to test a specific hypothesis based on theory or prior research. The hypothesis should ideally (1) identify the set of IVs that relate to the DV and (2) specify the form of the relationship between the IVs and the DV. In some studies the researcher may also wish to control statistically for other background variables (e.g., age, socioeconomic status [SES]) even though they may not be of central theoretical interest.

We begin with a simple artificial example. Suppose a researcher has a sample of 100 people from the community. For each person, she collects a measure of the number of stressful life events (LE) during the past year (e.g., rela-

tionship breakup, loss of job; range 0–10 events) and the number of friends who could provide support (SUP; range 0–5 friends) during these stressful times. The DV is each person's score on the Beck Depression Inventory (BDI; range 0–63). Finally, she collects a measure of each participant's SES (range 1 = lower class to 5 = upper class) as a control variable.

Table 33.1 presents the results of the analysis of three regression models that might be hypothesized to account for these data. In Model A (Panel A), the researcher proposes the simple hypothesis that stressful life events are associated with higher levels of depression. Model B represents a more complex hypothesis in which two IVs each have a unique effect on depression: An increase in life events is expected to increase depression, whereas support from friends is expected to decrease depression (see Wheaton, 1985). Finally, Model C investigates whether the hypothesized relationships in Model B will still hold even when each participant's SES is controlled.

Each hypothesis in Table 33.1 is represented by a regression equation. In these equations, b_0 is the intercept, the predicted value of BDI (BDI) when the value of each IV in the equation is 0. For Model A, $b_0 = 5.46$ is BDI when no stressful life events have occurred (LE = 0). In contrast, for Model C, $b_0 = -3.68$ is BDI when LE = 0, SUP = 0, and SES = 0. Note that in Model C $b_0 = -3.68$ is negative, an *impossible* value, given BDI ranges from 0 to 63. Although LE and SUP = 0 are plausible values, SES = 0 is not—SES can range only from 1 to 5. The problem of the intercept representing an impossible value can be avoided by mean centering each of the IVs. In Model C, we would create a new centered form of each IV, $LE_C = LE - M(LE)$, $SUP_C = SUP - M(SUP)$, and $SES_C = SES - M(SES)$, where $M()$ indicates the sample mean of the variable in parentheses and the subscript C indicates a centered variable. In the centered regression equation,

$$BDI = b_0 + b_1 LE_C + b_2 SUP_C + b_3 SES_C \quad (1)$$

centered $b_0 = 14.1$, the mean BDI score in the sample, often a useful value (see Wainer, 2000). The estimates of b_1, b_2, and b_3 do not change from those in Table 33.1(C). In the absence of centering, extreme care must be taken in interpreting intercepts (and other lower-order regression coefficients in complex regression models, as shown below).

TABLE 33.1. Three Possible Regression Models

A. Life Events Influence Depression: $BDI = b_0 + b_1 LE$

Term	Unstandardized estimate b	95% CI Lower	95% CI Upper	Standardized β	sr	pr	t	p
b_0: intercept	5.46	2.39	8.53	—	—	—	3.53	<.001
b_1: LE	1.77	1.19	2.35	.52	—	—	6.09	<.001

$R^2_{Y.1} = .274$
Overall Model Test: $F(1, 98) = 37.06$, $p < .001$

B. Life Events and Social Support Influence Depression: $BDI = b_0 + b_1 LE + b_2 SUP$

Term	Unstandardized estimate b	95% CI Lower	95% CI Upper	Standardized β	sr	pr	t	p
b_0: intercept	8.05	4.30	11.79	—	—	—	4.26	<.001
b_1: LE	1.99	1.39	2.58	.59	.56	.56	6.62	<.001
b_2: SUP	−1.41	−2.63	−0.19	−.20	−.19	−.23	−2.29	.024

$R^2_{Y.12} = .312$
Overall Model Test: $F(2, 97) = 21.95$, $p < .001$

C. Life Events, Social Support, and SES Influence Depression: $BDI = b_0 + b_1 LE + b_2 SUP + b_3 SES$

Term	Unstandardized estimate b	95% CI Lower	95% CI Upper	Standardized β	sr	pr	t	p
b_0: intercept	−3.68	−5.64	−1.72	—	—	—	−3.72	<.001
b_1: LE	0.09	−0.22	0.41	0.03	.02	.06	0.59	ns
b_2: SUP	−1.50	−2.02	−0.97	−0.22	−.20	−.50	−5.67	<.001
b_3: SES	−6.47	−5.85	−7.09	−0.94	−.75	−.90	−20.75	<.001

$R^2_{Y.123} = .875$
Overall Model Test: $F(3, 96) = 223.01$, $p < .001$

D. Correlation Matrix

	LE	SUP	SES	BDI
LE	1.00			.52
SUP	.31	1.00		−.02
SES	−.60	−.20	1.00	−.91

Note. Artificial data. *sr*, semipartial correlation; *pr*, partial correlation.

b_1, b_2, and b_3 represent the unstandardized partial regression coefficients for LE, SUP, and SES, respectively. In linear regression equations containing only first-order terms (e.g., $b_1 X$), the respective b_1, b_2, and b_3 coefficients are identical in the centered and uncentered case— only b_0 is affected by centering, as is explained below. We highlight here the interpretation of b_1 in the *uncentered* case presented in Table 33.1. In those equations in which they appear, b_2 and b_3 are interpreted in a manner analo-gous to b_1. In Model A in which there are no other predictors, $b_1 = 1.77$ is the predicted amount of increase in BDI for each 1-unit increase in the IV, here LE. In Model B, $b_1 = 1.99$ is now interpreted as the predicted amount of increase in BDI with the SUP variable held constant at a fixed value (e.g., 0). For example, if we sampled a special group of individuals with 0 friends who could provide support, their predicted value of BDI would increase by about 2 points for each additional stressful event.

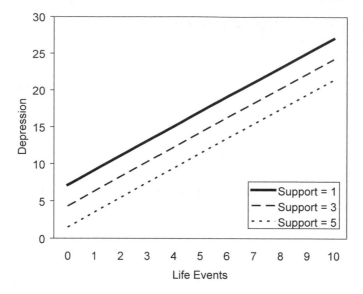

FIGURE 33.1A. Two-dimensional plot illustrating the additive effect of two IVs. The plot depicts the predicted relationship between Life Events and Depression for individuals having 1, 3, or 5 Supportive Friends. The relationship of Life Events to Depression is constant across number of Supportive Friends; adding Supportive Friends reduces Depression by a constant amount regardless of the number of Life Events. Artificial data.

Figure 33.1 provides two different graphical depictions of this relationship. Figure 33.1A illustrates the regression equation for Model B, $BDI = 8.05 + 1.99LE - 1.41SUP$, by substituting values into the equation corresponding to SUP = 1, 3, and 5 friends. This procedure results in the three parallel regression lines, one corresponding to each of the three levels of support. This same invariant relationship between LE and BDI will also hold at all other values of SUP. Figure 33.1B provides an alternative representation of this same information by treating both LE and SUP as continuous variables. The regression surface is a flat plane, as it will be in any regression model that includes only first-order terms. The right bottom corner of the plane represents the intercept $b_0 = 8.05$ when LE = 0 and SUP = 0. SUP increases from right to left on the graph. The lower edge of the plane represents the relation between BDI and SUP when LE = 0, $BDI = 8.05 - 1.41SUP$. Depression (BDI) is lowest when SUP is highest (5 friends, at the left edge of the graph) and increases as SUP decreases toward 0 friends. The right edge of the plane represents the relation between BDI and LE when SUP = 0, $BDI = 8.05 + 1.99LE$. The flat shape of the regression plane indicates that the slope of the

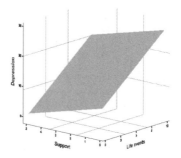

FIGURE 33.1B. Three-dimensional plot of regression surface for a model with addictive effects of two IVs. The regression surface depicts the relationship between Number of Supportive Friends (Support), Number of Life Events (Life Events), and predicted Beck Depression Inventory Scores (Depression). Notice that the origin where Support and Life Events both = 0 is the point at the lower right corner of the graph closest to the reader. The highest point in the surface (i.e., the highest predicted level of depression on the BDI) is at the upper right where Life Events = 10 and Support = 0. The plot is based on the same artificial data as in Figure 33.1A.

regression of *BDI* on SUP at different levels of LE, as well as the slope of the regression of *BDI* on LE at different levels of SUP, is constant.

Returning to Table 33.1, Model C shows that there is no longer a relationship between LE and BDI, $b_1 = 0.09$, when SUP and SES are both included in the regression equation. Examination of the correlation matrix in Table 33.1(D) helps explain this finding. Considered alone, LE has a strong positive relationship with BDI ($r = .52$) and SES has a strong negative relationship with BDI ($r = -.91$). However, LE and SES have a high negative correlation ($r = -.60$) and so are confounded. We cannot attribute the full effect uniquely to either LE or SES.

The columns of Table 33.1, labeled "Standardized β", "*sr*," and "*pr*," also illustrate other standardized metrics in which the same effects can be reported. Again, we focus on LE as an illustration. In Model A, $\beta_1 = .52$, is the standardized regression coefficient, the number of standard deviations (*SD*s) *BDI* changes for a 1 *SD* increase in LE. In Model B, $\beta_1 = .59$ is the number of *SD*s that *BDI* is expected to increase for a 1 *SD* increase in LE, now holding SUP constant. $sr = .56$ is the semipartial correlation coefficient. In Model B, *sr* is the correlation between LE and BDI holding SUP constant. $sr^2 = (.56)^2 = .3112$ is the proportion of unique variation in BDI accounted for by LE, over and above SUP. $pr = .56$ is the partial correlation. $pr^2 = .3113$ is the proportion of unexplained variation in BDI (i.e., not accounted for by the other predictors, here SUP) that is accounted for by LE. A comparison of the formulas in the two-IV case helps clarify the distinction between sr^2 and pr^2.

$$sr^2 = R_{y.12}^2 - r_{y2}^2$$

$$\text{and} \tag{2}$$

$$pr^2 = \frac{R_{y.12}^2 - r_{y2}^2}{1 - r_{y2}^2}$$

$R^2_{Y.12}$ is the multiple correlation of Y with X_1 and X_2, and r^2_{Y2} is the square of the correlation of X_2 with Y. The denominator of the equation for pr^2, $1 - r^2_{Y2}$, will be less than 1 except in the special case when r^2_{Y2} is 0, so that the magnitude of the partial correlation will generally exceed that of the semipartial correlation. sr^2 and pr^2 are important in the estimation of statistical power.

Comments about Standardized and Unstandardized Metrics

1. The *t*-test of significance and *p*-value for the corresponding unstandardized *b*, standardized β, *pr*, and *sr* are identical. Computer packages routinely report confidence intervals for *b*, and they can easily be constructed for β in linear models; they are far more difficult to construct for *sr* and *pr* because the value of the parameter affects the size of its standard error. Confidence intervals are increasingly preferred because they are more informative than significance tests about the potential range of the *magnitude* of the effect (Cumming & Finch, 2005; Reichardt & Gollub, 1999; Wilkinson & the APA Task Force for Statistical Significance, 1999).

2. The use of the unstandardized *b* with same IVs, DV, and regression model across different studies permits direct comparisons of their results. If the studies are carried out on different populations, restriction or expansion of range on the IVs does *not* affect the estimate of unstandardized *b*. For example, personality traits related to intelligence can show strikingly different correlations with other variables in studies conducted at highly selective versus nonselective colleges.

3. The use of standardized metrics permits a limited comparison of the relative importance of the unique contributions of IVs within a study. Such comparisons assume that all of the IVs in the regression equation have the same reliability and that the sampling procedure did not affect the range of the IVs. Other methods attempt to define importance without specifying a particular regression model. The methods use different definitions of the importance of IVs and consequently may produce different answers (e.g., dominance analysis) (Azen & Budescu, 2003; Budescu, 1993). Standardized metrics also permit some comparisons of relationships across studies using different measures of the same construct within the framework of meta-analysis (Hunter & Schmidt, 2004). Meta-analytic approaches generally assume that the same regression model is estimated across studies or that the full correlation matrix is reported.

4. In the next section we consider models involving interactions and curvilinear effects. In these more complicated models the interpretation of *b*, *sr*, and *pr* is straightforward. How-

ever, complexities arise in the interpretation of standardized β for the interaction term reported by computer programs. In regression analyses with the raw X_1X_2 product term as a predictor, the corresponding standardized regression coefficient is for the z-score of the product X_1X_2. However, the correct interaction term for the standardized solution is the product of the z-scores, $z_{X1}z_{X2}$. Aiken and West (1991, Chap. 3) describe a procedure involving the initial standardization of the predictor variables and formation of the product term $z_{X1}z_{X2}$ that produces the proper standardized regression coefficients.

Our review of the 2004 volumes of *JPSP:PPID* showed that standardized metrics are far more commonly reported than unstandardized coefficients—67% of the articles involving regression in *JPSP:PPID* reported standardized regression coefficients, whereas only 11% reported unstandardized coefficients.[2] Some researchers simply report correlations or standardized coefficients as a default. Other researchers argue that standardized coefficients are always preferable because measures in personality psychology are rarely in a meaningful metric (e.g., a 6-point Likert scale). We encourage researchers to carefully choose the best metric for their own unique research context. In many research contexts, the unstandardized regression coefficient is preferred. The primary

exception occurs when researchers wish to compare the magnitude of relationships between constructs that are measured in different units. Cohen, Cohen, Aiken, and West (1999) present a discussion of the interpretation of a variety of unstandardized scales commonly used in psychology.

More Complex Models: Interactions and Curvilinear Effects

Thus far we have made the default assumption that each IV has a linear relationship to the DV. However, this is a *strong* assumption that may not be correct. One or more of the IVs may have a curvilinear relationship to the DV. For example, increases in anxiety may lead to increases in performance up to a point beyond which further increases in anxiety interfere and test performance falls off (see Figure 33.2A). Or two or more IVs may interact to affect the DV. For example, one form of the stress-buffering hypothesis would predict that stress leads to increases in depression, but that as support from others increases, the strength of this relationship is weakened (see Figure 33.2B). At the end of this section we revisit the effects of centering, which become important in complex regression models.

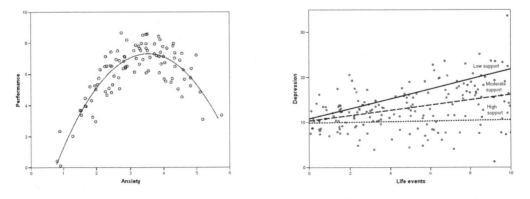

FIGURE 33.2. Plots illustrating curvilinear and interactive relationships. (A) This two-dimensional plot shows a quadratic relationship between Anxiety and Performance. The highest predicted value on the curve corresponds to a moderate level of Anxiety (between 3 and 4 on the scale). Artificial data. (B) This two-dimensional plot shows a stress-buffering interaction between Life Events and Support in predicting Depression. For high levels of Support (dotted line), the slope of the line representing the relationship between Life Events and Depression is close to 0. As support decreases to Low Support (solid line), the slope of the line becomes steeper, indicating a stronger relationship between Life Stress and Depression. Artificial data.

Curvilinear Effects

Curvilinear effects signify that the relation between the IV and DV follows a curved form rather than a straight line. Curvilinear relationships are most commonly represented by adding higher-order polynomial terms (X^2, X^3, etc.) to the regression equation. Special nonlinear regression models may provide a better representation of some relationships, particularly when the predicted value of Y approaches an (upper or lower) asymptote as X increases.

Polynomial (Quadratic) Models

In psychology, curvilinear relationships are most commonly represented using quadratic models. Returning to our example of anxiety (ANX) and performance (PERF), we could express the relationship as follows:

$$PERF = b_0 + b_1 ANX + b_2(ANX)^2 \qquad (3)$$

where $PERF$ is the predicted performance, b_0 is the predicted level of PERF when ANX = 0, and b_1 is the linear tangent line (the instantaneous linear slope) to the curve at the point where ANX = 0. Centering ANX endows b_1 with two useful interpretations. b_1 is now the overall average linear trend of the regression of PERF on ANX across all of the values of ANX. b_1 is also the coefficient for the regression of Y on X at the mean of X. b_2 is the rate of change of the instantaneous linear slope (acceleration), which is constant across all values of ANX in the quadratic model. The maximum (or minimum) of the quadratic curve will occur when $ANX = -2b_1/b_2$. The relationship between ANX and PERF will appear to be curved but will not reach the maximum value when this value falls outside the actual range of ANX in the dataset. This property gives quadratic models the ability to fit a wide variety of curvilinear datasets. The quadratic model can be extended by using higher-order polynomial terms, $PERF = b_0 + b_1 ANX + b_2(ANX)^2 + b_3(ANX)^3 + \ldots + b_p(ANX)^p$, where p denotes the order of the highest-order polynomial term. For example, when $p = 3$, it is a cubic model and when $p = 4$, it is a quartic model. Atkinson (1985) cautions that it is rarely of value to consider functions that are more complex than the quadratic unless (1) measurement is very precise and (2) values across the full potential range of the IV are represented, as in designed parametric experiments.

Special Nonlinear Models

More complex nonlinear models can be useful when measurement quality is high, particularly when growth or decline to an asymptote is occurring (Cohen et al., 2003, Chap. 6; Seber & Wild, 2003). As one illustration, consider a learning experiment in which memory (MEM) for new words increases toward an upper asymptote as the number of trials increases. Following Neter, Kutner, Nachtsheim, and Wasserman (1996), this relationship could be represented as exponential growth, $MEM = b_0 + b_2 e^{b_1 TRIALS}$. When b_1 and b_2 are both negative in this model, b_0 is the upper asymptote that MEM approaches as the number of TRIALS gets large, and b_1 and b_2 reflect different aspects of the speed of learning. More complex relationships can also be modeled by choosing a function that represents the desired nonlinear form (see Seber & Wild, 2003). Such nonlinear models can be difficult to estimate, and researchers may be unfamiliar with these computer routines even though they have long been available in standard statistical packages (e.g., SAS PROC NONLIN, SPSS NONLIN). Although these models have previously been little used in most areas of psychology, they are particularly attractive for the study of the growth and decline of abilities and personality traits over time, areas that are receiving increased attention.

Interactions

Interactions indicate that the effect of one IV on the DV depends on (or is moderated by) the value of one or more other IVs, as in the stress buffering example illustrated in Figure 33.2B. Otherwise stated, there is a difference between the combined effect of two (or more) IVs and the sum of their separate effects. Interactions are specified in regression models by including one or more product terms (e.g., $X_1 X_2$) to represent the combined effects of the two IVs. Space concerns here limit our presentation to interactions between two predictors (see Aiken & West, 1991, for a more complete presentation).

Linear by Linear Interactions

The simplest form of interaction is linear by linear. In this form, the regression of Y on X_1 is linear at all values of X_2 and the regression of Y on X_2 is linear at all values of X_1 (see Figure 33.2B). In personality psychology, linear by linear interactions are typically the only form of moderator effect that is investigated. Returning to our example of stress and social support, the stress buffering hypothesis presented in Figure 33.2B would be modeled as

$$BDI = b_0 + b_1 LE + b_2 SUP + b_3 LE*SUP \quad (4)$$

The partial regression coefficient b_3 for the product term LE*SUP represents the interaction effect in this equation. In a regression equation containing an interaction, the regression coefficient for each lower-order term involved in the interaction (here b_1, b_2) is *conditional*, that is, specific to one value of the other predictor. b_1 now represents the effect of LE on BDI when SUP = 0. b_2 now represents the effect of SUP on BDI when LE = 0. These *conditional* effects are testable *only* when the value of the other IV = 0. Given that SUP is the number of supporters, 0 supporters is a meaningful value in this example. However, with many other IVs (e.g., SES in our earlier example or Likert scales with a range of 1–6), 0 will not be a meaningful value so that b_1 and b_2 will also not be interpretable. We can rearrange the equation above to show the slope of the regression of LE on BDI at a particular value of SUP, the *simple slope*:

$$\text{Simple (conditional) slope} = (b_1 + b_3 SUP) \quad (5)$$

This equation indicates that the simple slope changes by b_3 for each 1-unit change in SUP. Only when SUP = 0 will this simple slope = b_1.

When we center the IVs, $SUP_C = 0$ at the mean value of support. Now b_1 represents the *average effect* of LE on DEP across the observed range of SUP, providing a meaningful interpretation of the results. In addition to the average effect, we recommend choosing a high and low value of the moderator at which to examine the simple slope. As a simple illustration, suppose in our example of the stress buffering hypothesis (Figure 33.2B), $b_1 = 2$, $b_3 = -1$ *for the solution in which all predictors are centered*. The original range of SUP is 0–5 friends, M = 2.5. We might examine the simple slopes at original values of SUP = 1 (low), 2.5 (moderate), and 4 (high), number of supportive friends. For $SUP_C = SUP - 2.5$, the corresponding values are −1.5 (low), 0 (average effect), and +1.5 (high). In this case, using Equation 5, the simple slopes would equal 3.5, 2, and 0.5, for the low, moderate, and high levels of support, respectively. This outcome supports the stress buffering hypothesis that social support weakens the impact of stress on health and mental health problems. Aiken and West (1991) provide an extensive discussion of the use of SPSS Regression to test simple slopes for statistical significance. Preacher, Curran, and Bauer (2006) offer tools for probing interactions, including a Web-based calculator. Of importance, note that for a linear × linear interaction, the simple slope changes by a constant amount for each 1-unit change on the moderator variable. Chaplin (Chapter 34, this volume) provides a fuller discussion of moderator models in personality research.

The choice of a priori meaningful values of the moderator is strongly encouraged when this IV has a clear meaning, as with SUP, or has clear interpretative guidelines, as with IQ or the BDI. For a less well understood variable, Cohen and colleagues (2003) recommend the default of choosing the values of the moderator variable equal to the mean, mean − 1 SD, and mean + 1 SD because these points fall within the actual range of the data in most datasets. With highly skewed moderator variables, other values that fall within the actual range of the data may be chosen.

Other Forms of Interactions

The linear × linear interaction specifies that the effect of the moderator is symmetric, so that the same amount of increase or decrease in the score on the moderator would lead to the same amount of change in the simple slope (see Equation 5). More complex forms of interactions may be needed in some cases to characterize the data. Aiken and West (1991, Chap. 5) discuss in detail the properties of full range of models containing higher-order interactions and present figures illustrating their forms. For example, the regression of Y on X may change in a curvilinear manner, which can be represented by

$$Y = b_0 + b_1 X_1 + b_2 X_2 + b_3 X_1 X_2 \\ + b_4 X_2^2 + b_5 X_1 X_2^2 \quad (6)$$

The last two terms add a quadratic effect of X_2 ($b_4 X_2^2$) and a quadratic (curvilinear) form of moderation of the X-Y relationship ($b_5 X_1 X_2^2$). Note that the equation for the interaction should include all of the lower-order terms that comprise the highest-order interaction, here $X_1 X_2^2$, as was done in the above equation. Otherwise, if the regression coefficients of these omitted terms are not equal to 0, they will confound the interpretation of each of the terms in the equation (Cleary & Kessler, 1982; Piexoto, 1987).

Comments about Interactions and Curvilinear Effects

1. We have emphasized the usefulness of centering in this section. In models involving quadratic effects or linear × linear interactions, centering can allow us to interpret lower-order coefficients as average effects. This advantage can be of critical importance in extensions of regression to more complex approaches such as multilevel analysis and growth modeling, where even the intercept may be of considerable theoretical importance. Centering also eliminates nonessential multicollinearity. Multicollinearity is an index of the relationship between one IV and the other IVs. In models involving interactions or quadratic effects, a part of this multicollinearity is "nonessential," as it results from the location of 0 in the scaling of each of the IVs. The standard diagnostics for multicollinearity, such as the variance inflation factor (VIF), reflect nonessential multicollinearity; centering provides a simple solution by eliminating it. Otherwise, special procedures described by Fox and Monette (1992) must be used in the calculation of multicollinearity diagnostics. The lower-order effects in the centered solution will have smaller standard errors than in the uncentered solution. In extensions to more complex procedures like structural equation models with interactions between latent variables, proper solutions are more likely to occur if the measured variables have been centered (Algina & Moulder, 2001).

2. In quadratic models and models with linear × linear interactions, centering produces immediately interpretable lower-order effects (average effects), so that the effects may be tested in a single regression analysis (Aiken & West, 1991; Cohen et al., 2003). Prior to the use of centering, hierarchical analysis strategies were proposed in which lower-order effects were tested and interpreted at step 1 and the interaction at step 2 (Cohen & Cohen, 1975). These lower-order effects are unconditional at step 1 when the interaction is not yet included in the equation. They become conditional and therefore change in meaning when the interaction is added at step 2. We recommend hierarchical step-down strategies for testing interactions involving more than one term when the interest is in the overall test of the effect. For example, in Equation 6, the interaction term is represented by the combination of the linear $b_3 X_1 X_2$ term and the quadratic $b_5 X_1 X_2^2$ term. To test the full (omnibus) interaction term, Equation 6 (the full model) must be compared with a reduced model without those terms, $Y = b_0 + b_1 X_1 + b_2 X_2 + b_4 X_2^2$, using the standard gain in prediction formula (see Cohen et al., 2003, Section 5.5).

3. The individual difference variables that are often the IVs in personality research may be correlated. In such cases it can be difficult to distinguish between models that include quadratic effects and those that include interactions (Kromrey & Foster-Johnson, 1999; MacCallum & Mar, 1995). The ability to make this distinction can be enhanced via three strategies: the use of large sample sizes, very reliable IVs, and optimal design strategies (McClelland, 1997). In personality research, optimal design involves oversampling cases in specific parts of the distribution on the IVs to maximize the statistical power to differentiate between the competing models (Pitts, 1993).

Categorical Predictors

In some cases IVs may be categorical, representing different natural groups such as gender (males, females) or personality types (e.g., attachment styles), or experimental treatment conditions. With categorical IVs, attention must be given to choosing a coding scheme that represents the researcher's hypothesis. An extensive discussion of coding schemes can be found in Cohen and colleagues (2003, Chap. 8), and a more technical development can be found in Serlin and Levin (1985). Here, we briefly review two coding schemes that are typically most useful in personality psychology: dummy codes and contrast codes. We illustrate these coding schemes by considering a three-group experiment in which there are two treatment conditions (T_1, T_2) and a control condition (C).

Dummy Codes

With the use of dummy codes, one group is designated as a reference group and each of the other groups is then compared with this group. For example, suppose an experiment is run with three conditions, in which T1 and T2 represent two different methods of unobtrusively priming a personality trait and NP is a no-prime condition. Y is a measure of memory of past experiences related to this trait. The $G = 3$ groups are represented by $(G - 1)$ code variables, here $3 - 1 = 2$. D_1 and D_2 represent the two dummy codes necessary to represent the three groups. Two possible dummy coding schemes are presented below, in which D_1 and D_2 represent the values of the two dummy codes for each group.

Dummy Coding Scheme 1		
Group	D_1	D_2
T1	1	0
T2	0	1
NP*	0	0

Dummy Coding Scheme 2		
Group	D_1	D_2
T1*	0	0
T2	0	1
NP	1	0

Note. The group marked with * is the reference group.

To understand the interpretation of regression equations with dummy codes, consider Equation 7:

$$\hat{Y} = b_0 + b_1 D_1 + b_2 D_2 \tag{7}$$

Using dummy coding scheme 1, b_0 is the mean of the NP reference group, b_1 is the difference between the mean of T1 and the mean of the reference group, and b_2 is the difference between the mean of T2 and the mean of the reference group. Coding scheme 1 might be used if the researcher were exploring two different potential priming techniques, desiring to see if they produced a difference from the no-prime control group. b_1 represents the difference of T1 from the reference group, and b_2 represents the difference of T2 from the reference group.

Using dummy coding scheme 2, T1 is the reference group. Coding scheme 2 might be used if T1 represented the standard priming manipulation used in the literature (e.g., a subliminal visual prime) and T2 represented a new enhanced manipulation (e.g., a combined subliminal visual + auditory prime). b_1 still represents the difference between the no-prime and standard prime conditions and tests the success of the replication of the standard effect. Now b_2 represents the difference between the standard and enhanced prime conditions. The test of b_2 answers the question of whether the enhanced prime led to any gain in memory over and above the standard prime. Depending on the research context and the questions of interest, the appropriate coding scheme would be chosen.

Contrast Codes

Contrast codes are used when a priori comparisons are desired that involve two or more group means. Returning to our illustration of the priming experiment, the researcher might be interested in comparing the mean of the tests of memory in the two prime groups with the mean of the no-prime control group. In this case, the researcher could use the following contrast (C) coding scheme.

Contrast Coding Scheme		
Group	C_1	C_2
T1	+0.33	+0.5
T2	+0.33	−0.5
NP	−0.67	0.0

In the regression equation $\hat{Y} = b_0 + b_1 C_1 + b_2 C_2$, b_0 is now the unweighted mean of the three treatment groups, $\overline{M} = (M_{T1} + M_{T2} + M_{NP})/3$. b_1 is the difference between $(M_{T1} + M_{T2})/2$ and M_{NP}. If it is believed that T1 and T2 should not differ from each other, but that they will differ from NP, then this contrast provides a focused test of the hypothesis. b_2 is the difference between M_{T1} and M_{T2}. This second contrast provides an important check on the assumption that T1 and T2 do *not* differ in their effects. If this assumption is *not* supported, then the interpretation of the C_1 contrast is seriously compromised. Abelson and Prentice (1997), Maxwell and Delaney (2004), and Rosenthal, Rosnow, and Rubin (2000) all argue for increased use of contrast codes to test the focused hypothesis of interest when more than two groups are involved. Such contrasts also have the advantage of having higher statistical power than tests of the multiple degree of freedom (df), omnibus hypothesis that there are overall mean differences among groups. Methods of constructing contrast codes to test specific hypotheses are described in Cohen and colleagues (2003, Section 8.5).

Comments about Coding Schemes

1. 1. Although the practice has decreased over the past two decades, some researchers still cut continuous variables into two or three categories for "ease of analysis." This practice typically makes it more difficult to detect true effects (i.e., decreased statistical power). In more complex regression models, such as models with interactions, this practice can easily lead to spurious first-order effects (Maxwell & Delaney, 1993). MacCallum, Zhang, Preacher, and Rucker (2002) present a detailed review of the effects of dichotomizing continuous variables, which are nearly always deleterious.

2. Unweighted effects and weighted effects coding schemes may also be used. These coding schemes compare the mean of one group to the unweighted or weighted mean of all of the groups, respectively. Although unweighted effects coding is preferred in most typical research contexts, weighted effects may be preferred when the proportion of cases in each group represents the proportion in the population, as in a (truly) random sample. For example, they are useful in comparing the means of different demographic groups with the overall mean.

3. We do *not* generally recommend reporting standardized effect sizes with categorical variables. Standardization (e.g., standardized β, sr, pr) is affected by the proportion of cases in each group. For example, a sample having 50% females will show a profoundly different standardized effect than a sample having 80% females, even if the unstandardized b for gender is identical in the two samples. In general, only if the proportion of cases in each group represents the corresponding proportion in the population should standardized effects be reported.

4. More complex regression equations including interactions between categorical and continuous variables can be constructed. Returning to our priming example using dummy code scheme 1 (NP as reference group), imagine that each participant's level on the personal-

ity trait of openness to experience (O) was also measured at baseline. As usual, we center O, $O_C = O - M(O)$, to facilitate interpretation of the effects. The regression equation $\hat{Y} = b_0 + b_1 D_1 + b_2 D_2 + b_3 O_C + b_4 D_1 O_C + b_5 D_2 O_C$ provides a test of the interaction. Of importance, if we use the first dummy coding scheme described above, b_3 is the slope of the regression of Y on O in the no-prime (NP) reference group, b_4 is the difference between the slopes in the NP and T1 groups, and b_5 is the difference between the slopes in the NP and T2 groups. West, Aiken, and Krull (1996) and Aguinis (2004) present fuller discussions of methods of testing and interpreting categorical × continuous variable interactions.

Model and Data Checking

The previous sections have shown how researchers can test hypothesized models in multiple regression. However, there is no guarantee that the tested model is the correct one. If an incorrect model has been specified, the results of the regression analysis can be seriously misleading. Nor is there any guarantee that the data do not contain errors or unusual data points. We now consider a variety of graphical and statistical procedures that can help researchers assess the adequacy of their models and their data. Use of these procedures can potentially lead to a more adequate model that is tested with greater statistical power. Here, space limitations allow only a brief introduction. Fuller presentations are available in Cleveland (1993), Cohen and colleagues (2003, Chap. 4), and Weisberg (2005). West (2006) provides illustrations of the use of these procedures in several datasets.

Graphical Model Checking

Detecting Problems with the Regression Model

The predicted regression line is known as the *mean function*. To determine whether we have chosen the correct mean function for the data, we initially examine scatterplots of Y against each IV separately. Figure 33.3A depicts a scatterplot of the outcome anxiety (Y) versus stress (X_1) in an artificial dataset. Three plot enhancements known as lowess lines (Cleveland, 1979; Cook & Weisberg, 1999) are added to facilitate interpretation. The middle (mean) lowess line is a smoothed function that closely tracks the actual data, showing the actual relationship between the IV and DV with no regression model imposed. In Figure 33.3A the middle lowess line is curved rather than straight, suggesting that the mean function is curvilinear in form. The upper line is the mean lowess line + 1 SD; the lower line is the mean lowess line – 1 SD. Lowess estimates the SD at each value of the IV (here, each value of stress), so these SDs may vary. The examination of the lowess ± 1 SD lines permit us to examine the *variance structure* of the data. In our illustration the variability of the residuals around the mean lowess line increases as the value of X_1 increases. This plot indicates that our standard assumption of constant variance (homoscedasticity) of the residuals is not met.

Further information is provided by plotting the residuals against X_1 (see Figure 33.3B). Residual plots *magnify* any problems with the regression model, making misspecifications in the mean and variance structure even more evident. In Figure 33.3B, anxiety residuals are plotted against stress. The straight horizontal line (at 0 on the Y-axis) shows that the *linear* relationship between stress and anxiety has been removed. We are examining the residuals from a linear regression analysis predicting anxiety from stress. The middle lowess line shows that the curvilinearity remains. The two outer lowess lines capture the increasing variance in the residuals as stress increases. The re-

siduals should be plotted against each of the IVs and especially against $\hat{Y}$. The residuals should also be plotted against potentially important variables *not* in the model. If systematic relationships are observed, such findings identify any omitted variables that should be included in the model.

Graphical methods can also help detect potential interactions by examining more than one IV at a time. Conditioning plots (coplots; Cleveland, 1993) use a series of two-dimensional graphs, all plotted using the same scaling of the X- and Y-axes. The series of plots shows how the relationship between X_1 and Y changes as a function of the value of another IV, here X_2. The panels of Figure 33.4 present a series of co-plots. Each panel represents a different, successive range of values of X_2. In Figure 33.4, the IV X_1 for each graph is life events. The data for each graph are selected based on X_2, level of support. Each of the three panels of Figure 33.4 contains approximately one-third of the cases: (1) highest third (support = 4 or 5 friends), (2) middle third (support = 2 or 3 friends), and (3) bottom third (support = 0 or 1 friend). As we move up the panels, we see that the lowess line is approximately linear within each panel and that the slope of the line becomes increasingly flatter as X_2 increases. This pattern suggests that a linear × linear interaction provides an adequate representation of the data. The two-dimensional plot of the linear × linear interaction for these data was presented earlier in Figure 33.2B. Possible interactions

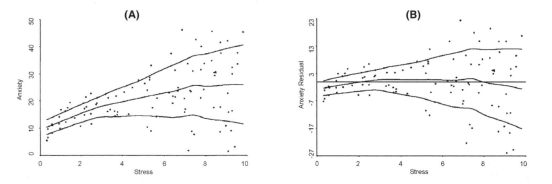

FIGURE 33.3. Scatterplots with superimposed lowess lines. (A). Raw data. Each point in the plot represents the scores on Stress and Anxiety for one participant. The three superimposed lines are lowess smooths. The middle line represents the best fitting nonparametric relationship between Stress and Anxiety (mean function). The upper and lower lines represent 1 SD above and below the mean function. They show that the variance increases as Stress increases. Artificial data. (B) Anxiety Residuals versus Stress. The points now represent the Residuals for each participant plotted against their value on Stress. Lowess lines representing the mean function and 1 SD above and below the mean function. The straight horizontal line in the center of the plot indicates where the residuals = 0.

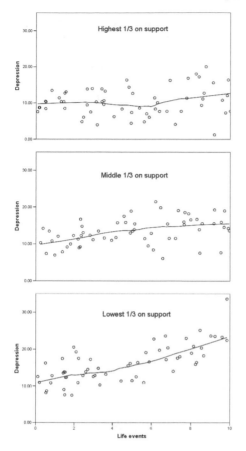

FIGURE 33.4. Three conditioning plots. Conditioning plots display the relationship between the focal IV (Life Events) and the DV (Depression) for different ranges on the moderator variable (Support). Each panel displays a scatterplot of the data for Life Events versus Depression for a different segment of the data. The lowess mean function representing the best nonparametric fit is superimposed. Panel (A) shows a nearly horizontal line for participants who have high scores on Support (4 or 5). Panel (B) shows an increasing relationship for participants who have moderate scores on Support (2 or 3). Panel (C) shows a more steeply increasing line for participants who have low scores on Support (0 or 1). The same artificial data are depicted as shown in Figure 33.2A.

can also be explored using three-dimensional plots. Lowess can be extended to provide a nonparametric surface that shows the relationship between two IVs and the outcome variable. When such nonparametric surfaces appear to be warped (not flat, as in Figure 33.1B), the warped pattern suggests the strong possibility of an interaction between the two variables. These plots are available using special interactive graphs (Igraph) in SPSS.

Remedies

When the mean function does not represent the data well, the researcher should explore the addition of other terms to the model (e.g., interaction, quadratic). These terms allow the model to more closely match the form of the mean structure in the data. In contrast, when problems with the variance structure are identified in large samples, the researcher should explore alternatives to OLS regression (e.g., weighted least squares) that specifically attempt to model nonconstant variance. When problems with both the mean structure and the variance structure are detected, the researcher should explore transformations of the data that may simplify the model or other extensions of regression analysis within the generalized linear model (see Cohen et al., 2003, Chap. 6, for an extensive treatment of transformations, and Chap. 13, for the generalized linear model). Cohen and colleagues (2003) and Weisberg (2005) present detailed discussions of these and other methods of detecting problems in regression models and their remedies. Graphical methods for model checking are now available in many major statistical packages (e.g., SPSS, S-Plus).

Data Checking

Detecting Errors and Unusual Cases

Initial examination of plots of each of the variables is an important and often overlooked aspect of MR. Univariate plots can depict the range of the data and areas in which data are sparse. This examination may suggest important limits in the inferences that may be drawn from the data. In addition, univariate plots can identify unusual cases known as *outliers*. For example, the BDI is often collected in studies of clinically depressed patients; scores within the range of roughly 20–50 may be expected (see

Figure 33.5). However, some patients may fall outside this range because of data entry errors (e.g., a BDI score of 30 is recorded as 3), the patient's inability to understand the questionnaire, or other reasons. Another example: Physiological measures of arousal such as galvanic skin response (GSR) have traditionally been collected in studies of reactions to emotional stimuli. However, unusual GSR responses will be obtained if the participant does not attend to the stimulus or hiccups immediately after its presentation. Such observations are known as "contaminated" cases. Although contaminated cases resulting from known failures of the experimental protocol should be flagged, such problems in the experimental protocol are not always observed by the researcher.

Cases with data entry errors or known failures of the experimental protocol must be corrected or dropped from the analysis. In other cases clear a priori rules can be developed for inclusion of data (say, a BDI score = 20–50 for a clinically depressed sample). The analysis is then limited to participants who meet the inclusion rules, and generalization of the findings is strictly limited to the population specified by the inclusion rules. But, not infrequently, the outlier may be a legitimate, but rare observation (e.g., clinically depressed, highly defensive individuals who have BDI scores in the range of 0–5; see Figure 33.5).

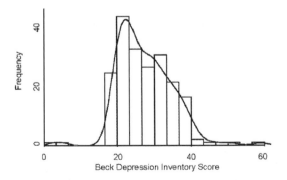

FIGURE 33.5. Histogram with superimposed kernel density estimate. The histogram depicts Beck Depression Inventory (BDI) Scores for a sample of clinical patients. The superimposed kernel density estimate line provides the optimal estimate of the distribution in this population. The data are clearly right skewed. Note the small clump of outliers with very low values on the BDI, which would not be expected in a clinical sample. Artificial data.

Special statistics have been developed that identify multivariate outliers and their effects in the MR model. These are *case statistics*, with each case having its own value on the statistic. For example, if there are 100 participants, there will be 100 of each of the different case statistics.

Leverage measures how extreme a case is in the set of IVs relative to the full sample. An extreme case in the IVs has the *potential* to distort the regression analysis—that is, to change the regression coefficients.[3] Leverage is useful in identifying cases of nonmeaningful responding (e.g., circling all 4's on a set of 5-point scales in which half of the items are reversed) or legitimate, but rare cases (e.g., a 12-year-old college freshman). Leverage measures the distance of the observed IVs for a case from the point representing the sample mean of all of the IVs. This measure is not affected by the regression model or the participants' scores on Y. As one very rough guideline, values of leverage greater than $2(p + 1)/n$, where p is the number of variables and n is the number of cases, identify roughly the most extreme 5% of cases in large samples.

Discrepancy refers to the difference between the predicted and the observed Y-values for each case. Because an extreme data point can strongly affect the regression line, the simple residual $(Y_i - \hat{Y}_i)$ is not the optimal measure of discrepancy. Instead, the *externally Studentized residual* t_i is typically preferred. For each case i in the dataset, a new regression equation is calculated based on all of the data, except that case i is deleted. The predicted value for case i is computed from the regression equation with case i deleted, $\hat{Y}(i)$. The deleted residual d_i is $(Y - \hat{Y}(i))$. This value is divided by the standard error SE_{di} of the deleted residual to yield the externally Studentized residual, $t_i = d_i/SE_{di}$. A value of t_i is calculated for each case in the dataset. Once again, cases with large values of t_i are outliers that have the *potential* to distort the results of the regression analysis. The values of the externally Studentized residual can be compared to a t-distribution. Because the number of cases identified as outliers increases as n increases, researchers typically use increasingly extreme cutoff values (or a Bonferoni correction of the critical t-value) to identify a reasonable number of the most important outliers for examination as the sample size gets larger. A value of ±3 may be used in a small sample, whereas ±5 may be used in a larger sample.

Influence refers to the effect that each case *actually* has on the results of the regression analysis. Influence is a function of the multiplicative product of both leverage and discrepancy. $DFFITS_{ij}$ provides a global measure of influence: How many standard deviations would the predicted value change if case i were deleted from the dataset? Values of $DFFITS_{ij} > 1$ for small or medium-size datasets are conventionally taken as identifying influential data points. $DFBETAS_{ij}$ provides a separate measure of how much the deletion of case i would affect each of the regression coefficients b_0, b_1, ... , b_p. Thus, including the intercept, $p + 1$ $DFBETAS_{ij}$ are calculated corresponding to each case. $DFBETAS_{ij}$ indicates the number of standard errors by which the regression coefficient for each IV (X_j) would change if case i were deleted. Values of $DFBETAS_{ij} > 1$ for small or medium-size datasets are often taken as identifying influential data points.

Remedies

When outliers representing an error or contaminated observation are detected, they should be corrected or deleted. When an outlier represents a legitimate but rare observation, the analyst is faced with a dilemma. Possible courses of action include taking no action, deleting the outlier, respecifying the regression model, or employing robust regression procedures that use alternatives to OLS estimation that are less sensitive to the influence of outliers (Wilcox, 2005). Each of these approaches has strengths and weaknesses (see Cohen et al., 2003, Chap. 10). For example, robust regression procedures use alternatives to OLS estimation that greatly reduce the influence of the outliers on the results of the regression analysis. In most cases, the results of robust regression procedures will be far more likely to be replicated in future samples. Robust regression procedures are now beginning to become available in standard statistical packages (e.g., SAS). However, robust regression can potentially hide misspecified models, the interpretation of the regression coefficients changes subtly, and alternative procedures may have to be used for significance testing, estimation of R^2, and the construction of confidence intervals (Cook, Hawkins, & Weisberg, 1992; Staudte & Sheather, 1990). It can be valuable to compare the results of multiple analyses. For example, the researchers may compare the results of

standard OLS regression, OLS regression with the outliers deleted, and robust regression. If the results of different approaches converge, as is often the case, it is extremely unlikely that the outliers are having a material influence on the results. However, if the results of different approaches diverge, then the researchers should report the results of multiple analyses and provide their best understanding of the source of the discrepancy.

Comments

1. Scatterplots with a lowess line for the mean function superimposed (implemented in SPSS Scatterplot) that depict the relationship between the IVs should also be plotted. Multiple regression analysis adjusts only for linear relationships between pairs of IVs. If the relationship between two different IVs deviates substantially from a straight line, then a transformation of the IVs that linearizes the relationship should be considered. In cases in which multiple terms are used to represent a single IV (e.g., X_1 and X_1^2 are used to represent the effects of X_1), the nonlinear relationship of the IV (here, X_1) to the DV is accounted for in the model.

2. Our presentation has emphasized graphical rather than statistical checking of model specification. Graphical data checking is more versatile and has the ability to detect a wider variety of problems than any statistical test. Many of the statistical tests are also very sensitive to violations of ancillary assumptions that may occur with real data (e.g., the Breusch-Pagan test of linear changes in residual variance is greatly affected by nonnormality of the residuals). More general statistical tests of violations of assumptions are often very low in statistical power. Thus, graphical methods appear to be more useful as a general approach to detecting problems with model specification, although statistical approaches may be more useful in cases in which a specific form of violation is hypothesized (e.g., linearly increasing variance of the residuals; see Weisberg, 2005).

3. The case statistics we have presented are useful in detecting single extreme cases (outliers) and are available in standard regression packages (e.g., SPSS, SAS). Graphical displays and specialized outlier statistics (e.g., Hadi & Simonoff, 1993) can be useful in detecting sets of multiple outliers ("clumps") that may be influencing the results. Such clumps may indicate

the existence of a small subgroup of cases from another population that is contained in the sample. For example, a clump of 14-year-old college freshmen may identify participants in a special university advanced placement program who are not part of the traditional freshman class.

Missing Data

In many areas of personality research, datasets with complete data on all participants are the rare exception rather than the rule. Participants may inadvertently fail to respond on an experimental trial, refuse to answer a question, fail to complete a timed test (e.g., Graduate Record Examination, GRE), not appear for a measurement session, or cease participation altogether in a longitudinal study. Standard multiple regression programs require complete data for analysis. Traditional methods of creating complete data such as mean substitution, listwise deletion, or pairwise deletion[4] typically produce less than optimal results. Far better results can be achieved through the use of modern missing data techniques. To understand these techniques, we need to distinguish among three types of missing data (Rubin, 1976). In practice, researchers typically do not know which type of missing data they have in their study.

Types of Missing Data

The first type of missing data is termed *missing completely at random* (MCAR). Imagine that 200 participants are randomly selected from a city and are measured on a quick self-report checklist of depression. The researcher then randomly selects 60 participants from the 200 who completed the self-report checklist and remeasures each of the 60 participants 1 month later, using an in-depth diagnostic interview (e.g., the Structured Clinical Interview for DSM-IV) that is believed to have much higher validity as a measure of clinical depression. The data on the interview are MCAR: No measured or unmeasured variable is expected to be related to whether a participant has or does not have an interview score.

The second type is termed *missing at random* (MAR). Imagine that the researcher selects the 60 participants scoring above a cut score on the checklist (high depressive symptomatology) and remeasures these individuals 1 month later

with the diagnostic interview. Now the data on the interview are missing at random. Once we adjust for the measured initial checklist score, no measured or unmeasured variable is expected to be related to whether a participant has an interview score.

The third type is termed *missing not at random* (MNAR). Imagine that the researcher invites all 200 participants to return for the diagnostic interview, but only 60 return. Now, the reasons for missingness of the diagnostic interview are no longer known and measured. Among many other possible reasons, participants may fail to appear because they have been hospitalized or have started abusing alcohol. The interview data obtained from the 60 returnees do not represent the population, but the explanation of the missingness and the nature of the needed adjustment of the data are unknown.

Modern Approaches to Missing Data

There are two modern approaches to missing data that provide unbiased estimates of parameters and correct standard errors when data are MCAR or MAR. Of importance, these methods also typically produce *less biased* results when data are MNAR. The two methods are *full information maximum likelihood* (FIML) estimation and *multiple imputation* (MI).

Full Information Maximum Likelihood

Conceptually, FIML identifies each pattern of missing data and estimates the means, variances, and correlations for each pattern. To illustrate conceptually how FIML works, consider a longitudinal study in which the researcher planned to measure the participants each year for 4 years. The table below depicts the patterns of data that were actually observed. Based on the 4 years of measurement (X1, X2, X3, X4) there are five patterns of missing data, where o = observed, M = missing, and *n* is the number of participants who show the pattern.

	X1	X2	X3	X4	*n*
Pattern 1	o	o	o	o	100
Pattern 2	o	o	o	M	40
Pattern 3	o	o	M	M	30
Pattern 4	o	M	o	o	20
Pattern 5	o	M	M	M	10

In this illustration, for pattern 1, in which the data are complete for all four measurements, estimates of the means and variances for X1, X2, X3, and X4 as well as the correlations between the six possible pairs of variables can be computed based on the 100 cases. In contrast, for pattern 3, only estimates of the means and variances for X1 and X2 and the X1-X2 correlation can be computed for the 30 cases. Finally, for pattern 5, only the mean and variance of X1 can be computed for the 10 cases. The estimates of the statistics for each pattern of data are computed and combined to produce overall estimates of the regression coefficients and their standard errors, based on all available data in the full sample. Unlike traditional approaches like pairwise deletion, FIML takes into account the number of cases associated with each missing data pattern. FIML produces estimates with standard errors that reflect all of the data that are actually observed. These estimates are unbiased, assuming that the data are MCAR or MAR. FIML estimation can now be easily implemented in many structural equation modeling programs (e.g., AMOS, EQS, MPLUS, MX).

Multiple Imputation

In MI (Rubin, 1987), m multiple copies of the dataset are created. Traditionally, $m = 5$ to 10 copies of the dataset were believed to be sufficient, but recent work suggests that more copies (e.g., 50) may be much better, particularly in small to moderate-size samples. If a value is observed for a participant for a given variable, that value is used in all copies of the dataset. If a value is missing, then a value is imputed from all other observed variables in the dataset. A key feature of MI is that random variation that matches the observed amount of random variation of the variable is added to each imputed value. For example, consider a participant who fails to complete X4 (pattern 2). Suppose that 6 is the predicted value for X4 for this participant, and, based on the observed cases for X4, the standard deviation of this estimate is 1.5. Rather than assigning a constant value of 6 across each copy of the dataset, values from roughly 3 to 9 [here, $6 \pm (2)(1.5)$, assuming normally distributed error] with an expected value of 6 would be assigned for this participant. This feature reproduces the original variability in the dataset. Each of the m copies of the dataset is then analyzed separately using standard regression analysis.

We now have m different estimates of each regression coefficient, each with a different standard error. To combine the different estimates, multiple imputation software (described below) is used. For each regression coefficient (e.g., b_1), the mean of the m estimates of that coefficient is calculated as the optimal value (e.g., M_{b_1}). The calculation of the standard error of each regression coefficient (e.g., s_{b_1}) is more complicated. First, the estimated standard errors are squared to convert these estimates to variances (e.g., $s_{b_1}^2$). Then the program uses a procedure that is essentially the opposite of the familiar decomposition used in analysis of variance. First, the mean of the m within imputation variance estimates is computed. Second, the between imputation variance is computed. These estimates are then appropriately weighted and combined to produce an estimate of the total variance. The square root of the total variance is the correct standard error. This standard error can be used to conduct significance tests[5] or to construct confidence intervals for the mean regression coefficient (e.g., M_{b_1}). Several excellent software packages, including both commercial (e.g., SAS PROC MI) and freeware versions (e.g., NORM [Schafer, 1997], a menu-driven program freely downloadable from Schafer's website (*www.stat.psu. edu/~jls/misoftwa.html*), are available to create multiple datasets. Other programs such as SAS PROC MIANALYZE and M-Plus combine the results of multiple analyses and compute hypothesis tests and confidence intervals.

The two modern approaches, FIML and MI, represent substantial advances over earlier approaches to regression analysis with missing data. Two of these, listwise deletion and pairwise deletion, which are the most easily available options in SAS and SPSS, continue to be fairly widely used in personality research, sometimes without acknowledgment of the existence of any missing data by authors. When data are MCAR, listwise deletion and pairwise deletion produce unbiased regression coefficients like MI and FIML. However, the standard errors are larger than with the modern approaches so that the power of the test will be reduced. When data are MAR, listwise deletion and especially pairwise deletion typically produce biased results. When data are MNAR, none of the methods may produce correct estimates, although the FIML and MI estimates are expected to be *less* biased representations of the population values than those based on listwise or pairwise deletion. However, listwise deletion does produce unbiased estimates of the regression coefficients *for the population who would provide complete data.* However, there is no guarantee that these individuals are representative of the population as a whole nor that a subsequent "exact replication" of the study could reproduce the same processes that led to the missing data in the initial study.

Excellent introductions to missing data analysis are available in Schafer and Graham (2002) and Allison (2002). More advanced statistical texts that provide thorough coverage of missing data issues are Little and Rubin (2002) and Schafer (1997).

Comments

1. FIML and MI are theoretically expected to produce identical results in very large samples. In sample sizes more representative of personality research, they typically produce very similar results.

2. Both methods assume multivariate normality. If some of the variables have markedly nonnormal distributions, a simple solution is to first transform the data so that they more closely approximate normality. Then MI can be used to create the copies of the transformed dataset. If desired, the copies of the transformed dataset can be transformed back to the original metric of each of the variables prior to analysis. In addition, if interactions (X_1X_2) or curvilinear effects (X_1^2) are hypothesized, these terms can be added to the dataset and their values imputed when data are missing. Otherwise, both FIML and MI may tend to underestimate interaction and curvilinear effects when data are missing.

3. The procedures described here apply most readily to data involving relatively continuous variables collected in a cross-sectional design. Other specialized procedures must be used with categorical variables and with longitudinal panel data. Presentations of these specialized procedures can be found in Little and Rubin (2002) and Schafer (1997). Advanced programs used in conjunction with S-Plus or R software that incorporate these specialized procedures are available at Schafer's (1997) website (given above). Recent advances in the understanding of missing data in longitudinal designs provide some ability to address data that are missing not at random.

4. MI has the advantage that all observed variables can be easily used to create the copies of the dataset, yielding more accurate imputed values. The IVs, DVs, and other background variables should all be included in the imputation process. This is a particular advantage if variables that predict missingness (e.g., distance from participant's home to measurement site) and demographic variables are included in the dataset. Once the multiple copies of the full dataset have been created, only the specific subset of variables that comprise the hypothesized regression model need be included in the analysis (see Collins, Schafer, & Kam, 2001).

5. When a large, rich dataset with hundreds of variables is collected, multiple imputation can become very cumbersome. Particularly when a large number of researchers are conducting different, overlapping analyses, keeping track of these multiple analyses involving multiple copies of the dataset can become overwhelming.

Statistical Power and Sample Size

Statistical power is the probability that an effect of a specified size in the population will be detected by a statistical test. Power depends on the specific statistical test, the effect size in the population, n (the sample size), and α (the Type I error rate). Power analyses should be routinely conducted prior to the beginning of a study to determine if there is sufficient sample size to detect the hypothesized effects; otherwise the study may not be worth conducting. Unfortunately, many researchers using multiple regression rely on misleading rules of thumb, such as 10 or 20 participants per predictor, rules that can often lead to the result that the study will *not* have sufficient power to detect the effect of interest even .50 of the time (Maxwell, 2000). Cohen (1969, 1988) proposed the convention that power = .80 is adequate; this convention has become the gold standard in the behavioral sciences.

Sample Size Estimation

When the population is large and easy to access, as is often the case with undergraduate populations, the typical question raised by researchers is, "How many participants are needed to detect the hypothesized effect with power = .80 using α = .05?" There are two separable sample size questions in multiple regression: (1) What is the n needed to detect a population R^2 of a specified value? (2) What is the n needed to detect a specified population regression coefficient (β). We focus on the second question here because it is typically of primary interest to personality researchers.

Central in the calculation of statistical power is the specification of an effect size in the population. Answering the question of what size effect is likely to occur can be challenging, but several practical strategies have emerged that may provide useful ideas. These are presented below, roughly ordered from best to worst in terms of the likely quality of the effect size estimate that will be obtained. But even a very rough estimate of the effect size can often provide a reasonable "ballpark estimate" of the sample size needed for a study (e.g., 500 rather than 100 cases). Such ballpark estimates are nearly always better than no estimate at all.

The quality of the effect size estimate will depend on the amount of data and the similarity of the proposed study to previous research. Meta-analyses often provide good estimates of the typical effect sizes and their variability in developed research areas, as well as information about potential factors that may modify those effect sizes. Standardized tests often provide good normative data about means, SDs, and correlations of scales (e.g., Costa & McCrae, 1992, offer norms for the NEO Personality Inventory [NEO-PI], based on very large samples). A series of previous studies (or even one) of the same or a related question in one's own or another laboratory can also be a good source of information about the size of effects. Pilot studies of the research question can also provide useful information, although the typical small size of pilot studies and changes in procedure between the pilot and planned studies can sometimes reduce the quality of the effect size information. Sometimes diverse sources of information about effect sizes can be combined, with the weight given to each source depending on the researcher's judgment about the similarity of the prior research context to that of the study currently being planned. When all else fails, Cohen (1988) has offered default normative values of small, medium, and large effect sizes based on his review of the behavioral science literature. Cohen suggested that the squared population correlation = .01, .09, and .25 and squared population partial correlations (pr^2) for individual IVs (or sets of IVs) of .02, .13, and .26 represent small, moderate, and large effects, respectively. Given uncertainty about the effect size, the sample size needed to detect a range of effect sizes can be computed (e.g., pr^2 = .10, .13, .16 for an effect expected to be approximately moderate in size). As we move from models involving linear relationships between the IVs and the DV to those involving interactive relationships, larger sample sizes are needed. Chaplin (1991; Chapter 34, this volume) reviews studies in personality psychology suggesting that interactions will typically have only small effect sizes; McClelland and Judd (1993) present theoretical analyses showing why small effects will characterize most research involving interactions in multiple regression. Although statisticians (e.g., Lenth, 2001) are justifiably skeptical of the generalization of such normative values to new research contexts, Cohen's moderate effect sizes tend to be similar to those that have been found in many meta-analyses in psychology and in the personality research area.

Estimation of Statistical Power

In other research contexts, there may be a more or less fixed number of participants that can be recruited. Examples include ongoing longitudinal studies in which the maximum number of potential participants is set by the number recruited at the beginning of the study, studies involving expensive measures such as magnetic resonance imaging (MRI), and studies involving rare populations such as individuals who experienced the death of a parent during early childhood. In such cases we can identify a feasible sample size, the effect size, and alpha, and then explore the statistical power of the tests. The question can be recast as, "What size effects can we detect with a given sample size based on the number of available participants or budgetary constraints?" In some cases it may turn out that important hypotheses cannot be addressed with anything approaching adequate statistical power. In those cases, it is important to explore other design and measurement approaches that may yield adequate statistical power.

Estimation of Sample Size and Statistical Power

Various approaches to computing power and sample size may be taken. Lenth (2001) prefers an approach based on using unstandardized effect sizes. His approach requires the specification of the number of predictors, the SD for each IV, the variance inflation factor (VIF, a measure of multicollinearity) for each IV, the standard deviation of the error ($\sqrt{MS_{error}}$), and the value of the unstandardized regression coefficient in the population. When reasonable values of all of these variables are known, Lenth's approach provides highly accurate estimates of sample size and power. However, in many research areas considerable uncertainty will be associated with the value of one or more of these inputs. A power calculator is available at his website, *www.stat.uiowa.edu/~rlenth/Power/*. In contrast, Cohen (1988) proposed using standardized effect sizes. As noted above, the researcher needs to specify the number of predictors in each set, the population R^2 for the first set of predictors, and the population squared semipartial or squared partial correlations (sr^2 or pr^2) for the predictor(s) of interest. This approach is somewhat less accurate than that of Lenth, but it is typically far easier for personality researchers to apply. Cohen's approach is implemented in commercial software (SPSS SamplePower) and in the freeware G-Power program (Erdfelder, Faul, & Buchner, 1996) available at *www.psycho.uni-duesseldorf.de/aap/projects/gpower/*). SAS has also recently implemented two different power analysis and sample size estimation programs relevant to multiple regression and the general linear model, PROC POWER and PROC GLMPOWER. We hope that the increasing awareness of available, easy-to-use power programs will reduce the proportion of underpowered studies in personality psychology.

Comments

1. Cohen's (1962) early review of the statistical power of articles published in the 1960 volume of the *Journal of Abnormal and Social Psychology* (*JASP*)[6] showed that power to detect moderate effect sizes that typify psychology was inadequate: mean power = .48. Rossi (1990) reported mean power = .55 for the 1982 volumes of *JPSP*, and Ward and Rossi (2005) reported mean power = .63 for the 2000 volumes of *JPSP*. This lack of sufficient power may reflect researchers' interests in studying more subtle effects (e.g., mediation, moderation) and their desire to control for additional IVs as research areas mature. More subtle effects imply smaller effect sizes, which require substantially larger sample sizes to achieve the desired level of statistical power. Unless other aspects of the design are changed, a 50% decrease in the effect size implies an approximate fourfold increase in the sample size to achieve the same level of statistical power. Statistical power to detect moderate effect sizes now does approach .80 in health psychology journals (Maddock & Rossi, 2001), perhaps reflecting the greater emphasis on adequate statistical power in health-related research.

2. Maxwell (2000) presents an alternative approach to power based on correlations. He warns that Cohen's choice of guidelines for small, moderate, and large pr^2 in the population often implies larger Pearson rs that we normally achieve in personality psychology. His own approach is limited, however, by the necessity to assume a common level of correlation (e.g., .3) between each pair of IVs other than the focal IV in the power analysis.

3. Following Wilkinson and colleagues' (1999) call for the use of confidence intervals instead of significance tests, Kelley and Maxwell (2003, in press) provide an excellent discussion of how to plan studies to have confidence intervals for regression coefficients with a specified width (precision). The SPSS add-on SamplePower and the freeware MBESS package (available from Ken Kelley's website, *www.indiana.edu/~kenkel/mbess/index.shtml*) that works in conjunction with R software will estimate the sample size needed to achieve a specified level of precision.

4. Nearly all discussions of statistical power emphasize increasing sample size as the primary method of increasing power. However, the effect size can also potentially be increased. In regression, sampling or manipulating the IVs so that their variance is increased (e.g., oversampling extreme values), sampling or manipulating the IVs so that their intercorrelations are decreased, using more reliable measures or other procedures that decrease the error variance, and minimizing the amount of missing data, coupled with applying FIML or MI to use all of the available data, can also increase statistical power. Of note, procedures that increase the variance of the distribution of the IVs, but leave the correlation between each pair of IVs unaltered, change the standardized coefficients and standardized effect sizes, but do not alter the estimates of the unstandardized regression coefficients.

In contrast, designs such as factorial experiments and sampling procedures that reduce the natural level of correlation between the IVs can also alter the unstandardized coefficients. The quantitative results of such designs can be generalized only to the hypothetical population created in the design. To illustrate, suppose we study participants' performance (PERF) as a function of their levels of anxiety (ANX) and depression (DEP), IVs that are normally highly correlated. We select participants so that anxiety and depression will be uncorrelated in our sample, then calculate the regression equation, $PERF = b_0 + b_1 ANX + b_2 DEP$. b_1 now represents the change in PERF for a 1-unit increase in ANX for a hypothetical population in which ANX and DEP are uncorrelated. Such analyses can provide important information about whether a theoretically important effect exists, but can tell us nothing about the magnitude of this effect in any real population.

Within-Subject Variables and Nonindependence

Standard multiple regression models assume that the data are collected independently from each participant. Although this assumption characterizes the majority of studies, new research areas have gained popularity in personality during the past decade in which this assumption will typically not be plausible. The same DV may be collected from the same participants over time, as in a daily diary study studying stress and coping over several weeks. Or the same DV may be measured in multiple situations, such as in a study of the mood reported in interactions with friends versus strangers. Or studies may involve intact groups such as families or classrooms, or artificial groups created in the laboratory that interact during the experimental session. In such applications in which independence is violated, regression models will yield proper estimates of the unstandardized effects. However, when the participants are not independent, the standard errors will be underestimated, often substantially. This result means that all hypothesis tests and confidence intervals will also be incorrect. We discuss extensions of multiple regression that address problems of nonindependence below. Some of these approaches go beyond simply modeling the dependency, allowing us to ask new and interesting research questions.

The Sum–Difference Approach

When there are two repeated measures conditions as in a pretest–posttest design, the sum–difference approach provides a simple solution. For example, imagine that a researcher collects a baseline measure of hostility (H) from participants. The participants then play an interactive game with a research assistant. The game is divided into two phases in which the researcher manipulates the interpersonal style of the assistant. During phase 1 of the game, the assistant is instructed to act in an agreeable manner. During phase 2 of the game, the assistant is instructed to act in a disagreeable manner. The DV is the participant's liking for the assistant after the completion of each phase of the game, Y_1 and Y_2.

We wish to construct a regression analogue to a between–within analysis of variance (ANOVA) To do this, two different composite DVs are constructed. The sum, $S = (Y_1 + Y_2)$ represents the participant's total liking of the assistant across the two phases of the game. The difference, $D = (Y_1 - Y_2)$ is the difference between the participant's ratings in the agreeable and disagreeable sessions. Following our usual practice, we would center hostility prior to the analysis, $H_C = H - M(H)$. Two separate regression equations are written that correspond to the between and within portions of the ANOVA, respectively. In the first equation (between subjects),

$$\hat{S} = b_0 + b_1 H_C \qquad (8A)$$

b_1 represents the main effect of hostility. In the second equation (within subjects),

$$\hat{D} = b_{0*} + b_{1*} H_C \qquad (8B)$$

b_{0*} represents the mean difference between the agreeable and disagreeable conditions and b_{1*} represents the hostility × partner style interaction. (In this notation * identifies a coefficient in the within-subjects equation that will generally differ from the corresponding coefficient in the between-subjects equation). Below we put the two equations together to create the multiple regression analogue of a between–within ANOVA in which hostility is a continuous between-subjects variable and assistant's style is a dichotomous within-subjects manipulation.

Between Subjects (Equation 8A)
  b_0—grand mean
  b_1—linear effect of hostility (H_C)
  Mean Square Residual (Equation 8A)
Within Subjects (Equation 8B)
  b_{0*}—main effect of assistant style
  b_{1*}—H_C × assistant style interaction
  Mean Square Residual (Equation 8B)

b_1, the effect of hostility, is tested against the appropriate between-subjects residual error term (mean square error) and b_{0*} and b_{1*} are both tested against the appropriate within-subjects error term. Although this approach can be extended to more than two within-subject treatment groups by creating $G - 1$ contrasts, such extensions can be more easily implemented within general linear model programs such as SAS PROC GLM and SPSS GLM.

To illustrate the GLM approach, imagine that the three priming conditions described in the previous section on categorical predictors were a within-subjects manipulation. Suppose that we had measured the IV Openness to Experience (O) and had created the centered Openness IV, $O_C = O - M(O)$. This IV would be specified as a continuous, between-subjects centered predictor. The three priming groups represent the IV, which would be specified as a within-subject variable. The software would provide (1) the 1 df test of the linear Openness main effect (tested with the between-subjects error term) and (2) the 2 df Priming main effect and the 2 df Openness × Priming interaction (both tested using the within-subjects error term). In addition, any of the dummy or contrast codes described previously could be used to create 1 df within-subjects hypothesis tests. Such tests have the advantage that they are focused on specific comparisons of interest rather than omnibus (overall) tests. These focused tests have more statistical power if the hypothesis of interest is true, and they do not require further consideration of the within-subject error structure. Except in rare cases in which the participants' residuals can be considered to be independent across the three repeated measures, an error structure (e.g., compound symmetry, autoregressive) must be specified. This error structure represents the form of the relationships between the residuals in the within-subjects conditions; it is specified in the form of a variance–covariance matrix of the residuals. We briefly consider this issue in our comments at the end of this section.

Multilevel Models

Multilevel models are used to address two typical forms of clustering in personality research.

1. The participants are grouped into higher-level units, as, for example, when participants are members of intact groups (e.g., classrooms) or experimental treatments are delivered to groups (e.g., different group psychotherapy treatments).
2. The participants are independent, but they are measured repeatedly, as in an event-sampling study of everyday experience (Reis & Gable, 2000). Here, participants are the higher-level units and observations within each participant are the lower-level units.

In both cases, the data analysis can conceptually be thought of as taking place at two levels of analysis. In practice, computer programs perform both levels of analysis simultaneously to optimize the estimates of all parameters.

Consider an event-sampling study in which observations are clustered within persons. We use as an illustration a study by Oishi, Diener, Scollon, and Biswas-Diener (2004), simplified for ease of presentation. Participants were randomly signaled several times a day for a week, resulting in about 40 observations per participant. When signaled, each participant identified the type of other people present in the situation [alone vs. friend(s) vs. family member(s)] and reported his or her current mood. The researchers also recorded the gender of each participant.

This is a multilevel data structure with two levels. Conceptually, we consider each level separately. At the lower, within-individual level, the IV is the type of other people present in the situation. One approach would be to use the following set of contrast codes.

	C1	C2
Alone	−0.67	0
Friend	+0.33	−0.5
Family	+0.33	+0.5

The first contrast, C1, compares the unweighted mean of the Friend and Family conditions with the mean of the Alone condition. The second contrast, C2, compares the mean of the Friend condition with the mean of the Family condition. We could then could write a separate equation to predict the mood of *each* participant at each observation:

$$MOOD_{ij} = b_{0i} + b_{1i}C1_{ij} + b_{2i}C2_{ij} \qquad (9)$$

Note the each of the variables now has two subscripts. $MOOD_{ij}$ is the reported mood for participant i on the jth observation. Similarly, $C1_{ij}$ and $C2_{ij}$ are the contrast codes that denote the type of other present for participant i at the jth observation. b_{0i} estimates the unweighted mean mood across all conditions, b_{1i} the magnitude of the first contrast, and b_{2i} the magnitude of the second contrast. We can imagine conducting this analysis separately for each participant, one for each of the i participants, resulting in a separate estimate of b_{0i}, b_{1i}, and b_{2i} for each of the 371 participants.

We then consider the higher level of the data structure; here the $n = 371$ individual participants. One individual difference variable, gender (-0.5 = male; $+0.5$ = female) was measured in our example. We can predict the three regression coefficients for the participants using three higher-level regression equations:

$$\hat{b}_{0j} = \gamma_{00} + \gamma_{01}Gender \qquad (10A)$$
$$\hat{b}_{1j} = \gamma_{10} + \gamma_{11}Gender \qquad (10B)$$
$$\hat{b}_{2j} = \gamma_{20} + \gamma_{21}Gender \qquad (10C)$$

In Equation 10A, γ_{00} is the mean of the 371 intercepts ("grand intercept"), which is the unweighted mean mood of the participants in the sample. γ_{01} is the difference in mean intercepts for females and males. In Equation 10B, γ_{10} is the mean of the 371 estimates of C1, the difference between the mean of the moods when participants were alone versus the unweighted mean of the moods when friends or family were present. γ_{11} is the difference between females and males on C1—that is, the discrepancy between males and females in how their moods varied when alone versus with others. This difference between differences represents a *cross level* interaction between Gender and C1 (described below). Note that Gender is at the higher level and C1 is at the lower level in our multilevel analysis. Finally, γ_{20} is the mean difference between the mean moods on C2, the contrast between the family and friends conditions, and γ_{21} is the difference between males and females on C2, again a cross level interaction.

To gain a greater understanding of the cross level interactions, we can write these equations in another way known as the *mixed model*. We do this by substituting the estimates of the regression coefficients at the higher level into the equation at the lower level of analysis.

$$\hat{MOOD}_{ij} = b_{0i} + b_{1i}C1_{ij} + b_{2i}C2_{ij} \qquad \text{(10A repeated)}$$

$$\hat{MOOD}_{ij} = (\gamma_{00} + \gamma_{01}Gender) + (\gamma_{10} + \gamma_{11}Gender)C1_{ij}$$
$$+ (\gamma_{20} + \gamma_{21}Gender)C2_{ij}$$

$$\hat{MOOD}_{ij} = \gamma_{00} + \gamma_{01}Gender + \gamma_{10}C1_{ij} + \gamma_{20}C2_{ij} \qquad (11)$$
$$+ \gamma_{11}GenderC1_{ij} + \gamma_{21}GenderC2_{ij}$$

In Equation 11 the Gender $\times$ C1 and Gender $\times$ C2 interactions become more apparent. The Gender $\times$ C1 interaction answers the question, "Do females show a larger (or smaller) difference in their moods when alone versus with others than do males?" The Gender $\times$ C2 interaction answers the question, "Do females show a larger (or smaller) difference in their moods when with family versus friends than do males?"

In our example, we only considered categorical predictors at the lower and higher levels of analysis. At the lower level, multilevel analysis can incorporate any categorical or continuous IV that varies across measurement occasions. For example, a measure of the current level of stress could be collected from each participant at each measurement occasion. At the higher level, multilevel analysis can incorporate any categorical or continuous IV that is stable over time (i.e., stable individual differences). For example, a measure of the Big Five variable of neuroticism might be collected from each participant at the beginning of the study. Cohen and colleagues (2003, Chap. 14) and Nezlek (Chapter 29, this volume) present an introduction to multilevel models, and Hox (2002), Raudenbush and Bryk (2002), and Snijders and Bosker (1999) provide more complete treatments. Multilevel analysis can be performed in packages such as SAS PROC Mixed, SPSS MIXED, and HLM (Raudenbush, Bryk, Cheong, & Congdon, 2004).

Growth-Curve Models

An important special case of multilevel data occurs for datasets in which *repeated* observations are collected from individuals over time. Researchers may have an interest in modeling the growth or decline of behaviors, abilities, or personality traits. In growth-curve models, a time-related variable becomes a key IV in the lower-level model for each individual. Typical examples of time-related IVs include the individual's age at each observation or the elapsed time at each observation since some significant event in the individual's life (e.g., college enrollment, marriage, divorce, retirement; see Biesanz, West, & Kwok, 2003, for a fuller presentation). These models are very flexible: All participants do not need to be measured at fixed time points or ages, and certain types of missing data (MCAR, MAR) can be accommodated without introducing bias (see the earlier section on missing data).

To illustrate: Imagine a researcher hypothesizes that there is growth in conscientiousness during early adulthood. During a two-decade period, she collects the same measure of conscientiousness (CON) every 3–5 years from a group of 100 participants. The participants are all in their early 20s at the beginning of the longitudinal study. The general form of the lower-level (within-individual) model including the error of prediction e_{ij} is

$$\hat{CON}_{ij} = b_{0i} + b_{1i}Age_{Sij} \qquad (12)$$

Care needs to be taken to scale Age to a metric Age_S (Age scaled), which has a meaningful 0 point. It makes little sense to interpret the level of conscientiousness at $Age = 0$ (birth). Consequently, the researcher may choose a value of $Age_S = Age - 21$ to represent the beginning of adulthood, a value of $Age_S = Age - 40$ to represent the end of the study and the approximate beginning of middle age, or some other theoretically meaningful value. We use $Age_S = Age - 21$ here. Using this model, we estimate a different line for each individual representing his or her linear change over the age period from 21 to 40. Figure 33.6 depicts the lines representing predicted linear change for each of a sample of 20 of the participants. Because we have $Age_S = 0$ when participants are 21 years of age, the intercept of the regression line for each individual depicts the conscientiousness of the individual at age 21.

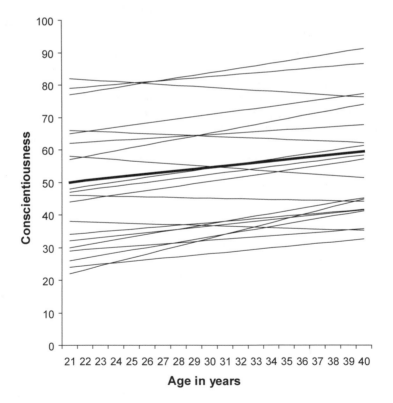

FIGURE 33.6. Individual growth lines. The estimated linear growth is depicted for 20 participants from the sample. Observations are collected between $Age = 21$ and $Age = 40$. Each light thin line represents a single participant. Note that the intercept and slope of the lines vary across participants. The dark thick line represents the mean line for all of the participants. In the analysis, scaled Age is used where $Age_S = Age - 21$, so that the intercepts represent conscientiousness at raw $Age = 21$.

We can now move to the higher level (between-subjects) and write equations for the intercept and slope. Suppose the researcher hypothesizes that the amount of parental discipline (DIS, 0–10 rating scale) that the participant received as a child will affect the development of conscientiousness. Following our usual practice, we initially center DIS, DIS_C = DIS – M(DIS). The following higher-level equations capture this hypothesis for the intercept (level at age 21) and slope.

$$b_{0i} = \gamma_{00} + \gamma_{01}DIS_{Ci} + r_{0i} \qquad (13A)$$
$$b_{1i} = \gamma_{10} + \gamma_{11}DIS_{Ci} + r_{1i} \qquad (13B)$$

In these equations, γ_{00} is the mean initial level of conscientiousness (at age 21) and γ_{01} is the increase in initial conscientiousness for each 1-unit increase in parental discipline. γ_{10} is the mean slope (growth rate) for all of the participants in the sample, and γ_{11} is the amount of change in the slope for each 1-unit increase in parental discipline. Once again, we observe that γ_{11} represents a cross level interaction of $DIS_C \times AGE_S$ (in Figure 33.6, the growth lines are not parallel). Finally, r_{0i} and r_{1i} represent the residual in predicting each individual's intercept and slope, respectively. The magnitude of the variance of the intercepts, $VAR(r_{0i})$ and the variance of the slopes $VAR(r_{1i})$ provide useful information for model development at the higher level. If substantial variance remains in the intercepts, slopes, or both, it may be possible to identify other stable individual difference variables that account for this variance.

Comments

1. We first return to our consideration of multilevel models in which participants are the lower-level units and groups are the higher-level units. The effect of clustering on the results of the analysis is a multiplicative function of the average group size and the intraclass correlation (ICC). If we define the variance of the intercepts as τ_{00} and the variance of the lower-level residuals as σ^2_e, then ICC = $\tau_{00}/(\tau_{00} + \sigma^2_e)$. The ICC may theoretically range from 0 to 1.0: Practical experience indicates that the values tend to range from 0 to roughly 0.2 in most research contexts, although higher values do occur. Suppose the researcher specifies α = .05 as the desired level of significance. With an ICC of .05 and group size = 10, the actual α = .11. If group size is increased to 20, the actual α = .28,

more than five times the stated α level. Another way to think about the effect of clustering is in terms of the design effect (Muthén & Satorra, 1995). The *design effect* = $1 + (n_g - 1)ICC$, where n_g is the average group size. The design effect indicates the factor by which the standard error will be too small. Thus, when the design effect is 2, this implies that the standard error will be one-half the proper size, or a 50% underestimate. When the group size is 1 or the ICC is 0, then the design effect is 1.0 and the observations are independent. Otherwise, the design effect will be larger than 1.0.

2. Hierarchical linear models can be extended to more than two levels. For example, a study that collected (a) repeated measures on (b) individuals interacting in (c) laboratory groups could be analyzed as a three-level model. Datasets in which there are very few units at the highest level (e.g., fewer than 20 groups) can lead to very low statistical power for the tests of the higher-level effects. Datasets in which the number of observations comprising each higher-level unit are small (e.g., three-person groups; three observation times) can sometimes lead to problems in estimation of some of the effects. Designs in which the number of observations per higher-level unit varies (e.g., group size averages three, but varies from two to five) can exacerbate these problems of small numbers of observations per unit.

3. Datasets in which the observations are made at different times (e.g., participant 1 is measured at ages 20, 24, 30, 33, 38; participant 2 is measured at ages 21, 24, 28, 35, 40) present no difficulties for estimating growth models using multilevel modeling software. Such data can also be properly analyzed using structural equation modeling packages (e.g., Amos, EQS, MX, M-Plus,) so long as they include full information maximum likelihood (direct maximum likelihood) estimation options (see Mehta & West, 2000).

4. A variety of exciting extensions of growth models are possible that include different forms of growth, growth in different life stages (e.g., Piagetian stages), and relationships between concomitant or sequential growth processes. These more advanced applications are discussed in Biesanz and colleagues (2003), Bollen and Curran (2006), Collins and Sayer (2001), McArdle and Nesselroade (2003), and Singer and Willett (2003).

5. The growth models discussed in this sec-

tion provide the proper adjustment for the clustering at the higher (individual participant) level. However, they do not provide an adjustment for the possibility that the $e_{ij}s$, the lower-level residuals taken from subject i across times j, may be correlated over time in a repeated measures design. In general, residuals that are closer together in time (e.g., adjacent mood ratings) tend to be more similar than those that are farther apart. Multilevel modeling packages permit specification of within-subject error structures that can help reduce or eliminate this problem and provide proper statistical tests (see Kwok, West, & Green, in press; Weiss, 2005). Utilization of many of these error structures requires a constant rather than a varying elapsed time period between observations (e.g., a fixed measurement interval of 4 hours rather than a mean interval length of 4 hours, with a range of 2–4 hours). Proper specification of the within-subject error structure avoids estimates of the standard errors that are too small and the resulting inappropriate hypothesis tests and confidence intervals.

6. A variety of other approaches, that answer different questions, may be taken to longitudinal data in personality. Biesanz and colleagues (2003), Ferrer and McArdle (2003), Khoo, West, Wu, and Kwok (2006), McArdle and Nesselroade (2003), Mroczek (Chapter 31, this volume), Muthén (2004), and West and Hepworth (1991) provide introductions to many of the available approaches and issues in this area.

Summary

In this chapter we have reviewed many of the applications of multiple regression to personality data. Theories in personality hypothesize a variety of forms of relationships involving diverse forms of data. We have considered how multiple regression can represent simple linear relationships, curvilinear relationships, and interactions between two or more independent variables. These independent variables may be qualitative (categorical), quantitative, or mixtures of the two. We also considered tools that help researchers assess problems in both the regression model and in the data, particularly outliers and missing data. We identified alternative analysis strategies that provide remedies to these problems. We also considered the often overlooked problem of ensuring that the

planned study has sufficient statistical power to detect the hypothesized effect. Finally, we considered extensions of multiple regression that address nonindependence of observations that result from clustering of the data in higher-level units or the collection of repeated measures over time from each individual. Some of these approaches are well represented in the personality research literature, whereas others are just beginning to appear. In each case, we tried to identify important issues that arise in the context of personality research, particularly those that are not well understood. These issues carry over to a number of other chapters in this volume. Multiple regression provides foundational understanding for many more advanced statistical techniques, such as multilevel modeling, structural equation modeling, and analyses such as logistic regression that consider other forms of dependent variables (e.g., binary variables, ordered categories) that do not approximate a continuous variable. Given its wide use by personality researchers, its ability to answer diverse research questions, and the foundation it provides for a number of important new statistical techniques, multiple regression has truly become the data-analytic workhorse of the personality researcher.

Notes

1. Textbooks such as Cohen et al. (2003, Chaps. 1–10), Fox (1997, Chaps. 1–13), and Pedhazur (1997, Chaps. 1–15) provide more in-depth presentations of these issues for a general behavioral science audience.
2. A substantial minority of the articles failed to include direct information about the magnitude of the relationship, reporting only the p-value, or stating that the relationship was significant, or reporting the overall R or R^2 for the regression equation.
3. As discussed later in this section, the extent to which a case with high leverage *actually* affects the regression coefficients is also dependent on the discrepancy between the predicted and observed values of the DV.
4. Mean imputation fills in missing data with the mean value of the variable to create a dataset with the original number of cases. Listwise deletion considers only those cases with complete data on *all* of the variables in the analysis. In pairwise deletion, a correlation is calculated based on the available data for each pair of variables. The resulting correlation matrix is analyzed by the program as if it were calculated from

complete data. Various rules have been proposed to estimate a sample size for regression analyses based on pairwise deletion, inasmuch as the number of cases associated with the computation of each correlation will typically differ.

5. The logic of the computation of the degrees of freedom (df) is also complex as they are based on a Satterthwaite approximation. dfs are provided by software packages.

6. *JASP* split in 1966 into the *Journal of Abnormal Psychology* and the *Journal of Personality and Social Psychology*. Cohen (1977) revised his normative guidelines for medium effect sizes slightly in 1977.

7. Sources on ANOVA (e.g., Maxwell & Delaney, 2004, pp. 504–597) consider between–within designs in which the between-subjects IV is a categorical grouping variable. Here, H is continuous. The analogous ANOVA error terms would be $MS_{\text{Subjects within H}}$ and $MS_{\text{Assistant Style} \times \text{Subjects within H}}$.

Recommended Readings

Aiken, L. S., & West, S. G. (1991). *Multiple regression: Testing and interpreting interactions*. Newbury Park, CA: Sage.

Cohen, J., Cohen, P. West, S. G., & Aiken, L. S. (2003). *Applied multiple regression/correlation analysis for the behavioral sciences* (3rd ed.). Mahwah, NJ: Erlbaum.

Cook, R. D., & Weisberg, S. (1999). *Applied regression including computing and graphics*. New York: Wiley.

Fox, J. (1997). *Applied regression analysis, linear models, and related methods*. Thousand Oaks, CA: Sage

Kelley, K., & Maxwell, S. E. (in press). Power and accuracy for omnibus and targeted effects: Issues of sample size planning with applications to multiple regression. In P. Alasuuta, J. Brannen, & L. Bickman (Eds.), *Handbook of social research methods*. Newbury Park, CA: Sage.

Schafer, J. L., & Graham, J. W. (2002). Missing data: Our view of the state of the art. *Psychological Methods*, 7, 144–177.

Snijders, T., & Bosker, R. (1999). *Multilevel analysis*. London: Sage.

Weisberg, S. (2005). *Applied linear regression* (3rd ed.). New York: Wiley.

References

Abelson, R. P., & Prentice, D. A. (1997). Contrast tests of interaction hypotheses. *Psychological Methods*, 2, 315–328.

Aguinis, H. (2004). *Regression analysis for categorical moderators*. New York: Guilford Press.

Aiken, L. S., & West, S. G. (1991). *Multiple regression: Testing and interpreting interactions*. Newbury Park, CA: Sage.

Aiken, L. S., West, S. G., & Pitts, S. C. (2003). Multiple linear regression. In J. Schinka & W. Velicer (Eds.), *Comprehensive handbook of psychology: Vol. 2. Research methods in psychology* (pp. 483–507). New York: Wiley.

Algina, J., & Moulder, B. C. (2001). A note on estimating the Jöreskog-Yang model for latent variable interactions using LISREL 8.3. *Structural Equation Modeling*, 8, 40–52.

Allison, P. D. (2002). *Missing data*. Thousand Oaks, CA: Sage.

Atkinson, A. C. (1985). *Plots, transformations and regression: An introduction to graphical methods of diagnostic regression analysis*. Oxford, UK: Clarendon Press.

Azen, R., & Budescu, D. V. (2003). The dominance analysis approach for comparing predictors in multiple regression. *Psychological Methods*, 8, 129–148.

Biesanz, J. C., West, S. G., & Kwok, O.-M. (2003). Personality over time: Methodological approaches to the study of short-term and long-term development and change. *Journal of Personality*, 71, 905–941.

Bollen, K. A., & Curran, P. J. (2006). *Latent curve models: A structural equation perspective*. New York: Wiley.

Budescu, D. V. (1993). Dominance analysis: A new approach to the problem of the relative importance of predictors in multiple regression. *Psychological Bulletin*, 114, 542–551.

Chaplin, W. F. (1991). The next generation of moderator research in personality. *Journal of Personality*, 59, 143–178.

Cleary, P. D., & Kessler, R. C. (1982). The estimation and interpretation of modifier effects. *Journal of Health and Social Behavior*, 23, 159–169.

Cleveland, W. S. (1979). Robust locally weighted regression and smoothing scatterplots. *Journal of the American Statistical Association*, 74, 829–836.

Cleveland, W. S. (1993). *Visualizing data*. Summit, NJ: Hobart Press.

Cohen, J. (1962). The statistical power of abnormal-social psychological research: A review. *Journal of Abnormal and Social Psychology*, 65, 145–153.

Cohen, J. (1969). *Statistical power analysis for the behavioral sciences*. New York: Academic Press.

Cohen, J. (1977). *Statistical power analysis for the behavioral sciences* (Rev. ed.). New York: Academic Press.

Cohen, J. (1988). *Statistical power analysis for the behavioral sciences* (2nd ed.). Mahwah, NJ: Erlbaum.

Cohen, J., & Cohen, P. (1975). *Applied multiple regression/correlation analysis for the behavioral sciences*. Hillsdale, NJ: Erlbaum.

Cohen, P., Cohen, J., Aiken, L. S., & West, S. G. (1999). The problem of units and the circumstance for POMP. *Multivariate Behavioral Research*, 34, 315–346.

Cohen, J., Cohen, P., West, S. G., & Aiken, L. S. (2003).

Applied multiple regression/correlation analysis for the behavioral sciences (3rd ed.). Mahwah, NJ: Erlbaum.

Collins, L. M., & Sayer, A. G. (Eds.). (2001). *New methods for the analysis of change*. Washington, DC: American Psychological Association.

Collins, L. M., Schafer, J. L., & Kam, C. M. (2001). A comparison of inclusive and restrictive strategies in modern missing-data procedures. *Psychological Methods, 6*, 330–351.

Cook, R. D., Hawkins, D. M., & Weisberg, S. (1992). Comparison of model misspecification diagnostics using residuals from least mean of squares and least median of squares fits. *Journal of the American Statistical Association, 87*, 419–424.

Cook, R. D., & Weisberg, S. (1999). *Applied regression including computing and graphics*. New York: Wiley.

Costa, P. T., Jr., & McCrae, R. R. (1992). *Revised NEO Personality Inventory and NEO Five Factor Inventory (NEO-FFI) professional manual*. Odessa, FL: Psychological Assessment Resources.

Cumming, G., & Finch, S. (2005). Inference by eye: Confidence intervals and how to read pictures of data. *American Psychologist, 60*, 170–180.

Erdfelder, E., Faul, F., & Buchner, A. (1996). GPOWER: An general power analysis program. *Behavior Research Methods, Instruments, and Computers, 28*, 1–11.

Ferrer, E., & McArdle, J. J. (2003). Alternative structural models for multivariate longitudinal data analysis. *Structural Equation Modeling, 10*, 493–504.

Fox, J. (1997). *Applied regression analysis, linear models, and related methods*. Thousand Oaks, CA: Sage.

Fox, J., & Monette, G. (1992). Generalized collinearity diagnostics. *Journal of the American Statistical Association, 87*, 178–183.

Hadi, A. S., & Simonoff, J. S. (1993). Procedures for the identification of multiple outliers in linear models. *Journal of the Royal Statistical Society, Series B, 54*, 761–777.

Hox, J. (2002). *Multilevel analysis: Techniques and applications*. Mahwah, NJ: Erlbaum.

Hunter, J. E., & Schmidt, F. L. (2004). *Methods of meta-analysis: Correcting error and bias in research findings*. Thousand Oaks, CA: Sage.

Kelley, K., & Maxwell, S. E. (2003). Sample size for multiple regression: Obtaining regression coefficients that are accurate, not simply significant. *Psychological Methods, 8*, 305–321.

Kelley, K., & Maxwell, S. E. (in press). Power and accuracy for omnibus and targeted effects: Issues of sample size planning with applications to multiple regression. In P. Alasuuta, J. Brannen, & L. Bickman (Eds.), *Handbook of social research methods*. London: Sage.

Khoo, S.-T., West, S. G., Wu, W., & Kwok, O.-M. (2006). Longitudinal methods. In M. Eid & E. Diener (Eds.), *Handbook of multimethod measurement in psychology* (pp. 301–317). Washington, DC: American Psychological Association.

Kromrey, J. D., & Foster-Johnson, L. (1999). Statis-

tically differentiating between interaction and nonlinearity in multiple regression analysis: A Monte Carlo investigation of a recommended strategy. *Educational and Psychological Measurement, 59*, 392–413.

Kwok, O.-M., West, S. G., & Green, S. B. (in press). The impact of misspecifying the within-subject covariance structure in multiwave longitudinal multilevel models: A Monte Carlo study. *Multivariate Behavioral Research*.

Lenth, R. V. (2001). Some practical guidelines for effective sample size determination. *American Statistician, 55*, 187–193.

Little, R. J. A., & Rubin, D. B. (2002). *Statistical analysis with missing data* (2nd ed.). New York: Wiley.

MacCallum, R. C., & Mar, C. M. (1995). Distinguishing between moderator and quadratic effects in multiple regression. *Psychological Bulletin, 118*, 405–421.

MacCallum, R. C., Zhang, S., Preacher, K. J., & Rucker, D. D. (2002). On the practice of dichotomization of quantitative variables. *Psychological Methods, 7*, 19–40.

Maddock, J. E., & Rossi, J. S. (2001). Statistical power of articles published in three health psychology-related journals. *Health Psychology, 20*, 76–78.

Maxwell, S. E. (2000). Sample size and multiple regression analysis. *Psychological Methods, 5*, 434–458.

Maxwell, S. E., & Delaney, H. D. (1993). Bivariate median splits and spurious statistical significance. *Psychological Bulletin, 113*, 181–190.

Maxwell, S. E., & Delaney, H. D. (2004). *Designing experiments and analyzing data: A model comparison perspective* (2nd ed.). Mahwah, NJ: Erlbaum.

McArdle, J. J., & Nesselroade, J. R. (2003). Growth curve analysis in contemporary psychological research. In J. Schinka & W. Velicer (Eds.), *Comprehensive handbook of psychology: Vol. 2. Research methods in psychology* (pp. 447–480). New York: Wiley.

McClelland, G. H. (1997). Optimal design in psychological research. *Psychological Methods, 2*, 3–19.

McClelland, G. H., & Judd, C. M. (1993). Statistical difficulties in detecting interactions and moderator effects. *Psychological Bulletin, 114*, 376–390.

Mehta, P., & West, S. G. (2000). Putting the individual back in individual growth curves. *Psychological Methods, 5*, 23–43.

Muthén, B. O. (2004). Latent variable analysis: Growth mixture modeling and related techniques for longitudinal data. In D. Kaplan (Ed.), *Handbook of quantitative methodology for the social sciences* (pp. 345–368). Newbury Park, CA: Sage.

Muthén, B. O., & Satorra, A. (1995). Complex sample data in structural equation modeling. *Sociological Methodology, 25*, 267–316.

Neter, J., Kutner, M. H., Nachtsheim, C. J., & Wasserman, W. (1996). *Applied linear regression models* (3rd ed.). Chicago: Irwin.

Oishi, S., Diener, E., Scollon, C. N., & Biswas-Diener, R. (2004). Cross-situational consistency of affective experiences across cultures. *Journal of Personality and Social Psychology, 86*, 460–472.

Pedhazur, E. J. (1997). *Multiple regression in behavioral research: Explanation and prediction* (3rd ed.). Fort Worth, TX: Harcourt Brace.

Piexoto, J. L. (1987). Hierarchical variable selection in polynomial regression models. *American Statistician, 41*, 311–313.

Pitts, S. C. (1993). *The utility of extreme groups analysis to detect interactions among correlated predictor variables*. Unpublished master's thesis, Arizona State University.

Preacher, K. J., Curran, P. J., & Bauer, D. J. (2006). Computational tools for probing interaction effects in multiple linear regression, multilevel modeling, and latent curve analysis. *Journal of Educational and Behavioral Statistics, 31*, 437–448.

Raudenbush, S. W., & Bryk, A. S. (2002). *Hierarchical linear models: Applications and data analysis* (2nd ed.). Thousand Oaks, CA: Sage.

Raudenbush, S. W., Bryk, A. S., Cheong, Y. F., & Congdon, R. (2004). *HLM 6: Hierarchical linear and nonlinear modeling*. Lincolnwood, IL: Scientific Software.

Reichardt, C. S., & Gollub, H. F. (1999). When confidence intervals should be used instead of statistical significance tests, and vice versa. In L. L. Harlow, S. A. Mulaik, & J. H. Steiger (Eds.), *What if there were no significance tests?* (pp. 259–284). Mahwah, NJ: Erlbaum.

Reis, H. T., & Gable, S. L. (2000). Event-sampling and other methods for studying everyday experience. In H. T. Reis & C. M. Judd (Eds.), *Handbook of research methods in social and personality psychology* (pp. 190–222). New York: Cambridge University Press.

Rosenthal, R., Rosnow, R. L., & Rubin, D. B. (2000). *Contrasts and effect sizes in behavioral research: A correlational approach*. New York: Cambridge University Press.

Rossi, J. S. (1990). Statistical power of psychological research: What have we gained in 20 years? *Journal of Consulting and Clinical Psychology, 58*, 646–656.

Rubin, D. B. (1976). Inference and missing data (with discussion). *Biometrika, 63*, 581–592.

Rubin, D. B. (1987). *Multiple imputation for nonresponse in surveys*. New York: Wiley.

Schafer, J. L. (1997). *Analysis of incomplete multivariate data*. New York: CRC Press.

Schafer, J. L., & Graham, J. W. (2002). Missing data: Our view of the state of the art. *Psychological Methods, 7*, 144–177.

Seber, G. A. F., & Wild, C. J. (2003). *Nonlinear regression* (2nd ed.). Hoboken, NJ: Wiley.

Serlin, R. C., & Levin, J. R. (1985). Teaching how to derive directly interpretable coding schemes for multiple regression analysis. *Journal of Educational Statistics, 10*, 223–238.

Singer, J. D., & Willett, J. B. (2003). *Applied longitudinal data analysis: Modeling change and event occurrence*. New York: Oxford University Press.

Snijders, T. A. B., & Bosker, R. J. (1999). *Multilevel analysis: An introduction to basic and advanced multilevel modeling*. Thousand Oaks, CA: Sage.

Staudte, R. J., & Sheather, S. J. (1990). *Robust estimation and testing*. New York: Wiley.

Wainer, H. (2000). The centercept: An estimable and meaningful regression parameter. *Psychological Science, 11*, 434–436.

Ward, R. M., & Rossi, J. S. (2005). *Are we there yet? Examining the statistical power and effect sizes in three psychology journals*. Unpublished manuscript, Miami University, Oxford, OH.

Weisberg, S. (2005). *Applied linear regression* (3rd ed.). New York: Wiley.

Weiss, R. E. (2005). *Modeling longitudinal data*. New York: Springer-Verlag.

West, S. G. (2006). Seeing your data: Using modern statistical graphics to display and detect relationships. In R. R. Bootzin & P. E. McKnight (Eds.), *Strengthening research methodology: Psychological measurement and evaluation* (pp. 159–182). Washington, DC: American Psychological Association.

West, S. G., Aiken, L. S., & Krull, J. L. (1996). Experimental personality designs: Analyzing categorical by continuous variable interactions. *Journal of Personality, 64*, 1–48.

West, S. G., & Hepworth, J. T. (1991). Data analytic strategies for temporal data and daily events. *Journal of Personality, 59*, 609–662.

Wheaton, B. (1985). Models for the stress-buffering functions of coping resources. *Journal of Health and Social Behavior, 26*, 352–364.

Wilcox, R. R. (2005). *Introduction to robust estimation and hypothesis testing* (2nd ed.). Burlington, MA: Elsevier Academic Press.

Wilkinson, L., & the APA Task Force for Statistical Significance. (1999). Statistical methods in psychology journals: Guidelines and explanations. *American Psychologist, 54*, 594–604.

## CHAPTER 34

Moderator and Mediator Models in Personality Research

A Basic Introduction

William F. Chaplin

The decades of the 1960s, 1970s, and 1980s were a traumatic time for the field of personality psychology. In 1968, Walter Mischel published his critique of the field and many otherwise thoughtful psychologists reached what is now recognized as the premature conclusion that individual differences were not useful *at all* for predicting and understanding behavior. During these decades funding for personality research was greatly reduced, *JPSP* was the *Journal of personality and SOCIAL Psychology*, and many psychology departments reduced their commitment to teaching personality and training personality psychologists. This era has been labeled the "Dark Ages" of personality, or even more fancifully, the Mischelian "ice age" (Westen, 1995), and the attitude of some scholars was that they could not wait until personality theories became "historical curiosities" (Farber, 1964).

For the past decade or so, the field of personality has been enjoying a renaissance (Swann &

Seyle, 2005). In part, this renaissance has been fueled by the recognition that the early critiques of personality were based on methodologically and statistically naive methods that included the use of unreliable behavioral measures (Epstein, 1983), the arbitrary (e.g., median split) dichotomization of continuous personality measures (Chaplin, 1991), the comparison of correlations rather than regression slopes in many analyses (Chaplin, 1997), and the tendency to report only significant results that confirmed hypothesis (Chaplin & Goldberg, 1984). However, the field of personality also learned some hard lessons from this experience (Kenrick & Funder, 1988) and the field's renaissance has also been influenced by applying these lessons to contemporary personality research.

Historically, the field of personality conducted research using what I have labeled the "*r*'s and stars approach" (Chaplin, 1994). In the extreme version of this approach, a relatively large number of self-report measures are administered to a modest sample of, typically, college students and the resulting data are used to compute correlations between the measures. One then inspects the output (usually in SPSS using the "Flag significant correlations" option) to see which correlations have a "*" next to them, indicating statistical significance at the .05 level. In some cases, multiple stars are used to indicate more profound significance levels (two stars for the .01 level, three stars for the .001 level, and so on). Thus, the "Paris Hilton" of correlations would be a five-star ($p <$ .00001) r, and investigators seldom see the need to go beyond this level.

Although this simple approach to personality research is still difficult to resist, the hard lesson the field has learned is that to be taken seriously, personality research must go beyond merely correlating self-report measures with self-report measures among college students and seeing what r's get stars. Much of the renaissance enjoyed by the field has resulted from testing hypotheses about the relation of personality to meaningful outcomes in samples of participants taken from relevant populations. Indeed, editorial guidelines (e.g., Funder, 1994) in major personality journals now tend to explicitly address this issue, and the fields of health psychology (e.g., Barefoot, Dahlstrom, & Williams, 1983), industrial/organizational psychology (Hogan, 2005), and forensic psychology (Krueger et al., 1994), among others, have proven to be fruitful areas for such research.

In addition to focusing on meaningful outcomes in relevant populations using different modes of assessment, the field of personality has also come to recognize that simple bivariate correlation and regression hypotheses involving personality variables are generally uninteresting and not useful for demonstrating either the scientific importance or practical utility of personality constructs. This chapter concentrates on the conceptual and data-analytic issues involved in testing models that go beyond the simple hypothesis that a personality variable is related to an outcome. Specifically, this chapter addresses the evaluation of hypotheses that (1) personality constructs combine (interact) to predict an outcome or that personality constructs impact (moderate) the effect of a treatment, risk factor, or experimental manipulation—what West, Aiken, and Krull (1996) referred to as "experimental per-

sonality designs," and (2) the relation between a personality variable and an outcome is mediated (explained) by other variables, or that personality variables may themselves mediate some relations. These models are presented primarily as specific applications within the general data-analytic platform of multiple regression analysis described by West, Aiken, Wu, and Taylor, Chapter 33, this volume.

Moderator Models

Basics

The specification of, rationale for, and statistical evaluation of moderator models have been well described in a large number of texts and articles for some time (e.g., Aiken & West, 1991; Baron & Kenny, 1986; Chaplin, 1997; James & Brett, 1984). Moreover, extensions of moderator analysis beyond the basic ordinary least squares regression to generalized linear models and mixed regression (multilevel) models have been clearly and compellingly described in the more recent literature (e.g., Cohen, Cohen, West, & Aiken, 2003; Judd, Kenny, & McClelland, 2001; Kenny, Mannetti, Pierro, Livi, & Kashy, 2002). In this section I summarily recapitulate the basics of moderator models. Far more detail is provided in the aforementioned references and most any graduate-level text on data analysis for the behavioral sciences.

A moderator model elaborates on a simple or simpler linear model by specifying a condition or conditions that may impact (increase, decrease, or otherwise change) the relation between an independent variable and a dependent variable. That is, moderator models provide the "it depends" answer to scientific questions. For example, when my child asks, "If I finish my homework, may I watch television?" the standard parental response "It depends" (e.g., on when you finish, on what you want to watch, and so on) is a moderator response. The relation between finishing homework and watching television is moderated by when the homework is finished and so on. As a less parental example, consider the hypothesis that conscientiousness is positively related to job performance. This simple hypothesis is certainly wrong, at least in the sense that it will not be universally true. Instead, the rational conclusion about the status of this hypothesis (and all other scientific hypotheses) is that "it depends" (e.g., on the nature of the job, the type of the performance measure, the neuroticism of the employee, and so on). As I (Chaplin, 1997) and others (e.g., Cronbach, 1975) have suggested, the certainty of the existence of moderator effects makes hypotheses about moderator effects scientifically treacherous. Simply hypothesizing that a relation between two or more variables is moderated by other variables is trivially true. The meaningful testing of moderator hypotheses requires, at a minimum, a clear specification of the moderator variables involved, the mechanisms of their action, and the specific effect a moderator has on the relation between the variables in question.

The statistical evaluation of a moderator hypothesis requires specifying a hierarchical regression (which can be ordinarily linear or generalized, such as logistic or mixed) model in which the initial model regresses the dependent variable (DV; often symbolized by Y) on the independent variable (IV; often symbolized by X) and moderator (M) and the second model adds the product of X and M (Cohen, 1978). There are few restrictions on the IV and/or the moderator; they can be either continuous or categorical (with appropriate coding using dummy, effects, or contrast coefficients), they can be represented by single variables or sets of variables, and lower-order (e.g., using two-way products) moderator effects can be further moderated by additional moderator variables (e.g., using three-way, four-way, etc., products). The most basic moderator model is shown in Equations 1 and 2. In SPSS, such hierarchical models can be specified by entering the IV(s) and M(s) in the first block and adding their product(s) in the second block; higher-order products can be added in later blocks.

$$Y = B_0 + B_1X + B_2M \qquad (1)$$
$$Y = B_0 + B_1X + B_2M + B_3M*X \qquad (2)$$

where B_0 is the model constant or intercept, and B_1, B_2, and B_3 are the unstandardized partial regression coefficients ("regression weights," "slopes") for X, M, and the $X*M$ product, respectively.

The statistical evaluation of the moderator effects represented in these models is based on the increment in the degree to which the model with the product term(s) fit the observed data over the degree to which the model without the product term fits the data. In standard (ordinary least squares, or OLS) regression, the increment in fit is the increase in the squared multiple correlation obtained by adding the product terms (also called the squared semipartial correlation between the product term and the Y—called a "part" correlation in SPSS). In situations where the DV is not appropriate for OLS regression, (the two most common situations in the study of personality are dichotomous outcomes and dependent (repeated measures) outcomes), the evaluation of hierarchical models is based on maximum likelihood (as opposed to least-squares) estimation, and log-likelihoods for the two hierarchical models are compared ("−2LL test") using a chi-square distribution.

As anyone who has ever seriously analyzed data knows, the devil of data analysis is in the details, and this brief overview contains almost no detail. Readers who need more detail are referred to the books and articles mentioned at the beginning of this section. Before turning to a discussion of moderator models in the more specific context of personality research, I close with three points that are sometimes overlooked in the analysis of moderator models.

1. The product term is *not* the moderator effect; rather, the term "carries" the effect, because product terms must be partialed with respect to all the lower-order terms they contain. So, a two-way product must have the two direct effects partialed from it before the two-way product becomes a moderator effect; a three-way product must have the three direct effects, as well as the three two-way products among those three variables, partialed before it becomes a moderator effect, and so on (Cohen, 1978). The reason that the partialed product represents the moderator effect is that such effects are statistically independent of the direct relations between the variables that form the product and the criterion. In the analysis of variance the interaction effect is a residual effect that is literally based on the between-cell sums of squares (SS) after the SS of the main effects are subtracted out. That is, $SS(A \times B) = SS(\text{between}) - SS(A) - SS(B)$. Extending this to regression analysis, the product term is generally correlated with the variables that are multiplied together to create the product. To make the product independent of the terms that create it, those terms are partialed from the product. Thus, it is the residualized product, just

like the residualized between groups sums of squares, that represents the moderator effect.

2. The lower-order effects should *not* be statistically evaluated in the context of the higher-order product terms. For example, the direct effects of X and M should not be evaluated statistically in the context of their product (X*M). As described above, product terms are generally correlated ("multicollinearity") with the terms that are multiplied together to create them. Although it is necessary to partial out this redundancy when evaluating the product, it is wrong to "back partial" the redundancy of the product from the terms that formed the product. If one were to evaluate a direct effect of variable X after partialing its created association with the product, one would essentially be evaluating X after controlling for X.

3. Tests of differences between correlations are not the same as tests of moderator effects. So, if the correlation between openness-to-experience and firmness of handshake is different for men and women (Chaplin, Phillips, Brown, Clanton, & Stein, 2000) this does not necessarily imply that gender moderates the relation between openness-to-experience and handshake firmness. As always, correlations index the fit of the model to the data, whereas the unstandardized partial regression weights *are* the model (slopes). Generally, a moderator effect concerns the model (is the change in handshake firmness for, say, a standard deviation change on openness different for men and women?) rather than the fit of the model (which may be influenced by, for example, greater range attenuation, measurement unreliability, or skewness in one group as compared with the other).

Applications to Personality Research

There are two main applications of moderator models that can be fruitful for testing hypotheses about the relation of personality to important outcomes. One application is based on using moderator models to combine individual personality constructs into two-, three-, (or even more) way interactive composites. The second application is treating personality constructs as moderators of the relation between situational factors, often experimentally manipulated, in a hybrid research design called "experimental personality research" (West et al., 1996).

Personality × Personality Interactions

Ask any person on the street, and he or she will readily tell you that there is a difference between the types of behaviors you can expect from an extravert you can trust and an extravert you cannot trust. Indeed, in our everyday lives we all know that our friends are not just extraverts, but undependable, agreeable, emotionally stable, and/or close-minded extraverts, and so on. Applied areas of psychology have also long shown an appreciation of the importance of viewing an individual client's personality as a constellation of personality traits that combine (interact) to produce an outcome. This is most readily seen in the use of diagnostic profiles that are provided by scoring services for the Minnesota Multiphasic Personality Inventory (MMPI), the 16 Personality Factors Inventory (16-PF), NEO Personality Inventory (NEO-PI), and other major multidimensional personality instruments. However, these profiles are typically interpreted at the level of the individual in the tradition of Gordon Allport (1961). In the nomothetic tradition of basic personality research, the incorporation of interactive combinations of personality characteristics into research questions and statistical models has been slower to catch on, although this appears to be changing (see, e.g., Morey et al., 2002; Warr, Bartram, & Martin, 2005; Witt, 2002; Witt, Burke, Barrick, & Mount, 2002).

CONCEPTUAL ISSUES

The fundamental idea behind the personality × personality research design is that the effect of personality constructs on important outcomes is more than the sum of those constructs. That is, a linear model such as the one shown in Equation 3 that simply includes more than one personality characteristic as independent variables does not capture the spirit of this approach.

$$\text{Sales performance} = B1(\text{extraversion}) \quad (3)$$
$$+ B2(\text{conscientiousness})$$

The issue is not merely whether different characteristics each make important unique additive contributions to the prediction of an outcome; rather, the issue is whether the synergistic (interactive) combination of personality characteristics contribute to the prediction of the outcome over and above the individual characteristics. Thus, it is possible that being extraverted predicts two sales/month because an extravert meets people to whom to sell the product, and being conscientious independently predicts another two sales/month because the conscientious salesperson ensures that items are in stock when people want them. Thus, using Equation 3, we would predict that a conscientious extravert would make four sales a month. This, however, is an additive prediction, not an interactive prediction. A conscientiousness × extraversion *interaction* would require an added unique increment for sales beyond the additive model. For example, there could also be the added benefit that a conscientious extravert will not only find people but will also write down pertinent information about these people, such as their children's names, and this *interaction* of extraverted and conscientious skills will add four more sales/month to the conscientious extravert's total sales because people buy from a person they feel they know. So the expected total monthly sales for a conscientious intravert would be two, for an unconscientious extravert the expected monthly sales would also be two, and for the conscientious extravert the expected monthly sales would be eight. This scenario is modeled in Equation 4.

$$\text{Sales performance} = B1(\text{extraversion}) \quad (4)$$
$$+ B2(\text{conscientiousness})$$
$$+ B3\,(\text{extraversion} \times \text{conscientiousness})$$

In formulating personality × personality interaction hypotheses, it is critical that one not confuse the idea that several different characteristics may add together to impact an outcome with the idea that the interactive combination of variables further impacts the outcome. It is perhaps easier to distinguish additive and interactive models when neither variable alone impacts the outcome and it is only the interactive combination that has the impact. Such situations, which would be represented by a fully disordinal or "crossed" interaction, are, however, likely to be difficult to find and harder to replicate because of the overwhelming evidence suggesting that direct linear relations tend to be more powerful than configural (interactive) ones (see Chaplin, 1997, for a summary of many examples in the literature). So it is critical that personality × personality interactive hypotheses not be confused with personality + personality additive ones, and this caution is particularly important because personality × personality hypotheses must always be framed with an understanding that they will almost certainly occur against a background of personality + personality additive ones.

Another important conceptual issue in approaching the personality × personality interactions is that the possible number of such interactions available from even a relatively small number of personality variables is quite large. For example, with just five personality variables there are 10 two-way interactions, 10 three-way interactions, 5 four-way interactions, and 1 five-way interaction, for a total of 26 interactions that could be evaluated. If an investigator wished to consider the 30 facets from the NEO-PI, the number of possible two-way interactions alone would be 435 and the number of possible three-way interactions would a staggering 4,060. Even the most adventurous of investigators would likely find the Type I error rate from "exploring" all these personality × personality interactions unacceptable. So to make the study of how personality variables interact to produce an effect tractable, it is critical to begin with a theory (Chaplin, 1997) and to be disciplined in one's approach (Cronbach, 1975; Epstein, 1983). Indeed, the technology available in today's high-speed computers make it possible to "mine" large numbers of moderator models for possible findings. Essentially, this exploratory tactic would be akin to the earlier r's and stars approach to personality research, taken to the next level. An interesting example of an approach to mining datasets for interactions that is perhaps acceptable can be found in O'Conner and Dvorak (2001).

STATISTICAL APPROACH

The data-analytic procedures for testing a personality × personality model are reasonably straightforward and are described in detail in Cohen and colleagues (2003) in their discussion of interactions among continuous variables. There are two preliminary steps to prepare the data for this analysis. First, all of the personality variables involved in the analyses as independent (predictor) variables (IV) should be centered around their means. Second, the products of the personality variables that will represent the relevant personality × personality interactions should be computed. These steps are illustrated (in SPSS) in Figure 34.1.

After the data have been prepared, the moderator model is evaluated using a series of regression models that have a hierarchical relation to each other. A hierarchical relation occurs when one model contains all the variables or sets of variables in a previous model plus an additional variable or set of variables.

Thus, Equation 4 in the preceding example is in a hierarchical relation to Equation 3, because Equation 4 contains all the variables in Equation 3 plus the product term. In SPSS, hierarchical regression is easily accomplished using the "Block" feature on the menus or with the syntax shown in Figure 34.2. Also shown in Figure 34.2 is the abridged output that is useful for evaluating the moderator model.

The example analyses in Figure 34.2 are based on actual data; however, the names of the variables have been changed to protect the

1. Calculate means of IVs.

```
DESCRIPTIVES
  VARIABLES=extrav agree consci neurot open
  /STATISTICS=MEAN STDDEV MIN MAX .
```

Descriptive Statistics

	N	Minimum	Maximum	Mean	Std. Deviation
extrav	650	1.3333	5.0000	3.274219	.6551735
agree	650	1.4444	5.0000	4.097949	.5919883
consci	650	2.0000	5.0000	4.057906	.5724961
neurot	650	1.0000	5.0000	2.738379	.8457092
open	650	1.6111	5.0000	3.470217	.5537930
Valid N (listwise)	650				

2. Center the IVs—for example:

```
COMPUTE cextrav = extrav-3.274291 .
EXECUTE .
```

And check the centering (Means all = 0; standard deviations unchanged)

Descriptive Statistics

	N	Minimum	Maximum	Mean	Std. Deviation
cextrav	650	−1.94	1.73	.0000	.65517
cagree	650	−2.65	.90	.0000	.59199
cconsci	650	−2.06	.94	.0000	.57250
cneurot	650	−1.74	2.26	.0000	.84571
copen	650	−1.86	1.53	.0000	.55379
Valid N (listwise)	650				

3. Compute the products to represent the relevant interactions.
For example, for a two-way (Extraversion × conscientiousness):

```
COMPUTE cexcc = cextrav * cconsci .
```

For a three-way (Extraversion × conscientiousness × agreeableness):

```
COMPUTE cexccxca = cextrav * cconsci * cagree .
EXECUTE .
```

FIGURE 34.1. Illustration of data preparation for testing personality × personality moderator models using SPSS.

Syntax

```
REGRESSION
/STATISTICS COEFF CI R CHANGE ZPP
/DEPENDENT leadership
/METHOD=ENTER cextrav cconsci /METHOD=ENTER cexcc.
```

Model Summary

Model	R	R Square	Adjusted R Square	Std. Error of the Estimate	Change Statistics				
					R Square Change	F Change	df1	df2	Sig. F Change
1	.526(a)	.277	.271	.4116874	.277	47.695	2	249	.000
2	.567(b)	.321	.313	.3996232	.044	16.261	1	248	.000

a Predictors: (Constant), cconsci, cextrav
b Predictors: (Constant), cconsci, cextrav, cexcc

Coefficients(a)

Model	Unstandardized Coefficients		Standardized Coefficients	t	Sig.	95% Confidence Interval for B		Correlations		
	B	Std. Error	Beta			Lower Bound	Upper Bound	Zero-order	Partial	Part
1 (Constant)	3.207	.026		123.652	.000	3.156	3.258			
cextrav	.501	.065	.461	7.724	.000	.374	.629	.514	.440	.416
cconsci	.148	.071	.123	2.063	.040	.007	.288	.322	.130	.111
2 (Constant)	3.173	.026		119.760	.000	3.121	3.226			
cextrav	.499	.063	.459	7.914	.000	.375	.623	.514	.449	.414
cconsci	.183	.070	.153	2.621	.009	.046	.321	.322	.164	.137
cexcc	.435	.108	.213	4.033	.000	.222	.647	.170	.248	.211

a Dependent Variable: leadership

FIGURE 34.2. Illustration of syntax and output to evaluate personality × personality interactions using hierarchical regression.

priority of substantive publications based on the results shown here. The two personality variables are extraversion and conscientiousness, and the dependent variable is a supervisor rating of leadership ability. The last line of the syntax presented in Figure 34.2 creates the hierarchical analysis. Specifically, the first METHOD = ENTER command creates the personality + personality (extraversion + conscientiousness) additive model that needs to be evaluated prior to, and, as argued above, in distinction from, the personality × personality interactive model, which is added in the second METHOD = ENTER command.

The first box of output provides the basic statistical evaluation of the personality × personality interaction as distinct from the personality + personality additive one. The critical column in this box is labeled "R Square Change." This column shows that the personality + personality model (Model 1) accounts for 27.7% of the variance in leadership and that the additional variance accounted for by the personality × personality interaction is 4.4%. The statistical test of these indices is provided by the F distribution, and for both the personality + personality model ($F_{2, 249} = 47.7$) and the increment from the personality × personality interaction ($F_{1, 248} = 16.3$) the size of these observed effects would be unlikely ($p < .001$) if the true effect size was zero (the standard null hypothesis test). Note that the 4.4% could be calculated directly from the Model R-Squares (second column) as $.321 - .277 = .044$.

The second box shows the model parameters for evaluating the personality + personality model (Model 1) and the personality × personality model (Model 2). The inferential tests (t-tests) are, of course, equivalent for both the unstandardized and the standardized (labeled "Beta" in SPSS) coefficients. However, interpretation of the models should generally be based on the unstandardized coefficients, as these provide information about how the independent variables in the model translate into the dependent variables in terms of the units of measurement of the variables. Many psychological measures are in units that seem to be arbitrary (e.g., 5-point or 7-point scales), and this has tended to lead investigators to focus on standardized model parameters (which are essentially unitless). The issue of the measurement of psychological constructs is a critical one for the behavioral sciences that goes well beyond the scope of this chapter (see, e.g.,

Blanton & Jaccard, 2006). However, Likert and other types of rating scales typically have labels on the response options, which can provide a guide for presenting and interpreting results, and the recommendation here is that model interpretation be based on the unstandardized coefficients.

In the present example, Extraversion and Conscientiousness and the Leadership ratings are based on 5-point scales ranging from 1 = Not at All to 5 = Highly. Thus, for the personality + personality model, an individual who is at the group average on Extraversion and Conscientiousness would be predicted to be slightly above the midpoint (3.207) on Leadership. For a person who was very high on both Extraversion and Conscientiousness (2 points above the midpoint) we would predict that this person would score about 1.3 scale points higher on Leadership ($.501 × 2 = 1.002$ and $.148 × 2 = .296$; $1.002 + .296 = 1.298$). Thus, the predicted level of Leadership for such an individual would be $3.207 + 1.298 = 4.505$, or indicating that he or she is between a moderately and highly effective leader. In contrast, a person who was Not at All Extraverted and Conscientious would be predicted to receive a rating of $3.207 - 1.298 = 1.909$, indicating a somewhat ineffective leader. Also shown in the second box are several alternatives for evaluating the relation of the IVs to the DV. These include the 95% confidence intervals around the unstandardized model parameters and the zero-order, partial, and semipartial (labeled "Part" by SPSS) correlations between the IVs and DV.

The parameter estimates in the second box in Figure 34.2 for Model 2 provide a means for evaluating the personality × personality model. The evaluation of interactions between two continuous variables has been thoroughly discussed in Aiken and West (1991) and Cohen and colleagues (2003), among other sources. The emphasis here is, again, using the unstandardized model parameters to predict scores on the DV and using these predicted scores as the basis for interpretation. Specifically, one can predict four scores from the model that correspond to the High-High, Low-Low, High-Low, and Low-High combinations of the two personality variables. These four scores can then be used to plot regression lines that reflect the interaction effect as well as the main effects (additive) in the data. The definition of "high" and "low" for continuous variables is somewhat arbitrary, but conventionally one uses +/–

1 standard deviation to indicate high and low values, respectively.

Based on the values shown in Figure 34.2, the following predicted values are computed, using +/–.66 (standard deviation of Extraversion) and +/–.57 (standard deviation of Conscientiousness) to define High and Low values on Extraversion and Conscientiousness, respectively.

High/High = 3.173 + .499(.66) + .183(.57)
+ .435(.66 × .57) = 3.173 + .33 + .10
+ .16 = **3.763**

High/Low = 3.173 + .499(.66) + .183(–.57)
+ .435 (.66 × –.57) = 3.173 + .33 – .10
– .16 = **3.243**

Low/High = 3.173 + .499(– .66) + .183(.57)
+ .435(–.66 × .57) = 3.173 – .33
+ .10 – .16 = **2.7**

Low/Low = 3.173 + .499(– .66) + .183(– .57)
+ .435(–.66 × –.57) = 3.173 – .33 – .10
+ .16 = **2.903**

Using the predicted values (**in bold**), we can construct the plots of predicted values shown in Figure 34.3. Two plots are shown in Figure 34.3 because it is arbitrary as to whether Extraversion or Conscientiousness appears on the *x*-axis and it is often helpful for interpretation to plot predicted values from both perspectives. Based on these plots, it is clear that Extraversion is the dominant characteristic in this model for predicting leadership. However, although Conscientiousness has a smaller overall effect, the combination of High Extraversion and High Conscientiousness does lead to more effective leadership (by about a half point (B = .435) for someone who is 1 point higher on both characteristics (say, a score of 4, as compared to 3)) than one would expect from simply adding the two together. Alternatively, one could couch the interpretation as a recommendation for someone seeking to hire individuals for positions requiring leadership. If faced with a choice between an extravert who is not so conscientious and a conscientious person who is not so extraverted, one should prefer the former candidate. However, holding out for a person who has both qualities would be optimal, depending on how high the person is on both characteristics.

SPSS again provides confidence intervals for the unstandardized parameter estimates as well as both zero-order and partial coefficients. These values provide alternative perspectives on evaluating the personality × personality models. It is perhaps useful to note that the squared Part correlation for the product term ($.211^2$ = .044) is the same as the R Square Change value in the first box. This is, of course, as it should be, as the increment in the R-square is the definition of the squared semi-partial correlation. Finally, although the printout provides parameter estimates, correlational effect sizes, and significance tests for the Extraversion and Conscientiousness in this model, these values are misleading as they reflect values partialed with respect to the product term. The personality + personality model parameters are appropriately evaluated in Model 1.

The personality × personality model can be extended to third-, fourth-, or higher-order models. The procedures for testing such higher-order models are logical extensions of the ones described here. That is, lower-order terms must be partialed from the higher-order ones so that personality × personality × personality models are evaluated independently of not only personality + personality models, but also the simpler personality × personality ones. Investigators embarking on formulating hypotheses about such models are cautioned that as interactions increase in complexity, the statistical power to detect them generally decreases owing to the reduction in degrees of freedom, the decreased reliability of the product terms (Chaplin, 1997), and the reduction in effect sizes that results from appropriately removing all variance associated with lower-order effects from the higher-order terms. In addition, the conceptual challenges of interpreting higher-order interactions should not be overlooked and neither should the computation of predicted scores for interpreting the models. For example, to interpret a four-way interaction one would have to predict 2^4 = 16 scores each from an equation containing 15 (4 direct effects, 6 two-way interactions, 4 three-way interactions, and 1 four-way interaction) weighted predictor variables plus a constant.

Personality × Treatment Interactions

The belief held by many, that situations are inherently more powerful than personality characteristics for predicting behavior, has not been supported by direct empirical evaluation (e.g., Funder & Ozer, 1983). Indeed, variance in behavior associated with person factors has been shown to be larger than the behavior vari-

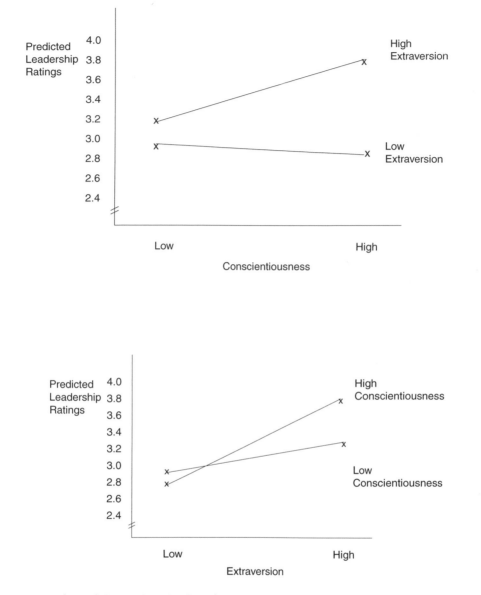

FIGURE 34.3. Plots of the predicted values from Model 2 to interpret the personality × personality interaction.

ance associated with either situations or person × situation interactions in some circumstances (Kenny, Mohr, & Levesque, 2001). Nonetheless, belief in the monolithic power of situations persists.

One reason for the persistence is that, historically, analyses that include both continuous person variables and categorical experimental ones tended to be done in an analysis of variance framework that required imposing (usually arbitrarily with a median split) categories on the person variables. Although the use of regression/correlation as a more general data-analytic platform has obviated the need to dichotomize continuous measures, the unfortunate categorization of continuous measures is still practiced in some literatures (e.g., Chen, Lee-Chai, & Bargh, 2001; Dechesne, Janssen, & van Knippenberg, 2000). The practice of dichotomizing personality measures strongly biases the analyses in favor of the experimental variables because of the attenuation in effect size, and therefore loss of statistical power, that occurs when a continuous variable is dichotomized (Cohen, 1983). In addition, imposing categories on continuous variables can lead to spurious detections of moderator effects (Maxwell & Delaney, 1993), and the practice is truly silly from a measurement perspective (see Figure 34.4). Thus, when person variables are forced to unfairly compete as dichotomies with situational variables, the finding that situational variables "win" is not particularly meaningful or interesting.

However, there is another reason for the persistent belief in the power of situations that has not been as widely acknowledged by personality psychologists. Under circumstances where situational variables are powerful, generally when they are experimentally manipulated to be so, those situational variables often have a stronger effect on outcomes than personality variables. Although this conclusion may seem to border on the heretical for an audience of personality psychologists, a little reflection suggests that it must be true. If we compare the utility of the experimental variable "run over by a truck" (dummy coded as 1 = run over and 0 = not) to a measure of conscientiousness for predicting mortality, the experimental variable will be a better predictor by any definition of *better* (e.g., statistical significance, effect sizes, likelihood ratios) we choose. Less fancifully (and more ethically), in an efficacy-focused clinical trial using an aggressive multistep treatment combining behavioral and pharmacological interventions to reduce depression, the effect of the treatment on reduction of depression symptoms over time will be better (by any definition) than a measure of conscientiousness at predicting reduction of symptoms. Figure 34.5 shows the pattern of individual differences among patients treated aggressively to lower depression (again, the data are real, the variable names are not). From baseline to 6 months, nearly everyone responds the same way to treatment. From Month 12 to Month 36, the patients are in a maintenance phase in which individual differences can play a more important role. For personality psychologists, searching for individual differences as moderators of the treatment response from Months 0 to 6 would be Quixotic, but searching for a role for individual differences in the maintenance phase would be, perhaps, fruitful.

Thus, experimental and treatment variables are under the control of the investigator and can be manipulated to be very powerful,

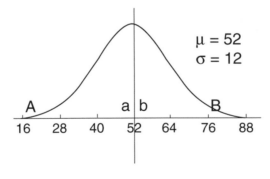

Extraversion

Using the median split as a measure, individuals below 52 all get a score of 0 on Extraversion and individuals above 52 get a score of 1. Thus, according to the median split measure person **b** (score = 53) has the identical level of Extraversion as person **B** (score of 77) and a ***different*** level of Extraversion than person **a** (score of 51), who, by the way is the same as person **A** (score of 17). This is just silly.

FIGURE 34.4. The silliness of the median split as a measurement operation on continuous variables such as extraversion.

Individual Patterns of Depression Symptoms Over Time

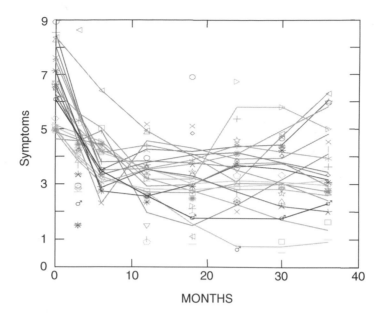

FIGURE 34.5. Illustration of individual differences (or lack thereof) in the context of strong treatment strategies.

whereas investigators cannot manipulate personality—research participants come as they are. The closest personality investigators can come to manipulating their variables is to select participants on the basis of extreme scores (e.g., contrast the upper and lower 10% of hostile people on some outcome), but such a strategy defeats a major strength of personality research, which is its naturalistic emphasis. The statistical, psychometric, and interpretive issues associated with the extreme groups approach have recently been explicated by Preacher, MacCallum, Rucker, and Nicewander (2005). This article is a critical reference for anyone considering using extreme groups approaches. Although experimental manipulation is often viewed as a stronger research method than naturalistic observation, experiments can be more cynically viewed as randomly doing unnatural things to people to see what happens. From this perspective it is not clear that naturalistic, but uncontrolled, personality research is inferior to unnatural, but controlled, experimentation. But the point here is not that one method is better than the other—rather, that both methods have their strengths and weaknesses. In fact, and in contrast to social psychologists who generally as-

sign no importance to individual differences, personality psychologists have always acknowledged that situations, and especially manipulated situations, can have strong influences on human behavior (Goldberg, 1972). That treatments have a potentially strong effect on human behavior is, of course, a positive conclusion. After all, a major goal of applied psychology is to effect positive change at both the individual and societal level, and we can perhaps best accomplish this via treatments and manipulations.

That experimental manipulations and treatments can have powerful effects on human behavior, and that such variables can generally be made to be more powerful predictors of human behavior than personality variables, is a realistic appraisal for the field of personality psychology to make. However, the extension of this appraisal to the conclusion that personality variables and other individual differences are unimportant, meaningless, or epiphenomenal would be a grave error for both basic research and applied interventions. It would be a grave error because as powerful as experimental manipulations can be, it is equally clear that not everyone responds to manipulations, risk factors, and treatments in the same way. Not all children raised in abusive homes become abusive parents, not all depressed patients respond to CBT (cognitive-behavioral therapy), not all people who smoke die young, not all people who receive motivational interviewing adhere to medication protocols, and not all participants in Milgram's (1963) demonstration of obedience killed the confederate (Blass, 1999). Indeed, in the field of medicine the tremendous breakthroughs in human genetics are creating much excitement about the possibility of tailoring pharmaceutical treatments based on individual genetic differences (see, e.g., Ross et al., 2004). So, a second major application of moderator models is in testing the role of personality as a moderator of treatment effects or risk factors.

CONCEPTUAL ISSUES

The search for individual differences that moderate the effects of treatments/manipulations and risk exposure is hardly new. From the very beginnings of the analysis of variance, the within-cell variation has proven seductive to personality psychologists. Historically, such variation was dismissed as "error," and this was justified because of the random assignment of people to experimental conditions. But such variation is "error" to those whose only interest is in the treatment's general or average effect on human behavior. For those interested in individual differences, this variation is a potential treasure trove of systematic individual differences. However, harnessing the within-cell variation to improve the efficacy of education via aptitude × treatment interactions (e.g., Cronbach, 1967) or psychotherapy via patient × treatment interactions (Dance & Neufeld, 1988) or to enhance our understanding of the consistency of human behavior (Chaplin & Goldberg, 1984) has proven to be one of the most elusive goals in behavioral science research (Chaplin, 1997).

So, why should we continue to pursue the search for person × situation (e.g., treatment, risk factor) interactions? One reason is simply that finding meaningful and replicable person × situation interactions would pay great dividends. The ability to explain why some people respond to one treatment but not another, or why risk factors work differently for different people, would allow the tailoring of treatments or prevention programs to patients. This, in

turn, would provide the health care system with greater credibility and cost-effectiveness, it would provide patients with sensible treatment and lifestyle options, and it would provide the field with the higher moral ground of providing the best empirically supported treatments for those patients empirically identified as the most likely to benefit.

A second reason is that the field of personality has become more sophisticated in formulating and testing hypotheses about personality variables as moderators of treatment effects. Indeed, although Dance and Neufeld (1988) reached a largely negative conclusion about patient × treatment interactions in clinical psychology, they suggested that the negative findings could well be attributed to naive methodology and data analysis. Through the efforts of Dance and Neufeld and others we now know better how to approach the study of personality × treatment or risk factor interactions. The recommendations include using adequately sized and substantively appropriate samples, well-constructed and appropriately applied measures of individual differences and research designs, and, perhaps most important, having a strong theory about the mechanism behind the interaction (Chaplin, 1997). In addition, the field of personality should now recognize that some treatments or manipulated situations will be so powerfully constructed that searching for individual difference moderators of those treatments will not be fruitful. In the language of RCTs (randomized clinical trials) personality moderators will be more likely to be important in *effectiveness* trials rather than *efficacy* trials. Effectiveness trials concern the question, "Does the treatment work if offered?" whereas efficacy trials concern the question, "Why does the treatment work?" In effectiveness trials, one reason that a treatment might not work is that some people will not adhere to it, and thus identifying the types of people who will and will not adhere to a particular treatment is an important research goal. In efficacy trials such as the one that generated the data shown in Figure 34.5, personality variables may be of less importance because the trial often requires that everyone respond to the treatment so that mechanisms and outcomes can be understood.

Finally, although it is elusive, the goal of identifying person × treatment (situation) interactions has from time to time been realized, generally in studies that exhibit a sophisticated understanding of the issues described above. For example, Revelle, Humphreys, Simon, and Gilliland (1980) relied on a strong biological theory of extraversion to predict a three-way interaction involving extraversion, time of day, and caffeine. Caspi and colleagues (2003) used a longitudinal sample and a well-established theory of the importance of specific alleles of the 5-HTT gene to demonstrate a gene × life stress interaction for predicting depression. Bolger and Patterson (2001) also used a large longitudinal sample and multiply measured outcomes to demonstrate the moderating effect of perceived control on the relation between abuse and internalizing problems in children. An example of a personality variable (sense of control) moderating the effects of a risk factor (social class) on health can be found in Lachman and Weaver (1998).

STATISTICAL APPROACH

Historically, the assessment of person × treatment interaction took place in an analysis of variance (ANOVA) framework using a categorized version of the continuous personality variable as one of the independent variables (IV). The categorization of the continuous variable was necessary because ANOVA models can "see" only categorical IVs. Thus, if one were to specify a continuous personality variable as an IV in an ANOVA, that variable would be treated as having upwards of 100 categories representing each individual score on the measure, generally with one observation per category. The results of such an analysis would be even sillier than one obtained by median splitting the continuous variable into two categories, because this measurement operation is even sillier. Linear regression analysis, however, recognizes continuous variables as continuous. Yet regression models do not naturally recognize categories, so if one has four treatment groups, say, Motivational Interviewing (MI), Pharmaceutical Treatment (PT), Psychoeducation (PE), and Usual Care (UC) nominally coded in a variable as 1, 2, 3, and 4, the regression software would treat this variable as continuous (4 > 3 > 2 > 1) and indeed as an interval scale (e.g., 4–3 = 2–1), and the results would again be silly. Fortunately, through appropriate coding and analytic strategies, nominal scales representing group membership can be sensibly included in a regression framework.

The details of representing qualitative groups in regression analyses and interpreting the results such analyses generate are available in Cohen and colleagues (2003) and other texts on regression analysis. Readers are encouraged to consult these more detailed resources, as the treatment of this issue here is cursory. Basically, one creates a set of variables that together, completely, unambiguously, and nonredundantly indicate to what group an individual belongs. It turns out that there are an infinite number of sets of variables that meet the aforementioned conditions, and all of these will be appropriate for statistically testing, in a regression framework, the hypothesis that there is a personality × treatment interaction. That is, all will generate the same p-values, multiple R's and squared semipartial correlations. However, all but a handful of these infinite sets will generate parameter estimates that are nonsense; indeed, these are discussed in Cohen and colleagues as "nonsense codes."

Figure 34.6 shows the three most commonly used sensible coding schemes and provides SPSS syntax to generate such codes from a nominal variable called "treatment." As shown in Figure 34.6, the coding schemes all consist of a set of three variables (e.g., D1, D2, D3) that together allow a person (or a regression equation) to unambiguously state which group a person is in. Thus, if one is told that a person scores 0, 1, 0 on D1, D2, and D3, respectively, one knows the person is in the PT group. If one is told the person scores 0, 0, 0 on D1, D2, and D3, one knows the person is in the UC group, and so on. It is critical to understand that it is the set of variables (three in this example) together that identifies group membership. The variable D1, by itself, indicates only whether a person is in the MI group (score of 1) or is in any one of the other three groups (score of 0). It is the combination of codes across D1, D2, and D3 that together completely and unambiguously represent group membership. The requirement of nonredundancy is met by using one less variable in the set than there are groups to represent. Many coding novices are bothered that one group seems to be "left out"; that is, in the dummy codes, for example, the MI, PT, and PD groups each get a variable with a "1" in it, whereas UC does not. But UC is uniquely identified precisely because it does not

Types of Sensible Codes

Group	Dummy			Effects			Contrast		
	D1	D2	D3	E1	E2	E3	C1	C2	C3
MI	1	0	0	1	0	0	1	1	1
PT	0	1	0	0	1	0	1	-2	0
PE	0	0	1	0	0	1	1	1	-1
UC	0	0	0	-1	-1	-1	-3	0	0

To create codes in SPSS from a nominal variable (called treatment) with values 1, 2, 3, 4 that stand for the MI to UC groups, respectively, one can use the following syntax (using dummy codes as an example):

```
IF (treatment=1) d1 = 1 .
EXECUTE .
IF (treatment>1) d1 = 0 .
EXECUTE .
IF (treatment = 1) d2 = 0.
EXECUTE
IF (treatment = 2) d2 = 1 .
EXECUTE .
IF (treatment > 2) d2 = 0 .
EXECUTE .
IF (treatment < 3) d3 = 0 .
EXECUTE .
IF (treatment = 3) d3 = 1 .
EXECUTE .
IF (treatment = 4) d3 = 0 .
EXECUTE .
```

FIGURE 34.6. Qualitative codes used to represent groups in regression analysis. MI, motivational interviewing; PT, pharmaceutical treatment; PE, psychoeducation; UC, usual care.

have a "1." That is, the pattern 0, 0, 0 uniquely identifies membership in UC. If a fourth variable, D4, with the pattern 0, 0, 0, 1 were included, any one variable would be completely predictable from the other three. Such complete multicollinearity among the predictors would prevent us from inverting the correlation matrix among the predictor variables, which would prevent solving for the partial regression coefficients.

Dummy, effects, and contrast codes (along with nonsense codes) all provide identical results with respect to the statistical tests of the hypotheses "Do the means of the dependent variable differ among the groups?" and "Is the effect of treatment moderated by a personality variable?" The differences between the codes are in the specific parameter (partial regression coefficients) estimates associated with the coded variables. For dummy codes, the parameter estimates reflect differences on the outcome variable between the group coded 1 on the D_i and the group coded 0 on all the D_i's.

Thus, dummy codes may be chosen for designs where there is a logical control group, as is the case for the example we have been using. Effects codes, however, get their name from the term *effect* in the analysis of variance, which refers to the difference between a group mean and the grand mean. The parameters for a set of effects coded variables reflect the difference between the mean of the group coded "1" on E_i and the overall grand mean. Finally, contrast codes are identical to the orthogonal contrast codes used in the analysis of variance to reflect specific hypotheses. In the example in Figure 34.6, C1 contrasts the three treatments with the control, C2 contrasts pharmaceutical treatment with the two behavioral treatments, and C3 contrasts the two behavioral treatments.

Once the qualitative treatment group has been appropriately represented for regression analysis, the personality × treatment model can be specified and evaluated. The logic of the analysis is the same as for the personality × personality analyses. That is, the analysis is hierarchical and the product of the set of variables representing the treatment groups and the personality variable is partialed by the set of variables and the personality measure that make up the product. In addition to coding the treatment variable, one should again center the personality variable and finally compute products between each of the set of code variables and the personality variable (creating a set of product variables).

Figure 34.7 illustrates a personality × treatment analysis. This analysis can be thought of as a test of the moderating effects of conscientiousness on the impact of treatment group on a clinical outcome, such as global clinical ratings of improvement on some outcome at posttreatment (1 = No Improvement, 3 = Modest Improvement, 5 = Substantial Improvement). Again, the data used to create this example are real; the variable names are hypothetical. At the top of Figure 34.7 is the syntax for creating the necessary set of three product terms to test the treatment × conscientiousness interaction. Next is a simple one-way ANOVA to compare the mean improvement ratings across the four groups. This step is shown to persuade those who remain skeptical about the equivalence of ANOVAs to compare group means with regression using coded sets to test the relation between treatment and outcome. Note that the value of F for the ANOVA of 7.134 is identical to the F to test the multiple R obtained by regressing the improvement ratings onto the set of three dummy coded variables to indicate group membership (Model 1 in the next step). Finally, the results of the hierarchical regression are shown in Step 3. The first step of the hierarchy is the set of three dummy coded variables representing group membership, and the test indicates that treatment accounts for 5% of the variance in improvement ratings (F = 7.134, $p < .001$). Next, the personality variable of conscientiousness is added, and doing so increases the variance accounted for in outcome from 5 to 12.2%, an increment (squared semipartial correlation) of 7.2% (F = 33.095, $p < .001$). Clearly (in this hypothetical example), it is better to have conscientious patients regardless of which treatment is used. Finally, and most critically, is the increment in model fit (e.g., R^2) from the moderating effects of conscientiousness on the effects of treatment on improvement. This increment (squared semipartial for the set of three variables) is 2.1% (F = 3.280, $p = .021$). Thus,

the effect of treatment on improvement differs, depending on the patient's level of conscientiousness. The model coefficients are shown at the bottom of Figure 34.7.

Of course, the finding of a significant moderator effect is largely meaningless until the nature of the interaction has been clarified. Two approaches to this clarification are shown in Figure 34.8. At the top of Figure 34.8 are the plots of the regression lines for all four groups, superimposed on a scatterplot of the data. These plots were obtained by predicting values using the unstandardized coefficients from Model 3 at the bottom of Figure 34.7. Specifically, values were predicted for each of the four patterns of the dummy coefficients for a value of conscientiousness that was 1 standard deviation above the mean, and again for a value of conscientiousness that was 1 standard deviation below the mean, in a manner essentially identical to that used to interpret the personality × personality interaction. Inspection of this plot and, perhaps more clearly, the parameter values for Model 1 in Figure 34.7 indicates some small overall differences between the treatment groups, with UC having the overall lowest mean improvement and PT the highest. The upward slope of all four lines indicates the overall positive effect of conscientiousness on improvement. However, of most importance is that the plot indicates that the effect of the different treatment groups on outcome was influenced by the level of conscientiousness of the patients. MI had the best outcomes for conscientious patients but the worst outcomes (even as compared with UC) for less conscientious patients. Alternatively, degree of conscientiousness mattered little for patients in UC. The analyses shown at the bottom of Figure 34.8 are simply the relation between conscientiousness and improvement separately for each group. This is a "simple main effects" analysis that follows up the significant interaction. The simple slopes shown in the four analyses can be derived from the overall analysis shown in Figure 34.7. For example, the slope of .506 for the MI group can be obtained from the slope of conscientiousness (.106) and the slope d1xc (.400); .106 + .400 = .506. Note also that the slope of conscientiousness (.106) is the slope of the UC group. However, it is perhaps easier, after obtaining an overall personality × treatment interaction, to split the file on the treatment group variable and run separate simple regressions as illustrated in Figure 34.8.

1. SPSS Syntax to the set of three personality × treatment products between the set of dummy coded
   variables to represent group membership (D1, D2, and D3) and a centered measure of Conscientiousness

```
COMPUTE d1xc = d1 * cconsci .
EXECUTE .
COMPUTE d2xc = d2 * cconsci .
EXECUTE .
COMPUTE d3xc = d3 * cconsci .
EXECUTE .
```

2. For comparison, a simple one-way ANOVA comparing the four treatment groups

```
ONEWAY
  extrav BY treatment
  /MISSING ANALYSIS .
```

ANOVA

extrav

	Sum of Squares	df	Mean Square	F	Sig.
Between Groups	4.109	3	1.370	7.134	.000
Within Groups	77.562	404	.192		
Total	81.671	407			

3. Hierarchical regression analysis to test the Conscientiousness × Treatment interaction

```
REGRESSION
  /MISSING LISTWISE
  /STATISTICS COEFF OUTS R ANOVA CHANGE
  /CRITERIA=PIN(.05) POUT(.10)
  /NOORIGIN
  /DEPENDENT extrav
  /METHOD=ENTER d1 d2 d3 /METHOD=ENTER cconsci /METHOD=ENTER d1xc d2xc d3xc .
```

Model Summary

Model	R	R Square	Adjusted R Square	Std. Error of the Estimate	Change Statistics R Square Change	F Change	df1	df2	Sig. F Change
1	.224(a)	.050	.043	.4381599	.050	7.134	3	404	.000
2	.350(b)	.122	.114	.4217285	.072	33.095	1	403	.000
3	.379(c)	.143	.128	.4181950	.021	3.280	3	400	.021

a Predictors: (Constant), d3, d2, d1
b Predictors: (Constant), d3, d2, d1, cconsci
c Predictors: (Constant), d3, d2, d1, cconsci, d1xc, d2xc, d3xc

(continued)

FIGURE 34.7. Illustrative analysis of a treatment × personality interaction.

Model		Unstandardized Coefficients		Standardized Coefficients	t	Sig.
		B	Std. Error	Beta		
1	(Constant)	3.371	.043		77.704	.000
	d1	.119	.061	.115	1.944	.053
	d2	.268	.061	.260	4.374	.000
	d3	.203	.061	.197	3.315	.001
2	(Constant)	3.382	.042		80.913	.000
	d1	.128	.059	.124	2.175	.030
	d2	.252	.059	.244	4.262	.000
	d3	.167	.059	.161	2.806	.005
	cconsci	.282	.049	.271	5.753	.000
3	(Constant)	3.375	.042		81.216	.000
	d1	.152	.059	.147	2.569	.011
	d2	.260	.059	.252	4.433	.000
	d3	.170	.059	.165	2.866	.004
	cconsci	.106	.089	.102	1.194	.233
	d1xc	.400	.131	.193	3.040	.003
	d2xc	.106	.139	.046	.765	.445

FIGURE 34.7. *(continued)*

Mediator Models

Basics

The concept of mediation, also referred to as "indirect effects," "intervening variables," or "intermediate effects," has been discussed in various forms in the behavioral sciences literature for quite some time (e.g., Judd & Kenny, 1981; MacCorquodale & Meehl, 1948; Rozeboom, 1956). However, the publication in 1986 of the classic article by Baron and Kenny on mediators and moderators probably marks the point at which mediator hypotheses and models became widely incorporated into behavioral science research. Since that time a host of refinements and alternatives to evaluating mediation models have been described (e.g., Collins, Graham, & Flaherty, 1998; Kenny, Kashy, & Bolger, 1998; Kraemer, Stice, Kazdin, Offord, & Kupfer, 2001; MacKinnon, Lockwood, Hoffman, West, & Sheets, 2002; Shrout & Bolger, 2002), including extensions to multilevel models (e.g., Kenny, Korchmaros, & Bolger, 2003; Krull & MacKinnon, 2001). The discussions and extensions of the evaluation of mediator models cited above are of critical importance, and readers who plan to venture into the realm of mediation are strongly encouraged to make use of these resources. However, the purpose of this section is to present the basic concept of mediation and to provide the data-analytic starting point for testing mediational models. Thus, the emphasis is on the basic regression approach outlined by Baron and Kenny (1986).

A mediator model elaborates on a simple linear model by specifying possible reasons for the relation between two variables. Thus, mediator models address the fundamental scientific goal of explanation. When I tell my children that they should eat vegetables, the dreaded question, "Why?" is nearly inevitable. When I respond, "Because you will grow up big and strong," the next "Why" is also inevitable. Usually, this explanatory chain gets one more response such as, "Because they have good vitamins," before the parental nuclear option of "Or you won't get dessert" is employed. This game of "Why" is an everyday example of mediation. The never-ending nature of the "Why" game is as true in science as it is at the dinner table, although the phrase "beyond the scope of this study," as opposed to the threat of no dessert, is generally the way the game ends in science.

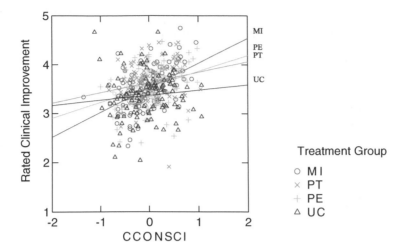

		Unstandardized Coefficients		Standardized Coefficients		
Model		B	Std. Error	Beta	t	Sig.
1	(Constant)	3.527	.039		90.876	.000
	cconsci	.506	.089	.493	5.665	.000

a Dependent Variable: improvement ratings
b Treatment = Motivational Interviewing

		Unstandardized Coefficients		Standardized Coefficients		
Model		B	Std. Error	Beta	t	Sig.
1	(Constant)	3.636	.040		90.712	.000
	cconsci	.213	.103	.202	2.063	.042

a Dependent Variable: improvement ratings
b Treatment = Pharmaceutical

FIGURE 34.8. Interpeting the conscientiousness × treatment interaction.

Thus, the distinction between moderation and mediation is that the former concerns the issue of "It depends," whereas the latter concerns the issue of "Why." More formally, moderator models address the issue of the conditions that will change the simple relations between an independent (predictor) and dependent (criterion) variable. Mediator models concern the issue of understanding why a relation exists.

Scientific hypotheses and the analysis of data are fundamentally about relations between variables. This is true regardless of whether the study is a "correlational" study or an "experimental" study. Indeed, showing that a treatment group scores significantly higher on an outcome variable than does the control group is equivalent to showing that there is a significant correlation between group and outcome. One can analyze such data using an independent samples t-test to compare the group means, or one can correlate outcome and group (often called a "point–biserial" correlation) and the results will be identical as shown

```
T-TEST
  GROPS = conttrt(0 1)
  /MISSING = ANALYSIS
  /VARIABLES = outcome
  /CRITERIA = CI(.95) .
```

Independent Samples Test

		Levene's Test for Equality of Variances		t-test for Equality of Means						
									95% Confidence Interval of the Difference	
		F	Sig.	t	df	Sig. (2-tailed)	Mean Difference	Std. Error Difference	Lower	Upper
outcome	Equal variances assumed	.817	.366	2.012	636	.045	.0382852	.0190276	.0009207	.0756497

```
CORRELATIONS
  /VARIABLES=conttrt outcome
  /PRINT=TWOTAIL NOSIG
  /MISSING=PAIRWISE .
```

Correlations

		conttrt	outcome
conttrt	Pearson Correlation	1	-.080(*)
	Sig. (2-tailed)		.045
	N	650	638
outcome	Pearson Correlation	-.080(*)	1
	Sig. (2-tailed)	.045	
	N	638	650

* Correlation is significant at the 0.05 level (2-tailed).

FIGURE 34.9. The equivalence of the comparison between experimental group means on the outcome and the correlation between group membership and outcome.

in Figure 34.9. In Figure 34.9 the p-value (.045) for the t-test of the null hypothesis that the outcome means of the two groups are equal, is equivalent to the p-value (.045) for the test of the null hypothesis that the correlation between group and outcome is 0. Thus, from a data-analytic standpoint, essentially all analyses are correlational.

The critical scientific issue, of course, is *why* a particular relation exists. As all of us learned at an early stage in our careers, "correlations do not imply causation." Perhaps of equal, but generally unstated, importance is the recognition that correlations also do not imply a *lack* of causation either. Put another way, a correlation between two variables is "caused" by something, it is just that the correlation, by itself, does not tell us what that cause is. It is here that the correlational–experimental distinction becomes relevant. *Correlational designs* are typically naturalistic in the sense that the research participants are not treated or otherwise put into manipulated situations, but most critically there is no random assignment of participants to experimental conditions. *Experimental designs*, however, are based on the random assignment of participants to treatments or manipulations. It is because of this random assignment that when a relation between experimental group and outcome is found in experimental designs, the investigator is in the position of saying that the relation is *caused* by how the participants were treated. This is the basis for the randomized clinical trial (RCT) in medicine, psychology, and other applied fields as the gold standard for empirically supported treatments.

However, as powerful as RCT and other experimental designs may be for showing cause, such designs (as do all designs) still beg the question of *why* the manipulation worked. In the language of RCTs, this issue is discussed as the distinction between "effectiveness" (did the treatment work?—who cares why) and "efficacy" (what is the mechanism behind the treatment; that is, "why" did the treatment work?) trials. Thus, in both experimental and correlational designs, the concept of mediation is relevant. In correlational designs, mediator variables can be proposed as hypothesized reasons for why two variables are related and mediational models can be tested to show support (or lack thereof) for the hypothesized reason. These designs, however, remain correlational,

so the causal foundation for inferences is not solid. In experimental designs such as RCTs the initial question, "Why do the groups differ?" has an answer: "Because of the different way they were treated." However, subsequent "Why did the treatment work?" questions again require proposed mediators and the testing of mediational models, which generally also have a weaker causal foundation because mediators are typically not experimentally manipulated.

Mediational models are generally represented by path diagrams as shown in Figure 34.10. The first model indicates the simple relation between an IV and a DV. It is generally accepted that the simple direct path (a) from the IV to the DV must be non-zero for any mediational analysis to proceed. After all, if there is no relation between the IV and DV, there is nothing to mediate. Exceptions to this perspective can be found in MacKinnon, Krull, and Lockwood (2000) and Shrout and Bolger (2002), who outline some circumstances where this requirement might be waived. The second model shown illustrates mediation. In this model, at least some of the direct IV–DV relation is diverted through the Mediator (M) via paths b and c. If all of the relation between the IV and DV travels through M, then path a' is zero and the relation between the IV and DV is said to be fully mediated by M. If path a' is not zero, but is smaller than path a, then the mediation is described as partial.

The basic statistical evaluation of mediation models using ordinary least squares (OLS) regression was outlined by Baron and Kenny (1986) and requires estimating and evaluating the parameters in the three linear models shown in Equations 5, 6, and 7.

$$DV = B_0 + B_1(IV) \tag{5}$$
$$M = B_0 + B_2(IV) \tag{6}$$
$$DV = B_0 + B_3(IV) + B_4(M) \tag{7}$$

Equation 5 concerns the basic relation between the IV and DV and estimates B_1, which is the path coefficient a in the first model shown in Figure 34.10. Equation 6 estimates B_2, which is path b in the second model shown in Figure 34.10, and Equation 7 estimates B_4, which is path c in Figure 34.10, and B_3, which is path a' in Figure 34.10.

After estimating the parameters, one conducts three statistical tests to determine

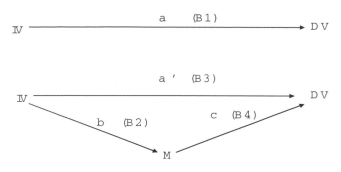

FIGURE 34.10. Path diagrams of basic mediation models. *Note.* B1, B2, B3, and B4 are the regression coefficients from equations 5, 6, and 7 used to estimate the paths.

whether the sample estimates of the parameters are sufficiently large that they are unlikely to be truly 0. Specifically, one tests B_1, B_2, and B_4 against 0. If all three tests suggest that 0 is an unlikely value for the tested parameter estimate, then the results are consistent with the hypothesis that M mediates, at least partially, the relation between the IV and DV. The evaluation of the model in Equation 7 is a *widely misunderstood* aspect of the evaluation of mediation. The critical parameter estimate to be evaluated in this model is B_4, the path (labeled *c* in Figure 34.10) from M to the DV. The parameter estimate B_3 does not need to be evaluated, and indeed its evaluation is irrelevant according to Baron and Kenny's (1986) original formulation. The misunderstanding of the evaluation of this model results when investigators focus on the path *a'* (which is estimated by B_3). The reason for "misfocusing" on path *a'* is understandable, as it is the relation of the IV to the DV that is the focus of the research, and investigators are inclined to want to show that *a'* is 0, or not significantly different from 0, or at least smaller than path *a*. However, the evaluation of mediation in the framework described here is indirect and based on the logic of path analysis (Wright, 1918). Specifically, if the tests of the path coefficient estimates B_1, B_2, and B_4 indicate that all three coefficients are unlikely to be truly 0, then it must be the case that B_3 will be smaller than B_1, implying *some* mediation of the IV–DV relation. Thus, there is no need to test B_3 unless one has hypothesized that the IV–DV relation will be completely mediated by M (Kenny et al., 1998).

Before discussing and illustrating mediator models in the context of personality research, I offer three points that deserve some emphasis.

1. The issue of evaluating path *a'* in mediator models is a source of some controversy. In the original formulation of mediator models (Baron & Kenny, 1986) this path is largely ignored, as the issue of full mediation (when this path is 0) versus partial mediation (when this path is not 0, but smaller than path *a*) is not emphasized. However, full mediation represents a stronger hypothesis and some have argued that it should be tested (e.g., Kenny et al., 1998; Rozeboom, 1956). A statistical issue associated with this position is that the test of B_3 for full mediation is based on the failure to reject a null model. This can result from low statistical power based on small sample size, range restriction, measurement unreliability, and other factors. Thus, concluding that the strong hypothesis, that mediation is full because one failed to reject the model that B_3 is 0, may be unwarranted. Indeed, from a conceptual standpoint full mediation would seem to be the exception rather than the rule, simply because most events have multiple effects and multiple causes.

2. Mediational models are generally viewed as having a causal structure that is implied by unidirectional arrows in the models. Thus, the IV is seen as causing, or at least influencing, the DV, the IV is seen as influencing the Mediator, and the Mediator is seen as influencing the DV. As noted above, unless the IV is experimental, the direction of the arrows is tenuous, and even then the direction of the arrow from M to the DV is tenuous. So the specification of the mediation model is more often justified on a conceptual or logical basis rather than an empirical one. That is, in some cases it is clear that an IV (such as gender) will have causal priority over another variable such as strength, which in

turn will have causal priority over another variable such as physical aggression. Being strong does not logically cause a person to be a man, and being physically aggressive does not cause a person to be strong. Thus, a mediational model that proposes to explain (at least partly) gender differences in physical aggression by appealing to differences in the strength of men and women is a far more reasonable model than proposing that physical aggression causes either strength or gender. But there is no experimental manipulation here, and the observed correlations between the variables do not empirically distinguish these models.

In many cases the causal priority of a proposed IV, M, and DV will be more difficult to sort out on conceptual grounds. For example, both arterial inflammation and depression are known to be related to coronary heart disease (CHD). In a review of this research, Shimbo, Chaplin, Crossman, Haas, and Davidson (2005) recently noted that a variety of models may be proposed to describe the interrelations among these variables. One of many possibilities is that inflammation mediates the relation between depression and CHD, but an alternative model in which depression is the mediator of the inflammation–CHD relation is also possible. In such cases the evaluation of mediational models will be most persuasively done using longitudinal datasets where temporal order can be used to enhance inferences of causal priority. That is, where the experimental manipulation of variables is not possible, the next best strategy is to have time on your side. Longitudinal mediational designs can be analyzed using latent growth models, autoregressive cross-lagged models, or perhaps most effectively, a combination of the two (Bollen & Curran, 2004; Curran & Bollen, 2001).

3. The evaluation of mediation models in the basic regression framework is based on testing the three parameter estimates, B_1, B_2, and B_4. If all three of these parameters are found to differ from 0, then it must be the case that path a' will be smaller than path a (Figure 34.10) and mediation exists. However, the mediating effect (the difference between a and a') may be trivial and not itself statistically significant. It is important to realize that the test of a' does not provide an adequate evaluation of the mediating effect, as this test speaks only to the issue of full versus partial mediation. Mediation does not need to be full or complete to be nontrivial and significant, but there is no direct

test of whether the decrease $a - a'$ is a significantly different from 0. The reason there is no direct test is that there is no standard error for the $a - a'$ difference. Fortunately, the mathematics of path analysis provides an indirect test of the $a - a'$ difference because the product of paths b and c (estimated by B_2 and B_4) is equal to the $a - a'$ difference and a standard error for that product is available from the standard errors for B_2 and B_4. The test of the product is usually called the "Sobel test" (Sobel, 1982) and is based on the standard unit normal ("z") distribution. There are several different variants (see, e.g., Aroian, 1947; Goodman, 1960) of this test that differ on how the standard error of the product is estimated. MacKinnon, Warsi, and Dwyer (1995) provide technical details about the variants as well as a comparative evaluation. The general consensus seems to be that the Aroian version is to be preferred. This test is shown in Equation 8.

$$z = [b * c]/[SQRT[(b^2 * sc^2) + (c^2 * sb^2) + (sc^2 * sb^2)]]$$

where b is the unstandardized regression coefficient (B_2) from Equation 6, c is the unstandardized regression coefficient (B_4) from Equation 7, sc is the standard error of c, sb is the standard error of b, and z is a "z-score" that is referred to the standard unit normal distribution. A Web-based calculator for performing this test, as well as programs for more contemporary approaches to mediational analyses and further discussion, may be found at *www.unc. edu/~preacher/sobel/sobel.htm*.

Applications to Personality Research

There are two possible roles for personality variables in mediational models: as the IV whose relation to the DV needs to be explained by a Mediator, and as the Mediator that will help explain an IV–DV relation.

Personality Variable as IV

CONCEPTUAL ISSUES

When a relation is found between a personality variable and an outcome, this is the beginning of the story, not the end. If we find that Extraversion is correlated with leadership styles (e.g., Johnson, Vernon, Harris, & Jang, 2004), or Hostility is correlated with coronary heart disease (e.g., Barefoot et al., 1983), or that Alienation is associated with delinquency (Krueger et al., 1994), the "why" question immediately comes to mind. Personality constructs may be useful predictor variables, but they are wretched as explanatory variables. They are wretched as explanatory variables because the mechanisms by which they operate are not specified, and this is frustrating both scientifically and practically.

Scientifically, the assertion "She is perceived by her staff as a good leader because she is extraverted" is both vacuous and unwarranted by the correlation on which the assertion is based. The assertion "She is a good leader because her extraverted personality leads her to seek out and talk over decisions with her staff" provides a more specific mechanism and is, in principle, testable. Of course, recall that "why" questions are never-ending. So one could continue with "Why does talking over decisions with staff members lead them to perceive her as a good leader?" and so on. But answering even one "why" question is an appropriate and often useful step in a program of research.

From a practical standpoint, the finding that Extraversion is related to leadership ability is also frustrating. It is frustrating because there is nothing in that finding that could be used to teach people how to improve their leadership. That is, to tell individuals wishing to become better leaders to "be more extraverted" is not helpful both because there is nothing specific in the advice to tell them how to do that, and because, based on personality theory, such advice cannot be followed. Extraversion is viewed as a stable trait that is not easily changed. However, telling the individual that she can be perceived as a better leader if she "discusses decisions with her staff" is advice that even an introvert can follow, although perhaps not easily. Thus, the specification of mechanisms that link the personality construct to the outcome provides a more satisfying and testable explanation of the relation and often facilitates the translation of a basic scientific finding into an application, in this case leadership training.

STATISTICAL APPROACH

The statistical evaluation of the mediator model discussed above requires a measure of extraversion (E) among a group of leaders, ratings of leadership by those leaders' staff (L), and a measure of the extent to which decisions were discussed with staff prior to being made (D). Three separate regression models would then be run, as shown in Figure 34.11. As shown in Figure 34.11, the tests provide support for the hypothesis that the relation of extraversion to leadership is mediated by engaging in staff discussions. (Again, the data used for this example are real, but the names of the variables have been changed to fit the example.) Specifically, E is related to L ($t = 2.012$, $p = .045$), E is related to D ($t = 3.731$, $p < .001$), and the partial relation between D and L is significant, controlling for E ($t = 7.105$, $p < .001$). The appropriate path coefficients from this analysis are displayed in Figure 34.12, as is the result of the Aroian test, which shows that the mediation effect is significant ($z = 3.225$, $p = .0006$). Displaying results from a mediation analysis in a path diagram is generally useful.

Personality Variable as Mediator

The use of mediational models to clarify why personality constructs are related to outcome variables is of critical importance to the field. However, hypotheses that use personality constructs as mediators are more tenuous. Generally, personality constructs are viewed as relatively stable and consistent entities that are not readily changed by treatments or other variables. Thus, placing those variables in the middle of a relation where the personality variable is caused or influenced by an IV may not always be sensible. Nonetheless, there are circumstances in which a personality variable can be sensibly placed in a mediating role.

One such circumstance is where the personality variable is viewed as a state rather than a trait variable, as state variables are viewed as being influenced by situational factors (Chaplin, John, & Goldberg, 1988). Thus, experimental manipulations to make people anxious or sad or angry, or for that matter relaxed, happy, and peaceful, can legitimately invoke such state variables as mediators. Another circumstance that may justify a personality construct as a mediator is where a variable that is with a person from birth—sex is the best example here—may have a personality variable that is in the mediating variable position. Indeed, although a person's sex is a powerful predictor of many outcomes, sex is probably even more wretched as an explanatory variable than personality constructs. Thus, a mediational model to test whether the relation between sex and vi-

1) Is Extroversion related to Leadership (Path a in Figure 34.10)?

```
REGRESSION
 /MISSING LISTWISE
 /STATISTICS COEFF OUTS R ANOVA
 /CRITERIA=PIN(.05) POUT(.10)
 /NOORIGIN
 /DEPENDENT Leadership
 /METHOD=ENTER Extroversion.
```

Coefficients (a)

Model		Unstandardized Coefficients		Standardized Coefficients	t	Sig.
		B	Std. Error	Beta		
1	(Constant)	.449	.012		38.448	.000
	Extroversion	.038	.019	.080	2.012	.045

a Dependent Variable: leadership

2) Is Extroversion related to Discussion (Path b in Figure 34.10)?

```
REGRESSION
 /MISSING LISTWISE
 /STATISTICS COEFF OUTS R ANOVA
 /CRITERIA=PIN(.05) POUT(.10)
 /NOORIGIN
 /DEPENDENT Discussion
 /METHOD=ENTER Extroversion .
```

Coefficients (a)

Model		Unstandardized Coefficients		Standardized Coefficients	t	Sig.
		B	Std. Error	Beta		
1	(Constant)	4.022	.030		134.548	.000
	Extroversion	.181	.048	.148	3.731	.000

a Dependent Variable: Discussion

3) Is Discussion related to Leadership with Extroversion partialed (Pat c in Figure 34.10)?

```
REGRESSION
 /MISSING LISTWISE
 /STATISTICS COEFF OUTS R ANOVA
 /CRITERIA=PIN(.05) POUT(.10)
 /NOORIGIN
 /DEPENDENT Leadership
 /METHOD=ENTER Extroversion Discussion .
```

Coefficients (a)

Model		Unstandardized Coefficients		Standardized Coefficients	t	Sig.
		B	Std. Error	Beta		
1	(Constant)	.880	.062		14.096	.000
	Extroversion	.019	.019	.040	1.017	.310
	Discussion	.108	.015	.278	7.105	.000

a Dependent Variable: leadership

FIGURE 34.11. Basic regression evaluation of a mediator model using SPSS.

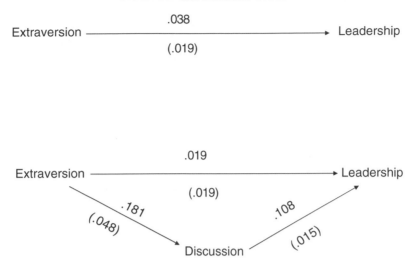

Note. The unstandardized regression coefficients from Figure 34.11 are the path coefficients shown above the lines. The standard errors of those coefficients (from Figure 34.11) are shown below the lines in parentheses. The decrease of .038–.019 is the path a – a' difference and this is the mediating effect.

As explained in the text, .181 × .108 = .019 That is, b × c = a – a'.
This is the basis of the Aroian version of the Sobel to test if the mediating effect of .019 is statistically significant. The calculations for that test are shown below.

$$Z = (.181 * .108)/SQRT[(.181^2 * .015^2) + (.108^2 + .048^2) + (.015^2 * .048^2)] =$$
$$.19/SQRT[.0000074 + .0000268 + .0000005] =$$
$$.19/.0058906 = 3.225 \; p = .0006$$

Note if the results are entered into Preacher's Web-based calculator, the result for the test is $Z = 3.3154364$ and $p = .000915$. The discrepancy is small and reflects greater rounding error in the hand calculation shown on this page.

FIGURE 34.12. Summary of the mediation analysis shown in Figure 34.11.

olent crime was mediated by the tendency of men to feel more alienated than women would not be unreasonable. Of course, a chain of "why" questions with further mediators between alienation and crime would likely be required before a satisfactory conclusion could be reached.

Finally, the fact that personality variables can be arranged into hierarchies ranging from broad to narrow (e.g., Hampson, John, & Goldberg, 1986) can be another basis for specifying mediational structures among personality variables. That is, the relation between a broad variable such as extraversion and an outcome may be mediated by a narrower manifestation of the broad variable, such as talkative. However, this represents a causal view of traits. Such a causal view is probably appropriate within the context of mediation models. Yet an alternative view of trait constructs sees them as

descriptive summaries, as in the act-frequency theory of Buss and Craik (1983). From this perspective, the narrower acts may be viewed as causing the person to be described as extraverted. This issue is similar to the distinction between components (descriptive) and factors (causal) in factor analysis (Chaplin, 2005). Ultimately, the structure specified by mediational models must be justified by theory, so the suggestions made here are certainly not rules; at best they are guidelines. Once specified, the statistical analyses of the models will proceed exactly as shown in Figures 34.11 and 34.12.

More Complex Extensions

The goal of this chapter has been to provide a basic and foundational introduction to moderator and mediator models, with special emphasis on the issues associated with their application to personality research. Within the past decade there has been an enormous increase in the complexity of these models and the sophistication with which data are analyzed to evaluate such models. These developments have resulted from the attention these models have received from quantitatively sophisticated psychologists, and this attention underscores the importance of these models in behavioral science research. It was beyond the scope of this chapter to track and discuss all of the developments that are occurring. Moreover, to appreciate these developments a foundation must be in place. In this section I briefly highlight some of the more important developments that have taken place.

1. The statistical approach emphasized in this chapter is OLS regression on observed variables. One of the most important advances in the study of moderator and mediator models has been the extension of the evaluation of these models to latent variables via structural equation modeling. For mediator models this extension is relatively straightforward, as the models are typically expressed in path diagrams, which can be readily extended to structural models through the multiple measurement of the constructs. For moderator models the extension to structural models has been a bit slower to develop. This is largely because one must impose constraints on the paths from the observed product terms to the latent construct that reflects the interaction. These constraints are necessary to ensure that the latent term reflects an interaction and not just a product variable—that is, the constraints are essentially akin to the partialing of the lower-order terms from the product in OLS regression. Unfortunately, determining the constraints is not generally straightforward, particularly for investigators whose forte is not quantitative methods. An excellent discussion of these issues that includes some different approaches to estimating and imposing constraints can be found in the edited volume by Schumacker and Marcoulides (1998). An alternative view about the importance of constraints can be found in Wen, Marsh, and Hau (2004), and an example of an approach to these issues in a substantive context is Johnson and Krueger (2005).

2. As the field of psychology has become more focused on applied research and the change and development of human behavior, the utility of pure experimental approaches has diminished and the emphasis on the use of longitudinal data for studying change and its causes has increased. This has been accompanied by a rapid increase in discussions of how to study change (e.g., Collins & Sayer, 2001) and the development of creative approaches for analyzing moderator and mediator models in longitudinal data (e.g., Bollen & Curran, 2004; Curran, Bauer, & Willoughby, 2004; Curran & Bollen, 2001). Indeed, in the view of some (Kraemer et al., 2001) moderator and mediator models can be appropriately evaluated only in longitudinal data, as such data provides the only basis for testing causal hypotheses in variables that are not amenable to experimental manipulation and randomization.

3. Although moderator and mediator models have been discussed separately in this chapter, these models can be combined into more complex moderated mediation models and mediated moderation models. In the former case the mediation of the IV–DV relation occurs only under some conditions (e.g., only for men, only for older individuals, and so on). Thus, the mediator effect is moderated by those conditioning variables. In mediated moderation the relation of the partialed product variable (interaction) is at least partly "carried by" or can be "explained by" a mediator. Such models can address questions such as "*Why* is the relation of hostility to coronary heart disease different for men and women?" (e.g., Haas et al., 2005). Finally, it is possible for a variable to serve as both a moderator and a mediator in the same analyses.

A Note on Suppressor Models

When I was initially invited to prepare this chapter, it was suggested that I also consider suppressor models. However, in reviewing the literature on suppressor models it generally appears that the concept of suppression has not been a particularly fruitful one in personality psychology. In contrast to mediator and moderator models, for which the literature has become vast, I found that this section would be based on two articles, one methodological (MacKinnon, Krull, & Lockwood, 2000) and one substantive (Paulhus, Robins, Trzesniewski, & Tracy, 2004). Essentially, suppressor models are those in which the inclusion of two IVs in a model *increases* the separate unique relation of one or both variables to the DV over the simple direct relations of either alone. This happens because the shared variance between the IVs is not shared with the DV. This is an uncommon situation, as, generally, variables in regression models all share variance, as at some level they all concern the same phenomena. Thus, when evidence of suppression is found, it tends to be difficult to interpret, hard to replicate, and possibly artifactual. As a result, suppressor models have not generally proven useful.

The MacKinnon, Krull, and Lochwood (2000) article discusses how the statistical evaluations, if not the conceptualizations, of mediator, confounding, and supressor variables are equivalent. Paulhus and colleagues (2004), after discussing the pessimistic past of suppressor research, report supressor results from a study on shame and guilt and another study on narcissism and self-esteem that are both substantively interpretable and that were empirically replicated. It may well be that these two articles will provide the impetus for the further development of supressor models as the next major growth area in personality psychology. If so, the next edition of this book will undoubtedly contain a larger section on this topic.

Conclusion

This chapter was written to introduce relative newcomers to the field of personality research to two important types of models, moderator models and mediator models, that are becoming widely used in research designed to further our understanding of how personality constructs can contribute to understanding important human behaviors and other outcomes. It is no longer the case that merely showing that there is a correlation between a measure of a personality construct and an outcome is a sufficient contribution. Instead, we must attempt to more deeply understand this relation by specifying the conditions under which it occurs and does not occur (moderator models) and/or by testing hypotheses about why the relation was found (mediator models). Just as the finding that a personality measure is related to an outcome is only the very beginning of a story, so too, this chapter is only the beginning of an introduction to these models. But all things must have a beginning and, for that matter, an end.

Recommended Readings

Baron, R. M., & Kenny, D. A. (1986). The moderator-mediator variable distinction in social psychological research: Conceptual, strategic, and statistical considerations. *Journal of Personality and Social Psychology, 51,* 1173–1182.

Chaplin, W. F. (1997). Personality, interactive relations, and applied psychology. In R. Hogan, J. Johnson, & S. Briggs (Eds.), *Handbook of personality psychology* (pp. 873–890). San Diego, CA: Academic Press.

Cohen, J., Cohen, P., West, S. G., & Aiken, L. S. (2003). *Applied multiple regression/correlation analysis for the behavioral sciences* (3rd ed.). Mahwah, NJ: Erlbaum.

Kraemer, H. C., Stice, E., Kazdin, A., Offord, D., & Kupfer, D. (2001). How do risk factors work together?: Mediators, moderators, and independent, overlapping, and proxy risk factors. *American Journal of Psychiatry, 158,* 848–856.

MacKinnon, D. P., Lockwood, C. M., Hoffman, J. M., West, S. G., & Sheets, V. (2002). A comparison of methods to test mediation and other intervening variable effects. *Psychological Methods, 7,* 83–104.

West, S. G., Aiken, L. S., & Krull, J. (1996). Experimental personality designs: Analyzing categorical by continuous variable interactions. *Journal of Personality, 64,* 1–47.

References

Aiken, L. S., & West, S. G. (1991). *Multiple regression: Testing and interpreting interactions*. Newbury Park, CA: Sage.

Allport, G. W. (1961). *Pattern and growth in personality*. New York: Holt, Rinehart & Winston.

Aroian, L. A. (1947). The probability function of the product of two normally distributed variables. *Annals of Mathematical Statistics, 18,* 265–271.

Barefoot, J. C., Dahlstrom, W. G., & Williams, R. B., Jr. (1983). Hostility, CHD incidence, and total mortality: A 25 year follow-up study of 255 physicians. *Psychosomatic Medicine, 45,* 59–63.

Baron, R. M., & Kenny, D. A. (1986). The moderator–mediator variable distinction in social psychological research: Conceptual, strategic, and statistical considerations. *Journal of Personality and Social Psychology, 51,* 1173–1182.

Blanton, H., & Jaccard, J. (2006). Arbitrary metrics in psychology. *American Psychologist, 61,* 27–41.

Blass, T. (1999). The Milgram paradigm after 35 years: Some things we know about obedience to authority. *Journal of Applied Social Psychology, 3,* 955–978.

Bolger, K. E., & Patterson, C. J. (2001). Pathways from child maltreatment to internalizing problems: Perceptions of control as mediators and moderators. *Development and Psychopathology, 13,* 913–940.

Bollen, K. A., & Curran, P. J. (2004). Autoregressive latent trajectory (ALT) models: A synthesis of two traditions. *Sociological Methods and Research, 32,* 336–383.

Buss, D. M., & Craik, K. H. (1983). The act frequency approach to personality. *Psychological Review, 90,* 105–126.

Caspi, A., Sugden, K., Moffitt, T. E., Taylor, A., Craig, I. W., Harrington, H., et al. (2003). Influence of life stress on depression: Moderation by a polymorphism in the 5-HTT gene. *Science, 301,* 386–389.

Chaplin, W. F. (1991). The next generation of moderator research in personality psychology. *Journal of Personality, 59,* 143–178.

Chaplin, W. F. (1994, June). *Methodological issues in reporting findings in personality.* Paper presented at the seventh annual Nags Head International Conference on Personality and Social Behavior, Highland Beach, FL.

Chaplin, W. F. (1997). Personality, interactive relations, and applied psychology. In R. Hogan, J. Johnson, & S. Briggs (Eds.), *Handbook of personality psychology* (pp. 873–890). San Diego, CA: Academic Press.

Chaplin, W. F. (2005). Factor analysis of personality measures. In B. Everitt & D. Howell (Eds.), *Encyclopedia of statistics in behavioral sciences* (pp. 219–230). London: Wiley.

Chaplin, W. F., & Goldberg, L. R. (1984). A failure to replicate the Bem and Allen study on individual differences in cross-situational consistencies. *Journal of Personality and Social Psychology, 47,* 1074–1090.

Chaplin, W. F., John, O. P., & Goldberg, L. R. (1988). Conceptions of traits and states: Dimensional attributes with ideals as prototypes. *Journal of Personality and Social Psychology, 54,* 541–557.

Chaplin, W. F., Phillips, J. B., Brown, J. D., Clanton, N. R., & Stein, J. L. (2000). Handshaking, gender, personality, and first impressions. *Journal of Personality and Social Psychology, 79,* 110–117.

Chen, S., Lee-Chai, A. Y., & Bargh, J. A. (2001). Relationship orientation as a moderator of the effects of social power. *Journal of Personality and Social Psychology, 80,* 173–187.

Cohen, J. (1978). Partialed products *are* interactions: Partialed powers are curve components. *Psychological Bulletin, 85,* 858–866.

Cohen, J. (1983). The cost of dichotomization. *Applied Psychological Measurement, 7,* 249–253.

Cohen, J., Cohen, P., West, S. G., & Aiken, L. S. (2003). *Applied multiple regression /correlation analysis for the behavioral sciences* (3rd ed.). Mahwah, NJ: Erlbaum.

Collins, L. M., Graham, J. W., & Flaherty, B. P. (1998). An alternative framework for defining mediation. *Multivariate Behavioral Research, 33,* 295–312.

Collins, L. M., & Sayer, A. G. (2001). *New methods for the analysis of change.* Washington, DC: American Psychological Association.

Cronbach, L. J. (1967). How can instruction be adapted to individual differences? In R. M. Gagne (Ed.), *Learning and individual differences* (pp. 23–43). Columbus, OH: Merrill.

Cronbach, L. J. (1975). Beyond the two disciplines of scientific psychology. *American Psychologist, 12,* 671–684.

Curran, P. J., Bauer, D. J., & Willoughby, M. T. (2004). Testing main effects and interactions in latent curve analysis. *Psychological Methods, 9,* 220–237.

Curran, P. J., & Bollen, K. A. (2001). The best of both worlds: Combining autoregressive and latent curve models. In L. M. Collins & A. G. Sayer (Eds.), *New methods for the analysis of change* (pp. 105–136). Washington, DC: American Psychological Association.

Dance, K. A., & Neufeld, R. W. J. (1988). Aptitude–treatment interaction research in the clinical setting: A review of attempts to deal with the "patient uniformity" myth. *Psychological Bulletin, 104,* 192–213.

Dechesne, M., Janssen, J., & van Knippenberg, A. (2000). Derogation and distancing as terror management strategies: The moderating role of need for closure and permeability of group boundaries. *Journal of Personality and Social Psychology, 79,* 923–932.

Epstein, S. (1983). Aggregation and beyond: Some basic issues on the prediction of behavior. *Journal of Personality, 51,* 360–392.

Farber, I. E. (1964). A framework for the study of personality as a behavioral science. In P. Worchel & D. Byrne (Eds.), *Personality change* (pp. 3–37). New York: Wiley.

Funder, D. C. (1994). Editorial. *Journal of Research in Personality, 28,* 1–3.

Funder, D. C., & Ozer, D. J. (1983). Behavior as a function of the situation. *Journal of Personality and Social Psychology, 44,* 107–112.

Goldberg, L. R. (1972). Some recent trends in personality assessment. *Journal of Personality Assessment, 36,* 547–560.

Goodman, L. A. (1960). On the exact variance of products. *Journal of the American Statistical Association, 55,* 708–713.

Haas, D. C., Chaplin, W. F., Shimbo, D., Pickering, T. G., Burg, M., & Davidson, K. W. (2005). Hostility is an independent predictor of recurrent coronary heart disease in men but not women: Results from a population based study. *Heart, 91,* 1609–1610.

Hampson, S. E., John, O. P., & Goldberg, L. R. (1986). Category breadth and hierarchical structure in personality: Studies of asymmetries in judgments and trait implications. *Journal of Personality and Social Psychology, 51,* 37–54.

Hogan, R. (2005). In defense of personality measurement: New wine for old whiners. *Human Performance, 18,* 331–341.

James, L. R., & Brett, J. M. (1984). Mediators, moderators, and tests for mediation. *Journal of Applied Psychology, 69,* 307–321.

Johnson, A. M., Vernon, P. A., Harris, J. A., & Jang, K. L. (2004). A behavior genetic investigation of the relationship between leadership and personality. *Twin Research, 7*, 27–32.

Johnson, W., & Krueger, R. F. (2005). Higher perceived life control decreases genetic variance in physical health: Evidence from a national twin study. *Journal of Personality and Social Psychology, 88*, 165–173.

Judd, C. M., & Kenny, D. A. (1981). Process analysis: Estimating mediation in treatment evaluations. *Evaluation Review, 5*, 602–619.

Judd, C. M., Kenny, D. A., & McClelland, G. H. (2001). Estimating and testing mediation and moderation in within-subjects designs. *Psychological Methods, 6*, 115–134.

Kenny, D. A., Kashy, D. A., & Bolger, N. (1998). Data analysis in social psychology. In D. Gilbert, S. T. Fiske, & Lindzey (Eds.), *Handbook of social psychology* (4th ed., Vol. 1, pp. 233–265). New York: McGraw-Hill.

Kenny, D. A., Korchmaros, J. D., & Bolger, N. (2003). Lower level mediation in multilevel models. *Psychological Methods, 8*, 115–128.

Kenny, D. A., Mannetti, L., Pierro, A., Livi, S., & Kashy, D. A. (2002). The statistical analysis of data from small groups. *Journal of Personality and social psychology, 83*, 126–137.

Kenny, D. A., Mohr, C. D., & Levesque, M. J. (2001). A social relations variance partitioning of dyadic behavior. *Psychological Bulletin, 127*, 128–141.

Kenrick, D. T., & Funder, D. C. (1988). Profiting from controversy: Lessons from the person–situation controversy. *American Psychologist, 43*, 23–34.

Kraemer, H. C., Stice, E., Kazdin, A., Offord, D., & Kupfer, D. (2001). How do risk factors work together? Mediators, moderators, and independent, overlapping, and proxy risk factors. *American Journal of Psychiatry, 158*, 848–856.

Krueger, R. F., Schmutte, P. S., Caspi, A., Moffitt, T. E., Campbell, K., & Silva, P. A. (1994). Personality traits are linked to crime among men and women: Evidence from a birth cohort. *Journal of Abnormal Psychology, 103*, 328–338.

Krull, J. L., & MacKinnon, D. P. (2001). Multilevel modeling of individual and group level mediated effects. *Multivariate Behavioral Research, 36*, 249–277.

Lachman, M. E., & Weaver, S. L. (1998). The sense of control as a moderator of social class differences in health and well-being. *Journal of Personality and Social Psychology, 74*, 763–773.

MacCorquodale, K., & Meehl, P. E. (1948). On a distinction between hypothetical constructs and intervening variables. *Psychological Review, 55*, 95–107.

MacKinnon, D. P., Krull, J. L., & Lockwood, C. M. (2000). Equivalence of the mediation, confounding, and suppression effects. *Prevention Science, 1*, 144–158.

MacKinnon, D. P., Lockwood, C. M., Hoffman, J. M., West, S. G., & Sheets, V. (2002). A comparison of methods to test mediation and other intervening variable effects. *Psychological Methods, 7*, 83–104.

MacKinnon, D. P., Warsi, G., & Dwyer, J. H. (1995). A simulation study of mediated effect measures. *Multivariate Behavioral Research, 30*, 41–62.

Marsh, H. W., Wen, Z., & Hau, K-T. (2004). Structural equation models of latent interactions: Evaluation of alternative estimation strategies and indicator construction. *Psychological Methods, 9*, 275–300.

Maxwell, S. E., & Delaney, H. D. (1993). Bivariate median splits and spurious statistical significance. *Psychological Bulletin, 113*, 181–190.

Milgram, S. (1963). Behavioral study of obedience. *Journal of Abnormal and Social Psychology, 67*, 371–378.

Mischel, W. (1968). *Personality and assessment.* New York: Wiley.

Morey, L. C., Gunderson, J. G., Quigley, B. D., Shea, M. T., Skodal, A. E., McGlashan, T. H., et al. (2002). The representation of borderline, avoidant, obsessive–compulsive and schizotypal personality disorders by the five-factor model. *Journal of Personality Disorders, 16*, 215–234.

O'Connor, B. P., & Dvorak, T. (2001). Conditional associations between parental behavior and adolescent problems: A search for personality–environment interactions. *Journal of Research in Personality, 35*, 1–26.

Paulhus, D. L., Robins, R. W., Trzesniewski, K. H., & Tracy, J. L. (2004). Two replicable supressor situations in personality research. *Multivariate Behavioral Research, 39*, 303–328.

Preacher, K. J., MacCallum, R. C., Rucker, D. D., & Nicewander, W. A. (2005). Use of extreme groups approach: A critical reexamination and new recommendations. *Psychological Methods, 10*, 178–192.

Revelle, W., Humphreys, M. S., Simon, L., & Gilliland, K. (1980) The interactive effect of personality, time of day, and caffeine: A test of the arousal model. *Journal of Experimental Psychology: General, 109*, 1–31.

Ross, M. E., Mahfouz, R., Onciu, M., Liu, H-C., Zhou, X., Song, G., et al. (2004). Gene expression profiling of pediatric acute myelogenous leukemia. *Blood, 104*, 3679–3687.

Rozeboom, W. W. (1956). Mediation variables in scientific theory. *Psychological Review, 63*, 249–264.

Schumacker, R. E., & Marcoulides, G. A. (1998). *Interaction and nonlinear effects in structural equation modeling.* Mahwah, NJ: Erlbaum.

Shimbo, D., Chaplin, W., Crossman, D., Haas, D., & Davidson, K. (2005). Role of depression and inflammation in incident coronary heart disease events. *American Journal of Cardiology, 96*, 1016–1021.

Shrout, P. E., & Bolger, N. (2002). Mediation in experimental and nonexperimental studies: New procedures and recommendations. *Psychological Methods, 7*, 422–425.

Sobel, M. E. (1982). Asymptotic intervals for indirect effects in structural equations models. In S. Leinhart (Ed.), *Sociological methodology 1982* (pp. 290–312). San Francisco: Jossey-Bass.

Swann, W. B., & Seyle, C. (2005). Personality psychology's comeback and its emerging symbiosis with social psychology. *Personality and Social Psychology Bulletin, 31,* 155–165.

Warr, P., Bartram, D., & Martin, T. (2005). Personality and sales performance: Situational variation and interactions between traits. *International Journal of Selection and Assessment, 13,* 87–91.

West, S. G., Aiken, L. S., & Krull, J. (1996). Experimental personality designs: Analyzing categorical by continuous variable interactions. *Journal of Personality, 64,* 1–47.

Westen, D. (1995). A clinical-empirical model of personality: Life after the Mischelian ice age and the NEO-lithic era. *Journal of Personality, 63,* 495–524.

Witt, L. A. (2002). The interactive effects of extroversion and conscientiousness on performance. *Journal of Management, 28,* 835–851.

Witt, L. A., Burke, L. A., Barrick, M. R., & Mount, M. K. (2002). The interactive effects of conscientiousness and agreeableness on job performance. *Journal of Applied Psychology, 87,* 164–169.

Wright, S. (1918). On the nature of size factors. *Genetics, 3,* 367–374.

## CHAPTER 35

Computational Modeling of Personality as a Dynamical System

Yuichi Shoda

> To escape from the sterile enumerations of the omnibus definitions it is
> necessary to stress active organization. The crucial problem of
> psychology has always been mental organizations (association).
> —ALLPORT (1937, p. 48)

There once was a time when psychologists looked up to physics as a model science. Psychologists sought the kinds of lawful relationships physicists were able to find in the natural world, allowing them to predict a variable of interest as a function of other variables.

The trouble is, physics does not do this. Or, stated more precisely, most laws in physics do not *directly* predict variables of interest. To illustrate, suppose one wants to predict, from a spacecraft's current location, speed, and the gravitational force operating on it, where it will be 30 minutes from now. This is a phenomenon that should precisely conform to Newton's law of motion. But, in fact, Newton's law does not directly predict the location of an object. Rather, it states that acceleration, which is the rate of change in speed, which itself is rate of change in location, should be proportional to force.

In the case of guiding the spacecraft, it turns out that it is possible to derive an equation that

closely approximates the location of a space-craft as a function of time, fortunately for the astronauts on board a spacecraft returning from the moon to the earth. But the approximation works only insofar as the size of a spacecraft is small compared to that of the earth and the moon, so that the influence of the spacecraft on the earth and the moon can be ignored for all practical purposes. What if the spacecraft were much bigger? Can one write an equation predicting the location of the space-craft, the earth, and the moon? Surprising as it may seem, this problem, called the *three-body problem*, has not yet been solved five centuries after Newton, and many physicists believe it may never be solved.

If the prediction of three objects interacting in space is difficult, it is not surprising that the prediction of more than three objects interacting with each other is exceedingly difficult. As object 1 influences object 2, it in turn affects object 3, which then affects objects 4, 5, 6 . . .

all of which in turn affect objects 1, 2, and so on. Generally, when multiple objects form a system of interacting components, or a *dynamical system*, the behavior of the system becomes very complex and it is virtually impossible to write an equation predicting it, in the form of $Y = f(X1, X2 \ldots)$.

Considering that the brain is a system of not a few, but billions of interacting neurons, and that the interactions between neurons are more complex than the gravitational forces between two objects, it is not at all surprising that it has proved quite difficult to predict people's behaviors, in the form of behavior = $f(X1, X2 \ldots)$. To complicate the matter further, the neurons' reactions to the input can be nonlinear, meaning that a unit increase on the input side does not result in a constant increase on the output side. Nonlinear reactions are in fact quite ubiquitous in nature. For example, as the membrane potential of a neuron changes, nothing visible happens until the potential reaches a threshold, and all of a sudden a floodgate (of ion channels, literally) opens for a host of cellular activities, known as the action potential. Or an increasing tension between the earth's tectonic plates often does not lead to any visible effect, until the plates can no longer tolerate the pressure and shift, in a short burst of activities known as earthquake.

What is a researcher to do? This is where computational approaches enter the picture. Meteorologists, for example, don't have an equation in which precipitation on a given day in the future is predicted by the current conditions. But they do know with some precision how the current condition in one location affects the conditions in nearby locations *in the near future*. With that knowledge, they can construct a computer model. To do so, they start with the current conditions at many locations and then compute the effect of each location on nearby locations. For any given location, they can compute the sum total of influences of its "neighbors" and then make a fairly accurate prediction of its condition in the near future, such as an hour later. With the aid of fast computers, they can do this for every location. Now they have a predicted weather map, indicating the likely conditions at all locations a few minutes later. They can then repeat the whole process to make a predicted map one more hour into the future, and so on.

But how might such an approach be useful to psychology, and what might it look like? This chapter considers two examples at different levels of analysis. The first example is a network of thoughts and affective reactions characterizing an individual. To the extent that thoughts and feelings that are typically activated constitute an aspect of the "personality" of a network, this simulates the processes through which aspects of an individual's personality develop as an "emergent property" of the underlying dynamical system.

This example illustrates computer simulations of a nonlinear dynamical system, a system of interacting components in which the effect of one component on another does not necessarily follow a linear function, similar to a biological neuron. The second example considers the long-term change that may occur when an individual and his or her environment mutually influence each other over a long time span. It illustrates an approach in which the functioning of a dynamical system is simplified by assuming linear effects from one component to another. This simplifying assumption allows predictions of the system's "behavior" without using, as the first example does, a "brute force" computer simulation of the effect of each interacting component over many, many small steps. Instead, the second example uses a statistical model, in particular a structural equation modeling, to predict the trajectory of change in a system. These different examples help to illustrate an important distinction in mathematical modeling, between systems of equations that can be solved *analytically* (i.e., via algebraic manipulation of terms) and those that require *computational approximations*, as in the case of complex, nonlinear systems.

Example 1: Individual Differences in the Dynamics of Thought, Feeling, and Action

Consider Figures 35.1 and 35.2. They depict thoughts and feelings that may become activated as women encounter recommendations to perform breast self-examinations (BSE), identified in an extensive literature review (Miller, Shoda, & Hurley, 1996). Each of the two figures represents the cognitive and affective dynamics of one type of individual, each with a distinctive pattern of cognitive and affective reactions to BSE. The term *dynamics* is used specifically to underscore the notion that the thoughts and affects are not static; they come and go. But individuals can differ mean-

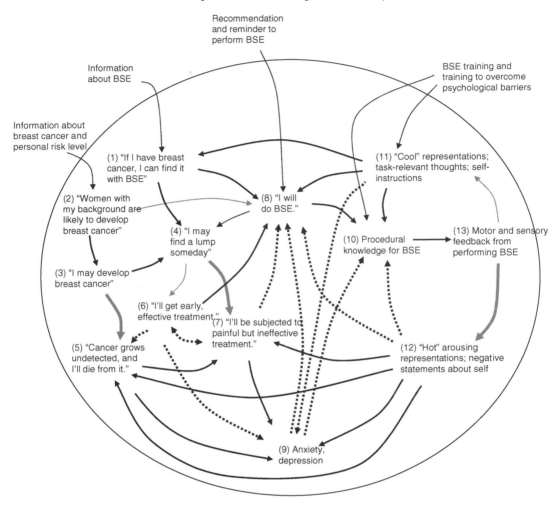

FIGURE 35.1. An illustrative CAPS network that undermines intention and performance of BSE. (Based on, and adapted from, Figure 5 of Miller et al., 1996.) Situational features activate specific subsets of the mediating units, which in turn activate other mediating units. The network of connections are considered stable and characterize the individual.

Arrows indicate activation relationships, such that when one unit is activated, other units that receive solid arrows from it will receive activation proportional to the weight associated with each arrow. The weight may be positive (solid arrows) or negative (dashed arrows).

ingfully in the kinds of thoughts and feelings that are likely to be activated, as well as in their temporal sequence. For example, one person may be characterized by a tendency for thought A to give rise to thought B, and thought C to give rise to thought D. But another person may be characterized by a tendency for thought A to give rise to thought C, and thought B often gives rise to thought D. The two individuals therefore may be equal in the overall frequencies of having each of these thoughts, but they differ reliably and meaningfully in the temporal patterns and sequences with which these thoughts come and go.

The arrows in Figures 35.1 and 35.2 represent these sequences. The figures contain examples of "cognitive and affective units" relevant to BSE. A solid arrow connecting one thought to another indicates that the activation of the first increases the activation of the second. Dashed arrows show that the activation of the first reduces the activation of the second. Each arrow therefore specifies how the activation level of one component of the system affects the other components (i.e., if an arrow goes from A to B, the type (solid or dashed) and thickness of the arrow indicate whether A increases or decreases the activation of B, and the

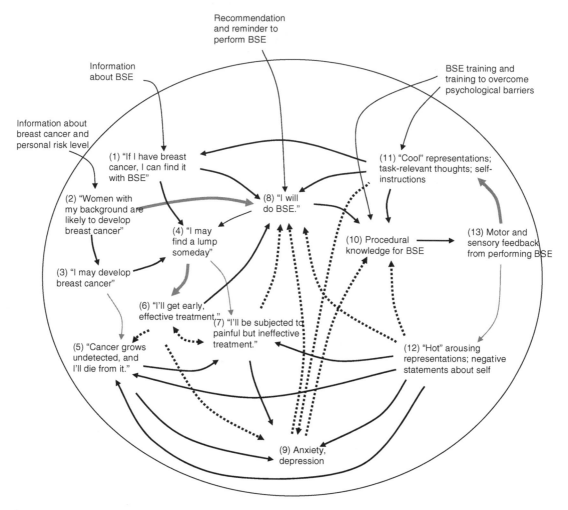

FIGURE 35.2. An illustrative CAPS network that enhances intention and performance of BSE. (Based on, and adapted from, Figure 6 of Miller et al., 1996.)

magnitude of such change. And if no arrow goes from *A* to *E*, *A* does not have a direct effect on *E*). With each arrow representing the dynamical (i.e., temporal) effect of one component of the system on another component, the whole network therefore constitutes the dynamical *system*.

The two figures are the same, except that the arrows connecting unit 3 to 5, 4 to 7, and 13 to 12 are thicker (i.e., more strongly connected) in Figure 35.1 than in Figure 35.2, whereas the arrows connecting unit 2 to 8, 4 to 6, and 13 to 11 are thicker in Figure 35.2 than in Figure 35.1. Thus, for a woman whose network resembles Figure 35.1, the thought, "I may find a lump someday" (unit 4) is more likely to activate the thought "I'll be subjected to painful but ineffective treatment" (unit 7). In contrast,

for a woman whose network resembles Figure 35.2, the first thought is more likely to activate the thought "I'll get early, effective treatment" (unit 6).

The difference between the two figures, in terms of the number of connections that are different (6, out of the 78 total potential connections between the units, or out of more than 30 non-zero connections drawn in Figures 35.1 and 35.2) is relatively minor. Would such small differences between the two networks result in appreciable differences in their responses to a health education program to increase women's awareness of breast cancer risks, for example, through genetic testing or pedigree analyses (Shoda et al., 1998)? The way the functioning of the systems is specified in Figures 35.1 and 35.2 is very much like the way a multiple-body system in physics or a weather system in meteorology is specified. Namely, what is known and specified is how one component of the system affects another component, as in the gravitational pull of one planet on another, or the movement of an air mass from one location to neighboring locations. The location of the planets, or the barometric pressure of each location, or the activation level of a thought at a given time, is not directly specified. Rather, what is specified is the change in location, barometric pressure, or the activation level of a thought in one part of the system as a result of the influence from another part of the system. Thus, just as in the prediction of the physical system, it is helpful, even necessary, to use a computational simulation to predict the functioning of psychological systems, such as those shown in Figures 35.1 and 35.2.

To simulate the network's functioning, it is assumed that cognitions and affects become activated, either by the salient "psychologically active" element in the situation (Shoda, Mischel, & Wright, 1994) or internally by other activated cognitions and affects. Activation then propagates through an individual's unique network of associations and ultimately results in thoughts or emotions the individual is aware of, or in a behavior that is observable.

An important characteristic of this model is that the network of associations between specific cognitions and affects (i.e., personality structure) that characterizes the person can be invariant across situations, but its behavioral output is expected to vary greatly, and predictably, from one situation to another. The cognitions and affects that are activated change from one time to the next, but the relations between the cognitions and affects activated at one time and those activated next are assumed to reflect the stable personality structure of the individual (Mischel & Shoda, 1995; Shoda & Mischel, 1998).

Another key aspect of the model is that potentially there may be connections between any given pair of processing units, resulting in multiple feedback loops in a network. Thus, "downstream" units can activate "upstream" units, generating a flow of thoughts, feelings, and even behaviors, without necessarily requiring an outside stimulus. That is, not only the external input, but also the thoughts and feelings at a given point, influence what happens next in the system. The result is something that may resemble a "stream of consciousness."

Network Simulations

To simulate the functioning of such a system, my colleagues and I conducted a computer simulation of personality dynamics, using the basic architecture reported more fully in Shoda, LeeTiernan, and Mischel (2002).

A hypothetical personality was simulated in a 13-unit network following a standard connectionist architecture (e.g., McClelland & Rumelhart, 1986).[1] In such a network, activation travels from one unit to another, according to the sign and magnitude of the "weight" of the connection between the units, which in the current simulation was assumed to be between -1 and $+1$. The connection weights were fixed for each person being simulated, analogous to the stability in personality over the short term. (In real life, of course, experiences, particularly intense or prolonged exposure to critical events, can change the connection weights, which in this simulation, represent *personality change*.)

Figure 35.3 illustrates the structure of associations between the units shown in Figure 35.1, but with the units arranged in a circle to facilitate a graphical representation. The numerical labels for the units correspond to those in Figure 35.1. Using the same notation as Figure 35.1, positive associations (shown by solid lines) indicate that when one unit becomes activated, it will increase the activation of the unit to which it is connected. Other associations are negative (shown by dashed lines), indicating that when one unit becomes activated, it will suppress the activation of the other unit. Figure 35.4 is a similar rearrangement of Figure 35.2, in preparation for a more compact representation needed to show temporal changes in Figures 35.5 to 35.8.

To understand the operation of such a system, we "stimulated" the dynamics of the network by temporarily increasing the activation of a subset of the units. This is analogous to what happens when a person is exposed to information about her genetic risk for breast cancer. Arrows show the paths through which activation spreads from one unit to another in the network.

Such spreading activation is not unlike the biological system that inspired the original connectionist modeling. However, in a biological system the activation levels of all the units change simultaneously, and more or less continuously. To simulate simultaneous and continuous changes with conventional computers, which operate serially (i.e., executing one oper-

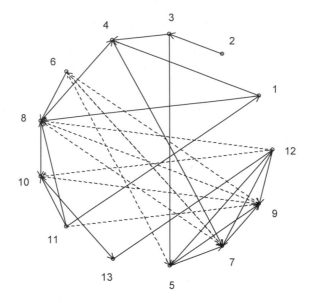

FIGURE 35.3. The 13 units from Figure 35.1 are rearranged in a circle to facilitate the condensed display format used in Figures 35.5–35.8. The connections shown are identical to those in Figure 35.1.

ation at a time, albeit extremely rapidly), many "cycles" of minute adjustments are made in the activation levels of each unit. Specifically, in one cycle, the input to each unit from all units to which it is connected are summed and added to 98% of its previous level of activation (i.e., activation of every unit is assumed to undergo a slow decay, such that 98% of its activation in

the previous cycle "carries over" to the next cycle; without any input to a unit, its activation value was 98% of its value in the previous cycle).

Then the adjustment process starts all over again in a new cycle. The configuration of activated units at a given moment represents the network's "state of mind." In the example of a

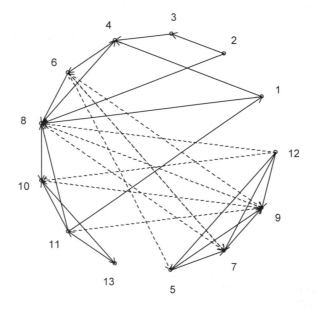

FIGURE 35.4. The 13 units from Figure 35.2 are rearranged in a circl, to facilitate the condensed display format used in Figures 35.5–35.8. The connections shown are identical those in Figure 35.2.

woman being advised to perform BSE, the state in which thought unit 8 is activated (by the external input, shown by an arrow in Figure 35.1, from an external event, "Recommendation and reminder to perform BSE," to unit 8, "I will do BSE") constitutes an initial state. The state of mind, as defined by the set of thought units activated a little while later, can be predicted by running the simulation from such an initial condition.

Figure 35.5 shows the results of a simulation. The top left panel, labeled "cycle 1," shows the initial state after unit 8 was activated. The graphs show each unit's activation level by drawing a circle around the unit, with the diameter proportional to the magnitude of activation. Thus, the large circle around unit 8 indicates that the unit is highly activated at this moment. The 13 units are arranged the same way as in Figure 35.3, except that the connections between the units are not shown. Instead, in Figure 35.5, arrows are used to indicate the actual amount of activation that is being spread, as shown in the panel labeled "cycle 2." Generally, an arrow from unit i to unit j is shown if the activation of unit i multiplied by the weight of the connection from unit i to unit j exceeded 0.4 in a given cycle.[2] This, in essence, selectively shows only those connections that are currently used to propagate activation.

This simulation shows the expected reaction of a network that is characterized by the connection patterns shown in Figure 35.1 (and Figure 35.3) after unit 8 is activated by external input—that is, the expected reaction to a recommendation and reminder to perform BSE by a person whose internal "structure" resembles Figure 35.1. The dynamic time course of thoughts and feelings activated after receiving the recommendation (hence activating unit 8, in the simulation) suggests the following: (1) Immediately after receiving the recommendation, procedural knowledge of BSE is activated (and hence actually performing BSE), as well as the thought "I may find a lump someday"; (2) soon (by cycle 16) the thought "I'll be subjected to painful but ineffective treatment" is activated, which in turn gives rise to anxiety and depression by cycle 32; (3) the expectation of painful and effective treatment and anxiety and depression remain the dominant thoughts and feelings for the next 100 or more cycles, which remain the most active even after cycle 256. In short, the expected reaction of a person characterized by a network shown in Figure 35.1 is one of initial performance of BSE followed by a prolonged period dominated by anxiety and depression.

What will happen when the same recommendation to perform BSE is given to a person characterized by a network shown in Figure 35.2? To find out, a simulation just like the one discussed was run, but this time using the network shown in Figure 35.2 (and Figure 35.4). Figure 35.6 shows the results. What happens soon after the initial activation of unit 8 is quite similar to the results of activating unit 8 in the first network (shown in Figures 35.1 and 35.3), as shown in the first few panels. But, as shown in subsequent panels, units 7 and 9 do not become activated. Instead, this network results in a stable, constant activation of many units, such as units 6, 8, and 10. They remain activated even after 256 cycles. This occurs because in a "recurrent" network such as the one used here, when a large enough number of units mutually activate each other, they can overcome the natural decay that is built in to the simulation. In the language of dynamical systems analysis, this network has settled into an "attractor state," a state toward which the system drifts and in which it remains (e.g., Anderson, Silverstein, Ritz, & Jones, 1977; Hopfield, 1982, 1984).

Psychologically, this simulation suggests that when a person characterized by the network shown in Figure 35.2 (and Figure 35.4) encounters a recommendation to perform BSE, the result is a successful maintenance of BSE practice and the thoughts and feelings that support it. Furthermore, anxiety and depression are unlikely to become activated.

What if the networks encounter different situational inputs? For example, how would the networks shown in Figures 35.1 and 35.2 respond when encountering information about breast cancer and personal risk level (i.e., activating unit 2—see Figures 35.1 and 35.2), information about BSE (i.e., activating unit 1), or BSE training and training to overcome psychological barriers (i.e., activating units 10 and 11)? Each row of Figure 35.7 shows the simulation results after stimulating the network shown in Figure 35.1 with each situational input. The first row of Figure 35.7, for example, shows that after encountering information about BSE, unit 1 was highly activated and the activation spread to units 4 and 8. By cycle 16, units 1, 4, 8, 10, 7 and 9 are activated. And by cycle 128, units 7 and 9 are activated. Note that even though the patterns of activation in cycles 2 and 16 are quite different from that shown in Figure 35.5, which was in response to

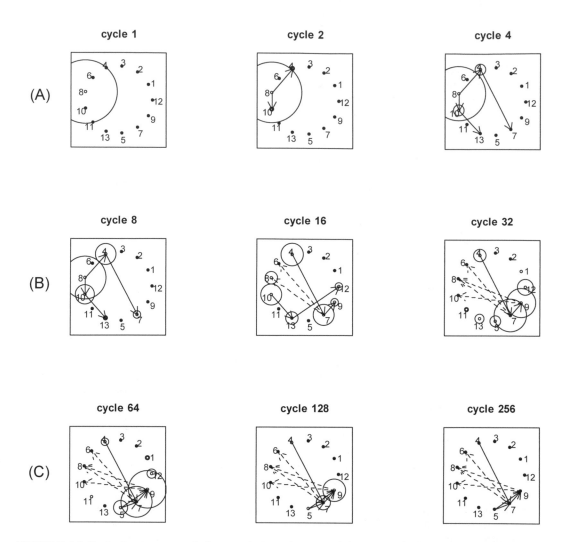

FIGURE 35.5. Activation spreads from unit 8 to the rest of the network shown in Figures 35.1 and 35.3. The network was exposed to a stimulus (e.g., recommendation and reminder to perform BSE) that activated unit 8 (intention to perform BSE). The level of activation of each unit is shown by the circle drawn on it, with the diameter proportional to the activation level. The "cycle 1" panel therefore shows that unit 8 (and only unit 8) is highly activated. The arrows in the "cycle 2" panel show that the activation is beginning to spread from unit 8 to units 4 and 10. The arrow is drawn when the amount of influence from the "sending" unit to the "receiving" unit exceeded 0.4. Thus, only the connection pathways that are actively influencing the activation levels of units are shown, which occurs when the sending unit is highly activated, and the connection weight between the sending unit and the receiving unit is large (to be more specific, this is proportional to the product of the activation of the sending unit and the connection weight). Dashed arrows seen in cycles 16, 32, 64, 128, and 256 show that the sending unit is actively reducing the activation level of the receiving unit.

The arrows in the panel labeled "cycle 2" show that the initial activation of unit 8 is beginning to spread to units 4 and 10, to which unit 8 has a positive connection. The "cycle 4" panel shows that the units 4 and 10 are now somewhat activated, and they are in turn propagating activation to units 7 and 13, respectively, to which they have positive connections. The "cycle 8" panel shows that units 7 and 13 are now slightly activated, while unit 8's original activation is beginning to fade (due to the spontaneous decay assumed to occur if a unit receives no further input). The "cycle 16" panel shows this trend continuing. It also shows that unit 7, which is by now activated fairly strongly, is propagating negative activation (i.e., inhibiting) to units 6 and 8, as shown by the dashed arrows from unit 7 to units 6 and 8. The "cycle 32" panel shows that activation of unit 8 has dissipated, while units 7 and 9 are strongly activated (along with units 13, 5, and 12). The "cycle 64" panel shows that the network remains virtually unchanged 32 cycles later. The "cycle 128" panel shows this continues to be the case, 64 more cycles later, although somewhat diminished. One hundred twenty-eight cycles later, the "cycle 256" panel shows that activation levels of units 7 and 9 are finally approaching 0, through natural decay, but they are still non-zero and are actively inhibiting units 6, 8, and 10, after 256 cycles.

a recommendation and reminder to perform BSE, by cycle 128, the pattern of activation in this network is virtually identical to what happened in Figure 35.5.

Similarly, the second row of Figure 35.7 shows that after encountering information about breast cancer and personal risk level, even though the initial pattern of activation is quite different from the simulation shown in Figure 35.5 and in the top row of Figure 35.7, by cycle 128, the network has settled into a pattern of activation that is virtually identical to that of Figure 35.5 and the top row of Figure 35.7. The third row of Figure 35.7, showing what happens when the network encounters BSE training and training to overcome psychological barriers, reveals a similar result. Thus, the pattern of activation after cycle 128, shown

in Figures 35.5 and 35.7, represents a characteristic pattern of activation for this network, a state in which it is often found. Specifically, this state is characterized by the activation of unit 7, "I'll be subjected to painful but ineffective treatment," and unit 9, representing anxiety and depression. That is, it may be reasonable to characterize the "personality" of this network as prone to depression and anxiety and to pessimistic thoughts.

In contrast, Figure 35.8 shows the results of simulating the reaction of the network shown in Figure 35.2 (and Figures 35.4 and 35.6) to the same set of stimuli as shown in Figure 35.7. The result shows, again, that despite the initial pattern of activation that depends greatly on the stimuli, the network has settled into its characteristic pattern of activation by cycle

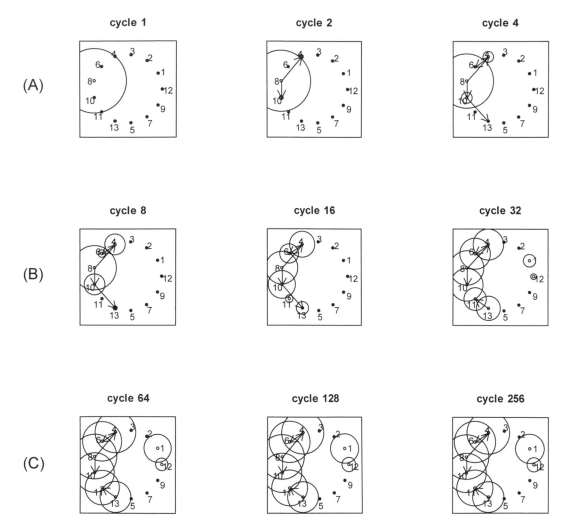

FIGURE 35.6. Activation spreads from unit 8 to the rest of the network shown in Figures 35.2 and 35.4.

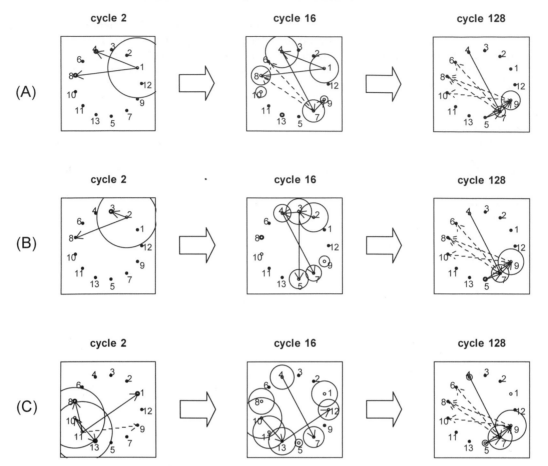

FIGURE 35.7. Spreading activation after the network shown in Figure 35.1 (and Figures 35.3 and 35.5) was exposed to stimuli that activated unit 1 (shown in the first row), unit 2 (shown in the second row), and units 10 and 11 (shown in the third row).

128. And this characteristic pattern is quite different from that shown in Figure 35.7 (and Figure 35.5). Depression and anxiety are not activated. Instead, the pattern is characterized by optimism and a constellation of thoughts and procedural knowledge that together support continued performance of BSE.

Note that the two networks differed only in the pattern of connectivity between the units, and no assumption was made about differences in the chronic levels of activation of any of the units in the two simulated persons. Furthermore, the initial condition of the simulations was identical, and there was no initial difference between the two simulated personalities in the activation levels of the units. Yet the expected reactions by the two networks were dramatically different. One resulted in a rapid extinction of BSE performance and a prolonged activation of anxiety and depression. The other

resulted in sustained BSE performance and little activation of anxiety and depression.

This observation is of some significance for personality psychology. Although many theorists, starting with Gordon Allport (1937), have stressed the importance of focusing on intra-individual dynamics, personality psychology has often focused on behaviors that are characteristic of an individual "over all" or chronic differences in the likelihood of a given set of behaviors, thoughts, or feelings. This can naturally lead to models that represent individual differences in chronic activation levels of certain cognitions and affects as underlying stable differences in behavioral tendencies. The simulations show, however, that models that focus on the dynamical properties are relevant not only for accounting for temporal changes, but also for accounting for "overall" or chronic differences, an aspect of individual functioning that has often been the focus of personality psychology.

Most relevant for the purpose of this chapter, this observation was made possible through the use of computational methods. That is because, as discussed earlier, properties of a dynamical system are often "emergent," meaning that they are not reflected directly in the property of any of the components of the system, but emerge out of the mutual interactions between the components. Thus, when a system is described by showing how each component interacts with others, such as in the network diagram shown in Figures 35.1 and 35.2, or in meteorologists' weather models or astronomers' models of the solar system, the prediction and understanding of the behavior of the system require a computational approach.

The type of network used in these simulations is called a *recurrent* network, referring to the fact that the flow of activation is not unidirectional from input to output, but, rather, can have many feedback loops, such that a downstream unit can activate upstream units. This type of network is also called a *parallel constraint satisfaction network*, because one of the most notable properties of such networks is that they settle into a set of activation patterns that satisfy multiple simultaneous constraints represented by the patterns of connections between the units in the network. The use of a recurrent, or parallel constraint satisfaction, network is consistent with models of human information processing in the broader cognitive sciences, including analogical reasoning (Holyoak & Thagard, 2002; Hummel & Holyoak, 2003; Spellman & Holyoak, 1992), attitude change (Spellman, Ullman, & Holyoak, 1994), explanatory coherence (Read & Marcus-Newhall, 1993; Thagard, 1989), dis-

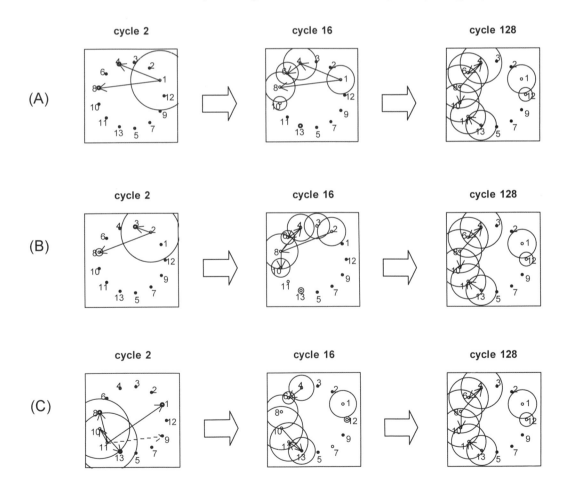

FIGURE 35.8. Spreading activation after the network shown in Figure 35.2 (and Figures 35.4 and 35.6) was exposed to stimuli that activated unit 1 (shown in the first row), unit 2 (shown in the second row), and units 10 and 11 (shown in the third row).

sonance reduction (Read & Miller, 1994; Shultz & Lepper, 1996; Simon, Snow, & Read, 2004), and impression formation and dispositional inference (Kashima & Kerekes, 1994; Kunda & Thagard, 1996; Read & Miller, 1993). Read and Miller (1998) describe some of the most important characteristics of neural network models, and Thagard and Kunda (1998) provide an introduction to the use of constraint satisfaction networks for modeling social cognition, particularly the function of schemas.

These methods can also be used to model coupled systems in which the behavior of one system becomes the context for another and vice versa—for example, a married couple in which one person's behavioral output becomes the other person's situational input. In the simulations of intra-individual dynamics discussed earlier, it was assumed that after an initial exposure to situations, the subsequent processing of the initial stimulus was carried out by the network in isolation, without further external inputs or constraints. Such a process may account for what may happen, for example, when an individual is watching a TV news program alone, in which the recommendation for BSE is given. When the next news story is presented, the process repeats, this time activating a different set of thoughts. Note that in this example, the situations (i.e., the news stories) are determined by factors outside the individual's influence. That is, the thoughts, feelings, and behaviors of the individual do not (under usual circumstances) influence the next item featured on the news.

In a dyadic interaction, however, what one person says, the tone of voice, or even the quick glimpse of a facial expression, can significantly affect the other person's thoughts, feelings, and behavior, which in turn constitutes the next situation encountered by the first person. Computationally, a dyadic system therefore can be modeled by a system that combines two networks, each representing a person (Figure 35.9). Each individual network becomes part of a larger parallel constraint satisfaction system. This coupling of individual networks is conceptually akin to work on coupled dynamical systems (see Nowak & Vallacher, 1998), which modeled the properties of dyads such as relationship synchronization and the manner in which a dyad reaches equilibrium (see also Gottman, Swanson, & Swanson, 2002).

One application of a dyadic system (Shoda et al., 2002) showed how each interpersonal sys-

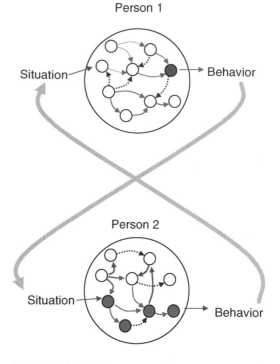

FIGURE 35.9. A conceptual representation of a dyadic system, in which the behavior of one partner (represented by an interconnected network of cognitive and affective units, labeled "Person 1") becomes the situational input for the other partner, whose behavioral output in turn becomes the situational input for the first partner.

tem formed by a combination of two individuals has predictable and distinctive behaviors and patterns of interactions. By comparing the properties of each of the individuals and the property of the interpersonal system made up of the individuals, this application illustrated the intuitive and theoretical observation that every interpersonal relationship has its own personality. Most important, the qualities of an interpersonal relationship are not simply an average of the personalities of the individuals that form it. For example, the marriage of two generally agreeable individuals may turn out to be full of discord and unhappiness, and the opposite can also occur, in which two generally disagreeable individuals form a happy and invigorating, if not quiet, partnership.

The possibility is not unlike that of chemistry, in which the "behaviors" of substance A in reaction to substance B are predicted by knowing the molecular structures of both. Modeling each individual's cognitive-affective system may help us get one step closer to being able to predict the "chemistry" of interpersonal systems. Computational approaches facilitate building models of human behavior capable of making such predictions.

Example 2: Stability and Change in Personality

The first example focused on the intra-individual dynamics of thoughts, feelings, and actions over a time span short enough to warrant the assumption that the personality structure itself is constant. But just as the terrain that guides the flow of water through streams, lakes, and rivers can change over time, the internal psychological terrain that guides the flow of thoughts, feelings, and actions in response to a situation may also change over time.

Such long-term gradual changes occur in a dynamical system consisting of the individual and the environment. That is, people influence their own environment through choice (e.g., of partners, friends, jobs) or through reactions by others (e.g., to one's appearance, behaviors, or social status), as reviewed by Caspi and Roberts (1999). The environment, in turn, can influence the individual's personality. Fraley and Roberts (2005) refer to the mutual influences of the person and the environment as transactional processes. These are characterized by how an individual's personality today influences the expected *change* in the environment tomorrow and how the environment today influences the expected *change* in personality tomorrow.

Fraley and Roberts (2005) modeled personality change in such dynamic transaction processes using a set of difference equations. They built a model in which change in the personality of an individual from time t to time $t + 1$ is determined by the environment at time t. Similarly, they assumed that change in an individual's environment from time t to time $t + 1$ is determined by the individual's personality at time t. The model also assumed the operation of a factor that remains constant throughout a person's life and that continues to exert an influence on personality (e.g., genetic variation in the neurotransmitter receptors). The model is shown in Figure 35.10.

The three circles on the left, labeled C, P, and E, represent an individual's "developmental constancy factor," "personality," and "environment," respectively, at time t_0. Following the conventional structural equation modeling

notation, the curved double-ended arrows show initial levels of correlation that may exist between the three variables. To the right of these three are personality and environment at time t_1. The C factor is, by definition, unchanging over time, so rather than repeating it at every time, it is shown only once at time t_0. Arrows going from the variables at time t_0 indicate that personality and environment at time t_1 are influenced by personality and environment at time t_0, as well as by the developmental constancy factor. The short arrows pointing to personality and environment at time t_1 indicate the influence of random factors uncorrelated with any of the other variables. Personality and environment at time t_2 are determined similarly by personality and environment at time t_1, as well as the developmental constancy factor.

By treating time in discrete units (they used a year as a unit) rather than as a continuous variable, Fraley and Roberts (2005) were able to use a structural equation modeling framework to make the predictions. Namely, personality at time $t + 1$ is modeled as a linear function of personality at time t, environment at time t, and the developmental constancy factor, each of which are in turn modeled as a linear function of personality and environment at time $t - 1$ and the constancy factor. To be sure, it is an approximation and a simplification to treat time in discrete steps and to assume that the influence of variables at time t on the variables at $t + 1$ is linear. But that made it possible to make direct predictions of the expected correlations between any ages, without resorting to "brute

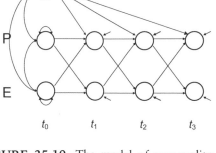

FIGURE 35.10. The model of personality development used in simulations of developmental dynamics conducted by Fraley and Roberts (2005). P represents the personality of an individual, E represents the individual's environment, and C, the developmentally constant factor (e.g., the individual's genome).

force" computational simulations that would have required massive computational power.

With this model, Fraley and Roberts (2005) asked, If one is to do a longitudinal study, following up people every year from age X, how will the longitudinal stability in personality change as years go by? Suppose the stability, measured by a test–retest correlation coefficient, was 0.6 between ages X and $X + 1$. What will the stability coefficient between ages X and $X + 2$ be? What about the stability between ages X and $X + 10$? It would make sense that the stability will diminish as the span of time

between the two assessments increases. But will it eventually reach 0? They also asked a number of other questions, such as, Will the stability between ages X and $X + 10$ be the same as the stability between ages $X - 10$ and X, both spanning 10 years, but one 10-year span following, and the other preceding, age X?

The answers provided by their model are shown in Figure 35.11. A line in each graph plots the longitudinal (test–retest) stability coefficient between age X and other ages represented by the horizontal axis, where X is 1 year old for the graphs in the left column, 10 for the

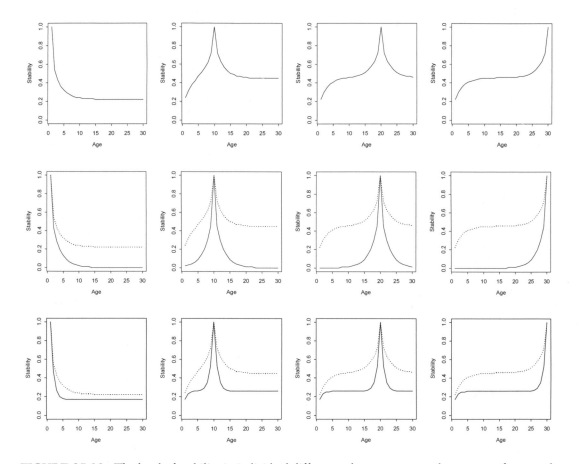

FIGURE 35.11. The level of stability in individual differences between repeated measures of personality at different ages, predicted by the model shown in Figure 35.10 (top row), as well as a model that removed the developmental constants from the model in Figure 35.10 (middle row), and a model that removed the transactional process from the model shown in Figure 35.10 (bottom row). The panels in the left column show the predicted stabilities between age 1 and a variety of ages shown on the horizontal axis. The panels in the second column show the predicted stabilities between age 10 and a variety of ages shown on the horizontal axis. The panels in the third column show the predicted stabilities between age 20 and other ages, and the panels in the rightmost column show the predicted stabilities between age 30 and the other ages. The dotted lines in the second and third columns duplicate the graph shown in the first row, to aid the comparison and assess the effect of removing the developmental constant from the model (second row) and that of removing the transactional processes form the model (third row).

second column, 20 for the third column, and 30 for the fourth column. The lines in the graphs in the first row show the predictions from their model, and the graphs in the second and third rows show what is expected if various parts of the model are removed, allowing one to see the role these removed components play in the full model shown in the first row.

Let us first focus on the graphs in the first row. The line in the top left graph shows that the expected longitudinal stability between age 0 and subsequent ages is expected to decline steeply from the initial theoretical same-age value of 1.0 (assuming a perfectly reliable measure) to an expected stability of about $r = 0.3$ between ages 0 and 5. From there on, stability is expected to decline further but it does not approach 0. Rather, it reaches an asymptote of about 0.2.

The second graph in the top row shows the expected longitudinal stability between age 10 and various other ages. Like the top left graph, it shows that the longitudinal stability between age 10 and $10 + Y$ years declines rapidly as Y increases. For example, the longitudinal stability between ages 10 and 11 is expected to be quite high (above 0.8). But when the time span ranges from ages 10 to 15, the expected stability is only about 0.4, and from there on the expected stability does not decline much, appearing to reach an asymptote.

To the left of the peak in this (second in the top row) graph, one can see a curve that is significantly different from what is seen to the right of the peak. Just as seen to the right of the peak, the longitudinal stability is expected to be high when the age span is short, such as predicting age 10 from age 9, and this declines steeply as the time span increases, reaching about 0.4 when predicting age 10 from age 5. However, rather than reaching an asymptote, as seen on the right side of the peak, the predicted stability continues to decline as the age span increases. For example, the stability from age 1 to age 10 is only about 0.2 and does not appear to be reaching an asymptote at all.

Why might this happen? An answer lies in the graphs in the second and third rows. The solid line in the graphs in the second row show the longitudinal stabilities expected when the effect of the development constant factor (C in Figure 35.10) is set to 0, in effect removing this factor from the model. (The dotted lines are the lines from the top row, copied here to facilitate comparison.) The effect is that predicted stability does not reach an asymptote as the target age is increased, so that eventually it will approach 0. The developmental constancy factor therefore is critical for producing the non-zero asymptote to the right of the peak. Why might *this* be the case? It can be thought of as the system reaching an equilibrium point between two opposing influences. On one hand, at every time period, the random influence (e.g., chance events in life) on personality and environment will accumulate and decrease predictability as the time span increases. On the other hand, the developmental constancy factor influences personality and environment steadily and consistently, year after year. Thus, this effect, although small, will accumulate to increase predictability as the time span increases. The two influences therefore reach an equilibrium point, and in the simulation, the equilibrium point when predicting from age 10 (the second graph in the top row) is about 0.4.

The third row of graphs shows what happens when the transactional processes are removed from the model. This was accomplished by setting the influence of personality on environment to 0, as well as setting the influence of environment on personality to 0. Comparing these graphs to the ones in the top row, it becomes evident that the transactional process contributed to the higher stability predicted by the intact model shown in the first row (i.e., without it, the stability is expected to be lower). This is because the transactional process can increase the "fit" between personality and environment. For example, a person who behaves abrasively may tend to create an environment that is not as accepting, which in turn may increase the person's abrasive manner, perhaps setting up a cycle of self-fulfilling prophecy such that an erroneous perception of the world as malevolent becomes a reality as time progresses. Fraley and Roberts (2005) examined this aspect by plotting the expected correlation between personality and environment, as shown in Figure 35.12.

The figure shows that even when the model assumed no correlation at birth between personality and environment, the correlation increases every year, which may be expected if infants' personalities (e.g., how difficult it is to soothe them) influenced their caretakers' attitudes toward them, which in turn influenced the developing infants' personalities. The person–environment correlation reaches a plateau of about 0.37 at about age 8, presumably when the cumulative stability-enhancing person–environment transaction is matched by the cumulative stability-reducing effect of random factors.

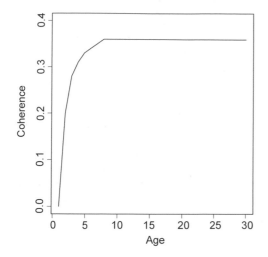

FIGURE 35.12. The correlation between personality and environment at different ages, as predicted by the full model shown in Figure 35.10 and the top row of Figure 35.11. The model assumes no correlation between personality and environment at birth. But the transactional processes increase the correlation during the first years, until it reaches an asymptote of about $r = 0.37$ at about age 8.

Interestingly, the stability-enhancing effect of the transactional process differs from that of the developmental constancy factor in one regard. That is, whereas the developmental constancy factor predicts a non-zero asymptote in the stability coefficient, the predicted stability from a model with a transactional process will eventually approach 0 if there is no developmental constancy factor (Fraley & Roberts, 2005).

Concluding Remarks

The first example discussed in this chapter illustrates one of the primary reasons for computational modeling. That is, when the model specifies how the current state affects the *changes* expected in the system, which is true of most dynamical systems, it is often not possible to make direct predictions about the state of the system later on. Just as in the case of a weather forecast model, all one can predict with confidence, based on the current state, is the state of the system in the very near future. And, as the multibody problem in physics illustrates, and as discussed often in the literature on the "chaotic" nature of dynamical systems, this difficulty in prediction is not necessarily due to random factors. It is because of the com-

plexity of mutual interactions that compound and increase exponentially as the time span for prediction increases.

Nonetheless, dynamical systems often show predictable patterns of behavior. One can make the prediction that hurricanes emerge in the Caribbean Sea several times a year, even though it is not possible to predict exactly when and where. Similarly, computational approaches allow one to gain insight into the behavior of a dynamical system. The insight gained by modeling a dyadic system by coupling dynamical models of two individuals, as discussed in the first example above, is a good example. It clearly shows that the "personality" of a dyad can be an emergent quality, in that it is not a simple combination of the personalities of the two people that make up the system. Thus, the dynamical model could provide an insight into such real-life occurrences as two generally agreeable individuals displaying malicious behaviors in their marriage (to one another) even though they rarely display such behaviors alone or when they interact with others.

Whereas the first example sought to model the dynamics underlying the thoughts, feelings, and behavior in response to immediate situations, the second example's goal was to model the long-term change in the personality–environment system over individuals' lifespans. The dynamics of such changes are likely to be several orders of magnitude more complex than the dynamics of personality, which is itself a dynamical system. Fraley and Roberts (2005), from whose work the second example is drawn, approached this task by treating time in discrete steps, namely year by year, and by assuming that the influences of the relevant variables are linear. This approximation allowed them to express the dynamics within the framework of structural equation modeling, avoiding the necessity for a massive, brute force modeling of moment-to-moment changes.

Using such an approach, they were able to conduct "experiments" on the system, by removing certain assumptions built into the model (as the second example illustrates). This led to an insight that is usually inaccessible without a formal model. Furthermore, the novel phenomena predicted by the model specifies the kinds of empirical data that are necessary to differentiate between models and to evaluate the importance of different assumptions on which a model is built.

Finally, a critical decision one needs to make when building a model of complex phenomena is, just how complex should the model be? First, increasing the complexity of models, even though doing so almost always allows one to explain more details of any phenomena, risks *overfitting*, or fitting data points that are not reliable. The history of science is replete with examples in which a theory or a model, which later turns out to be the "right" one, could not account for "an awful lot of chaotic data [for which] we even went so far as to state that the experiment was in error" (Feynman & Leighton, 1985, p. 253). In fact, considering experimental errors, a theory, even an ultimately correct one, is not expected to account for all existing data, as some of the conclusions from empirical data are erroneous (e.g., with the $p < .05$ convention, 5% of the statistically significant results can arise under null hypothesis). In fact, it *should not* account for all data, as some of them are likely to be in error. (The problem faced by scientists, of course, is that they don't know which of the existing results are errors!)

Second, even though any behavioral phenomenon is likely to reflect complex interactions between multiple structures and processes, trying to model every wrinkle in the data by incorporating an increasing number of factors can be self-defeating. Arguably, one of the goals of modeling is to gain basic insight into the workings of the dynamical processes underlying the phenomenon. In fact, the beauty of constructing a model is that it allows one to understand the implications of the theory that it implements. In other words, models allow one to gain insight in the form, "IF a dynamical system is built according to this principle, THEN the system will display the following behavior." The informativeness of such a statement would be greatly reduced if the model incorporated numerous principles. In a similar vein, Nowak (2004) proposed a principle of *dynamical minimalism*: constructing a system of interacting elements with a minimal set of assumptions necessary to produce the phenomenon of interest.

In conclusion, the ebb and flow in a person's experience has long been the core interest of personality psychology. Every person thinks, feels, and does different things in different situations. But the changes from situation to situation are not all random. There is a stable pattern in the stream of experiences that is unique to each individual. Understanding the nature of such variations, of course, is one of the main missions of personality psychology. In fact,

Allport (1937, p. 48) defined personality as follows: "Personality is the dynamic organization within the individual of those psychophysical systems that determine his unique adjustments to his environment." In other words, Allport's definition comes very close to defining personality as a dynamical system that underlies an individual's unique way of responding to different situations.

The goal of studying personality as a dynamical system has long been elusive because of the very nature of the phenomena in question: they are dynamic. To understand them requires more than reliably obtaining a person's position on a trait dimension. It requires conceptual and methodological tools that can model each person's "neuropsychic system (peculiar to the individual) with the capacity to render many stimuli functionally equivalent, and to initiate and guide consistent (equivalent) forms of adaptive and expressive behavior" (Allport, 1937, p. 295). And it requires "dense" data, about how a person lives his or her life in a variety of situations, reflecting the system at work, linking, in unique ways, each functionally equivalent set of stimuli to each functionally equivalent form of adaptive and expressive behaviors.

Human behavior reflects the operation of a highly complex dynamical system—the brain itself, the interpersonal systems, and the system of person–environment interactions of which the person is a part. Models of dynamical systems therefore seem to be essential for achieving the goal of psychological science. The last two decades have witnessed a significant advancement in the conceptual and methodological tools for building and testing dynamical models, some of which are illustrated in this chapter.

Further Reading and the Pragmatics of Computational Modeling

Computational modeling of dynamical systems is fast emerging in many areas of psychology. To learn more about the varieties of computational approaches being used and their theoretical underpinnings, as well as more detailed descriptions of specific examples of computational approaches beyond the two discussed in this chapter, consult publications such as those in "Recommended Readings."

In cases in which complex, nonlinear dynamics are being studied, computers are essential for approximating the processes being modeled. Programming languages and software packages that are commonly used in computational modeling include a freely available statistical language *R* (*www.r-project.org*; see Venables & Ripley, 2000) and its commercial counterpart, S-Plus (*www.insightful.com/products/splus*); Matlab (*www.mathworks.com/products/matlab*); PDP++ (*www.kcl.ac.uk/neuronet/products*; see also O'Reilly & Munakata, 2000); and Stella (*www.hps-inc.com/softwares/Education/StellaSoftware.aspx*). For a more comprehensive list of available neural network packages, see *www.kcl.ac.uk/neuronet/products* and *www.ncrg.aston.ac.uk/NN/software. html*.

Notes

1. The activation level of each unit was updated following the "squashing" function (e.g., McClelland & Rumelhart, 1986; Shultz & Lepper, 1996), which scaled the effect of net input into each unit in proportion to the distance left to the ceiling (when activation < 0) or to the floor (when activation > 0) of the possible range of activation, which was set from −1 to +1. Specifically, when $net_i > 0$,

$$a_i(t + 1) = d * a_i(t) + net_i * \{ceiling - a_i(t)\}$$

When $net_i < 0$,

$$a_i(t + 1) = d * a_i(t) + net_i * \{a_i(t) - floor\}$$

Net input into unit i was computed as

$$net_i = \sum_{i \neq j} (w_{ji} * f(a_j(t)))$$

where $a_j(t)$ is the activation level of unit j at time t and w_{ji} is the weight of the connection between unit j and unit i. The weights were symmetrical, so that $w_{ij} = w_{ji}$. $f(a_j(t)) = 1/(1 + e^{(-\lambda * (aj(t)-\theta))})$, which is a sigmoid function of $a_j(t)$ over −1 to +1. Constants are set as follows: $c = 1.0$, $d = .98$, ceiling = 1.0, floor = −1.0, $\lambda = 10$, $\theta = 0$.
2. Using the notation in the previous note, an arrow is drawn from unit i to unit j when $w_{ji} * f(a_j(t)) > 0.4$.

Recommended Readings

Application of Computational Models in Social and Personality Psychology

Liebrand, W., Nowak, A., & Hegselman, R. (1998). *Computer modeling and the study of dynamic social processes*. New York: Sage.

Polk, T. A., & Seifert, C. M. (2002). *Cognitive modeling*. Cambridge, MA: MIT Press.

Smith, E. R. (1996). What do connectionism and social psychology offer each other? *Journal of Personality and Social Psychology, 70*, 893–912.

Vallacher, R. R., & Nowak, A. (2007). Dynamical social psychology: Finding order in the flow of human experience. In A. W. Kruglanski & E. T. Higgins (Eds.), *Social psychology: Handbook of basic principles* (2nd ed., pp. 734–758). New York: Guilford Press.

Examples of Computational Models in Social and Personality Psychology

Carver, C. S., & Scheier, M. F. (2002). Control processes and self-organization as complementary principles underlying behavior. *Personality and Social Psychology Review, 6*, 304–315.

Gottman, J., Swanson, C., & Swanson, K. (2002). A general systems theory of marriage: Nonlinear difference equation modeling of marital interaction. *Personality and Social Psychology Review, 6*, 326–340.

Nowak, A., Vallacher, R. R., & Zochowski, M. (2002). The emergence of personality: Personality stability through interpersonal synchronization. In D. Cervone & W. Mischel (Eds.), *Advances in personality science* (pp. 292–331). New York: Guilford Press.

Read, S. J., & Miller, L. C. (2002). Virtual personalities: A neural network model of personality. *Personality and Social psychology Review, 6*, 357–369.

References

Allport, G. W. (1937). *Personality: A psychological interpretation.* New York: Holt, Rinehart and Winston.

Anderson, J. A., Silverstein, J. W., Ritz, S. A., & Jones, R. S. (1977). Distinctive features, categorical perception, and probability learning: Some applications of a neural model. *Psychological Review, 84*, 413–451.

Caspi, A., & Roberts, B. W. (1999). Personality continuity and change across the life course. In L. A. Pervin & O. P. John (Eds.), *Handbook of personality: Theory and research* (2nd ed., pp. 300–326). New York: Guilford Press.

Caspi, A., & Roberts, B. W. (2001). Personality development across the life course: The argument for change and continuity. *Psychological Inquiry, 12*, 49–66.

Feynman, R. P., & Leighton, R. (1985). *Surely you're joking, Mr. Feynman!* New York: Norton.

Fraley, R. C., & Roberts, B. W. (2005). Patterns of continuity: A dynamic model for conceptualizing the stability of individual differences in psychological constructs across the life course. *Psychological Review, 112*, 60–74.

Gottman, J., Swanson, C., & Swanson, K. (2002). A general systems theory of marriage: Nonlinear difference equation modeling of marital interaction. *Personality and Social Psychology Review, 6*, 326–340.

Holyoak, K. J., & Thagard, P. (2002). Analogical mapping by constraint satisfaction. In T. A. Polk & C. M.

Seifert (Eds.), *Cognitive modeling* (pp. 849–909). Cambridge, MA: MIT Press.

Hopfield, J. J. (1982). Neural networks and physical systems with emergent collective computational abilities. *Proceedings of the National Academy of Sciences, 79*, 2554–2558.

Hopfield, J. J. (1984). Neurons with graded responses have collective computational properties like those of two-state neurons. *Proceedings of the National Academy of Sciences, 81*, 3088–3092.

Hummel, J. E., & Holyoak, K. J. (2003). A symbolic-connectionist theory of relational inference and generalization. *Psychological Review, 110*, 220–264.

Kashima, Y., & Kerekes, A. R. Z. (1994). A distributed memory model of averaging phenomena in person impression formation. *Journal of Experimental Social Psychology, 30*, 407–455.

Kunda, Z., & Thagard, P. (1996). Forming impressions from stereotypes, traits, and behaviors: A parallel-constraint-satisfaction theory. *Psychological Review, 103*, 284–308.

McClelland, J. L., & Rumelhart, D. E. (1986). A distributed model of human learning and memory. In J. L. McClelland & D. E. Rumelhart (Eds.), *Parallel distributed processing: Explorations in the microstructures of cognition: Vol. II. Psychological and Biological Models* (pp. 170–215). Cambridge, MA: MIT Press/Bradford Books.

Miller, S. M., Shoda, Y., & Hurley, K. (1996). Applying cognitive social theory to health protective behavior: Breast self-examination in cancer screening. *Psychological Bulletin, 119*, 70–94.

Mischel, W., & Shoda, Y. (1995). A cognitive-affective system theory of personality: Reconceptualizing situations, dispositions, dynamics, and invariance in personality structure. *Psychological Review, 102*, 246–268.

Nowak, A. (2004). Dynamical minimalism: Why less is more in psychology. *Personality and Social Psychology Review, 8*, 183–192.

Nowak, A., & Vallacher, R. R. (1998). *Dynamical social psychology.* New York: Guilford Press.

O'Reilly, R. C., & Munakata, Y. (2000). *Computational explorations in cognitive neuroscience: Understanding the mind by simulating the brain.* Cambridge, MA: MIT Press.

Read, S. J., & Marcus-Newhall, A. (1993). Explanatory coherence in social explanations: A parallel distributed processing account. *Journal of Personality and Social Psychology, 65*, 429–447.

Read, S. J., & Miller, L. C. (1994). Dissonance and balance in belief systems: The promise of parallel constraint satisfaction processes and connectionist modeling approaches. In R. C. Schank & E. Langer (Eds.), *Beliefs, reasoning, and decision making: Psycho-logic in honor of Bob Abelson* (pp. 209–235). Hillsdale, NJ: Erlbaum.

Read, S. J., & Miller, L. C. (998). On the dynamic construction of meaning: An interactive activation and competition model of social perception. In S. J. Read

& L. C. Miller (Eds.), *Connectionist models of social reasoning and social behavior* (pp. 27–68). Mahwah, NJ: Erlbaum.

Rumelhart, D. E., & McClelland, J. L. (Eds.). (1986). *Parallel distributed processing: Explorations in the microstructure of cognition: Vol. I. Foundations.* Cambridge, MA: MIT Press/Bradford Books.

Shoda, Y., LeeTiernan, S., & Mischel, W. (2002). Personality as a dynamical system: Emergence of stability and constancy from intra- and inter-personal interactions. *Personality and Social Psychology Review, 6*, 316–325.

Shoda, Y., & Mischel, W. (1998). Personality as a stable cognitive-affective activation network: Characteristic patterns of behavior variation emerge from a stable personality structure. In S. J. Read & L. C. Miller (Eds.), *Connectionist and PDP models of social reasoning and social behavior* (pp. 175–208). Mahwah, NJ: Erlbaum.

Shoda, Y., Mischel, W., Miller, S. M., Daly, M. B., & Engstrom, P. F. (1998). Facilitating well-informed decisions for BRCA1/2 testing. *Journal of Clinical Psychology in Medical Settings, 5*, 3–17.

Shoda, Y., Mischel, W., Miller, S. M., Diefenbach, M., Daly, M. B., & Engstrom, P. F. (1998). Psychological interventions and genetic testing: Facilitating informed decisions about BRCA1/2 cancer susceptibility. *Journal of Clinical Psychology in Medical Settings, 5*, 3–17.

Shoda, Y., Mischel, W., & Wright, J. C. (1994). Intra-individual stability in the organization and patterning of behavior: Incorporating psychological situations into the idiographic analysis of personality. *Journal of Personality and Social Psychology, 67*, 674–687.

Shultz, T. R., & Lepper, M. R. (1996). Cognitive dissonance reduction as constraint satisfaction. *Psychological Review, 103*, 219–240.

Simon, D., Snow, C. J., & Read, S. J. (2004). The redux of cognitive consistency theories: Evidence judgments by constraint satisfaction. *Journal of Personality and Social Psychology, 86*, 814–837.

Spellman, B. A., & Holyoak, K. J. (1992). If Saddam is Hitler then who is George Bush? Analogical mapping between systems of social roles. *Journal of Personality and Social Psychology, 62*, 913–933.

Spellman, B. A., Ullman, J. B., & Holyoak, K. J. (1994). A coherence model of cognitive consistency: Dynamics of attitude change during the Persian Gulf War. *Journal of Social Issues, 49*, 147–165.

Thagard, P. (1989). Explanatory coherence. *Behavioral and Brain Sciences, 12*, 435–467.

Thagard, P., & Kunda, Z. (1998). Making sense of people: Coherence mechanisms. In S. J. Read & L. C. Miller (Eds.), *Connectionist models of social reasoning and social behavior* (pp. 3–26). Mahwah, NJ: Erlbaum.

Venables, W. N., & Ripley, B. D. (2000). *S Programming.* New York: Springer.

## CHAPTER 36

Meta-Analysis in Personality Psychology

A Primer

Brent W. Roberts
Nathan R. Kuncel
Wolfgang Viechtbauer
Tim Bogg

We assume that if you are reading this chapter, you are interested in doing a meta-analysis. Good for you. We believe more researchers should take advantage of this technique. In fact, if you have ever done a literature review, then you probably have examined enough studies to conduct a meta-analysis. Moreover, analytically speaking, meta-analyses are not unusually difficult. The fact that two of us (B. W. R. and T. B.) have published meta-analyses is testament to the fact that the technique can be mastered by the mathematically challenged. That is not to say that they are easy to do. A good meta-analysis usually takes more time and effort than a typical study, despite the fact that you seldom collect your own data. Just don't let the analytical barriers faze you.

In this chapter we provide an overview of the steps one should take in performing a meta-analysis. Our treatment is by no means exhaustive and does not replace one of the numerous in-depth descriptions of the technique

(see "Recommended Readings"; Cooper & Hedges, 1994; Hedges & Olkin, 1985; Hunter & Schmidt, 2004; Lipsey & Wilson, 2001; Rosenthal, 1991). Our goal is to provide the reader with a decipherable overview of the steps taken in most meta-analyses within personality psychology. In addition, we point out more authoritative sources for the specifics of meta-analysis. The reader should be forewarned: There will be a few formulas along the way, but these are no more complicated than those found in elementary discussions of classical test theory, and when examined closely, can actually illuminate several key issues.

The chapter is organized around the steps typically taken in conceptualizing and performing a meta-analysis. In the first section we discuss why meta-analysis is useful. The second section deals with aspects of data collection. Inasmuch as the data for a meta-analysis are derived from a set of related studies, issues in conducting a thorough literature review are considered in some detail. The third section focuses on a critical stage of the meta-analysis—organizing and coding the studies before analyzing them. The fourth section describes the varied approaches to analyzing meta-analytic data. Finally, the fifth section touches on some of the issues that we have been confronted with in our own meta-analytic work and that may be particularly germane to personality psychologists.

Why Do a Meta-Analysis?

Imagine the following scenario. An investigator is interested in linking the trait of conscientiousness to tobacco consumption (e.g., Bogg & Roberts, 2004). Across three studies she finds correlations of −0.33, −0.15, and −0.25, suggesting that higher levels of conscientiousness are related to less tobacco consumption. However, with modest sample sizes of 75 participants in each study, one would find only the −.33 correlation to be statistically significant. What should the researcher conclude on the basis of these findings? Should the three studies be written up as one rejection of the null hypothesis and two failures to reject? If this approach is taken, how likely is this researcher's article to be published? Given our reliance on null hypothesis significance testing for determining the existence of an effect, the reviewers would inevitably conclude that the original study failed to replicate, twice.

This scenario is all too common. One can find countless examples of researchers concluding that either their newly collected data or already published findings are contradictory because some effects are statistically significant whereas others are not. We often rely on this apparently contradictory pattern to justify new research, as we believe that through some ingenious methodological innovation of our own we will be able to rectify the discrepancy. Unfortunately, the conclusion that the results are contradictory is often erroneous for one specific reason. Most of our studies are woefully underpowered (Cohen, 1992). For better or worse, personality psychologists tend to study small groups (e.g., 50–150 participants). Given the modal effect size of our research and the low power of studies in personality psychology, we often have only a 50:50 chance of determining that a small or medium-size effect is statistically significant. Such odds are not particularly

comforting. The tragedy is that we continue to design studies in this way despite knowing better (see Fraley, Chapter 8, this volume).

This problem highlights one of the first and most fundamental reasons to do a meta-analysis—to ask the question, "Is there an effect?" or, more accurately, "What is the magnitude of the effect?" given the fact that the effect is seldom "nill." In the case of our example, when combined meta-analytically, the effect size is −.24, and voilà, it is statistically significant. Is this a small effect? Not in terms of the normal range of effect sizes found across psychology and medicine (Meyer et al., 2001). Thus, it would have been an inferential error to conclude that there was no effect. The preponderance of underpowered studies in personality psychology alone is sufficient justification for combining the results from several commensurable studies with meta-analytic methods. And, as noted above, rather than conducting a narrative review of the literature that comes to the inevitable conclusion that the research is contradictory, why not run a small meta-analysis and derive a point estimate that might frame the results of your study more concretely and precisely?

Alternatively, if a domain has a rich history, then one can perform a more exhaustive meta-analysis in order to determine whether an effect exists and how large it is. This is exactly what we did with our meta-analysis of the relationship between conscientiousness and health behaviors (Bogg & Roberts, 2004). We were optimistic that conscientiousness would be related to at least some of the leading behavioral contributors to premature mortality. What we were truly interested in was whether it was related to *all* of the behaviors, which it was. Thus, we did a relatively straightforward "is there an effect here" meta-analysis that resulted in profoundly important results—conscientiousness has pervasive relationships to all of the reasons people die prematurely.

The second reason to do a meta-analysis is exactly the same reason we do any study—to test hypotheses or compare models. Just like any other analytical technique, such as regression, analysis of variance, or even the simple correlation coefficient, meta-analysis can be used to test specific hypotheses derived from different theories. For example, in our two meta-analyses of longitudinal personality trait development, we tested the theory that personality traits stop changing after age 30 and found convincing evidence leading us to reject the "no change after 30" hypothesis in both cases (Roberts & DelVecchio, 2000; Roberts, Walton, & Viechtbauer, 2006a). Here, we used meta-analysis like any other statistical technique—as a hypothesis-testing tool.

Once you have decided to conduct a meta-analysis, what are the basic steps and issues to consider at each of these stages? If the devil is in the details, then conducting a meta-analysis is surely fraught with danger. Executing a large-scale meta-analysis involves considerable management of information to minimize wasted effort, ensure precision, and avoiding the agony of needing to redo parts of the study. Although work on each of these phases may overlap, it is valuable to think of a meta-analysis as being broken into five key phases: Conceptualizing the problem to be studied, identifying and obtaining articles, coding and proofing the data, and analyzing data and reporting the results. Table 36.1 provides a checklist of issues to consider at each of these stages. This is not a hard-and-fast checklist, as several decisions made along the way will affect which steps are actually taken. Nonetheless, we believe that most of the important and pragmatic issues are highlighted.

Conceptualizing the Problem to Be Studied

It is critical to clearly specify the research question to be answered before the literature search is actually conducted. Doing so will be invaluable for the same reasons this step is critical for primary research. Most important, having a clear conceptualization of the primary research questions helps one to make better decisions with respect to the relevant information one should gather. This, in turn, will focus the literature search and ensure that the project does not spin out of control.

As in any study, the primary issue is the tradeoff between breadth and specificity. If the research question is too broad, the resulting meta-analysis may be too diffuse to answer the original research question well. For example, meta-analytic research is often criticized for mixing "apples and oranges" because the studies being aggregated are different from one another in some key way. Of course, if you are interested in fruit, then the broader level of conceptualization is appropriate. Conversely, if

TABLE 36.1. Meta-Analysis Checklist

I. *Conceptualizing the problem*
  1. Research question/hypothesis
  2. Level of analysis

II. *Identifying and collecting articles*
  1. Search databases and journals
    a. PsychLit, PubMed, etc.
    b. Conference proceedings and programs
    c. Technical reports
    d. Relevant journals
    e. Review articles
    f. Dissertations
  2. Search out fugitive literature
  3. Snowballing
    a. Search references in articles in the database
    b. Citation index search of all articles

III. *Coding articles*
  1. Create coding protocol
  2. Coder training
  3. Coding and periodic coding checks

IV. *Preparing the data*
  1. Transforming effect sizes
  2. Directionalizing effect sizes
  3. Aggregating nonindependent effect sizes
  4. Consider correcting for artifacts

V. *Analyzing your data and reporting results*
  1. Choose a model: fixed effects, random effects, mixed effects
  2. Test for publication bias
  3. Test for moderators
  4. Aggregating effect sizes and reporting your results

the research question is too narrow, there may be too few studies to analyze and the question may be of little interest to all but a few readers. Striking the right balance between breadth and specificity by an appropriately formulated research question is one of the most critical issues when doing a meta-analysis.

The key arbiter of getting the tradeoff right is experience. The entire meta-analytic enterprise, and especially the conceptualization of the research question, will be much easier for those who have long toiled in the back alleys of primary data collection and know a research area well. Approaching a new area for meta-analytic investigation with little experience is fraught with numerous conceptual and procedural potholes. The idea may not be sound. The key studies may escape the search. A meta-analysis on the topic may already have been published. These issues should not stop a new researcher from doing a meta-analysis. What it should do is motivate the researcher to do his or her homework and to talk the issues through with people actively involved in the particular area of research. Once a clear plan for a meta-analysis has been acquired through hard work or high-quality consultation, you are ready to start identifying and collecting articles (i.e., "data collection").

Identifying and Collecting Articles

Given the advent of the personal computer and the ever improving databases and search engines, one might conclude that identifying the relevant articles is as easy as doing a PsychLit search. This is not the case. A thorough and valid search of the literature encompasses using electronic databases and journals, searching for the fugitive literature, and then "snowballing" existing articles. We describe each of these techniques in turn.

When it comes to electronic database searches, we recommend the following procedure. First, generate a list of key words and conduct searches with the key words used in various combinations. It is critical to remember that many social science domains are studied by more than one discipline. Conducting searches using the databases and jargon of these fields is valuable for creating a thorough search. If the resulting lists are too large, restrict key words to the title of the paper. In general, it is far better to conduct a too broad search rather than one that is too narrow. In addition, detailed notes regarding the key words used and the steps followed during the search process will be invaluable for rerunning searches at a later point.

All searches should then be imported into a bibliographic database (e.g., Endnote, Reference Manager, Refworks). These searches can be supplemented by searching conference programs, conference proceedings, and technical report lists for relevant organizations. Many bibliographic database programs allow for the identification of identical references. After duplicates are deleted, the database can be further edited by examining each abstract to make a judgment about its relevance. References *should not* be deleted; rather, they should be labeled as rejected, using another field in the bibliographic database manager.

Data for some topics can be found in journal articles without being the central focus of the study. This makes electronic searches challenging. For example, in a meta-analysis on the validity of self-reported grade point averages (Kuncel, Credé, & Thomas, 2005) it became apparent that the pertinent data were often mentioned in a method section about the outcomes measured without being the actual focus of the study. A combination of approaches can be used to address this common problem. The first is to identify specific topics that seem to frequently contain the desired information even if it is not the central focus of the study. Such ancillary topics can then be searched using typical methods described above. Second, one can identify journals that seem to most commonly contain the necessary information and conduct hand searches of those journals.[1] Third, reading review articles, like those found in the *Annual Review of Psychology* or in the constantly proliferating handbooks now being published every week may reveal articles that are not found in a typical electronic database search. Note that these techniques could be used for any meta-analytic topic to enhance the comprehensiveness of the search.

Once a database of desired articles has been constructed, the items need to be collected. The bibliographic database software can be used to generate a compact list of articles to be collected. It is important at this stage to be kind to your interlibrary loan personnel as they can make this stage far easier. Fortunately, many documents are now available in electronic format and can be directly downloaded, including dissertations and technical reports. Key researchers that show up frequently in the database can also be contacted at this stage to see if they have other published studies that were overlooked during the literature search or unpublished studies they would be willing to share.

As the articles enter the laboratory, the bibliographic database needs to be updated to note that the articles are now "in house." A filing system can be created that facilitates the processing of articles. At a minimum, there should be space for new articles, articles that have been coded, articles that have been processed (data and "snowballs" entered), and articles that have been proofed and are ready for more long-term storage.

The next to last step in the search is concerned with the "fugitive literature." This step in the search process is especially important in that it may result in the inclusion of a number of studies that report null effects, as the field is nearly uniformly biased against publishing null findings.[2] The inclusion of these studies should provide more accurate estimates of effect sizes. These studies can be discovered through requests to list serves. Another technique we have found useful is to send the initial list of studies included in the meta-analysis to key individuals who have studied the phenomena of interest. These researchers can often identify unpublished studies and studies that have unusual titles that do not show up in the typical search procedures.

The last step taken, once the initial database has been compiled, is to snowball the preliminary database. First, the references of articles included in the meta-analysis or the references found in review articles should be examined for studies that were missed during the electronic search. Second, papers that reference the studies in the meta-analytic database should be examined to see if they report similar data (i.e., a citation index search). Review articles and dissertations, owing to their lengthy review sections, are especially helpful for snowballing. The easiest approach is to simply mark in the reference lists of the articles that look promising. To avoid duplicate collection of articles, these noted references should be compared against the updated bibliographic database to see if an article has already been identified and collected. New articles can be added and flagged using a separate field. Depending on the topic, snowballs can easily increase a database by 30–50%. Efficiently collecting this information is dependent on having a well-managed bibliographic database.

As indicated by the GIGO acronym used to deride factor analysis (i.e., garbage in, garbage out), a meta-analysis is only as good as the studies it examines. In addition to being one of the most critical stages of the process, literature identification will also take much longer than typically expected. Its importance should not be underestimated. To use a sports metaphor, it is like getting the footwork right for a tennis shot. If the feet are not in the right place, it matters little how well the person swings; the player will still miss the shot. Don't make your meta-analysis a swing and a miss. Put the necessary time and effort into the data collection stage, and you will be rewarded with a definitive study.

Coding Articles

Once a suitable body of literature has been identified and collected, the next task is to extract information from each study that will be used in the subsequent analyses. The most common means of extracting information from research reports and other data sources is a coding protocol. A coding protocol (sometimes initially guided by a coding manual) is a form used by coders to document two distinct types of information from data sources: (1) study descriptors—information regarding the characteristics of the study, also called *moderators*; and (2) effect sizes—information regarding the actual findings of the study (Lipsey & Wilson, 2001).

The key to the successful development of any coding protocol is planning. Decisions need to be made early on regarding study descriptor and effect size information that is relevant for the meta-analysis. Some of these decisions will be guided by the a priori investigative goals of the meta-analyst (e.g., gender is expected to moderate the effect of interest). Other decisions will require a review of the collected body of literature (or a representative subsample thereof) to determine which study descriptor and effect size information occurs with sufficient frequency to warrant inclusion in the coding protocol. Even if a particular study descriptor (e.g., ethnicity) is of interest, a review of the collected literature may reveal it to be reported so infrequently that requiring coders to document it across studies would be unproductive.

A list of potential moderators and outcomes should be identified at the beginning of the project. We should note that the term *moderator* is analogous to *independent variable* in primary data collection. In meta-analytic jargon this reflects the fact that an independent variable that is related to variability in meta-analytic outcomes is directly analogous to a moderator effect in a typical study. As coding proceeds, it is often the case that new variables may appear that are interesting. For example, a new outcome may appear in a few studies that had not been considered before. New fields or codes should be created for these variables in the coding sheet, and previous studies should be reexamined. However, it is important to note that moderator analyses can be overdone. It is valuable to think of a database as having a limited amount of information value. A vast number of thoughtless moderator tests can, by chance, yield an apparently important moderator. It is best to avoid this shotgun approach to research.

A moderator that is common to many meta-analyses is the "study quality" moderator, in which the researcher makes a global evaluation of whether a study is of high quality or not. In practice, this is often a subjective judgment made by those coding the studies. This approach can easily fall prey to the coder's biases regarding theories, journals, methods, and even other scientists. It is our position that such a subjective approach should be avoided. Given the vast number of books and articles on experimental, correlational, and quasi-experimental design, study quality can be thoughtfully and specifically operationalized. That is, as scientists we should be able to clearly specify how and why one study is of lower quality than another. In many cases, multiple study characteristic codes will be necessary to capture this information.

As mentioned above, the types of study descriptors coded for each study are dependent on the declarative and exploratory interests of the meta-analyst. At the broadest level is information about the source of the study (i.e., journal, dissertation, book, etc.) and its year of publication. Information about the study's author(s) may also be of interest, as well as any sources of funding for the research (Lipsey & Wilson, 2001). Of more substantive interest are study characteristics that have a direct or an indirect bearing on the relationship being investigated. These characteristics include the source of the sample (e.g., a long-standing national or regional study), demographic information about the sample (e.g., gender, age, ethnicity, socioeconomic status), and other identifying features of the sample (e.g., clinical versus nonclinical, inpatient versus outpatient, delinquent, criminal).

Perhaps the most important study descriptors are those related to the independent and dependent variables. These characteristics include the types of independent and dependent variables employed (usually described in terms of constructs and their forms of operationalization) and the quality of the measures used (e.g., reliability). For example, in a meta-analysis investigating the relationship between extraversion (independent variable) and exercise (dependent variable), the coding protocol would provide options for which construct related to extraversion was investigated in the study (e.g.,

extraversion, social dominance, sociability, activity) as well as how it was measured (e.g., NEO-FFI, California Psychological Inventory). Similarly, options for specifying the exercise-related construct (e.g., strength, flexibility, endurance, cardiorespiratory fitness) as well as the means of measurement (e.g., maximal bench press, VO_2 maximal treadmill test) would be provided. In this way, the coding protocol behaves as a survey, providing the coder with response options or the ability to provide an "open" response.

In terms of the actual statistical analyses of the studies, effect size information must be carefully considered and coded. At the very least, there are two statistics that must be entered into the coding protocol for each study—the effect size statistic and the sample size specific to that effect size. This information is crucial for meta-analytic calculations. There are also other features—some statistical, some conceptual—that are desirable to code. Additional effect size information includes a description of the variables that comprise the effect size (described by construct labels, measures, or both), subsample information (relevant when multiple effect sizes are coded across different configurations of a sample or multiple samples in a study), standard deviations, reliability of variables comprising the effect size, dichotomization of variables comprising the effect size, statistical transformation procedure (how an effect size was calculated if the desired metric was not available in the study, e.g., using means and standard deviations to calculate a correlation coefficient), a confidence rating for the effect size (coder-rated level of surety in the integrity of the coded effect, usually lower for crude estimations), and a page number or other location information (e.g., table) where the effect size information (or any other characteristic of the study) can be double-checked for accuracy. As with the study descriptors, decisions regarding the inclusion of effect size information should be made based on an understanding of which information is desired and typically available in the collected body of studies.

As effect sizes are so important to the meta-analytic approach, we now discuss in detail some effect size measures frequently found in the personality research literature, namely the standardized mean difference for two independent groups, the standardized mean difference for two dependent groups, the raw product–moment correlation coefficient, and the correlation coefficient after applying Fisher's variance stabilizing transformation. It should be noted that the effect size measures discussed are just a selection of a large number of effect size indices that can be calculated. They were chosen for a more detailed description because of their ubiquitous use in personality research and for illustrative purposes, but not as an argument for their superiority to other effect size indices. The choice of an effect size measure is partly dependent on the types of studies being meta-analyzed and on the reporting practices within a research community. Because the types of studies and reporting practices can differ widely, a large variety of effect size indices are available and have been described in detail in the existing literature (e.g., Fleiss, 1994; Lipsey & Wilson, 2001; Rosenthal, 1994).

Standardized Mean Difference for Two Independent Groups

The standardized mean difference (SMD) measures the mean difference between two independent groups on some continuous outcome measure, in which one group can be considered the experimental (E) and one the control group (C). Because the raw units of outcome measures across studies are typically not commensurable (e.g., a 5-point mean difference between two groups on the California Psychological Inventory (CPI) Dominance scale may reflect a larger/smaller difference than a 5-point difference on the Jackson Personality Inventory (JPI) Dominance scale), we must first find a way to make different scales comparable across the studies. This can be accomplished by dividing (standardizing) the raw mean difference by the pooled standard deviation of the two groups.

Therefore, assume that for each study, the scores within the two groups are normally distributed with means μ^E_i and μ^C_i and common variance σ^2_i. Then the effect size in the ith study is given by

$$\theta_i = \frac{\mu^E_i - \mu^C_i}{\sigma_i}$$

which we can estimate with

$$d_i = \frac{\overline{x}^E_i - \overline{x}^C_i}{s^P_i}$$

where $\overline{x}^E_i$ and $\overline{x}^C_i$ are the observed sample means and s^P_i is the pooled standard deviation of the two groups. However, d_i tends to be

slightly too large on average (it overestimates θ_i). One can easily correct this bias by computing

$$ES_i = \left(1 - \frac{3}{4m_i - 1}\right)d_i$$

where $m_i = n^E_i + n^C_i - 2$ and n^E_i and n^C_i are the sample sizes of the two experimental groups (Hedges, 1981).

The sampling variance of ES_i can be calculated with

$$vi = \frac{n^E_i + n^C_i}{n^E_i n^C_i} + \frac{ES^2_i}{2(n^E_i + n^C_i)}$$

Therefore, v_i denotes the amount of variance expected in the effect size estimate due to sampling fluctuations alone. As the sample sizes (n^E_i and n^C_i) of the two experimental groups increase, v_i becomes smaller, reflecting the fact that effect size estimates based on larger samples tend to be closer to their corresponding θ_i value.

Standardized Mean Difference for Dependent Samples

The SMD can also be used when the same group of subjects is measured at two points in time, such as before and after receiving some kind of treatment or as part of a longitudinal study to examine changes across time. Because the same group of subjects is measured twice, the subjects' scores can no longer be assumed to be independent. Specifically, when $j = 1, \ldots, n_i$ subjects are tested at two time points, T1 and T2, and the scores at the two time points are normally distributed with means μ^{T1}_i and μ^{T2}_i and common variance σ^2_i, then we expect there to be a certain amount of correlation between the scores at T1 and T2, which we denote with ρ_i.

The raw change across time, given by $\mu^{T2}_i - \mu^{T1}_i$, is typically not a useful effect size measure in meta-analysis, because the units of the various outcome measures across the studies are not directly comparable. The solution again is to standardize the raw mean difference in some way, and two options for doing so have been suggested in the literature (Morris & DeShon, 2002).

Raw Score Metric

The first option is to standardize the mean change by the standard deviation of the raw scores, yielding the effect size

$$\theta_i = \frac{\mu_i^{T2} - \mu_i^{T1}}{\sigma_i}$$

An estimate of θ_i is given by

$$ES_i = \left(1 - \frac{3}{4m_i - 1}\right)\frac{\overline{x}_i^{T2} - \overline{x}_i^{T1}}{s_i^{T1}}$$

where $m_i = n_i - 1$, $\overline{x}_i^{T1}$ and $\overline{x}_i^{T2}$ are the observed sample means at the two time points, and s_i^{T1} is the observed standard deviation of the scores at time T1. The sampling variance of ES_i can be calculated with

$$v_i = \frac{2(1 - r_i)}{n_i} + \frac{ES_i^2}{2n_i}$$

where r_i is the observed correlation of the scores at times T1 and T2. Note that standardization in the raw score metric yields an effect size that is *not* influenced by the degree of correlation between the scores at T1 and T2 (although the sampling variance of the effect size estimate is).

Change Score Metric

A second option is to standardize the mean change by the standard deviation of the change scores, yielding the effect size

$$\theta_i = \frac{\mu_i^{T2} - \mu_i^{T1}}{\sigma_i^D}$$

where σ_i^D denotes the standard deviation of the change scores. The corresponding effect size estimate is given by

$$ES_i = \left(1 - \frac{3}{4m_i - 1}\right)\frac{\overline{x}_i^{T2} - \overline{x}_i^{T2=1}}{s_i^D}$$

where s_i^D is the observed standard deviation of the change scores (i.e., the standard deviation in the scores after subtracting the T1 score from the T2 score). The sampling variance can be calculated with

$$v_i = \frac{1}{n_i} + \frac{ES_i^2}{2n_i}$$

It can be shown that

$$\theta_i = \frac{\mu_i^{T2} - \mu_i^{T1}}{\sigma_i^D} = \frac{\mu_i^{T2} - \mu_i^{T1}}{\sigma_i\sqrt{2(1 - \rho)}}$$

which reveals that standardization in the change score metric yields an effect size that *is* influenced by the degree of correlation between the scores at T1 and T2. Specifically, when the correlation is greater than .5, then standardization in the change score metric yields a larger effect size than that obtained through standardization in the raw score metric, and vice

versa. For more details on the different methods of standardization in the dependent samples case, see Morris and DeShon (2002).

Correlation Coefficient

The SMD is typically used as the effect size index when interest is centered on the mean difference between two sets of scores (whether from two independent groups or from the same group at two time points). However, in other cases, interest is focused on the strength of the relationship between two continuous variables, in which case the correlation coefficient is usually employed as the effect size measure. Suppose that pairs of scores are obtained within each of the k studies and let ρ_i denote the correlation between the two sets of scores. Now the effect size is defined simply as

$$\theta_i = \rho_i$$

An estimate of θ_i is given by the raw product–moment correlation coefficient observed in the ith study, denoted by r_i. It turns out that r_i actually underestimates θ_i slightly, but this bias can be easily corrected (Olkin & Pratt, 1958) by using

$$ES_i = r_i + \frac{r_i(1 - r_i^2)}{2(n_i - 4)}$$

as the effect size estimate. The sampling variance of ES_i can be computed with

$$v_i = \frac{(1 - ES_i^2)^2}{n_i - 1}$$

The distribution of the raw correlation coefficient becomes increasingly nonnormal as r_i increases. Therefore, several researchers (e.g., Hedges & Olkin, 1985; Lipsey & Wilson, 2001; Rosenthal, 1991) have recommended the use of Fisher's variance stabilizing transformation when meta-analyzing correlation coefficients. Specifically, one computes

$$ES_i = \frac{1}{2}\ln\left[\frac{1 + r_i}{1 - r_i}\right]$$

where ln[ ] denotes the natural logarithm. The sampling variance of ES_i is now given by

$$v_i = \frac{1}{n_i - 3}$$

The advantage of the transformed correlation coefficient is that its distribution is much closer to that of a normal distribution.

Given our experiences in coding studies and attempting to extract effect size information from studies, we cannot help but editorialize a bit at this stage. We would like to appeal to researchers to be more giving of their data and not to forget the archival role of journals. Too many researchers fail to report basic descriptive statistics. These are critical to the meta-analyst and the future researcher interested in comparing your sample to subsequent samples focusing on similar issues. Furthermore, too many researchers report incomplete statistics. For example, one bad habit is to report that the effects were "statistically significant (all p's < .05)." This style of reporting typically leaves the meta-analyst no choice but to throw your article out of the database. Another egregious example is to report findings in graphical form without providing accompanying statistics (means *and* standard deviations). Our least favorite example of this approach is for some authors to report differences as pluses, minuses, or zeros, depending on their idiosyncratic interpretation of the effect size and whether it was positive or negative. Please, please, please report your descriptive statistics and point estimates.

On the surface, coding appears to be a straightforward task. Unfortunately, it is very complicated for some topics and requires extensive coder training. A process we have found useful is to initially have all coders code the same set of five to seven articles and then come together in a meeting to discuss coding discrepancies. The training articles should be selected to have codeable data. This process continues until the structure and content of the coding sheet has stabilized and the number of coding errors reaches an acceptable lower limit. During the process a coding manual is created that specifies how coding decisions are to be made. Random checks of coding then occur after the initial training meetings. These checks can be done by independently coding the article in question and comparing those results with the initial coded results.

To summarize, a coding protocol is a standardized tool that imposes some order on a process that can be rather unruly. The success of a protocol (and a meta-analysis) requires careful planning and an examination of the collected body of studies to determine which information is consistently available for coding. Clear decisions must be made early on to avoid confusion and missed analytic opportunities.

Preparing the Data for Analysis

Now that you have a database in hand, there are a few additional details to consider. Typically, the data are not in a form that can be readily analyzed, for a variety of reasons that need to be addressed. In particular, the effect sizes most likely need to be converted into a common metric. They may also need to be "directionalized," as, depending on the way a predictor is scored (e.g., as neuroticism or emotional stability), two effects may mean the same thing but have the opposite signs. It is also common to have multiple effect sizes from each sample, and this raises nonindependence issues. Finally, you will need to decide whether to correct for artifacts. We discuss each of these issues in turn.

It is frequently the case that studies report results using a wide range of statistics. Many effect sizes can be converted from one form to another. These include correlation coefficients, standardized mean differences, chi-square statistics obtained from 2×2 tables, odds ratios, frequency tables, t-tests, F-tests, phi coefficients, point-biserial correlations, and means and standard deviations. Moreover, exact p-values can be transformed into an effect size if the sample size is known (Rosenthal & Rubin, 2003). There is almost no case in which a bivariate test statistic or outcome measure cannot be transformed into a standard effect size. Your goal at this stage is to simply transform the plethora of effect sizes and test statistics into one common effect size for the analysis stage. To facilitate this process, we have reproduced the formulas for transforming the most common test statistics reported in personality research (see Table 36.2; Rosenthal, 1991).

Certain types of effect sizes may be more difficult to incorporate into a meta-analytic framework. Specifically, partial correlations and beta-weights from complex multiple regression analyses pose a significant challenge. The problem lies in the fact that sampling distributions for each particular type of model would need to be known and converted to a common metric. One solution is to use the $r_{equivalent}$ statistic in which the p-value associated with the test statistic is transformed into a correlation coefficient (Rosenthal & Rubin,

TABLE 36.2. Common Statistical Transformations in Meta-Analytic Research

Statistical score(s)	Transformation

Transformation to Cohen's d

Means and standard deviations of two groups	$d = \dfrac{M_1 - M_2}{\sigma_{pooled}}$, $\sigma_{pooled} = \sqrt{\left[\dfrac{(\sigma_1^2 + \sigma_2^2)}{2}\right]}$, or when $\sigma_1 \approx \sigma_2$, then $\sigma_{pooled} \approx \dfrac{\sigma_1 + \sigma_2}{2}$, i.e., the simple average
t score with df	$d = \dfrac{2t}{\sqrt{df}}$, when $n_1 = n_2$; or when $n_1 \neq n_2$ $d = \dfrac{t(n_1 + n_2)}{\left[\sqrt{(df)}\sqrt{(n_1 n_2)}\right]}$
F with $df = 1$ in numerator	$r = \sqrt{\dfrac{F(1,-)}{F(1,-) + df_{error}}}$
r	$d = \dfrac{2r}{\sqrt{1 - r^2}}$

Transformation to r

d with two known group sizes	$r = \dfrac{d}{\sqrt{\left[d^2 + \left(\dfrac{1}{pq}\right)\right]}}$, where $p = \dfrac{n_1}{N}$ and $q = 1 - p$, or when $p \approx q$, use $r = \dfrac{d}{\sqrt{d^2 + 4}}$
p, converted with Z-value table	$r = \dfrac{Z}{\sqrt{N}}$

Note. p is the proportion of the total sample (N) in the first of two groups (n_1) being compared.

2003). In some cases, the test statistics from these more complex, multivariate models can be broken into bivariate effect sizes. For example, forward or backward regression analyses often provide sufficient information to permit recovery of the original correlation matrix. A second consideration is using correlations to represent relationships from dichotomous variables as the magnitude of the correlation is sensitive to cell frequencies or base rates. As a result, it is often critical to consider base rates or cell frequencies when converting effect sizes. Another option would be to use odds ratios as a common metric, as they are not biased by base rates or cell frequencies. Two helpful works are Cohen (1988) and Rosenthal (1994).

Another data transformation issue common to personality psychology is the *direction of the effect* problem. For example, one researcher may report the relationship between neuroticism and positive emotionality as −0.50. A second researcher may report the relationship between emotional stability and positive emotionality as 0.50. These correlations, though opposite, reflect the same relationship. Yet, if combined without consideration of the effect

direction, the resulting average effect size would be zero and we would erroneously conclude that the domain of neuroticism/emotional stability was unrelated to positive emotionality. The solution to this very common dilemma is to "directionalize" one's effect sizes. In this case, the analyst chooses one particular direction for the relationship and makes sure, by changing the sign where necessary, that the effect size estimates properly represent the appropriate direction. For example, the analyst could choose to represent the relationship as "positive" with "positive" or emotional stability with positive emotionality. This would mean that the effect sizes from any study that reported the relationship between neuroticism and positive emotionality would have to be multiplied by −1 to reverse the sign of the effect size. The meta-analyst will need to be careful about using this method when there is disagreement about the nature of a trait (e.g., positive and negative affect).

In personality psychology one is often confronted with the problem that multiple effect sizes are derived from a single sample. It is quite common for researchers to report the correlation between a simple outcome, such as tobacco consumption, and the entire set of scales drawn from a personality inventory. Even if you are interested in just one domain, such as conscientiousness, most personality inventories contain at least a handful of scales tapping that and other domains. It is problematic to ignore the dependency between these measures drawn from the same sample and can lead to biased estimates of the population parameters.

There are several strategies that can be used to address the dependency between effect sizes. One can randomly select effect sizes from each study, so that any given sample contributes only one effect size to the meta-analysis. Sometimes more systematic selection may be in order. For example, when examining the effect of study moderators on mean-level change in personality traits, we used a strategy in which underrepresented age periods were emphasized rather than randomly selecting from the database (Roberts et al., 2006a). A third solution is to aggregate effect sizes within the sample. We have used this strategy several times to good effect (Bogg & Roberts, 2004; Kuncel, Hezlett, & Ones, 2001; Roberts & DelVecchio, 2000). Although a tremendous number of specific data points are thrown out when using one of these methods, doing so typically yields a more conservative estimate of the population effect sizes. The critical ingredient to a successful aggregation is how studies, samples, and moderator variables are coded, as described above. You will want to anticipate having to rely on one of these strategies by incorporating numbered codes for all of these variables, which can then be used to aggregate the data.

The ideal technique for addressing stochastically dependent effect sizes is to run some form of multivariate analysis in which the correlation among the effects taken from the same sample is accounted for (Gleser & Olkin, 1994). In principle, this is a relatively straightforward procedure. In the example given above in which four conscientiousness measures are used to predict tobacco consumption, all one would need is the correlation among those four conscientiousness measures in that sample. Unfortunately, as we have noted, most researchers fail to include the descriptive statistics relevant to their analyses, and almost no researchers include ancillary analyses, such as the entire correlation matrix of the measures used in the study. One hopes that with the advent of more fluid online publishing of scientific articles and

the availability of increased computer storage capacity, supplementary information such as this can be included with research reports as appendixes. Nonetheless, if this information can be acquired, the multivariate approach should be attempted in order to maximize the use of all the information available from each study.

The effect of sampling error on the variability of effect sizes is widely recognized across meta-analytic methods. Less frequently considered is the role of other statistical artifacts. Two loosely defined schools of thought have developed around this issue. The first school is agnostic. The decision of whether to account for artifacts besides sampling error is left up to the researcher (see Cooper & Hedges, 1994). The second school prescribes that as many artifacts as possible should be accounted for because ignoring them may lead to the erroneous conclusion that moderators exist and that the effects vary systematically (Hunter & Schmidt, 2004).

When addressed, the most common of these statistical artifacts are independent variable (IV) and dependent variable (DV) measurement unreliability, IV and DV range restriction, and dichotomization of study variables. All of these artifacts have two important effects on meta-analytic findings. The first is a reduction or attenuation of effects except in the case of range enhancement, which increases the effect. In other words, unreliability, range restriction, and dichotomization of variables reduce the magnitude of observed effects, leading to the conclusion that personality variables have weaker relations with other variables than is actually the case. The second effect is an increase in observed study variability. This has the undesirable effect of potentially leading researchers to believe that results are inconsistent across studies for substantive rather than artifactual reasons. When unaddressed, these artifacts can also make comparisons from study to study, and even meta-analysis to meta-analysis, difficult. A few examples may help to illustrate common situations in which these effects might occur in personality psychology.

The most common scenario is a meta-analysis of the association between a common trait, say, Harm Avoidance, and job performance across a number of different personality measures that all seem to capture the trait. Two problems would arise when some of these measures are markedly less reliable than others. First, the average correlation obtained will tend to be lower than what would be obtained had all of the studies employed highly reliable measures. Second, the variability across studies will be larger, owing to the measurement properties of the studies rather than substantive moderators.

Another common scenario is a meta-analysis in which the samples differ in their variability on the trait of interest. For example, a meta-analysis of the personality trait of socialization may contain studies done on National Merit Scholar finalists, criminals, and high school students. We would expect the first two samples to be less variable than the third. As in the reliability situation, we will have attenuated effects and increased effect size variability. That is, we might conclude that socialization is not as strongly associated with, say, grades in a course, simply because we have studies that have samples with relatively narrow ranges of socialization.

Artificially dichotomizing a variable, for example, by splitting a sample into a high and low socialization group, results in a loss of information and also tends to reduce the overall observed effect (Cohen, 1990). When samples are dichotomized, all individuals in each half are effectively treated as having equal scores on the dichotomized variable. Again, the meta-analysis would contain estimates of artifactually small effects and increased variability.

The most complete set of methods for addressing these issues was suggested by Hunter and Schmidt (2004) as part of their psychometric meta-analytic approach. This method is especially useful for meta-analytic work when the study samples have been restricted in range owing to direct or indirect selection on the independent variable and/or when the measures across studies vary considerably in reliability. Both of these situations are quite common in personality research, and it is no surprise that the Hunter and Schmidt method has seen extensive use in studies on personality (e.g., Barrick & Mount, 1991; Bono & Judge, 2004; Ones, Viswesvaran, & Schmidt, 1993).

Statistical artifacts can be handled with one of two different approaches. The first is to directly correct each study for its artifacts (i.e., range restriction, unreliability, and dichotomization) and then conduct a meta-analysis with the corrected correlations or standardized mean differences. This approach is ideal in theory but nearly impossible in practice. Rare is the literature in which all studies provide complete information including reliability and variance information. We often feel lucky if a study presents an effect size and information regarding the sample size, let alone local reliability and variance information.

Instead, artifact distributions are commonly used to correct for artifacts. Artifact distributions make use of available information to correct all of the effects in the meta-analysis. The underlying assumption is that the available artifact data represent a reasonable random sample of all the artifact data for all of the studies. This assumption is, of course, more or less tenable across literatures. There are several technical treatments of the artifact distribution method.

In the artifact distribution method, all artifacts and their frequencies are compiled and each study effect is corrected by all possible combinations of the statistical artifacts weighted by their relative frequencies. For example, if the unreliability estimate of 0.70 occurs four times in the database because four studies used the same measure, whereas the unreliability estimate of 0.80 occurs eight times because eight studies used a different measure, the study effects will be corrected by both reliability estimates but the 0.80 corrections will receive twice the weight because they occur twice as often. This method makes maximum use of the available information and allows the researcher to account for the simultaneous effects of both range restriction and unreliability. Unfortunately, this is a more complicated process than simply creating columns of study artifacts. The details become perilous when we need to decide which artifact data to use and how best to use them.[3]

Should you or should you not correct for artifacts? As is true of many methodological choices we make, there are tradeoffs for both approaches. If you choose not to correct for artifacts, it would be prudent to keep in mind that the resulting variability in effect sizes may not be due to moderators. In other words, you should not imbue estimates of heterogeneity with too much significance. However, correcting for artifacts provides somewhat idealized estimates. That is, the corrected estimates reflect what would happen in a world in which we used perfectly reliable measures, optimal sampling techniques, and appropriate measurement models (i.e., not dichotomizing our measures). In this case, one should not imbue the actual magnitude of the population estimates with too much significance, as researchers in the trenches of flawed primary data collection will most likely never encounter the effect sizes reported in these meta-analyses. Of course, the obvious and common compromise is to report both types of estimates so that the readers can judge for themselves whether an effect exists and what it would look like in an optimal situation.

How to Analyze Your Data

When conducting a meta-analysis, most of the time will be spent on literature searches, the retrieval of studies, assessing the relevance and quality of the retrieved studies, extraction of effect size estimates, and coding of moderator variables. In this section we discuss how to analyze the data once all of the previous steps have been completed. Although the data analysis takes comparatively little time, some important decisions must be made at this point that can greatly influence the results obtained from the meta-analysis. In particular, there has been an ongoing debate in the literature about the appropriate model to adopt when conducting a meta-analysis, and this is the first issue we address.

Fixed Effects, Random Effects, Mixed Effects: Which Model Do I Use?

Assume that a collection of k studies has been selected for inclusion in the meta-analysis and that a single (independent) effect size estimate is extracted from each study. Let ES_i denote the ith effect size estimate ($i = 1, \ldots, k$). The ES_i values may be, for example, standardized mean differences, raw correlation coefficients, or correlation coefficients after using Fisher's variance stabilizing (r to z) transformation. Regardless of the effect size measure used, it is important to recognize that each effect size estimate ES_i is an *estimate* of a corresponding parameter θ_i, which indicates the true effect size in the ith study. Therefore, we must draw a clear distinction between the actual or true "effect size" θ_i and the corresponding "effect size estimate" ES_i. Symbolically, this can be expressed by writing

$$ES_i = \theta_i + \varepsilon_i$$

where ε_i is the sampling error for the ith study. In other words, ES_i, the effect size estimate we actually observe in the ith study, differs from the true effect size θ_i by some unknown amount ε_i simply due to sampling fluctuations. It is usually reasonable to assume that the sampling error ε_i is normally distributed with mean zero and variance v_i.

Not surprisingly, effect size estimates based on larger samples tend to be closer to their corresponding θ_i values. In other words, effect size estimates based on larger samples have, all else being equal, smaller sampling variances (i.e., smaller v_i values) and therefore should receive proportionally more weight in the analysis because they provide more accurate information. As shown below, we can easily calculate the amount of sampling variance in an effect size estimate. Therefore, corresponding to each ES_i value, we also compute v_i, which indicates the amount of sampling variability in the effect size estimate.

Because of the sampling errors, the ES_i values will not coincide across studies. When all of the differences among the effect size estimates can be assumed to be a result of such sampling fluctuations, then the so-called *fixed-effects model* is appropriate. Here, the assumption is that the true effect sizes are exactly the same for all k studies (i.e., $\theta_1 = \theta_2 = \ldots = \theta_k = \theta$), and in this case the effect sizes are said to be *homogeneous*.

However, it is possible (and usually quite likely) that the true effect sizes (i.e., $\theta_1, \theta_2, \ldots, \theta_k$) differ from each other. In that case, the effect sizes are said to be *heterogeneous*. Heterogeneity can be the result of systematic moderator effects, random differences between the true effect sizes, or a combination of both. Depending on the presence of these effects, a more complex model applies.

First, consider the case in which moderators are introducing systematic differences between the effect sizes. For example, in a meta-analysis on social loafing (the tendency of individuals to reduce their effort when working in a group), it was found that the effect size (the difference in performance when effort was evaluated individually versus collectively) depended on the size of the group, with more social loafing occurring as group size increased (Karau & Williams, 1993). Group size, therefore, was a relevant moderator, which differed between the various studies included in the meta-analysis, and therefore should be taken into consideration in the analysis. The appropriate model in this case is the *fixed-effects with moderators model*.

Effect sizes may also differ from each other not because of systematic differences introduced by moderator variables, but owing to random heterogeneity. In this case, the typical assumption is that the θ_i values are randomly drawn from a normal distribution with mean μ_θ and variance τ^2. The size of τ^2 then indicates the amount of random heterogeneity among the effect sizes, and μ_θ indicates the average true effect size. The appropriate model in this case is the *random-effects model*.

Finally, it is possible that a combination of systematic moderator effects plus some additional random (residual) heterogeneity are jointly introducing differences into the θ_i values. In other words, the effect sizes vary systematically with some study-level characteristics and additional heterogeneity exists among the effect sizes that is purely random. The appropriate model in this case is the *mixed-effects model*.

A summary of these four models is given in Table 36.3. To reemphasize the main implications of the various models, imagine that each study included in the meta-analysis on social loafing used a very large sample size (e.g., thousands of subjects). As discussed earlier, the amount of sampling variability in an effect size estimate decreases with the sample size. Consequently, when sample sizes are very large, the sampling variability in each effect size estimate will be so small as to be almost negligible. Therefore, if the fixed-effects model holds, then each ES_i value should be essentially equal to each other and equal to the true population effect size θ. This idea is illustrated in Figure 36.1(a), which shows a plot of 10 hypothetical effect size estimates under the fixed-effects model where θ is assumed to be .44 (the average effect size found by Karau & Williams,

1993, in their meta-analysis). The figure illustrates how the effect size estimates are clustered around θ, the homogeneous effect size for all 10 studies.

However, when sample sizes are very large and heterogeneity is present, then each effect size estimate will narrow in on its corresponding θ_i value. In other words, if the θ_i values are not all equal to each other because they depend on some moderator (such as group size), then the ES_i values should also not be equal to each other, even if the sample size of each study is very large. Figure 36.1(b) shows effect size estimates for 10 hypothetical studies in which the studies are ordered by group size (with study 1 examining the amount of social loafing in small groups and study 10 examining the amount of social loafing in large groups). Because the sample sizes are very large, the sampling variability of the effect size estimates is very small and the pattern created by the moderator variable becomes clearly visible. Calculating a single overall effect size estimate would be meaningless here, because it would reflect neither the amount of social loafing in small groups, nor the amount of social loafing in large groups.

In the random-effects model, variability also will remain in the effect size estimates when sample sizes become very large. However, the variability will not be systematic, as in the fixed-effects with moderators model. Instead, the θ_i values will simply differ randomly from each other. Consider Figure 36.1(c), which shows a plot of effect size estimates for 10 hypothetical studies with very large sample sizes. The effect sizes were randomly drawn from a normal distribution with $\mu_\theta = .44$ and variance $\tau^2 = .01$. Note that the individual effect size estimates no longer narrow in on a single value, even though the amount of sampling variability is negligible. Instead, the ES_i values narrow in on their corresponding θ_i values, which in turn fluctuate randomly around μ_θ.

Finally, large sample sizes will also fail to remove all of the variability from the effect size estimates when the mixed-effects model holds. Consider Figure 36.1(d), which shows a plot of effect size estimates from 10 hypothetical studies under the mixed-effects model, assuming very large sample sizes. Here, the effect sizes depend on a single moderator (group size) plus an additional source of random variability. Therefore, we do recognize the increasing trend in the effect sizes as a function of the moderator, but the effect size estimates still fluctuate

TABLE 36.3. Four Meta-Analytic Models

Model	Moderators present	Random heterogeneity
Fixed effects	No	No
Fixed effects with moderators	Yes	No
Random effects	No	Yes
Mixed effects	Yes	Yes

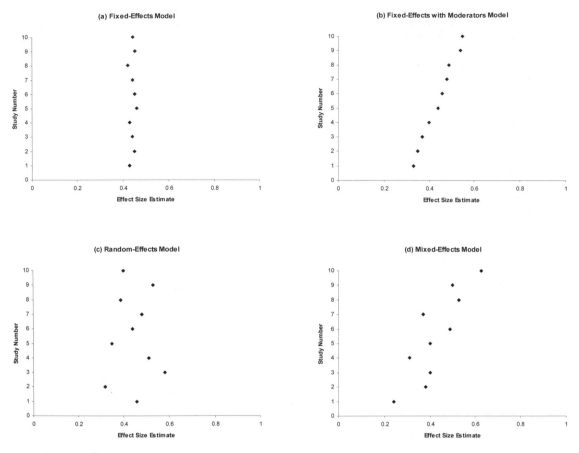

FIGURE 36.1. Plot of 10 hypothetical effect-size estimates under fixed-effects model, fixed-effects with moderator model, random-effects model, and mixed-effects model.

noticeably, despite the fact that the amount of sampling variability is negligible.

In practice, the sample sizes of studies included in a meta-analysis are typically not so large that the sampling errors can be disregarded. Patterns like those shown in Figures 36.1(b) and 36.1(d) may then become less discernible to the naked eye. Therefore, it is generally more difficult to determine which of the models is appropriate. We return to this issue below, where we discuss how to approach the model selection task.

Detecting Publication Bias

Despite his or her best efforts during a literature search, the studies an analyst retrieves from the published literature usually constitutes a subset of all studies that have been conducted on a particular topic. Not surprisingly, studies of higher quality are more likely to be

published than those suffering from design flaws or other shortcomings. Although little fault can be found with restricting the published literature to studies of higher quality, the analyst needs to be concerned with the consistent finding that highly statistically significant findings are much more likely to appear in the literature than results that do not reach statistical significance (e.g., Sterling, Rosenbaum, & Weinkam, 1995). For example, researchers may selectively report only those findings that reach significance and/or journal editors/reviewers may favor studies with significance findings. The net effect of this publication bias is that the effect size estimates obtained from the published literature may overestimate the actual effect size. Therefore, publication bias (also called the "file drawer problem") can be a major problem in meta-analysis.

The simplest method for detecting publication bias is by means of a funnel plot. For this, one plots the effect size estimates against the corresponding sample sizes or variances of the studies. An example of such a plot is shown in Figure 36.2a. Assuming that the fixed-effects model holds, studies with very large sample sizes should fluctuate negligibly around the true θ value. Yet studies with smaller sample sizes should fluctuate more substantially around the true θ value. The figure therefore should look like an inverted funnel (e.g., Figure 36.2b). However, if studies with small effect sizes and small sample sizes (and therefore studies that are unlikely to reach statistical significance) are not published, then the funnel will lack symmetry or will include a hollow area for effect size estimates near zero and small sample sizes. Figure 36.3 illustrates this clearly. This latter shape reflects the fact that as sample size increases the effect sizes move closer to zero, creating the peak of the distribution close to zero. The fact that small studies with small or null effects seldom get published leaves the left portion of the funnel missing. What the researcher must watch out for is the situation in which many small studies with medium effects have been published along with a handful of large studies with very small effects. The small studies with larger effects may lead to mistakenly large population estimates of effect sizes that are due to publication bias, rather than the result of a true effect's occurring.

Visual inspection of funnel plots for publication bias often leaves considerable room for conflicting interpretations, and therefore systematic methods for detecting publication bias have been suggested. Rosenthal (1979), for example, proposed a simple method for calculat-

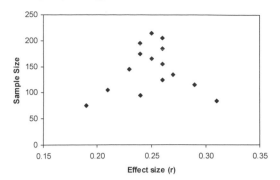

FIGURE 36.2b. Example funnel plot for studies with moderate sample sizes (true $r = 0.25$).

ing the number of unpublished studies averaging null results required to bring the overall level of significance in a research synthesis down to *just significant*. If only a few additional studies with nonsignificant results would be sufficient to do so, then the overall conclusions are argued to be sensitive to publication bias and should be interpreted with caution. However, if hundreds or thousands of studies with null results would be needed, then the findings can be considered robust to publication bias.

More advanced approaches for dealing with publication bias have also been developed. For example, the "trim and fill" method by Duval and Tweedie (2000a, 2000b) allows researchers to estimate the number of studies missing from the published literature due to their not having reached statistical significance and then provides adjusted estimates of the overall effect that account for the missing studies.

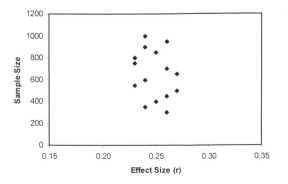

FIGURE 36.2a. Example funnel plot for studies with large sample size (true r 0.25).

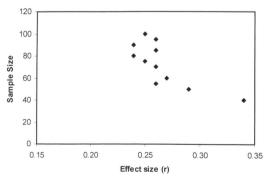

FIGURE 36.3. Example funnel plot for studies with small sample sizes (true $r = 0.25$).

Of course, the most important thing a meta-analyst can do to deal with publication bias is to make a concerted effort to locate the fugitive literature. Statistical adjustments are less than ideal replacements for actual data.

Testing for Moderators

As indicated earlier, the goal during the data analysis step is to determine which of the four models introduced earlier is most appropriate. Based on recent findings (Viechtbauer, 2004), we advocate starting out with the assumption that the most complex (i.e., the mixed-effects model) is actually the most appropriate model, followed by an examination of possible reductions in model complexity. Therefore, one starts out with the assumption that moderators are present and allows for the possibility that the moderators to be included in the analysis may not account for all of the heterogeneity among the effect sizes.

If no moderators are found to influence the effect sizes, then the question remains whether all of the differences among the effect size estimates are due to sampling fluctuations (in which case we would adopt the fixed-effects model) or whether random heterogeneity is present (in which case, we would adopt the random-effects model). If moderators are found to influence the effect sizes, however, then the question remains whether we can account for all of the differences among the effect sizes based on the moderators (in which case we would adopt the fixed-effects with moderators model) or whether there is residual heterogeneity in the effect sizes (in which case, we would adopt the mixed-effects model).

Fitting the mixed-effects model requires specifying a model for the relationship between the effect sizes and the moderators, estimating the parameters of this model, and estimating the amount of residual heterogeneity in the effect sizes (i.e., the amount of heterogeneity in the effect sizes that is not accounted for by the moderators). Methods for fitting the mixed-effects model have been described in the literature (e.g., Konstantopoulos & Hedges, 2004; Overton, 1998; Raudenbush, 1994; Raudenbush & Bryk, 1985, 2002; Sheu & Suzuki, 2001; Viechtbauer, 2004) and are beyond the scope of this chapter. Although working with mixed-effects models requires more statistical expertise on the part of the meta-analyst than using the still popular fixed-effects

models, we want to stress here that moderator tests should be conducted in the context of a mixed-effects model. It can be shown (Viechtbauer, 2004) that the Type I error of moderator tests in the context of fixed-effects models can become severely inflated, leading researchers to discover spurious moderators (i.e., moderators that are actually unrelated to the effect sizes often turn out to be significant when tested with fixed-effects models). However, the mixed-effects model adequately controls the Type I error rate and therefore should be preferred.

If none of the moderators turn out to be significant, then a single overall effect size can be provided. A random-effects model should be preferred in this case over the fixed-effects model, unless the evidence suggests (usually by means of a homogeneity test) that the effect sizes are truly homogeneous. For more details, see Shadish and Haddock (1994).

Aggregating Effect Sizes

If the effect sizes are not influenced by moderators, then a single aggregated effect size estimate provides an adequate summary of the data.[4] In that case, we must still distinguish between two cases, namely, whether the effect sizes are heterogeneous because of random differences (i.e., the effect sizes are assumed to be randomly drawn from a normal distribution with mean μ_θ and variance τ^2) or homogeneous (i.e., all the effect sizes are equal to each other: $\theta_1 = \theta_2 = \ldots = \theta_k = \theta$). The random-effects model is appropriate in the former case and the aggregated effect size estimates μ_θ. However, the fixed-effects model applies to the latter case and we estimate θ.

If the effect sizes are homogeneous, then an estimate of θ is given by

$$\hat{\theta} = \frac{\sum w_i ES_i}{\sum w_i}$$

where $w_i = 1/v_i$. Therefore, studies with larger sample sizes (and consequently smaller sampling variances) are given more weight, as they provide more accurate information about the true effect size θ. One can also obtain an approximate 95% confidence interval for θ with

$$\hat{\theta} \pm 1.96 \sqrt{\frac{1}{\sum w_i}}$$

as a way to gauge the precision of the estimate of θ. If the confidence interval includes zero, then this is equivalent to testing $H_0: \theta = 0$ at $\alpha = .05$ and failing to reject the null hypothesis that the effect size is equal to zero.

One can test whether the effect sizes are actually homogeneous (i.e., whether the fixed-effects model is appropriate for the data) with the so-called Q-test by computing

$$Q = \sum w_i (ES_i - \hat{\theta})^2$$

If Q exceeds the critical value of a chi-square distribution with $k - 1$ degrees of freedom, then this suggests the presence of heterogeneity among the effect sizes. An estimate of the amount of heterogeneity among the effect sizes (DerSimonian & Laird, 1986) is then given by

$$\hat{\tau}^2 = \frac{Q - (k-1)}{c}$$

where

$$c = \sum w_i - \frac{\sum w_i^2}{\sum w_i}$$

An estimate of μ_θ is then obtained with

$$\hat{\mu}_\theta = \frac{\sum w_i ES_i}{\sum w_i}$$

where $w_i = 1/(v_i + \hat{\tau}^2)$. An approximate 95% confidence interval for μ_θ is given by

$$\hat{\mu}_\theta \pm 1.96 \sqrt{\frac{1}{\sum w_i}}$$

again with $w_i = 1/(v_i + \hat{\tau}^2)$. This confidence interval will always be wider than the one computed under the fixed-effects model, reflecting the additional variability introduced by the heterogeneity among the effect sizes. Inclusion of zero in the interval indicates that we cannot reject $H_0: \mu_\theta = 0$ at $\alpha = 0.05$.

Because the Q-test is not infallible, it is generally advisable to automatically adopt the random-effects model and to estimate the amount of heterogeneity as described above. Should the effect sizes be homogeneous, then $\hat{\tau}^2$ will tend to be close to zero or even negative, in which case $\hat{\tau}^2$ is truncated to zero and the random-effects model reduces to the fixed-effects model (note that the equations for estimating θ and μ_θ differ only in the weights used, which are identical when $\hat{\tau}^2 = 0$). A pragmatic approach would be to compute the aggregated effect size and corresponding confidence inter-

val under both the fixed- and the random-effects model, as part of a sensitivity analysis.

In sum, analysis of the meta-analytic database proceeds very quickly once the appropriate model is chosen. The key choices are whether one believes that the population effect sizes are heterogeneous and how to account for moderators. Once the analyses have been computed, then the appropriate findings should be reported. Common approaches to this step of the process are described in Halvorsen (1994).

Lessons Learned

Although we are by no means the most prolific users of meta-analytic techniques, we have done enough of them now to provide some insights and lessons that may help the budding personality meta-analyst.

First, the most important lesson we have learned is that meta-analyses are a lot of work. The ignorant sap that maligns your meta-analytic efforts as easy because they entail secondary analyses of already collected data should be scolded. To do an exhaustive and therefore authoritative meta-analytic review will typically take a few years, minimum. Keep this in mind when planning your meta-analysis.

A second lesson we have learned concerns the blessings and banes of the Big Five taxonomy of personality traits. In some ways the Big Five are a godsend to meta-analysts. The ability to organize the dizzying array of personality measures post hoc into five basic domains has allowed for key findings in many areas of psychology and related fields. Without the Big Five we would not understand which personality traits are most important for specific types of job outcomes (Hogan & Holland, 2003), creativity (Feist, 1998), and criminal behavior (Miller & Lynam, 2001). The pre-Big Five meta-analyst was forced to provide an estimate for "personality," rather than for different traits within the personality trait taxonomy, which essentially washed out differential relationships. In this respect, the Big Five is a wonderful tool and has provided invaluable clarity on the role of personality traits in numerous domains.

We are also acutely aware of the limitation of the global categorization of traits into these five domains. In many regards, the Big Five are too broad, and very specific facets of each domain are more interesting and theoretically relevant. In our study tying conscientiousness to health behaviors, for instance, we found certain facets to be much more important than others in predicting health behaviors. For example, the traditionalism and impulse control facets had much more pervasive effects across health domains, whereas the organization facet did not. We demonstrated similar refinements in our analysis of mean-level change in personality. Based on the work of Helson and Kwan (2000), we reorganized the domain of extraversion into the subdomains of social dominance and social vitality. This led to starkly different findings. People increased substantially on measures of social dominance and showed little or no change on measures of social vitality. If we had simply merged the two facets into one overall domain of extraversion, these patterns would have gone undetected. To refine our categorization of traits, we need a taxonomy of personality traits that is more specific than the Big Five (see Roberts, Walton, & Viechtbauer, 2006b). Unfortunately, there exists no empirically supported lower-order taxonomy of personality traits. We hope that this taxonomy is identified in the near future so we can further refine our measurement of personality and our organization of meta-analyses of personality traits.

One of the key lessons we have learned from doing meta-analysis is the insanity of null hypothesis significance testing. Doing a meta-analysis makes one acutely aware of the importance of effect sizes and the capricious nature of statistical significance as an arbiter of whether someone claims an effect is present or not. By looking across studies that vary in terms of their sample size, you are automatically confronted with the fact that the studies with 50–100 people have to contain medium to large effects in order to satisfy the typical null hypothesis significance testing (NHST) standards. In turn, these same studies essentially throw away effect sizes below 0.20. At the same time, researchers who bother to collect a respectable number of data points lay claim to effects as statistically significant that are below 0.20. The beauty of meta-analytic techniques is that by combining data across multiple studies, statistical significance becomes a moot point. Everything is statistically significant from zero, making statistical significance an uninteresting and uninformative standard by which to judge whether an effect is real.

In terms of the typical approach to designing our studies, we would like to get in line behind the many researchers who have noted that our studies lack the power to detect the effects we are interested in. Too often, we use rules of thumb to determine how many participants to include in our research without planning or thinking about the number that would be appropriate, given the magnitude of the effects we expect to find. We have a sweeping recommendation to make. Regardless of the number of participants you are planning to incorporate in your study, double it. That way, like meta-analysis, poor power will not deter the science of personality from accumulating meaningful patterns of results.

In conclusion, we hope that our overview of meta-analysis in personality psychology is both helpful and informative. As we noted at the beginning of this chapter, meta-analyses can bring clarity to research domains that often appear at first blush to be muddled and confused. They also tend to shift the question ever so slightly from "Is there an effect?" to "What size is the effect?"—a shift that we believe can better lead to a science of personality psychology that stands much more firmly in the face of criticism and that cumulates findings in a more productive fashion.

Acknowledgment

Preparation of this chapter was supported by Grant No. R01 AG21178 from the National Institute on Aging.

Notes

1. This task is preferably carried out by a highly motivated researcher/graduate student or an assistant with obsessive–compulsive tendencies.
2. We have found one special circumstance when null findings have been preferred. Specifically, researchers have been prone to overreport null findings for the validity of achievement tests such as the SAT (Hezlet et al., 2001), whereas positive results tend not to be published.
3. For an in-depth treatment of these issues, see Hunter and Schmidt (2004).
4. It is important to realize that a single aggregated effect size estimate can be misleading when moderators are actually present. Take, for example, the situation in which the effect sizes depend on a single dichotomous moderator and the effect sizes

are negative (e.g., –0.5) for half of the set of studies and positive (e.g., +0.5) for the other half. An aggregated effect size estimate would then be close to zero, suggesting the absence of an effect.

Recommended Readings

Cooper, H. M., & Hedges, L. V. (Eds.). (1994). *The handbook of research synthesis*. New York: Sage.

Duval, S. J., & Tweedie, R. L. (2000a). Trim and fill: A simple funnel-plot-based method of testing and adjusting for publication bias in meta-analysis. *Biometrics, 56*, 455–463.

Hedges, L. V., & Olkin, I. (1985). *Statistical methods for meta-analysis*. San Diego, CA: Academic Press.

Lipsey, M. W., & Wilson, D. B. (2001). *Practical meta-analysis*. Thousand Oaks, CA: Sage.

Rosenthal, R. (1991). *Meta-analytic procedures for social research*. Newbury Park, CA: Sage.

References

Barrick, M. R., & Mount, M. K. (1991). The Big Five personality dimensions and job performance: A meta-analysis. *Personnel Psychology, 44*, 1–26.

Bogg, T., & Roberts, B. W. (2004). Conscientiousness and health behaviors: A meta-analysis of the leading behavioral contributors to mortality. *Psychological Bulletin, 130*, 887–919.

Bono, J. E., & Judge, T. (2004). Personality and transformational and transactional leadership: A meta-analysis. *Journal of Applied Psychology, 89*, 901–910.

Cohen, J. (1988). *Statistical power analysis for the behavioral sciences* (2nd ed.). Hillsdale, NJ: Erlbaum.

Cohen, J. (1990). Things I have learned (so far). *American Psychologist, 45*, 1304–1312.

Cohen, J. (1992). A power primer. *Psychological Bulletin, 112*, 155–159.

Cooper, H. M., & Hedges, L. V. (Eds.). (1994). *The handbook of research synthesis*. New York: Sage.

DerSimonian, R., & Laird, N. (1986). Meta-analysis in clinical trials. *Controlled Clinical Trials, 7*, 177–188.

Duval, S. J., & Tweedie, R. L. (2000a). A nonparametric "trim and fill" method of accounting for publication bias in meta-analysis. *Journal of the American Statistical Association, 95*, 89–98.

Duval, S. J., & Tweedie, R. L. (2000b). Trim and fill: A simple funnel-plot-based method of testing and adjusting for publication bias in meta-analysis. *Biometrics, 56*, 455–463.

Feist, G. J. (1998). A meta-analysis of personality in scientific and artistic creativity. *Personality and Social Psychology Review, 2*, 290–309.

Fleiss, J. L. (1994). Measures of effect size for categorical data. In H. M. Cooper & L. V. Hedges (Eds.), *The handbook of research synthesis* (pp. 245–260). New York: Sage.

Gleser, L. J., & Olkin, I. (1994). Stochastically dependent effect sizes. In H. M. Cooper & L. V. Hedges (Eds.), *The handbook of research synthesis* (pp. 339–356). New York: Sage.

Halvorson, K. T. (1924). The reporting format. In H. M. Cooper & L. V. Hodges (Eds.), *The handbook of research synthesis* (pp. 425–438). New York: Russell Sage.

Hedges, L. V. (1981). Distribution theory for Glass's estimator of effect size and related estimators. *Journal of Educational Statistics, 6*, 107–128.

Hedges, L. V., & Olkin, I. (1985). *Statistical methods for meta-analysis*. San Diego, CA: Academic Press.

Helson, R., & Kwan, V. S. Y. (2000). Personality development in adulthood: The broad picture and processes in one longitudinal sample. In S. Hampson (Ed.), *Advances in personality psychology* (Vol. 1, pp. 77–106). London: Routledge.

Hezlett, S. A., Kuncel, N. R., Vey, M. A., Ahart, A., Ones, D. S., Campbell, J. P., et al. (2001, April). The predictive validity of the SAT: A comprehensive meta-analysis. In D. S. Ones & S. A. Hezlett (Chairs), *Predicting Performance: The Interface of I/O Psychology and Educational Research*. Symposia presented at the annual conference of the Society for Industrial and Organizational Psychology, San Diego, CA.

Hogan, J., & Holland, B. (2003). Using theory to evaluate personality and job-performance relations: A socioanalytic perspective. *Journal of Applied Psychology, 88*, 100–112.

Hunter, J. E., & Schmidt, F. L. (2004). *Methods of meta-analysis* (2nd ed.). Newbury Park, CA: Sage.

Karau, S. J., & Williams, K. D. (1993). Social loafing: A meta-analytic review and theoretical integration. *Journal of Personality and Social Psychology, 65*, 681–706.

Konstantopoulos, S., & Hedges, L. V. (2004). Meta-analysis. In D. Kaplan (Ed.), *The Sage handbook of quantitative methodology for the social sciences* (pp. 281–297). Thousand Oaks, CA: Sage.

Kuncel, N. R., Credé, M., & Thomas, L. L. (2005). The reliability of self-reported grade point averages, class ranks, and test scores. *Review of Educational Research, 75*, 63–87.

Kuncel, N. R., Hezlett, S. A., & Ones, D. S. (2001). A comprehensive meta-analysis of the predictive validity of the graduate record examinations: Implications for graduate student selection and performance. *Psychological Bulletin, 127*, 162–181.

Lipsey, M. W., & Wilson, D. B. (2001). *Practical meta-analysis*. Thousand Oaks, CA: Sage.

Meyer, G. J., Finn, S. E., Eyde, L. D., Kay, G. G., Moreland, K. L., Dies, R. R., et al. (2001). Psychological testing and psychological assessment. *American Psychologist, 56*, 128–165.

Miller, J. D., & Lynam, D. (2001). Structural models

of personality and their relation to antisocial behavior: A meta-analytic review. *Criminology, 39*, 765–798.

Morris, S. B., & DeShon, R. P. (2002). Combining effect size estimates in meta-analysis with repeated measures and independent-groups designs. *Psychological Methods, 7*, 105–125.

Olkin, I., & Pratt, J. W. (1958). Unbiased estimation of certain correlation coefficients. *Annals of Mathematical Statistics, 29*, 201–211.

Ones, D. S., Viswesvaran, C., & Schmidt, F. L. (1993). Comprehensive meta-analysis of integrity test validities: Findings and implications for personnel selection and theories of job performance. *Journal of Applied Psychology, 78*, 679–703.

Overton, R. C. (1998). A comparison of fixed-effects and mixed (random-effects) models for meta-analysis tests of moderator variable effects. *Psychological Methods, 3*, 354–379.

Raudenbush, S. W. (1994). Random effects models. In H. M. Cooper & L. V. Hedges (Eds.), *The handbook of research synthesis* (pp. 301–321). New York: Sage.

Raudenbush, S. W., & Bryk, A. S. (1985). Empirical Bayes meta-analysis. *Journal of Educational Statistics, 10*, 75–98.

Raudenbush, S. W., & Bryk, A. S. (2002). *Hierarchical linear models: Applications and data analysis methods.* Thousand Oaks, CA: Sage.

Roberts, B. W., & DelVecchio, W. F. (2000). The rank-order consistency of personality from childhood to old age: A quantitative review of longitudinal studies. *Psychological Bulletin, 126*, 3–25.

Roberts, B. W., Walton, K. E., & Viechtbauer, W. (2006a). Patterns of mean-level change in personality traits across the life course: A meta-analysis of longitudinal studies. *Psychological Bulletin, 132*, 1–25.

Roberts, B. W., Walton, K. E., & Viechtbauer, W. (2006b). Personality traits change in adulthood: Reply to Costa & McCrae (2006). *Psychological Bulletin, 132*, 29–32.

Rosenthal, R. (1979). The "file drawer problem" and tolerance for null results. *Psychological Bulletin, 86*, 638–641.

Rosenthal, R. (1991). *Meta-analytic procedures for social research.* Newbury Park, CA: Sage.

Rosenthal, R. (1994). Parametric measures of effect size. In H. M. Cooper & L. V. Hedges (Eds.), *The handbook of research synthesis* (pp. 231–244). New York: Sage.

Rosenthal, R., & Rubin, D. B. (2003). R-equivalent: A simple effect size indicator. *Psychological Methods, 8*, 492–496.

Shadish, W. R., & Haddock, C. K. (1994). Combining estimates of effect size. In H. M. Cooper & L. V. Hedges (Eds.), *The handbook of research synthesis* (pp. 261–281). New York: Sage.

Sheu, C.-F., & Suzuki, S. (2001). Meta-analysis using linear mixed models. *Behavior Research Methods, Instruments, and Computers, 33*, 102–107.

Sterling, T. D., Rosenbaum, W. L., & Weinkam, J. J. (1995). Publication decisions revisited: The effect of the outcome of statistical tests on the decision to publish and vice versa. *American Statistician, 49*, 108–112.

Viechtbauer, W. (2004). *Model selection strategies in meta-analysis: Choosing between the fixed-, random-, and mixed-effects model.* Manuscript submitted for publication.

## CHAPTER 37

What Kinds of Methods Do Personality Psychologists Use?

A Survey of Journal Editors and Editorial Board Members

Richard W. Robins
Jessica L. Tracy
Jeffrey W. Sherman

Of all the fields of psychology, personality is, arguably, the most methodologically diverse. Indeed, methodological pluralism is a cornerstone of the field. Thumbing through a typical issue of a personality journal will reveal a rich array of methods, including longitudinal and experimental designs; studies of typical and atypical populations; and a wide range of assessment procedures, including self-report scales, informant reports, projective tests, observational assessment, and DNA analyses. This methodological diversity reflects, and is in fact compelled by, the breadth and complexity of the substantive questions personality researchers seek to address. It is not surprising that a field that aims to understand everything from genetic to cultural influences on the person involves a wide range of methods.

But what exactly are the most common methods in contemporary personality research? That is, what is the best way to characterize the personality approach to psychology? Despite lively discussions at conferences and in the halls of psychology departments about which methods are rising or falling in popularity, there have been virtually no systematic studies of this issue.[1] This raises the question, Does the reality match the stereotype? Do personality researchers actually use a diverse range of methods? What exactly are the research designs, assessment methods, and statistics in the methodological tool kit of the 21st-century personality researcher?

To address these questions, we conducted a survey of prominent personality researchers; specifically, members of the editorial boards of the leading journals in the field. We asked our respondents to answer a comprehensive set of questions about the way they design their studies, assess their key constructs, and analyze their data. The aim of the survey was to gauge the frequency with which personality researchers use each method and, by doing so, provide an empirical snapshot of the current state of personality research.

Method

Respondents and Procedure

Our sample consists of editors, associate editors, and other members of the editorial boards of three of the leading journals in personality psychology: the *European Journal of Personality*, the *Journal of Personality*, and the *Journal of Personality and Social Psychology: Personality Processes and Individual Differences*.[2] We selected members of personality editorial boards for several reasons. First, these individuals are very likely to conduct research on personality and to perceive themselves as personality psychologists. Second, these individuals are typically among the most productive researchers working the field, so they are collectively responsible for a large body of personality research. Third, members of editorial boards cover a broad range of career stages, so the sample would include individuals who are at the early, middle, and late stages of their scientific careers. Fourth, members of editorial boards decide what is and is not accepted for publication in personality journals and thus are the "gatekeepers" of personality psychology. These individuals are highly knowledgeable about what constitutes personality research; in fact, one could argue that they set the standards for the field.

Participants were contacted by electronic mail and were told, "The goal of the survey is to learn more about the kinds of research conducted by prominent personality psychologists." If they agreed to participate, they were directed to a World Wide Web address where they could access the survey and complete it online. Of the 142 individuals contacted, 72 completed the survey, for a response rate of 51%.

Respondents were assured complete anonymity; they were informed that their survey responses were completely confidential and could not be tied to their names or e-mail addresses.

Survey Questionnaire

The survey was constructed through an iterative process. As a starting point, we asked a focus group of seven leading personality researchers to generate a set of methodological features that could be used to describe the prototypical personality approach. We then supplemented this list by reviewing recent journals, edited volumes, and textbooks to identify methods used in personality research. This led to an initial pool of survey items. We sent this set of items to a small group of personality researchers and solicited feedback on ambiguities, omissions, and redundancies in the survey. Based on their feedback, we eliminated and rephrased many items and added new items to fill gaps in the item pool.

This procedure resulted in a final survey that included multiple sections and more than 200 items. In this chapter, we report findings related to the first three sections, which map onto the major sections of this volume (research designs, assessment methods, statistical procedures), and thus provide a useful reference point.

In the first section of the survey, respondents were asked to rate the frequency with which they used each of 12 research designs and approaches in their research (e.g., experimental, correlational, longitudinal, etc.); in the second section, respondents rated the frequency with which they used each of 17 assessment methods/measures (e.g., self-report, informant report, behavioral observation, etc.); and in the third section respondents rated the frequency with which they used each of 21 statistical procedures and data-analytic strategies (e.g., analysis of variance, correlation, factor analysis, etc.). All ratings were made on a 7-point scale, ranging from 1 ("never") to 7 ("always"), with 4 ("sometimes") as the midpoint of the scale.

After completing these ratings, respondents were asked to rate the extent to which they "study issues and topics related to the field of personality psychology," using a 7-point scale ranging from 1 ("not at all") to 7 ("very much"), with 4 ("somewhat") as the midpoint of the scale.

Finally, at the end of the survey, participants provided demographic information about their gender, age, type of workplace (small college, non-PhD-granting university, PhD-granting university, research institute/government agency, business/corporation), and country in which their workplace is located. Participants were also asked to indicate the journals on which they serve as editors or editorial board members.

Results

Characteristics of Sample

Of the 72 respondents, 75% were male ($n = 54$) and 25% were female ($n = 18$). The median age of respondents was 43 years ($SD = 9.3$). Most respondents worked in the United States ($n = 52$, 74%), and the majority of the rest worked in Europe ($n = 14$, 20%) or Canada ($n = 3$, 4%). Eighty percent of respondents worked in PhD-granting research universities ($n = 57$) and the rest in non-PhD-granting universities ($n = 5$, 7%), small colleges ($n = 4$, 6%), research institutes/government agencies ($n = 4$, 6%), and businesses/corporations ($n = 1$, 1%).

Research Designs and Approaches

We analyze and report the survey data in two ways. First, we treat the personality psychologists in our sample as a group and report their mean responses across each survey item. Second, we examine individual differences in the degree to which respondents indicated that they study topics and issues related to personality; by correlating this item with survey responses, we can determine whether, even within this select sample of personality psychologists, the degree of immersion in the field is associated with the use of particular designs, statistics, and measures.

The first column of Table 37.1 shows mean responses for each of the 12 research designs, as well as the percentage of participants who indicated that they had ever used that design (i.e., who gave any rating other than 1, "never"). The simple correlational design remains by far the most frequently used in personality research, followed by the longitudinal, cross-sectional, and experimental designs. Thus, contrary to many people's intuitions, the experimental design is relatively common in personality research; in fact, 86% of our participants indicated that they use the design more than "never" in their research (39% use experimental designs "sometimes" to "always").

Cross-species comparisons and case studies are the least frequently used designs in personality research. In the former case, the low frequency may reflect, at least in part, the fact that researchers who do comparative studies of animal personality typically identify themselves as comparative psychologists, primatologists, animal behaviorists, and so on, rather than as personality psychologists, and thus are not well represented in our sample. The low frequency of case studies, in contrast, may reflect a more general trend in the field away from case studies, psychobiographies, and other person-centered approaches (see Craik, Chapter 12, this volume; Elms, Chapter 6, this volume; Grice, Chapter 32, this volume). Despite the low overall level of use of cross-species and case studies, they are nonetheless used at least somewhat by a nontrivial percentage of researchers (10% and 18%, respectively).

The second column of Table 37.1 shows correlations of the individual difference variable (the extent to which individuals study personality) with frequency of using each design. Consistent with the pattern of means, individuals who describe their research as focusing on issues and topics that are central to the field of personality psychology are more likely to use correlational, cross-sectional, and longitudinal designs. Interestingly, these individuals are less likely to use experimental designs, despite the high overall mean for experimental research. Thus, experimental methods are frequently used by most personality psychologists, but those individuals who use them most tend to see their research as less strictly about "personality" topics.

Statistical Procedures and Data-Analytic Strategies

As Table 37.1 shows, the statistical procedures used most frequently by personality researchers are correlation, reliability analyses, multiple regression, factor/component analysis, t-tests, ANOVA, and partial correlation; these procedures are used by virtually all personality researchers. The least frequently used statistical procedures are mathematical modeling, multidimensional scaling, computer simulations, item response theory (IRT) analyses, and time-series analyses.

These results may simply reflect the most frequently (and least frequently) used statistical procedures in the broader field of psychology (Aiken, West, Sechrest, & Reno, 1990), rather than being particularly characteristic of personality research. However, the results shown in column 2 of Table 37.1 provide converging evidence for the pattern of means, at least for procedures that involve correlation and other indices of association between or among variables. Specifically, the degree to which

TABLE 37.1. The Methodological Tool Kit of the Personality Psychologist: An Analysis of Research Designs, Statistical Procedures, and Assessment Methods

Survey question	Mean (SD)	% ever used[a]	r with personality research orientation[b]
Research design/approach			
Correlational	5.76 (1.03)	100%	.44*
Longitudinal	4.10 (1.59)	93%	.26*
Cross-sectional	4.03 (1.50)	96%	.40*
Experimental	.76 (1.80)	86%	−.41*
Quasi-experimental	3.60 (1.75)	86%	−.08
Field studies	3.44 (1.73)	83%	.09
Cross-cultural	2.86 (1.51)	76%	.04
Dyadic or group interactions	2.82 (1.61)	71%	−.05
Patient studies	2.36 (1.56)	58%	−.03
Twin and adoption studies	1.69 (1.49)	22%	.14
Psychobiography/case studies	1.42 (1.14)	18%	.17
Cross-species	1.33 (1.10)	10%	−.10
Statistical/data-analytic procedure			
Reliability analyses	5.96 (1.09)	100%	.36*
Correlation	5.94 (1.03)	100%	.52*
Multiple regression	5.60 (0.96)	100%	.36*
Factor/component analysis	4.76 (1.25)	100%	.35*
t-tests	4.73 (1.48)	100%	.13
ANOVA	4.72 (1.44)	97%	−.14
Partial correlation	4.67 (1.48)	99%	.26*
Convergent/discriminant validity	4.26 (1.64)	93%	.30*
Mediation analyses	4.10 (1.36)	94%	.00
Structural equation modeling	3.79 (1.74)	87%	.17
Power analyses	3.72 (1.73)	89%	−.04
Hierarchical/multilevel modeling	3.44 (1.79)	79%	.15
Growth-curve modeling	2.57 (1.78)	56%	.02
Computer simulations	1.73 (1.22)	36%	.09
Cluster analysis	2.40 (1.41)	68%	.33*
Meta-analysis	2.36 (1.42)	60%	−.00
Discriminant function analysis	2.12 (1.21)	61%	.18
Time-series analyses	1.79 (1.23)	40%	.13
IRT analyses	1.76 (1.26)	37%	.16
Multidimensional scaling	1.72 (1.23)	36%	.16
Mathematical modeling	1.65 (1.23)	32%	.10
Assessment methods/measures			
Self-report scales and questionnaires	6.17 (0.93)	100%	.43*
Judgments of self and others	5.07 (1.57)	99%	.26*
Informant reports	3.68 (1.82)	86%	.26*
Behavioral observation	3.58 (1.47)	89%	−.09
Structured interviews	3.15 (1.89)	76%	.14
Behavioral responses	3.11 (1.55)	81%	−.13
Other judgment tasks (e.g., of stimuli)	3.10 (1.61)	79%	−.07
Narrative/open-ended questionnaires	3.03 (1.69)	74%	.11
Reaction time measures	2.93 (1.90)	61%	−.14
Experience sampling	2.89 (1.90)	65%	.14
Implicit measures	2.76 (1.87)	64%	−.12
Memory tasks	2.52 (1.58)	62%	−.13
Autonomic arousal	2.22 (1.42)	57%	−.30*
Judgments of groups/nations/cultures	2.19 (1.68)	43%	−.05
Hormone levels	1.94 (1.59)	36%	−.18
Neuroimaging (fMRI, ERP, etc.)	1.75 (1.44)	32%	−.11
Molecular genetics/DNA testing	1.60 (1.21)	26%	.07

Note. N = 72. All items were rated on a 7-point scale ranging from 1 ("not at all") to 7 ("very much"), with 4 ("somewhat") as the midpoint of the scale.

[a] Percentage of respondents who indicated that they ever use the method in their research (i.e., who gave any rating other than 1, "never").

[b] Extent to which respondents indicated that they "study issues and topics related to the field of personality psychology."

* $p < .05$.

researchers study topics central to the field of personality psychology is associated with greater use of correlation, reliability analyses, multiple regression, factor/component analysis, convergent/discriminant validity, and partial correlations. The relatively greater prevalence of these methods in personality research may reflect their application to the study of individual, rather than group, differences. In contrast, the two procedures that are more typically applied to the study of group differences—ANOVA and *t*-tests—are not especially common among those who study personality-relevant research topics, although they are still quite common overall.

It is also worth noting that despite their well-known advantages, the interrelated procedures of structural equation modeling, hierarchical/multilevel modeling, and growth-curve modeling have yet to reach the "frequent use" level in personality research (and, no doubt, in other areas of research as well). However, although they may not be used frequently, the majority of personality researchers do use these methods to some extent (56%, 79%, and 87% for growth-curve modeling, hierarchical modeling, and structural equation modeling, respectively).

Assessment Methods/Measures

Finally, we examined the specific assessment methods and measures used by personality researchers. By far the most frequently used method is, not surprisingly, self-report scales and questionnaires, followed by the related category of "judgments of self and other"; these methods are ubiquitous in personality research, and virtually everyone in our sample uses them at least some of the time. Less common, but still relatively frequently used methods include informant reports, behavioral observation, and structured interviews; these methods are also used by the vast majority of personality researchers, reflecting the multimethod approach that predominates in the field.

Despite widespread discussion of the rise of neuroscience and other biologically oriented approaches to personality, the use of such methods, including DNA testing, functional magnetic resonance imaging/event-related potential (fMRI/ERP), and measures of hormone levels and autonomic arousal, remains quite infrequent. At the same time, these methods are used on occasion by a fairly large percentage of researchers (26%, 32%, 36%, and 57% for

DNA, fMRI/ERP, hormone levels, and autonomic arousal, respectively). In general, this pattern may reflect a trend in the field as a whole; research on citation rates and dissertation topics suggests that the neuroscientific approach to psychology is becoming more prominent, but has not yet begun to approach the levels of prominence seen by other major approaches to psychology (e.g., the cognitive perspective; Tracy, Robins, & Gosling, 2004).

Consistent with the pattern of means, the correlational analyses show that individuals who study issues and topics that are central to the field of personality psychology are particularly likely to use self-report scales, judgments of self and others, and informant reports, and less likely to use measures of autonomic arousal.

Discussion

In this chapter, we reported findings from a survey of leading personality researchers. Our goal was simple: To peer inside their methodological tool kit and see what we find. Overall, the picture that emerged is one of extreme methodological pluralism. There is no particular research design, data-analytic approach, or assessment method that characterizes our sample of elite personality researchers. Instead, the field seems to adopt a "by any means necessary" approach to research, using a wide range of approaches and techniques.

The findings generally converge with our intuitions about the prototypical personality approach, but they nonetheless reveal some interesting discrepancies and nuance. Certainly, one can find support in these data for the prevalence of the stereotypical personality study, in which self-report measures are administered and intercorrelated. Yet our data also show that this is just one of many kinds of studies that are common in the personality literature. Indeed, most personality researchers conduct experiments and use ANOVA to analyze their data. Many also conduct cross-cultural and field research; they study twins and patient populations; they use sophisticated statistical techniques such as hierarchical modeling; and they assess personality not only through self-reports but also through informant reports, behavioral observation, cognitive tasks, and biological indicators. Thus, our findings paint a picture of personality psychology as a vibrant field, characterized by a rich array of methods and procedures.

We would like to point out two important limitations of our research. First, there may be a discrepancy between the methods that respondents report using and the methods that they actually use in their research. For example, respondents may exaggerate the degree to which they use a diverse set of methods and procedures, either because of self-deception or impression management (Paulhus & Vazire, Chapter 13, this volume). One way to address this concern would be to content-code articles published in leading personality journals, to determine the actual frequency with which each design, statistical procedure, and assessment method is used in personality studies (Fraley & Marks, 2005).

Second, our sampling procedure—focusing on members of editorial boards—may limit the generalizability of the findings beyond this elite group of personality researchers. It is possible that less prominent and productive researchers use a more restricted range of methods.

Finally, we would like to note that our results are necessarily limited to this particular snapshot in time. As Craik (Chapter 12, this volume) points out, the field of personality psychology has gone through dramatic shifts in the prevalence of different research methods and approaches. What the future may hold for the field remains to be seen. But, at least based on the present analyses, we see a field well positioned to respond to the challenges and opportunities posed by the recent shift in psychology toward multilevel analyses of complex aspects of human behavior.

Acknowledgment

We would like to thank the respondents who participated in the survey and the seven individuals who participated in our focus group.

Notes

1. Fraley and Marks (2005) assessed the frequency with which a number of statistical procedures were used in 259 articles published in two of the leading personality journals (*Journal of Personality* and *Journal of Personality and Social Psychology: Personality Processes and Individual Differences*) between 2000 and 2002. The correlation, ANOVA, *t*-test, and multiple regression were the most frequent data-analytic techniques, but a wide range of other procedures were also used. This study provided an interesting snapshot of the personality researchers' statistical tools, but the researchers did not ask broader questions about research approach, design, or assessment methods. Vazire (2006), in an article on the informant method in personality research, analyzed all studies published in the *Journal of Research in Personality* in 2003 and found that 98% used self-reports but only 24% collected informant reports (i.e., ratings of the targets by well-acquainted others, such as friends, spouses, or co-workers). Aiken, West, Sechrest, and Reno (1990) conducted a survey to determine how frequently PhD programs in psychology offer courses that cover a wide range of statistical procedures and methods, but they did not break their results down into subprograms such as personality psychology. Finally, Baumeister and Vohs (2006), in an article published in *Dialogue*, the Society for Personality and Social Psychology newsletter, content coded recent issues of *JPSP* and found that only a very small subset of studies included direct assessments of behavior; the vast majority of studies relied on ratings and reports of some kind.

2. Many survey respondents were on multiple editorial boards, including some nonpersonality journals.

References

Aiken, L. S., West, S. G., Sechrest, L., & Reno, R. R. (1990). Graduate training in statistics, methodology, and measurement in psychology: A survey of PhD programs in North America. *American Psychologist, 45,* 721–734.

Baumeister, R. F., & Vohs, K. D. (2006). Are personality and social psychologists behaving themselves? *Dialogue: Newsletter of the Society for Personality and Social Psychology,* pp. 3, 7.

Fraley, R. C., & Marks, M. J. (2005). Quantitative methods in personality research. In B. S. Everitt & D. C. Howell (Eds.), *Encyclopedia of statistics in behavioral science* (Vol. 3, pp. 1637–1645). Chichester, UK: Wiley.

Tracy, J. L., Robins, R. W., & Gosling, S. D. (2004). Exploring the roots of contemporary psychology: Using empirical indices to identify scientific trends. In T. C. Dalton & R. B. Evans (Eds.), *The life cycle of psychological ideas: Understanding prominence and the dynamics of intellectual change* (pp. 105–130). New York: Plenum Press.

Vazire, S. (2006). Informant reports: A cheap, fast, and easy method for personality assessment. *Journal of Research in Personality, 40,* 472–481.

Author Index

Subject Index